Donald School
Atlas of
Clinical Application of
Ultrasound in
Obstetrics & Gynecology

Donald School

Atlas of Clinical Application of Ultrasound in Obstetrics & Gynecology

Editors

JM Carrera MD PhD
Head, Fetal Medicine Service
Department of Obstetrics and Gynecology
University Institute "Dexeus"
Barcelona, Spain

Asim Kurjak MD PhD
Professor and Chairman
Department of Obstetrics and Gynecology
Medical School University of Zagreb
Sveti Duh Hospital, Zagreb
Croatia

JAYPEE BROTHERS
MEDICAL PUBLISHERS (P) LTD
New Delhi

Anshan
Tunbridge Wells
UK

First published in the UK by

Anshan Ltd.
in 2006
6 Newlands Road
Tunbridge Wells
Kent TN4 9AT, UK

Tel/Fax: +44 (0)1892 557767
E-mail: info@anshan.co.uk
www.anshan.co.uk

ISBN-10 1 904798 780
ISBN-13 978 1 904798 78 1

British Library Cataloguing in Publication Data
A catalogue record for this book is available from the British Library

Printed in India by Sanat Printers, Kundli

Many of the designations used by manufacturers and sellers to distinguish their products are
claimed as trademarks. Where those designations appear in this book and where the publisher
was aware of a trademark claim, the designations have been printed in initial capital letters.

Dedicated to
Our Children and
Grand Children

CONTRIBUTORS

W Andonotopo
Department of Obstetrics and Gynecology
Medical School University of Zagreb
Sveti Duh Hospital, Sveti Duh 64, 10000 Zagreb, Croatia

F Astudillo
Fetal Medicine Service
Department of Obstetrics and Gynecology
University Institute "Dexeus"
Passeig Bonanova, 67, 08017 Barcelona, Spain

G Azumendi
Clinica Gutenberg
C/ Gutenberg-1, 29016 Malaga, Spain

MJ Barco
University Clinic "Lozano Blesa"
50004 Zaragoza, Spain

PN Barri
Head of the Department of Obstetrics and Gynecology
University Institute "Dexeus"
Passeig Bonanova, 67, 08017 Barcelona, Spain

S Bau
Assisted Reproduction Unit
International Ruber Hospital
La Maso 38, 28034 Madrid, Spain

R Bauman
Department of Obstetrics and Gynecology
Medical School University of Zagreb
Sveti Duh Hospital, Sveti Duh 64
10000 Zagreb, Croatia

D Bjelos
Department of Obstetrics and Gynecology
Medical School University of Zagreb
Sveti Duh Hospital, Zagreb, Croatia

JM Carrera
Fetal Medicine Service
Department of Obstetrics and Gynecology
University Institute "Dexeus"
Passeig Bonanova, 67, 08017 Barcelona, Spain

C Comas
Prenatal Diagnosis Unit
Centro Gutenberg
C/ Gutenberg-1, Málaga 29016, Spain

S Dexeus
University Institute "Dexeus"
Passeig Bonanova, 67
08017 Barcelona, Spain

M Echevarria
Fetal Medicine Service
Department of Obstetrics and Gynecology
University Institute "Dexeus"
Passeig Bonanova, 67, 08017 Barcelona, Spain

B Funduk
Polyclinic "Modern Medical Center"
Zvonimirova 26, 10000 Zagreb, Croatia

S Gajovic
Department of Histology and Embryology
School of Medicine, University of Zagreb
Salata 3, 10000 Zagreb, Croatia

A Galindo
Ultrasound and Fetal Physiopathology Unit
Department of Obstetrics and Gynaecology
Hospital Universitario "12 De Octubre"
28041 Madrid, Spain

M Kos
Polyclinic "Vili"
Gjure Dezelica 32
10000 Zagreb, Croatia

Lj Kostovic-Knezevic
Department of Histology and Embryology
School of Medicine, University of Zagreb
Salata 3, 10000 Zagreb, Croatia

S Kupesic
Department of Obstetrics and Gynecology
Medical School University of Zagreb
Sveti Duh Hospital, Sveti Duh 64
10000 Zagreb, Croatia

A Kurjak
Department of Obstetrics and Gynecology
Medical School University of Zagreb
Sveti Duh Hospital, Sveti Duh 64
10000 Zagreb, Croatia

V Latin
Polyclinic "Vili"
Gjure Dezelica 32, 10000 Zagreb, Croatia

N Maiz
Fetal Medicine Service
Department of Obstetrics and Gynecology
University Institute "Dexeus"
Passeig Bonanova, 67, 08017 Barcelona, Spain

JM Martínez
Institut Clínic De Ginecologia
Obstetricícia I Neonatologia (Icgon)
Hospital Clínic, Universitat De Barcelona
Villarroel 170, 08036 Barcelona, Spain

U Marton
Polyclinic for Gynecology and Obstetrics "Dr Marton"
Andrije Hebranga 20, 10000 Zagreb, Croatia

LT Merce
Assisted Reproduction Unit
International Ruber Hospital
La Maso 38, 28034 Madrid, Spain

C Millán
Fetal Medicine Service
Department of Obstetrics and Gynecology
University Institute "Dexeus", Passeig Bonanova, 67
08017 Barcelona, Spain

A Muñoz
Fetal Medicine Service
Department of Obstetrics and Gynecology
University Institute "Dexeus"
Passeig Bonanova, 67, 08017 Barcelona, Spain

MA Pascual
Gynecologic Ecography
Department of Obstetrics and Gynecology
University Institute "Dexeus"
Passeig Bonanova, 67, 08017 Barcelona, Spain

P Prats
Fetal Medicine Service
Department of Obstetrics and Gynecology
University Institute "Dexeus"
Passeig Bonanova, 67
08017 Barcelona, Spain

M Prka
Department of Obstetrics and Gynecology
Medical School University of Zagreb
Sveti Duh Hospital, Sveti Duh 64, 10000 Zagreb, Croatia

MA Rodriguéz
Fetal Medicine Service
Department of Obstetrics and Gynecology
University Institute "Dexeus"
Passeig Bonanova, 67, 08017 Barcelona, Spain

M Ruiz
Fetal Medicine Service
Department of Obstetrics and Gynecology
University Institute "Dexeus"
Passeig Bonanova, 67, 08017 Barcelona, Spain

L Sanchez
Department of Obstetrics and Gynecology
University Institute "Dexeus"
Passeig Bonanova, 67
08017 Barcelona, Spain

E Scazzocchio
Fetal Medicine Service
Department of Obstetrics and Gynecology
University Institute "Dexeus"
Passeig Bonanova, 67, 08017 Barcelona, Spain

M Stanojevic
Department of Obstetrics and Gynecology
Medical School University of Zagreb
Sveti Duh Hospital, Sveti Duh 64
10000 Zagreb, Croatia

M Torrents
Fetal Medicine Service
Department of Obstetrics and Gynecology
University Institute "Dexeus"
Passeig Bonanova, 67, 08017 Barcelona, Spain

D Varga
Insurance Zagreb Nemetova Polyclinic
Nemetova-2, 10000 Zagreb, Croatia

N Vecek
Department of Obstetrics and Gynecology
Medical School University of Zagreb
Sveti Duh Hospital, Sveti Duh 64
10000 Zagreb, Croatia

FOREWORD

It has been claimed that the three greatest breakthroughs in obstetrics and gynecology during the past 50 years have been ultrasound, ultrasound, and ultrasound. The DONALD SCHOOL ATLAS shows that this bold claim is not an exaggeration—but clinical reality. The editors, Carrera and Kurjak, are both pioneers in the use of ultrasound who have made significant contributions year after year. They draw on their vast experience to craft a textbook that is comprehensive with state of the art images. This work documents the beauty and clinical application of ultrasound at its best.

The book starts with a description of normal fetal development and anatomy. Detailed illustrations then document fetal anomalies which can be detected. Other aspects of obstetric ultrasound are illustrated including abnormal growth, multiple gestation, and the placenta. The latest breakthroughs in 3- and 4-dimensional ultrasound, fetal behavior, and power Doppler are elucidated. The section on clinical gynecology then covers the vital topics of adnexal masses, infertility, sonohysterography, and ectopic pregnancy.

Some of us are old enough to remember the "dark ages" before the advent of ultrasound, when twins and fetal anomalies were a surprise at delivery and ectopic pregnancies presented as maternal deaths. The editors, Carrera and Kurjak, are two of the visionaries that have lead the profession of obstetrics and gynecology into a Renaissance: the constantly evolving clinical application of ultrasound with the result of continuous improvements in the care of our female and fetal patients.

Frank A Chervenak MD
Given Foundation Professor and Chairman
Department of Obstetrics and Gynecology
Weill Medical College of Cornell University
New York, USA

CONTENTS

SECTION 1—OBSTETRICS

Section 2—GYNECOLOGY and Infertility

Section 1
Obstetrics

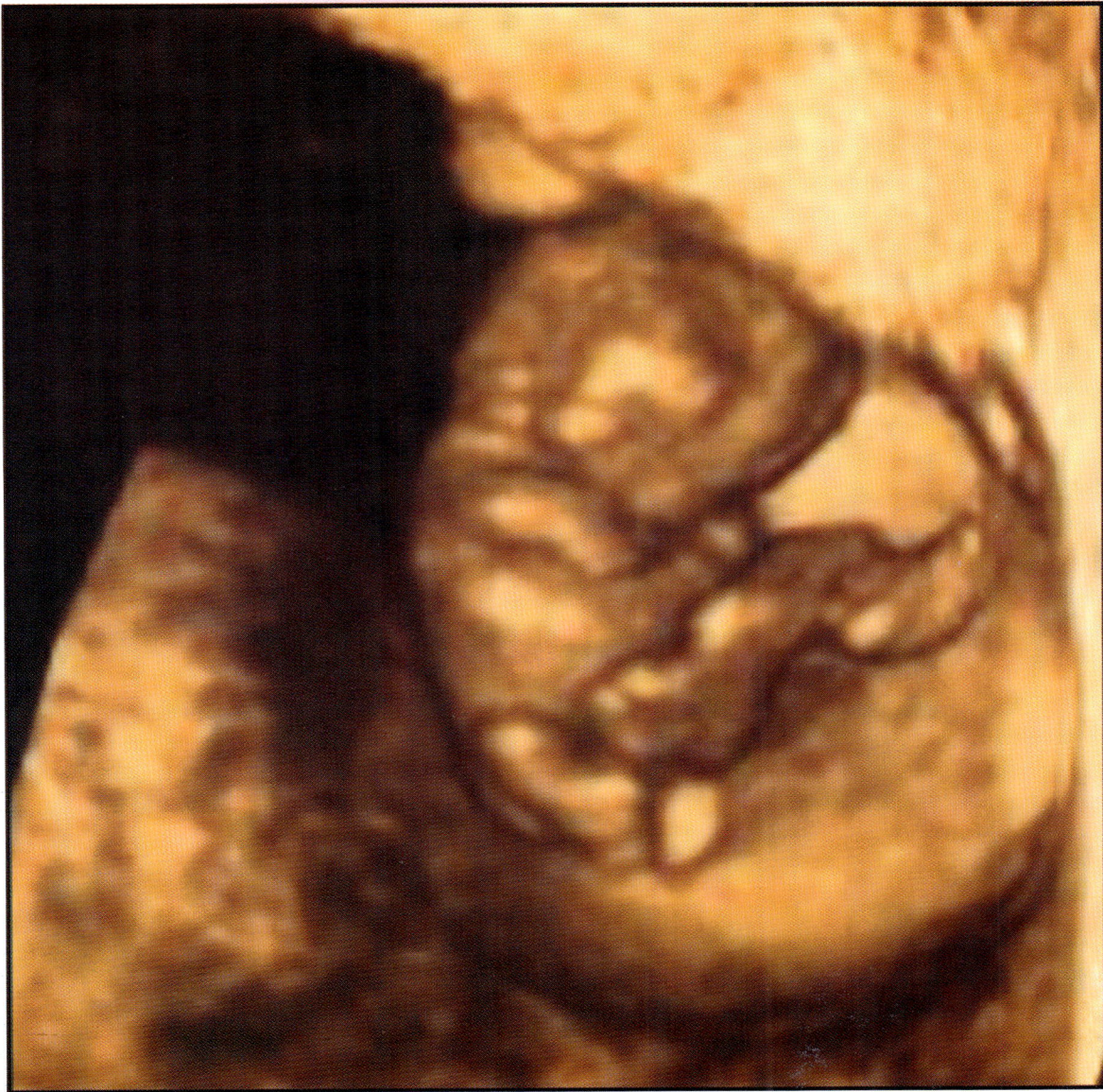

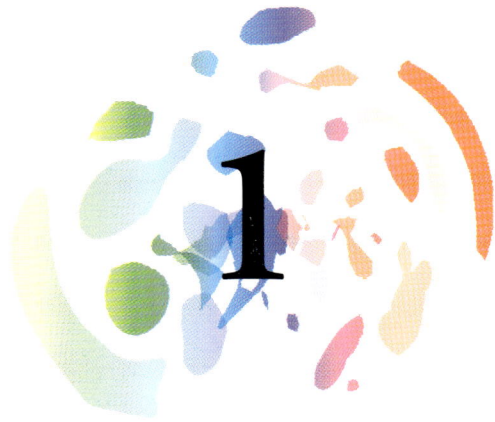

Ljiljana Kostovic-Knezevic
Srecko Gajovic

Human Embryo before Ultrasound Visualization

INTRODUCTION

The mystery of development is the question of how the fertilized egg under right conditions gives rise to a complex multicellular organism consisting of differentiated cells arranged in a precise pattern. The first month of the human embryo development is characterized by two main morphogenetic processes: gastrulation and neurulation. During this period the embryo is in the intimate contact with the endometrial wall and therefore hidden from the view of ultrasound.

In the early embryonic development period, dating of pregnancy in humans is very imprecise. From this reason Carnegie staging system was established. It uses precise criteria based on groups of morphological characteristics classified into 23 stages determined on specimens from Carnegie collection of human embryos. The Carnegie staging system is also very commonly used in comparative and experimental investigations of early mammalian development.

EARLY EMBRYONIC DEVELOPMENT

First Week of Development: Pre-embryonic Period

Fertilization

Human development as a repeating process from generation to generation starts by fertilization, which usually takes place in the ampulla of the uterine tube. Fertilization is a complex process (not a moment) that involves some preparations as well as set of interactions between sperm and egg.

The ejaculated sperm first must undergo a process of maturation, known as capacitation, which is the alteration of the glycoprotein surface of sperm under the influence of secretion products of the femal reproductive tract.

The ovulated oocyte is a large cell approximatelly 80 μm in diameter, surrounded by folicular granulosa cells called corona radiata, and by a 13 μm thick, transparent acellular glycoprotein envelope—zona pellucida. The zona is composed of three glycoproteins: ZP1, ZP2 and ZP3. ZP3 functions as a species-specific receptor for complementary molecules on the head of the sperm and it influences sperm binding to the zona pellucida. After process of binding, ZP3 is also responsible to induce the acrosomal reaction of the sperm.[1, 2] The acrosome membrane fuses with the outer sperm membrane and releases enzymes, which start to digest the zona. In this way sperm reaches the oocyte membrane, binds and fuses with it. After initial fusion of sperm's and egg's plasma membranes, the head and tail of the sperm sink into the egg. Once the sperm has fused with the egg, the polyspermy is prevented by the cortical reaction of the egg. The sperm-egg syngamy propagates a number of sequential events, i.e.:

- Metabolic activation of the egg
- Decondensation of the sperm nucleus
- Completion of second meiotic division of the egg
- Development and fusion of male and female pronuclei
- Restoration of the normal diploid number of chromosomes
- Formation of a zygote
- Determination of the sex of the future embryo.

Cleavage

The process of fertilization results in the zygote formation. Zygote divides after 24 to 36 hours into two cells and begins the process of cleavage. During cleavage, through subsequent divisions, the daughter cells called blastomeres are gradually smaller in diameter, and they form the morula. The size of the morula is

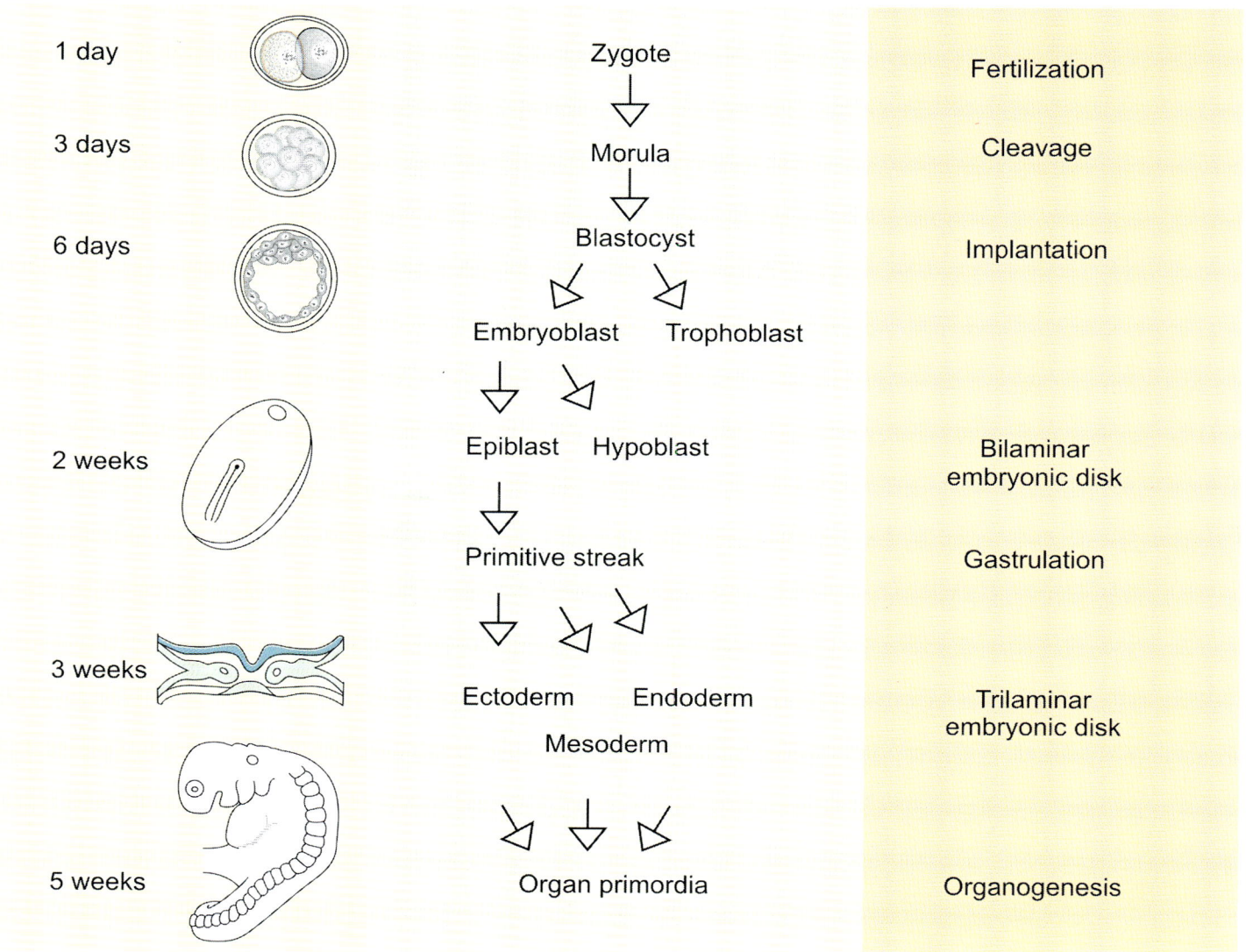

Fig. 1.1: Sequence of events during early embryonic development

constant because it is still enclosed within zona pellucida. In the two- and four-cell stage the blastomeres are identical in their capabilities expressing totipotency (Fig. 1.1). That indicates one of possibilities of twin formation. At the eight-cell stage the first communications between cells appear through formation of the intercellular contacts. This process is called compaction.[3,4] The densely packed cells form a continuous epithelial layer, thus defining inside and outside of the embryo. When the morula reaches 32- to 58-cell number it is referred as free (early) blastocyst. Inside it contains a cavity with secreted fluid known as blastocele. The cells segregate into an internally situated inner cell mass or embryoblast and surrounding, outer trophoblast cells (see Fig. 1.1)

The events described above belong to the first week (preimplantation) period during which the transportation of zygote, morula and early blastocyst occurs from ampullar tube region to the uterus.

Second Week of Development: Implantation and Differentation of Bilaminar Embryonic (Germ) Disk

Implantation

Human implantation is difficult to identify in the uterus. The evidence is based on morphological studies of human and animal embryos, and on experimental data mostly in the mouse.

Successful implantation depends on coordination of both the blastocyst and the endometrium. The complex preparation for the implantation (dialog between mother and embryo) starts during the preimplantation period, soon after fertilization. It includes secretion of hormones, numerous signal molecules, factors and receptors from both blastocyst and endometrium. By that time the endometrium undergoes hormonaly induced preparation—decidualization. This process is characterized by series of changes in glandular and surface epithelium, stromal cells, stromal vessels and extracellular matrix components. The changes are known as "the window of implantation," which corresponds to a range of morphological and biochemical modifications of the endometrium during its maximal receptivity of blastocyst, which are favorable to the further development of the embryo and enable immunological tolerance.[5-7]

After the blastocyst reaches the uterine cavity the first step in preparing implantation is "hatching" from the zona pellucida by enzymes secreted by trophoblastic cells.

Approximately 5 to 6 days after fertilization, the blastocyst begins the "attachment" to the surface epithelia of the endometrium (Fig. 1.2). The apical surface of the endometrial cells expresses a variety of adhesion molecules called integrins.

Both in vivo and in vitro studies have shown that attachment of the blastocyst occurs at the area above the embryoblast (inner cell mass) referred as embryonic pole. In this area the trophoblast proliferates and differentiates into inner cellular cytotrophoblast and outer multinucleated syncytiotrophoblast, where cells loose border membranes, and coalesce to form syncytium.

The next step of implantation is penetration (invasion) of the uterine epithelium by highly invasive syncytiotrophoblastic projections. By days 9 after fertilization, they expand and erode quickly into the endometrial stroma. Within the syncytiotrophoblast lacunae appear. On day 10, the embryo is embedded in the endometrium, and syncytiotrophoblast erodes

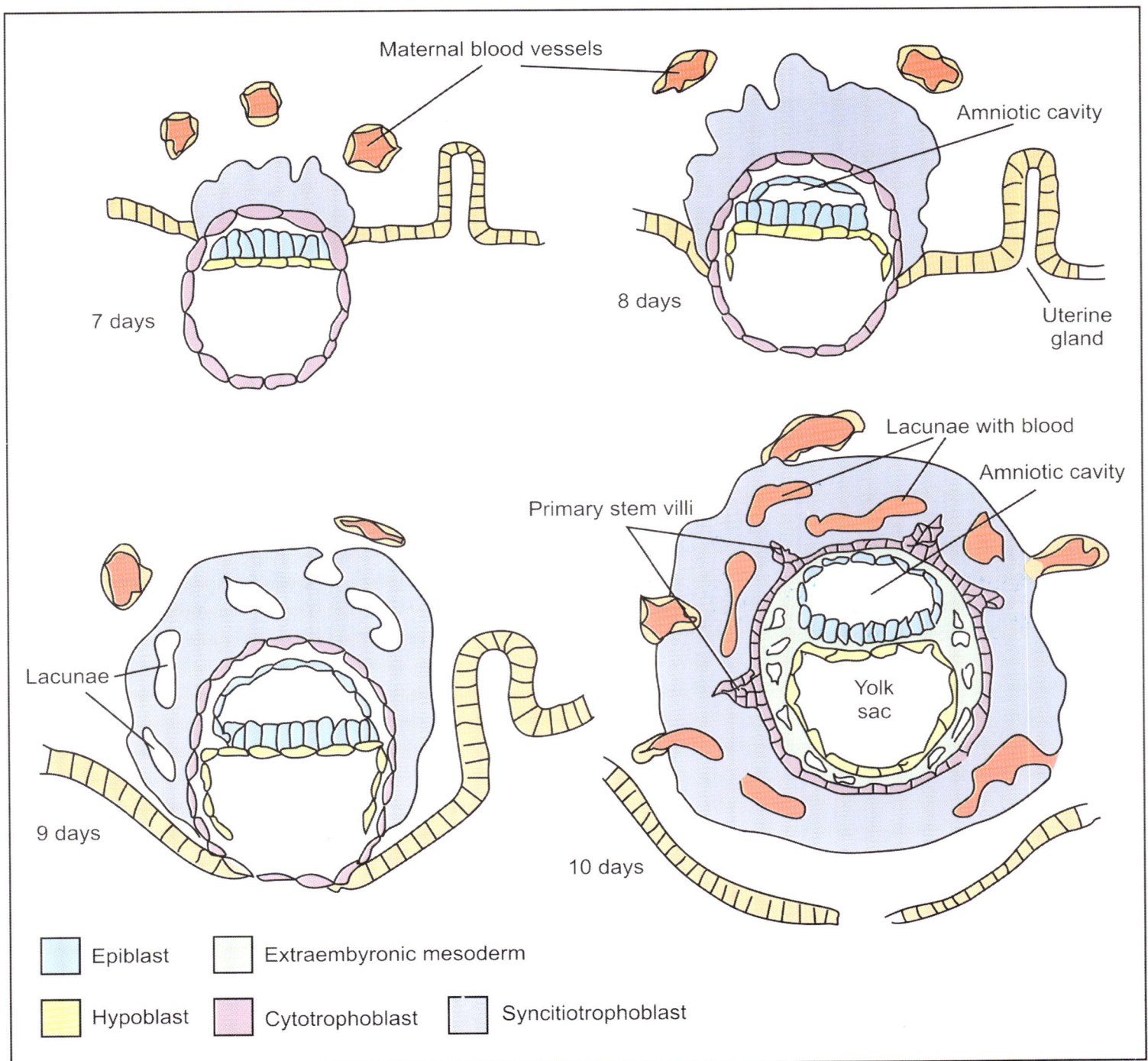

Fig. 1.2: Implantation period and bilaminar embryonic disk with the amniotic cavity and yolk sac formation

endometrial blood vessels walls. The maternal blood begins to fill the lacunae that have been forming in the trophoblast (Fig. 1.2). Maternal capillaries near the syncytiotrophoblast expand to form maternal sinusoids that rapidly anastomose with the trophoblastic lacunae, and the primitive uteroplacental circulation is established.

Bilaminar Embryonic (Germ) Disk

During the implantation period and differentiation of the trophoblast, the cells of the embryoblast (inner cell mass) split into two layers, i.e. the upper epiblast or primary ectoderm, and the lower hypoblast, primary or primitive endoderm. These two layers form the bilaminar germ disk, which develops into the embryo proper. A cavity called amniotic cavity or amnion develops within the epiblast. The cells that form the amniotic membrane are amnioblasts. The amniotic cavity is very small, but by the time it expands steadily (by the 8th week it encloses the whole embryo). The hypoblast gives rise to the endodermal lining of the primary yolk sac. On day 8, cells at the periphery of the hypoblast migrate out over the inner surface of the cytotrophoblast. On day 10, the flattened hypoblastic cells form exocelomic (Heuser's) membrane, lining the cavity called primary yolk sac or exocelomic cavity. At that stage the bilaminar germ disk is located between the primary yolk sac on ventral side and the amniotic cavity on its dorsal surface (see Fig. 1.2).

By day 12 the cells of hypoblast proliferate and migrate again forming a secondary or definitive yolk sac, while the primary yolk sac becomes constricted and pushed in front of it. The secondary yolk sac remains as an important structure through the fourth week giving rise to endothelial and hematopoietic stem cells (blood islands), as well to the primordial germ cells that migrate to the gonads.

Starting at about days 12 some cells of the hypoblast give rise to another extraembryonic tissue, the extraembryonic mesoderm. This mesoderm becomes the first connective tissue that supports the epithelium of amnion and yolk sac as well as the chorion (chorionic villi), which arises from the trophoblast.

Third Week of Development: Gastrulation

Formation of the Trilaminar Embryonic (Germ) Disk

At the end of the second week the primitive streak appears as a thickening on the dorsal surface of the epiblast near the caudal end of the bilaminar germ disk. The superior end of the primitive streak contains small elevation called primitive or Hensen's node. On day 16, the cells of epiblast proliferate, migrate and form a groove along the midline of the region of the primitive streak.

As the cells of epiblast reach the primitive streak, they change the shape and migrate down between the epiblast and hypoblast. Some of them displace the hypoblast cells replacing them with a layer of definitive or secondary endoderm. Others migrate laterally and cranially between epiblast and hypoblast and form a new germ layer, the intraembryonic or secondary mesoderm. The bilaminar embryonic disk is converted into trilaminar embryonic disk consisting of three definitive germ layers, i.e. ectoderm, mesoderm and endoderm. This process called gastrulation is the most important event in the early development establishing the main body axis and the source of embryo tissues and organs.

The cells passing through the primitive streak change their structure and organization. While the epiblast cells have typical epithelial structure and properties, upon invagination cells elongate, loose basal lamina and take a characteristic bottle shaped morphology. Reaching the space between epiblast and hypoblast, the bottle cells assume the structure of mesenchymal cells (Fig. 1.3).

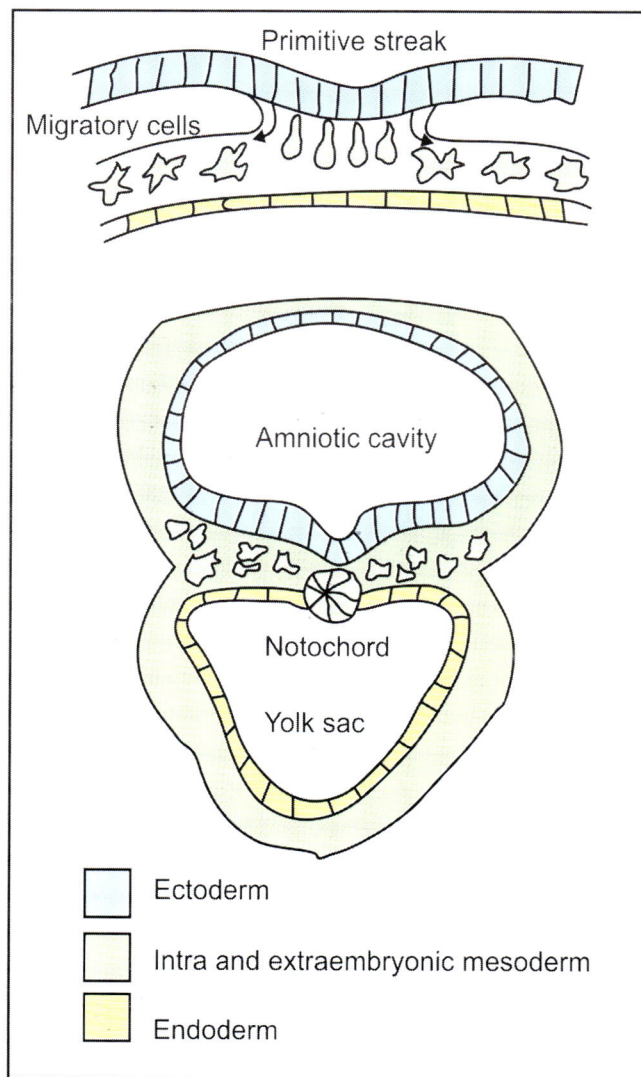

Fig. 1.3: Gastrulation period and notochord formation

Regression of the Primitive Streak

As mentioned before the primitive streak appears on day 16 and expands cranially until day 18. After that time it regresses caudally and soon disappears. The remains of primitive streak cells can produce tumors in sacrococcygeal region, referred as teratomas. Teratomas consist of many different tissues (cartilage, muscle, hair, fat glands epithelial tissue) as they contain cells, which can give rise to derivatives of all three germ layers.

Notochord

The epiblast cells in the area of the primitive node invaginate and migrate in midline and cranial direction (day 16 to 17) and give rise to the notochordal plate and notochordal process, which differentiate in the definitive notochord completed at day 31. The notochordal cells produce extracellular matrix molecules including collagen and form the primitive axial skeleton of the embryo (see Fig. 1.3). The notochord plays an important role in the induction of the overlying ectoderm in early development of the nervous tissue, a process called neurulation. The notochord also induces the vertebral body formation. The failure of these inductive interactions results in various vertebral column and spinal cord abnormalities, including spina bifida.

Abnormal Gastrulation

The period between 3 and 8 weeks of development is the critical period for abnormal development of the embryo, as this is the time when organs and systems are being established. The defects in gastrulation can have wide consequences and could influence a body plan. For example, abnormal mesoderm formation in the third week may cause several syndromes affecting caudal part of the body referred to as caudal agenesis, sacral agenesis and caudal dysplasia. Syrenomelia is severe reduction of the caudal structures, which results in fusion of the lower extremity limb buds. Milder anomalies of this type exhibit varying degrees of neurologic deficit particularly in the caudal regions. Some caudal malformations are associated with cranial abnormalities called **VATER**, including some or all of these: vertebral defects, anal atresia, tracheal-esophageal fistula and renal defects.

Differentiation of Germ Layers

Differentiation of Ectoderm: Neurulation

Upon influence of the notochord the above ectoderm starts the process of neurulation, i.e. formation of the neural tube (Fig. 1.4). This process consists of series of steps. First the ectoderm positioned in the midline, which corresponds to the region above the underlying notochord, thickens and forms the neural plate. The formation of neural plate is a sign for division of ectoderm in two separate regions, i.e. neuroectoderm in the midline which will give rise to the nervous system, and surface ectoderm laterally which will give rise of the epidermis of the skin. Lateral parts of the neural plate start to bend and form neural folds surrounding the neural groove in the middle. The neural folds approach dorsally in the midline and close the structure in the neural tube. The closure of the neural tube starts at the hindbrain/spinal cord boundary and then proceeds in anterior and posterior directions. Therefore until neurulation is completed two openings are present at the both sides of the closing neural tube: anterior neuropore and posterior neuropore. During the process of the neural tube closure cells located at the border between neuroectoderm and surface ectoderm migrate out and form the neural crest. The neural crest cells migrate to variety of destination throughout the body and give rise to the range of derivatives including those belonging to the nervous system like spinal and autonomous ganglia, but as well those not related to the nervous system like mesenchymal cells of head and neck, or melanocytes of the skin.

The process of neurulation is rather complex and it involves a cascade of events generated both inside the neuroectoderm, as well as in the surrounding tissues. One of the forces that influence change of shape of neuroectodermal cells is a constriction of apical part of the cells mediated by microfilament bundles. In addition one medial and two lateral hinge points within the neuroectoderm aid the elevation of neural folds. The bending of neural plate is as well supported by expansion of the neighboring mesodermal cells. Cell-cell affinities and cell-cell communications are important for the final fusion of the neural folds when the neural folds have approached each other.[7,8]

The failure of neural tube to close or its reopening leads to neural tube defects (NTDs), which are among the most common congenital defects in human. The NTDs are manifested as anencephaly in the cranial region or spina bifida in the lumbosacral region.

Differentiation of Mesoderm

During the third week the mesoderm cells which migrate through the primitive streak and laterally from it begin to condense into sheet-like structure. After notochord formation the mesoderm forms paired cylindrical condensations called the paraxial mesoderm. Paraxial mesoderm condenses in groups of cells positioned along the notochord and the neural tube and forms somites. Continuous with the paraxial mesoderm is a lateral region of the intermediate mesoderm which laterally splits into

Neural plate

Neural groove

Neural folds

Neural tube

■ Neuroepithelial cells

□ Neural crest cells

□ Surface ectoderm

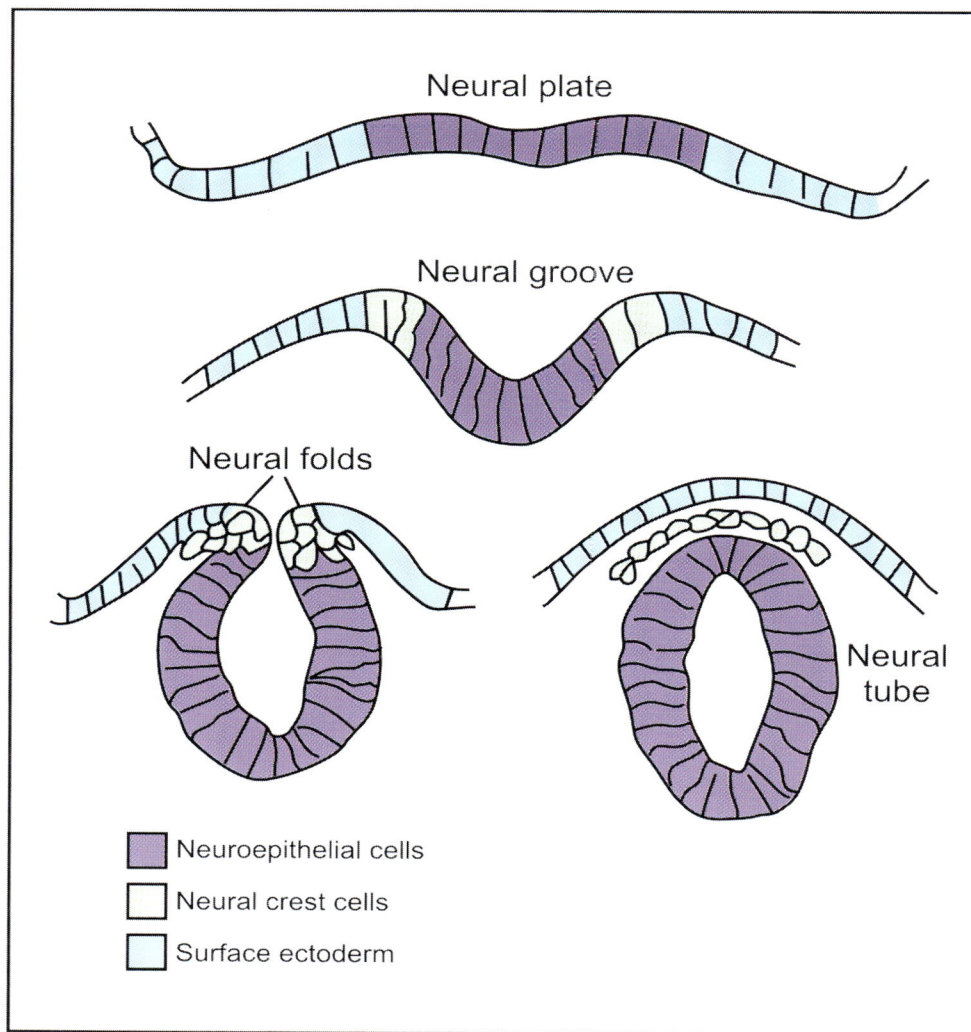

Fig. 1.4: Cross-sections through the stages in formation of the neural tube

lateral plate mesoderm forming two layers: the parietal (somatic), and visceral (splanchnic) sheath (Fig. 1.5). Between them the intraembyonic celom develops.

The paraxial mesoderm differentiates into the axial skeletal structures, voluntary musculature, and connective tissue (dermis) of the skin. The intermediate mesoderm produces urinary system and part of the genital system. The lateral mesoderm (somatic and splanchnic) forms the bulk of the body wall, the wall of the digestive tube and limbs (Fig. 1.6).

Differentiation of Endoderm

Endoderm gives rise to the epithelial lining of the gastrointestinal and respiratory tracts and some glands (Fig. 1.6).

Development of the intraembryonic endoderm germ layer is connected with the folding of the embryo in the craniocaudal direction forming a C-shaped structure. Early in the third week the roof of the yolk sac constitutes future intraembryonic part. By the folding of embryo this flat part transforms into a tubular primitive gut delineated from the yolk sac. The primitive gut

differentiates into the foregut, midgut and hindgut. The midgut remains open to the yolk sac ventrally. The anterior end of the embryo foregut is temporarily connected to the surface ectoderm forming a bilayer called oropharyngeal membrane, which separates the future mouth - stomodeum. The caudal part of hindgut — cloaca forms another endodermal-ectodermal attachment referred as the cloacal membrane.

At the end of the fourth week the region of the yolk sac is reduced to form the yolk stalk (omphalomesenteric or vitelline duct).

EARLY CIRCULATION DEVELOPMENT

Starting on day 17, first vessels primordia begin to develop in the extraembryonic mesoderm of yolk sac wall forming aggregations of cells called blood islands. This process occurs under inductive interaction of endoderm of yolk sac. On the day 18 vasculogenesis (blood vessels formation) begins. The blood island cells are pluripotent stem cells—hemangioblasts,

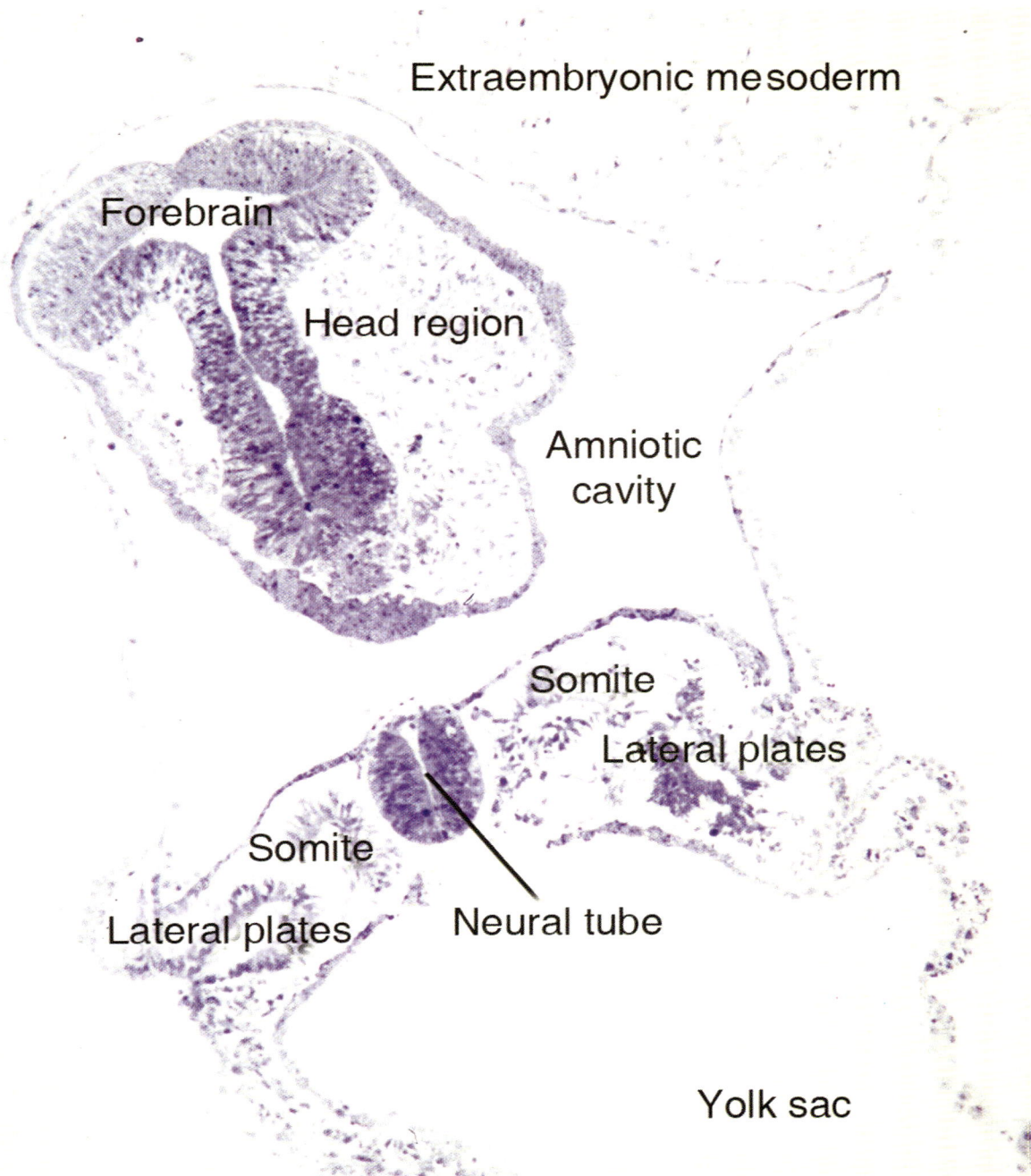

Fig. 1.5: Transverse 1 μm thick section stained by toluidine blue of the human embryo (2 mm crown-rump length, 21 to 22 days)

peripherally differentiating into the endothelial vascular wall and centrally into primitive hematopoietic cells. The vessels fuse to form networks of endothelial channels. The primitive blood vessels by the same time extend into the mesenhyme of the connecting stalk (allantoic) and chorionic villi, and by the end of the third week the vascular extraembryonic network is established.

On days 18, vasculogenesis in the embryo begins in the splanchnic mesoderm and it does not involve any more formation of blood cells. The mesenchymal cells differentiate in the angioblasts, which develop into the flattened endothelial cells forming angiocysts. Later angioblastic cords develop by the fusion of the angiocysts forming a network of angioblastic plexuses that establish the initial circulatory system of the embryo. The yolk sac is the first supplier of blood cells to the embryonic circulation. Later in the week 5, the blood cell production (hematopoiesis) starts in embryonic organs, including liver, spleen, thymus and bone marrow. The source of these cells is unclear.

The primitive heart forms in a similar manner from mesenchymal cells in the cardiogenic area. The cardiac primordium is located in the front of the head fold. Paired endocardial heart tubes develop before the end of the third week. Soon after these tubes approach each other and fuse into a

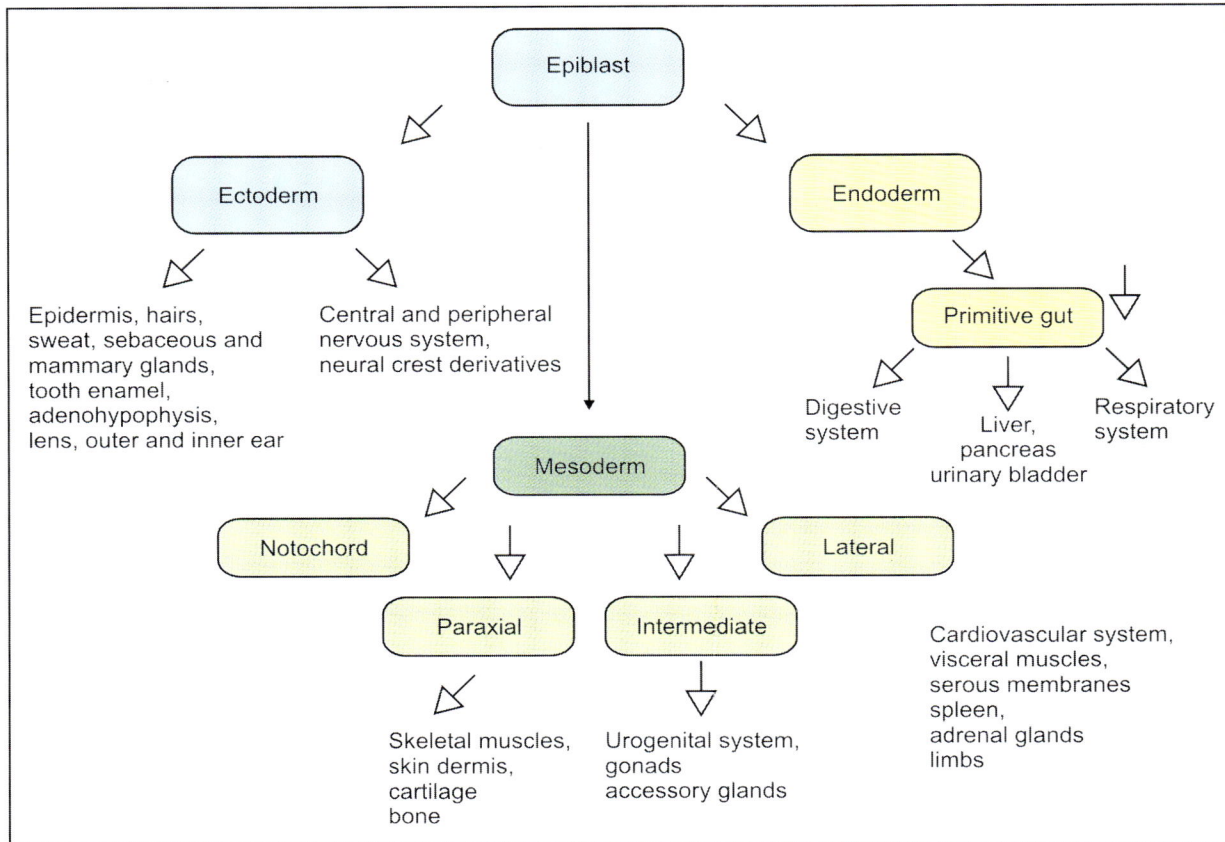

Fig. 1.6: Presentation of the germ layer origin of the organs and tissues

primitive heart tube. The heart elongates and develops dilatations and constrictions: the truncus aretriosus, bulbus cordis, primitive ventricle, primitive atrium and sinus venosus.

By the end of the third week the heart tubes are linked up with blood vessels in the embryo, connecting stalk, chorion, and yolk sac to form a primitive cardiovascular system. The circulation of blood starts by the end of the third week when contractions of the primitive heart begins (day 22). The cardiovascular system is the first organ system to reach a functional state.

The blood from the primitive heart is distributed by aortic arches to the tissue of branchial arches (future head and neck region), and by the aortae and their branches to the caudal part of the embryo body.

REFERENCES

1. Cohen N, Wasserman PM. Association of egg zona pellucida glycoprotein mZP3 with sperm protein sp56 during fertilization in mice. Int J Dev Biol 2001; 45:569-76
2. Esterhuizen AD, Franken DR, Luorens JGH, van Royen LH. Clinical importance of zona pellucida-induced acrosome reaction and its predictive value for IVF. Hum Reprod 2001; 16:138-44
3. Carlson BC. Human Embryology & Developmental Biology, Mosby 1999.
4. Tao J, Tamis R, Fink K, Williams B, Nelson-White T, Graig R. The neglected morula/compact stage embryo transfer. Hum Reprod 2002; 17:1513-8.
5. Ma WG, Song H, Das SK, Paria BC, Dey SK. Estrogen is a determinant that specifies the duration of the window of uterine receptivity for implantation. Proc Natl Acad Sci USA. 2003; 100:2963-8.
6. Lukassen HG, Joosten I, van Cranenbroek B, van Lierop MJ, Bulten J, Braat DD, van Der Meer A. Hormonal stimulation for IVF treatment positively affects the CD56bright/CD56dim NK cell ratio of the endometrium during the window of implantation. Mol Hum Reprod 2004; 10:513-20.
7. Colas JF, Schoenwolf GC. Towards a cellular and molecular understanding of neurulation. Dev Dyn 2001;221:117-45.
8. Melton KR, Iulianella A, Trainor PA. Gene expression and regulation of hindbrain and spinal cord development. Front Biosci 2004;9:117-38.

2

MA Rodríguez, E Scazzocchio, M Echevarria, JM Carrera

Fetal Anatomy

INTRODUCTION

The study of fetal anatomy is at present absolute priority of the diagnostic ultrasonography. Only exceptionally it is necessary to use other complementary imaging tools such as Magnetic Resonance. Many illustrative photos are shown in separate chapters of this book, but it is useful to discuss fetal anatomy in detail before the reader reaches chapters of fetal abnormalities.

FETAL HEAD: ANATOMY OF ENCEPHALUM

Transabdominal Approach

Today, as a consequence of recommendation of the American Institute of Ultrasound in Medicine, American College of Radiology and the American College of Obstetricians and Gynecologists,[1-4] it is usual, as a part of all obstetric ultrasonography exploration, to make three standard axial views: transthalamic, transventricular and transcerebellar (Fig. 2.1).[5]

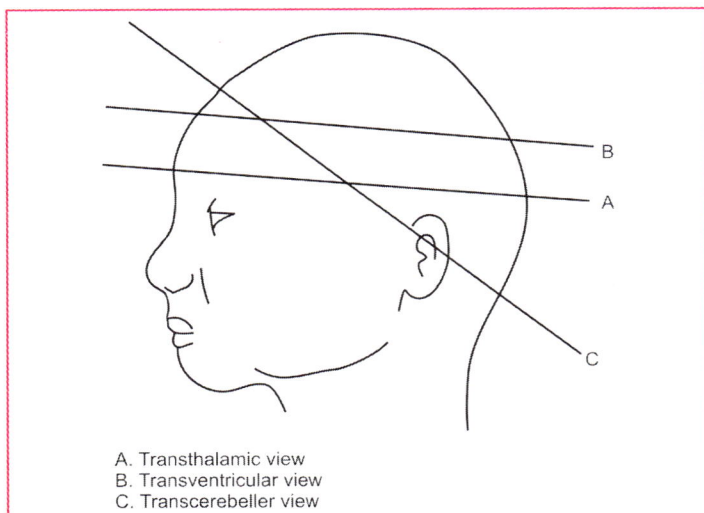

A. Transthalamic view
B. Transventricular view
C. Transcerebeller view

Fig. 2.1: Head axial views: A. Transthalamic view, B. Transventricular view, C. Transcerebellar view

The introduction of three-dimensional (3D) ultrasound in obstetrics produced objective imaging, not only of fetal superficial structure but also bony structure, multiplanar analysis of morphology, sono-angiography and volume calculation of target organ.[6,7]

Transthalamic View

This is the standard plane used for obtaining the measure of biparietal diameter and also head circumference. Traditionally was known as a medium scan plane.

In this plane it is possible to observe the frontal horns of the lateral ventricles, the cavum, the septum pellucidum (between the frontal horns), the third ventricle and the sylvian cisterna (Fig. 2.2).[8]

On both sides of third ventricle it is possible to observe the thalamohipogenic structure which size increases along the gestation. In favorable circumstances it is also possible to observe the nucleus caudado and putamen.

Transventricular View

Transventricular view corresponds to medium-high scan plan of the classic descriptions. It is obtained at a plane just superior to the transthalamic view. The aim of this plane is the observation of the lateral cerebral ventricles (Fig. 2.3). From 12th to 13th weeks, the choroid plexus (very echogenic) fills all the lateral ventricles (from side-to-side), and for this reason is the aspect more gaudy of the cerebral hemispheres. The frontal horn does not occupy for choroid plexus, but however, are well visible and prominent. In front of frontal horn, the corpus callosum knee is situated, and for back of occipital horn, the splenium of corpus

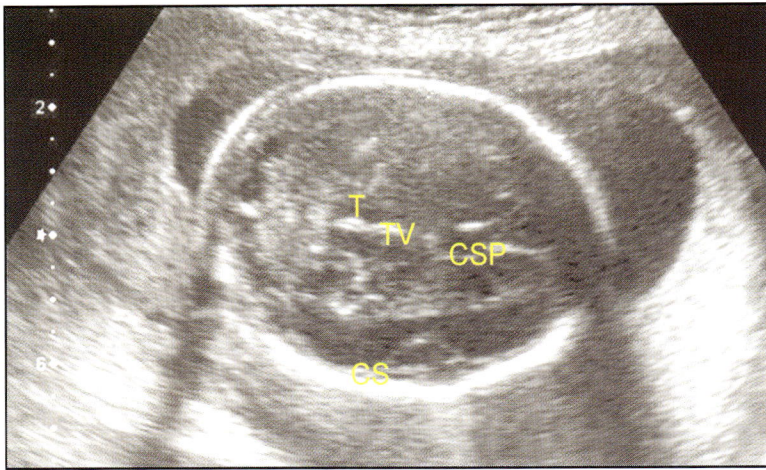

Fig. 2.2: Transthalamic view
T : Thalamo
CSP : Cavum septum pellucidum
TV : Third ventricle
CS : Silvian cisterna

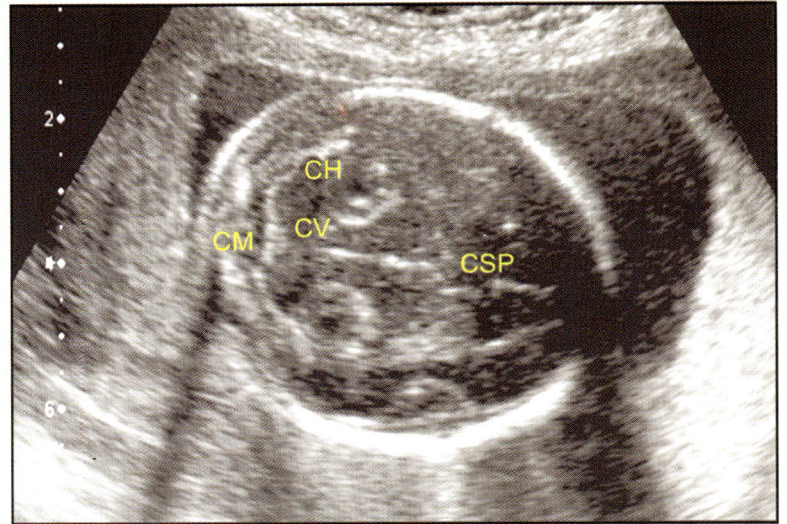

Fig. 2.4: Transcerebellar view
CH: Cerebellar hemispheres
CV: Cerebelar vermix
CM: Cisterna magna
CSP: Cavum septum pellucidum

callosum.

The lateral and medial walls of the lateral ventricles run nearly parallel to the midline interhemispheric fissure until 18th week, but, from this moment, as a consequence of the development of the temporal horns, the lateral ventricles are drawn laterally. At the same time, progressively, the ventricles and choroid are minus pronounced and minus gaudy.

During the third trimester, the axial sonograms to this level show a parallel line (periventricular lines) in the far ventricle that is thought to represent intracerebral veins or fibers within the cerebral white matter. In either case, the periventricular line

The cisterna magna is a fluid space, situated between the dorsum of the cerebellar hemisphere and the inner calvarium. It is perfectly visible in all cases, during second and early third trimesters. The depth of the cisterna magna gradually increases with gestational age.[9]

The cerebellum usually is more echogenic than the cerebral hemispheres and is separated of the tentorium from supratentorial structures.

The coronal and sagittal scan planes, (Fig. 2.5) relatively easily obtained in neonates, are the most difficult for identification in fetuses, except in special circumstances, as a podalic presentation.

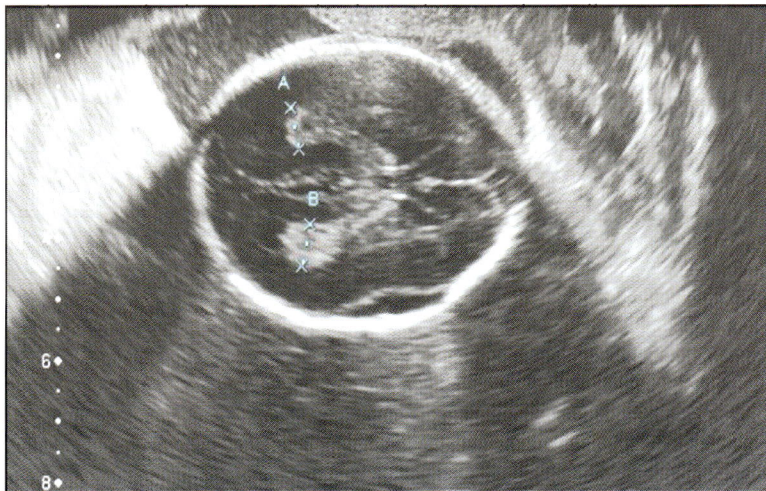

Fig. 2.3: Transventricular view at the ventricular atrium level

Transcerebellar View

This plane includes the cerebellar hemispheres and cisterna magna. This is an angled view through the posterior fossa (Fig. 2.4).[5]

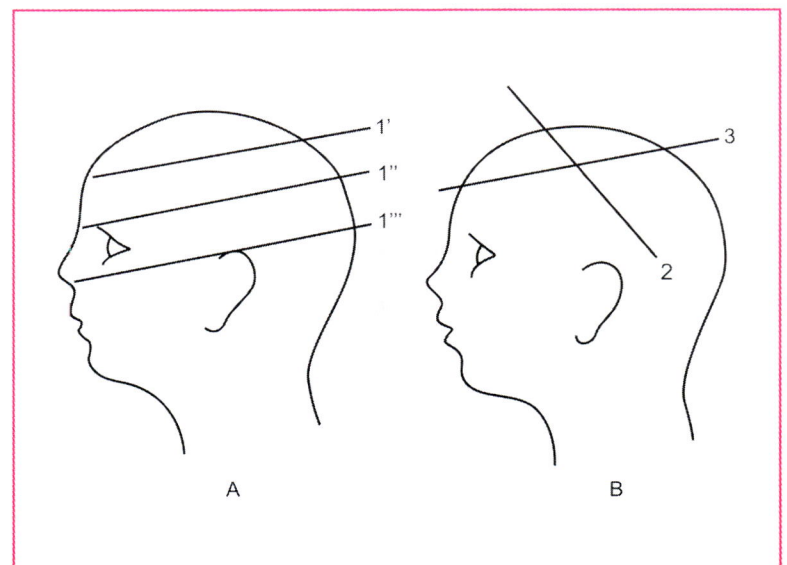

Fig. 2.5: A. Horizontal scans (1), B. Coronal (2) and sagittal (3) scans

Transvaginal Approach

Transvaginal approach of the fetal brain during the second and third trimesters was introduced by Monteagudo et al.[10] This technique permits the assessment of sagittal and coronal views of fetal brain, through the fontanelles and sagittal suture.[11-13] With serial oblique reactions the same ultrasound window shows a very detailed image of the intracranial morphology (Figs 2.6 and 2.7).[11]

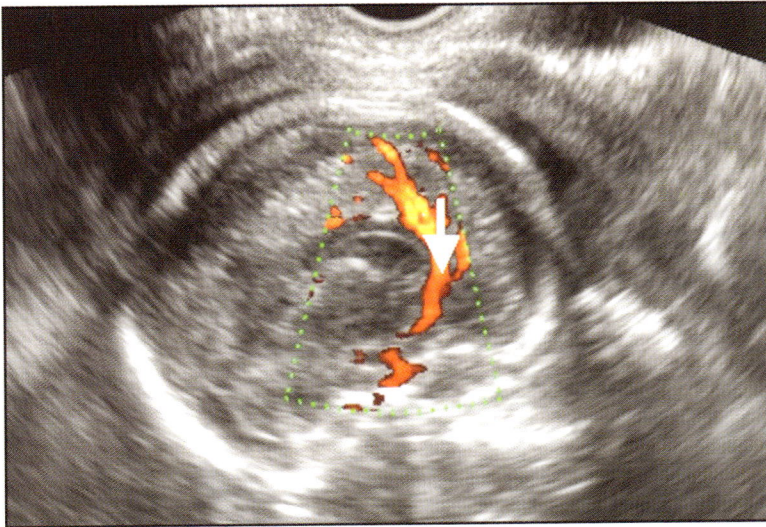

Fig. 2.6: Parasagittal view shows the corpus callosum as an hypoechoic semicircular image (arrow). Color Doppler shows the pericallosal artery

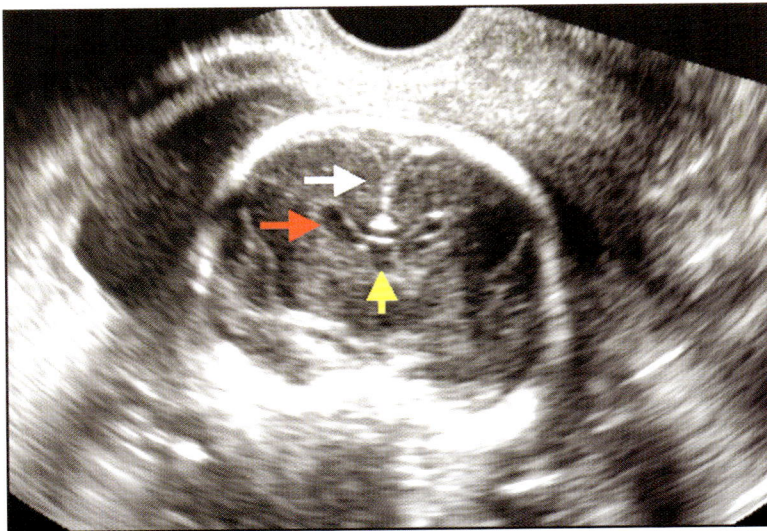

Fig. 2.7: Coronal scan: the white arrow shows the echogenic falx, surronding subarachnoid spaces. The red arrow indicates the lateral ventricle and the yellow ones show the cavum of the septum pelucidum

FACE AND NECK

The evaluation of the face and neck can be made by means of 2D and 3D ultrasonography.

Evaluation of the Face by 2D Ultrasonography

By means of 2D ultrasonography it is possible to visualize the face quite well as early as 12th to 13th weeks. Specially indicated are those scan planes that permit visualization of the silhouette of the face.

Contrary to what was usually considered, the study of the face structures is easier in the first half of the gestation due to absence of the flexion of the head, and the continuous movement of the fetus. This fact permits to make all the types of sections in a short time.

Very early it is possible to evaluate the profile of the fetal face, to provide the diagnosis of several malformations of the facial mass, but also the suspicion of determined encephalic malformation syndromes distinguished by facial dysplasias (Fig. 2.8).

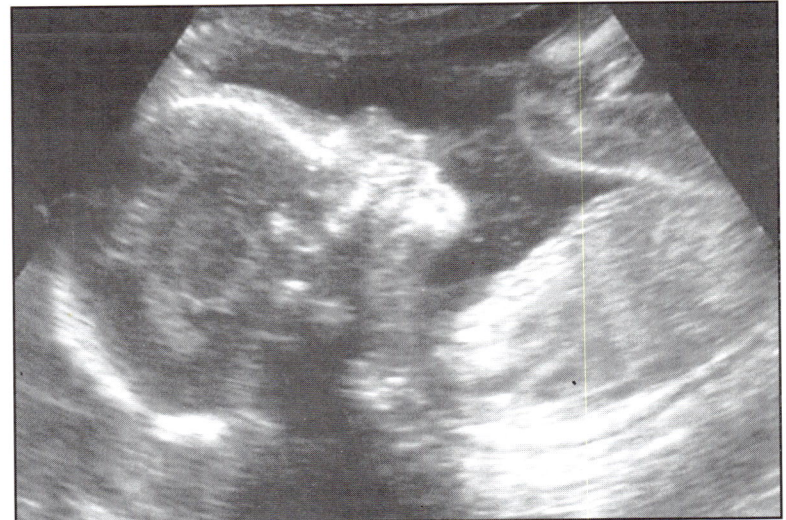

Fig. 2.8: Normal fetal profile: 20th weeks

Effectively, the facial dysmorpheas are usually associated with one encephalic malformation or one polymalformative genetic syndrome.[14]

There are four specific scan planes for recognition of the profile and the fetal face: (Fig. 2.9)[15]

1. Lambda-orbitary scan, that permits the visualization of the orbits.

2. Chin-frontal scan, which aim is the same, plus more observation into the mouth (tongue, etc).

3. Vertex-nose, permits the visualization of the nasal cavities and also external ear, and

4. Nose-chin scan, which objective is the identification of nasal cavities, nasal bridge, nose, and lips.

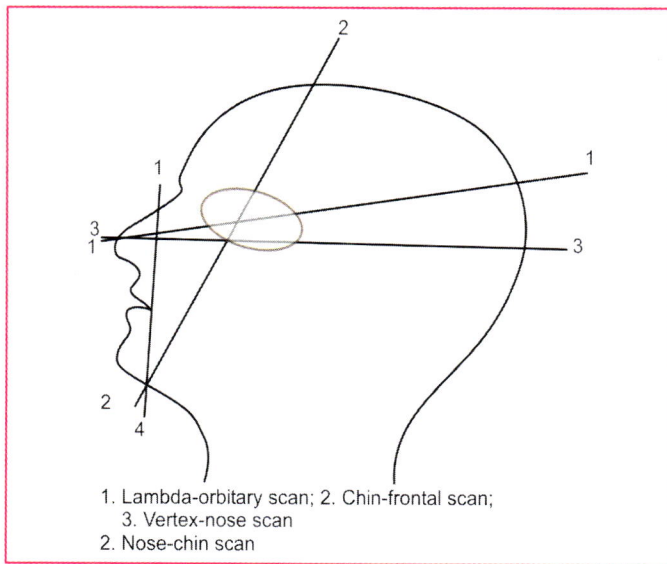

Fig. 2.9: Scan planes for recognition of the profile and the fetal face: 1. Lambda-orbitary scan. 2. Chin-frontal scan. 3. Vertex-nose scan. 4. Nose-chin scan

These planes of section make possible the visualization of the following.

Orbital Region

The orbital cavities appear as two rounded areas, echonegative but with very refringent limits. In cases of suspected anomalies, it is important to measure binocular distance. This parameter provides information regarding hypotelorism and hypertelorism (Fig. 2.10).

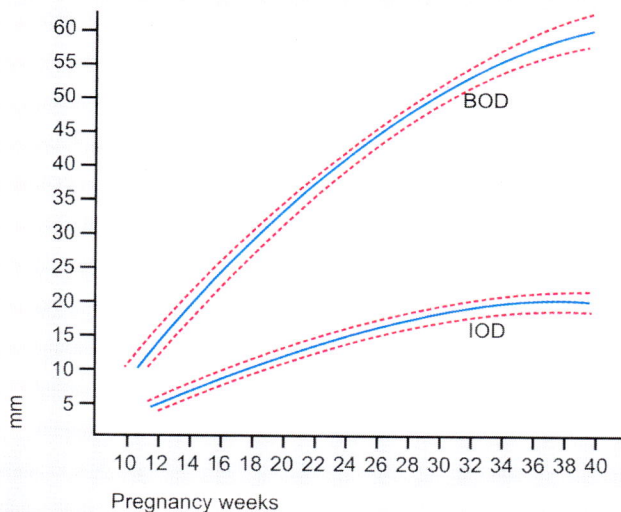

Fig. 2.10: Growth of the ocular parameters. BOD: Binocular distance; IOD: Interocular distance

In each orbital cavity we can visualize the lens (crystalline) which adopt the form to the lineal echo, very refringent. From 17 to 19th weeks until 6th month of gestation, this lineal image usually is perpendicular to anterior wall of the orbit. On the

contrary, from 28 to 29th weeks it is located in a parallel way to that one (Fig. 2.11).[16]

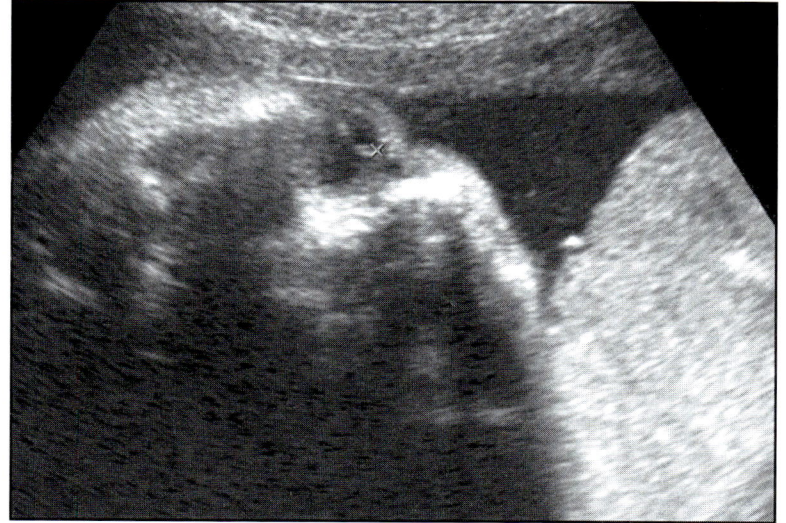

Fig. 2.11: Fetal crystalline: 30th week

The lens vision allows studying of the eyes movements and confirms an active ocular cinetic. The eyes movements can be up-down (vertical) or lateral (horizontal), being possible to move both eyes at the same time (synchronic) or each one by his side (asynchronic). During the fetal sleep (state of REM) it is possible to observe circular movements of the lens[48,49] which are accompanied by breathing movements rhythmic and very quick, swallowing movements and diaphragmatic activity.

Nasal Area

Between the orbital cavities, it is possible to recognize, especially in transversal sections, one very refringent area that corresponds to nose base. Inside of this area it is possible to identify clearly two parallel echonegative zones, which belong to the nasal cavities (choanas) and are placed on both sides of a medial structure, considerably echogenic, which corresponds to nasal bridge (Fig. 2.12).

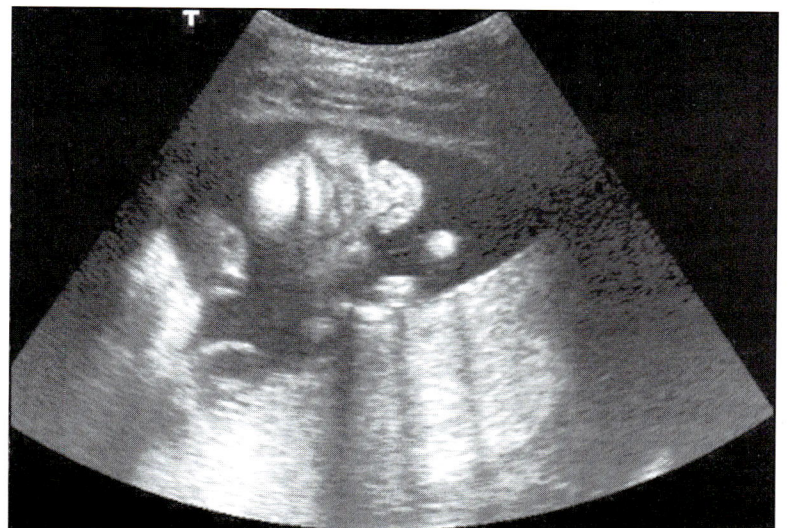

Fig. 2.12: Nose-chin scan

Mouth Area

By means of frontal view, it is possible to identify the upper lip, mouth, lower lip, and the tongue. Evaluation of these structures provides useful information regarding several malformations: cleft lip, macroglosia, etc.

Ears

By means of parasagittal scans, it is very easy to visualize the external ear shape, making possible the identification of lobule, cruz antihelices, helix, anti-helix and also scaphoid fossa. It is important to decide if the size of ear is correct, if the position is low, and if the ears are deformed.

Evaluation of the Face by Means of 3D and 4D

It is described in a separate chapter in this book.

Fetal Neck

The visualization of the fetal neck is possible only when the section plane does not run over the shoulders since in that case these structures give a shadow area which makes difficult the visualization of the spine.

In a favorable longitudinal scan it is possible to see perfectly the cervical spine with its very hyperechogenic double line and medullar canal (the anechogenic area located between both lines), which is somewhat more thick in this level than in the lower segments. Besides, it is possible to observe the neck vessels (braquiocephalic trunk, etc). Its sonographic examination is easier in podalic than in cephalic presentation, especially if there is a plentiful of amniotic fluid.

SPINE

The spine can be sonographically evaluated with three types of scans: transversal, sagittal or longitudinal and coronal.

In the transversal scans, the neural canal appears as an anechogenic area, surrounded by a ring which is formed in front by the vertebral body, and behind and on the sides by lateral masses and posterior arch (Fig. 2.13).[17]

In longitudinal scan, (Fig. 2.14) two parallel lines limit the neural tube, which correspond to vertebral body and posterior arch. In some circumstances it is possible to see even three lines, corresponding to anterior ossification center and two dorsal ossification centers. The two lines are ended in the sacral region.

During sonographic examination it is possible to observe the perimedular dura madre from 25th week. It appears in longitudinal section as a lineal and hyperechogenic echo placed

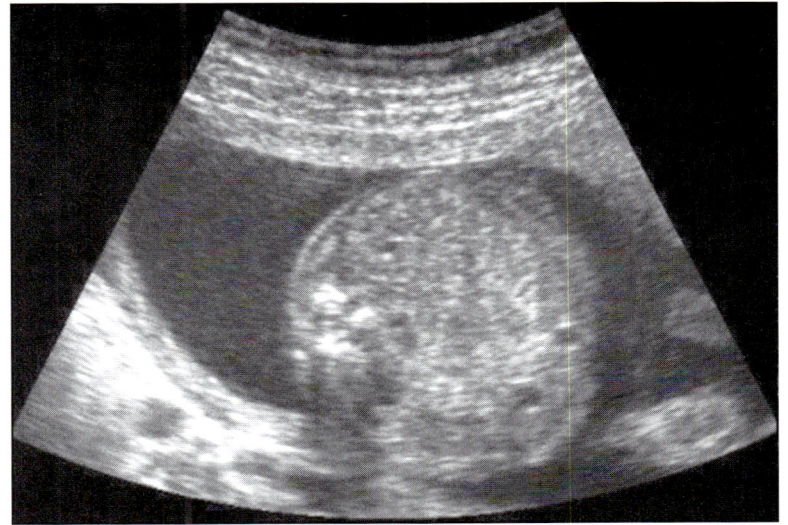

Fig. 2.13: Spine transversal scan on the lumbar area

in the interior of the spinal cord. It is usually observed with special clarity in the terminal cone of the spine.

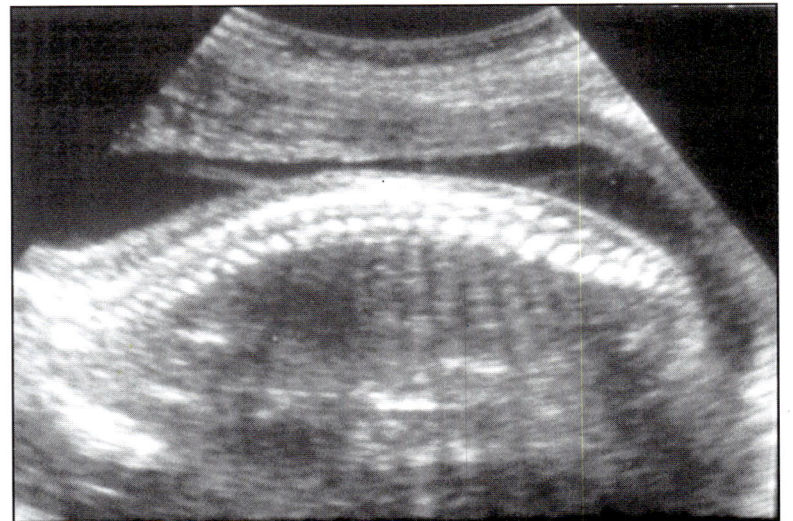

Fig. 2.14: Spine longitudinal scan

The coronal scan passes by vertebral laminas generating like in the longitudinal scans, two parallel echogenic lines delineating the vertebral space (Fig. 2.15).

Three-dimensional ultrasound permits to evaluate the spine in multiple planes.[18]

THORAX

In the *transverse scan,* the fetal thorax appears as a circular structure, limited by spine on the back, by the sternum ahead and the ribs on sides.

In the thorax, besides the heart and the anterior timic mass located in central position, two lung images located laterally can be observed. The lung limits are very clear since lungs are situated between the amniotic fluid (that surrounds the thorax) and the anechogenic images of the cardiac cavities (Fig. 2.16).[15]

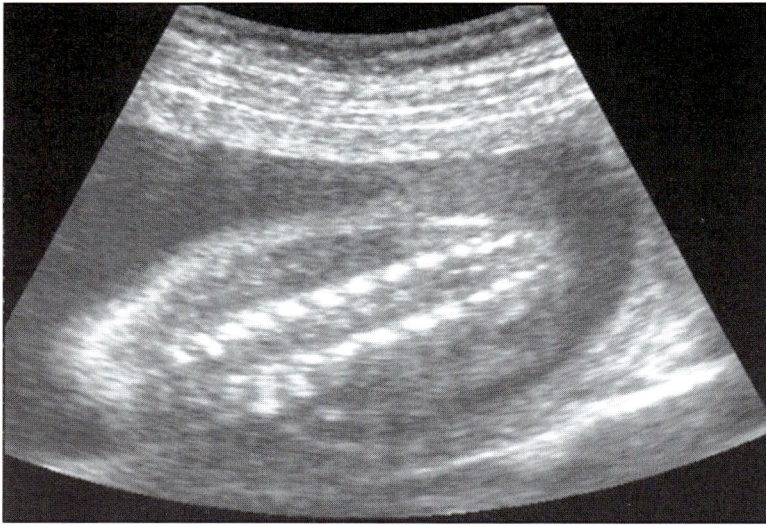

Fig. 2.15: Spine coronal scan

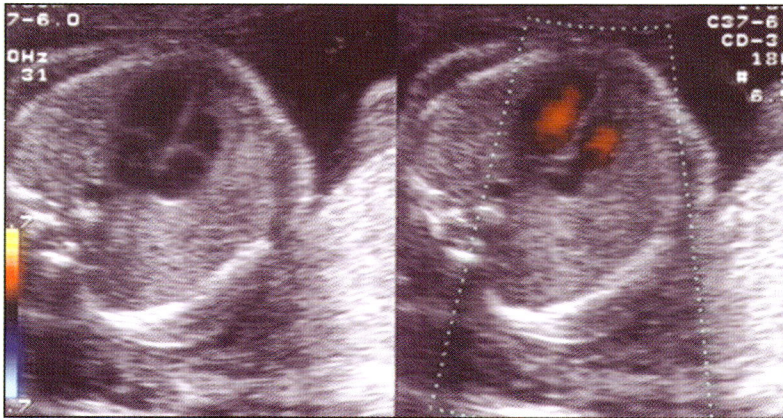

Fig. 2.16: Apical four-chamber view. Color Doppler allows the atrio-ventricular flow

In the *longitudinal scan,* the thorax adopts the form of conus trunk, limited by the spine and the rib cage.

The lungs during fetal life are visualized as solid structures. Examination of the lungs, using the same section as for the four-chamber view of the fetal heart, is sufficient.[16] The echogenicity of the lungs is uniform. Usually the central third of the thoracic area is occupied by the heart and the remaining two-thirds by the lungs.

The respiratory ways are at present visible, thanks to the high definition of equipments.

The *trachea* is recognizable for its central localization between the soft anterior tissues and the spine. Appears as a tubular anechogenic structure, very clearly limited, differentiated from the other neighboring structures (carotid, jugular, etc) for the fact that it has no pulsatility. In occasions, it is possible to observe its bifurcation.

The characteristic image of the pyriformis sinus in the coronal sections is the reference point for the identification and limitation of the hypopharynx.

It is possible to observe the larynx, thanks to the breathing movements, but the visualization of the vocal cords is very difficult. The movements of swallowing and breathing modify considerably the aspect of these structures.

Utsu et al[19] have studied the dynamic of tracheal fluid my means of Doppler.

From 13 to 14th weeks it is possible to observe the *diaphragm,* especially in the longitudinal scan. It appears as an echo-negative line, with a tick of 2 to 3 mm, located between the base of the heart and fetal liver. It is lightly incurved and with the breathing movements moves up and down (Figs 2.17 and 2.18).

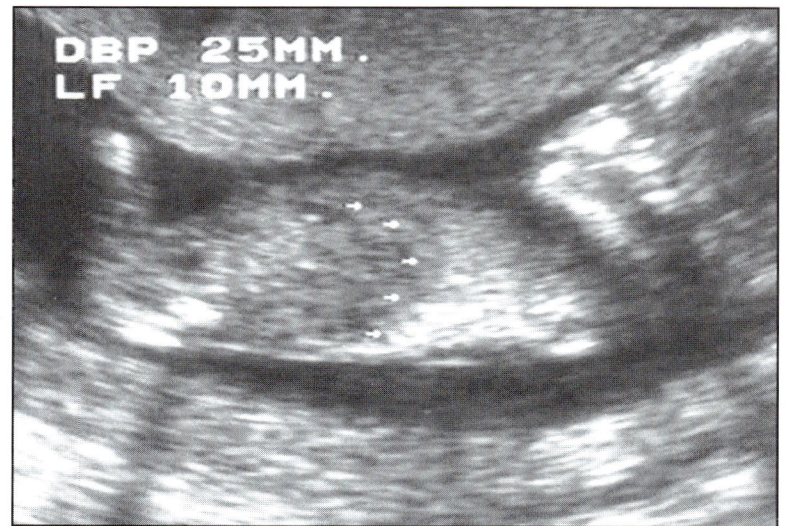

Fig. 2.17: Fetal diaphragm at 13th week

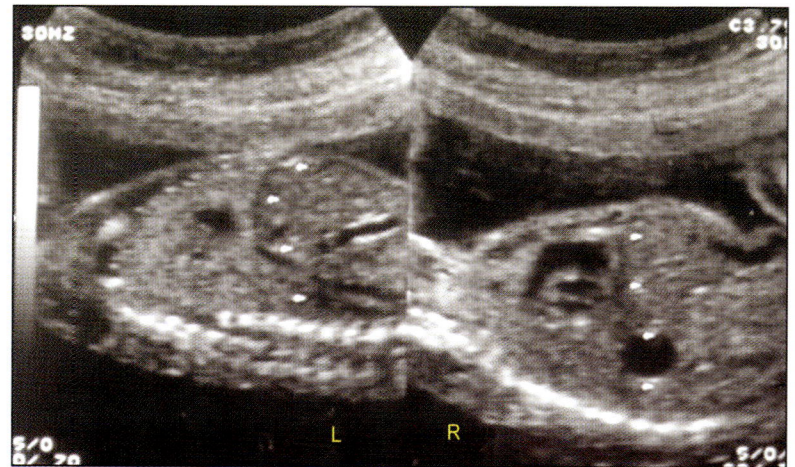

Fig. 2.18: R: Right hemidiaphragm; L: Left hemidiaphragm

HEART

The anatomic study of the fetal heart requires the *combination of several ultrasound techniques:*[20]

1. Two-dimensional echocardiography identifies anatomical structures, spatial relationships, the position of the heart, the myocardial thickness and myocardial function.

2. Doppler and color Doppler. Color Doppler opacifies cardiac activities and vessels.

3. M-mode is used to measure accurately the size of cavities and vessels.
4. Fetal position within the uterus may be used to evaluate different heart structures. Anterior dorsum is usually the best fetal position to study the aortic arch and the aorta, as well as the ductus arteriosum arch. Posterior dorsum is the most favorable position to obtain the four-chambers view, and to evaluate the ventricular size and anatomy of the inlet septum, the A-V valves and the atrioventricular connections. Lateral dorsum best identifies the right and left outflow tracts and the outlet septum, as well as ventriculoarterial connections.

Fetal Heart Scanning

The standard scanning to be obtained for a complete evaluation of the fetal heart includes:

1. *The four-chamber view*. Since the fetal heart lies horizontally in the thorax, to obtain a four-chamber view, it is necessary to slide the transducer toward the fetal chest, maintaining the transverse plane.[21]

There are three types of a four-chamber view, according to the fetal position. If the left anterior chest wall is closest to the transducer, then an apical four-chamber is obtained. When the fetal spine is anterior and closest to the transducer, then a basal four-chamber is obtained. Finally, when the fetal spine is lateral, closer to the lateral uterine walls, then it is possible to obtain a transverse four-chamber view.

A number of normal features should be identified in the four-chamber view: (i) Two equal-sized atria; (ii) the right ventricle is major than the left; (iii) two atrioventricular valves with complete leaflet excursion and different insertion on the ventricular septum; (iv) the pulmonary veins should be seen entering the left atrium; (v) septal integrity should be present; (vi) the foramen oval occupying the middle third of the atrial septum, with a detectable moving membrane; (vii) the right ventricle can be identified, apart the major size, by the presence of a moderator band.

2. *Longitudinal view*. These scan planes cut the heart along longitudinal or major axis. Included are: (i) the long axis view of the left cavities; (ii) the long axis view of the right cavities, and (ii) the long axis view of the inferior and superior venae cavae.

3. *Transversal view*. In this case the section planes go transversally through the fetal heart. There are three main scans: (i) the scan of the great vessels (Fig. 2.19A); (ii) the medium transversal scan (includes the A-V valves); and (iii) the apical scan.

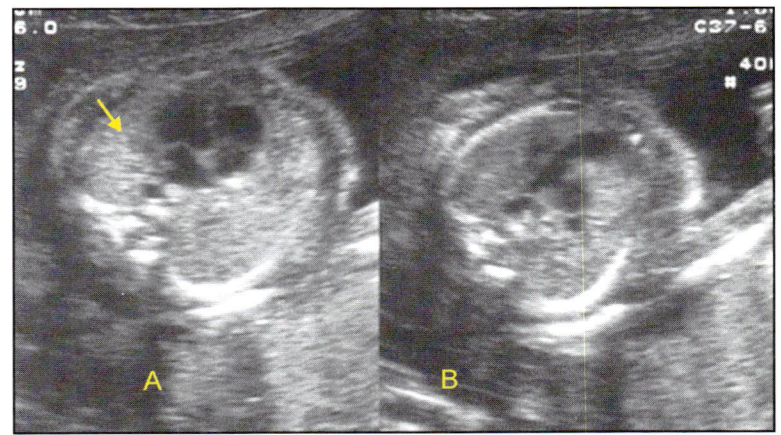

Fig. 2.19: A. Aortic root of the left ventricle. B.Great vessels outflow

4. *Subdiaphragmatic view*. Thanks to this scan it is possible to observe both ventricles and the normal (or abnormal) relationship of the aorta and pulmonary artery (Fig. 2.19.B).
5. *Special scans*. Include the aortic arch scan, the ductus arteriosum scan (ductal arch) (Fig. 2.20).

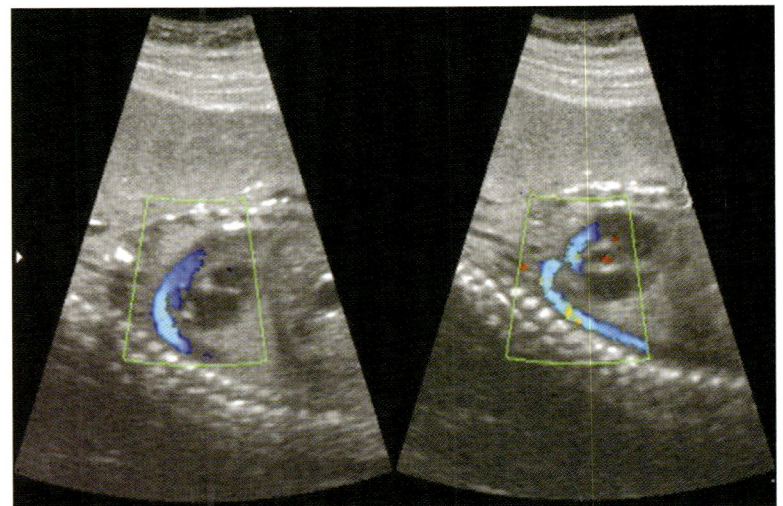

Fig. 2.20: Aortic and pulmonary arches

GASTROINTESTINAL TRACT

The *oesophagus* can be observed only when the exploration is made in the moment when the fetus is swallowing the amniotic fluid. In this case it appears as a thick anechogenic line that runs up and down in the thorax.

The fetal *stomach* is visible from 11 to 12th weeks, moment that the fetus is capable of swallowing sufficient amounts of amniotic fluid to permit the sonographic visualization. It adopts the aspect of a cystic formation, rounded, without echoes and the limits well defined. The stomach size depends on the gestational age, but especially on the grade of repletion. Non-visualization of the stomach may require repeated scanning a few hours or even days later.[22] By 15 to 16th weeks the fetal stomach should be demonstrated early in all normal fetuses (Fig. 2.21).

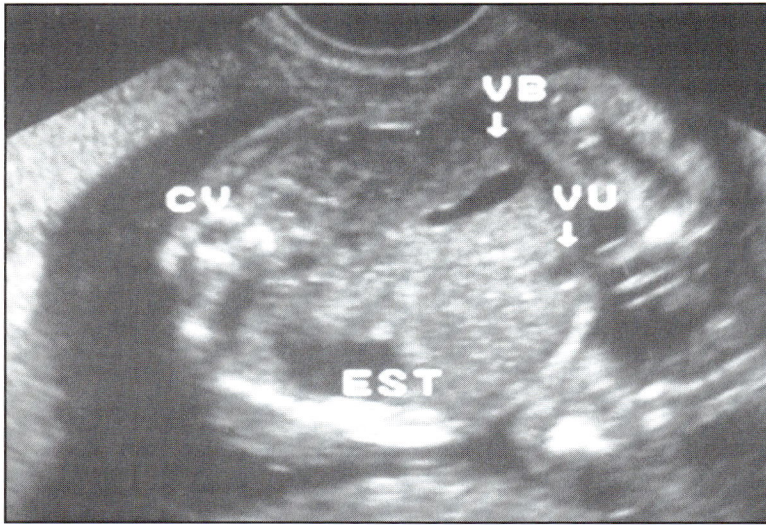

Fig. 2.21: Transverse scan of the fetal abdomen.CV: Spine; EST: Stomach; VB: Gallblader, VU: Umbilical vein

In the first half of the gestation, the *bowel* is usually visualized as an ill-defined area of the increased echogenicity in the mid to lower abdomen. Individual segments of bowel are not identified at this time.

After 20th week, distinguishing large bowel from small one is possible. While the large bowel appears as a continuous tubular structure located in the periphery of abdomen, the small bowel is located centrally. On the other hand, while the large bowel is filled with hypoechoic meconium, the small bowel remains more echogenic. There are four grades of the bowel maturation: according to the echogenicity of the contents, the limit aspect, multiple small bowel loops, and the presence of active peristaltis.[23]

The large bowel progressively enlarges with meconium. In some fetuses, one sonolucent image appears in colon presumably due to increased water content of meconium (Fig. 2.22).

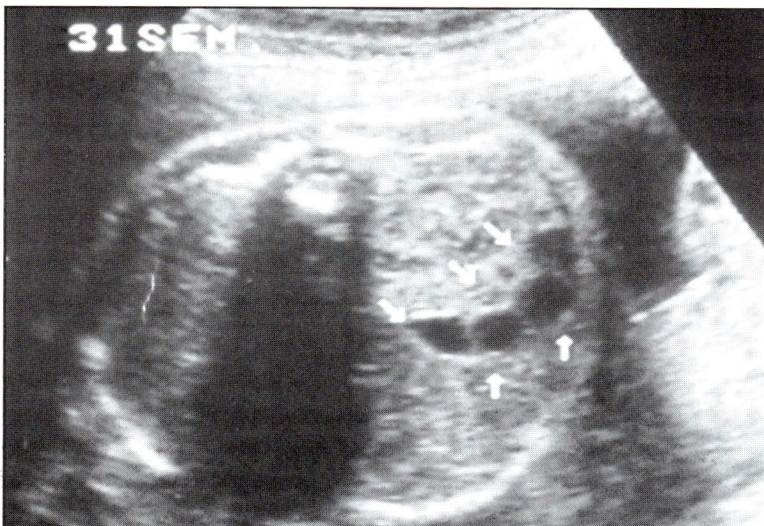

Fig. 2.22: Bowell loop at 31st week

The *fetal liver* is located in the third superior of the abdomen. The aspect is different from that of the lung, because it has a major echogenicity, and also because the bowel has a homogeneous structure. The observation of the liver is possible from 16 to 17th weeks (Fig. 2.23).

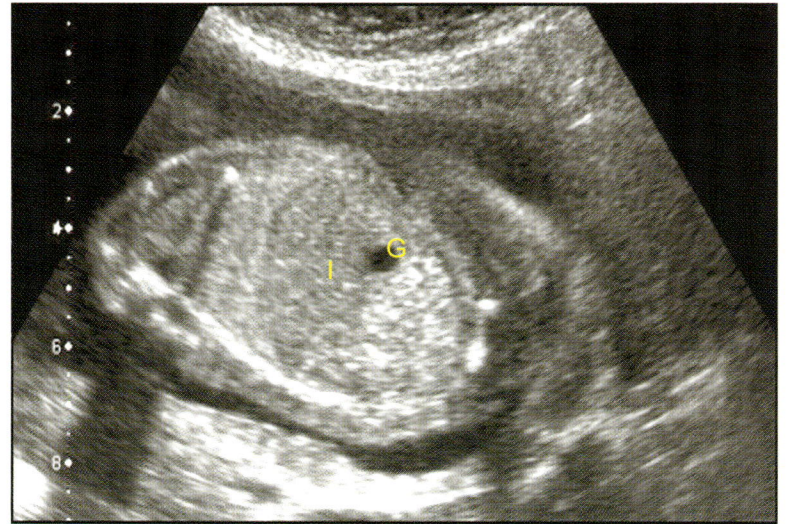

Fig. 2.23: L: Liver; G: Gallbladder

The *gallbladder* is usually visualized as an ovoid or rounded fluid-filled structure to the right and inferior to the intrahepatic portion of the umbilical vein (Figs 2.21 and 2.23).

KIDNEY AND URINARY TRACT

The *fetal kidneys* are visible as early as 9th week,[24] but the observation and accurate statement about their internal architecture usually cannot be made until 15 to 16th weeks. Grignon[25] and Mahoney et al[26] consider that the correct sonographic exploration of the kidney depends, basically, of the fetal position. The kidneys are especially visible when the fetus is in dorsum-anterior position and the transversal scan is absolutely perpendicular to spine (Fig. 2.24).

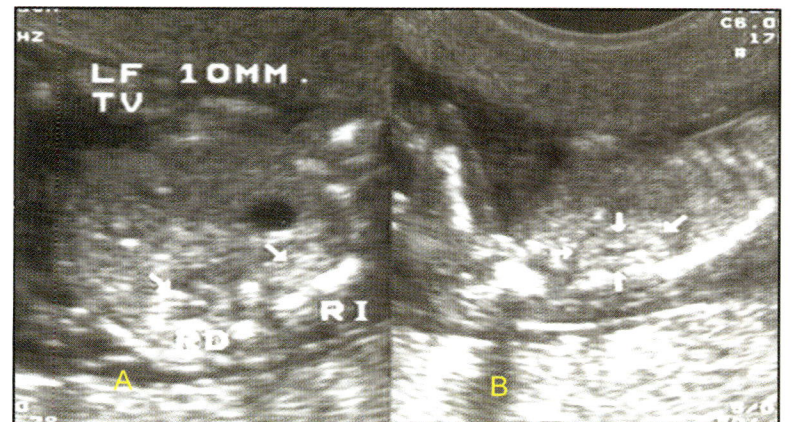

Fig. 2.24: A: Transverse section of the fetal abdomen at 13th week. RD: Right kidney, RI: Left kidney. B: Longitudinal view

Until 16 to 18th weeks, the kidneys appear as bilateral paraspinous structures, with an elliptical or circular shape. Variations in fetal position and scarce difference of echogenicity between the kidney and surrounding tissues can make the identification of both fetal kidneys difficult. Sometimes it is possible to observe the para-vertebral muscles, to both sides of kidneys. In this period it is not possible to recognize the structure of fetal kidneys.

After 17 to 18th weeks it is possible to recognize some structures but at 20th week the sonographic architecture of the kidney is very clear. Then, the identification of the following details is possible:

1. *Renal cortex:* Is a thin line, considerably echorefringent that delimits the organ.
2. *Renal parenchyma:* The medullae usually appear hypoechoic, and the renal sinus, with the aspect of sonolucent "slit" within the central portion of kidneys.
3. *Pielocaliciliar zone*: Appears as one central and irregular structure of very variable impedance due to alternasy of hyperechogenic tracts with other hypoechogenics (calyces). In occasions it is possible to observe areas without echoes that correspond to pelvis or calyces full or urine. The size of these areas never surpasses 10 mm and adopts an ovoid or tubular form (Fig. 2.25).
4. *Renal hilus:* Renal vessels that are beating are visible. This is the place more adequate to make the measures of kidney because it constitutes an excellent point of reference.

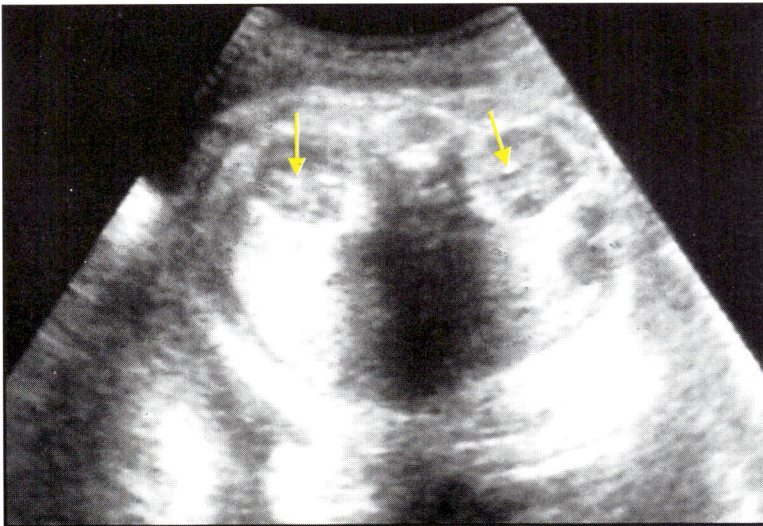

Fig. 2.25: Transversal scan. The pielocaliciliar zone are visible

In the longitudinal scan sections, the view is of a low quality. The kidney adopts an elliptical form, with structural characteristic described for transversal scan, and located very near to aorta, and parallel to this vessel (Fig. 2.26).

The kidneys grow along the gestation. The standard measurements of diameters, renal circumference, volume, etc. are in relation to gestational age. Apparently in IUGR the renal size is affected earlier than BPD.

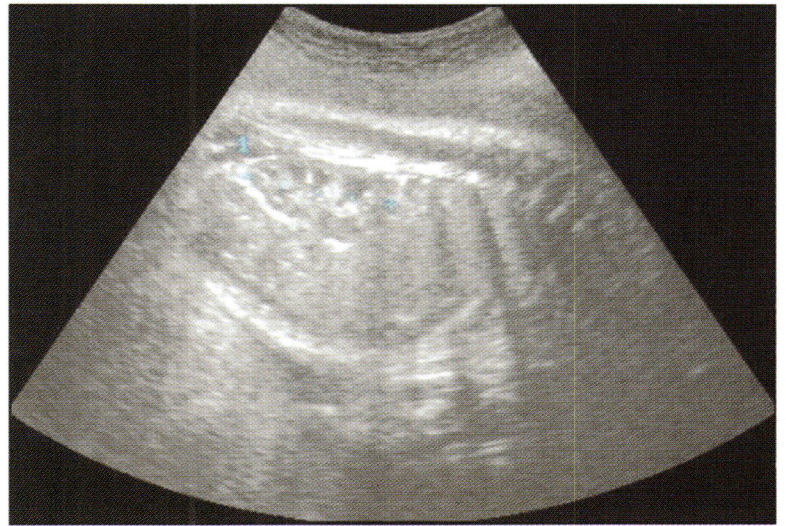

Fig. 2.26: Kidney longitudinal scan at 39th week

The *fetal bladder* can be identified at 10 to 12th weeks, shortly after the beginning of fetal urine production. It adopts the form of cystic space, without echoes, located in the third lower of abdomen. The volume is variable according to the grade of repletion. The fetus normally fills and empties the bladder every 20 to 30 minutes and produces an average of 25 to 30 ml/hr or urine near term.

By means of color Doppler the visualization of internal iliac arteries which embrace the bladder, is possible. Thanks to this anatomic detail it is possible to make the differential diagnosis with other cystic pathologic structures (Fig. 2.27).

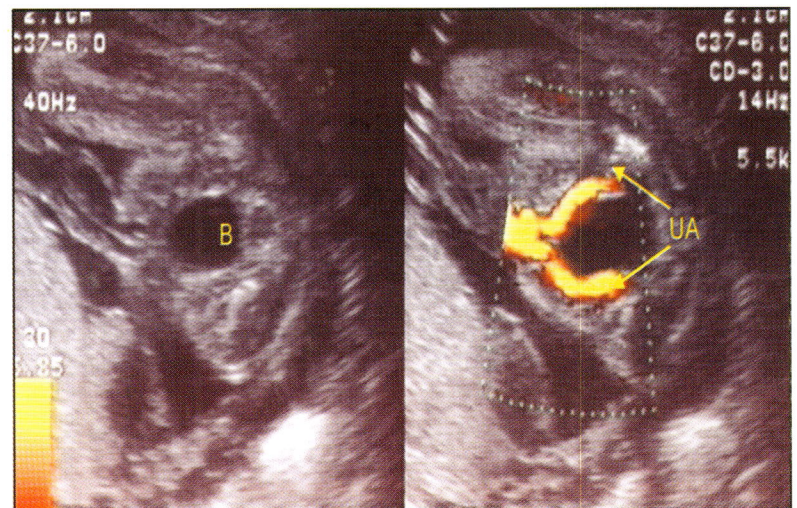

Fig. 2.27: Fetal bladder (B). Umbilical arteries surrounding the bladder (UA)

The *ureters* are not usually visualized except when a pathological dilatation exists. But, with high-resolution scanner it is possible in some occasions to visualize ureters if measuring 1 mm in diameter.[18]

The American Institute of Ultrasound in Medicine recommends that the second and third trimesters ultrasonography exploration includes information about the fetal urinary bladder, fetal kidneys and assessment of amniotic fluid volume. Assessment of amniotic fluid represents an important aspect of the evaluation of the urinary tract, because in the majority of the disorders associated with poor renal function the oligohydramnios is observed.

FETAL GENDER

The identification of the fetal gender is important, not only by giving this information to parents, but also for diagnosis of ambiguous genitalia, intersex state (discrepant sonography and karyotype), confirmation of dizygocity in twins, etc.

Before 11th week of gestation, male and female genitalia are identical, but from thismoment it is possible to determine the fetal gender.[27]

Clearly, there are two sonographic patterns.

Male Pattern

To detect the male pattern, the identification of scrotum and penis image is necessary.

The scrotum appears as a bilobuloid excrecency with limits very clear that protrude of the fetal ventral wall. Thanks to the amniotic fluid the contours are very precise. The testicles normally descend into the scrotum between 28th and 34th weeks of gestation. The visualization of testicles (more or less refringent) within the scrotum provides 100 percent reliability in gender assessment.[28] Usually, it is possible to distinguish both scrotal bags.

About the penis, the solitary image of the scrotum and penis is similar to a tortoise or snail. It is possible, if the penis is erected, to observe the urethra (Figs 2.28 and 2.29).

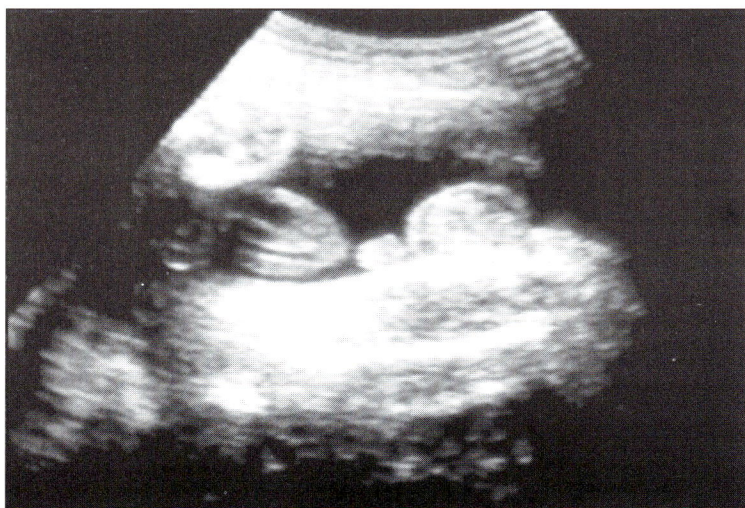
Fig. 2.29: Male genitalia at 35th week

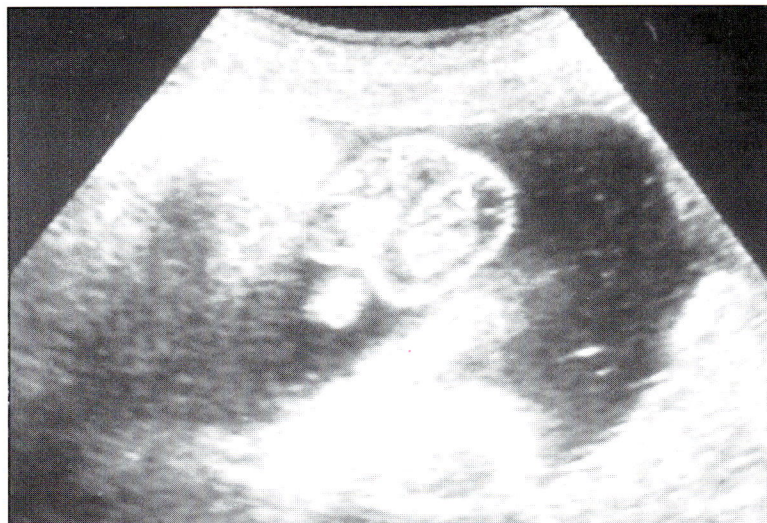
Fig. 2.30: Female genitalia at 20th week

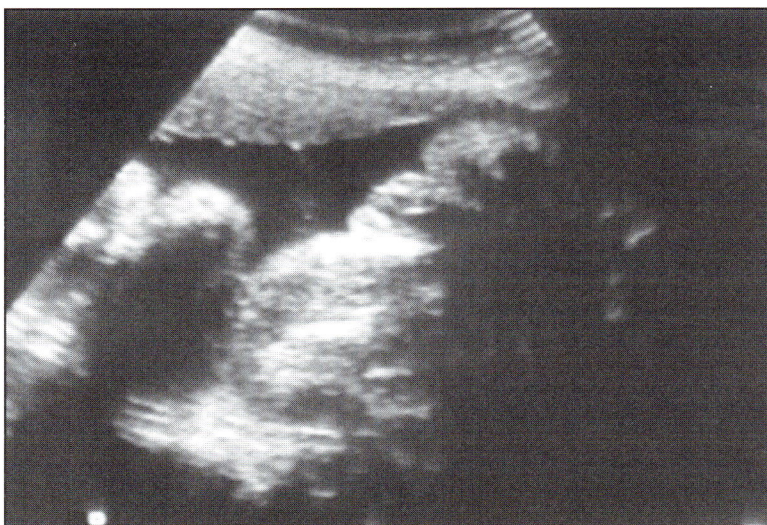
Fig. 2.31: Female genitalia at 40th week

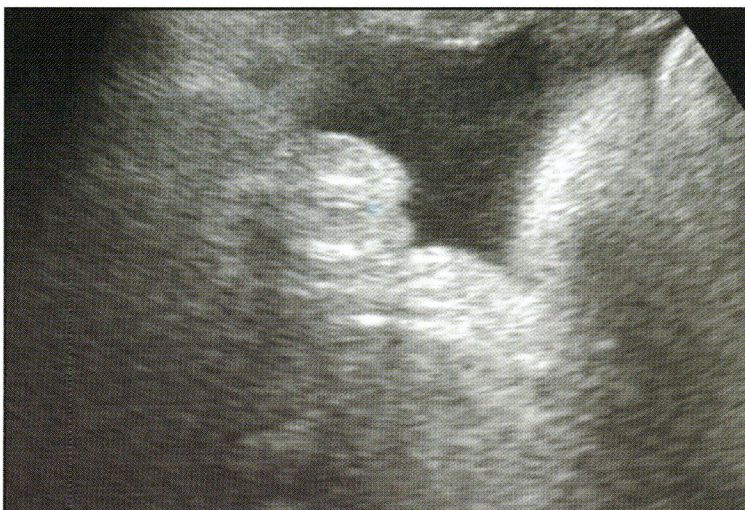
Fig. 2.28: Male genitalia at 20th week

Female Pattern

The sections more adequate for identifying the female gender are the perpendicular to femoral axis, and also that which coincide with the so called perineal axis (Figs 2.30 and 2.31).

In these scans the identification of three elements of easy visualization is possible:

1. *Fetal hips*; These are two ovoid images with very echogenic echoes. They correspond to femur.
2. *Vaginal space*: Between the images of hips, a space free of echoes can be observed, with a triangular or rectangular shape

(triangle of Le Lann et al). The vertex is internal. Sometimes it is possible to observe one central lineal echo.

3. *Major labia:* Appear as two small mamelons considerably hyperechogenic, behind the triangle of Le Lann. The borders are very nitid, due to the contact with amniotic fluid. Between the major labia in occasions the identification of the minor labia and clitoris is possible.
4. *The fetal uterus:* The uterus observation is sometimes possible if the fetal bladder is full.

The visualization of the fetal miction, through the genitalia, is very easy especially with the use of color Doppler. It adopts the form of the jet that moves and displaces the near amniotic fluid.

EXTREMITIES

The fetal extremities appear in the longitudinal scans as cylindrical structures and in the transversal scans as circular or round images, with a great activity.

At present we have ultrasonographic patterns by all the large bones. Tables 2.1 correlates the length of each bone with the gestational age.

The visualization of the bones of the extremities starts between 10th and 13th weeks, and from 14 to 15th weeks the observation of three segments of each extremity is possible.

The *femur* adopts the typical image of stick golf club. This image can be observed from 10th week. The femur appears to curve slightly until 18th week, but after it is progressively rectilinear until term of gestation. The femur growth is very uniform (1, 25 cm each 5th week) (Fig. 2.32).

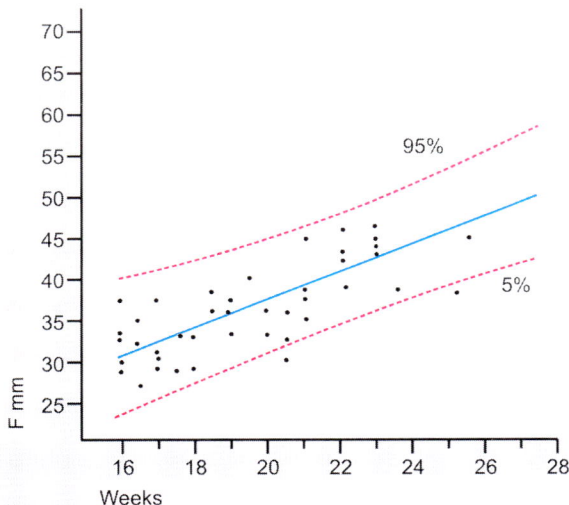
Fig. 2.32: Normal femur growth

Usually the sonographic femur length measures include only the ossified femoral diaphysis or greater tuberosity.[29] The shadowing from the ossified diaphysis makes the femur look narrower than it is (Fig. 2.33).

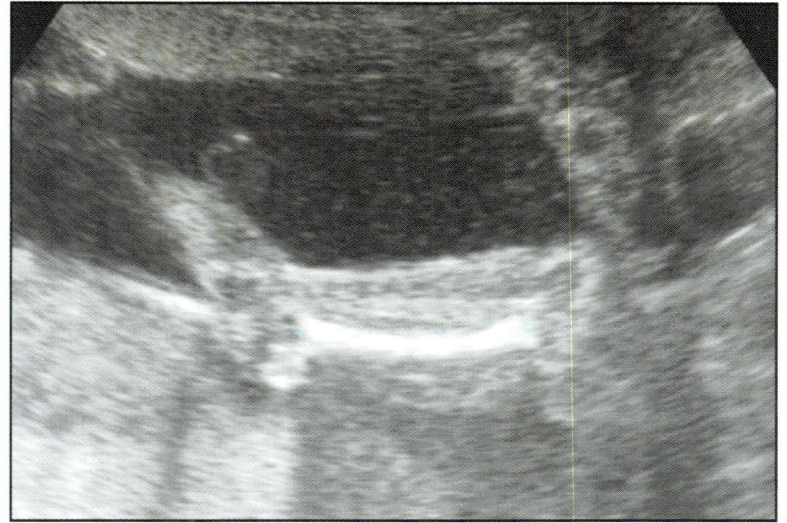
Fig. 2.33: Fetal femur at 20th week

A sagittal scan of the extended knee shows the femoral diaphysis, quadriceps tendon, patella, patella ligament and proximal tibial epiphyseal cartilage. During the third trimester, the secondary epiphyseal ossification centers of the distal femur and the proximal tibia, become visible centrally located within their respective cartilages (Fig. 2.34).[29]

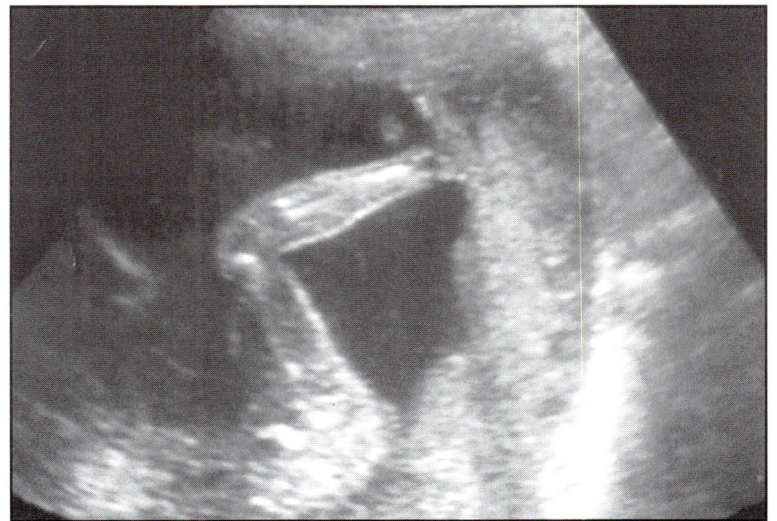
Fig. 2.34: Sagittal scan of the extended leg

The *tibia* and *fibula* appear as two parallel lines very hyperechogenic, visible from 12th week. The tibia line is thicker, but the longer correspond to fibula. The growth of these bones is more or less 1.5 cm each 5th week (Figs 2.35 to 2.37).

The *coxal* bone can also be visualized.

The cartilaginous types of the bones create echogenic gaps between the ossified diaphyses of these bones as well as of the ossification metatarsals and phalanges (Mahoney).

The non-ossified tarsal bones are less visible than matatarsal bones.

The *clavicle* and *scapula* represent the shoulder girdle. In long axis coronally, the scapula has a characteristic shape

Table 2.1: Development of extremities as per gestational age

mm	TIBIA Percentile			FEMUR Percentile			ULNA Percentile			HUMERUS Percentile		
	P-5	P-50	P-95	P-5	P-50	P-95	P-5	P-50	P-95	P-5	P-50	P-95
10	10 + 4	13 + 3	16 + 2	10 + 3	12 + 4	14 + 6	10 + 1	13 + 1	16 + 1	9 + 6	12 + 4	15 + 2
11	10 + 6	13 + 5	16 + 4	10 + 5	12 + 6	15 + 1	10 + 4	13 + 4	16 + 4	10 + 1	12 + 6	15 + 4
12	11 + 1	14 + 1	17	11	13 + 2	15 + 4	10 + 6	13 + 6	16 + 6	10 + 3	13 + 1	15 + 6
13	11 + 4	14 + 3	17 + 2	11 + 2	13 + 4	15 + 6	11 + 1	14 + 1	17 + 2	10 + 6	13 + 4	16 + 1
14	11 + 6	14 + 6	17 + 5	11 + 5	13 + 6	16 + 1	11 + 4	14 + 4	17 + 5	11 + 1	13 + 6	16 + 4
15	12 + 1	15 + 1	18	12	14 + 1	16 + 4	11 + 6	15	18	11 + 3	14 + 1	16 + 6
16	12 + 4	15 + 4	18 + 3	12 + 2	14 + 4	16 + 6	12 + 2	15 + 3	18 + 3	11 + 6	14 + 4	17 + 2
17	13	15 + 6	18 + 6	12 + 5	14 + 6	17 + 1	12 + 5	15 + 5	18 + 6	12 + 1	14 + 6	17 + 4
18	13 + 2	16 + 1	13	15 + 1	17 + 4	13 + 1	16 + 1	19 + 1	12 + 4	15 + 1	18	
19	13 + 5	16 + 4	19 + 4	13 + 2	16 + 4	17 + 6	13 + 4	16 + 4	19 + 4	12 + 6	15 + 4	18 + 2
20	14 + 1	17	19 + 6	13 + 5	15 + 6	18 + 1	13 + 6	16 + 6	20	13 + 1	15 + 6	18 + 5
21	14 + 4	17 + 3	20 + 2	14	16 + 2	18 + 4	14 + 2	17 + 2	20 + 3	13 + 4	16 + 2	19 + 1
22	14 + 6	17 + 6	20 + 5	14 + 2	16 + 4	18 + 6	14 + 5	17 + 5	20 + 6	13 + 6	16 + 5	19 + 3
23	15 + 1	18 + 1	21 + 1	14 + 6	16 + 6	19 + 1	15 + 1	18 + 1	21 + 1	14 + 2	17 + 1	19 + 6
24	15 + 4	18 + 4	21 + 3	15	17 + 2	19 + 4	15 + 4	18 + 4	21 + 4	14 + 5	17 + 3	20 + 1
25	16	18 + 6	21 + 6	15 + 3	17 + 4	19 + 6	16	19	22 + 1	15 + 1	17 + 6	20 + 4
26	16 + 3	19 + 2	22 + 1	15 + 5	18	20 + 1	16 + 3	19 + 3	22 + 4	15 + 4	18 + 1	21
27	16 + 6	19 + 5	22 + 4	16 + 1	18 + 2	20 + 4	16 + 6	19 + 6	22 + 5	15 + 6	18 + 4	21 + 3
28	17 + 1	20 + 1	23	16 + 3	18 + 5	20 + 6	17 + 2	20 + 2	23 + 3	16 + 2	19	21 + 6
29	17 + 4	20 + 4	23 + 4	16 + 6	19	21 + 2	17 + 5	20 + 6	23 + 6	16 + 5	19 + 3	22 + 1
30	18 + 1	21	23 + 6	17 + 1	19 + 3	21 + 5	18 + 1	21 + 1	24 + 2	17 + 1	19 + 6	22 + 4
31	18 + 4	21 + 3	24 + 2	17 + 4	19 + 6	22	18 + 4	21 + 5	24 + 6	17 + 4	20 + 2	23
32	18 + 6	21 + 6	24 + 5	17 + 6	20 + 1	22 + 3	19 + 1	22 + 1	25 + 1	18	20 + 5	23 + 4
33	19 + 2	22 + 1	25 + 1	18 + 1	20 + 4	22 + 5	19 + 4	22 + 5	25 + 5	18 + 3	21 + 1	23 + 6
34	19 + 5	22 + 4	25 + 4	18 + 4	20 + 6	23 + 1	20 + 1	23 + 1	26 + 1	18 + 6	21 + 4	24 + 2
35	20 + 4	23 + 4	26 + 3	19 + 3	21 + 4	23 + 6	21 + 1	24 + 1	27 + 1	19 + 5	22 + 4	25 + 1
37	21	23 + 6	26 + 6	19 + 5	22	24 + 1	21 + 4	24 + 4	27 + 5	20 + 1	22 + 6	25 + 5
38	21 + 4	24 + 3	27 + 2	20 + 1	22 + 3	24 + 4	22 + 1	25 + 1	28 + 1	20 + 4	23 + 3	26 + 1
39	21 + 6	24 + 6	27 + 5	20 + 4	22 + 5	25	22 + 4	25 + 4	28 + 5	21 + 1	23 + 6	26 + 4
40	22 + 3	25 + 2	28 + 1	20 + 6	23 + 1	25 + 3	23 + 1	26 + 1	29 + 1	21 + 4	24 + 2	27 + 1
41	22 + 6	25 + 5	28 + 4	21 + 1	23 + 4	25 + 5	23 + 4	26 + 5	29 + 5	22	24 + 6	27 + 4
42	23 + 2	26 + 1	29 + 1	21 + 4	23 + 6	26 + 1	24 + 1	27 + 1	30 + 2	22 + 4	25 + 2	28
43	23 + 5	27 + 4	29 + 4	22	24 + 2	26 + 4	24 + 5	27 + 5	30 + 6	23	25 + 5	28 + 4
44	24 + 1	27 + 1	30	22 + 3	24 + 5	26 + 6	25 + 1	28 + 2	31 + 2	23 + 4	26 + 1	29
45	24 + 4	27 + 4	30 + 4	22 + 6	25	27 + 2	25 + 6	28 + 6	31 + 6	24	26 + 5	29 + 4
46	25 + 1	28	30 + 6	23 + 1	25 + 3	27 + 5	26 + 2	29 + 3	32 + 3	24 + 4	27 + 1	30
47	25 + 4	28 + 4	31 + 3	23 + 4	25 + 6	28 + 1	26 + 6	29 + 6	33	25	27 + 5	30 + 4
48	26 + 1	29	31 + 6	24	26 + 1	28 + 4	27 + 3	30 + 4	33 + 4	25 + 4	25 + 4	28 + 1
49	26 + 4	29 + 3	32 + 2	24 + 3	26 + 4	28 + 6	28	31 + 1	34 + 1	26	28 + 6	31 + 4
50	27	29 + 6	32 + 6	24 + 6	27	29 + 2	28 + 4	31 + 4	34 + 5	26 + 4	29 + 2	32
51	27 + 4	30 + 3	33 + 2	25 + 1	27 + 3	29 + 5	29 + 1	32 + 1	35 + 2	27 + 1	29 + 6	32 + 4
52	28	30 + 6	25 + 4	27 + 6	30 + 1	29 + 5	32 + 6	35 + 6	27 + 4	30 + 2	33 + 1	
53	28 + 4	31 + 3	34 + 2	26	28 + 1	30 + 4	30 + 2	33 + 3	36 + 3	28 + 1	30 + 6	33 + 4
54	29	31 + 6	34 + 6	26 + 3	28 + 4	30 + 6	30 + 6	34	37	28 + 5	31 + 3	34 + 1
55	29 + 4	32 + 3	35 + 2	26 + 6	29 + 1	31 + 2	31 + 4	34 + 4	37 + 5	29 + 1	32	34 + 5
56	30	32 + 6	35 + 6	27 + 1	29 + 4	31 + 5	32 + 1	35 + 1	38 + 2	29 + 6	32 + 4	35 + 2
57	30 + 4	33 + 3	36 + 2	27 + 4	29 + 6	32 + 1	32 + 6	35 + 6	38 + 6	30 + 2	33 + 1	35 + 6
58	31	33 + 6	36 + 6	28 + 1	30 + 2	32 + 4	33 + 3	36 + 3	39 + 4	30 + 6	33 + 4	36 + 3
59	31 + 4	34 + 3	37 + 2	28 + 4	30 + 5	33	34	37 + 1	40 + 1	31 + 3	34 + 1	36 + 6
60	32	34 + 6	37 + 6	28 + 6	31 + 1	33 + 3	34 + 4	37 + 5	40 + 6	32	34 + 6	37 + 4
61	32 + 4	35 + 3	28 + 2	29 + 2	31 + 4	33 + 6	35 + 2	38 + 2	41 + 3	32 + 4	35 + 2	38 + 1
62	33	35 + 6	38 + 6	29 + 5	32	34 + 1	35 + 6	39	42	33 + 1	35 + 6	38 + 5
63	33 + 4	36 + 4	39 + 3	30 + 1	32 + 3	34 + 5	36 + 4	39 + 4	42 + 5	33 + 6	36 + 4	39 + 2
64	34 + 1	37	39 + 6	30 + 4	32 + 6	35 + 1	37 + 1	40 + 2	43 + 2	34 + 3	37 + 1	39 + 6
65	34 + 4	37 + 4	40 + 3	31	33 + 2	35 + 4	—	—	—	35	37 + 5	40 + 4
66	35 + 1	38	41	31 + 4	33 + 5	36	—	—	—	35 + 4	39 + 2	41 + 1
67	35 + 5	38 + 4	41 + 4	31 + 6	34 + 1	36 + 3	—	—	—	36 + 1	39 + 6	41 + 5
68	36 + 1	39 + 1	42	32 + 2	34 + 4	36 + 6	—	—	—	36 + 6	39 + 4	42 + 2
69	36 + 6	39 + 5	42 + 4	32 + 6	35	37 + 2	—	—	—	37 + 3	40 + 1	42 + 6
70	37 + 2	40 + 1	43 + 1	33 + 1	35 + 4	37 + 5	—	—	—	38	40 + 6	43 + 4
71	—	—	—	33 + 5	35 + 6	38 + 1						
72	—	—	—	34 + 1	36 + 3	38 + 4						
73	—	—	—	34 + 4	36 + 6	39 + 1						
74	—	—	—	35	37 + 2	39 + 4						
75	—	—	—	35 + 4	37 + 5	40						
76	—	—	—	35 + 6	38 + 1	40 + 3						
77	—	—	—	36 + 3	38 + 4	40 + 6						
78	—	—	—	36 + 6	39 + 1	41 + 2						
79	—	—	—	37 + 2	39 + 4	41 + 5						
80	—	—	—	37 + 6	40	42 + 2						

* Gestational Age (Weeks and Days)

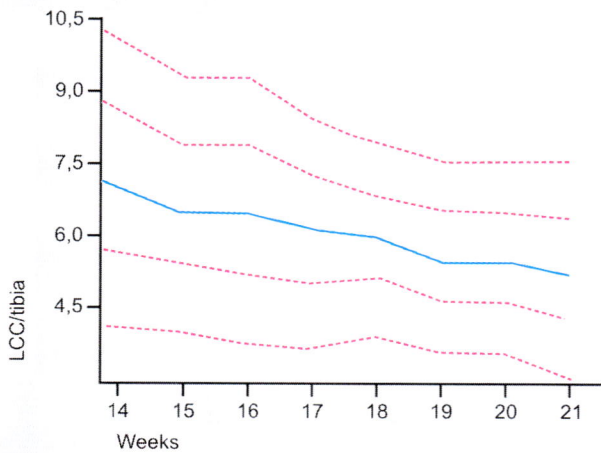

Fig. 2.35: Relationship between CRL/tibia

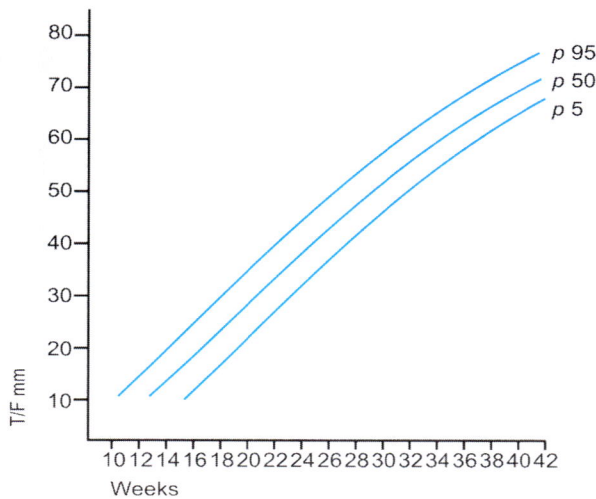

Fig. 2.36: Curve of the longitudinal growth of tibia/fibula

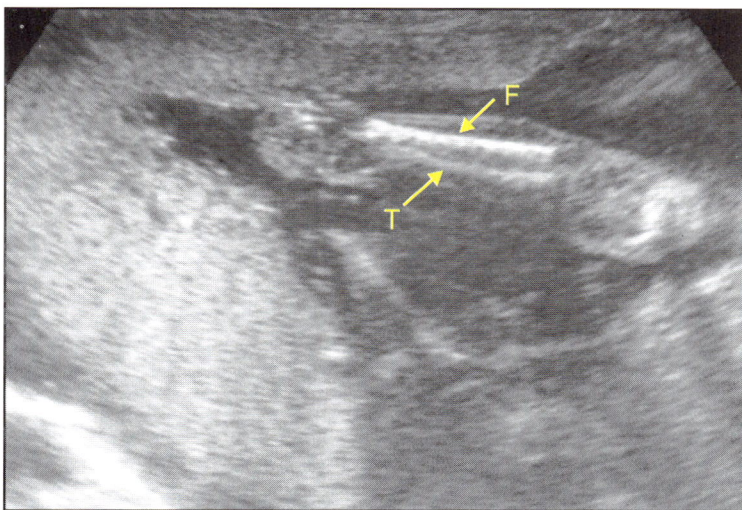

Fig. 2.37: Tibia (T), and Fibula (F)

resembling a "Y" with the supraspinatus, subscapularis and infraspinatus muscles in their respective fossae (Fig. 2.38).[30]

The oblique scan through the fetal shoulder identifies clearly the scapula that adopts a triangular shape.

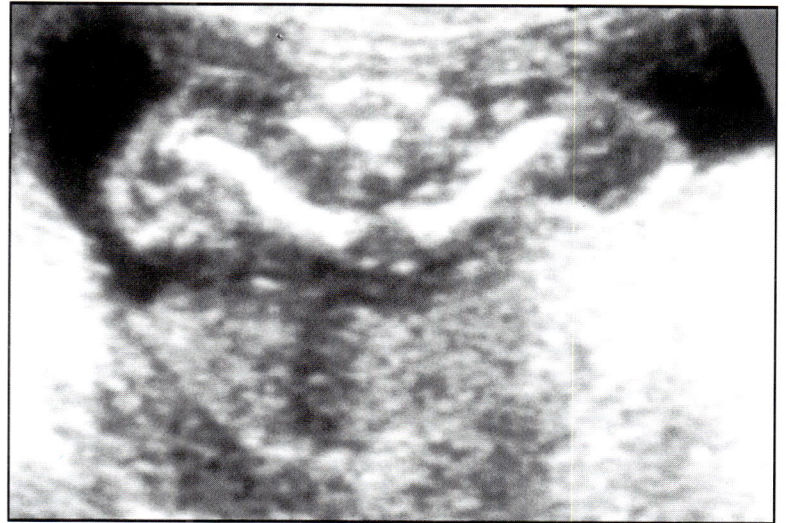

Fig. 2.38: Fetal clavicle

It is also possible to observe the clavicle, if not obscured by flexion of the fetal head. The gestational age in weeks is approximately the same of length of the clavicle in mm (Fig. 2.39).

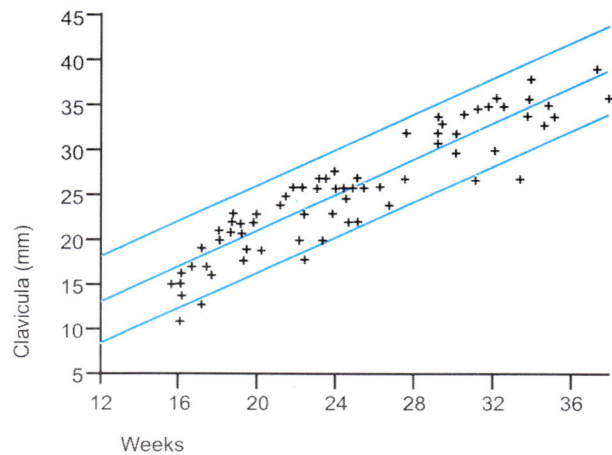

Fig. 2.39: Percentilar curve of the clavicle length

The *humerus* can be visualized from 10th week. It adopts the shape of the rectilinear image, grows at velocity of 10 mm each 5th week. Until 20th week the length of the humerus and femur is very similar. Scan of the humerus shows the secondary ossification center to proximal humeral epiphysis, which appears near term centrally within the epiphyseal cartilage (Fig. 2.40).

The *ulna* and *radius* appear as two parallel lines, the major and more caudal of which is the ulna. The growth of both bones is similar to the humerus (Fig. 2.41).

The *bones of the hands* can be clearly visible from 15 to16th weeks but the identification of each phalanx is not possible until 18th week (Fig. 2.42).

The visualization of the small bones of *metacarpal* is also possible due to the correct ossification. On the contrary the non-ossified carpals produce a conglomerate zone of gray echoe.

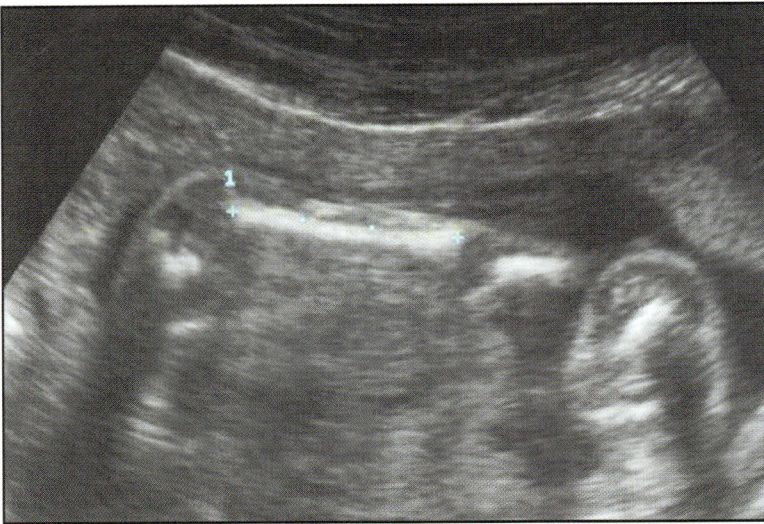

Fig. 2.40: Fetal humerus

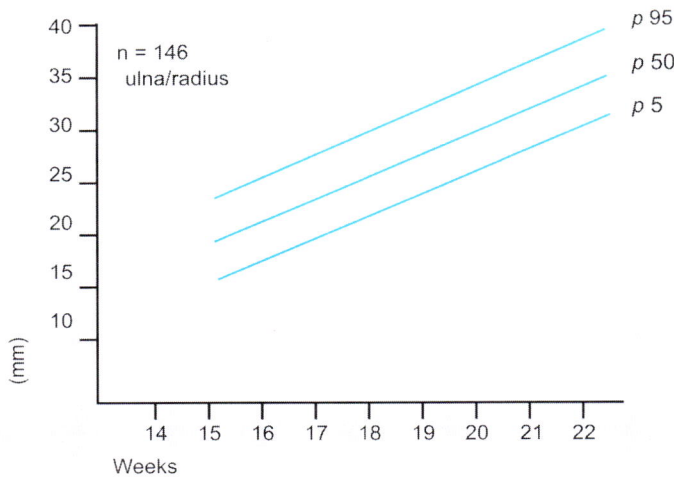

Fig. 2.41: Growth (percentilar) of the ulna/radius length

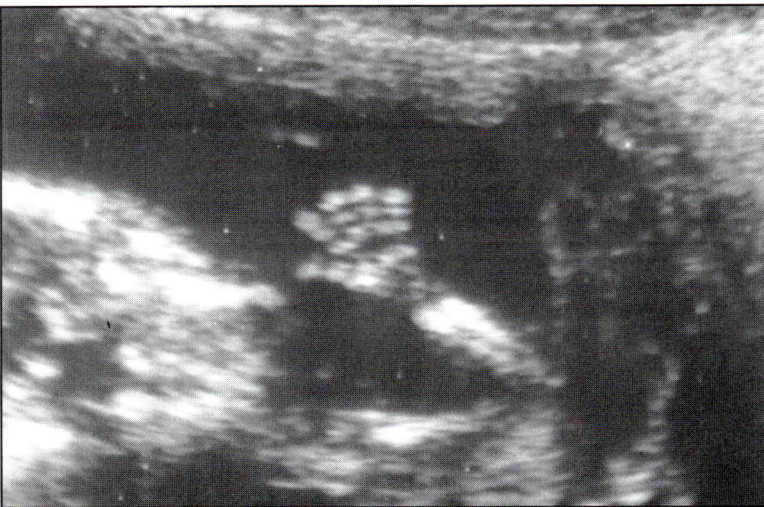

Fig. 2.42: Fetal hand at 19 weeks

Both extremities are important for the study of the movements and also the interrelation between different segments of the extremities. In suspected cases the position of the hand in relation to forearm, and the feet in relation to the legs is necessary for accurate and reliable separation from normal findings.

REFERENCES

1. ACOG, Technical Bulletin No 116. Washington DC. ACOG, May 1988.
2. American Institute of Ultrasound in Medicine. Newsletter, October 1988.
3. Leopold GR. Antepartum obstetrical ultrasound examinations guidelines. J Ultrasound Med 1986;5:241-2.
4. Pretorius DH, Mahony BS. The role of obstetrical ultrasound. In: Nyberg DA, Mahony BS, Pretorius DH (Eds). Diagnostic Ultrasound of Fetal Anomalies. Text and Atlas. Mosby: St. Louis 1990, pp 1-20.
5. Filly RA, Cardoza JD, Goldstein RB, et al. Detection of fetal CNS anomalies. A practical level of effort a "routine" sonogram. Radiology 1989;172:403-8.
6. Pooh RK, Pooh KH. Fetal central nervous system. In: Kurjak A, Chervenak FA (Eds). Textbook of Ultrasond in Obstetrics and Gynecology. Jaypee Brothers: New Delhi 2004, pp 250-70.
7. Pooh RK, Maeda K, Pooh RH, Kurjak A. Sonographic assessment of the fetal brain morphology. Prenat Neonat Med 1999;4:18-38.
8. Johnson ML, Dunne M, Mack I, et al. Evaluation of fetal intracranial anatomy by static and real-time ultrasound. J Clin Ultrasound 1980;8:311-8.
9. Mahony B, Callen P, Filly R, et al. The fetal cisterna magna. Radiology 1984;153:773-6.
10. Monteagudo A, Reuss ML, Timor-Tritsch IE. Imaging the fetal brain in the second and third trimesters using transvaginal sonography. Obstet Gynecol 1991;77:27-32.
11. Timor-Tritsch IE, Monteagudo A. Transvaginal fetal neurosonography: standardization of the planes and sections by anatomic landmarks. Ultrasound Obstet Gynecol 1996;8:42-7.
12. Monteagudo A, Timor-Tritsch IE. Development of fetal gyri, sulci and fissures: A transvaginal sonographic study. Ultrasound Obstet Gynecol 1997;9:222-8.
13. Pooh RK, Nakagawa Y, Nagamachi N, Pooh KH, et al. Transvaginal sonography of the fetal brain: detection of abnormal morphology and circulation. Croat Med J 1998;39:145-7.
14. Mahony BS, Hegge FN. The face and neck. In: Nyberg DA, Mahony BS, Pretorius DH, (Eds). Diagnostic Ultrasound of Fetal Anomalies. Text and Atlas. Mosby: St. Louis 1990; pp 203-61.
15. Carrera JM, Torrents M, Munoz A. Anatomia ecografica fetal. In: Kurjak A, Carrera JM, (Eds). Ecografia en Medicina Materno-Fetal. Masson SA: Barcelona 2000; pp 367-97.
16. Papp Z. Cervical, thoracic and abdominal malformations. In: Papp Z, (Ed). Atlas of Fetal Diagnosis. Elsevier: Amsterdam 1992; pp 139-42.
17. Gray DL, Crane JP, Rudloff MA. Prenatal diagnosis of neural tube defects: Origin of midtrimester vertebral ossification centers as determined by sonographic water-bath studies. J Ultrasound Med 1988;7:421-7.
18. Nyberg DA, McGahan JP, Pretorius DH, Pilu G. Neural tube defects and the spine. In: Nyberg DA, McGahan JA, Pretorius DH, Pilu G (Eds). Diagnostic Imaging of Fetal Anomalies. Lippincot Williams and Wilkins: Philadelphia 2003; pp 289-94.
19. Utsu M, Sakakibarg S, Ishida J, et al. Dynamics oftracheal fluid flow in the human fetus, studied with pulsed doppler ultrasound. Acta Obstet Gynecol Jap 1983;35:2017.
20. Mortera C, Carrera JM. Fetal echocardiography. In: Kurjak A (Ed). Textbook of Perinatal Medicine. Parthenon Publishing: London 1998; pp 305-45.
21. Volpe P, Rustico MA, Gentile M. Ultrasound evaluation of the fetal heart. In: Kurjak A, Chervenak FA (Eds). Textbook of Ultrasound in Obstetrics and Gynecology. Jaypee Brothers: New Delhi 2004; pp 280-9.
22. Pretorius DH, Gosink BB, Clautice-Engle T, et al. Sonographic evaluation of the fetal stomach: Significance of non-visualization. AJR 1988;151:987-9.
23. Zilanti M, Fernandez S. Correlation of ultrasonic images of fetal intestine with gestational age and fetal maturity. Obstet Gynecol 1983;62:569-73.
24. Bronshtein M, Zoffe N, Brandes JM, Blumenfeld Z. First and early second-trimester diagnosis of fetal urinary tract anomalies using transvaginal sonography. Prenat Diagn 1990;10:653-66.
25. Grignon A, Fillon R, Filitrault D. Urinary tract dilatation in utero-classification and clinical applications. Radiology 1986;160:645-7.
26. Mahony BS, Filly R, Callen PW, Hricak H, Golbus M, Harrison MR. Fetal renal dysplasia: Sonographic evaluation. Radiology 1984;152:143-6.
27. Benoit B. Opinion: early fetal gender determination. Ultrasound Obstet Gynecol 1999;13:299-300.
28. Nyberg DA, McGahan JP, Pretorius DH, Pilu G. Genitourinary malformations. In: Nyberg DA, McGahan JP, Pretorius DH, Pilu G (Eds). Diagnosis Imaging of Fetal Anomalies. Lippincot Williams and Wilkins: Philadelphia 2003; pp 603-60.
29. Lessoway VA, Schulzer M, Wittmann BK. Sonographic measurement of the fetal femur: factors affecting accuracy. J Clin Ultrasound 1990;18:171-5.
30. Mahony BS, Filly RA. High resolution sonographic assessment of the fetal extremities. J Ultrasound Med 1984;3:489-98.

W Andonotopo, A Kurjak
S Kupesic, G Azumendi, M Torrents

3

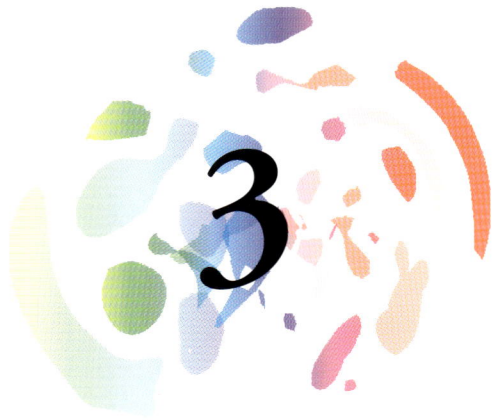

Early Normal Pregnancy

INTRODUCTION

Diagnostic ultrasound has played an important role in a better understanding of early human development. This diagnostic tool has opened up unparalleled possibilities to study morphology and physiology from conception to the end of first trimester. A large number of biochemical, morphological and vascular changes occur during early human development and most of them can be studied by different ultrasonic methods. After fertilization, the embryo is transported into the uterus where, under favorable hormonal and environmental conditions, it will implant and develop into a new and unique individual. The introduction of transvaginal color Doppler has enabled the detection of blood vessels and the analysis of the direction and velocity of blood flow.[1] Thus, transvaginal color Doppler allows detailed examinations of small arteries, such as the vessels that supply the preovulatory follicle, the corpus luteum and the endometrium. Failure of the vascular factors contributes significantly to the failure of current techniques of assisted reproduction and causes the high percentage of occult reproductive losses. Here we review data from our own and other published studies of the use of ultrasound in the morphological and functional assessment of the normal early pregnancy.

Major advances in the diagnosis of early pregnancy have been made with the technical development of transvaginal three-dimensional (3D) and four-dimensional ultrasound (4D) equipment.[1,2] The use of the transvaginal technique has improved the image quality to such an extent that a detailed anatomical description of the developing embryo and early fetus has become possible. The possibility to describe the embryonic anatomy using the new technique has initiated a field called sonoembryology[3] (Fig. 3.1). It has been possible to produce images of such quality that interest has gone beyond the practical diagnostic level and towards using sonoembryology as a research tool in the basic evaluation of the growing embryo.[3-13]

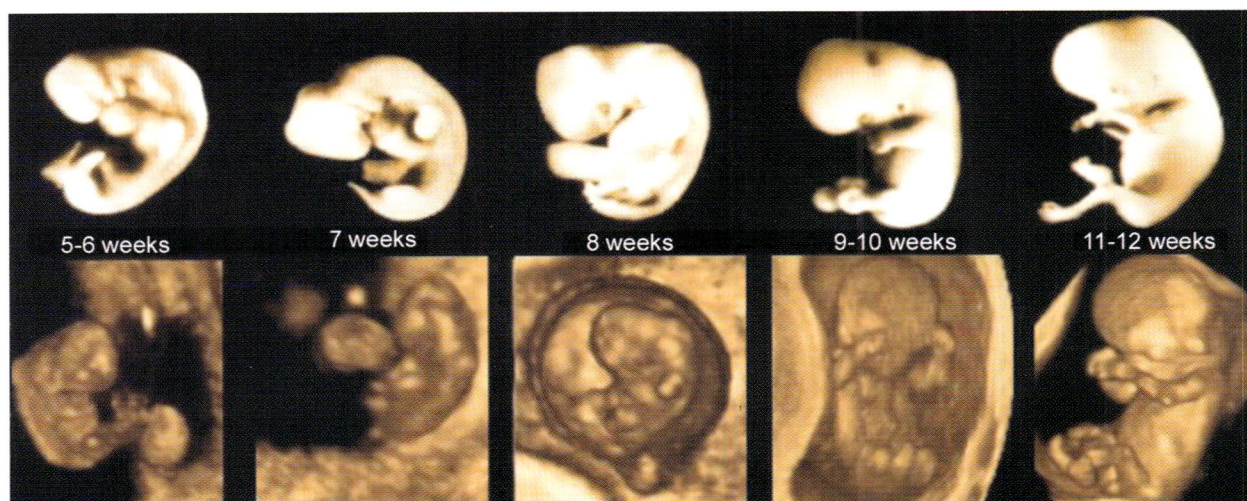

Fig. 3.1: Comparison between computer animation model of embryonal development and a series of in vivo obtained images of the human embryo by 3D sonography, emphasizing development of the embryo in the early pregnancy

ULTRASOUND FINDINGS FROM OVULATION TO IMPLANTATION

Uterus

Implantation is the penetration of the blastocyst through the endometrium with erosion of epithelial cells, probably due to proteolytic enzymes of the external cellular mass of the blastocyst or trophoblast. This process is very complex and needs precise synchronization between the stage of development of the embryo and uterine receptivity, which is known as the "window of implantation". However, at present, the determining factors of the uterine receptivity in women are not yet fully known.

Doppler Studies of the Uterine Receptivity

Blood flow, as an important factor of the uterine receptivity has been studied mainly in stimulated cycles of the patients undergoing in vitro fertilization or in patients receiving hormone replacement treatment. This appears to be the most appropriate model since it allows assessment of all the variables that can affect the result of the procedure before transfer.

Kupesic and Kurjak measured the flow velocity of the uterine, radial and spiral arteries during the periovulatory period in 78 patients with spontaneous and induced ovarian cycles with confirmed ovulation. In spontaneous cycles, the uterine flow velocity had a pulsatility index (PI) of 3.16 two days before ovulation, and started to decrease the day before ovulation (PI=2.22). In stimulated cycles, these changes did not occur, and the mean PI of 3.06 remained at that level during the periovulatory period.

Clear flow velocity waveforms were obtained from myometrium and endometrium at around the time of ovulation. The pulsatility indices of radial and spiral arteries showed significantly higher values in stimulated than in spontaneous cycles. The authors found a strong correlation between endometrial thickness and flow velocities. However, this did not apply to the group of patients stimulated with clomiphene citrate in combination with human menopausal gonadotropins and normal endometrial growth, where the authors demonstrated the absence of diastolic flow in spiral arteries in 55.6 percent of patients.

The main clinical application of assessing the uterine perfusion is to obtain reliable parameters that indicate when it is advisable to postpone the transfer, cryopreserve the embryos and/or improve the uterine vascular receptivity conditions in order to increase the implantation and pregnancy rates. If an upper limit is established, the prediction of a non-receptive uterus has high specificity (96 to 100 percent) and positive predictive

value (88 to 100 percent), although the sensitivity (13 to 35 percent) and negative predictive values (44 to 56 percent) are low. Therefore, Doppler evaluation seems to be better than other sonographic parameters such as endometrial thickness. Inadequate uterine blood flow impedes pregnancy, although adequate uterine perfusion is not an isolated predictor of the likelihood of pregnancy.

Biophysical Uterine Profile: Scores for Uterine Receptivity Evaluation

It has been proposed to study the uterus in the mid-luteal phase to evaluate different parameters indicative of uterine receptivity by biophysical uterine profile. Amongst these are the following: (i) endometrial thickness, (ii) endometrial layering, (iii) myometrial contractions, (iv) myometrial echogenicity, (v) uterine artery blood flow, (vi) endometrial blood flow, and (vii) myometrial blood flow. Taking into consideration all these parameters, a uterine score for reproduction techniques has been developed. A perfect score of 20 is associated with conception in all cases. Scores between 17 and 19 were associated with pregnancy in 77 percent of cases, and between 14 and 16 in 60 percent. Scores of 13 or below suggested poor uterine receptivity.

It is obvious that normal early human development is determined by uterine perfusion, implantation process and chromosomal structure of the fetus. Insufficient implantation and inadequate uterine blood flow can be noninvasively perceived by Doppler technique (Fig. 3.2). Consequently, entire set of new undiscovered circumstances concerning this matter is accessible for research.

After ovulation, there is a brief interval throughout which endometrial receptivity is at its maximum. During these few days, a blastocyst traveling to the uterine cavity can achieve a physical contact with the endothelial lining and eventually—implant. At the beginning of its attachment, the blastocyst is directed with the inner cell mass toward the endometrium. Furthermore, the trophoblast produced action of the proteolysis enzymes which enabled penetration and erosion of the uterine mucosa. During implantation, the trophoblast erodes lying near maternal capillaries, and maternal blood enters to a direct contact with the conceptus. The intercommunicating lacunar network begins to be the intervillous space of the placenta (Fig. 3.3).

Throughout the 4th week the migrating trophoblast penetrates the uterine wall and invades venous sinusoids of increasing size and superficial arterioles. Trophoblastic cells can be discovered inside the spiral arteries at approximately the 6th week following fertilization. Increasing blood flow produces progressive

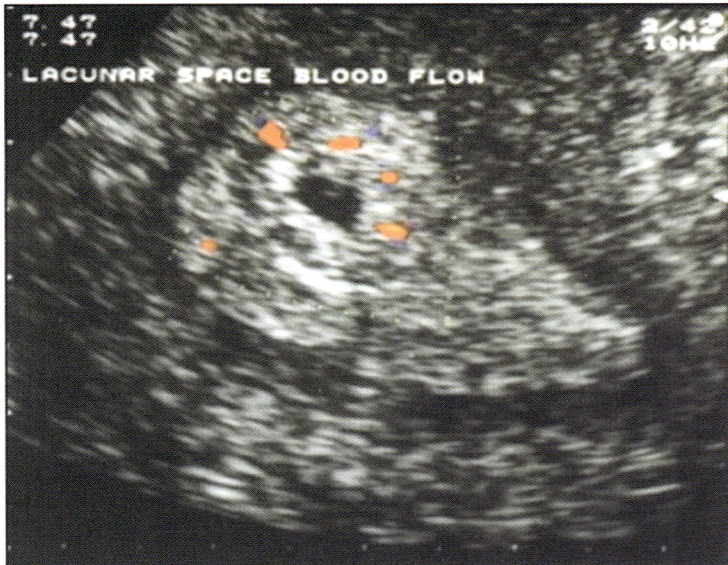

Fig. 3.2: Blood flow in the lacunar space as seen by color Doppler at the periphery of an early gestational sac

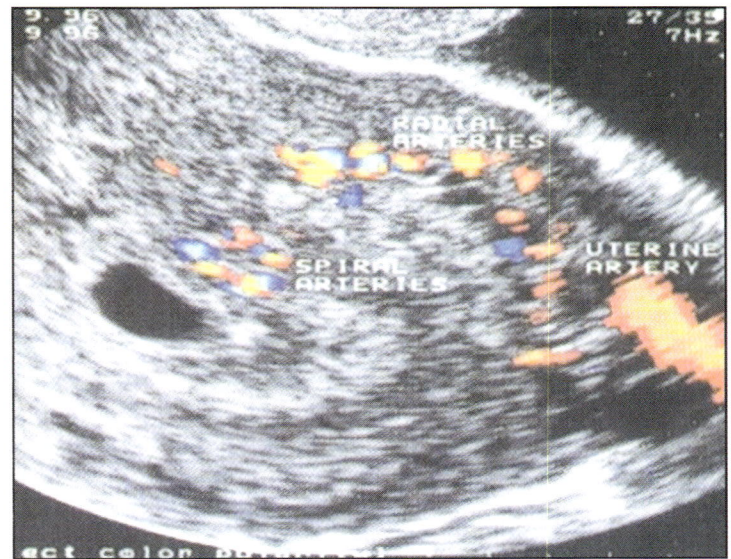

Fig. 3.4: Transvaginal Doppler imaging at 5th to 6th weeks of gestation. Dominant color signals demonstrate the uterine vascular network

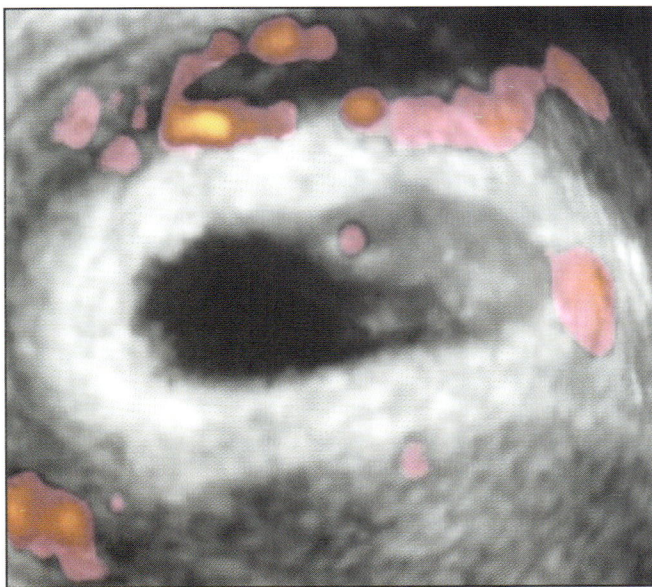

Fig. 3.3: 3D power Doppler showing uterine perfusion during implantation, the trophoblast erodes lying near maternal capillaries and maternal blood enters to a direct contact with the conceptus

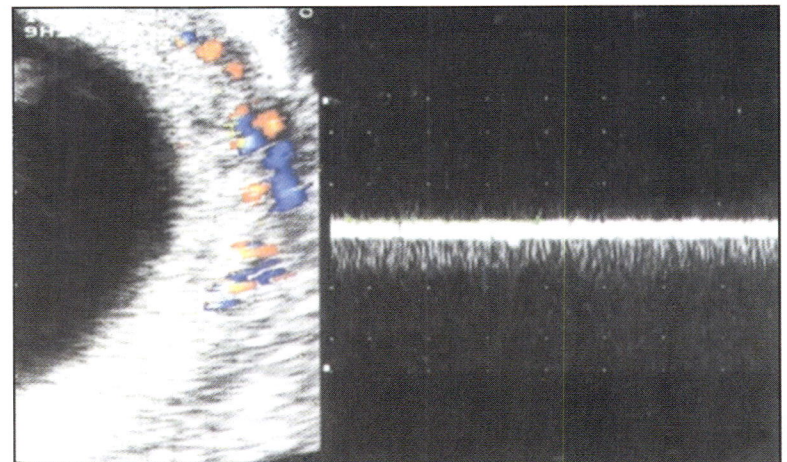

Fig. 3.5: Continuous flow of a venous type, venous blood is easily detectable from the intervillous space

distention of these arteries into the uteroplacental arteries having the ability of adapting the increasing blood supply (Figs 3.4 and 3.5).

Ovaries

Preovulatory Follicle and Follicular Blood Flow during Ovulation

With transvaginal sonography and color flow imaging, it is possible to study minor vascular changes during the ovarian cycle in physiological as well as pathophysiological conditions. The ovary receives its arterial vascularization from two sources: the ovarian artery and the uteroovarian branch of the uterine artery. These arteries anastomose, forming an arch parallel to the ovarian hilus, and constitute the vascular arcade.

Signals from the ovarian artery are characterized by the low Doppler shifts of small vessels with low blood velocity. The waveform varies with the state of activity of the ovary. Studies of ovarian artery blood flow velocity waveforms show the difference in the vascular impedance between the two ovarian arteries, depending on the presence of the dominant follicle or corpus luteum. Our study of the ovarian artery over the ovarian cycle suggested decreased pulsatility and resistance indices, reflecting decreased vascular impedance and increased flow to the ovary containing the dominant follicle or corpus luteum. The ovarian artery of the inactive ovary showed low end-diastolic flow or absence of diastolic flow. A rise in end-diastolic flow velocity of the active ovary is most obvious on day 21. The ovarian artery is a high-pressure system with flow velocity waveforms very different from intraovarian waveforms.

The ovary has an arterial supply known for its special pattern and obvious functional changes. From the ovarian hilus, arterial branches penetrate the stroma and acquire a tortuous and helicoid pathway. Because of their characteristic shape, they are named spiral or helical arteries. This type of vascularity demonstrates a high-resistance to blood flow. Such vessel structure also facilitates accommodation to changes in ovarian size, due to development of the follicle and the corpus luteum. As they grow, the arteries unwind and become larger, returning to the basal state during follicular atresia or luteal regression. This is vitally important for the understanding of changes in intraovarian Doppler velocimetry. The assessment of follicular growth and ovulation is used in routine clinical practice starting from the 9th or the 10th day of a regular 28-day menstrual cycle. The dominant follicle is seen as an anechoic cystic structure with sharp borders usually measuring 8 to10 mm in diameter. It grows at a rate of 2 to 3 mm/day. When a dominant follicle attains 10 mm in diameter, follicular flow velocity waveforms are usually detected at the follicular rim. A few days preceding ovulation, the resistance index (RI) is about 0.54. A decline in resistance to flow usually starts 2 days prior to ovulation, reaching its nadir at ovulation 0.44 ± 0.04. As the blood flow velocity increases before ovulation, it is considered that, apart from hormonal factors, angiogenesis is also involved. Even in the presence of a relatively constant resistance index, the imminent ovulation might be revealed by a significant increase in the peak systolic blood flow velocity. This may be due to angiogenesis and dilatation of these newly formed vessels between the vascular theca cell layer and the hypoxic granulosa cell layer of the follicle. Disruption of these vascular changes may have profound effects on the oxygen concentration across the follicular epithelium. In 12 cases of luteinized unruptured follicles, we have observed a failure of blood velocity to peak in the preovulatory period. These data support the hypothesis that changes in oxygen tension within the follicular wall may be necessary for follicular rupture. We hope that information on ovarian perfusion may be used in the future to predict ovulation, and to investigate ovulatory dysfunction. In patients with polycystic ovarian syndrome, the characteristic changes in resistance to flow in the ovarian arteries and intraovarian parenchymal vessels during the menstrual cycle were lacking. High diastolic flow patterns were followed continuously by the ovarian stroma, resulting in a mean RI of 0.54. These vascular changes have possible effects of local hyperandrogenism and/or stimulus by luteinizing hormone (LH) to (vascular) theca cells. We have also studied ovarian flow velocity in both the group with spontaneous cycles and the group with stimulated cycles during the periovulatory period, but no significant differences were found. The data on intrafollicular flow may have important implications for the management of women wishing to achieve conception.

Luteal Blood Flow

Following ovulation, the corpus luteum is formed, as the result of many structural, functional and vascular changes in the former follicular wall. Transvaginal color Doppler can detect luteal flow early in the second half of the ovarian cycle and also in normal and abnormal early pregnancy. Such noninvasive assessment of luteal blood flow velocities gives direct information about the active ovarian arterial circulation. The mature corpus luteum shows increased blood flow velocity in relation to the preovulatory follicle with a mean RI of 0.43 ± 0.4. In the non-pregnant state the regression of the corpus luteum begins at about the 23rd day of the menstrual cycle and can be recognized by an increased RI of 0.49 ± 0.02. In pregnancy, the corpus luteum is maintained by the hormone, human chorionic gonadotropin (hCG) produced by the trophoblast.

We have studied corpus luteum vascularization in 127 pregnancies between the 5th and 12th weeks of gestation. The resistance and pulsatility indices did not change significantly between 6th and 12th weeks of gestation ($p > 0.05$) and none of the patients studied had a corpus luteum RI of <0.50. Beyond 12 weeks of gestation, it is thought that these luteal velocity waveforms disappear, following the regression of the corpus luteum. It was found that corpus luteum function in early pregnancy was mainly determined by the rate of change in hCG levels.

A significantly lower rate of change was found with ectopic pregnancy and spontaneous abortion when compared with normal intrauterine pregnancy. Analyzing corpus luteum blood flow in normal and abnormal pregnancies, our group found that in the first trimester of pregnancy resistance and pulsatility indices were similar to those in the non-pregnant state during the early luteal phase. In ectopic pregnancies, these indices showed similar values to those in the non-pregnant state during the late luteal phase. Almost no difference was found when luteal blood flow in ectopic pregnancy was compared with normal early pregnancy.

However, in threatened, incomplete and missed abortions the resistance and pulsatility indices were significantly higher than in normal pregnancy ($p < 0.01$). Follow-up of the luteal flow might have prognostic value in a group of patients with threatened abortion and so contribute to clinical work. It seems that an RI increase reduces the chance for an embryo to survive.

Studies on luteal blood flow velocities suggest the possiblity of factors other than hCG to influence the functioning of the corpus luteum in early pregnancy. When the placenta takes over the role of production of progesterone, the corpus luteum starts regressing. The regression begins after the 10th week and the corpus luteum completely resolves by the 16th week. Luteal flow might be used as a parameter of corpus luteum regression, which could be correlated with progesterone, relaxin, prostaglandin or angiogenic growth peptide factors that influence its function. Prostaglandin (PGF2a) produced locally near the regression time may, as a powerful vasoconstrictor, increase the impedance to flow in blood vessels within the corpus luteum. Since inadequate vascularization seems to play the role in luteal phase defect, transvaginal color Doppler may potentially help clarifying this issue in the future.

EVENTS FOLLOWING IMPLANTATION

The gestational sac can be visualized with transvaginal ultrasound at around 4.4 to 4.6 weeks (32 to 34 days) following the onset of the last menstruation, when it reaches a size of 2 to 4 mm, corresponding to a maternals serum β-human chorionic gonadotropin (β-hCG) level of > 1000 ml U/ml.[14] Ultrasonographically it is presented as a hypoechoic oval structure, surrounded by a hyperechoic ring, situated asymmetrically in the uterine cavity (Fig. 3.6 and 3.7). The gestational sac representing the deciduoplacental interface and the exocelomic cavity is the first sonographic evidence of a pregnancy. In normal pregnancies between the 5th and 6th weeks, the gestational sac grows at a rate of 1 mm/day in mean diameter.

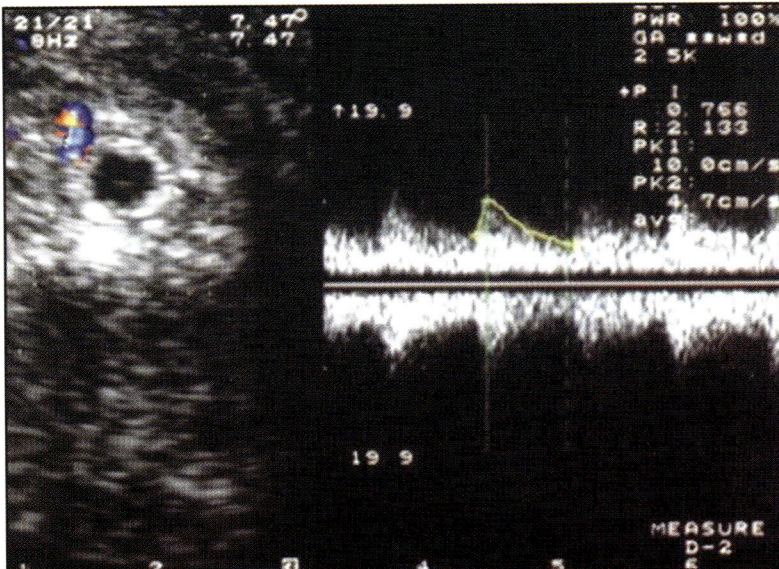

Fig. 3.6: Blood flow signal can be derived from the intervillous space starting from 5 to 6 weeks gestation

As the fetal and placental structures develop, their vascular network becomes more pronounced. Hence, it is possible to observe three separate and yet unified units: the maternal, placental and fetal portions of the vascular network.

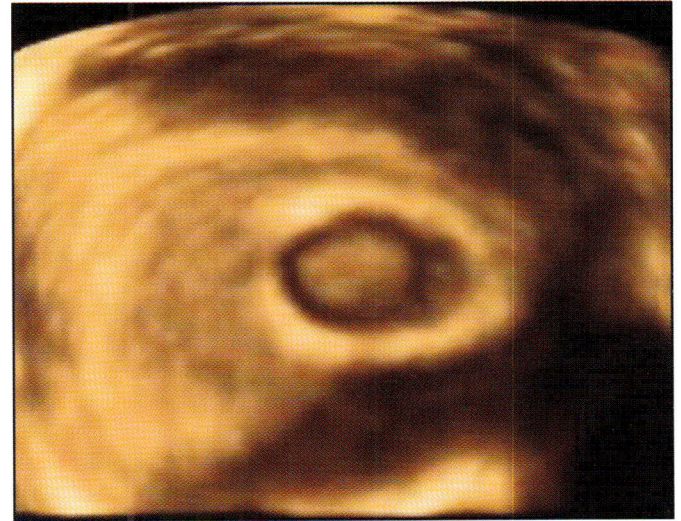

Fig. 3.7: 3D images of gestational sac during 5th week of pregnancy

Maternal Portion

The maternal portion of the placental circulation consists of the main uterine arteries and their branches that spread throughout the uterus until they reach the decidual plate of placenta. The main uterine arteries originate from the internal iliac arteries, and they give off branches, which extend inward for about a third of the myometrium thickness without significant branching. At this point, they subdivide into an arcuate wreath encircling the uterus. From this network, smaller branches called the radial arteries, arise and are directed towards the uterine lumen. The radial arteries branch into basal arteries and endometrial spiral arteries as they pass the myometrial-endometrial border. Basal arteries, that are relatively short, terminate in a capillary bed that serves the stratum basale of the endometrium. The spiral arteries project further into the endometrium and terminate in a vast capillary network that serves the functional layer of the endometrium. All of them can be clearly identified in the pregnant uterus by their anatomical position and characteristic waveform profile.

Intrauterine placental development requires adaptive changes of the uterine vascular environment. The fact that the uterine vascular network elongates and dilates throughout the pregnancy is well known from anatomical study view point.[15]

Doppler Findings

Flow velocity waveforms from small arteries show significantly lower pulsatility and blood velocity as compared to the main uterine artery. The branching of the uterine circulation and the increased total vascular cross-sectional area, which results in lower impedance to blood flow, is the background of this phenomenon. Most authors have demonstrated that the progressive decrement in the impedance to blood flow observed in the main uterine artery during early pregnancy occurs in all the segments of the uteroplacental circulation.[16-19]

Transvaginal color and pulsed Doppler allow identification of the uterine vascular transformation. Furthermore, the invasion of larger maternal blood vessels of higher pressure results in higher velocity and larger diastolic component of Doppler signal.

Kurjak and colleagues have pointed to vascular changes in early pregnancy even before visualization of the gestational sac (Figs 3.8 and 3.9).[20] With advancing gestational age, impedance to blood flow decreases from the main uterine to spiral arteries. At the same time, an increase in blood flow by means of peak systolic velocity has a decreasing trend from the uterine, through the arcuate to the radial arteries. The increment in blood flow through the uterine network is probably caused by an urgent need of the placenta and fetus for nourishment.

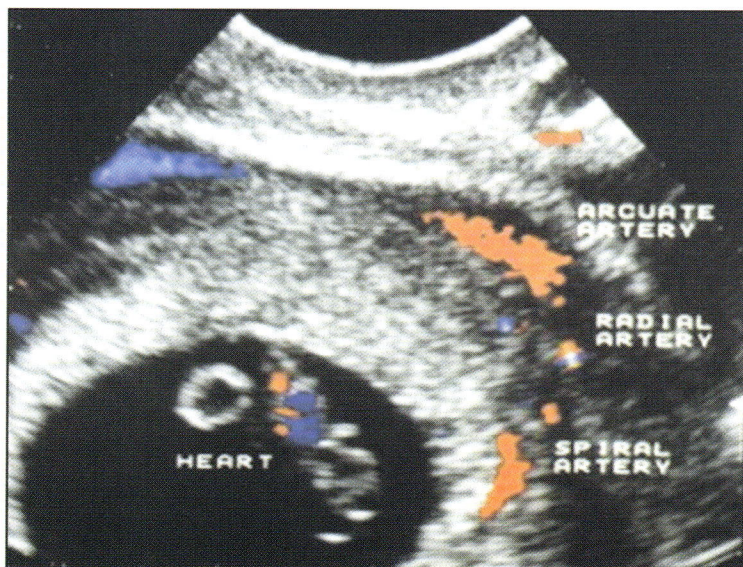

Fig. 3.9: Transvaginal color Doppler from the fetus at 9 weeks of gestation demonstrated blood flow signal from vitelline duct and the yolk sac

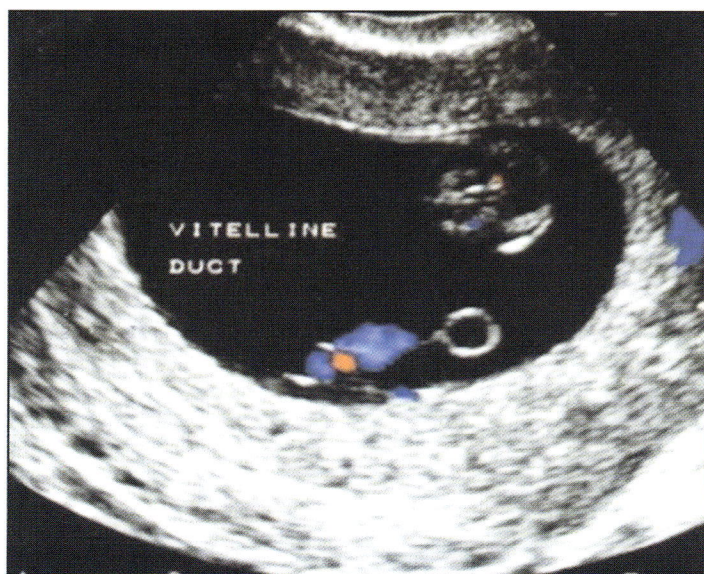

Fig. 3.8: Transvaginal Doppler can obtained signal from the uteroplacental blood flow and from the fetus at the same time

development of pregnancy (trophoblast invasion). Obviously, this decrement continues during the second trimester of pregnancy and can be observed in all the segments of the uteroplacental circulation.

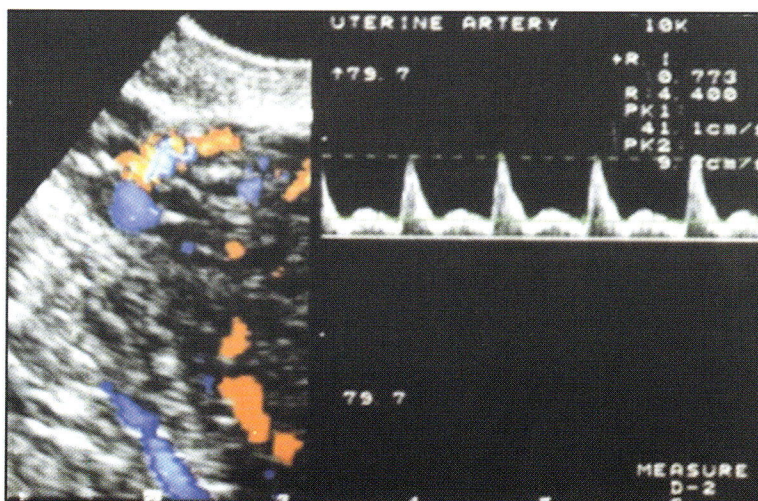

Fig. 3.10: Uterine artery blood flow signal can be obtained by Doppler technique laterally to the cervix at the level of cervicorporeal junction

Uterine Artery Blood Flow in Early Pregnancy

The main uterine artery can be visualized at the level of cervicorporeal junction (Fig. 3.10), as it approaches the uterus laterally and curves upward alongside the uterine body. Pulsed Doppler waveform profiles of the main uterine artery are characteristic, comprising a high peak systolic component with a characteristic notch in the protodiastolic part and very low end-diastolic flow. Numerous Doppler studies have demonstrated a gradual decrement in the uterine artery resistance index during the first trimester of pregnancy.[16-19]

Characteristic notch in the protodiastolic part of sonogram is gradually disappearing; diastolic flow is characterized by high velocity, and difference between systolic and diastolic flow velocities decreases. This kind of changes indicates normal

Arcuate and Radial Arteries Blood Flow

Arcuate arteries may be seen within the outer third of the myometrium, while the radial arteries are identified within the two inner thirds of the myometrium (Figs 3.11 and 3.12). Doppler sonograms of the arcuate and radial arteries are very similar, with moderate peak systolic and diastolic components of blood flow. However, differences exist in the values of the resistance (RI) or pulsatility (PI) indices. These are lower in the radial than in the arcuate arteries, corresponding to the lower peripheral impedance to blood flow.

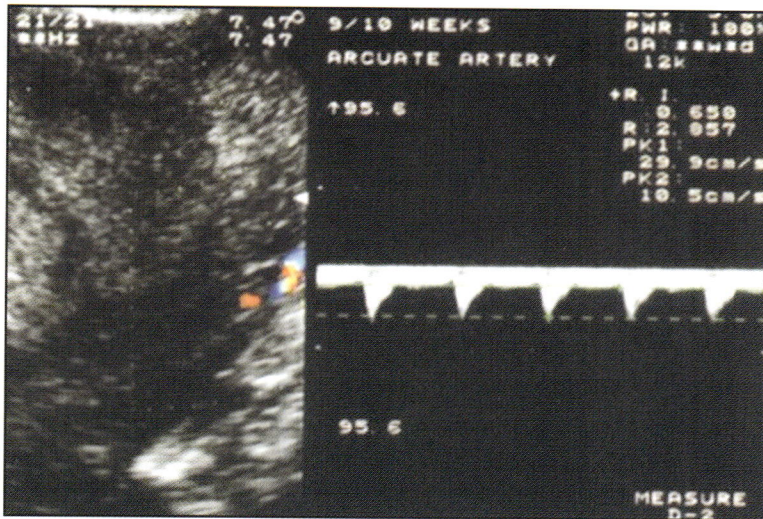

Fig. 3.11: Arcuate artery blood flow demonstrates moderate vascular resistance index, lower than that obtained in the main uterine artery

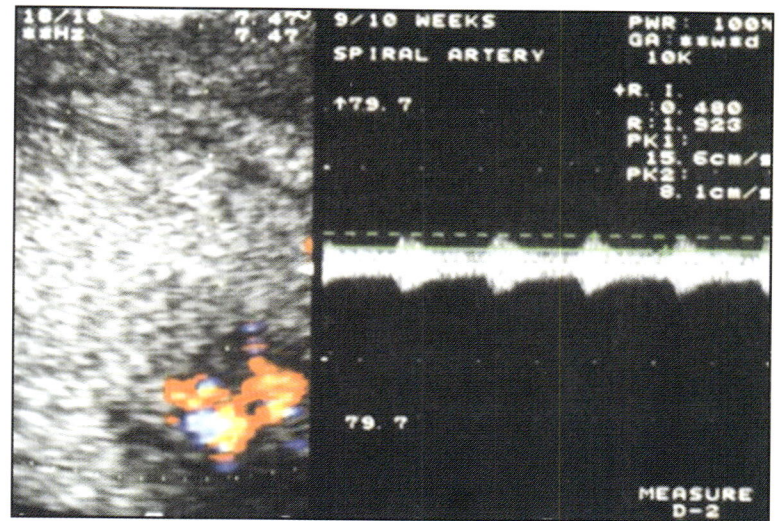

Fig. 3.13: Blood flow velocity waveforms of the spiral arteries demonstrate turbulent flow and a low resistance index

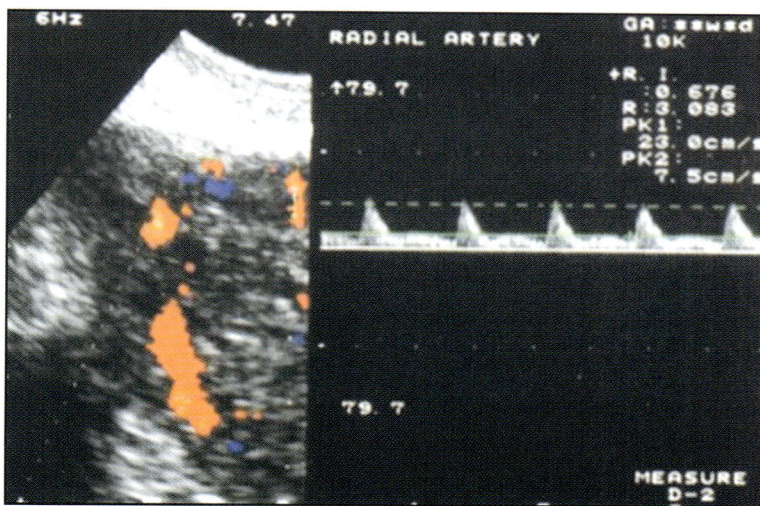

Fig. 3.12: Blood flow velocity waveforms of the radial artery. Note the lower velocity and lower impedance are detected in the examined vessels

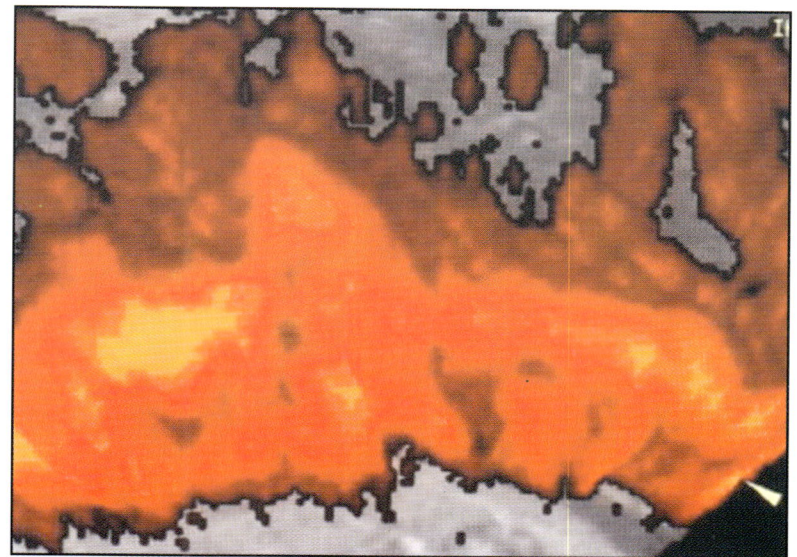

Fig. 3.14: Transvaginal 3D power Doppler image on early pregnancy demonstrates blood flow signal derived from spiral arteries

Normal Finding of Spiral Arteries in Early Pregnancy

During early pregnancy, the spiral arteries are progressively converted to non-muscular dilated tortuous channels. The normal musculoelastic wall is replaced with a mixture of fibrinoid material and fibrous tissue. Easy to be detected above the chorion (near the placental implantation site), spiral arteries are characterized by lower resistance index and higher peak systolic velocities followed by turbulent flow (Figs 3.13 and 3.14). This kind of flow is typical for wide tortuous blood vessels and has hemodynamic characteristics of an arteriovenous shunt. The active trophoblast induces vascular adaptation, which ensures adequate blood supply to the growing embryo.

Pulsed Doppler waveform signals obtained from spiral arteries show low impedance to blood flow and a characteristic spiky outline. The sonogram presents the blood flow from more than one spiral artery. The spiral arteries change their wall structure with gestation and become vessels with completely different hemodynamics in relation to other arteries of the uteroplacental circulation.

Placenta

Development and the Ultrasound Imaging

Primary chorionic villi develop between 13th and 15th days after the ovulation (during 4th week of gestation) and mark the beginning of the placental development (Fig. 3.15). At the same time, the formation of blood vessels starts in the extraembryonic mesoderm of the yolk sac, the connecting stalk and the chorion.[21] By 18th to 21st days (during 5th week of gestation), the villi have become branched and the mesenchymal cells within the villi have differentiated into blood capillaries and formed an arteriocapillary venous network. Chorionic villi cover the entire surface of the gestational sac until the end of the 8th week. At that time, the villi on the side of the chorion proliferate towards the decidua basalis to form the chorion frondosum, which develops into the definitive placenta. The villi in contact with the decidua capsularis begin to degenerate and form an avascular shell, known as the chorion laeve or smooth chorion. The placenta is mostly derived from fetal tissues, when maternal component contributes little to the architecture of the definitive placenta.

Normal placentation requires a progressive transformation of the spiral arteries and an infiltration of trophoblastic cells into the placental bed. These physiological changes normally extend into the inner third of the myometrium, and in normal pregnancies, all the spiral arteries are transformed into uteroplacental arteries before 20th week of gestation.[33] In some cases of early pregnancy failure and pregnancy-induced hypertension, there is an adequate placentation with a defective transformation of spiral arteries.[22]

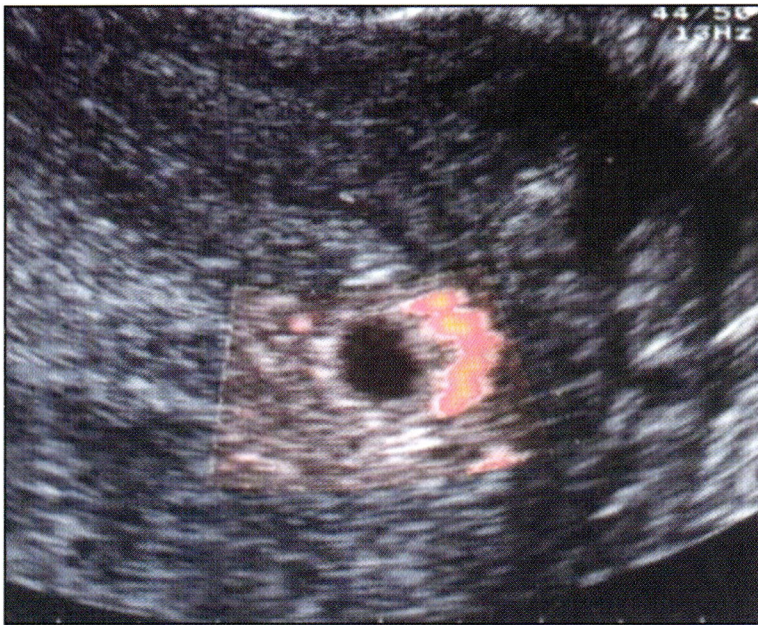

Fig. 3.15: Transvaginal power Doppler scan of early gestational sac shows early chorionic vascularization

Power Doppler Studies in Assessment of Early Chorionic Circulation

New developments on the cutting edge of the ultrasound technology enabled us to expand investigations of early placental vascular supply. 3D power Doppler is able to depict the integral 3D image of placenta and embryo and their vascular network.[3,23] Additionally, it is possible to quantify and express numerically data related to vascular signals in the investigated volume.

Development of the process of placentation begins after the first contact between trophoblast and decidua has been established. There are two waves of trophoblastic invasion. First occurs at 8th week of gestation. It is characterized by invasion

of interstitial trophoblast invasion into the myometrium and cytotrophoblast (endothelial trophoblast) into complete decidua, but not myometrium. Second wave is characterized just by invasion of endothelial trophoblast into the myometrium and occurs between 16th and 18th weeks of gestation.[24]

Uteroplacental arteries are not responsive to the autonomous nervous system. In the second lunar month, the intervillous space increases as the result of the extensive branching of the villi. The intervillous space, combined with the villi, is the functional unit of the human placenta, where maternal-fetal metabolic exchange occurs.[25] In this period, many terminal parts of the spiral arteries near the intervillous space contain plugs of cytotrophoblastic cells. At the same time, centrally placed communications between the decidual veins are numerous and large. After 40 days spiral arteries show direct openings into the intervillous space and the cytotrophoblastic cells appear within their lumen. The maternal blood reaches the intervillous space through the gaps between the cells of the endovascular trophoblast. These events can be nicely studied by 3D color and power Doppler ultrasound (Figs 3.16A to D).

During pulsed Doppler analysis two types of waveform can be visualized: pulsatile arterial-like, and continuous venous-like flow. Lumen of the spiral arteries is never completely obstructed by the trophoblastic plugs. These data indicate that establishment of the intervillous circulation is a continuous process rather than an abrupt event at the end of the first trimester. Hafner et al did cross-sectional study in a group of patients in gestational age 5th to 11th weeks. After acquirement of the volume containing 3D power Doppler data of the pregnant uterus, the signals belonging to the chorion were isolated. Vascular 3D measurements were undertaken and expressed by Vascularization Index (VI) and Vascularization Flow Index (VFI). Volume of the chorion increased exponentially throughout observation period. The VI and VFI positively correlated with the crown-rump length (CRL) and chorion volume, and showed gradual increment through the investigation period (Figs 3.17A to E).

Fetal Portion

The assessment of the fetal portion of circulation includes the umbilical and fetal circulation (Fig. 3.18). Hemodynamic changes in the umbilical artery represent the placental side of the uteroplacental circulation. Signals from the umbilical artery may be clearly visualized at the embryo's lateral edge connected to the placenta. The fetal circulation is usually analyzed through assessment of the fetal heart, fetal aorta, carotid arteries and intracranial circulation (middle cerebral artery in particular) (Fig. 3.19).

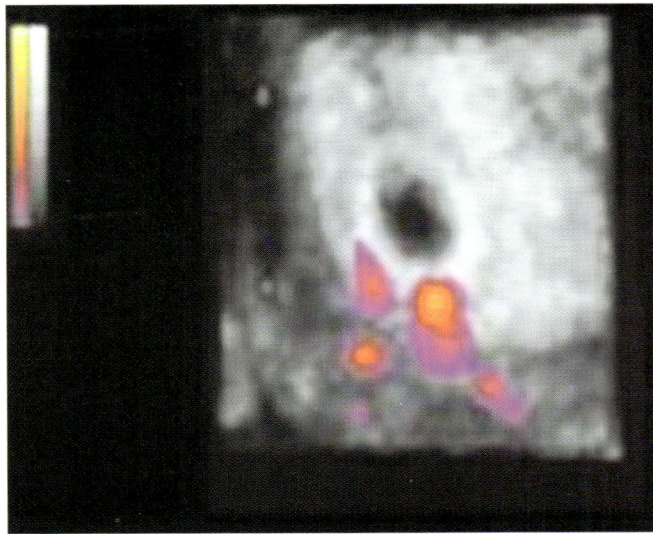

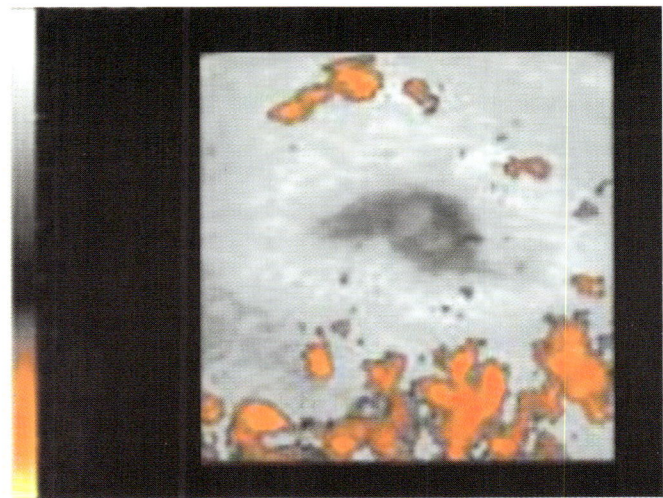

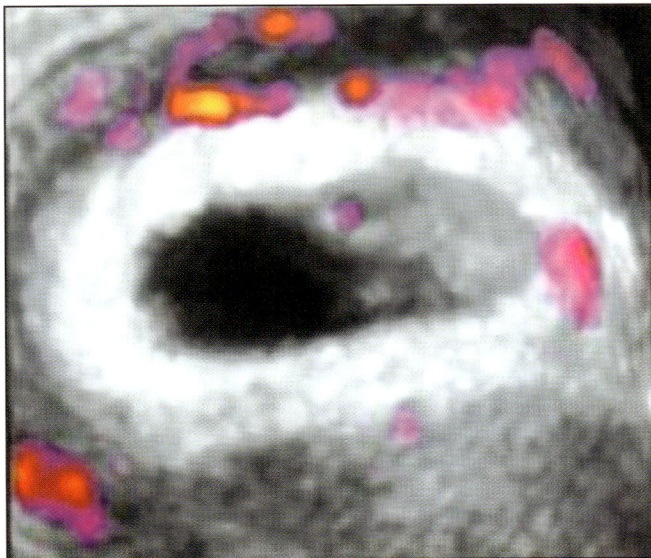

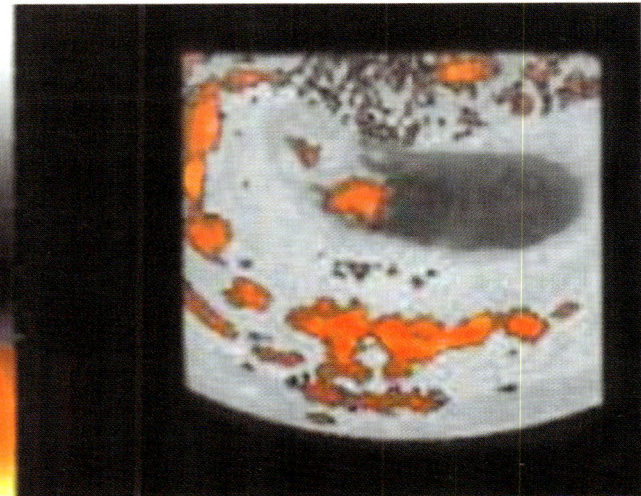

Figs 3.16A to D: 3D power Doppler image of early gestation and its vascular supply: A. 5th week, B. 6th week, C. 8th week, D. 9th week

The appearance of blood flow in these arteries is described separately for each gestational week and compared to the main histological and conventional gray scale ultrasound findings. Kurjak and Kupesic used combined B-mode and power Doppler imaging in order to evaluate fetal growth and development of fetal circulation.[26] Different rendering modalities were used in color-coded data processing and presentation. A minimum-intensity projection of the vascular network was used to create a translucent image, and a maximum-intensity projection was applied for a surface rendered vascular image. The former was superior in assessment of the spatial interrelationship of the vascular structures, and the latter was useful in the assessment of the morphology and outer surface of a confined vascular structure.

The 5th Week

Characteristic embryological findings: The deep neural groove and the first somites are present. The embryo is almost straight and somites produce conspicuous surface elevation. The heart prominence is distinct and the optic pits are present.

The attenuated tail with its somites is also a characteristic feature.

Ultrasound findings: Gestational sac can be visualized as a small spherical anechoic structure placed inside one of the endometrial leafs. 3D sonography enables precise measurement of exponentially expanding gestational sac volume during the first trimester (Fig. 3.20). Kupesic and co-workers found that 3D measurement of yolk sac volume and vascularity may be predictive of a pregnancy outcome.[27] Using this noninvasive modality one can obtain multiplanar and surface images in reduced scanning time. Surface images seem to be beneficial in the evaluation of the yolk sac echogenicity and detection of the hyperechoic yolk sac which may indicate chromosomal abnormality. Automatic and manual volume calculation allows analysis of the precise relationship between the yolk sac and gestational sac volumes, as well as assessment of the correlation

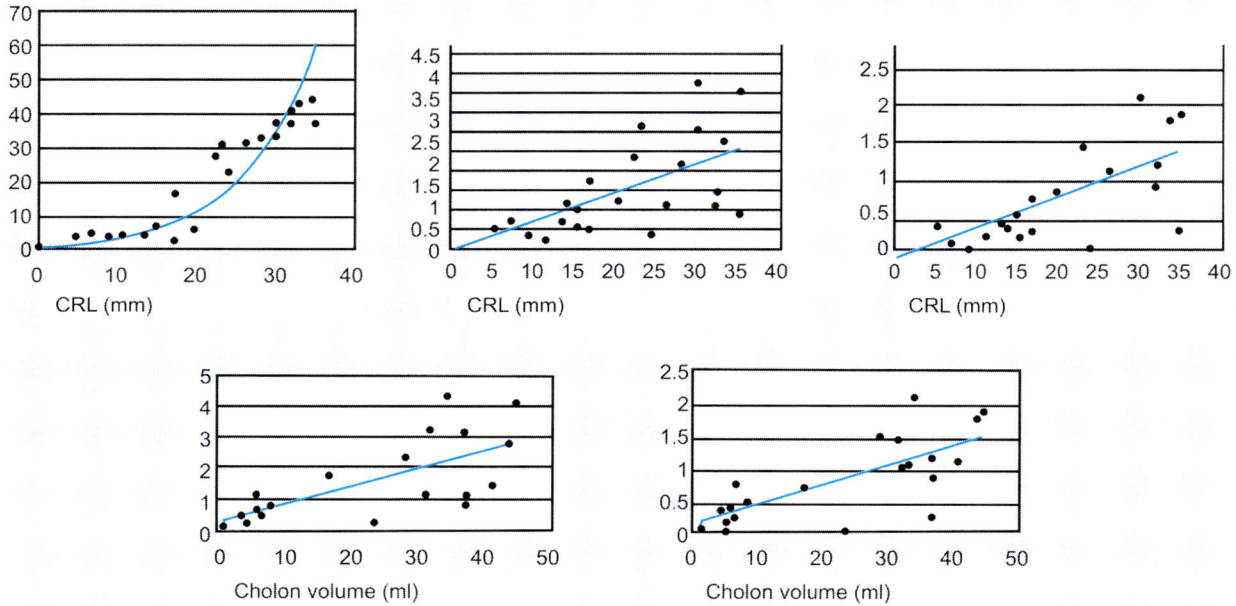

Figs 3.17A to E: Correlation between vascular activity in the chorion detected by 3D power Doppler:
A. Chorionic volume (Vch) related to the crown-rump length (CRL)
B. Chorionic vascularization index (VI) related to the crown-rump length (CRL)
C. Chorionic vascularization flow index (VFI) related to the crown-rump length (CRL)
D. Chorionic vascularization index (VI) related to the chorionic volume
E. Chorionic vascularization flow index (VFI) related to the chorionic volume

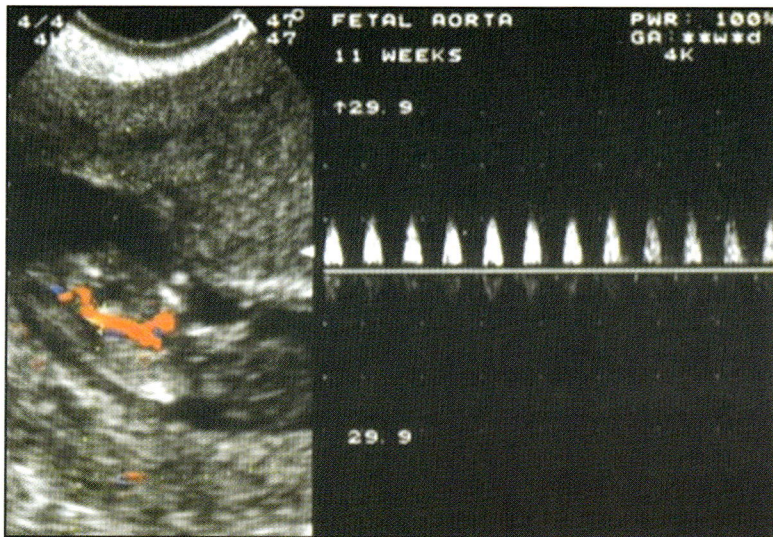

Fig. 3.18: Doppler signal derived from the fetal aorta. Note absent of the end-diastolic from the signal

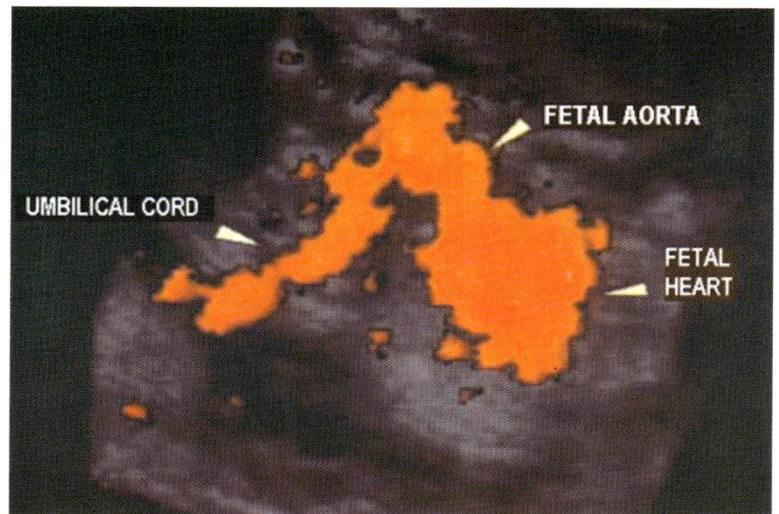

Fig. 3.19: 3D power Doppler demonstrated signals from the umbilical artery, fetal heart, fetal aorta at the embryo's lateral edge connected to the placenta

between yolk sac volume and CRL measurements. Planar mode tomograms are useful for detecting the embryonic pole inside the gestational sac. The embryo itself can be seen 24 to 48 hr after visualization of the yolk sac, at approximately 33 days after menstruation, at which is 2 to 3 mm long.[28] Adjacent to the yolk sac, embryo can be seen as a small straight line measuring by the end of 5th gestational week.

Power Doppler findings: 3D power Doppler reveals intensive vascular activity surrounding the chorionic shell starting from the first sonographic evidence of the developing pregnancy during the 5th week of gestation (Fig. 3.21). Gestational sac can be detected as a tiny ring shaped structure at the beginning of gestational age of 5th week (Fig. 3.22). 3D power Doppler reveals intense vascular activity surrounding it. A hyperechoic chorionic

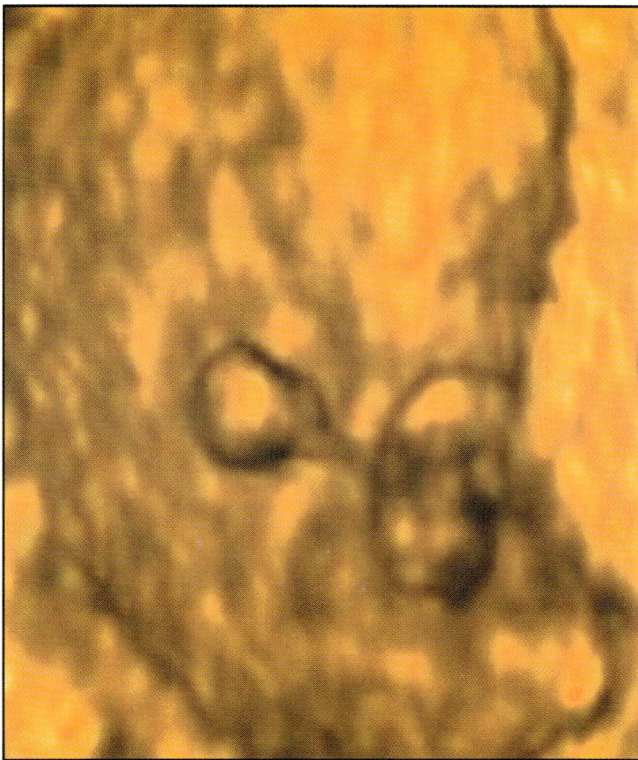

Fig. 3.20: 3D ultrasond at 5th weeks of gestation. The deep neural groove and the first somites are present. The embryo is almost straight and somites produce conspicuous surface elevation. Gestational sac can be visualized as a small spherical anechoic structure placed inside one of the endometrial leafs

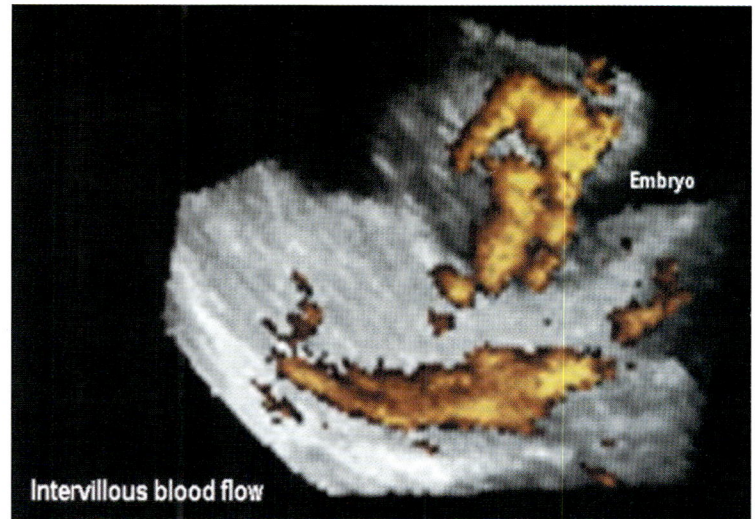

Fig. 3.21: 3D power Doppler reveals intensive vascular activity surrounding the chorionic shell starting from the first sonographic evidence of the developing pregnancy during the 5th week of gestation

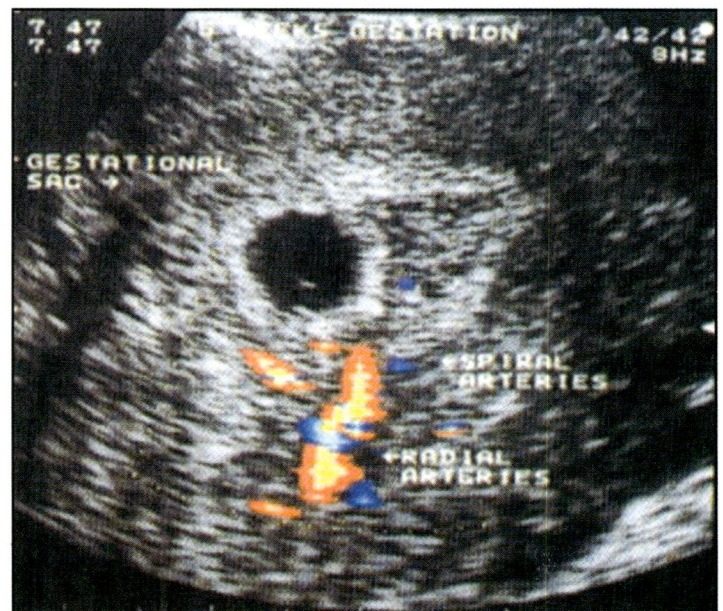

Fig. 3.22: Transvaginal color Doppler scan of the gestational sac at 5th week of gestation. Note the prominent vascularity at the periphery of the sac indicative of trophoblastic penetration

ring is interrupted by color-coded sprouts of early intervillous and spiral artery blood flow. At the end of the fifth week, when the gestational sac exceeds 8 mm, the small secondary yolk sac is visible as the earliest sign of the developing embryo.

The 6th Week

Characteristic embryological findings: The embryo has a C-shaped curve. The growth of the head (caused by the rapid development of the brain) exceeds that of the other regions.

Ultrasound findings: Rounded bulky head and thinner body characterize 3D image of an embryo during the 6th week of gestation (Figs 3.23 and 3.24). The head is prominent due to the developing forebrain. Limb buds are rarely visible in this stage of pregnancy. However, umbilical cord and vitelline duct are always clearly seen. At 6th week of gestation ductus omphalomesentericus can be as much as three to four times the length of the embryo itself. The amniotic membrane is also visible, initially at the dorsal part of the embryo. A few days later it surrounds the embryo but not the yolk sac, which remains in the extracelomic cavity.

CNS development: At the end of 6th week, the first part of the embryonic brain, the rhombencephalic cavity, appears as a tiny hypoechogenic area in the cranial pole of the embryo. In the sagittal section, it is seen as a shallow hypoechogenic area, cranial in the embryonic body. Anterior to it, the narrow tube of the midbrain may be detected.[4]

Power Doppler findings: Aortic and umbilical blood flow is well depicted. Initial branches of the umbilical vessels are visible at the placental umbilical insertion (Fig. 3.25). 3D power Doppler detects embryonic heartbeats as early as five weeks and four days menstrual age (Fig. 3.26), at the embryo CRL of 3 ± 4 mm. At this very early stage, this finding may help clinicians to diagnose the viability of the pregnancy. Near the end of the 6th week first signs of aortic and umbilical blood flow within the embryo's trunk are visible. The initial branches of the umbilical vessels are visible at the placental umbilical insertion.

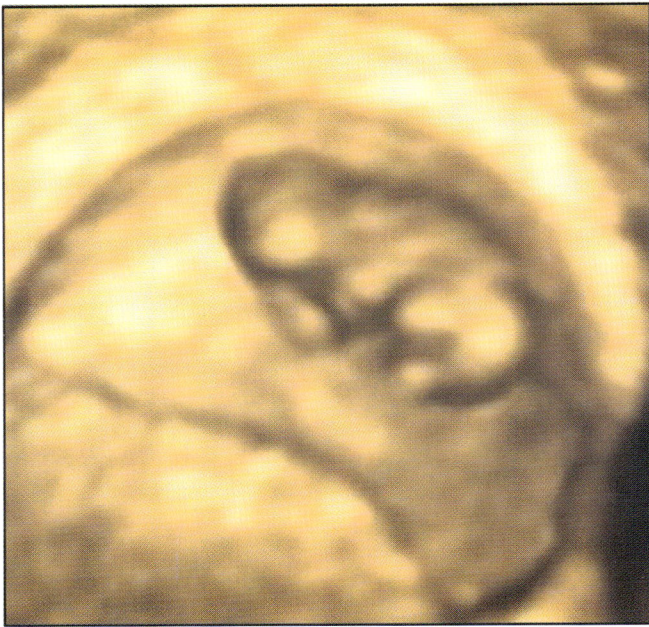

Fig. 3.23: Rounded bulky head and thinner body characterize 3D image of an embryo during the 6th week of gestation. The head is prominent due to the developing forebrain. Limb buds are rarely visible in this stage of gestation

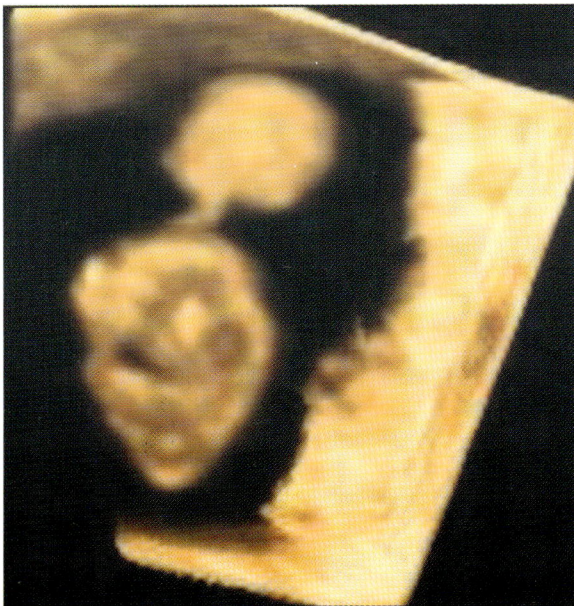

Fig. 3.24: 3D surface rendering demonstrates embryo and yolk sac structure at the 6th week of gestation

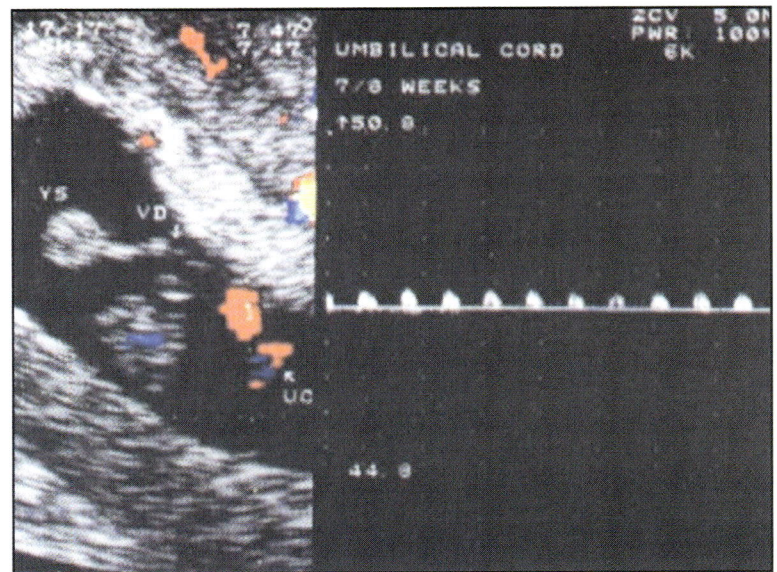

Fig. 3.25: Blood flow signals derived from the umbilical cord, demonstrating the absence of diastolic flow

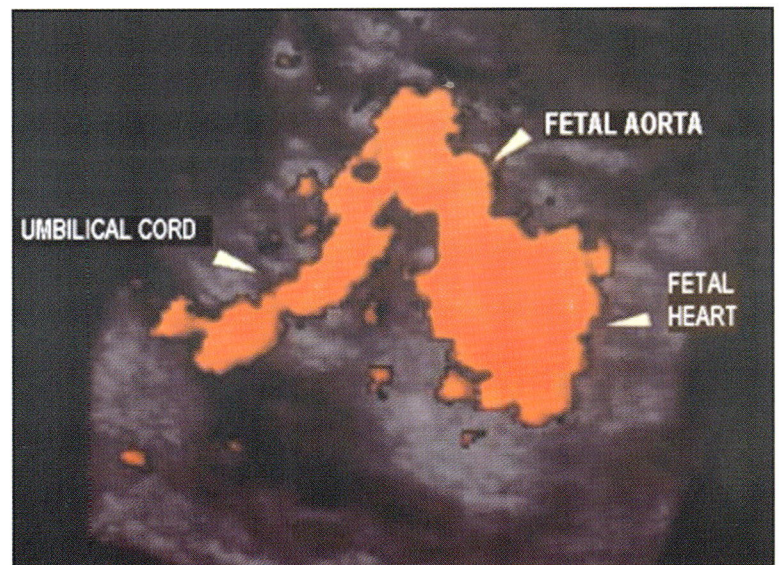

Fig. 3.26: 3D power Doppler image of an embryo during the 6th week of gestation: Aortic and umbilical blood flow is well depicted. Initial branches of the umbilical vessels are visible at the placental-umbilical insertion

The 7th Week

Characteristic embryological findings: The head is now much larger in relation to the trunk and is more bent over the cardiac prominence. The trunk and neck have begun to straighten. Hand and foot plates are formed and digital or finger rays started to appear.

Ultrasound findings: During the 7th gestational week spine gradually becomes visible, as well as limb buds, lateral to the body. Amnion can be seen as a spherical hyperechoic membrane, still close to the embryo. Chorion frondosum can be distinguished from the chorion laeve. Fast development of rhombencephalon (hind-brain) occurs. This process gives even more prominence to the head. Head becomes the dominant embryonic structure. Using the multiplanar mode, developing vesicles of the brain can be depicted as anechoic structures inside the head. The biggest, and usually the only visible, is rhombencephalon placed on the top of the head (vertex). The head is strongly flexed anterior being in contact with the chest. (Figs 3.27 and 3.28).

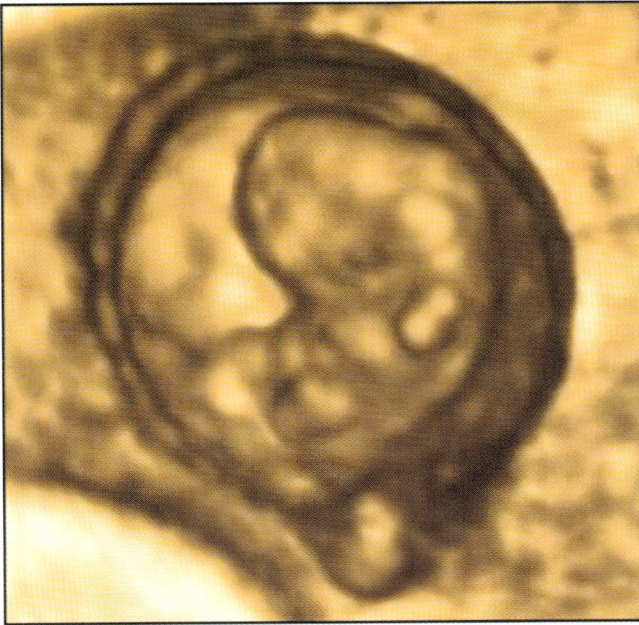

Fig. 3.27: 3D image during the 7th gestational week, spine gradually becomes visible, as well as limb buds, lateral to the body. Amnion can be seen as a spherical hyperechoic membrane, still close to the embryo

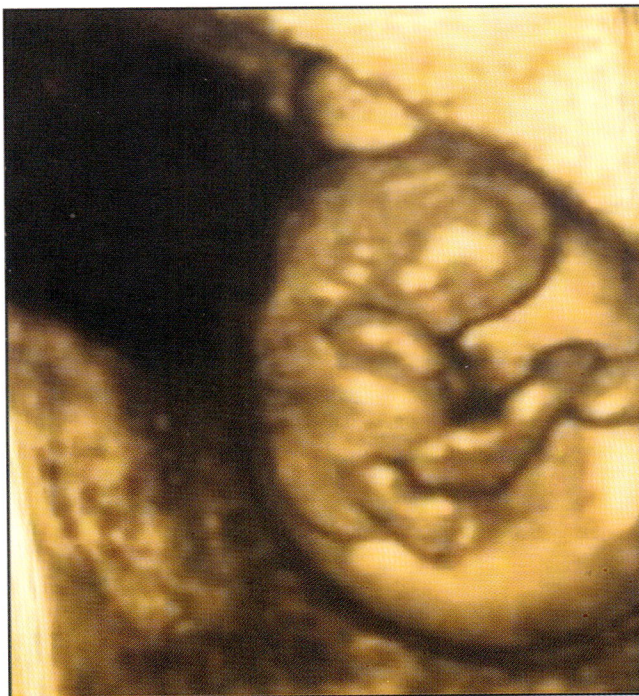

Fig. 3.28: 3D surface rendering from the embryo at 7th week of gestation showing the umbilical cord in its full length. Note the head is strongly flexed

CNS development: During 7th week the hypoechogenic brain cavities could be identified, including the separated cerebral hemispheres (Fig. 3.29). The lateral ventricles are shaped like small round vesicles. The cavity of the diencephalon (future third ventricle) runs posteriorly. In the smallest embryos, the medial telencephalon forms a continuous cavity between the lateral ventricles. The future foramina of Monro are wide. In the sagittal plane, the height of the cavity of the diencephalon (future third ventricle) is slightly greater than that of the mesencephalon. Thus,

the wide border between the cavities of the diencephalon and the mesencephalon is indicated. The curved tube-like mesencephalic cavity (future sylvian aqueduct) lies anterior, its rostral part pointing caudal. It straightens considerably during the following weeks. The telencephalon impar represents the broad area between the hemispheres. At this stage the telencephalon lies very close to the beating heart. The spine appears as a double line.[4]

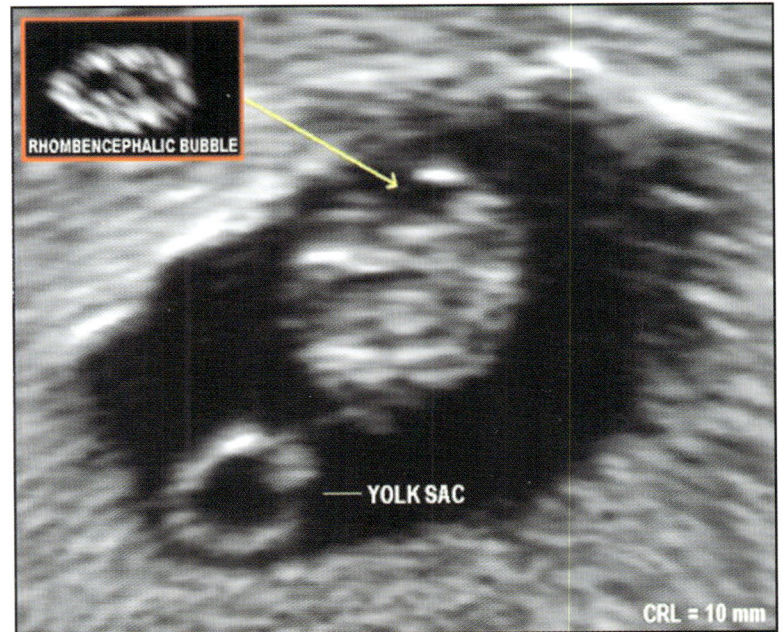

Fig. 3.29: Horizontal section through the head of a 7-week embryo, crown-rump length 10 mm. The cavity of the rhombencephalon is visualized

Power Doppler findings: Besides the aorta and umbilical blood flow, at the end of the 7th week 3D power Doppler depicts features of early vascular anatomy on the base of the skull. Vessels are evolving laterally to the mesencephalon and cephalic flexure. Apart from embryonic circulation, 3D power Doppler can obtain blood flow signals from the intervillous space. The gestational sac occupies about one-third of the uterine volume. The main landmark now is an echogenic fetal pole consisting of embryo adjacent to a cystic yolk sac. The intracranial circulation becomes visible during the seventh week of gestation. At this time discrete pulsations of the internal carotid arteries are detectable at the base of the skull (Figs 3.30 and 3.31).

The 8th Week

Characteristic embryological findings: By the beginning of the 8th week, the embryo has developed a skeleton, which is mostly cartilaginous and gives a form to its body. The communication between the primitive gut and the yolk sac has been reduced to a relatively small duct (the yolk stalk).

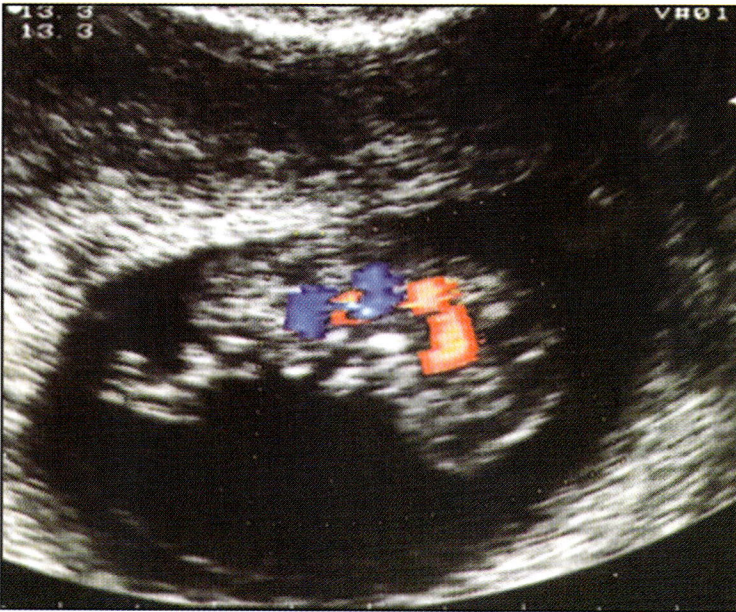

Fig. 3.30: Transvaginal color Doppler scan of an embryo at 7th to 8th weeks of gestation. Lower limb buds are clearly seen, while upper limb buds are discretely visualized. Note the blood flow signals obtained from the fetal heart and intracranial vessels

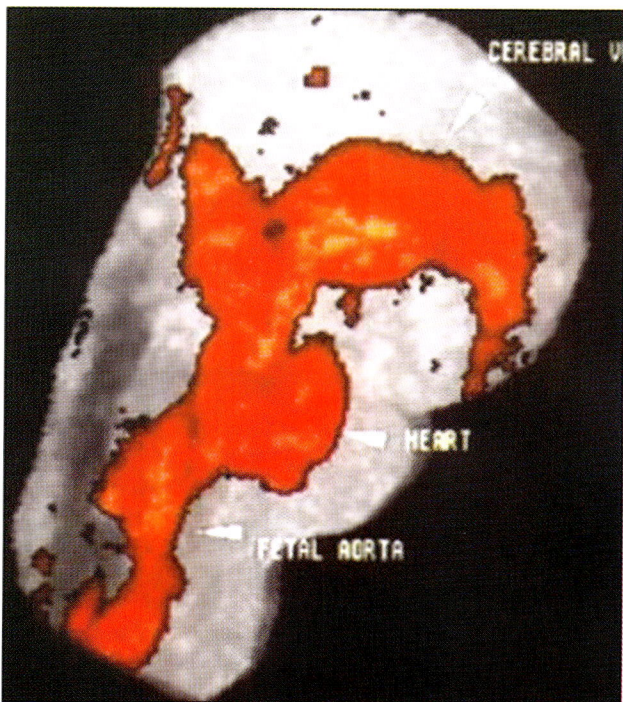

Fig. 3.31: 3D power Doppler findings demonstrated the aortic and umbilical blood flow, at the end of the 7th weeks. 3D power Doppler depicts features of early vascular anatomy on the base of the skull. The intracranial circulation becomes visible during this gestational age

Ultrasound findings: The most characteristic finding is a complete visualization of the limbs, which end in thicker areas that correspond to the future hands and feet. The shape of the face begins to appear but is not clearly seen (Figs 3.32 and 3.33). The great majority of embryos show a cranial pole flexion that makes it almost impossible to see the face. Insertion of the umbilical cord is visible on the anterior abdominal wall. During

the 8th week of gestation there is expansion of the ventricular system of the brain (lateral, third and midbrain ventricles). Due to these processes the head erects from the anterior flexion. The vertex is now located over the position of the midbrain. Structures of the viscerocranium are not visible due to their small size. Arms and feet are clearly visible. Insertion of the umbilical cord is visible on the anterior abdominal wall. During the 8th and 9th weeks the developing intestine is being herniated into the proximal umbilical cord.

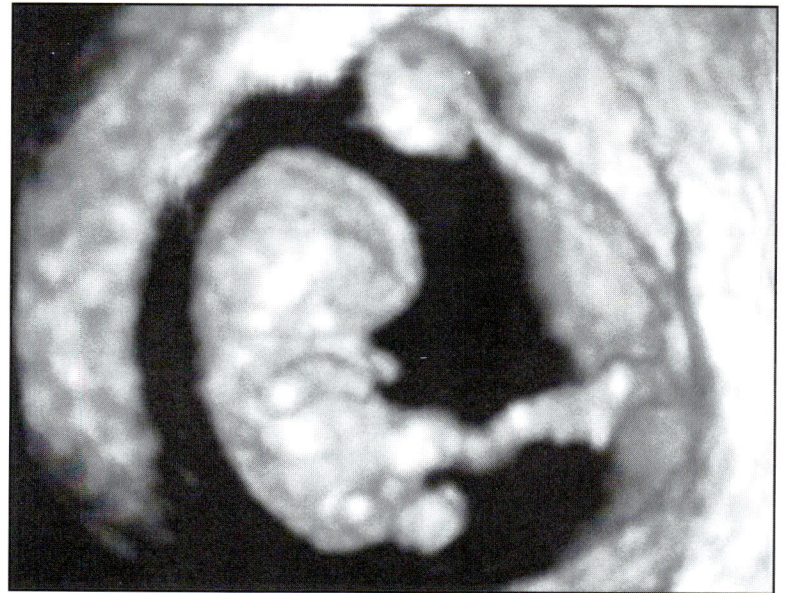

Fig. 3.32: 3D Ultrasound findings demonstrated complete visualization of the limbs, which end in thicker areas that correspond to the future hands and feet. The shape of the face begins to appear but is not clearly seen. The communication between the primitive gut and the yolk sac has been reduced to a relatively small duct (the yolk stalk)

CNS development: Blaas and co-workers reported on a 7th weeks and 5 days gestational age embryo whose brain structures were analyzed in detail by 3D ultrasound.[29] They described distinct hemispheres how the rhombencephalic cavity (future fourth ventricle) deepens gradually with the growth of the embryos, at the same time decreasing its length.[29] At this time, it has a pyramid-like shape with the central deepening of the pontine flexure as the peak of the pyramid.[30]

The hemispheres enlarge; the foramina of Monro become distinct. Care should be taken so that the hemispheres are not mistaken for the orbits. The mesencephalic cavity is connected with the rhombencephalic cavity by the narrow isthmus rhombencephaly (Fig. 3.34). The increased growth of the rostral brain structures and the deepening of the pontine flexure lead to the deflection of the brain, which becomes obvious during 8th week, the mesencephalon lies superior in the head of the embryo, and the length of the rhombencephalic cavity decreases.[4] Slight body movements become visible at the beginning of week 8, and some days later limb movements can be seen. The

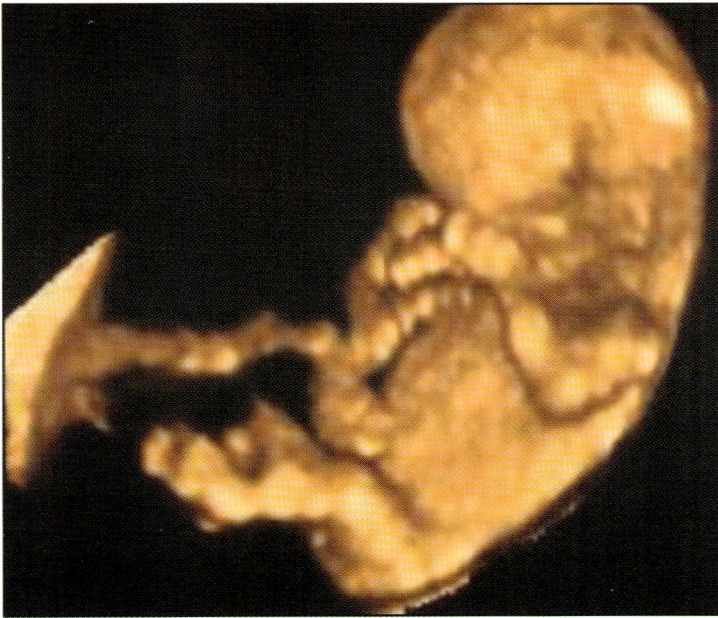

Fig. 3.33: The fetus at 8th to 9th weeks of gestation. 3D surface rendering shows visualization of the limbs, hands and feet. The shape of the face appeared is clearly seen. The primitive gut has been totally retracted

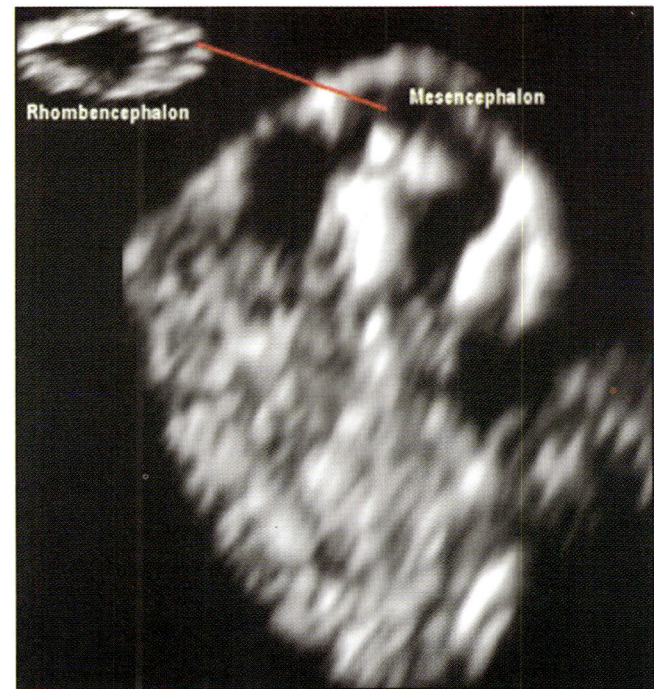

Fig. 3.34: This image shows the mesencephalic cavity connected with the rhombencephalic cavity by the narrow isthmus rhombencephaly

thickenings of the anterior rhombic lips, which will later develop into the cerebellar hemispheres, become evident. The choroid plexuses in the fourth ventricle become detectable as hyperechogenic structures in the roof of the rhombencephalon. At the end of week 8, the primordia to the choroid plexuses of the lateral ventricles are seen as small hyperechogenic areas within the lateral ventricles. In a slightly oblique sagittal section, the continuity of the brain cavities from the hemisphere on one side of the diencephalon, the mesencephalon and the rhombencephalon may be imaged.[4]

Power Doppler findings: During the 8th and 9th weeks, developing intestine is being herniated into the proximal umbilical cord, which can be assessed using this technique (Figs 3.35 and 3.36). By the eighth week, an embryo's length is between 10 and 16 mm, and the CRL is easily measured. The visualization rate of the fetal aorta and umbilical artery is higher. Blood flow in the fetal heart and aorta as well as in the umbilical artery and intracranial is clearly visualized. At this stage of pregnancy 3D power Doppler imaging allows visualization of the entire fetal circulation.

The 9th to 10th Weeks

Characteristic embryological findings: The head is more rounded and constitutes almost half of the embryo (Fig. 3.37). The hands and feet approach each other. The upper limbs develop faster that the lower limbs, and toward the end of the 9th week, the fingers are almost entirely formed. The intestines are in the umbilical cord (physiological mid-gut herniation).

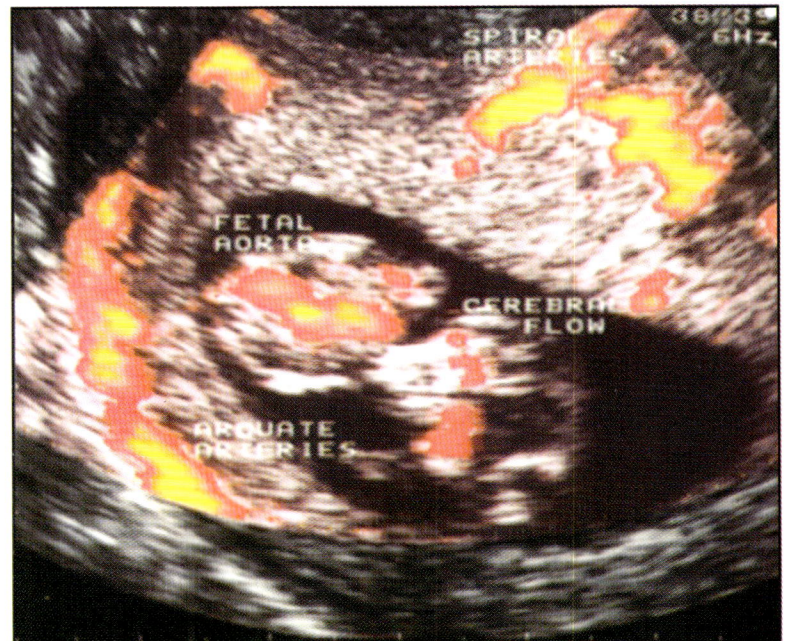

Fig. 3.35: Power Doppler further enhances the visualization of the vascular signals from the living fetus

Ultrasound findings: Merz and co-workers were able to provide striking images of the fetal face at this gestational age.[31] They reported cases in which transvaginal 3D ultrasound produced remarkably well-defined facial images as early as 9th week of gestation. Sometimes even the external ear can be depicted using 3D surface imaging. Herniation of the mid-gut is still present as it is a consequence of the rapid growth of the bowel and liver before closure of the abdominal wall. Although this is a physiologic phenomenon, it does not appear in each fetus.

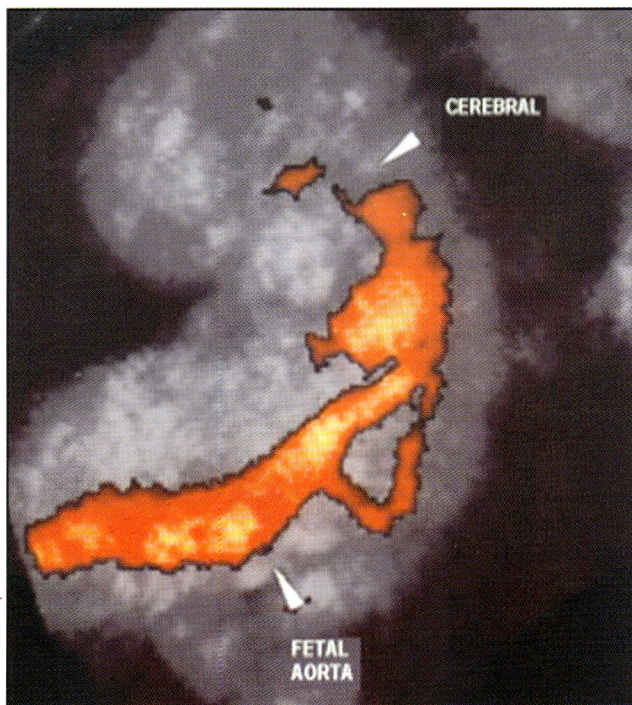

Fig. 3.36: 3D power Doppler visualized the fetal aorta and umbilical artery. Developing intestine is being herniated into the proximal umbilical cord, which can be assessed using this technique

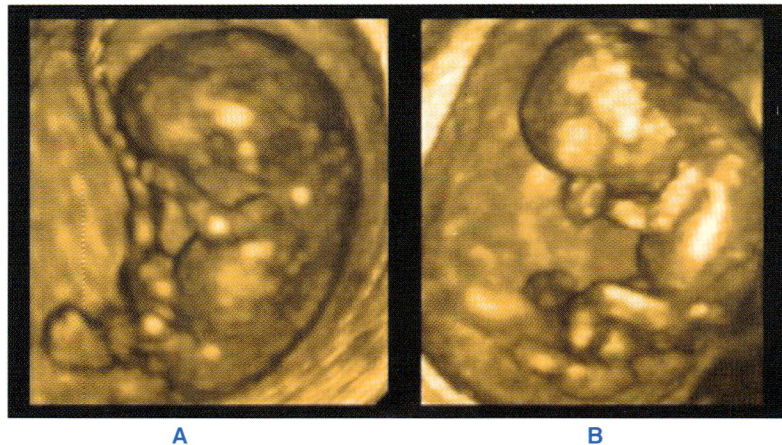

Fig. 3.37: 3D image at A. 9th week and B.10th weeks of gestation. The head is more rounded and constitutes almost half of the embryo. The hands and feet approach each other. The upper limbs develop faster than the lower limbs, and toward the end of the 9th week the fingers are almost entirely formed

Possibly, we cannot, visualize it, or else its size may vary. At 10th week, the bowel undergoes two turns of 180 degrees, returning to its original position, at the same time that closure and development of the abdominal wall end. Cerebral hemispheres continue to develop during the 9th and 10th weeks of gestation. Visible are lateral ventricles containing hyperechoic choroid plexuses. The head is clearly divided from the body by the neck. External ear is sometimes depicted in the 3D surface image. Herniation of the midgut is present. Dorsal column, the early spine, can be examined in its whole length. The arms with elbow and legs with knees are clearly visible. Feet can be seen approaching the midline.

CNS development: The size of the lateral ventricles increases rapidly and the cerebral hemispheres begin to show the typical C-shape. While the third ventricle is still relatively wide at the beginning of this week, its anteromedial part narrows due to the growth of the thalami. In the fetuses of 25 mm CRL and more, there is a clear gap between the rhombencephalic and the mesencephalic cavity due to the growing cerebellum. The isthmus rhombencephaly is narrow and in most cases, it is not visible in its complete length. The cavity of the diencephalon decreases in the larger fetuses (CRL = 25 mm), and becomes narrow especially at its upper anterior part. The spine is still characterized by two echogenic parallel lines.

The choroid plexuses are echogenic structures. During 9th week, the eyes may become distinguishable. They are small, the distance between them is large. At the beginning of 9th week, the third ventricle can still be broad, but later it becomes narrow, due to the growth of the thalamus. The cavity of the mesencephalon, the future aqueduct, is still a large cavity. The cerebellar hemispheres have enlarged, narrowing the lateral recesses. The choroid plexuses of the fourth ventricle traverse the roof and separate it into the areae membranaceae superior and inferior.[4]

At the 10th week of gestation the cerebral hemispheres cover the diencephalon. Cranially they meet at the midline. The ventricles are almost filled with the large choroid plexuses, but some fluid is seen in the frontal horns. The walls of the hemispheres are about 1 mm thick. The hypoechogenic walls of the diencephalon have thickened, the third ventricle is narrow. The dorsal evaginations of the mesencephalic cavity become detectable. Due to the growth of the cerebellum, the distance from the choroid plexuses of the fourth ventricle to the cerebellum now becomes shorter.[4]

Power Doppler findings: Fetal structures are now clearly discernible and they are represented by distinct parts of the fetal body—head, trunk and limbs. The head measures two-thirds of the entire body and becomes a distinct anatomical structure (Figs 3.38 to 3.41). The common and internal carotid arteries may be visualized at the end of the eighth gestational week and the beginning of the ninth week. A cerebral circulation (circle of Willis and its major branches) can be documented at eighth week in the form of discrete pulsations of the intracerebral part of the internal carotid artery. From the ninth gestational week, arterial pulsations can be detected on transverse section, lateral to the mesencephalon and cephalic flexure.

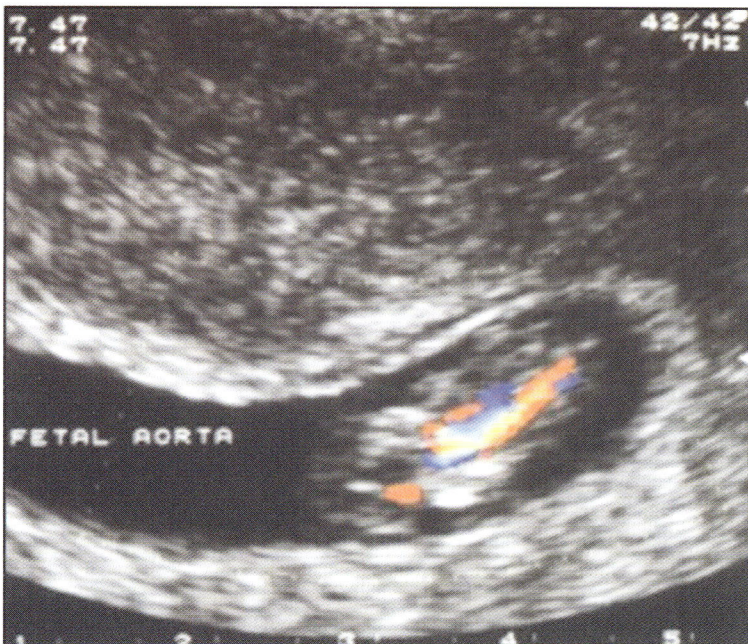

Fig. 3.38: Transvaginal color Doppler scan at 9th to 10th weeks of gestation. Note the full length of the fetal aorta

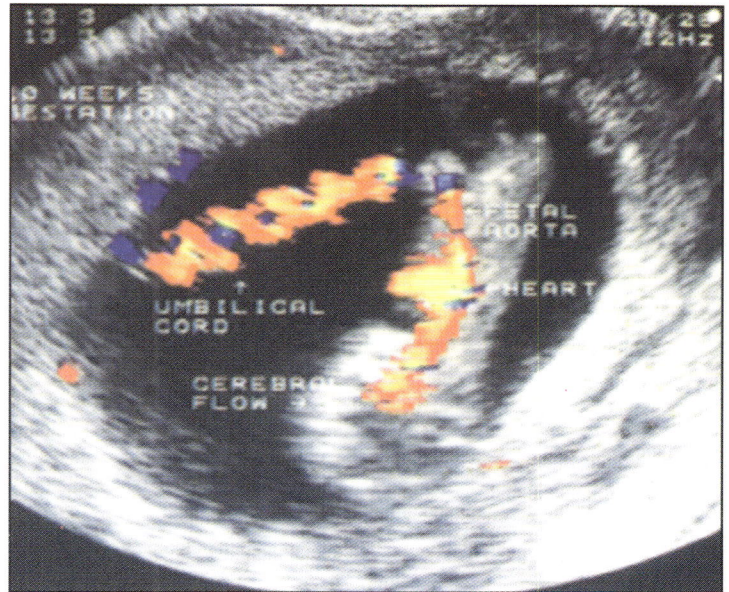

Fig. 3.40: Color Doppler displays the fetal and umbilical circulations

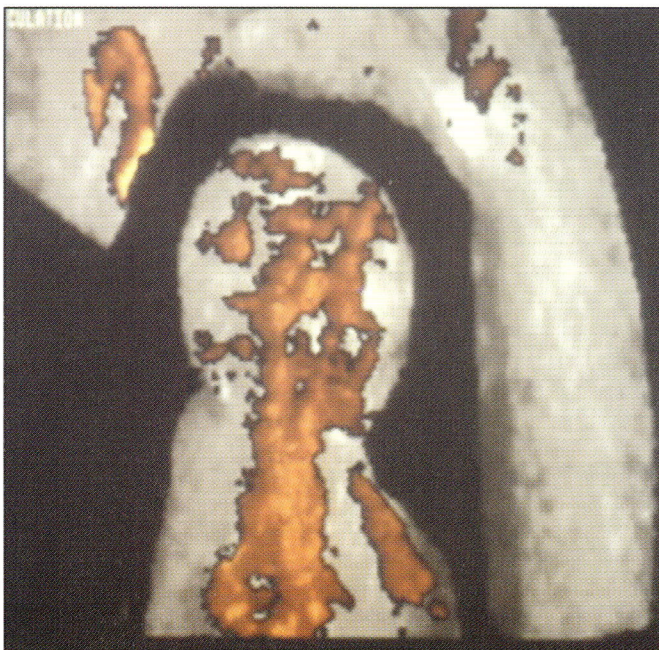

Fig. 3.39: 3D power Doppler image showed the cerebral circulation (circle of Willis and its major branches) in the form of discrete pulsations of the intracerebral part of the internal carotid artery

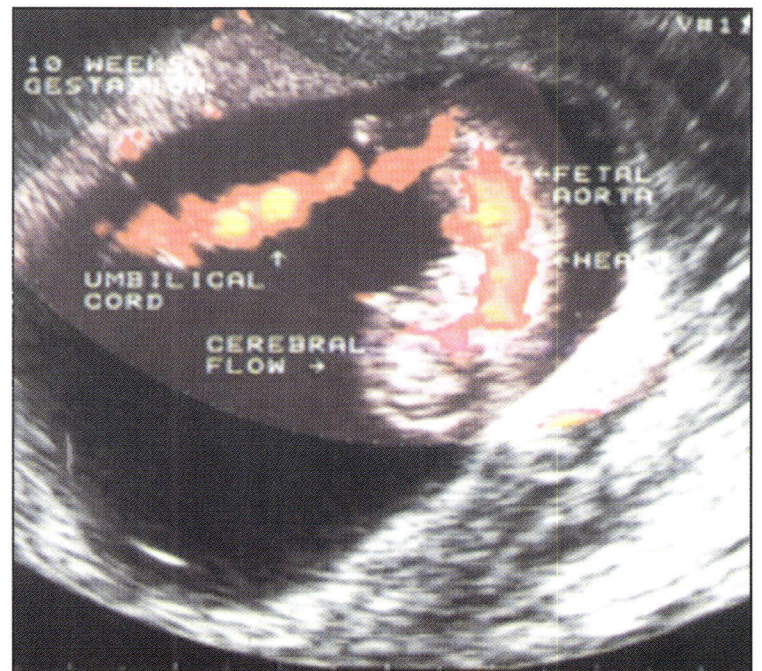

Fig. 3.41: The same fetus as in Figure 3.40 examined by power Doppler technique

The 11th Week

Characteristic embryological findings: The mid-gut herniation disappears and fetal kidneys produce urine that is excreted into the amniotic fluid.

Ultrasound findings: During the 11th week of gestation development of the head and neck continues. Facial details such as nose, orbits, maxilla and mandibles are often visible (Fig. 3.42A). Herniated mid-gut returns into the abdominal cavity. Its persistence after 11th week of gestation is presumptive of an omphalocele. Planar mode enables detailed analysis of the embryonic body with visualization of the stomach and urinary bladder. Kidneys are often visible. Arms and legs continue with development. The ability to visualize fetal hands/fingers and feet/toes was better with 3D that with 2D ultrasonography in the late first trimester (detection rates were 65 percent and 41 percent by 3D ultrasonography for hands and feet, respectively and 41 percent and 12 percent, by 2D ultrasonograpliy). Long bones can be visualized as hyperechoic elongated structures inside upper and lower extremities. Detailed 3D analysis of the fetal spine, chest and limbs is obtainable by using the transparent, X-ray-like-mode (Fig. 3.42B). With the use of the transparency X-ray system, starting at 13th week, the medullar channel, each vertebra and rib can be visualized and even the intervertebral disks can be measured. This opens unexpected possibilities for early diagnosis of skeletal malformations.

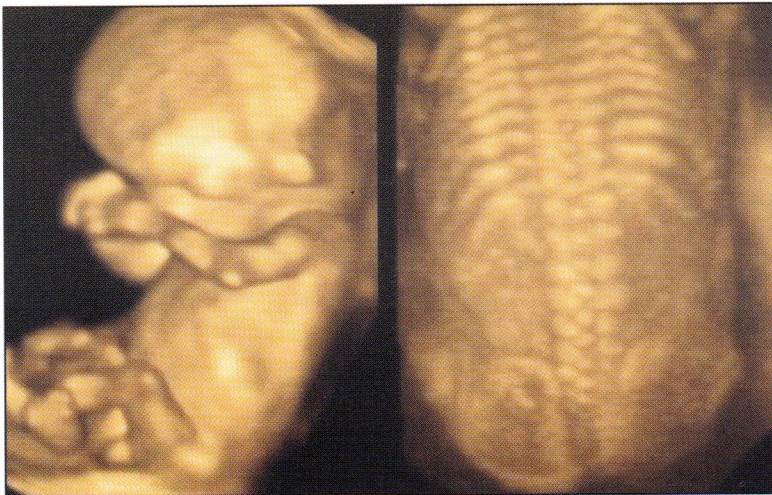

Figs 3.42A and B: 3D image during the 11th week of gestation showing development of the head and neck. A. Facial details such as nose, orbits, maxilla and mandibles are often visible. B. Detailed 3D analysis of the fetal spine, chest and limbs is obtainable by using the transparent, X-ray-like-mode

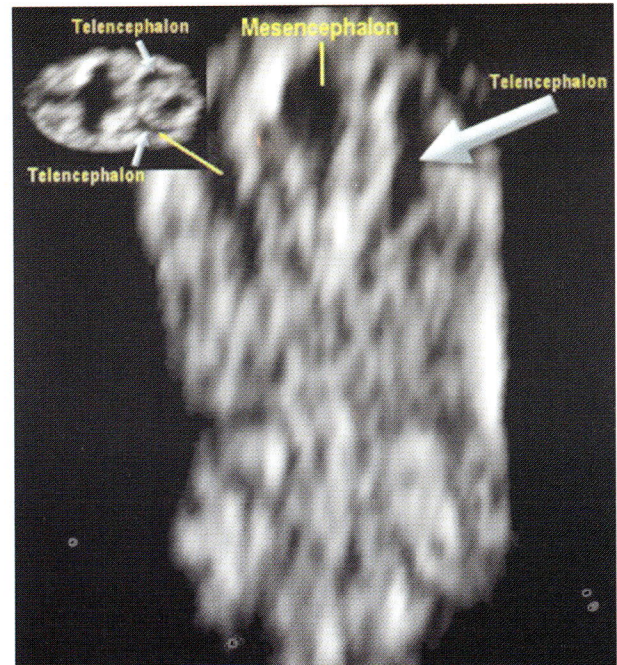

Fig. 3.43: The brain structures such as mesencephalon and telencephalon are visualized, the cerebral hemispheres dominate the brain, but the brain is still immature

CNS development: It is possible to differentiate between many of the brain structures such as mesencephalon and telencephalon (Fig. 3.43), but the brain is still immature. The cerebral hemispheres dominate the brain. The anterior and inferior horns are easily seen, but the posterior horns have not yet developed. The third ventricle is a narrow slit. The corpus callosum has not yet developed. The cavity of the mesencephalon is still wide. The choroid plexuses of the fourth ventricle lie just beneath the caudal border of the cerebellar hemispheres, which now meet in the midline.

The 12th Week

Characteristic embryological findings: Fetal sex is clearly distinguishable by 12th week. The neck is well defined, the face is broad and the eyes are widely separated. By the end of the 12th week, erythropoiesis decreases in the liver and begins in the spleen. The decidua capsularis adheres to the decidua parietalis.

Ultrasound findings: Visualization by 3D ultrasound in 12th week of gestation enables more detailed analysis of fetal anatomy, especially limbs. It is possible to count fingers and toes (Figs 3.44 and 3.45). Growing cerebellum is clearly visible. Lateral ventricles dominate the brain.[32]

Power Doppler findings at 11th and 12th weeks of gestation: With the use of the 3D power Doppler, it is possible to depict major branches of the aorta (Figs 3.46 to 3.50) such as common

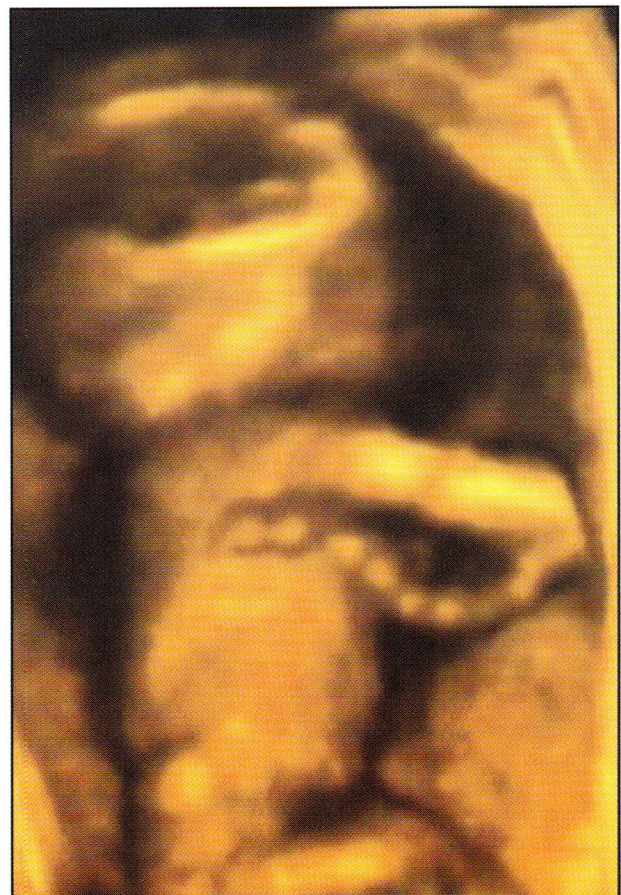

Fig. 3.44: Active movement of the fetus at 12th week of gestation. The fetus seems to be pulling on the umbilical cord

iliac and renal arteries. Circle of Willis and its branches are easily visible (Fig. 3.49). From this week a more detailed anatomical survey can be obtained, including the cerebral and cardiovascular systems and the digestive and urinary tracts. At

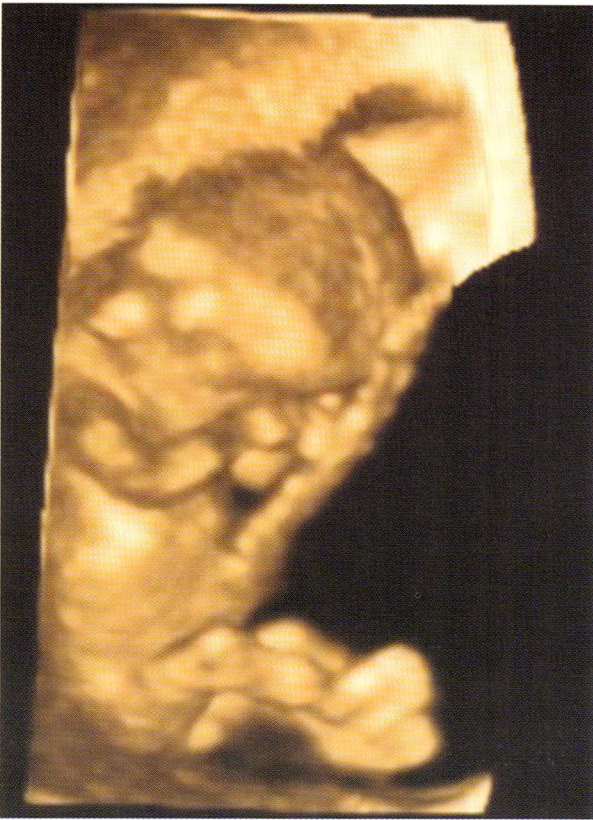

Fig. 3.45: Visualization by 3D ultrasound in 12th week of gestation enables more detailed analysis of fetal anatomy, especially limbs

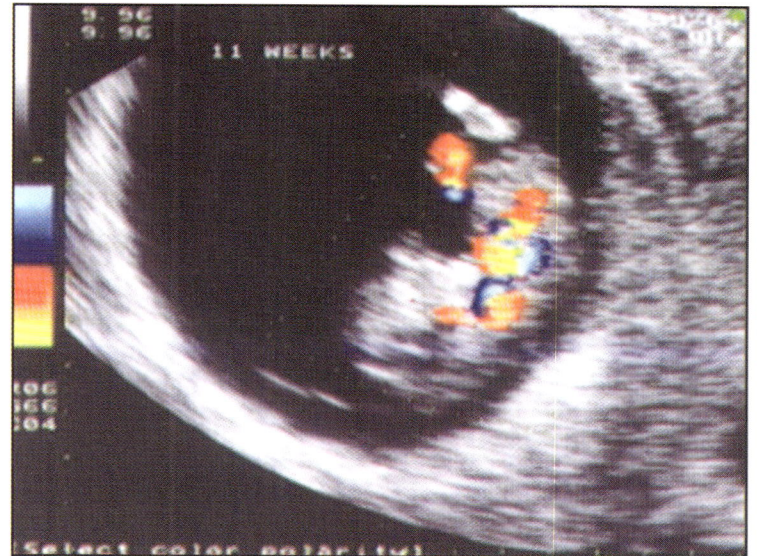

Fig. 3.46: Transvaginal color Doppler scan of the fetal circulatory system at 11th week of gestation

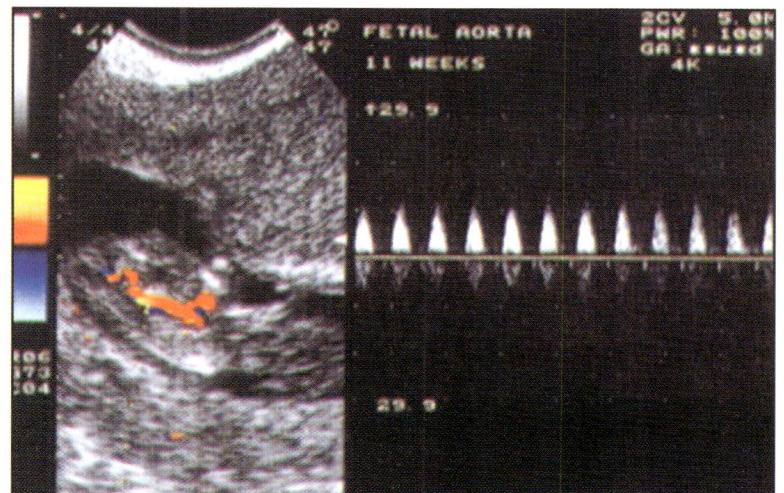

Fig. 3.47: Fetal aorta at 11th week of gestation, demonstrating absence of diastolic flow; this is considered to be physiological at this gestational age

this stage, the pulsations of the middle cerebral artery can be easily discerned as a separate vessel. However, until the end of the tenth gestational week the ultrasonically detected vascular network should be called intracranial circulation (Fig. 3.48). Until the end of the first trimester, the absence of end-diastolic blood flow in fetal and placental components of the circulation is a normal physiological finding.

YOLK SAC AND 3D ULTRASOUND

3D ultrasound imaging may give additional data to functional Doppler studies for research in developmental anatomy and embryology. This method allows a detailed morphologic and volumetric analysis of extraembryonal static structures. Conventional methods for measuring volumes of fluid-filled spaces include modeling of shapes (e.g. using an ellipsoidal approximation).

Using 3D planar mode, the position of the yolk sac wall is accurately spatially assessed. Measurement of the volume, rather than estimation from a simple geometric model, increases the accuracy of the measurement. Growth and appearance of the yolk sac have been correlated with the outcome of the pregnancy.[33] Kupesic and Kurjak measured gestational sac volume (Fig. 3.51) and yolk sac volume and vascularity in pregnancy between 5th and 12th week of gestation (Fig. 3.52).[34] Regression analysis revealed exponential growth of the gestational volume throughout the first trimester of pregnancy.

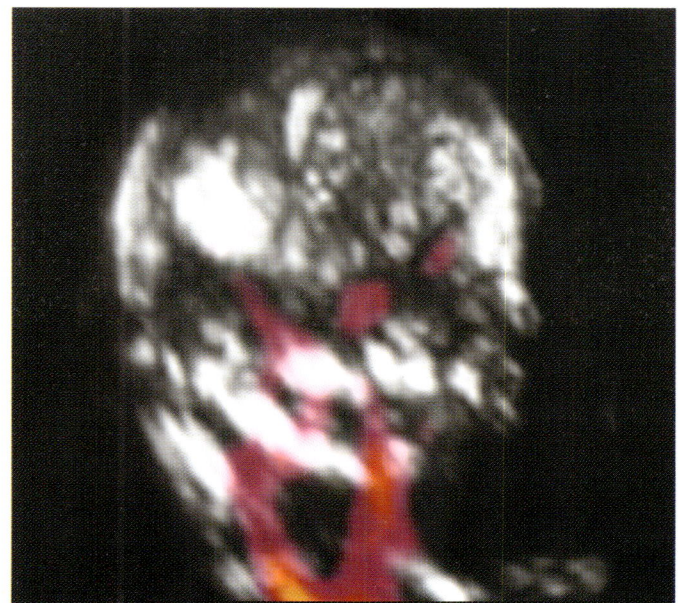

Fig. 3.48: 3D power Doppler image demonstrated the pulsations of the middle cerebral artery as a separate vessel. However, until the end of the tenth gestational week the ultrasonically detected vascular network should be called intracranial circulation

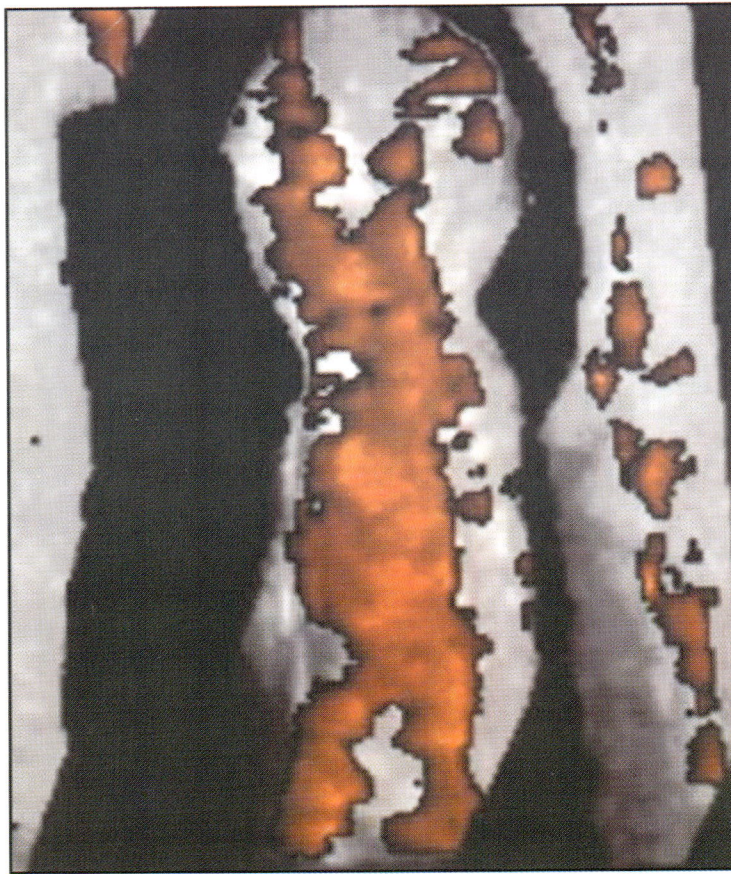

Fig. 3.49: By using 3D power Doppler technique, it is possible to depict major branches of the aorta: common iliac and renal arteries. Circle of Willis and its branches are easily visible

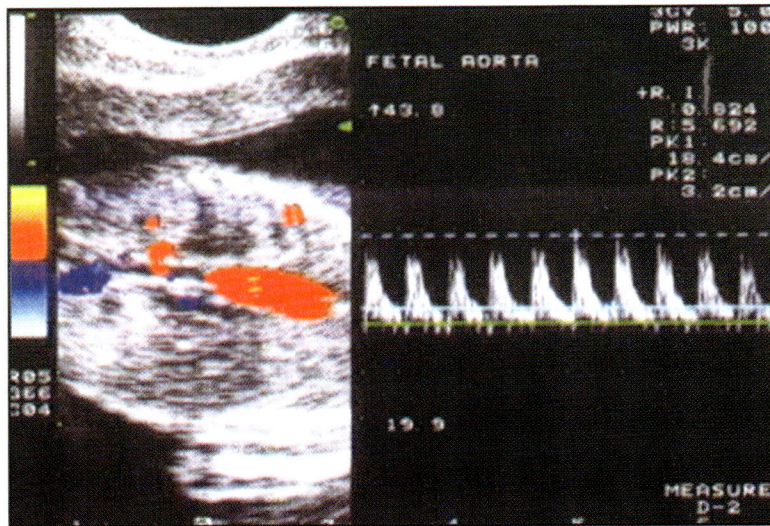

Fig. 3.50: Color Doppler scan of the fetal aorta at 12th week of gestation. Note the appearance of the continuous diastolic flow and significant reduction of the vascular resistance

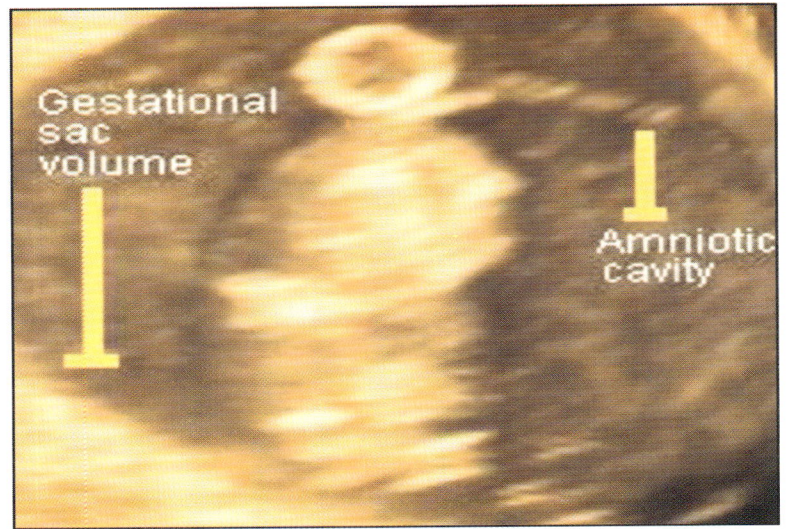

Fig. 3.51: 3D embryonic structure demonstrated gestational sac and amniotic cavity. Growth and appearance of the yolk sac have been correlated with the outcome of the pregnancy. Regression analysis displayed exponential growth of the gestational volume during the first trimester of pregnancy

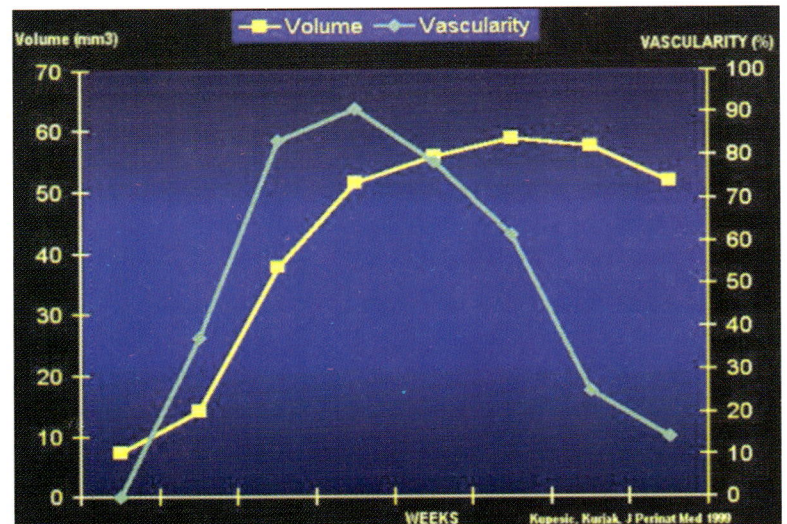

Fig. 3.52: Vascularity in pregnancy between 5th and 12th weeks of gestation. Regression analysis revealed exponential growth of the gestational sac volume throughout the first trimester of pregnancy

With the formation of the extraembryonic celomic cavity at the end of the 4th week, the primary yolk sac is replaced with newly-formed secondary yolk sac. During organogenesis and before the placental circulation is established, the yolk sac is the primary source of exchange between the mother and the embryo. It has nutritive, metabolic, endocrine, immunological, excretory and hematopoietic functions. At the beginning of the 5th week, it becomes visible as the first structure inside the chorionic cavity. At this time, a circular, well-defined, echo free area measures 3 to 4 mm in diameter,[35] while the gestational sac measures about 8 to 10 mm. The yolk sac grows slowly until it reaches a maximum diameter of approximately 5 to 6 mm at 10th week. Its stalk can be followed from its origin all the way to the embryonic abdomen. As the gestational sac grows and the amniotic cavity expands, the yolk sac as an extraembryonic structure is gradually separated from the embryo. Different theories exist about the destiny of the yolk sac. Until recently, it was assumed that it gets caught and compressed between amnion and chorion and then ultimately disappears by the end of the 11th week.

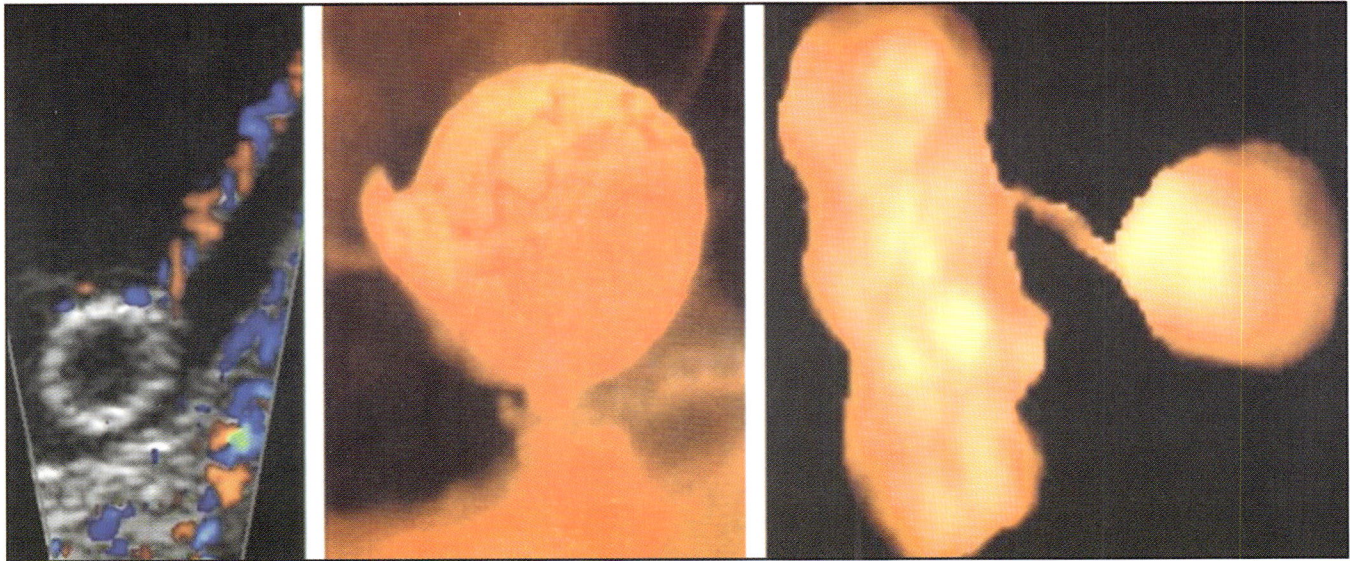

Fig. 3.53: The yolk sac is the primary source of exchange between the mother and the embryo. It has nutritive, metabolic, endocrine, immunological, excretory and hematopoietic functions. A. At the beginning of the 5th week, using 2D ultrasound it becomes visible as the first structure inside the chorionic cavity. B. Vizualisation of yolk sac vascularization with fetoscopy. C. Visualization of yolk sac using 3D technique

Recent studies emphasized that instead of getting compressed the yolk sac degenerates first and then consequently disappears. The ultrasound appearance of the yolk sac (Figs 3.53A to C) has already been proposed as a prognostic parameter for the outcome of pregnancy. Kurjak and co-workers established some criteria for distinguishing between normal and abnormal yolk sac appearance.[36] In their experience, yolk sac should always be visible before the viable embryo; it measures 4.0 to 5.0 mm in diameter until 7th to 8th weeks of gestation and reaches 6.0 to 6.5 mm by the end of the 9th week. It is evident that sonographic detection of abnormal yolk sac morphology may predict abnormal fetal outcome. Absence of yolk sac, its abnormal size, echogenicity, shape and number are predictive indicators of early pregnancy failure. All these parameters should be defined and assessed prior to 10th gestational week. Abnormal yolk sac size may be the first sonographic indicator of associated failure. Primarily, the presence of an embryo without the visible yolk sac before the 10th gestational week is mostly an abnormal finding.

According to some authors, the inner diameter of the yolk sac is always less than 5.6 mm in a normal pregnancy before the 10th week of gestational age. Lyons[37] established that for a mean gestational sac diameter of less than 10 mm, the yolk sac diameter should be less than 4 mm. In 15 patients who had abnormally large sacs, six had no embryo, five aborted spontaneously and only one conceptus survived. Out of nine others with embryo and large yolk sac, eight patients aborted and in one patient trisomy 21 was detected at the 24th gestational week. The yolk sac can be too small, and this is accepted as a marker of poor pregnancy outcome. Green and Hobbins[38] reported a group of patients distributed between 8th and 12th weeks gestational age, with a yolk sac diameter less than 2 mm associated with an adverse outcome.

It is unknown whether abnormalities of the yolk sac are related primarily to the yolk sac or secondary to the embryonic maldevelopment. According to the present data it seems that the yolk sac plays an important role in maternofetal transportation in early pregnancy. Changes in size and shape could indicate or reflect the significant dysfunction of this system, and therefore could influence early embryonic development. Currently, major benefits of the sonographic evaluation of the yolk sac are:

1. Differentiation of potentially viable and non-viable gestations,
2. Confirmation of the presence of an intrauterine pregnancy against a decidual cast, and
3. Indication of a possible fetal abnormality.

Recently, Kupesic and associates[39] performed a transvaginal color Doppler study of yolk sac vascularization and volume estimation by 3D ultrasound. They examined 150 patients whose gestational age ranged from 6th to 10th weeks from the last menstrual period during normal uncomplicated pregnancy. Transvaginal 3D and power Doppler examination was performed before the termination of pregnancy for psychosocial reasons. The highest visualization rates for yolk sac vessels were in the 7th and 8th weeks of gestation, reaching value of 90.71 percent. A characteristic waveform profile included low velocity (5.8±1.7 cms), and the absence of diastolic flow was found in all the examined yolk sacs (Figs 3.54 and 3.55). The pulsatility index showed a mean value of 3.24 ± 0.94 without significant changes between subgroups. The authors found a positive correlation between gestational age and volumes of the yolk sac until 10th week of gestation. At the end of the first trimester, yolk sac volume remained constant, while gestational sac volume continued to grow. 3D ultrasound may significantly contribute to in vivo observation of the yolk sac's "honeycomb" surface pattern (Fig. 3.56).

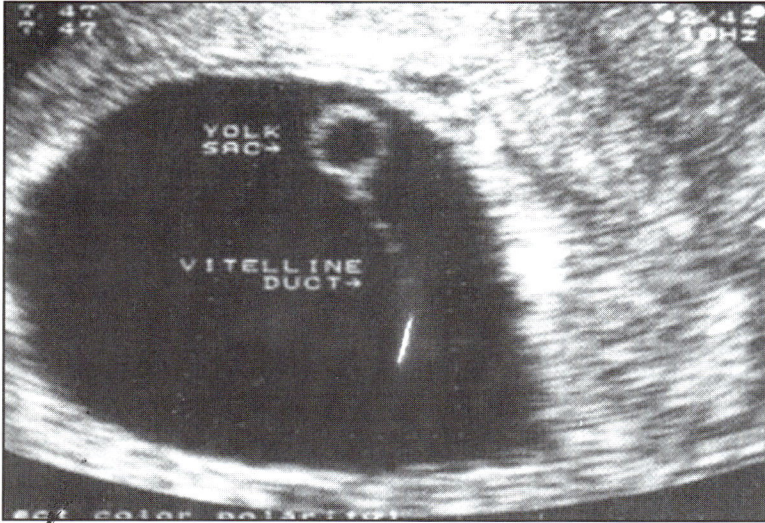

Fig. 3.54: Elongation of the vitelline duct and removal of the yolk sac from the fetal body, one can detect a decrease in the vascularity of the yolk sac and vitelline duct

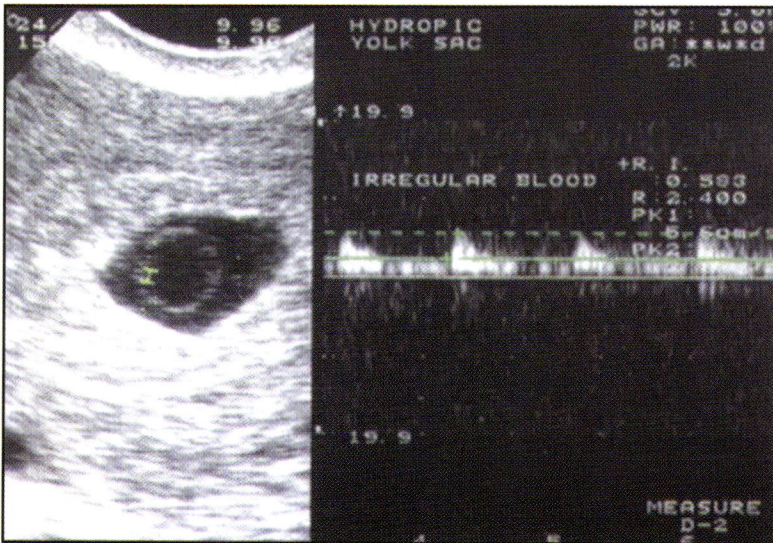

Fig. 3.55: Pulsed Doppler signals derived from the yolk sac. Note the continuous diastolic flow is easily detected from the yolk sac

Increased echogenicity of the yolk sac walls were reported as a sign of dystrophic changes that occur in a non-viable cellular material indicating early pregnancy loss.[40] Automatic volume calculation will allow us to estimate precise relationship between the yolk sac and gestational sac volumes, as well as to obtain the correlation between yolk sac volume and CRL measurements. Kupesic and co-workers[41] measured gestational sac volume and yolk sac volume and vascularity in eighty women with uncomplicated pregnancy between 5th and 12th weeks of gestation. Regression analysis revealed an exponential growth of the gestational sac volume throughout the first trimester of pregnancy. Gestational sac volume measurements can be used for estimation of the gestational age in early pregnancy. Abnormal gestational sac volume measurement could potentially be used as a prognostic marker for pregnancy outcome. The

yolk sac volume was found to increase from 5th to 10th weeks of gestation. However, when the yolk sac reaches its maximum volume at around 10th week it has already started to degenerate, which can be indirectly proved by a significant reduction in visualization rates of the yolk sac vascularity.

As suggested earlier, the disappearance of the yolk sac in normal pregnancies is probably the result of yolk sac degeneration rather than of a mechanical compression of the expanding amniotic cavity. These events suggest that the evaluation of the biological function of the yolk sac by measuring the diameter and/or the volume is limited. Therefore, a combination of functional and volumetric studies is necessary to identify some of the more important moments during early pregnancy.

Kurjak et al[36] reported vascularization of the yolk sac in normal pregnancies between 6th and 10th weeks of gestation. Pulsed Doppler signals characterized by low velocity and high pulsatility, were obtained in 85.71 percent of the yolk sacs during 7th and 8th gestational weeks. Although the reports on yolk sac and vitelline circulation are very exciting, it should be noted that such studies are not ethically feasible in ongoing human pregnancies since the secondary yolk sac is a source of primary germ cells and blood stem cells.[42]

3D ultrasound and power Doppler will allow us to study turgescent blood vessels withstanding from the surface of the yolk sac (Fig. 3.56). The same technique can be used to study the evolution from the embryovitelline towards embryoplacental circulation. Since yolk sac and vitelline blood vessels are prerequisites for the oxygen transfer, absorptive and transfer processes during the first trimester, alterations in this early circulatory system may have some prognostic value for predicting pregnancy outcome.

3D ULTRASOUND AS A TOOL FOR MEASUREMENT OF THE NUCHAL TRANSLUCENCY

The decade of the 1990s has announced in the prospect of first trimester ultrasound screening for fetal chromosomal abnormalities. The technique of measuring nuchal translucency, which gave rise to the remarkably higher detection rate of chromosomal abnormalities, still has to overcome some technical difficulties. The unsuccessful nuchal translucency (NT) measurements were reported in many studies.[43,44] It seems that establishment of the training regimen for NT measurement as reported by Monni et al[45] and Braithwaite et al[46] may overcome some of these methodological problems. Kurjak and coworkers[47] demonstrated that 3D transvaginal ultrasound (Fig. 3.57) enables the depiction of the successful mid-sagittal section of the fetus, allowing precise NT measurements. This is possible due to the

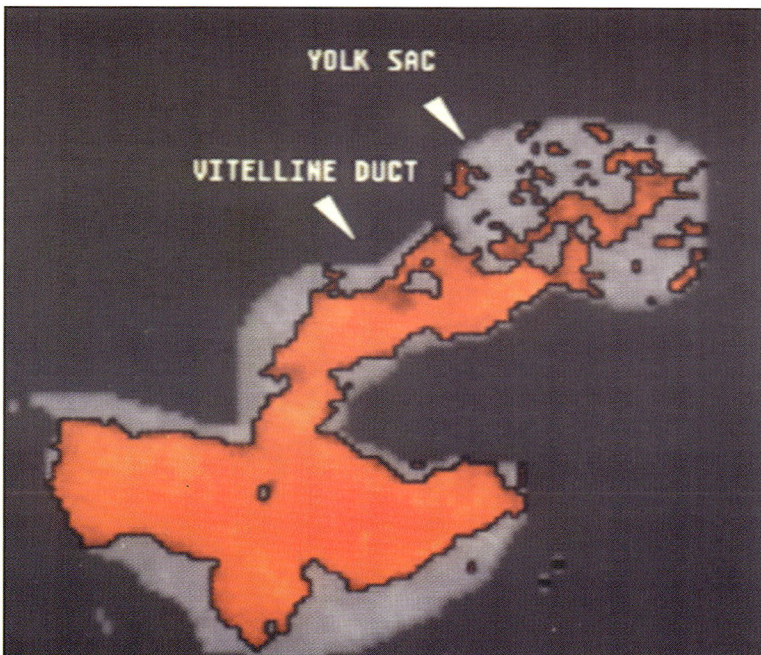

Fig. 3.56: 3D color Doppler study of yolk sac vascularization demonstrated the yolk sac's "honeycomb" surface pattern. 3D ultrasound and power Doppler will allow us to study turgescent blood vessels withstanding from the surface of the yolk sac

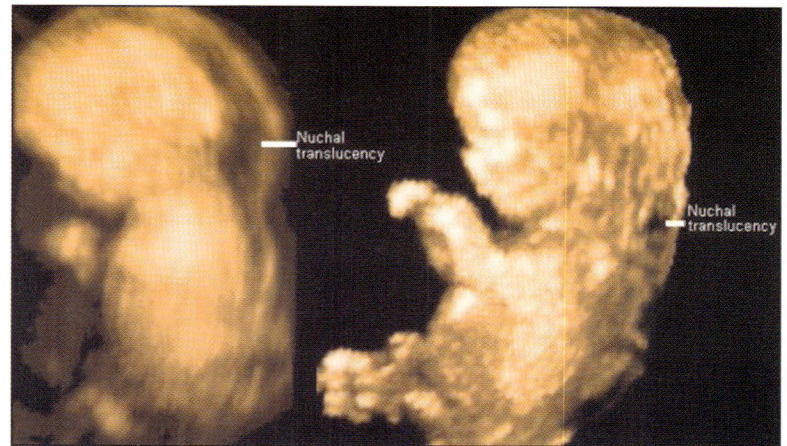

Fig. 3.57: 3D transvaginal ultrasound enables the depiction of the mid-sagittal section of the fetus, allowing precise NT measurements

ability of 3D ultrasound to reorient the fetal position using multiplanar imaging. Better intraobserver reproducibility was obtained for 3D than for 2D ultrasound. 3D transvaginal ultrasound improves accuracy of nuchal translucency measurement allowing appropriate mid-sagittal section of the fetus and clear distinction of the nuchal region from the amniotic membrane.

4D SONOGRAPHY AS A TOOL FOR ASSESSMENT OF FETAL BEHAVIOR IN EARLY PREGNANCY

4D sonography has become the new standard in prenatal diagnosis. This technique enables detailed examination of the fetal anatomy and higher quality depiction of some anomalies. Until recently, the main drawback of 4D sonography was its inability to present a realtime motional image. Furthermore, motoric activity of the fetus yielded with significant artifacts in the image, making it inadequate for diagnostic purposes. 4D depiction is technologically based on high velocity processing of the data. Development of the computer processors was the essential prerogative for 4D ultrasound devices. The latest development of calculating units enables 3D reconstruction at a frame rate of up to 20 images per second. In the human eye this frame rate produces quite smooth dynamic realtime 3D images, also known as 4D image.[1, 48]

The first trimester of pregnancy is a period of early human development of incomparable intensity. Before the 'ultrasound era' investigation of this field was reserved for postmortem

embryological analysis. However, transvaginal realtime B-mode, color Doppler, and, in the last few years, different forms of 3D sonography have enabled noninvasive and safe investigation in vivo. Due to the size of the pregnant uterus and relatively large amount of fluid surrounding the embryo, the first trimester is very suitable for 4D sonography. We already investigated embryonic or fetal movements and several movements were classified as following (Fig. 3.58):

- Gross body movements consisted of changing the position of the head towards the body
- Limb movements consisted of changes in position of extremities towards the body without extension or flexion in elbow or knee
- Complex limb movements consisted of changes in position of the limb segments towards each other, such as extension or flexion in elbow or knee.

According to CRL the pregnant women were divided into four groups:

- Group 1: CRL < 9 mm (less than 7th weeks of gestation)
- Group 2: CRL > 9 mm and < 15 mm (between 7th and 8th weeks)
- Group 3: CRL > 16 mm and < 30 mm (between 8th and 10th weeks)
- Group 4: CRL > 31 mm and < 50 mm (between 10th and 12th weeks).

Matters of interest were the gestational age at which each of these three kinds of movements appeared, and their visualization with advanced technology. A total of 98 pregnant women were analyzed. In the first group no movements were found. In the other groups, the incidence of each type of embryonic or fetal movements is presented in Table 3.1.

At the seventh week 38 percent embryos had spontaneous gross body movements. At this gestational age we found no limb movements. In 42 percent of fetuses from the third group

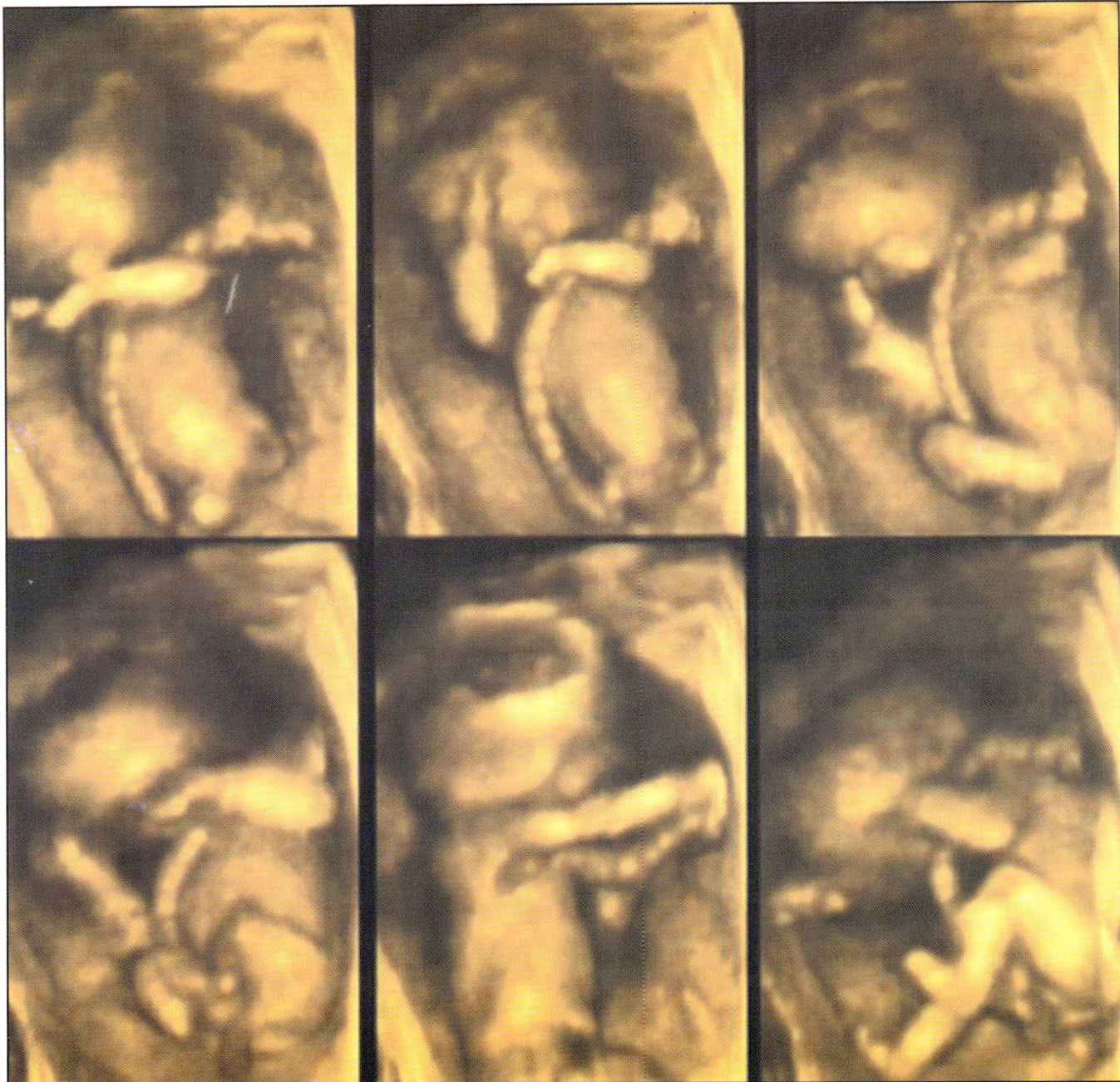

Fig. 3.58: 4D ultrasound sequence of the fetus at 12th week of gestation showing general movements. The complex movements of the limb, trunk and head are clearly visible and cause a shift in fetal position. In the first sequence, the right hand is flexed in elbow joint. In the next sequence, the fetus raised the hand and began to deflect in elbow joint. In the last sequence, further elevation of hand is seen

Table 3.1: The incidence of spontaneous embryonic/fetal movement according to gestational age

Gestational age (weeks)	CRL (mm)	No movements	Gross body movements	Limb movements	Complex limb movements
7-8	0 – 15	31	12	0	0
9-10	16 – 30	26	11	7	0
11-12	31 – 50	19	16	12	8

Source: Adapted from Reference 1

spontaneous gross body movements were presented. Furthermore, in 26 percent of fetuses only simple limb movements were visualized at this gestational age. In 84 percent of fetuses from the fourth group gross body movements and in 63 percent limb movements were presented. Additionally, in 42 percent spontaneous complex limb movements were visualized.

The straightforward development of 3D ultrasound has led to the possibility of performing 3D imaging in a realtime mode. This modality has been named 4D sonography. This improvement greatly facilitates the assessment of fetal movements because they can be visualized in three dimensions. Thus it is much easier to assess fetal motoric status than with 2D. For each embryonic structure there is a period between genesis and ultrasonic visualization.[49] As technology advances the period becomes shorter. Limbs begin to move from week seven onwards.[50] Using 2D transvaginal ultrasound technique body movements are visualized between weeks eight and nine, and limb movements are visualized between weeks 9th and 10th.[51] The embryo body movements, which were absent before seven weeks of gestation, were observed after eight weeks with a sensitivity of 100 percent, specificity of 92.8 percent, positive predictive value of 94.3 percent, and negative predictive value of 100 percent.[78] With 4D we found gross body movement at seven weeks, and limb movements at weeks eight to nine. New technology enables the visualization of the moving phenomenon a week earlier than 2D transvaginal ultrasound. The use of 4D technology should thus enable the diagnosis of motoric development failure at the end of the first trimester. It also makes possible the evaluation of complex limb movement, the visualization of simultaneous movement of all extremities and the spatial evaluation of movements.

At seventh gestational week the dominant embryonic feature is the head that is strongly flectioned anteriorily. Upper and lower limb buds are visible on the lateral aspects of the embryo. However, embryonic movements are not frequent and consist mainly of moving the head towards the rest of the body, while fetal limb movements are absent.[1]

At eighth to ninth weeks the embryo has different body features to be observed. The head is less flectioned and limbs are elongated. Segments of the arms and legs are distinguishable. Embryonic movements can be divided in two main groups: gross body movements that consist of changes of the position of the head towards the body and movements of the extremities: arms and legs are moved vigorously. However no flexion or extension in elbow or knee can be seen.[1]

At 10th to 12th weeks of gestation complex body and limb movements can be seen. At this gestational age there was a great resemblance of fetal movements to those in neonates.

Using the advantages of 4D technology a physiologic pattern of embryonic or fetal motor development was made. Any alteration from the pattern should be an indication for further diagnostic engagement. Development of the limbs is a complex process that consists of tissue differentiation (cartilage, muscle, nerves, blood vessels and tendons). An insult on each tissue in the differentiation process can alter the developmental pattern. An alteration of motor development can be a consequence of delayed or aborted motor development.

REFERENCES

1. Kurjak A, Vecek N, Hafner T, Bozek T, Kurjak BF, Ujevic B: Prenatal diagnosis: what does four-dimensional ultrasound add? J. Perinat. Med. 2002; 30: 57-62
2. Andonotopo W, Stanojevic M, Kurjak A, et al. Assessment of fetal behavior and general movements by four-dimensional sonography. Ultrasound Rev Obstet Gynecol (In press).
3. Benoit B, Hafner T, Bekavac I, Kurjak A. Three dimensional sonoembryology. Ultrasound Rev Obstet Gynecol 2001;1:111.
4. Blaas HG, Eik-Nes SH. Ultrasound assessment of early brain development. In Jurkovic D and Jauniaux E (Ed): Ultrasound and Early Pregnancy. London: The Parthenon Publishing Groups, 1996; pp 3–17.
5. Kurjak A, Kupesic S. Three-dimensional transvaginal ultrasound improves measurement of nuchal translucency. J Perinat Med 1999;27:91.
6. Bonilla-Musoles F. Three-dimensional visualization of the human embryo: a potential revolution in prenatal diagnosis. Editorial. Ultrasound Obstet Gynecol 1996;7: 393.
7. Bonilla-Musoles F, Raga F, Osborne N, Blanes J. The use of three-dimensional (3D) ultrasound for study of normal pathologic morphology of the human embryo and fetus: preliminary report. J Ultrasound Med 1995;14: 757.
8. Lee A, Deutinger J, Bernaschek G. Three-dimensional ultrasound: abnormalities of the fetal face in surface and volume rendering mode. Br J Obstet Gynaecol 1995;102: 40.
9. Lee A, Deutinger J, Bernaschek G. Voluvision: three-dimensional ultrasonography of fetal malformations. Am J Obstet Gynecol 1994;170: 1312.
10. Lee A, Kratochwil A, Deutinger J, et al. Three-dimensional ultrasound in diagnosing phocomelia. Ultrasound Obstet Gynecol 1995;5: 238.
11. Maymon J, Halperin Z, Weinraub A, Herman A, Schneider D. Three-dimensional sonography of conjoined twins at 10 weeks: a case report. Ultrasound Obstet Gynecol 1998;11: 292.
12. Pretorius DH, Nelson TR: Three-dimensional ultrasound of fetal surface features. Ultrasound Obstet Gynecol 1992;2:166.
13. Blaas HG, Eik-Nes SH, Berg S, Torp H. In-vivo three-dimensional ultrasound reconstructions of embryos and early fetuses. Lancet 1998;352: 1182.
14. Bree RL, Marn CS. Transvaginal sonography in the first trimested: embryology, anatomy, and hCG correlation. Semin Ultrasound CT and MR 1990;11:12-21.
15. Itskovitz J, Lindenbaum ES, Brandes JM. Arterial anastomosis in the pregnant human uterus. Obstet Gynecol 1980; 1:3-19.
16. Kurjak A, Zudenigo D, Funduk-Kurjak B, Shalan H, Predanic M, Sosic A. Transvaginal color Doppler in the assessment of the uteroplacental circulation in normal early pregnancy. J Perinat Med 1993;21:25-34.
17. Kurjak A, Kupesic S, Predanic M, Salihagic A. Transvaginal color Doppler assessment of the uteroplacental circulation 111 normal and abnormal early pregnancy. Early Human Dev 1992; 29(1-3):385-9.
18. Jauniaux E, Jurkovic D, Campbell S. In vivo investigations of anatomy and physiology of early human placental circulation. Ultrasound Obstet Gynecol 1991; 1:435-45.
19. Jaffe R, Warsof SL. Transvaginal color Doppler imaging in the assessment ofuteroplacental blood flow in the normal first trimester pregnancy. Am J Obstet Gynecol 1991; 164:781-5.
20. Kurjak A, Kupesic-Urek S, Predanic M, Zudenigo D, Matijevic R, Salihagic A. Transvaginal color Doppler in the study of early pregnancies associated with fibroids. J. Matern. Fetal. Invest. 1992; 2:81-7.
21. Pijnenborg R, Bland JM, Robertson WB, Brosens I. Utero-placental arterial changes related to interstitial trophoblast-migration in early human pregnancy. Placenta 1983; 4: 397-414.
22. Kanayama N. Trophoblast injury: A new etiological and pathological concept of preeclampsia. Croat Med J. 2003; 44 (2):148-56.
23. Kossof G, Griffiths KA, Warren PS et al. Three-dimensional volume imaging in obstetrics. Ultrasound Obstet Gynecol 1994; 4:196.
24. Kurjak A, Kupesic S. Doppler proof of the presence of intervillous circulation (Letter). Ultrasound Obstet Gynecol 1996;7: 463.
25. Kurjak A, Laurini R, Kupesic S, Kos M, Latin V, Bulic K: A combined Doppler and morphopathological study of intervillous circulation. Book of Abstracts. The Fifth World Congress of Ultrasound in Obstetrics and Gynecology, Kyoto, 25-29 November, 1995. Ultrasound Obstet Gynecol 1195; 6 (Suppl): 116.
26. Kurjak A, Kupesic S, Banovic I, Hafner T, Kos M. The study of morphology and circulation of early embryo by three-dimensional ultrasound and power Doppler. J Perinat Med 1999;27:145-57.
27. Kupesic S, Kurjak A, Ivancic-Kosuta M. Volume and vascularity of the yolk sac studied by three-dimfinsional ultrasound and color Doppler. J Perinat Med 1999; 27: 91-6.
28. Bonilla-Musoles et al. Demonstration of Early Pregnancy with Three-Dimensional Ultrasound. In Merz E (Ed): 3D Ultrasound in Obstetrics and Gynecology. Lippincott Williams & Wilkins, Philadelphia, New York, Baltimore 1998;31-7.
29. Blaas HG, Eik-Nes SH, Kiserud T, Berg B, Angelsen B, Olstad B. Three-dimensional imaging of the brain cavities in human embryos. Ultrasound Obstet. Gynecol. 1995; 5:228-32.
30. O'Rahilly R, Mueller F. Ventricular system and choroid plexuses of the human brain during the embryonic period proper. Am J Anat 1990; 189:285-302.
31. Merz E, Weber G, Bahlmann F, Miric-Tesanic D. Application of transvaginal and abdominal three-dimensional ultrasound for the detection or exclusion of fetal malformations of the fetal face. Ultrasound Obstet Gynecol 1997; 9:2373.
32. Kurjak A, Zodan T, Kupesic S. Three-dimensional sonoembryology of the first trimester. In Kurjak A, Kupesic S. (Eds): Clinical Application of 3D Sonography. The Parthenon Publishing. NY, London, 2000,109-21.

33. Lindsay DJ, Lyons EA, Levi CS, Zheng XH. Endovaginal appearance of the yolk sac in early pregnancy: normal growth and usefulness as a predictor of abnormal pregnancy outcome. Radiology 1988;166:109.
34. Kupesic S, Kurjak A. Volume and vascularity of the yolk sac studied by three-dimensional ultrasound and color Doppler. J Perinat Med 1999;27: 97.
35. Lindsay DJ, Lovett IS, Lyons EA, Levi CS, Zheng XH, Holt. SC, Dashefsky SM. Endovaginal appearance of the yolk sac in pregnancy: normal growth and usefulness as a predictor of abnormal pregnancy outcome. Radiology 1992; 183: 115-8.
36. Kurjak A, Kupesic S, Kostovic L. Vascularization of yolk sac and vitelline duct in normal pregnancies studied by transvaginal color Doppler. J Perinat Med 1994; 22:443.
37. Lyons EA. Endovaginal sonography of the first trimester of pregnancy. Proceedings of the 3rd International Perinatal and Gyynecological Ultrasound Symposiuni Ottawa, Ontario, 1994; pp1-25.
38. Green JJ, Hobbins JC. Abdominal ultrasound examination of the first trimester fetus. Am J Obstet Gynecol 1988; 159: 165-75.
39. Kupesic S., Kurjak A. Volume and vascularity of yolk sac assessed by three-dimensional and power doppler ultrasound; Early Pregnancy 2001; 5 (1): 40-1.
40. Harris RD, Fvincent LM, Askin FB. Yolk sac calcification: A sonographic finding associated with inlrauterine embryonic demise in the first trimester. Radiology 1988;166:109.
41. Kupesic S, Kurjak A, Ivancic-Kosuta M. Volume and vascularity of the yolk sac studied by three-dimfinsional ultrasound and color Doppler. J Perinat Med 1999; 27: 91-6.
42. Witschi E. Migration of the germ cells of human embryos from the yolk sac to the primitive gonadal folds. Contrib Embryol Carnegie Inst 1948; 32:67.
43. Roberts LJ, Bewley S, Mackinson AM, Rodeck CH. First trimester nuchal translucency: Problems with screening the general population I. Br J Obstet Gynaecol 1995; 102:381.
44. Haddow JE, Palomokie GE. Down's syndrome screening. Lancet 1996; 347:1625.
45. Monni G, Zoppi MA, Ibba RM, Floris M. Fetal nuchal translucency test for Down's syndrome. Lancet 1997;350:1631.
46. Braithwaite JM, Economides DL. The assessment of nuchal translucency with transabdominal and transvaginal sonography—success rates, repeatability and level of agreement. Br J Obstet Gynaecol 1995;68:720.
47. Kurjak A, Kupesic S, Ivancic-Kosuta M. Three-dimensional transvaginal ultrasound improves measurement of nuchal translucency. J Perinat Med 1999; 27:97-102.
48. Lee A. Four-dimensional ultrasound in prenatal diagnosis: leading edge in imaging technology. Ultrasound Rev Obstet Gynecol 2001;1: 144.
49. Kurjak A, S Kupesic, I Banovic, T Hafner, M Kos. The study of morphology and circulation of early embryo by three-dimensional ultrasound and Power Doppler. J Perinat Med 1999;27:145.
50. McLachlan J. Medical embryology. Addison-Wesley 1994.
51. Timor-Tritsch IE, D Farine,Rosen. Closes look at early embryonic development with high frequency transvaginal transducer. Am J Obstet Gynecol 1988;159: 676.

A Kurjak, S Kupesic, JM Carrera, B Funduk, N Maiz

4

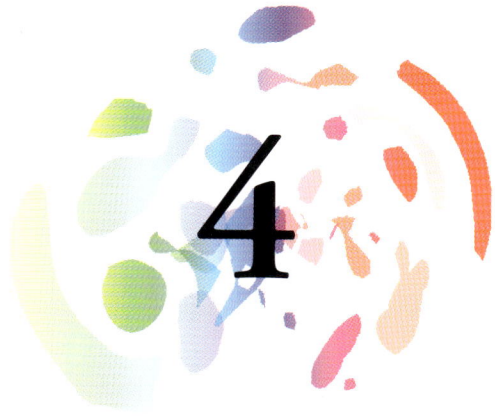

Ultrasound Evaluation of Abnormal Early Pregnancy

INTRODUCTION

The first trimester is characterized by many important landmarks with regard to the ultimate outcome of pregnancy and is mostly defined by the first 100 days of pregnancy. Woman becomes aware of her pregnancy after missing her last period and in that time she is already at least 4 weeks pregnant.[1]

A positive pregnancy test opens Pandora's box, offering more questions than answers. Although, a positive pregnancy test most likely suggests an intrauterine pregnancy. Production of human chorionic gonadotropin (hCG) occurs also by tumors (dysgerminoma, choricarcinoma) or maldevelopment of pregnancy (ectopic pregnancy or molal hydatidosa).[2] Falsely-positive results are mainly obtained in the case of proteinuria, erythrocyturia or some drug intake (e.g. tranquilizers). The role of the ultrasonographer in these situations is to help the practising clinician evaluate pregnancy and determine the exact pregnancy status. Ultrasound evaluation of an early pregnancy includes detection of the pregnancy location (extrauterine or intrauterine), the type of pregnancy (one fetus pregnancy, multiple pregnancy, molar pregnancy), the viability of the pregnancy and establishment of the gestational age. In evaluating pregnancy the ultrasonographer also recognizes the complications that may occur in first trimester. Ultrasound examination has become the "gold standard" in follow-up of the development and complications of early pregnancy. With introduction of transvaginal sonography (TVS) a possibility for early morphological and biometrical ultrasound examinations has been significantly improved. Application of color Doppler ultrasound has enabled functional hemodynamic presentation and evaluation soon after implantation.

Basic ultrasound markers for normal pregnancy are intrauterine gestational sac, morphologically normal embryo and its heart action. Normal embryonic echo, in 90 percent of the cases suggests normal pregnancy. The possibility of early pregnancy loss is very high and can be related to fetal biometry:[3]

- CRL is < 5 mm .... possibility for pregnancy loss is around 8 percent
- CRL measures 6 to 10 mm ...... possibility for pregnancy loss is around 3 to 4 percent, and
- CRL is > 10 mm. .... possibility for pregnancy loss is below 1 percent.

At present, ultrasonography is considered to be the best diagnostic method in detecting early pregnancy complications.

There is discordance between the clinicians' and embryologists' statements in determining the gestational age. Clinicians define gestational age from the first day of the last menstrual period. Embryologists do not agree with clinicians, and define the gestational age from the time of conception. Therefore, when talking about embryonic period embryologists define it as a period of organogenesis from the 3rd to the 8th weeks after conception, while obstetricians define it as a period from 5th to 10th weeks after first day of the last menstrual period.[4] Fetal period begins after 8th week according to embryologists, i.e. after 10th week according to clinicians. As the onset of marrow formation in the humerus (the end of embryonic period according to the embryologists that occurs 56th to 57th days after ovulation)[5] is not visible by the ultrasound, for ultrasound examination and evaluation of the embryo/fetus, Blass[6] suggests that disappearance of the physiological midgut herniation could be orientation as the end of embryonic period. The physiological midgut herniation is a macroscopically visible process, which starts after 7 completed weeks. The retraction of the bowel into the abdominal cavity occurs between approximately 10.5 to 12 completed weeks.[7] Application of 3D and 4D ultrasound seems to be advantageous in determining the points for differentiation of the embryo and the fetus.

EARLY PREGNANCY FAILURE AND VAGINAL BLEEDING

Early pregnancy failure is defined as a pregnancy that ends spontaneously before the embryo has reached by ultrasound detectible viable gestational age. The most common pathological symptom of the early pregnancy failure is the vaginal bleeding. One of the main problems in diagnosis of early pregnancy failure is why vaginal bleeding occurs. When vaginal bleeding occurs any clinician should ask several questions that can radically alter the management:

1. Is the patient pregnant?
2. Is the embryo viable or not?
3. What is the gestational age?
4. Is there any evidence to suggest that the pregnancy is ectopic?
5. If an abortion occurs, is it complete or incomplete?
6. Is there any associated pelvic mass?

Only differentiation and accurate estimation of the pregnancy status and embryo/fetus status make it possible to obtain appropriate therapeutic measures to cases where a normal outcome of the pregnancy can be expected. At this moment, ultrasonography is considered to be the best diagnostic method for detection of early pregnancy complications. For these patients the skill of the ultrasonographer is very important, since the accurate diagnosis of pregnancy failure will often result in surgical intervention.

Clinical presentation of the symptoms such as vaginal bleeding and abdominal pain, with or without the expulsion of products of conception[8] is suspected of a spontaneous abortion. For ultrasound evaluation, it is important to distinguish threatened, complete and incomplete abortion.

Threatened Abortion (Abnormal Vaginal Bleeding)

Threatened abortion is the clinical term used to describe symptom such as vaginal bleeding during the first 20 weeks of pregnancy in women who, on the basis of clinical evaluation, are considered to have a potentially living embryo/fetus. The main problem in the management of these patients is in confirming the accurate diagnosis. The threatened and spontaneous abortions together present the most common complications of early pregnancy. Sometimes we are not even

aware that a woman has been pregnant and that she aborted. If we take into the consideration these cases also, incidence of spontaneous abortions is estimated up to 70 percent.[9] Only 1/3rd of embryos continue further development, and 50 percent of abortions occur before the term of expected menstruation.[9,10] These types of abortion usually cause the symptoms of sterility rather than infertility, because it seems that a woman is not even able to conceive. Thirty to forty percent of pregnancies fail after implantation, and only 10 to 15 percent manifest with clinical symptoms.[10,11]

In patients with a normal intrauterine pregnancy, bleeding from the chorion frondosum is undoubtedly the most common source of vaginal bleeding during the first trimester.

The development of transvaginal sonography has allowed the improved assessment of patients presenting vaginal bleeding during the first half of pregnancy, clarifying the differential diagnosis of missed abortion, ectopic pregnancy, blighted ovum and threatened abortion with a living embryo. Embryo vitality can be established reliably by documenting cardiac activity on realtime, B-mode or color Doppler ultrasonography.

Sonographic evidence of vaginal bleeding can be identified as a perigestational hemorrhage in 5 to 22 percent of women with symptoms of threatened abortion. However, some precautions must be taken, because the perigestational hemorrhage is occasionally difficult to distinguish from a blighted twin. The prognostic significance of identifying perigestational hemorrhage during the first trimester remains uncertain. Most of the small hemorrhages resolve without clinical sequelae, while in some cases spontaneous abortion may occur.

Incomplete and Complete Spontaneous Abortion

As a definition, incomplete abortion is the passage of some, but not all fetal or placental tissue through the cervical canal. In complete abortion, all products of conception are expelled through the cervix.[12] In incomplete abortion, the uterine debris may consist of a combination of products of conception, blood and decidua.[13]

Transvaginal ultrasonography plays important role in evaluating uterine cavity in spontaneous abortion due to detection of the retained products of conception. Retained products of conception after abortion may cause bleeding or chorioamnionitis.[14] An echogenic and vascularized mass within the uterine cavity supports the diagnosis of retained products of conception.[15] Wong and coworkers[16] reported 100 percent sensitivity and 80 percent specificity of the transvaginal sonographic examination in differentiation of the complete from incomplete spontaneous abortions. The sonographic definition of incomplete abortion is a bilayer endometrial thickness of more than 8 mm. In 29 percent of patients with incomplete abortion transvaginal sonography obviated the need for surgical intervention, but in 30 percent of patients with complete abortion detected retained products of conception. Adding color Doppler examination to basic transvaginal 2D ultrasound examination increases detection rate of the retained trophoblastic tissue.[17-19] In their recent paper, Alcázar and co-workers[20] suggested that transvaginal color Doppler is a helpful method for detecting retained trophoblastic tissue in patients with first-trimester spontaneous abortion. They analyzed 62 patients with positive urine pregnancy test and history of heavy vaginal bleeding whose gestational age was lass than 14 weeks. In each patient transvaginal ultrasound (TV US) and βHCG serum measurements were performed at the time of admission to the hospital. Retained trophoblastic tissue was suspected in the presence of low resistance index (RI < 0.45) within the myometrium or just beneath the endometrial-myometrial interface. In 29 percent of women retained trophoblastic tissue was suspected and in 88.9 percent of these patients pathological analysis was positive for retained trophoblastic tissue. The authors suggested to perform B mode and color Doppler examination when there is suspicion on retained trophoblastic tissue (Fig. 4.1).

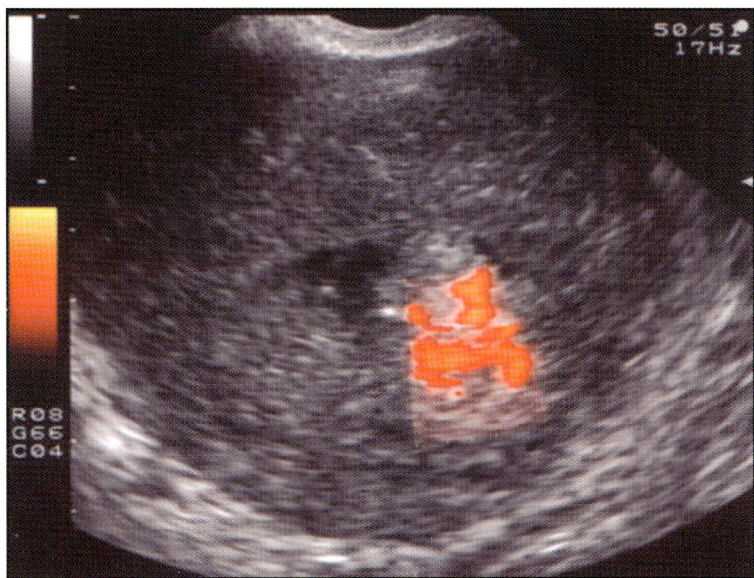

Fig. 4.1: Transvaginal power Doppler image of an irregular uterine cavity. Note abundant vascularity demonstrating residual placental tissue

Recent studies demonstrate that risk for repeated spontaneous abortion depends exclusively on the number of previous spontaneous abortions and their cause. Even though, many different risk factors have been thoroughly researched, around 60 percent of unsuccessful pregnancies remain a "causa ignota".[21] The important criteria for evaluation of pregnancy loss are:[22]

- Always to keep in mind that the risk of spontaneous miscarriage is higher in older women
- Try to uncover causes for repetitive first-trimester miscarriages. Karyotyping of couples will reveal that 3 to 8 percent have some abnormality, most frequently balanced chromosomal rearrangement, a translocation (other abnormalities: sex chromosome mosaicism, chromosome inversions or ring chromosomes). Besides spontaneous miscarriages, these abnormalities are associated with high risk of malformations and mental retardation. Karyotyping is especially vital if the couple has had a malformed infant or fetus in addition to miscarriages in previous pregnancies
- Smoking, alcohol, and heavy coffee consumption have been reported to be associated with an increased risk of recurrent pregnancy losses[23]
- Patients with thyroid disease or uncontrolled diabetes mellitus may suffer spontaneous miscarriages although these diseases are not causes of recurrent miscarriages
- Uterine abnormalities can result in impaired vascularization of a pregnancy, limited space for a fetus due to distortion of the uterine cavity, and incoordinate uterine contractility
- Looking at the first trimester miscarriage, a firm correlation with bacterial vaginosis-associated microorganisms was found in the study of Donders and colleagues[24]
- The major cause of thrombosis in pregnancy is an inherited predisposition for clotting, especially the factor V Leiden mutation.

Immunological problems can be classified into two groups: autoimmunity (self antigens), and alloimmunity (foreign antigens). In the autoimmunity, a humoral or cellular response is directed against a specific component of the host. The lupus anticoagulant and anticardiolipin antibodies are antiphospholipid antibodies, which arise as the result of an autoimmune disease. Several series demonstrated that 10 to 16 percent of women with recurrent miscarriages have had antiphospholipid antibodies.[9, 25] These antibodies are also associated with growth retardation and fetal death in addition to recurrent miscarriages. Preferred treatment for significant titers of antiphospholipid antibodies consists of the combination of low-dose aspirin (80 mg daily) and low-dose heparin as soon as pregnancy is diagnosed.[26, 27] Unfortunately, treatment is not always successful. Alloimmunity refers to all causes of pregnancy losses related to an abnormal maternal immune response to antigens on placental or fetal tissues.

MISSED ABORTION

The diagnosis of missed abortion is determined by the ultrasound identification of an embryo/fetus without any heart activity. It is relatively easy to make this diagnosis by means of the transvaginal color Doppler ultrasound. The main parameter is the absence of the heartbeats and the lack of color flow signals at its expected position after the 6th gestational week (Fig. 4.2).

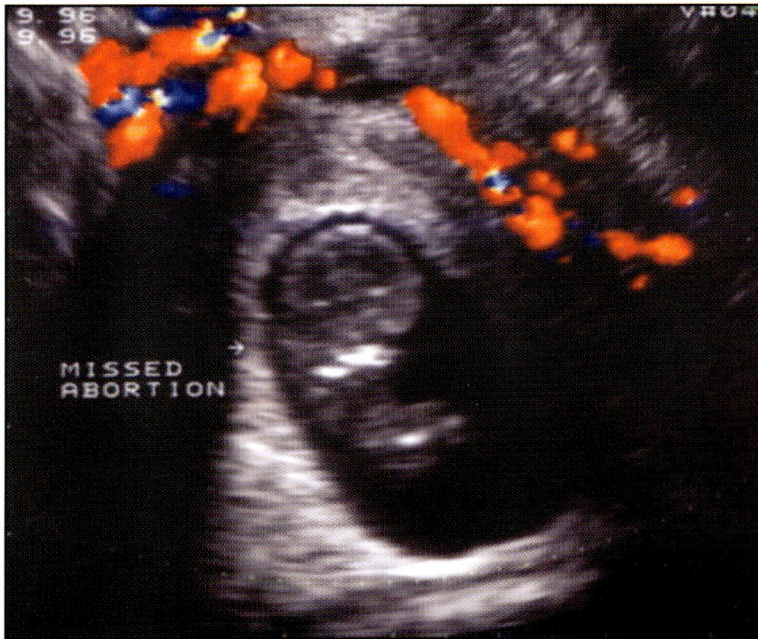

Fig. 4.2: Transvaginal color Doppler scan of a missed abortion. Prominent blood flow signals are obtained from the spiral arteries, while absence of heart activity is noted by color Doppler

With the aid of sensitive color Doppler equipment it is possible to demonstrate two types of blood flow velocity waveforms from the intervillous[28] space (pulsatile arterial-like and continuous venous-like patterns) in both, normal and abnormal early pregnancies. Studies did not show any difference in terms of RI and PI of the intervillous arterial blood flow between women with missed abortion and those with normally developing pregnancy. In long-standing demise, the cessation of the embryonic portion of placental circulation leaves the fluid pumping action of the trophoblast unaffected, as it remains nourished by the maternal side of circulation. As a consequence, the embryonic circulation no longer drains a trophoblast-conveyed fluid in the villous stroma. Progressive accumulation of the fluid may result in a significant reduction of the intervillous blood flow impedance. Lower impedance to blood flow, observed in spiral arteries, indicates that a massive ,and continuous infiltration of the maternal blood without effective drainage causes further disruption of the maternal embryonic interface resulting in abortion. These changes can be effectively studied by 2D and 3D power Doppler.

Histological studies of the material obtained after spontaneous abortions have shown insufficient trophoblastic invasion into the spiral arteries. Such findings suggest defective transformation of spiral arteries as a possible cause of spontaneous abortion in these cases. Being aware that chromosomal abnormalities are one of the most important factors for spontaneous abortion occurring in more than 50 percent it is not surprising that Doppler studies do not demonstrate any significant difference in terms of vascular resistance between normal pregnancies and those with missed abortions. Pellizzari and coworkers.[29] pointed out that blood flow analysis of uterine artery does not have any clinical role in the management of early pregnancies complicated by uterine bleeding.

Acharya and Morgan[30] compared 2D and 3D ultrasound findings in the first-trimester normal and abnormal pregnancies. 3D ultrasound volume measurements of intrauterine contents in normal and failed pregnancies correlated well with conventional 2D ultrasound. 3D volumetric assessment does not improve the diagnosis of abortion, but it can help in predicting pregnancies that will fail and gives possibility to determine the appropriate management regime.

BLIGHTED OVUM (ANEMBRYONIC PREGNANCY)

Blighted ovum (anembryonic pregnancy) refers to a gestational sac in which the embryo either failed to develop or died at a stage too early to visualize. The diagnosis of anembryonic pregnancy is based on the absence of embryonic echoes within the gestational sac, large enough for such structures to be visualized, independent of the clinical data or menstrual cycle. Advances in transvaginal sonography allow us to detect this kind of abnormality at a mean sac diameter of 1.5 cm.[31] If the volume of the sac is less than 2.5 ml and is not increasing in size by at least 75 percent over a period of 1st week, the definition of this pathological condition in early pregnancy is a blighted ovum. A large empty sac usually measures between 12 and 18 mm in mean diameter. To confirm the diagnosis, these findings should be correlated with other clinical and sonographic data including the presence of a yolk sac.

Transvaginal sonography can clearly detect existing, but a non-living embryo (embryonic demise) in some cases that undoubtedly would have been diagnosed as a blighted ovum if transabdominal sonography was the only examination performed. What the ultrasonographer would detect on his screen depends on gestational age and when the resorption process begun.

In anembryonic pregnancy, a fertilized ovum develops into a blastocyst, but the inner cell mass and resultant embryonic pole never develops. The gestational sac invades the endometrium and acts partly like a normally developing pregnancy. The sincytiotrophoblast invades the endometrium and produces human chorionic gonadotropin. Therefore, the results of a pregnancy test are positive and clinical signs of the pregnancy occur. But, the gestational sac fails to grow and develop normally, and the uterus fails to develop as expected. In this condition, the incidence of chromosomal abnormality is high. Generally, one can estimate that about 15 to 20 percent of all human pregnancies diagnosed before the end of the first trimester terminate in spontaneous abortion.

With falling levels of human chorionic gonadotropin, progesterone and estrogen, the feeling of being pregnant and the associated clinical signs of pregnancy that occurred earlier are lost. The diagnosis of a blighted ovum is in 100 percent of cases by 2D real-time ultrasonography examinations when performed a week apart after absence of embryo development has been confirmed.

Using color Doppler ultrasound in evaluation of the normal and abnormal pregnancies, Kurjak and Kupesic[32] hypothesized that lower PI from the intervillous space of the anembryonic pregnancy may reflect changes in the placental stroma, where individual villi are prone to edema. Sometimes even the embryos that measure 1 cm by transvaginal sonography may be absorbed totally after prolonged retention. Consequently, a trophoblast conveyed embryonic circulation no longer drains fluid in the villous stroma. Ongoing processes result in disruption of the maternal-embryonic interface, and finally abortion (Fig. 4.3).

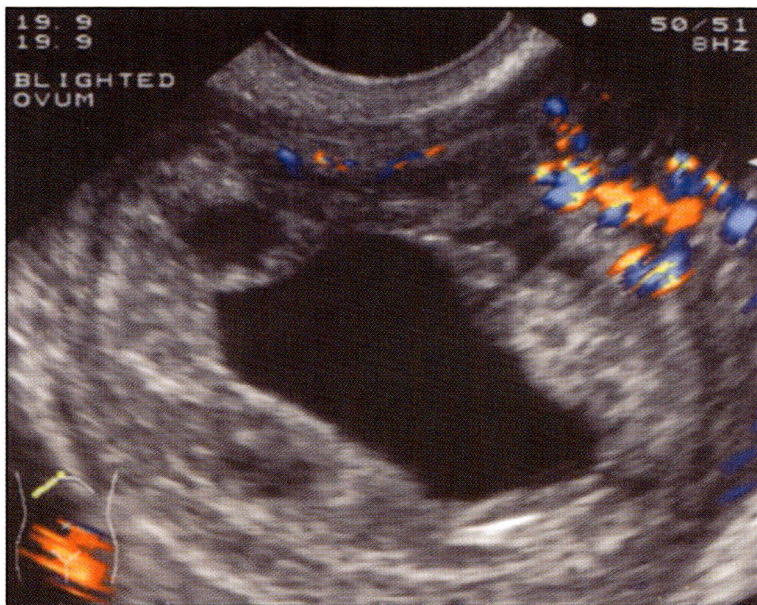

Fig. 4.3: Transvaginal sonogram of an anembryonic pregnancy. Note the absence of the living embryo and the yolk sac indicative of an anembryonic pregnancy. Color Doppler image presents signals obtained from the spiral arteries and other maternal vessels

Analyzing intervillous circulation as one of the first ultrasonographic signs of the pregnancy, studies demonstrated lower vascular resistance of the arterial-like signals in the patients with blighted ovum when compared with the normal pregnancies.

INTRAUTERINE HEMATOMAS

Intrauterine hematomas are defined as sonolucent crescent or wedge-shaped structures between chorionic tissue and uterine wall, or fetal membranes.[33] By localization we can divide them into retroplacental, subchorionic, marginal and supracervical. The most severe are large, central, retroplacental hematomas in which separation of chorionic tissue from basal deciduas occurs by mechanism similar to a mechanism of abruption of the placenta.

The most common causes of intrauterine hematoma are:
- Disturbed trophoblast invasion and defect in spiral arteries transformation
- Infection
- Mechanical factors
- Autoimmune factors
- Hematological factors.

It is important to stress that finding of an intrauterine hematoma does not immediately indicate the likelihood of a spontaneous abortion. As the measure of precaution rather classify this pregnancy into a high-risk group with additional necessity for further intensive monitoring.

Prognostically, there are two main elements, which determine the pregnancy outcome. First one is the location of the hematoma. According to Kurjak and associates, location is more predictive sign than the volume of hematoma.[33, 34] It is likely that if the bleeding occurs at the level of the definitive placenta (under the cord insertion), it may result in placental separation and subsequent abortion.[35] Conversely, a subchorionic hematoma detaching only a membrane opposite to the cord insertion could probably reach a significant volume before it affects normal pregnancy development.[36] Supracervical hematoma has much better prognosis because it is easily drained into the vagina and for this reason it does not represent mechanical factor for compression of the uteroplacental vessels. Higher incidence of spontaneous abortions has been reported in the cases where hematoma has been localized in the fundal or corporal region, which could be attributed to placental location in that area.[33] Retroplacental or central hematomas have the worst prognosis because they cause the largest incident of the uteroplacental circulation and placental tissue[37] (Fig. 4.4). The pathological mechanism is probably placental abruption, in which retroplacental clots are located between the placenta and myometrium, and preplacental clots are found between the amniotic fluid and the placenta later in the second trimester.

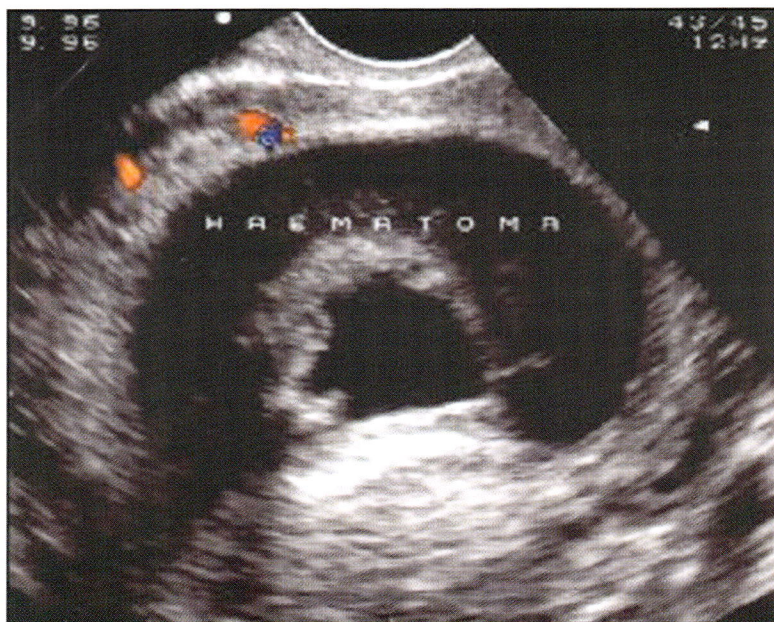

Fig. 4.4: Transvaginal sonogram of a large-volume hematoma located in fundal-corporeal region. Note the uterine blood flow signals on the side of the hematoma

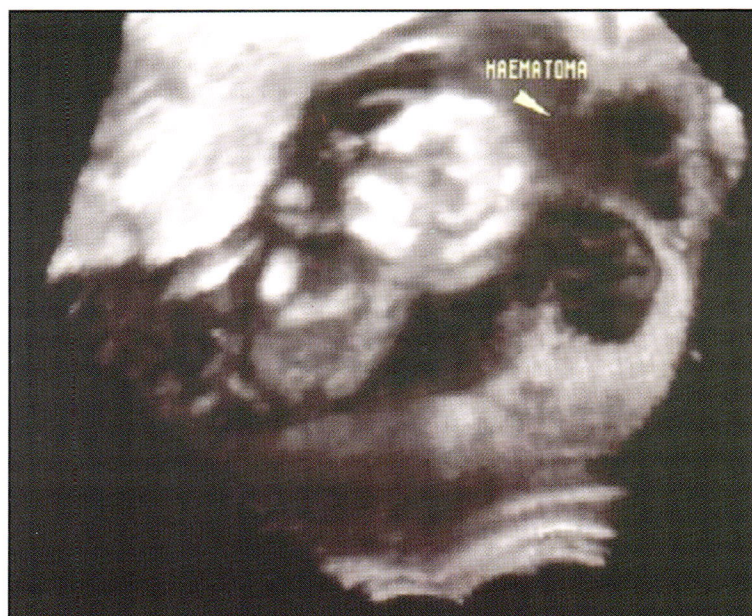

Fig. 4.5: Three-dimensional transvaginal sonogram of the subchorionic hematoma in a close proximity to the gestational sac

Table 4.1 presents data on hematoma site and pregnancy outcome.[33] Kurjak and coworkers reported on increased resistance to blood flow and decrease in velocity through spiral arteries on the side of subchorionic hematoma, which is a consequence of mechanical compression of hematoma itself.[33,38] With the progression of pregnancy and growth of the trophoblastic tissue most of the hematomas gradually disappear, and circulation normalizes, but the pregnancy remains in the high-risk group with necessity for intensive monitoring.

Table 4.1: Hematoma site and pregnancy outcome

Hematoma site		Spontaneous abortion		Preterm delivery	
Site	N	n	%	n	%
Supracervical	30	2	6.7	2	6.7
Fundus-corpus	29	8	27.5	1	3.4
Total	59	10	17.5	3	5

Fisher exact test: one-tail P = 0.01, two-tail P = 0.03.
From ref. 33 with permission

Second element in diagnosis of intrauterine hematoma is its size. The modern ultrasonographic machines with transvaginal approach enable accurate evaluation of the size of the intrauterine hematoma. Intrauterine hematoma should be analyzed in relation to the trophoblast tissue, and its distance from the internal cervical os.[39] Furthermore, software of the newest machines makes possible the spatial three-dimensional image of hematomas and surrounding structures as well as measuring their volume and dynamic follow-up of biometric changes (Fig. 4.5). At the same time Doppler measurements can evaluate compression effect on adjacent uteroplacental circulation.[33, 34]

Kupesic and coworkers[40] used color Doppler to visualize the spiral arteries in the patients affected with intrauterine hematoma. Blood flow velocity waveforms were analyzed by means of pulsed Doppler. Parameters used in the study were the resistance index (RI) and peak-systolic velocity (PVS). Table 4.2 presents the effect of the subchorionic hematoma on the local hemodynamics.[40]

Table 4.2: Clinical outcome of pregnancies complicated by subchorionic hematoma. Correlation among variables

Variable	Gestational weeks	Resistance index	Peak systolic velocity	Volume
GW	1.000			
RI	−0.304	1.000		
PS	0.702	−0.791	1.000	
V	0.157	0.527	-0.276	1.000

From ref. 40 with permission.
GW: Gestational weeks; RI: Resistance index; PS: Peak systolic; V: Volume.

The essential finding is that in the presence of hematomas, RI in the ipsilateral spiral arteries was increased and blood flow was decreased. Doppler measurements showed lack of the diastolic flow (RI=1.0) in most of the patients (Fig. 4.6). The subchorionic hematoma compresses the spiral arteries and reduces the peak-systolic velocity. With continuation of pregnancy and reabsorption of the hematoma, impedance to blood flow returns to normal values. This statistical relationship suggests that the changes in blood flow velocity are secondary, and not the cause of subchorionic hematoma. It means that the improvement of blood flow is predictive for normal pregnancy outcome, while decreased spiral artery perfusion indicates increased risk of first- and early second-trimester loss. Since no increased risk for preterm delivery was found in patients with subchorionic hematoma, it is expected that the elevated impedance to blood flow is a transitory consequence of a compression of the arterial walls by the hemorrhage itself.

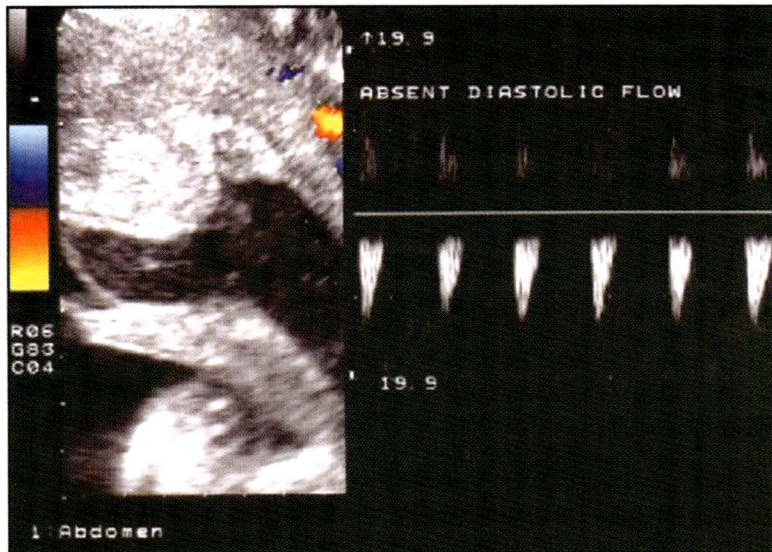

Fig. 4.6: Transvaginal color Doppler scan of a hematoma. Note the absence of diastolic flow (RI=1.0) detected in spiral arteries close to the perigestational hemorrhage

ECTOPIC PREGNANCY

When the endometrium is abnormally thick or has irregular echogenicity, and intrauterine sac is not detected in the patient with the positive urinary pregnancy test, one should always think of an ectopic pregnancy.

EARLY PREGNANCY LOSS

Gestational sac

The first visible structure within the uterus is a gestational sac. During the 5th gestational week, it measures 2 to 3 mm in diameter[41,42] as estimated by transvaginal ultrasound. The measurement should be obtained from the inner-to-inner part of the gestational sac. The gestational sac grows approximately 1 to 2 mm in size per day.[43]

Biometric and morphological characteristics of gestational sac and embryonic echo can be used as a predictive factor in diagnosis of abnormal early pregnancy. Decreased values of gestational sac diameter and/or its irregular shape can suggest upcoming incident and may be used as a marker for chromosomopathies. For example, early spontaneous abortion as one of the complications in early pregnancy usually connected with triploidy and trisomy is followed by abnormal gestational sac growth.[44, 45]

By transabdominal approach abnormal gestational sac criteria include:
- Impossibility to detect double decidual sac when sac diameter is 10 mm or greater,
- Impossibility to detect yolk sac when sac diameter is 20 mm or greater, and/or
- Impossibility to detect an embryo with cardiac activity when sac diameter is 25 mm or greater.[46 ,47]

By transvaginal approach abnormal gestational sac criteria include:
- Impossibility to detect yolk sac when sac diameter is 8 mm or greater, or
- Impossibility to detect cardiac activity when sac diameter is 16 mm or greater.[48]

When growth rate fails to increase at least 0.7 mm/d abnormal sac and early embryo failure should be considered.[49]

Color Doppler evaluation of the supposed gestational sac is important for obtaining additional information and differentiation between the pseudogestational sac and intrauterine gestational sac. Pseudogestational sac is characterized by either absent flow around it or very low velocity flow (< 8 cm/s peak systolic velocity) and moderate resistance to blood flow (RI> 0.50).[50] Normal or abnormal intrauterine gestational sac is characterized by high velocity and low resistance pattern (RI< 0.45) (Fig. 4.7). As mentioned, there is no difference in blood flow between normal and abnormal gestational sac.[51, 52]

Measurement of the gestational sac volume by 3D US can be used for the estimation of gestational age in the early pregnancy. An abnormal measurement of gestational sac could potentially be used as a prognostic marker for pregnancy outcome.[53]

Yolk sac

Yolk sac is the first recognizable structure inside the gestational sac and should be obtained as a regularly rounded extra-amniotic structure when gestational sac reaches 8 to 10 mm.[54] Normal biometric values of yolk sac diameter during the first trimester are 3 to 6 mm (inner diameter) (Fig. 4.8).

Following changes assessed by 2D US are related to spontaneous abortion prediction.[54]
- Absence of the yolk sac
- Too large—more than 6 mm (over 2SD, sensitivity 16 percent, specificity 97 percent, PPV 60 percent)
- Too small—less than 3 mm (below 2SD, sensitivity 15 percent, specificity 95 percent, PPV 44 percent)
- Irregular shape—mainly wrinkled with indented walls
- Degenerative changes—abundant calcifications with decreased translucency of the yolk sac, (Fig. 4.9) and

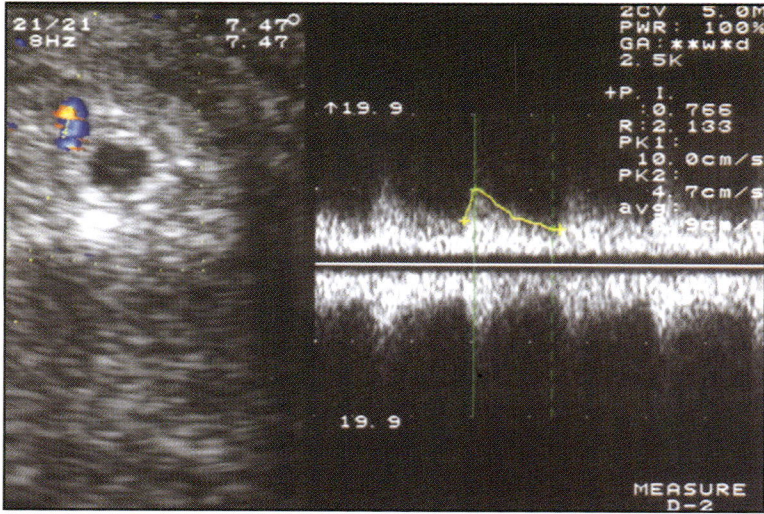

Fig. 4.7: Transvaginal color Doppler image of an early gestational sac. Blood flow signals derived from spiral arteries demonstrate low vascular resistance (PI=0.77)

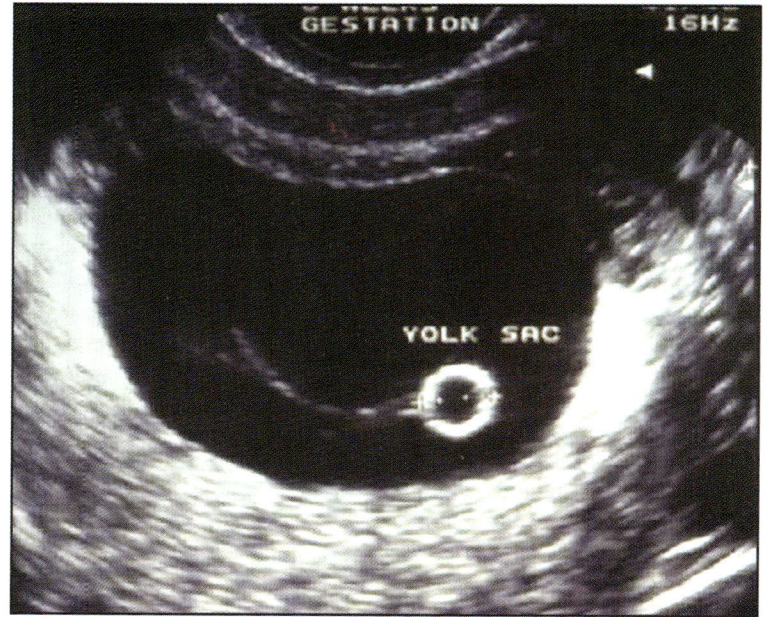

Fig. 4.9: Transvaginal sonogram of vitelline duct and yolk sac characterized with increased echogenicity

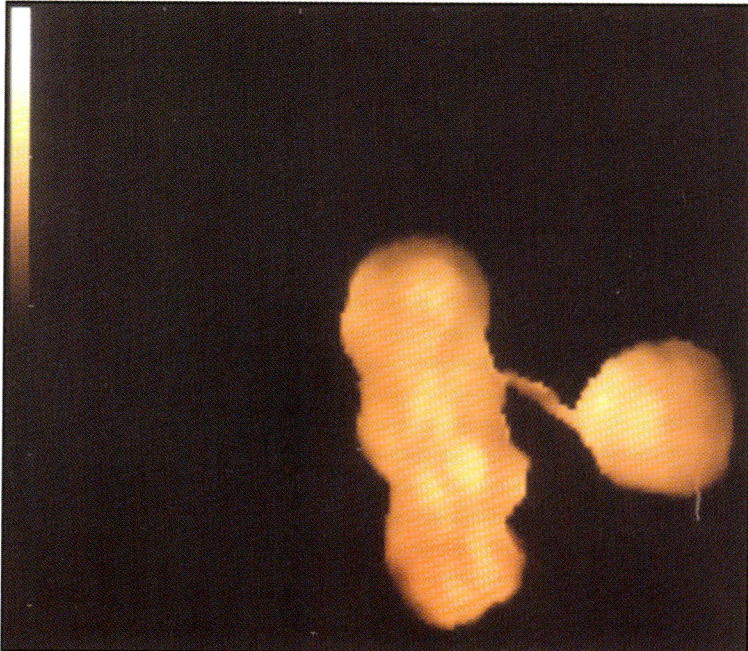

Fig. 4.8: Three-dimensional transvaginal imaging at 7th to 8th weeks of gestation by surface mode. Note regular shape of the yolk sac

Table 4.3: Yolk sac diameter and vascularity between 6th and 10th weeks of gestation in normal pregnancies

Gestational age (weeks)	N	Yolk sac diameter Mean (range) (mm)	Significance	Yolk sac vascularity N	%	Significance
6	9	3.1 (2.5-3.8)		3	33.33	$p<0.005$
7	15	3.6 (2.9-4.4)	$p<0.05$	12	80.00	$p<0.05$
8	19	4.1 (3.6-5.1)	$p<0.05$	17	89.47	$p<0.05$
9	18	4.5 (4.1-5.9)	$p<0.05$	15	83.33	$p<0.001$
10	14	5.3 (4.3-6.0)	$p<0.001$	8	57.14	$p<0.005$
11	12	5.0 (4.1-5.9)	$p<0.05$	3	25.00	$p<0.001$
12	10	4.3 (3.4-4.9)	$p<0.001$	0	0	
Total	87	4.2 (2.5-6.0)		58	66.67	

From ref. 55, with permission

- Number of yolk sacs—has to be equal to the number of the embryos.

It is, nowadays, supposed that yolk sac abnormalities are rather the consequence than the cause of altered embryonic development.[55, 56] Table 4.3 refers on yolk sac diameter and vascularity between 6th and 12th weeks of gestation in normal pregnancies.[55]

The ultrasound appearance of the yolk sac has already been proposed as a prognostic parameter for the outcome of pregnancy. Kurjak[33] and coworkers established sonographic criteria for distinguishing between "normal" and "abnormal" yolk sac appearance. In their experience, yolk sac should always be visible before the viable embryo; yolk sac measures 4.0 to 5.0 mm in diameter until 7 to 8 weeks of gestation and reaches

6.0 to 6.5 mm by the end of the 9th week. After that period yolk sac starts its regression and disappears at 12th week of gestation.[57]

The sonographic detection of abnormal yolk sac morphology may predict abnormal fetal outcome. Attempts have been made to identify abnormal parameters. Parameters of abnormal yolk sac findings listed above are predictive indicators of early pregnancy failure. All these parameters should be defined and assessed prior to 10th gestational week.

Abnormal yolk sac size may be the first sonographic indicator of associated failure. Primarily, the presence of an embryo without the visible yolk sac before the 10th gestational week is mostly an abnormal finding. According to some authors, the inner diameter of the yolk sac is always less than 5.6 mm in a normal pregnancy before the 10th week of gestational age. Lyons[58] established that for a mean gestational sac diameter of less than 10 mm, the yolk sac diameter should be less than

4 mm. In 15 patients who had abnormally large sacs, six had no embryo, five aborted spontaneously and only one conceptus survived. Out of nine others with embryo and large yolk sac, eight patients aborted and in one patient trisomy 21 was detected at the 24th gestational week.

The yolk sac can be too small, and this is accepted as a marker of poor pregnancy outcome. Green and Hobbins[59] analyzed a group of patients between 8th and 12th weeks of gestational age, and found out that patients with a yolk sac diameter less than 2 mm were associated with an adverse pregnancy outcome.

Most often, the shape of the yolk sac is changed when compressed by an enlarging fetus after the 10th gestational week. The normal spherical shape of the yolk sac could be distorted even earlier, requiring intensive follow-up within the next few weeks. The most difficult diagnostic puzzle is the double yolk sac (Fig. 4.10). Each singleton pregnancy should have a single yolk sac. A double yolk sac is an extremely rare finding. The diagnostic puzzle includes the morphological differentiation of a retarded disappearance of physiological midgut herniation or an early abdominal wall defect.

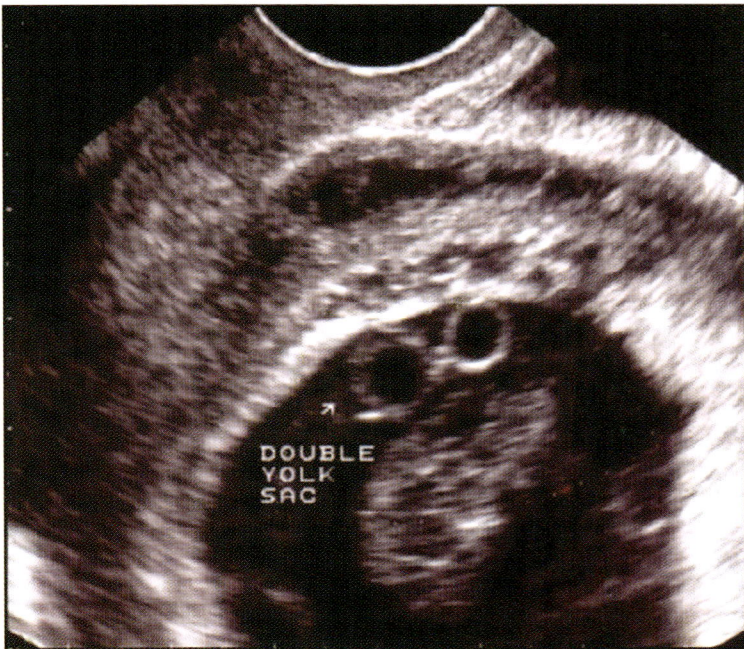

Fig. 4.10: Transvaginal color Doppler scan of an 8th week embryo. Note the double yolk sac close to the embryonic body

It is unknown whether abnormalities of the yolk sac are related primarily to the yolk sac or secondary to embryonic maldevelopment. According to the present data it seems that the yolk sac plays an important role in maternofetal transportation in early pregnancy. Changes in size and shape could indicate or reflect the significant dysfunction of this system, and therefore could influence early embryonic development. Currently, the major benefits of the sonographic evaluation of the yolk sac are:

1. Differentiation of potentially viable and nonviable gestations.
2. Confirmation of the presence of an intrauterine pregnancy vs. a decidual cast.
3. Indication of a possible fetal abnormality.

Kurjak and associates[55] performed a transvaginal color Doppler study of yolk sac vascularization. They examined 105 patients whose gestational age ranged from 6 to 10 weeks from the last menstrual period. Transvaginal color and pulsed Doppler examination was performed before the termination of pregnancy for psychosocial reasons. The overall visualization rate for yolk sac vessels was 72.38 percent. A characteristic waveform profile included low velocity (5.8 ± 1.7 cm/s), and the absence of diastolic flow was found in all examined yolk sacs. The pulsatility index showed a mean value of 3.24 ± 0.94 without significant changes between the subgroups.

Kurjak and coworkers[60, 61] also analyzed the vascularization of yolk sac in abnormal pregnancies. Study included 48 patients with missed abortion between 6th and 12th weeks of gestation. Yolk sac blood flow was detected in 18.54 percent of missed abortions. Three types of abnormal vascular signals were obtained from the yolk sac: irregular blood flow, permanent diastolic flow and venous blood flow signals. Changes in vascularization of the yolk sac noticed in missed abortions in this study are probably a consequence of embryonic death and reabsorption of the embryo through the vitelline duct. Abnormal patterns of the yolk sac vascularity can be related to decreased vitelline blood flow, which may cause progressive accumulation of nutritive secretions not utilized by the embryo. This process ends with enlargement of the yolk sac indicative of an early pregnancy failure. In 28.57 percent of missed abortions yolk sac vascularity was detected with large diameter of the yolk sac, and 20.00 percent with normal yolk sac diameter.

Yolk sac calcification was reported to result from the typical dystrophic changes that occur in nonviable cellular material.[62] Recognition of a calcified yolk sac without blood flow signals suggests long-standing demise in the first trimester, which directs the clinician for further diagnostic work-up.

Kurjak and Kupesic[61] presented data indicating that there is an interaction between the yolk sac vascularity and intervillous circulation in patients with missed abortion. In patients with long-standing demise, vascular signals could not have been extracted from the hyperechoic walls of the yolk sac. Parallel assessment of the intervillous circulation demonstrated numerous color-coded areas within the intervillous space indicating low mesenchymal turgor and progressive disruption of the materno-embryonic interface. Therefore, the changes in the intervillous circulation noticed in some missed abortions are rather the consequence of embryonic death and inadequate drainage than being the primary cause of early pregnancy failure. Independent Doppler studies from three institutions using sensitive conventional and power Doppler velocimetry found that continuous and pulsatile blood flow can be extracted from intervillous space in both normal pregnancies and those with adverse outcome.[63, 64, 65]

Data presented by Kurjak and Kupesic[61] support the concept that establishment of the intervillous circulation is a progressive process during the first trimester of pregnancy. Between the 6th and 10th weeks of gestation clear blood flow signals are derived from the walls of the yolk sac supporting the hypothesis that yolk sac is responsible for optimal delivery of nutrients and oxygen to developing embryo up to 10th week of gestation. Later on intervillous circulation becomes more prominent indicating a possible switch from the vitelline towards intervillous circulation.

Three-dimensional ultrasound (3D US) significantly contributes to "in vivo" observation of the yolk sac surface pattern, enabling reduced scanning time and observation of the honeycomb surface pattern of the yolk sac. Automatic volume calculation allows us to estimate precise relationship between the yolk sac and gestational sac volumes, as well as to obtain the correlation between yolk sac volume and CRL measurements.[66] Distinguishing the yolk sac and embryo in 6th and 7th weeks of gestation decreases possibility of CRL measurement error (see Fig. 4.10). Table 4.4 reveals normal and abnormal yolk sac features.[67]

Table 4.4: Normal and abnormal yolk sac characteristics

	Yolk sac characteristics	
	Normal yolk sac	Abnormal yolk sac
Size	5-6 mm up to 9th week of gestation	❖ < 2mm in 8 to 12 weeks (to small) ❖ > 6mm after 10th week (to large)
Shape	Round	Oval, distorted
Ultrasound finding	Echoic rim, hypoechoic center	Hyperechoic
Doppler	Absence of diastolic flow	❖Irregular blood flow ❖Permanent diastolic flow ❖Venous blood flow

From ref. 67, with permission

Crown-rump Length (CRL)

Crown-rump length is used to estimate growth of the embryo and define exact gestational age. Measurement of CRL is performed in midsagittal section from the top of the head (crown) to the end of the rump of embryo by transvaginal probe.

Reliability of CRL measurements depends on embryo size and the fact that the measurements are only precise when the greatest long axis reaches 18 to 22 mm. In smaller embryos, a mistake in few millimeters means a large deviation. In embryos

over 18 mm, when the real CRL is measured and the anatomic structures are visible, the possibility of a mistake is smaller.

The median CRL in fetuses with trisomies 21 and 13 or sex chromosome aneuploidies is not significantly different from the normal fetuses as reported by Kuhn and coworkers.[68] This is the reason why routine pregnancy dating should be by measurement of CRL as well as interpretation of the results from nuchal translucency or biochemical screening.

However, some results suggest that the measurement of fetal CRL may be useful predictor of spontaneous miscarriage and SGA in pregnancies with threatened abortion.[69]

Embryonic Heart Rate

The cut-off CRL for detecting cardiac activity by transvaginal probe is 4 mm,[70] and by transabdominal 9 mm.[71] Heart rate progressively increases to 120 to 160 beats/minute after 6 to 7 weeks.[72] Embryonic heart rate demonstrates certain physiologic variability within its normal range of frequencies that is 150 to 190 beats/minute for embryos bigger than 10 mm at 8th to 12th weeks of gestation. An embryonic heart rate less than 100 beats per minute (bpm) 7th week is recognized as embryonic bradycardia.[73] An embryonic heart rate less than 70 bpm has been reported to result in a fetal demise in 100 percent patients.[74] Bradycardia or arrhythmia could be considered as predictors for heart action cessation. In these cases, an early hemodynamic heart failure was noticed with consequential gestational sac enlargement, yolk sac enlargement (more than 6 mm) and initial generalized hydrops. This type of hemodynamic disturbances can occur in patients presenting with massive intrauterine hematomas prior to fetal demise.[75] Doubilet[76] reported that pregnancies in which the embryos have a slow heart rate at or before 7th week of gestation and which continue beyond the first trimester, have a high likelihood (90 percent) of congenital anomalies, but than embryos with normal heart rates. Reduced body movements of the embryo during first and second trimester are also considered possible predictors of early pregnancy complications.[75]

Amnion Evaluation

At 6th to 8th weeks of gestation by transvaginal probe, amniotic membrane is visualized as a thin rounded structure encircling embryo. It could appear before 6th week of gestation as a linear echogenic interface projected within the gestational sac in proximity to the embryo.[42]

When the amniotic membrane is clearly visualized or its thickness and echogenicity approach that of yolk sac, it should be always suspicious to abnormal amnion development.[77] Mean amniotic sac diameter is approximately equal to the CRL in normal early pregnancy. Enlarged amniotic cavity related to the CRL suggests early pregnancy abnormality.[77]

Horrow[78] presented data on the difference between the CRL and amniotic cavity diameter and stated that in normal pregnancies was approximately 1 mm but reached almost 9 mm in abnormal pregnancies.

In normal early pregnancy embryo is usually detected before amniotic membrane. Cases of "empty amnion" with gestational sac greater than 16 mm are highly suggestive of abnormal pregnancy and require further analysis.[79]

OBJECTS IN FIRST TRIMESTER SCREENING FOR CHROMOSOMOPATHIES

Nuchal Translucency

Increased nuchal translucency (NT) thickness at 10th to 14th weeks of gestation is associated with fetal chromosomal defects and many genetic syndromes and abnormalities.[80, 81] Measurement of NT may be obtained by transvaginal or transabdominal approach. The elements that should be kept in mind during NT measurement are:

- Embryo/fetus presented in sagittal section
- Magnification of the embryo/fetus image occupies at least 75 percent of the screen
- Ability to distinguish between fetal skin and amnion
- Measurement of the maximum thickness of the subcutaneous translucency, between the skin and the soft tissues overlying the cervical spine[80]
- CRL between 38 and 84 mm.

Pajkrt and coworkers[82] determined the normal range for the NT measurement in chromosomal and phenotypically normal fetuses. They demonstrated normal physiological variation in the NT thickness between 9th and 14th weeks of gestation. Cross-sectional data in Braithwhite's study[83] demonstrated an increase in NT measurement between 9th and 12th weeks, followed by the decrease at 13th and 14th weeks of gestation. Because of the change of the value of NT with CRL fixed cut off value is inappropriate and each measurement of the NT should be compared with adequate CRL value.[84] According to results of many studies NT measurement in first trimester presents one of the best ultrasonographic markers for detection of chromosomal abnormalities.[85, 86]

Limitations of NT measurement by 2D US are:
- Suboptimal fetal position
- Observation of inappropriate median sagittal section of the embryo

- Attachment of the nuchal region to the amniotic membrane
- Small size of the structure to be measured[87] and
- Long lasting examination.

Performing 3D US seems to overcome some of these limitations. After storing the volume data examiner may repeat volume scanning and perform the assessment of the nuchal region from all directions[88] (Fig. 4.11). Correlation of the 2D and 3D transvaginal ultrasound examinations indicated that 3D ultrasound is superior to 2D US, since using 3D US technique the midsagittal section of the fetus can be visualized with 100 percent success rate. Further more, the initial scan of the patient may be preformed by a less experienced ultrasonographer and stored values analyzed by an expert in settled conditions. 3D US improves the accuracy of NT measurement, producing an appropriate midsagittal section of the fetus and making a clear distinction of the nuchal region from the amniotic membrane. Similarly, 3D US measurements of the NT present better intraobserver reproducibility than that conventional 2D US, increasing the effectiveness of the screening programs.[87, 89]

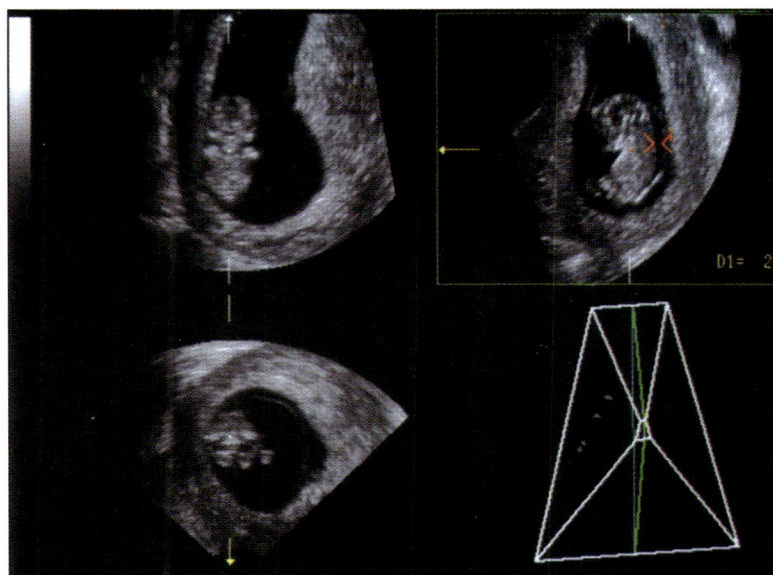

Fig. 4.11: Three dimensional scan of a fetus at 12th week gestation. Three perpendicular planes: plane A allows a frontal view of the fetal nuchal region; plane B shows an ideal mid-sagittal view of the fetus; plane C gives a symmetrical transverse section of the fetus. These planes make measurement of the nuchal translucency much easier and more accurate

Ductus Venosus and Heart Failure

Ductus Venosus (DV), Foramen Ovale and Ductus Arteriosus

Botali presents specific shunts during the intrauterine life. Function of ductus venosus is connecting to umbilical circulation with inferior vena cava. DV originates from the umbilical vein and enters the inferior vena cava at the level of the hepatic veins, just below the diaphragm, forming the subdiaphragmatic venous vestibulum.[90] The main function of DV is distribution of the oxygenated blood through foramen ovale into the left atrium. In normal conditions approximately 53 percent of the umbilical blood flows into the DV,[91] but during the state of hypoxia rises to 70 percent with decrease in intrahepatic hepatic blood flow.[92] Ductus venosus blood flow signals can be depicted in the right sagittal section of the fetal abdomen as a continuation of the umbilical vein towards inferior vena cava.[93]

In normal fetuses the DV waveform shows a peak velocity during ventricular systole, another peak during ventricular diastole and a nadir during atrial contraction. The DV pulsatility index is independent of the insonation angle and proved to be the most reproducible parameter.[94] Changes in the DV waveform have been reported in different hemodynamic situations. In cardiac failure without structural defects, reversed flow during atrial contraction has been detected.[95] Similar findings have been reported in growth-restricted fetuses.[96, 97] An abnormally increased DV pulsatility index may indicate a chromosomal defect.[59] Because NT is independent ultrasonographic marker, authors combined NT and DV measurement. The results from Antolín et al[98] demonstrated the usefulness of DV pulsatility index in an unselected population. Combining DV pulsatility index and NT measurement, overall sensitivity decreased to 55 percent, but specificity reached 99.3 percent, with a negative predictive value of 99.3 percent. When only autosomal trisomies were considered, the detection rate was similar to NT with decrease in the false-positive rate. Similar effectiveness was found during the early gestational age period. These results suggest that NT may be used as a first line-screening test in order to maintain the sensitivity, while examination of the DV waveforms is useful as a second line test in order to decrease the false-positive rate, reducing the need for invasive testing to less than 1 percent.[99] Increased DV pulsatility index (using 95th centile) can be explained by an early cardiac failure.[100] Transient changes in DV waveform have been noted in chromosomally abnormal fetuses in early pregnancy, with a reversed flow during atrial contraction. Suggesting a temporary phenomenon Huisman and Bilardo[100] found a twin pregnancy discordant for trisomy 18 where the affected fetus at 13th week of gestation had an increased nuchal translucency thickness and reversed end-diastolic DV flow.[100] Transient cardiac failure has been involved in the physiology of the NT thickness. It can be hypothesized that the same early cardiac dysfunction can produce a transient fluid accumulation in the back of the neck and a temporary increase in DV pulsatility index.[101] Normal DV hemodynamics has been reported in the pathology involving the left atrium or ventricle, although blood flow from this vessel is preferentially directed across the foramen ovale into the left heart. Abnormal DV parameters have been demonstrated in association with right ventricular pathology.[102] Malformations involving the right

ventricular inlet or outlet are more commonly associated with changes in the DV waveform during atrial contraction than isolated septal defects.[94] Zoppi and all[102] found reduced absent or reversed flow in the DV during late diastole, coinciding with atrial contraction. This was considered a sign of early fetal cardiac function impairment and was observed in the first trimester fetuses with chromosomal abnormalities that are expected to carry a more frequent rate of cardiac defects than normal. Because of the prevalence of the cardiac defects in fetuses carrying chromosomal abnormalities, it is clear that some signs of heart failure may be evident in the first trimester, and DV seems to be an essential site where this impairment could be manifested. The conclusion of this study is that DV pulsatility index should not be used as a first line screening test at 10th to 16th weeks of gestation because it does not increase the number of cases detected by NT, but can be useful as a second line test in screen-positive cases with increased NT thickness in order to increase the specificity, reducing the need for invasive testing. In chromosomally normal fetuses with an abnormal DV waveform pattern, a careful follow-up scan, including fetal echocardiography, should be mandatory.

Umbilical Artery Assessment

Analysis of the embryo/fetal umbilical artery flow shows variable results. While Zoppi and coworkers[103] demonstrated no alterations in the umbilical artery flow in embryo/fetuses with increased NT and normal karyotype and those with increased NT and trisomy 21, Borrell and co-workers[104] presented alarming data that Doppler ultrasound finding of a reversed end-diastolic flow in the umbilical artery during the first trimester of pregnancy may indicate structural and/or chromosomal defect. However, the importance of the umbilical artery flow measurements has yet to be established.

Nasal Bone

2D-ultrasound evaluation of the nasal bone in first trimester day-by-day becomes more important but also encourages academic discussion. In combination with NT, DV and biochemical markers, absence of the nasal bone indicates possibility of a chromosomal anomaly. The most common chromosomal anomaly connected with absence of the nasal bone is Down syndrome (trisomy 21). Screening regarding to this problem takes place between 11th and 14th weeks.[105] Visualization of the nasal bone should be done by transabdominal ultrasound in mid-sagittal view of the embryo/fetal profile, in an adequately magnified image, with an angle of insonation about 45 or 135° between the ultrasound beam and the line traced from the top of the chin of the embryo/fetus.[105, 106]

Most recent observations suggest it is the best to visualize nasal bone in sagittal section in medial orbital angle. Cicero and coworkers in their study analyzed nasal bone at 11th to 14th week of gestation.[105]

In 99.5 percent of chromosomally normal fetuses nasal bone was visible. In 73 percent of cases with trisomy 21 nasal bone was not found. Cicero and coworkers suggests that nasal bone screening in combination with NT thickness and maternal serum biochemical analysis sensitivity could achieve 90 percent.[105]

Heart Analysis

Simpson and Sharland[107] analyzed association between congenital heart defects and increased NT. Their data indicate that a normal nuchal scan in no way excludes karyotype abnormalities or serious cardiac malformations. For fetuses with increased nuchal translucency, the median gestational age at time of the diagnosis of the congenital heart disease was 20th weeks. Bronshtein and Zimmer[108] suggest that transvaginal ultrasound examination of the heart in at least two main planes of four chambers and three specific images of the vessels (X, P, Y) in a period between 14th and 16th weeks of gestation increases possibility of detecting heart defects. Earlier diagnosis preserves entire spectra of diagnostic and therapeutic options including genetic studies when indicated or therapeutic abortion. In cases of severe fetal malformations, early detection may prevent unnecessary invasive procedures.[108]

Umbilical Cord Diameter

Ghezzi and coworkers[109] analyzed NT and umbilical cord diameter in 784 patients between 10th and 14th weeks of gestation. The umbilical cord diameter was measured as outer to outer border at the maximal magnification. As the umbilical cord diameter increases with gestational age, 95th centile was cut off for enlarged diameter. The proportion of fetuses with enlarged umbilical cord diameter was higher in presence of fetal or placental chromosomal abnormalities.

Introduction of umbilical cord diameter as the ultrasonographic marker for chromosomal abnormalities slowly enters in every day practice.

COMBINED STRATEGIES FOR ANEUPLOIDY SCREENING

Unfortunately, definitive diagnosis of the aneuploidy still can only be accomplished by invasive procedures. Certain ultrasonographic markers (such as abnormal NT, DV and nasal bone) refer to possibility of existence of chromosomal abnormality. Trying to create an efficient noninvasive screening test clinicians combined ultrasonographic and non-

ultrasonographic markers. Sabria and coworkers[110] presented data from their 13 years long experience in prenatal screening with detection rate of 90.0 percent at 5.5 percent false-positive rate for trisomy 21, detection rate of 75.0 percent at 1.0 percent false-positive rate for trisomy 18 and detection rate of 87.5 percent at 5.2 percent false-positive rate for all aneuploidies. Their suggestion for first trimester ultrasound screening is to combine:

- Maternal age
- NT as ultrasound marker, and
- PAPP-A and free βHCG as biochemical markers.

This combination detects between 85 and 90 percent of Down's syndrome, at the 5 percent false positive rate.[111-113] Similar results are presented in retrospective studies for trisomy 13 and Turner's syndrome, while sex trisomies are usually not detectable.[114,115]

Introducing nasal bone as the independent ultrasonographic marker and using color Doppler evaluation of DV, as a second line marker Sabria suggests that detection rate for trisomy 21 will be 98 percent at 5 percent false-positive rate. Comas and coworkers[116] suggested for low-risk population single NT measurement or selective screening by NT and DV assessment, and for the high risk population combined simultaneous screening (including all sonographic, Doppler and biochemical parameters), all in sense of reducing invasive testing procedures.

CONCLUSIONS

Ultrasound examination has become the "gold standard" in follow-up of the development and complications in early pregnancy. With introduction of transvaginal sonography a possibility for early morphological and biometrical ultrasound examinations has been significantly improved. The essential aim of an early pregnancy ultrasound is not only to diagnose a pregnancy, but also to differentiate between normal and abnormal pregnancy. Application of color Doppler ultrasound has enabled functional hemodynamic presentation and evaluation soon after implantation.

Early pregnancy failure is defined as a pregnancy that ends spontaneously before the embryo has reached by ultrasound detectible viable gestational age. The most common pathological symptom of the early pregnancy failure is the vaginal bleeding. Only differentiation and accurate estimation of the pregnancy status and embryo/fetus make it possible to obtain therapeutic measures to cases where a normal outcome of the pregnancy can be expected.

The development of transvaginal sonography has allowed improved assessment of the patients presenting vaginal bleeding during the first half of pregnancy, clarifying the differential diagnosis of missed abortion, ectopic pregnancy, blighted ovum and threatened abortion with a living embryo. Embryo vitality can be established reliably by documenting cardiac activity on realtime, B-mode and/or color Doppler ultrasonography.

Threatened abortion is the clinical term used to describe vaginal bleeding during the first 20th weeks of pregnancy in women who, on the basis of clinical evaluation are considered to have a potentially living embryo/fetus. With a normal intrauterine pregnancy, bleeding from the chorion frondosum is undoubtedly the most common source of vaginal bleeding during the first trimester and should be considered in the diagnosis of threatened abortion.

As a definition, incomplete abortion is the passage of some, but not all fetal or placental tissue through the cervical canal. In complete abortion, all products of conception are expelled through the cervix. Transvaginal ultrasonography plays an important role in evaluating uterine cavity in spontaneous abortion since it enables detection of the retained products of conception. Retained products of conception after abortion may cause bleeding or endometritis. Recent studies demonstrate that the risk for repeated spontaneous abortion depends exclusively on the number of previous spontaneous abortions, their cause, maternal age, chromosomal abnormalities, uterine anomalies, etc. Even though many different risk factor have been thoroughly researched around 60 percent of unsuccessful pregnancies remain unknown. In patients with a suspicion on a spontaneous abortion it is suggested to perform not only 2D but also color Doppler sonographic evaluation of the retained trophoblastic tissue.

The diagnosis of missed abortion is determined by the ultrasound identification of an embryo/fetus without any heart activity. It is relatively easy to make this diagnosis by means of the transvaginal color Doppler ultrasound. The main parameter is the absence of the heartbeats and the lack of a color flow signals at its expected position after the 6th gestational week.

Blighted ovum (anembryonic pregnancy) refers to a gestational sac in which the embryo either failed to develop or died at a stage to early to visualize. The diagnosis of anembryonic pregnancy is based on the absence of embryonic echoes within the gestational sac large enough for such structures to be visualized independent of the clinical data or menstrual cycle. Advances in transvaginal sonography allow us to detect this kind of abnormality at a mean sac diameter of 1.5 cm. To confirm the diagnosis, these findings should be correlated with other clinical and sonographic data including the presence of a yolk sac.

Intrauterine hematomas are defined as sonolucent crescent or wedge-shaped structure between chorionic tissue and uterine wall, or fetal membranes. By localization intrauterine hematomas can be divided into retroplacental, subchorionic, marginal and supracervical. The most severe are large, central, retroplacental hematomas.

Prognostically, there are two main elements which determine the pregnancy outcome: location and the size of the hematoma. The essential color Doppler finding is that in the presence of hematomas, vascular resistance in the ipsilateral spiral arteries is increased and blood flow is decreased. Doppler measurements showed lack of the diastolic flow in most of hematomas resulting in RI of 1.0. Since no increased risk for preterm delivery was found in patients with subchorionic hematoma, it is expected that the elevated impedance to blood flow is a transitory consequence of a compression of the spiral arterial walls by the hemorrhage itself.

Biometric and morphological characteristics of gestational sac and embryonic echo can be used as predictive factors in diagnosis of abnormal early pregnancy. Decreased values of gestational sac diameter and/or its irregular shape can suggest upcoming incident and could be used as markers for chromosomopathies. When growth rate fails to increase at least 0.7 mm/d an early embryo failure should be considered.

Yolk sac is the first recognizable structure inside the gestational sac in early pregnancy. Following changes assessed by 2D US are related to the prediction of the spontaneous abortion: absence of yolk sac, too large yolk sac (more than 6 mm), too small yolk sac (less than 3 mm), irregular shape of the yolk sac (mainly wrinkled with indented walls), degenerative changes of the yolk sac (abundant calcifications with decreased translucency of yolk sac), and number of yolk sacs (has to be equal to the number of the embryos).

Crown-rump length (CRL) is used to estimate growth of the embryo and define exact gestational age. The median CRL in fetuses with trisomies 21 and 13 or sex chromosome aneuploidies is not significantly different from that of the normal fetuses. An embryonic heart rate less than 100 beats per minute (bpm) before 7 weeks is recognized as embryonic bradycardia. Bradycardia or arrhythmia could be considered as predictors for heart action cessation. In these cases, an early hemodynamic heart failure is usually noticed with consequential gestational sac enlargement, yolk sac enlargement (more than 6 mm) and initial generalized hydrops.

Mean amniotic sac diameter is approximately equal to the CRL in normal early pregnancy. Enlarged amniotic cavity related to the CRL suggests early pregnancy abnormality.

Increased NT thickness at 10th to 14th weeks of gestation is associated with fetal chromosomal defects, many genetic syndromes and abnormalities. Because of the change of the value of NT with CRL, each measurement of the NT should be compared with adequate CRL value. First trimester ultrasound screening should include: maternal age, NT as ultrasound marker and PAPP-A and free ßHCG as biochemical markers. These parameters have detection rate of 90.0 percent at 5.5 percent false-positive rate for trisomy 21, detection rate of 75.0 percent at 1.0 percent false-positive rate for trisomy 18 and detection rate of 87.5 percent at 5.2 percent false-positive rate for all aneuploidies.

In normal fetuses the DV waveform shows a peak velocity during ventricular systole, another peak during ventricular diastole and a nadir during atrial contraction. Results of different studies suggest that NT should be used as a first line-screening test in order to maintain the sensitivity, while examination of the DV waveforms can be useful as a second line test in order to decrease the false-positive rate, reducing the need for invasive testing to less than 1 percent.

In combination with NT, DV and biochemical markers absence of the nasal bone indicates possibility of a chromosomal anomaly. Introducing nasal bone as the independent additional ultrasonographic marker and using color Doppler evaluation of DV, as a second line markers it is suspected that detection rate will be 98 percent at 5 percent false-positive rate for trisomy 21.

REFERENCES

1. Kurjak A. Ultrasound in early pregnancy In Kurjak A (Ed): Diagnostic Ultrasound in Developing Countries. Mladost, 1986; pp 65-75.
2. Jukic J. Pathology of women's reproductive system. AGM: Zagreb, 1999.
3. Goldstein SR. Embryonic death in early pregnancy: a new look at the first trimester. Obstet Gynecol 1994; 84: 294-7.
4. Sadler TW. Langman's Medical Embriology, 7th edn. Williams and Wilkins, 1994.
5. Streeter GL. Developmental horizons in human embryo (4th issue). A review of the histogenesis of cartilage and bone. Contr Embryol Carneg Inst 1949;220:150-73.
6. Blaas HGK. The examination of the embryo and early fetus: how and by whom? Ultrasound Obstet Gynecol 1999; 14:153-8.
7. Blaas HG, Eik-Nes SH, Kiserud T, Hellevik LR. Early development of the abdominal wall, stomach and heart from the 7th to 12th weeks of gestation: a longitudinal study. Ultrasound Obstetr Gynecol 1995;6:240-9.
8. Cetin A, Cetin M. Diagnostic and therapeutical decision-making with transvaginal sonography for first trimester spontaneous abortion, clinically thought to be complete or incomplete. Contraception 1998; 57:393-7.
9. Edmonds DK, Lindsky KS, Miller JF. Early embryonic mortality in women. Fertil Steril 1982; 38: 447-53.
10. Hakim RB, Gray RH, Zacur H. Infertility and early pregnancy loss. Am J Obstet Gynecol 1995;172: 1510-7.
11. Alberman E. The epidemiology of repeated abortion. In Beard RW and Bishop F. (Eds.): Early Pregnancy Loss: Mechanism and Treatment. New York: Springer-Verlag. 1988; 9-17.
12. Kurtz AB, Shlansky-Goldberg BB. Detection of retained products of conception following spontaneous abortion in the first trimester. J Ultrasound Med 1991;10: 387-95.
13. Chung TKH, Cheung LP, Sahota DS, Haines CJ, Chang AM. Z. Evaluation of the accuracy of transvaginal sonography for the assessment of retained products of conception after spontaneous abortion. Gynecol Obstet Invest 1998; 45:190-3.
14. Kaakaji Y, Nghiem HV, Nodel C. Sonography of obstetric and gynecologic emergencies. AJR Am J Roentgenol 2000;174:641.
15. Moore L, Wilson SR. Ultrasonography in obstetric and gynecologic emergencies. Radiol Clin North Am 1994;32:1005.
16. Wong SF, Lam MO, Ho LC. Transvaginal sonography in the detection of retained products of conception after first-trimester spontaneous abortion. J Clin Ultrasound 2002; 30:428-32.
17. Achiron R, Goldenberg M, Lipitzs, Mashiach S. Transvaginal duplex Doppler sonography in bleeding patients suspected on having residual trophoblastic tissue. Obstet Gynecol 1993; 81:507-11.
18. Dillon EH, Case CQ, Ramos IM, Holland CK, Taylor KJW. Endovaginal ultrasound and Doppler findings after first-trimester abortion. Radiology 1993;186:87-91.
19. Tal J, Timor-Tritsch Y, Degani S. Accurate diagnosis of postabortial placental remanant by sonohysterography and color Doppler sonographic studies. Gynecol Obstet Invest 1997;43:131-4.
20. Alcázar JL, Ortiz CA. Transvaginal color Doppler ultrasonography in the management of first-trimester spontaneous abortion. Eu J Obstet Gynecol Reprod Bio 2002; 102:83-7.
21. Kos M, Kupesic, S Latin V. Diagnostics of spontaneous abortion. In Kurjak A (Ed): Ultrasound in Gynecology and Obstetrics. Zagreb: Art Studio Azinovic. 2000; pp 314-21.
22. Reccurent early pregnancy loss. In Speroff L, Glass R H, Kase NG. (Eds): Clinical Gynecologic Endocrinology and Infertility. London: Williams and Wilkins.1999; pp 1043-55
23. Windham GC, von Behren J, Fenster L, Schaefer C, Swan SH. Moderate maternal alcohol consumption and risk of spontaneous abortion. Epidemiology.1997; 8:509-14.
24. Donders GGG, Odds A, Veercken A, van Bulck B, Caudron J, Londers L, et al. Abnormal vaginal flora in the first trimester, but not full blown bacterial vaginosis, is associated with preterm birth. Prenat Neonat Med, 1998; 3: 558-93.
25. Kupesic S, Kurjak A, Chervenak F. Doppler studies of subchorionic hematomas in early pregnancy. In Chervenak F, Kurjak A, (Eds): Current Perspectives on the Fetus as a Patient. Carnforth, UK: Parthenon Publishing. 1996; 33-9.
26. Cowchock FS, Reece EA, Balaban D, Branch DW, Plouffe L. Repeated fetal losses associated with antiphospholipid antibodies: a collaborative randomized trial comparing prednizone with low-dose heparin treatment. Am J Obstet Gynecol 1992;166:1318-23.
27. Rai R, Cohen H, Dave M, Regan L. Randomized controlled trial of aspirin and aspirin plus heparin in pregnant women with recurrent miscarriage associated with phospholipid antibodies. Br Med 1997; 314, 253-7.
28. Kurjak A, Kupesic S. Doppler assessment of the intervillous blood flow in normal and abnormal early pregnancy. Ultrasound Obstet Gynecol 1997; 89:252-6.
29. Pellizari P, Pozzan C, Marchiori S, Zen T, Gangemi M. Assessment of uterine artery blood flow in normal first trimester pregnancies and those complicated by uterine bleeding. Ultrasound Obstet Gynecol 2002;19(4):366-70.
30. Acharya G, Morgan H. First-trimester, three-dimensional transvaginal ultrasound volumetry in normal pregnancies and spontaneous miscarriages. Ultrasound Obstet Gynecol 2002;19:575-9.
31. De Crepigni L. Early diagnosis of pregnancy failure with transvaginal sonography. Am J Obstet Gynecol 1988; 159-408.
32. Kurjak A, Kupesic S. Doppler Assessment of the intervillous blood flow in normal and abnormal early pregnancy. Ultrasound Obstet Gynecol 1997; 2:252-6.
33. Kurjak A, Schulman H, Kupesic S, Zudenigo D, Kos M, Goldenberg M. Subchorionic hematomas in early pregnancy: Clinical outcome and blood flow patterns. J Matern Fetal Med 1996;5: 41-4.
34. Kurjak A, Chervenak F, Zudenigo D, Kupesic S. Early pregnancy hemodynamics assessed by transvaginal color Doppler. In Chervenak F, Kurjak A (Eds): The Fetus as a Patient. Carnforth UK: Parthenon Publishing.1994; 435:55.
35. Jauniaux E, Gavril P, Nicolaides KH. Ultrasonographic assessment of early pregnancy complication. In Jurkovic D, Jauniaux E (Eds): Ultrasound and Early Pregnancy. Carnforth, UK: Parthenon Publishing. 1995; pp 53-64.
36. Kurjak A and Kupesic S. Blood flow studies in normal and abnormal pregnancy. In Kurjak A, Kupesic S (Eds): An Atlas of Transvaginal Color Doppler. London: Parthenon Publishing. 2000; pp 41-51.
37. Laurini, RN. Abruptio placentae: from early pregnancy to term. In Chervenak F, Kurjak A (Ed): The Fetus as a Patient. Carnforth UK: Parthenon Publishing. 1996; pp 433-44.
38. Mantoni M, Pedersen JF. Intrauterine hematoma: an ultrasound study of threatened abortion. Br J Obstet Gynecol 1981; 88:47-50.
39. Falco P, Milano V, Pilu G, David C, Grisolia G, Rizzo N, Bovicelli L. Sonography of pregnancies with first-trimester bleeding and viable embryo: a study of prognostic indicators by logistic regression analysis. Ultrasound Obstet Gynecol 1996;7: 65-9.
40. Kupesic S, Kurjak A. Physiology of uteroplacental and embryonic circulation. In Kurjak A (Ed): Textbook of Perinatal Medicine. Parthenon Publishing. 1998; 482-90.
41. Timor-Tritsch IE, Farine D, Rosen MG. A close look at the embryonic development with the high frequency transvaginal transducer. Am J Obstet Gynecol 1988;159:676-81.

42. de Crespigny LC, Cooper D, McKenna M. Early detection of intrauterine pregnancy with ultrasound. 1988; 10.

43. Fleischer AC, Kepple DM. Transvaginal sonography of Early intrauterine pregnancy. In Fleischer AC, Manning FA, Jeanty P, Romero R, (Eds): Sonography in Obstetrics and Gynecology Principles & Practice (sixth edition) The McGraw-Hill Companies. 2001; pp 61-88.

44. Bromley B, Harlow BL, Laboda LA, Benacerraf BR. Small sac size in the first trimester: a predictor of poor fetal outcome. Radiology.1991;178: 375-7.

45. Dickey RP, GasserR, Oltar TT, Taylor SN. Relationship of initial chorionic sac diameter to abortion and abortus karyotype based in new growth curves for the 16th to 49th postovulation day. Hum Reprod 1994; 9: 559-65.

46. Nyberg DA, Laing FC, Filly RA.Treatened abortion: sonographic distinction of normal and abnormal gestational sac. Radiology 1986;158:397-400.

47. Nyberg DA, Laing FC, Filly RA. Ultrasonographic differentiation of the gestational sac of early intrauterine pregnancy and pseudogestational sac of ectopic pregnancy. Radiology 1983;146:755-9.

48. Levi CS, Lyons EA, Lindsay DJ. Early diagnosis of normal pregnancy with transvaginal ultrasound. Radiology. 1988; 167: 383-5.

49. Nyberg DA, Mack LA, Laing FC, Patten RM. Distinguishing normal from abnormal gestational sac growth in early pregnancy. J Ultrasound Med 1987; 6:23-7.

50. Dillon EH, Feyock AL, Taylor KJW. Pseudogestational sacs: Doppler US differentiation from normal or abnormal intrauterine pregnancies. Radiology 1990;176:359-64.

51. Kurjak A, Zalud I, Predanic M, Kupesic S. Transvaginal and pulsed Doppler study of uterine blood flow in the first and early second trimesters of pregnancy: Normal versus abnormal. J Ultrasound Med 1994; 13:43-7.

52. Jaffe R, Warsof SL. Color Doppler imaging in the assessment of uteroplacental blood flow in the abnormal first trimester intrauterine pregnancies: an attempt to define etiologic mechanisms. J Ultrasound Med 1992; 11:41-4.

53. Benoit B, Hafner T, Bekavac I, Kurjak A.Three-dimensional sonoembryology. Ultrasound Rev Obstet Gynecol 2001;1:111-9.

54. Lindsay DJ, Lovett IS, Lyons EA. Endovaginal appearance of the yolk sac in pregnancy: normal growth and usefulness as a predictor of abnormal pregnancy. Radiology1992; 183, 115-8.

55. Kurjak A, Kupesic S, Kostovic LJ. Vascularization of yolk sac and vitteline duct in normal pregnancy studied by transvaginal color Doppler. J Perinat Med 1994; 22: 433-40.

56. Kurjak A, Kupesic S, Kos M, Latin V, Kos, Ma. Ultrasonic and Doppler studies of human yolk sac. In Chervenak F, Kurjak A (Eds): The Fetus as a Patient. Carnforth UK: Parthenon Publishing.1996; 345-7.

57. Jauniaux E, Moscoso JG. Morphology and significance of the human yolk sac. In Barnea E, (Ed): The First Twelve Weeks of Gestation. Heidelberg: Springer, 1992; pp192-216.

58. Lyons EA. Endovaginal sonography of the first trimester of pregnancy. Proceedings of the 3rd International Perinatal and Gyynecological Ultrasound Symposium Ottawa, Ontario; 1994;1-25.

59. Green JJ, Hobbins JC. Abdominal ultrasound examination of the first trimester fetus. Am J Obstet Gynecol 1988;159:165-75.

60. Kurjak A, Kupesic S. Parallel Doppler assessment of yolk sac and intervillous circulation in normal pregnancy and missed abortion. Placenta 1998;19:619-23.

61. Kurjak A, Kupesic S, Kos M. Early hemodynamics studied by transvaginal color Doppler. Prenatal and Neonatal Medicine 1996;1:38-49.

62. Harris RD, Vincent LM, Askin FB. Yolk sac calcification: a sonographic finding associated with intrauterine embryonic demise in the first trimester. Radiology 1988;166:109-16.

63. Merce LT, Barco MJ, Bau S. Color Doppler sonographic assessment of placental circulation in the first trimester of normal pregnancy. J Ultrasound Med 1996;15:135-42.

64. Valentin L, Sladkevicius P, Laurini R. Uteroplacental and luteal circulation in normal first-trimester pregnancies: Doppler ultrasonographic and morphologic study. Am J Obstet Gynecol 1996;174:768-75.

65. Kurjak A, Dudenhausen JW, Hafner T, et al. Intervillous circulation in all three trimesters of normal pregnancy assessed by color Doppler. J Perinat Med 1997;25:373-80.

66. Kurjak A, Kupesic S, Kos M. Three-dimensional sonography for assessment of morphology and vascularization of the fetus and placenta. J Soc Gynecol Investig 2002; 9:186-202.

67. Kurjak A, Kupesic S. Blood flow studies in early pregnancy. In Kurjak A, Kupesic S. (Eds): Color Doppler in Obstetrics, Gynecology and Infertility. Art Studio Azinovic-Medison Zagreb-Seoul 1999; 87-108.

68. Kuhn P, Brizot M, Pandya PP, Snijders RJ, Nicolaides KH. Crown-rump length in the chromosomally abnormal fetuses at 10th to 13th weeks of gestation. Am J Obstet Gynecol 1995;172:32-5.

69. Reljic, M. The significance of crown-rump length measurement for predicting adverse pregnancy outcome of threatened abortion. Ultrasound Obstet Gynecol 2001;17: 510-2.

70. Levi CS, Lyons EA, Zheng XH. Transvaginal US: demonstration of cardiac activity in embryos less than 5.0 mm in crown-rump length. Radiology 1990;176:71-74.

71. Pennell RG,Needelman L,Pajak T. Prospective comparison of vaginal and abdominal sonography in normal early pregnancy. J Ultrasound Med 1991; 10:63-7.

72. Laboda LA, Estroff JA, Benacerraf BR. First trimester bradycardia: a sign of impending fetal loss. J Ultrasound Med 1989;8:561-3.

73. Albayram F, Hamper UM. First-trimester obstetric emergencies: spectrum of sonographic findings. J Clin Ultrasound 2002; 3:161-77.

74. Benson CB, Doubilet PM. Slow embryonic heart rate in early first trimester: indicator of poor pregnancy outcome. Radiology 1994; 192:343.

75. Birnholz JC, Kent FB The embryo as a patient: early pregnancy loss. In Chervenak F, Kurjak A (Eds): The Fetus as a Patient. Carnforth UK: Parthenon Publishing.1996;345-7.

76. Doubilet PM, Benson CB, Chow JS. Long-term prognosis of pregnancies complicated by slow embryonic heart rates in early first trimester. J Ultrasound Med 1999; 18:537-541.

77. Laing FC, Frates MC. Ultrasound evaluation during the first trimester of pregnancy. In Callen PW (Ed): Ultrasound in Obstetrics and Gynecology 4th edition. Sunders Company. 2000; 105-45.

78. Horrow MM. Enlarged amniotic cavity: A new sonographic sign of early embryonic death. AJR Am J Roentgenol 1992;158:359-62.

79. McKenna KM, Feldstein VA, Goldstein RB, Filly RA. The "empty amnion": a sign of early pregnancy failure. J Ultrasound Med 1995;14:117-21.

80. Nicolaides KH, Azar G, Byrne D, Mansur C, Marks K. Fetal nuchal translucency screening for chromosomal defects in first trimester of pregnancy. Br Med J 1992; 034:867-69.

81. Pandya PP, Snijders RJM, Johnson SP, Brizot ML, Nicolaides KH. Screening for fetal trisomies by maternal age and fetal nuchal translucency thickness at 10th to 14th weeks of gestation. Br J Obstet Gynecol 1995; 102:957-62.

82. Pajkrt E, Bilardo CM, van Lith JMM. Nuchal translucency measurement in normal fetuses. Obstet Gynecol 1995; 86:994.

83. Braithwhite JM, Kadir RA, Economides DL. Nuchal translucency measurements: frequency distribution and changes with gestation in a general population. Br J Obstet Gynecol 1995;103:1201.

84. Taipale P, Hiilesma V, Salonen R, Ylostalo P. Increased nuchal translucency as a marker for fetal chromosomal defects. N Eng J Med 1997; 337:1654-8.

85. Monni G, Ibba RM, Zoppi MA. Antenatal screening for Down's syndrome. Lancet 1998;352:1631-2.

86. Zoppi MA, Ibba RM, Putzolu M, Floris M, Monni G. Nuchal translucency and the acceptance of invasive prenatal chromosomal diagnosis in women aged 35 and older. Obstet Gynecol 2001; 97:916-20.

87. Kurjak A, Kupesic S, Kosuta-Ivancevic M. Three-dimensional transvaginal ultrasound improves measurement of nuchal translucency. J Perinat Med 1999; 27:97-102.

88. Kurjak A, Matijevic R. Three-dimensional ultrasound markers of chromosomal anomalies. In Kurjak A, Kupesic S (Eds): Clinical Application of 3D Sonography. Parthenon Publishing London NY. 2000; 143-50.

89. Chung BL, Kim YP, Nam. Three-dimensional ultrasound for nuchal translucency measurement at 10-14 weeks of gestation. In Kurjak A, Kupesic S. (Eds): Clinical Application of 3D Sonography. Parthenon Publishing London NY. 2000;151-4.

90. Huisman TWA, Gittenberger-De Groot AC, Wladimiroff JW. Recognition of fetal subdiaphragmatic venous vestibulum essential for fetal venous Doppler assessment. Pediatr Res 1992; 32:338-41.

91. Edelstone DI. Regulation of blood flow through the ductus venosus. J Dev Physiol 1980;2:219-38.

92. Meyers RL, Paulick LP, Rudolph CD, Rudolph AM. Cardiovascular responses to acute, severe hemorrhage in fetal sheep. J Dev Physiol 1991;15:189-97.

93. Antolin E, Comas C, Carrera JM. Doppler velocimetry of the ductus venosus in the first trimester of pregnancy. In Kurjak A, Chervenak FA, Carrera JM (Eds): The Embryo as a Patient. Parthenon Publishing Group: New York London, 2001;181-85.

94. Hecher K, Campbell S, Snijders R, Nicolaides K. Reference ranges for fetal venous and atrioventricular blood flow parameters. Ultrasound Obstet Gynecol 1994;4:381-90.

95. Kiserud T, Eik-Nes SH, Hellevik LR, Blaas HG. Ductus venosus blood velocity changes in fetal cardiac diseases. J Matern Fetal Invest 1993;3:15-20.

96. Kiserud T, Eik-Nes SH, Blaas HG, Hellevik LR, Simensen B. Ductus venosus blood velocity and the umbilical circulation in seriously growth-retarded fetus. Ultrasound Obstet Gynecol 1994;4:109-14.

97. Hecher K, Campbell S, Doyle P, Harrington K, Nicolaides KH. Assessment of fetal compromise by Doppler ultrasound investigation on the fetal circulation. Arterial, intracardiac and venous blood flow velocity studies. Circulation 1995; 91:129-38.

98. Antolion E, Comas C, Torrents M, Munoz A, Figueras F, Echevarría M, et al. The role of ductus venosus blood flow assessment in screening for chromosomal abnormalities at 10th to 16th weeks of gestation. Ultrasound Obstet Gynecol 2001;17:295-300.

99. Montenegro N, Matias A, Areias JC, Castedo S, Barros H. Increased nuchal translucency: possible involvement of early cardiac failure. Ultrasound Obstet Gynecol 1997;10:265-8.

100. Huisman TWA and Bilardo CM. Transient increase in nuchal translucency thickness and reversed end-diastolic ductus venosus flow in a fetus with trisomy 18. Ultrasound Obstet Gynecol 1997;10:397-9.

101. DeVore GR, Horenstein J. Ductus venosus index: a new method for evaluating right ventricular preload in the second trimester fetus. Ultrasound Obstet Gynecol 1993;3:338-42.

102. Zoppi MA, Putzolu M, Ibba RM, Floris M, Monni G. First trimester ductus venosus velocimetry in relation to nuchal translucency thickness and fetal karyotype. Fetal Diagn Ther 2002;17:52-7.

103. Zoppi MA, Ibba RM, Putzolu M, Floris Marcella, Monni G. First trimester umbilical artery pulsatility index in fetuses presenting enlarged nuchal translucency. Prenat Diagn 2000; 20:701-4.

104. Borrell A, Martinez JM, Farre T, Azulay M, Cararach V, Fortuny A. Reversed end-diastolic flow in first trimester umbilical artery: An ominous new sign for fetal outcome. Am J Obstet Gynecol 2001;185:204-7.

105. Cicero, S. Curcio, Papageorghiou A, Sonek J, Nicolaides K. Absence of nasal bone in fetuses with trisomy 21 at 11th to 14th weeks of gestation: an observational study. Lancet 2001; 358(9294):1665-7.

106. Sonek J, Nicolaides K. Prenatal ultrasound diagnosis of nasal bone abnormalities in the three fetuses with Down syndrome. Am J Obstet Gynecol 2002;186:139-41.

107. Simpson JM, Sharland GK. Nuchal translucancy and congenital heart defects: Heart failure or not? Ultrasound Obstet Gynecol 2000; 16: 30-6.

108. Bronshtein M, Zimmer EZ. The sonographic approach to the detection of fetal cardiac anomalies in the early pregnancy. Ultrasound Obstet Gynecol 2002; 19: 360-5.

109. Ghezzi F, Raio L, di Naro E, Franchi M, Buttarelli M, Schneider H. First trimester umbilical cord diameter: a novel marker of fetal aneuploidy. Ultrasound Obstet Gynecol 2002;19:235-9.

110. Sabria J, Cabrero D, Bach C. Aneuploidy screening: ultrasound versus biochemistry. Ultrasound Rev Gynecol 2002; 2:221-8.

111. Wald NJ, Hacksaw AK. Combining ultrasound and biochemistry in first trimester screening for Down's syndrome. Prenat Diagn 1997;17:821-9.

112. De Graaf IM, Pajkrt E, Bilardo CM. Early pregnancy screening for fetal aneuploidy with serum markers and nuchal translucency. Prenat Diagn 1999; 19:458.62.

113. Spencer K, Souter V, Tul N. A screening program for trisomy 21 at 10th to 14th weeks using fetal nuchal translucency, maternal serum free ß-human chorionic gonadotropin and pregnancy-associated plasma protein- A. Ultrasound Obstet Gynecol 1999;13:231-7.

114. Spencer K, Ong C, Skentou H. Screening for trisomy 13 by fetal nuchal translucency, maternal serum free ß-HCG and PAPP-A at 10th to 14th weeks of gestation. Prenat Diagn 2000;20:411-16

115. Spencer K, Tul N, Nicolaides KH. Maternal serum free ß-HCG and PAPP- A in fetal sex chromosome defects in first trimester. Prenat Diagn 2000;20:390-4.

116. Comas C, Antolin E, Torrents M, Munoz A, Figueras F, Echevarria, et al. Early screening for chromosomal abnormalities: new strategies combining biochemical, sonographic and Doppler parameters. Prenat Neonat Med 2001; 6:95-102.

M Echevarria, JM Carrera,
M Torrents, C Millán

5

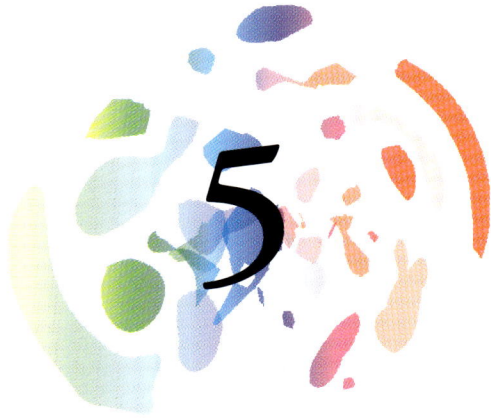

Ultrasonographic Detection of Aneuploidies

INTRODUCTION

The current implications of prenatal diagnosis on the public and society have been one of the reasons for obstetric techniques to evolve towards earlier and less aggressive methods. In this context, we assess the usefulness of ultrasonography and Doppler studies as markers of chromosomal defects in the first and second trimesters of gestation and, accordingly, their use as an early and noninvasive screening method for chromosome abnormalities in clinical practice. Several forceful arguments in favor of the indication of these procedures include the harmlessness of the method, the optimal cost/benefit ratio, the improved image resolution, better knowledge of embryological development, the chronological advance in the possibility of making a diagnosis and the high percentage of detection of chromosomal defects.

The importance of early ultrasound studies is related to the fact that early sonographic anomalies found in aneuploid fetuses are transient in about 50 percent of the cases and disappear spontaneously at more advanced gestational ages.

FIRST TRIMESTER

Increased fetal nuchal translucency (NT) (Figs 5.1 and 5.2) seems to be a well established ultrasonographic marker for aneuploidy screening, particularly when it is measured during the first trimester[1-5] (Fig. 5.3). Recently, Doppler parameters have been included in the fetal aneuploidy screening in order to improve the test performance. Increased impedance to flow in the umbilical artery[6-10] (Figs 5.4 and 5.5) and abnormal fetal heart rate[11-13] (Fig. 5.6) have been described as a potential marker of chromosomal abnormalities, although with variable results in

the literature. Scanty information is available about the venous circulation. Recent data suggest a relationship between early high resistance in the ductus venosus (DV) (Fig. 5.7) and aneuploidy[14-20] or cardiac defects.[21,22] Usually the resistance of DV is studied by means of evaluation of the ductus venosus pulsatility index for veins (DVPIV) (Fig. 5.8).

Table 5.1 summarizes the effectiveness of each single parameter as a marker for chromosomal abnormalities. Detection rate (DR) and specificity (S) chromosomal abnormalities are shown for each parameter. Results are displayed for the overall group and then broken down according to maternal age (<35 or 35 years), gestational age (10 to 13 weeks or 14 to 16 weeks) and type of chromosomal abnormality (main autosomal trisomies—trisomies 21, 18, 13—or other abnormalities). Using NT measurement, the overall DR was 68.8 percent for a S of 96 percent. NT effectiveness was better in the early gestational period (DR of 76%) and for predicting autosomal trisomies (DR of 90%), these differences being statistically significant (p<0.05). UAPI allowed an overall detection of about 21 percent with a 4 percent false-positive rate (FPR), also getting better in the earlier period (DR of 23%) and for lethal autosomal trisomies (DR of 40% for T18 and T13). FHR provided an overall detection of 15 percent, also getting better in the earlier period and for lethal autosomal trisomies (DR of 29% for T18 and T13), with a 4 percent FPR. Using the DVPIV, the overall DR was 70 percent with a S of 95 percent. Statistical parameters reflected an increase of effectiveness in the early gestational period and when predicting for autosomal trisomies, with a DR of 76 percent and 88 percent, respectively. We also evaluated the effectiveness of combined strategies for chromosomal abnormalities. Using NT and DVPIV,

Table 5.1: Effectiveness of individual parameters

	NT		UAPI		FHR		DVPIV		BR*	
	DR %	S %	DR %	S %	DR %	S %	DR %	S %	DR %	S %
Overall	68.8	96.0	21.4	96.4	14.7	96.1	70.4	95.3	66.7	91.8
MA<35y	67.7	96.2	19.2	96.2	10.9	96.5	71.4	95.3	50.0	92.9
35-37y	70.0	95.5	15.0	97.3	23.8	94.9	60.0	95.0	100	83.7
>37y	68.0	95.4	29.2	96.7	16.7	95.0	75.0	95.5	100	64.0
GA 10-13w	75.6	96.1	23.2	96.8	15.5	96.4	76.3	95.2	64.7	91.8
14-16w	51.6	95.9	17.2	95.8	12.9	95.5	56.3	95.3	100	92.0
T21,18,13	89.1	96.0	22.4	96.4	16.4	96.1	87.9	95.3	–	–
Others	40	96.0	20.0	96.4	12.2	96.1	42.9	95.3	–	–

DR: Detection rate
S: Specificity
Overall: Overall population
MA: Maternal age (in years)
GA: Gestational age (in weeks)
T (21,18,13): Trisomies 21, 18 and 13
Others: Other chromosomal abnormalities
*: Referred to trisomy 21

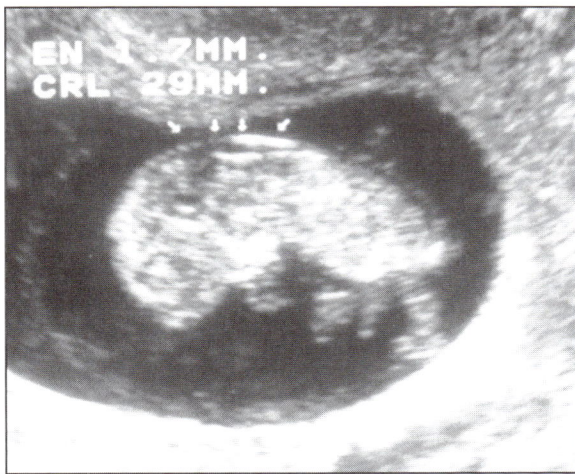

A

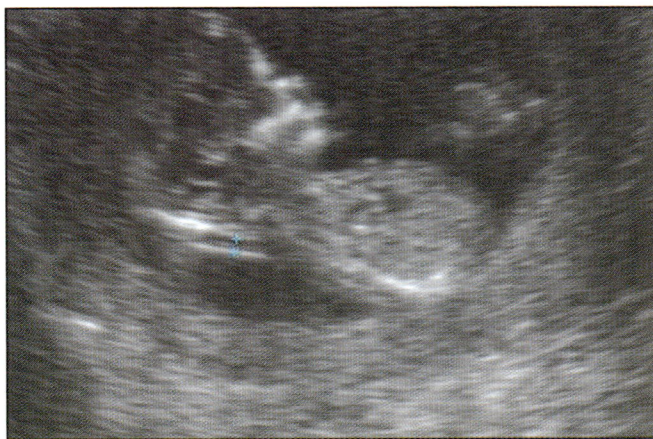

B

Figs 5.1A and B: Sagittal section of a (A) 10 weeks embryo and (B) 12 weeks fetus with normal nuchal translucency

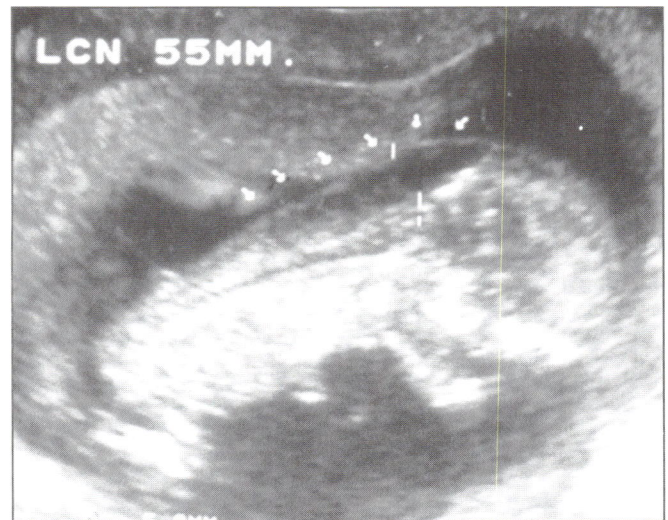

A

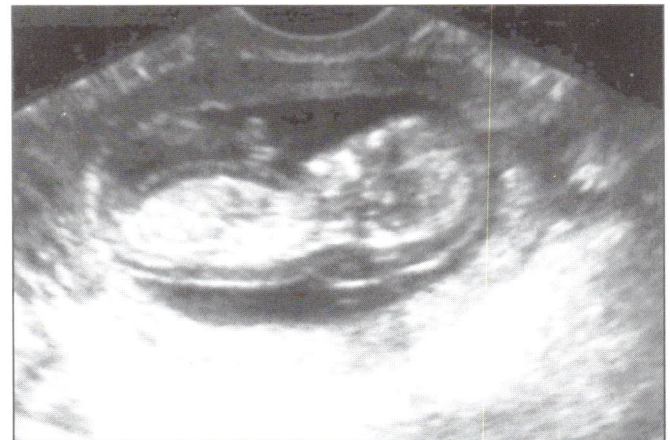

B

Figs 5.2A and B: Sagittal section of a (A) 11 weeks and (B) 12 weeks fetus with increased nuchal translucency

the DR was 44 percent with a S of 99.8 percent for all chromosomal abnormalities, while the DR increased to 71 percent for autosomal trisomies while maintaining the FPR. Combining simultaneously all sonographic and Doppler parameters and considering any abnormal result, we reached a DR of 99 percent with a S of 59 percent (64% under 35). In the trisomy 21 (T21) selected group, the effectiveness of different strategies were compared, especially between biochemical and sonographic screening. Finally, we compared the PPV of each marker. Under 35, we highlight the NT PPV (13%) and DVPIV PPV (10%), especially their combination (50%), in comparison with the low PPV of serum screening and the remaining Doppler parameters (3.8% for UAPI and 2.5% for FHR). Over 37, DVPIV

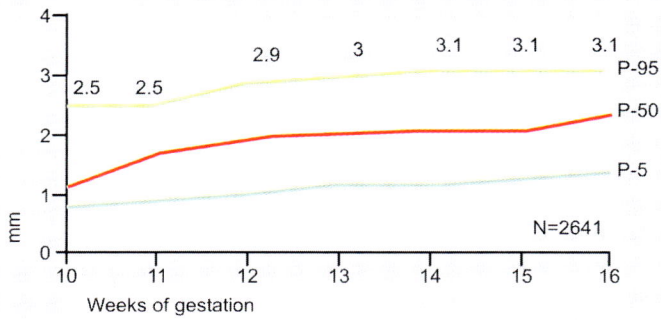

Fig. 5.3: Nuchal translucency: 10 to16 weeks

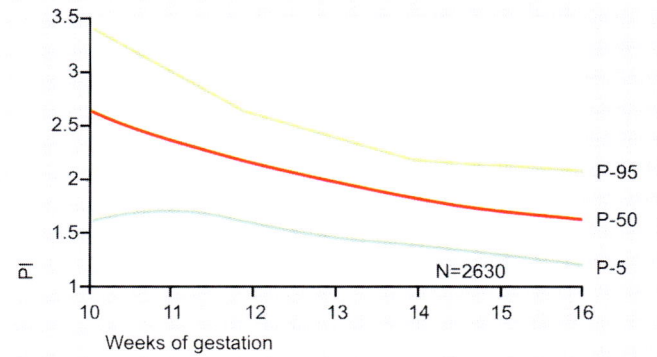

Fig. 5.5: Pulsatility index; umbilical artery: 10 to16 weeks

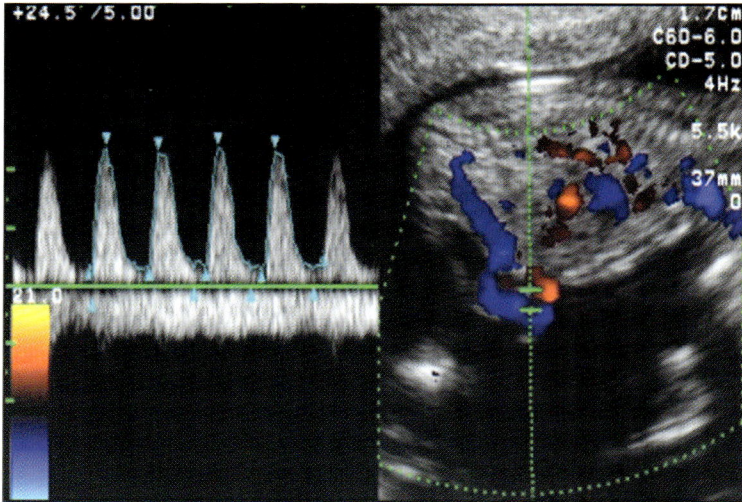

Fig. 5.6: Embryonic heart rate: 10 to16 weeks

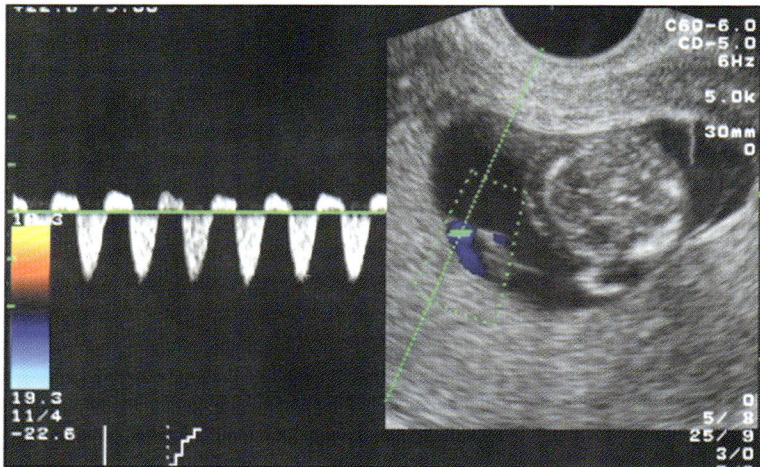

A

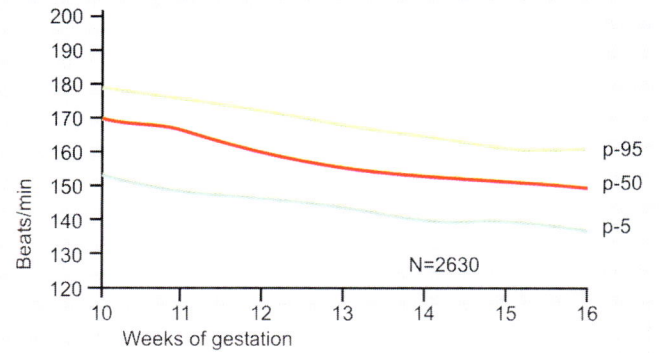

B

Figs 5.4A and B: Pulsed color Doppler of the umbilical artery, normal flow velocity waveform (A) and reversed end diastolic flow (REDF) (B)

yielded a PPV of 39 percent, followed by NT (32%), rising to 90 percent when combining both together. Serum screening had a PPV for T21 of 1.5 and 5.1 percent, under and over 35, respectively.

It is very important to make the measurement of NT with a standard method.[1] The main criteria are:

1. CRL between 45 and 84 mm.
2. Optimal gestational age: 11 to 13.6 weeks.
3. Sagittal section.

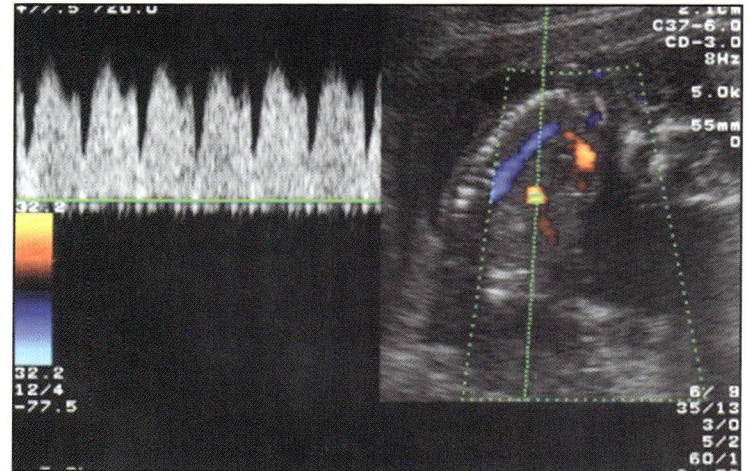

A

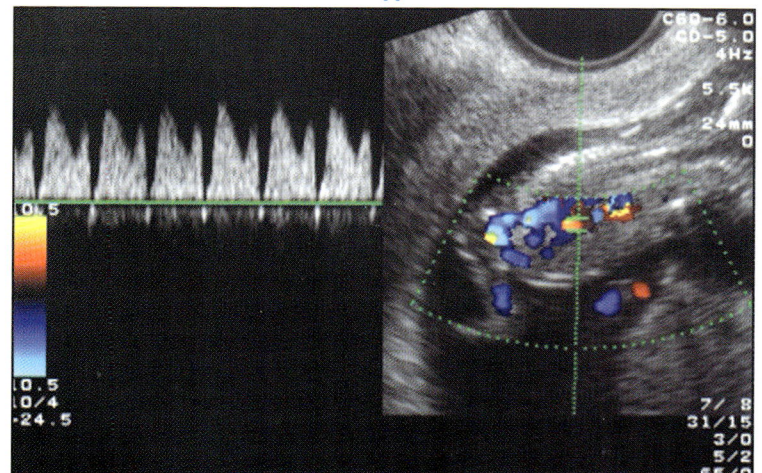

B

Figs 5.7A and B: Sagittal section of a 12 weeks fetus with a normal flow velocity waveform of the fetal ductus venosus (A) and abnormal a-wave (B)

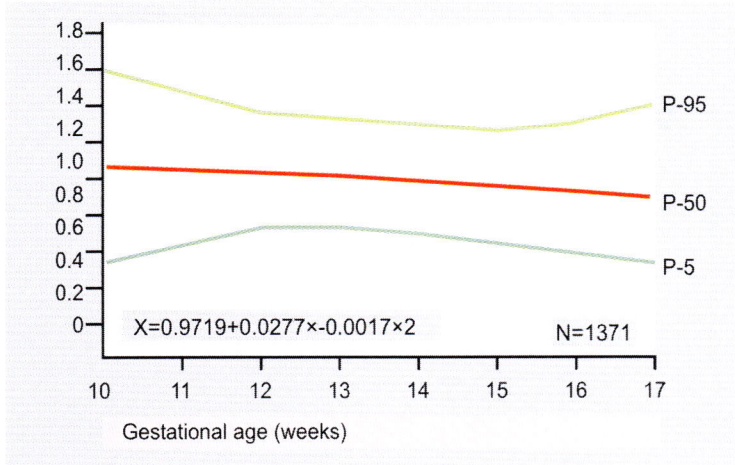

$$X = 0.9719 + 0.0277 \times -0.0017 \times 2 \qquad N = 1371$$

Fig. 5.8: Ductus venosus. Pulsatility index (PI)

4. Magnification: The fetus occupies at least three quarters of the image.
5. To distinguish between fetal skin and amnion.
6. Fetus in the neutral position.
7. Correct position of callipers: In-to-in.

For the measurement of pulsatility index of DV it is important to consider following aspects. It is necessary to locate the window of the Doppler probe in the distal portion of the umbilical venous sinus, in a mid-sagital view of the fetal body. Color Doppler identifying in this place one yellow or orange point due to aliasing phenomenon.

Contamination of the waveform with close venous structures should be avoided. Fetal quiescence is also important as well as that the insonation angle is less than 50 grades.

We summarize with the following conclusions:

1. Combined strategies which include independent parameters (biochemical, sonographic and Doppler) improve the test performance compared to individual screening programs.
2. Early screening programs for chromosomal abnormalities (10 to 13 weeks) are at least as effective as later strategies.
3. NT is the most sensitive and specific marker for autosomal trisomies, being the most powerful marker of aneuploidy under 35, in terms of PPV.
4. DVPIV is the most sensitive and specific marker for chromosomal abnormalities as a whole, being the most powerful marker of aneuploidy over 35, in terms of PPV.
5. UAPI and FHR are not effective single markers for chromosomal abnormalities. However, they may have a role in combined strategies, as markers of lethal autosomal trisomies.
6. The effectiveness of all sonographic and Doppler markers is higher than the earlier we make the measurements.

Three main aspects of early sonographic diagnosis of chromosome abnormalities are distinguished. These include indirect sonographic signs, detection of associated malformations and identification of sonographic markers.

FIRST AND SECOND TRIMESTERS

In the sonographic study of the second trimester of pregnancy, different methods have been proposed in order to make an overall assessment of a number of qualitative and quantitative sonographic parameters. The role of 3D and 4D sonography is discussed in detail in separate chapter in this book.

Indirect Signs

It has been traditionally considered that the presence of some indirect ultrasonographic signs of chromosomal defects would suggest the need for fetal cytogenetic studies. Although these signs are usually detected during the second half of pregnancy, some of them may be useful for early antenatal screening for aneuploidy.

Placental sonographic findings suggestive of polyploidy are usually found during the second half of gestation, although they have been recently documented at earlier stages. The paternal origin of the extra chromosome is responsible for degeneration of the placenta, with increased thickness and cystic images (from small and multiple sonolucent areas to a single cyst), and a tendency to increase in volume and echogenicity as pregnancy progresses.

The presence of a *single umbilical* artery (Fig. 5.9) is an ultrasound sign associated with a large number of syndromes, perinatal complications, intrauterine growth retardation and fetal malformations, accompanied by chromosomal defects in a variable percentage (between 12 and 47%) of cases. Its detection is facilitated by the use of transvaginal color Doppler. However, early assessment of this parameter is associated with a higher rate of false-positive results, so that it is recommended to confirm the diagnosis during the second half of pregnancy.

An *umbilical cord pseudocyst* has recently been associated with fetal chromosome abnormalities, particularly trisomies 18 and 13.[23-25] The indication of fetal cytogenetic studies is controversial when this is an early and single finding, since in cases of chromosomal defects it is usually associated with other signs, malformations, or ultrasound markers. Although in the series published in the literature,[23-25] umbilical cord pseudocyst is usually diagnosed during the second half of gestation, the use of transvaginal ultrasonography and color Doppler allows diagnosis at earlier stages.

Measurement of an *increased resistance index of the umbilical circulation is a warning sign*, usually reported in the second half

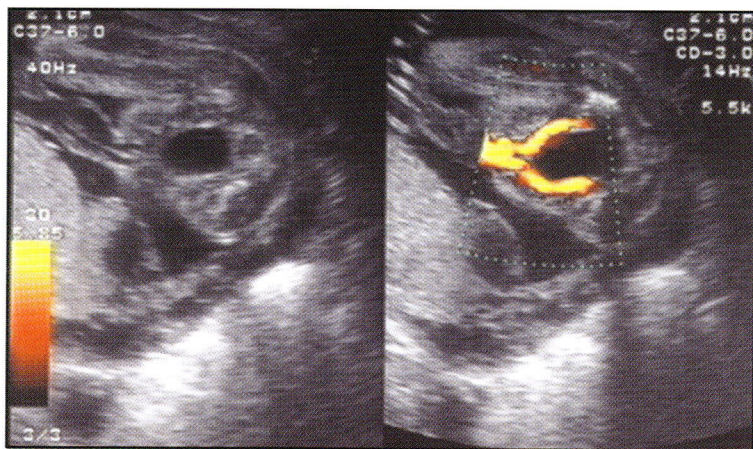

A

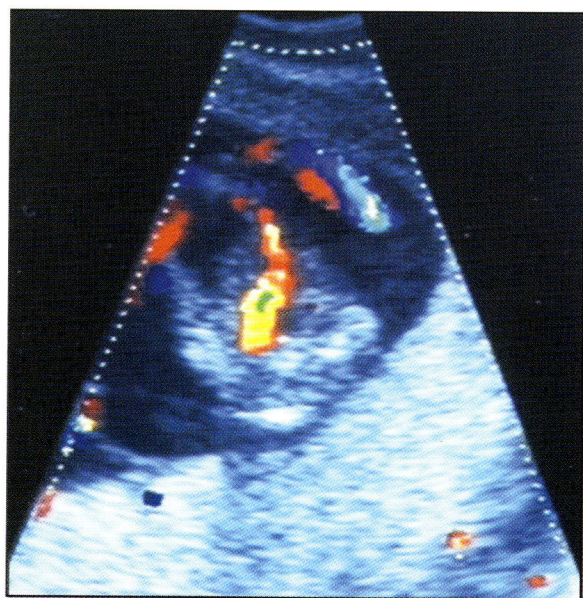

B

Figs 5.9A and B: (A) This represents a view of two umbilical arteries (orange) coursing around the fetal bladder by color Doppler ultrasound. (B) Another axial color Doppler scan at the level of the fetal bladder which is associated with single umbilical artery

of pregnancy, related to the appearance of perinatal complications and fetal chromosome abnormalities. The applicability of this finding for predicting aneuploidy and/or imminent fetal death at earlier stages of gestation has recently been reported.[6,8-10] Increased resistance to the umbilical-placental circulation has been suggested as a useful predictor of chromosomal defects, especially of autosomal trisomies in early pregnancy, although the predictive value of this parameter as a screening test in the general population remains to be evaluated.

Early detection of an *abnormal embryonic and/or fetal heart rate* pattern has been associated with spontaneous pregnancy failure, although in most studies the fetal karyotype was not analyzed. Abnormal heart rate activity has recently been associated with chromosome abnormalities, although the number of cases reported is small and results of the different series are not always consistent.[11-13]

Malformations

The association of fetal malformations detected in the second trimester of gestation and chromosome abnormalities is well documented. However, the clinical implications of the same congenital defects found in early pregnancy are uncertain and controversial. There are a large number of fetal malformations of which an early ultrasonographic diagnosis is not possible, because of the natural history of embryonic development. Accordingly, anatomical and physiological development of the embryo and the fetus throughout the gestational period should be taken into account in the assessment of fetal malformations, particularly when this evaluation is being performed in the context of the first trimester of pregnancy. Thus, some congenital anomalies are expressed late, because they develop as pregnancy progresses, requiring a certain silent period until detection. This group of malformations, including skull and face (cleft lip), neck (cystic hygromata) (Fig. 5.10), renal (obstructive uropathy), cardiac (myocardial hypertrophy), abdominal wall (exomphalos), intestinal (duodenal atresia) and central nervous system (hydrocephalus and haloprosencephaly) anomalies, constitute an important source of misdiagnoses. Some facial characteristics of the fetus (retrognathism, dysplasic ear), or characteristics of the hand (polydactily, clinodactily, overlapping index finger, sandal gap (Fig. 5.11), fifth finger hypoplasia, etc.) should rise suspicion of chromosomapaties. Other findings that have been related to trisomy are: pyelectasis (Fig. 5.12), megacystitis, reduction of the transversal diameter of the cerebellum, etc.

Currently there is no unanimous agreement on the value of every indicator. Some indicators appear very late in pregnancy and other don't provide statistical evidences of their profitability in low risk populations, even though they proved to be somewhat efficient in high risk populations.

Ultrasonographic Markers

During past years, different research groups have reported the presence of phenotypic sonographic features suggestive of chromosome abnormalities, named "sonographic markers". Although evidence provide by these findings is not sufficient to make the diagnosis of aneuploidy, they are useful for screening purposes. It has been shown that sonographic markers contribute to precise identification early in pregnancy of a group of high-risk women, independently of maternal age, family or personal history and results of biochemical tests. On the other hand, as a result of the clinical use of transvaginal ultrasonography, new subtle variations from normality are continuously added to the list of anatomical and/or biometrical anomalies indicative of aneuploidy. Since the overall incidence

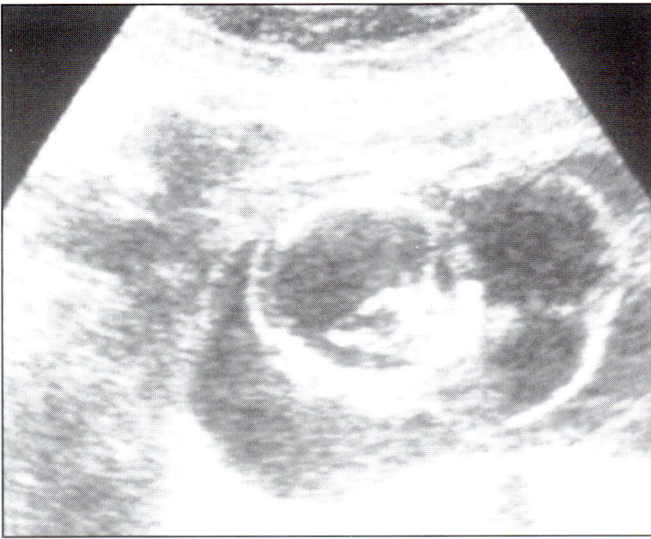

A

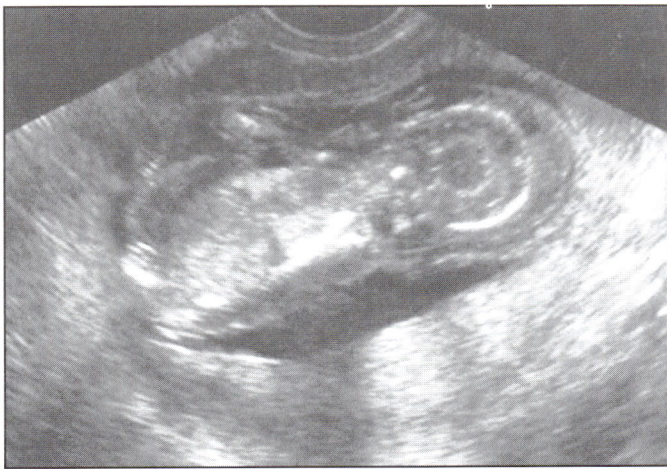

B

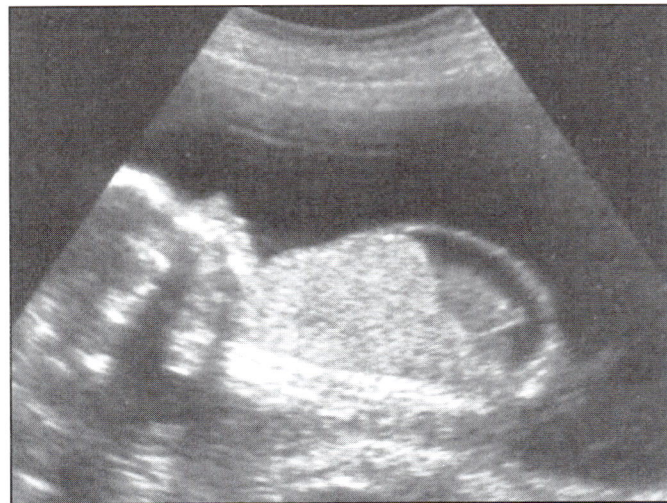

C

Figs 5.10A to C: Cystic hygroma, generalised edema and ascites (A to C)

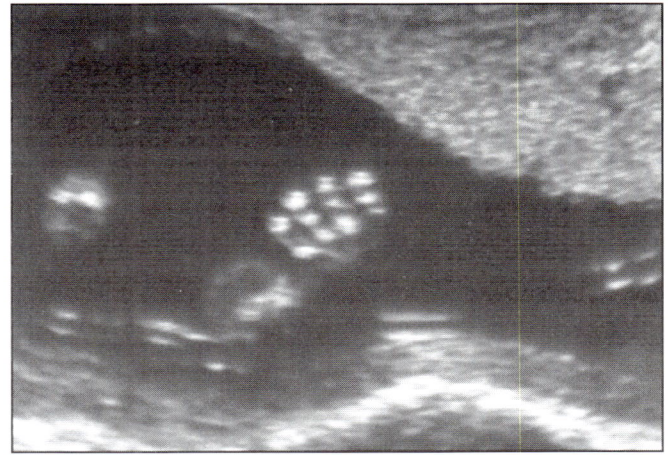

A

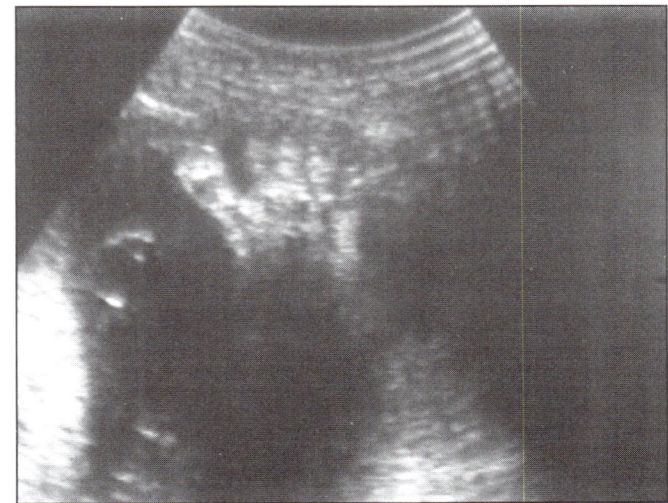

B

Figs 5.11A and B: (A) Mid-phalanx hypoplasia of the fifth finger; (B) Sandal gap

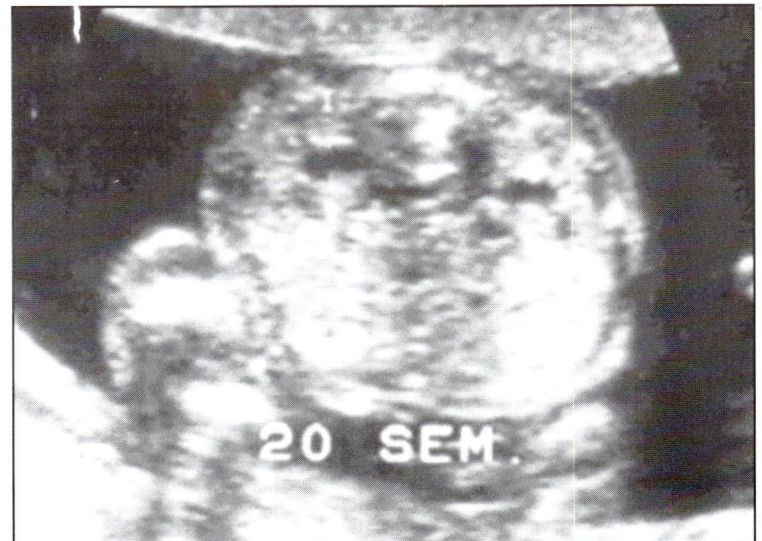

Fig. 5.12: Transverse sonogram of the fetal kidneys shows fluid-filled renal pelvis

of these markers is high, ranging between 1 and 5 percent, with a predictive value around 1 percent, their implications in terms of the couple's anxiety and costs should be re-evaluated.

Biometrical Markers

Some embryonic and fetal biometrical abnormalities associated with chromosomal defects are detectable early in the prenatal period (anomalies of yolk sac size, increase in the extraembryonic celom, reduction in the length of the umbilical cord) but others are usually diagnosed during the second half of pregnancy as a choroid plexus cysts (Fig. 5.13), although it is relevant if there are other anomalies.

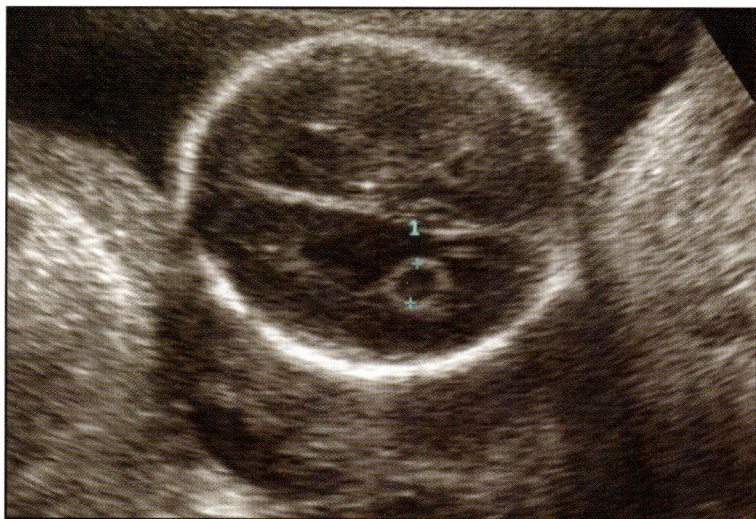

Fig. 5.13: Transverse axial sonogram of a fetus with choroid plexus cysts

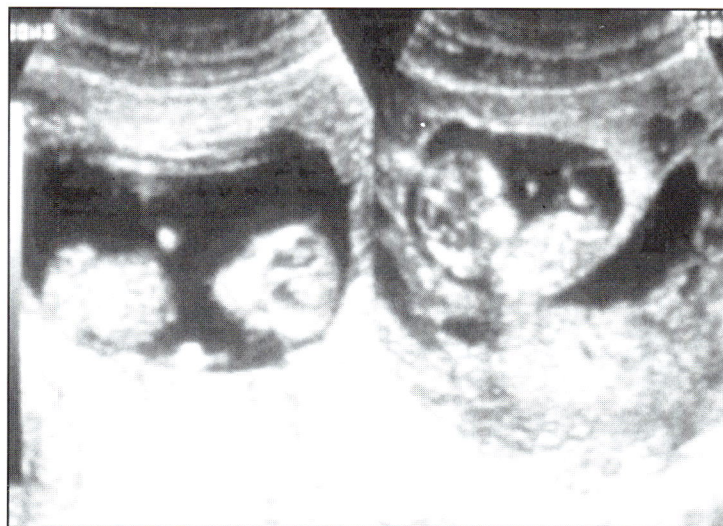

Fig. 5.14: Ultrasound appearance of dichorionic twins with early fetal growth restriction

Yolk sac size is a prognostic factor in the assessment of correct evolution of pregnancy, although the effectiveness of this marker is reduced by the large biological variation of its measurement. On the other hand, a *decrease in yolk sac size* has been suggested as an ultrasound marker of aneuploidy in relation to decreased maternal serum levels of α-fetoprotein in trisomic fetuses, although results are still inconclusive. [26,27] In addition, *increase in the extraembyonic celom* and *reduced length of the umbilical cord* have been reported as early screening markers of aneuploidy, but the usefulness of these findings is still controversial and further studies are needed to confirm their accuracy in clinical practice.[28]

Severe and symmetrical intrauterine growth retardation in the second trimester of pregnancy is an indication for karyotype analysis due to the incidence of aneuploidy in approximately 25 percent of fetuses (Fig. 5.14). The aneuploid placenta provides inadequate respiratory and nutritional support, which prevents normal embryofetal development. The impact of aneuploidy on fetal growth can be documented at earlier stages of gestation, probably due to the inherent effect of the chromosomal defect on cellular growth and proliferation, which is manifested by a reduction in the parameters defining embryonic growth. Measurement of the crown-rump length as evidence of early intrauterine growth impairment, and proportional to the degree of severity of the chromosomal defect, has been proposed as an early ultrasound sign for the detection of aneuploidies.[29-32] In fact, crown-rump length is a sensitive parameter for the prediction of embryonic death, risk of fetal malformations and chromosome anomalies.

Also other parameters as *short femur* indicated the presence of aneuploidies.

Nuchal Markers

Ultrasound markers related to abnormal fluid accumulation in the nuchal fold are very useful in the early prenatal screening of aneuploidies and merit special consideration. Thickening of the nuchal fold in the second trimester of gestation as a sonographic marker of trisomy 21 was initially suggested by Szabo and Gellen in 1990.[33] The usefulness of this sign was subsequently confirmed by these authors[28,33] and others,[1,2,4,34-36] although there is no consensus in the current literature regarding its predictive value. In general, nuchal translucency of ≤ 3 mm between 10 and 14 weeks has a sensitivity of 28 to 100 percent and a specificity of 48 to 99 percent in the diagnosis of trisomy 21. At present, however, it seems more appropriate to use a variable cut-off value in relation to gestational age, usually the 95 centile of the normal curve, instead of a predetermined fixed cut-off point. The effectiveness of this parameter in the overall screening of common autosomal trisomies (trisomies 18, 21 and 13) and less common disorders (trisomy 10), sex-linked chromosomal defects and polyploidies has been demonstrated.[1,4,13,26,34-38]

Absent Nasal Bone

About two-thirds of fetuses with trisomy 21 show an absent nasal bone (Fig. 5.15), and this anomaly is recognizable by ultrasonography in first and second trimester of gestation.

Other Markers

This group includes a series of ultrasound markers that cannot be classified into the aforementioned categories and that are mostly reported in the second half of pregnancy, although some of them may be useful at earlier stages.

The increase in the *echogenicity of the yolk sac* has recently been reported as an early ultrasound marker of trisomy 21, although data are still preliminary. *Ventricular echogenic foci* (Fig. 5.16) have been associated with cardiac tumors and chromosomal defects, although in most cases this is a benign

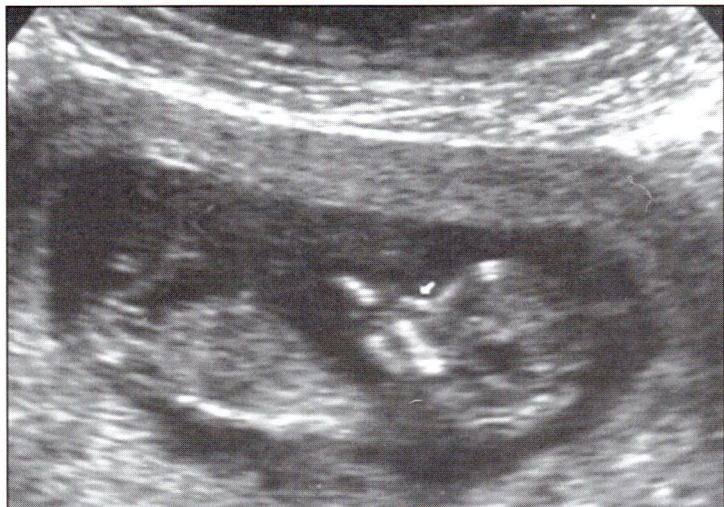

A

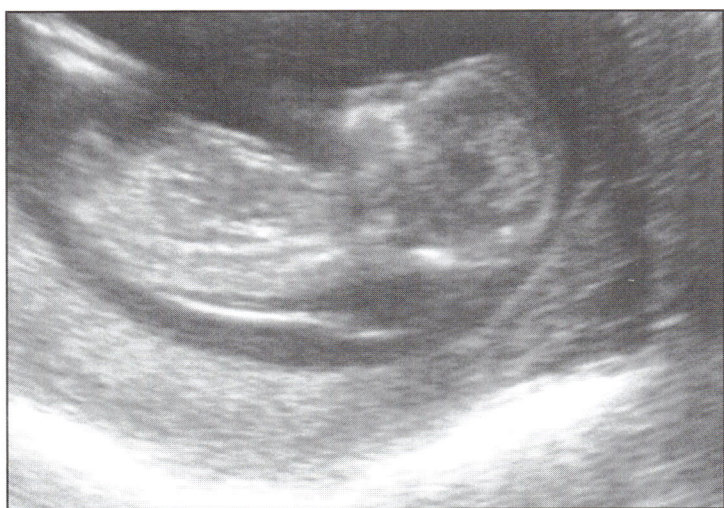

B

Figs 5.15A and B: Sagittal section of a 12 weeks fetus with present nasal bone (A) and a 12 weeks fetus with absent nasal bone (B)

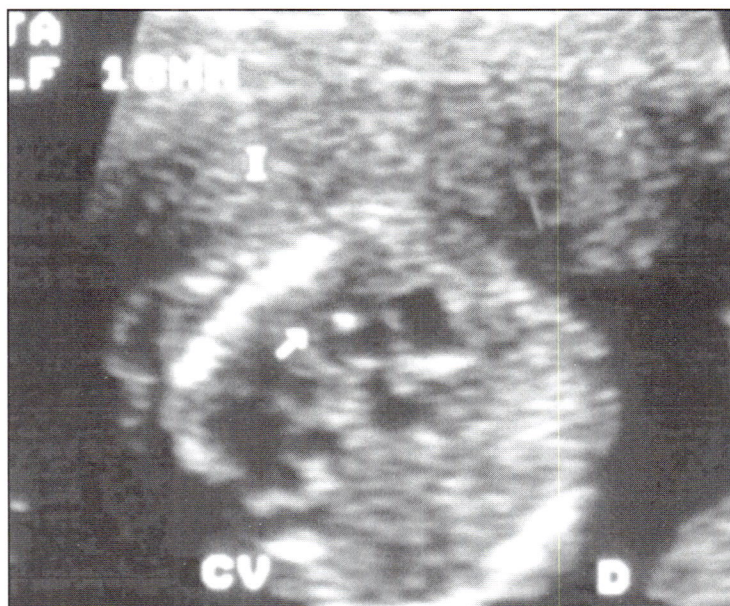

Fig. 5.16: Four chamber view of the heart with a cardiac echogenic foci in the left ventricle

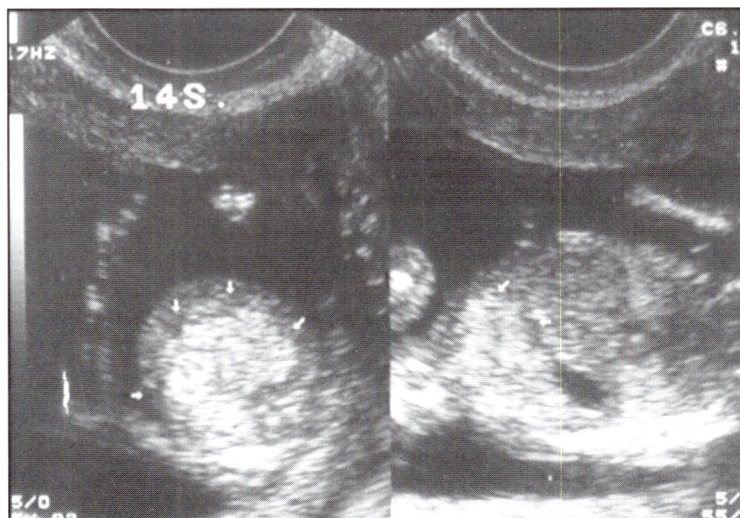

A

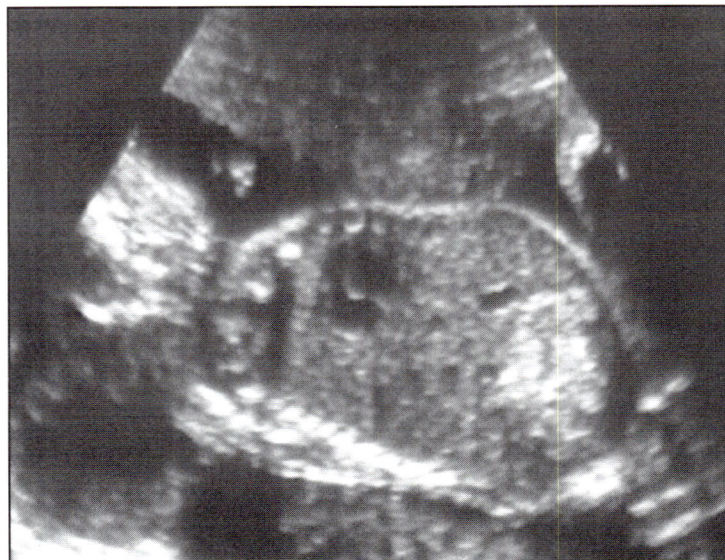

B

Figs 5.17A and B: Transverse and sagital section of a fetus with echogenic bowel (A and B)

sign, detected late and secondary to a variation from normality in the development of papillary muscles and chordae tendineae. *Bilateral ectasia* of the renal pelvis can be used as an additional sign in the ultrasound screening for trisomy 21. *Hyperechogenicity in the hemiabdomen* (Fig. 5.17) is associated with a significant increase in the risk of aneuploidy, although it can be attributed to other clinical conditions and may be a finding present in euploid fetuses or those of high perinatal risk. The usefulness of this observation has been mostly defined in the second trimester of pregnancy, but recent studies support its value as an early sign of trisomy 21.

REFERENCES

1. Nicolaides KH, Azar G, Byrne D, Mansur C, Marks K. Fetal nuchal translucency; ultrasound screening for chromosomal defects in first trimester of pregnancy. BMJ 1992;304:867-9.
2. Pandya PP, Kondylios A, Hilbert L, Snijders RJM, Nicolaides KH. Chromosomal defects and outcome in 1015 fetuses with increased nuchal translucency. Ultrasound Obstet Ginecol 1995;5:15-9.
3. Pandya PP, Snijders RJM, Johnson SP, Brizot ML, Nicolaides KH. Screening for fetal trisomies by maternal age and fetal nuchal translucency thickness at 10 to 14 weeks of gestation. Br J Obstet Gynaecol 1995;102:957-62.

4. Comas C, Martinez JM, Ojuel J, Casals E, Puerto E, Borrell A, Fortuny A. First-trimester nuchal edema as a marker of aneuploidy. Ultrasound Obstet Gynecol 1995;5:26-9.

5. Ville Y, Lalondrelle, Doumerc S, Daffos F, Frydman R, Oury JF, Dumez Y. First-trimester diagnosis of nuchal anomalies: significance and fetal outcome. Ultrasound Obstet Gynecol 1992;2:314-6.

6. Martinez JM, Comas C, Ojuel J, Puerto B, Borrell A, Fortuny A. Umbilical artery pulsatility index in early pregnancies with chromosome anomalies. Br J Obstet Gynaecol 1996;103:330-4.

7. Brown R, Di Luzio L, Gomes C, Nicolaides KH. The umbilical artery pulsatility index in the first trimester: is there an association with increased nuchal translucency or chromosomal abnormality? Ultrasound Obstet Gynecol 1998;12:244-7.

8. Martinez JM, Borrell A, Antolin E, Puerto B, Casals E, Ojuel J, Fortuny A. Combining nuchal translucency with umbilical Doppler velocimetry for detecting fetal chromosomal abnormalities. Br J Obstet Gynecol 1997;104:11-4.

9. Montenegro N, Beires J, Pereira Leite L. Reverse end diastolic umbilical artery blood flow at 11 weeks' gestation. Ultrasound Obstet Gynecol 1995;5:141-2.

10. Martinez JM, Comas C, Borrell A, Puerto B, Antolin E, Ojuel J, Fortuny A. Reversed end-diastolic umbilical artery velocity in two cases of trisomy 18 at 10 weeks' gestation. Ultrasound Obstet Gynecol 1996;7:447-9.

11. Jauniaux E, Gavrill P, Khun P, Kurdi W, Hyett J, Nicolaides KH. Fetal heart rate and umbilicoplacental Doppler flow velocity waveforms in early pregnancies with a chromosomal abnormality and/or increased nuchal translucency thickness. Hum Reprod 1996;11:435-9.

12. Hyett JA, Noble PL, Sinjders RJM, Montenegro N, Nicolaides KH. Fetal heart rate in trisomy 21 and other chromosomal abnormalities at 10-14 weeks of gestation. Ultrasound Obstet Gynecol 1996;7:239-44.

13. Martinez JM, Comas C, Ojuel P, Puerto B, Borrell A, Fortuny A. Fetal heart rate patterns in pregnancies with chromosomal disorders or subsequent fetal loss. Obstet Gynecol 1996;87:118-21.

14. Montenegro N, Matias A, Areias JC, Castedo S, Barros H. Increased nuchal translucency: possible involvement of early cardiac failure. Ultrasound Obstet Gynecol 1997;10:265-8.

15. Matias A, Montenegro N, Areias JC, Brandao O. Anomalous fetal venous return associated with major chromosomopathies in late first trimester of pregnancy. Ultrasound Obstet Gynecol 1998;11:209-13.

16. Borrell A, Antolin E, Costa D, Farre T, Martinez JM, Fortuny A. Abnormal ductus venosus blood flow in trisomy 21 fetuses during early pregnancy. Am J Obstet Gynecol 1998;179:1612-7.

17. Matias A, Gomes C, Flack N, Montenegro N, Nicolaides KH. Screening for chromosomal abnormalities at 10-14 weeks: the role of ductus venosus blood flow. Ultrasound Obstet Gynecol 1998;12:380-4.

18. Huisman TWA, Bilardo CM. Transient increase in nuchal translucency thickness and reversed end-diastolic ductus venosus flow in a fetus with trisomy 18. Ultrasound Obstet Gynecol 1997;10:397-9.

19. Antolin E, Comas C, Torrents M, Munoz A, Figueras F, Echevarria M, et al. The role of ductus venosus blood flow assessment in screening for chromosomal abnormalities at 10-16 weeks of gestation. Ultrasound Obstet Gynecol 2001;17:295-300.

20. Comas C, Antolin E, Torrents M, Munoz A, Figueras F, Echevarria M, et al. Early screening for chromosomal abnormalities: new strategies combining biochemical, sonographic and Doppler parameters. Prenat Neonat Med 2001;6:95-102.

21. Matias A, Huggon I, Areias JC, Montenegro N, Nicolaides KH. Cardiac defects in chromosomally normal fetuses with abnormal ductus venosus blood flow at 10-14 weeks. Ultrasound Obstet Gynecol 1999;14:307-10.

22. Bilardo CM, Müller MA, Zikulnig L, Schipper M, Hecher K. Ductus venosus studies in fetuses at high risk for chromosomal or heart abnormalities: relationship with nuchal translucency measurement and fetal outcome. Ultrasound Obstet Gynecol 2001;17:288-94.

23. Sepulveda W, Pryde PG, Greb AE, Romero R, Evans MI. Prenatal diagnosis of umbilical cord pseudocyst. Ultrasound Obstet Gynecol 1994;4:147-50.

24. Jauniaux E, Donner C, Thomas C, Francotte J, Rodesh F, Avni FE. Umbilical cord pseudocyst in trisomy 18. Prenat Diagn 1988;8:557-63.

25. Rizzo G, Arduini D. Umbilical cord pseudocyst in trisomy 13. Ultrasound Obstet Gynecol 1994;4:438.

26. Comas C, Martinez JM, Puerto B, et al. Estudio ecografico transvaginal en el primer trimestre de la gestacion. Valorpredictivo de los marcadores ecograficos en el diagnostico prenatal de aneuploidias. Resultados preliminares. Prog Diagn Prenatal 1994;6:225-35.

27. Wathen NC, Cass PL, Campbell DJ, Wald N, Chard T. Alpha-fetoprotein levels and yolk sac size in the first trimester of pregnancy. Prenat Diagn 1992;12:649-52.

28. Szabo J, Gellen J, Szemere G. Nuchal edema as an ultrasonic sign of trisomy 21 during the first trimester of pregnancy (Letter). Orv Hetil 1992;133:3167-8.

29. Drugan A, Johnson MP, Isada NB, et al. The smaller than expected first-trimester fetus is at increased risk for chromosome anomalies. Am J Obstet Gynecol 1992;167:1525-8.

30. Benacerraf BR. Intrauterine growth retardation in the first trimester associated with triploidy. J Ultrasound Med 1988;7:153-4.

31. Pedersen JF, Molsted-Pedersen L. Early fetal growth delay detected by ultrasound marks increased risk of congenital malformation in diabetic pregnancy. Br Med J 1981;283:269-71.

32. Pedersen JF. Ultrasound studies on fetal crown-rump length in early normal and diabetic pregnancies. Dan Med Bull 1986;33:296-304.

33. Szabo J, Gellen J. Nuchal fluid accumulation in trisomy 21 detected by vaginosonography in the first trimester. Lancet 1990;3:1133.

34. Brun JL, Saura R, Horovitz J, et al. First trimester diagnosis of fetal nuchal edema. Report of 29 cases. Fetal Diagn Ther 1994;9:246-51.

35. Schulte-Vallentin M, Schindler H. Non-echogenic nuchal oedema as a marker of aneuploidy. Ultrasound Obstet Gynecol 1995;5:26-9.

36. Brambati B, Cislaghi C, Tului L, et al. First-trimester Down's syndrome screening using nuchal translucency : a prospective study in patients undergoing chorionic villus sampling. Ultrasound Obstet Gynecol 1995;5:9-14.

37. Pandya PP, Goldberg H, Walton B, et al. The implementation of first-trimester scanning at 10-13 weeks' gestation and the measurement of fetal nuchal translucency thickness in two maternity units. Ultrasound Obstet Gynecol 1995;5:20-5.

38. Savoldelli G, Binkert F, Achermann J, Schmid W. Ultrasound screening for chromosomal anomalies in the first trimester of pregnancy. Prenat Diagn 1993;13:513-8.

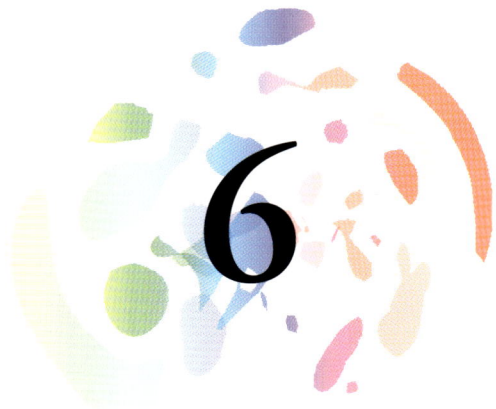

**N Maiz, JM Carrera,
MA Rodriguez, M Ruiz**

6

Fetal Growth:
Ultrasound Biometry

INTRODUCTION

"Growth" is usually defined as the process whereby the body mass of a living being increases in size as a result of the increase in number (hyperplasia) and size (hypertrophy) of its cells and intracellular matrix. "Development", on the other hand, should be understood as the process by which organs and their regulatory mechanisms gradually assume their functions in living beings. Broadly speaking, the term "growth" is preferred when referring to measurable anatomical changes; "development" is used to refer to the gradual acquisition of certain specific physiological functions.

The fetal growth rate is mainly determined by the intrinsic potential of fetal growth, which is primarily genetically controlled ("genetic factor"). However, the influence of this genetic factor is considerably modified by two other intrauterine regulating factors of fetal growth, the "hormone factor", fetal and growth promoting, and the "environmental factor," maternal and usually growth restraining.

BASIC PRINCIPLES

Fetal anthropometry is based on the biometric assessment of different fetal parameters according to which the clinical course of fetal growth can be studied. At present, ultrasonography is the only suitable technique for in utero evaluation of fetal anthropometry. Ultrasound scanning permits an accurate estimation to be made of dimensions of different body segments, long bones and particular organs. The availability of normal growth curves and tables for all these structures facilitates, for a properly trained echographer, the follow-up of fetal growth throughout the gestational period as well as the diagnosis of either excessive or defective pathological changes in fetal growth.

Curves or tables used should be appropriate for the studied population (Fig. 6.1) and as far as possible derived from a longitudinal rather than from a cross-sectional study.

ULTRASOUND FOR ASSESSMENT OF GESTATIONAL AGE

In order to perform a correct fetal ultrasound biometric study, a fundamental aspect is to know the gestational age as exactly as possible. Early ultrasound examination carried out during the first trimester of pregnancy permits determination of gestational age with remarkable precision on the basis of gestational sac, but especially by assessing the crown-rump length (CRL).

The CRL is a particularly sensitive biometric parameter that can be measured in the early stages of gestation.[1] The only technical limitation is the progressive bending of the embryo, which makes measurements less reliable after weeks 10 to12 of gestation. Between weeks 6 and 12 of gestation, there is an exponential increase in CRL, although this increase later appears to be linear (Fig. 6.2). A rough error at early stages consists of adding yolk sac diameter to CRL. The maximum error obtained when calculating this parameter with respect to gestational age is +/- 5 days in 95 percent of cases, because between weeks 6 and 14 fetal growth is rapid and the limits of confidence are very narrow. According to this parameter it would be possible to establish an early assessment of abnormal embryonic growth. CRL can be measured from week 6 of gestation with the use of transvaginal transducers and from week 7 of gestation using transabdominal transducers.

As shown in Table 6.1, there are no significant differences when results obtained by different authors using either transabdominal or transvaginal transducers are compared.[1-4]

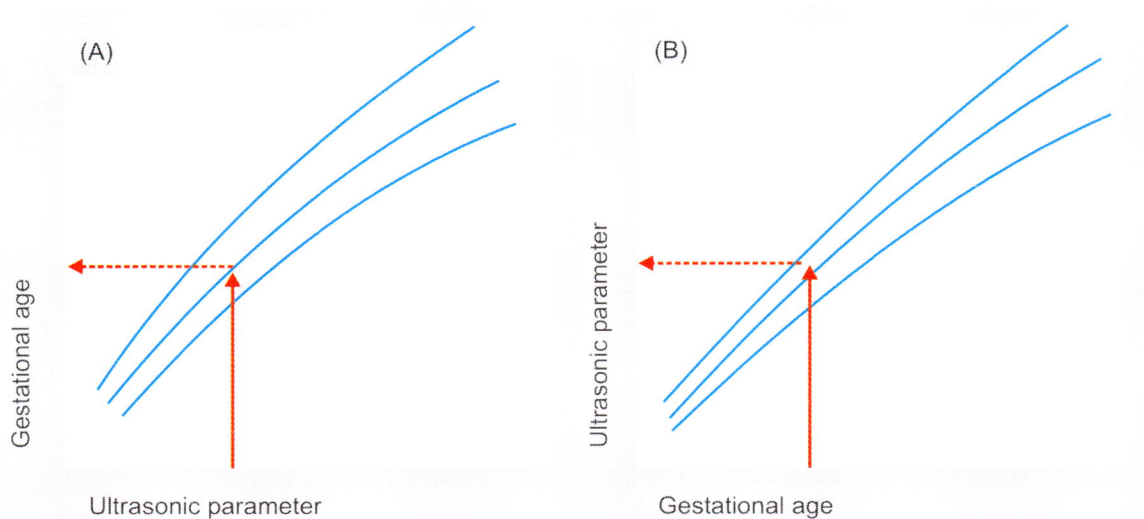

Fig. 6.1: With curve (A) the gestational age can be deduced from an independent variable (utrasonic parameter), but if the aim is to study fetal growth, the appropriate curve is (B), where the independent variable is gestational age

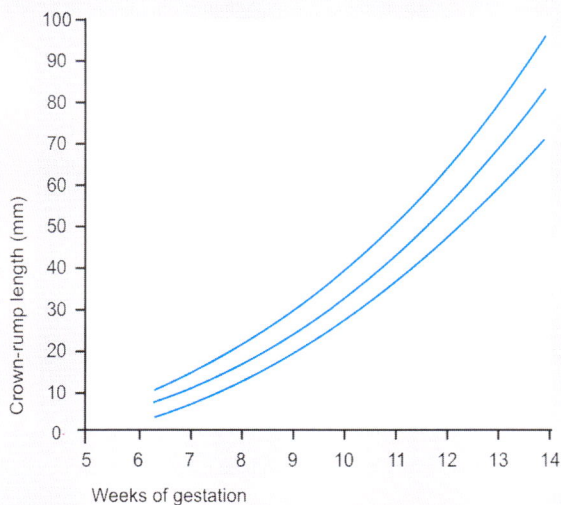

Fig. 6.2: Fetal crown-rump length against gestational age

Table 6.1: Assessment of gestational age from crown-rump length (CRL). There were no significant differences when results obtained by different authors using either transabdominal or transvaginal transducers were compared

CRL (mm)	Gestational age (weeks)			
	Robinson[1] (transabdominal)	Nelson[2] (transabdominal)	Drumm et al[3] (transabdominal)	Hadlock et al[4] (transvaginal)
10	7.0	8.1	6.9	7.1
12	7.4	8.3	7.3	7.4
14	7.7	8.5	7.6	7.7
16	8.0	8.6	7.9	8.0
18	8.3	8.8	8.2	8.3
20	8.5	9.0	8.5	8.6
22	8.8	9.2	8.7	8.9
24	9.0	9.3	9.0	9.1
26	9.3	9.5	9.2	9.4
28	9.5	9.7	9.5	9.6
30	9.7	9.9	9.7	9.9
32	9.9	10.0	9.9	10.1
34	10.0	10.2	10.1	10.3
36	10.3	10.4	10.4	10.5
38	10.5	10.5	10.6	10.7
40	10.7	10.7	10.8	10.9
42	10.8	10.9	11.0	11.1
44	11.0	11.1	11.2	11.2
46	11.2	11.2	11.3	11.4
48	11.4	11.4	11.5	11.6
50	11.5	11.6	11.7	11.7
52	11.7	11.7	11.9	11.9
54	11.8	11.9	12.1	12.0
56	12.0	12.1	12.2	12.2
58	12.1	12.3	12.4	12.3
60	12.3	12.4	12.6	12.5
62	12.4	12.6	12.7	12.6
64	12.6	12.8	12.9	12.8
66	12.7	12.9	13.0	12.9
68	12.9	13.1	13.2	13.1
70	13.0	13.3	13.4	13.2
72	13.1	13.5	13.5	13.4
74	13.3	13.6	13.7	13.5
76	13.4	13.8	13.8	13.7
78	13.5	14.0	14.0	13.8
80	13.7	14.1	14.1	14.00

Most authors have not found statistically significant differences according to race or gender[5,6] except for the series of Pedersen,[7] who reported a significantly larger CRL in male fetuses than in females (mean value of gender difference: 2 mm).

FETAL ULTRASOUND BIOMETRY FOR EVALUATING FETAL GROWTH

Accurate surveillance of fetal growth is the most important task of antenatal care. Timely detection of growth abnormalities is a challenge at the best of times but even more so in multicultural population.[8] It is well known that there are ethnic differences in fetal growth among populations. A number of studies have described ethnic differences in birth weight.[9-13]

With recent advances in ultrasound imaging, especially improvements in resolution and focusing, fetal intracranial, intrathoracic, and intra-abdominal organs can now be clearly identified.[14] Numerous reports on fetal organ measurements such as liver, spleen, and adrenal gland have been presented.[15-18]

Recent technical development of 3D ultrasound machine has led to a self-contained imaging system that can both produce conventional 2D images and generate within seconds a high-quality 3D image without a need for an external work-station or other additional, costly equipment.

This chapter presents the state-of-the-art on fetal growth and biometry with the use of conventional 2D and 3D ultrasonography.

The assessment of fetal growth is an integral part of obstetric management, because fetuses that do not grow properly have a higher mortality rate, usually show a variety of problems in the perinatal period and are at high risk for long-term neurological problems. The clinical methods of assessing fetal size and growth—maternal weight gain, fundal height, abdominal circumference—are relatively imprecise, whereas the measurements of an image of the fetus obtained by ultrasound have been demonstrated to have a better capacity to detect abnormalities in fetal growth.[19]

We focus, for the most used parameters, on technical aspects and possible errors in measurements, deriving the data from a review of the literature.

Head Size

A series of scans should be performed to find the long axis of the fetus. The probe should then be rotated through 90° to this axis, and angled so that the beam is along a transverse plane through the fetal head.[20] A series of parallel sections should be obtained in order to identify the following landmarks (Fig. 6.3):

1. Short midline;
2. Cavum septum pellucidum;
3. Thalami;
4. Basal cisternae.

Inclusion of all four features means that the section includes both biparietal diameter (BPD) and occipitofrontal diameter (OFD) and can also be used to measure head circumference (HC).

Having identified an appropriate section, measurements are made on a frozen image. For BPD, measurement is made from the leading edge of the echo from the proximal skull surface to the leading edge of the echo from the distal skull surface "outer to outer". Other authors use "outer to inner", "inner to outer" or "middle to middle" measurement according to the positioning of electronic calipers with respect to the skull (Fig. 6.4). It is important always to measure in the same fashion, comparing the results with curves obtained using the same method of measurement in order to avoid errors in over- or underestimations (up to 3 to 4% of obtained values).

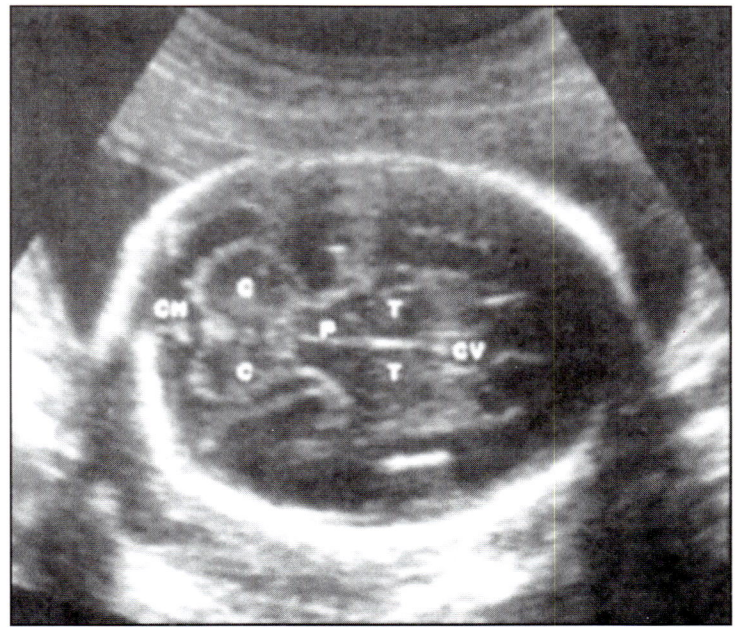

Fig. 6.3: Section of the fetal head including the biparietal diameter (BPD) and the occipitofrontal diameter (the line perpendicular to the BPD). CV: Cavum septum pellucidum; T: Thalamus; C: Cerebellum; CM: Cisterna magna

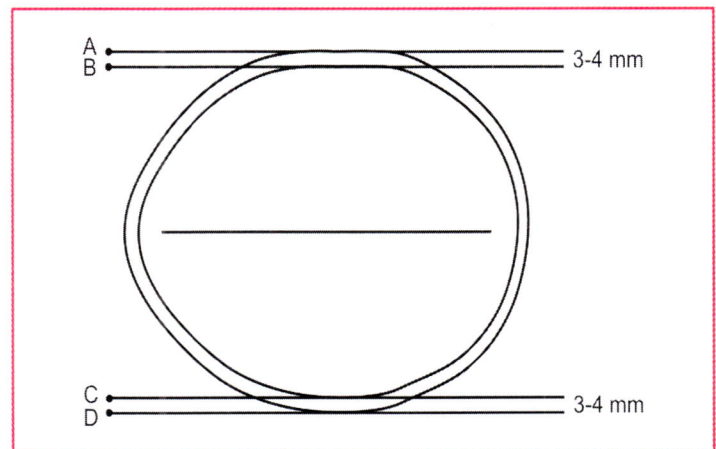

Fig. 6.4: Line diagram showing several possibilities of positioning the electronic calipers to measure the biparietal diameter (BPD). If we measure from A (outer) to D (outer), the measurement will be 3 to 4 mm (or 3 to 4 percent) greater than that obtained by poisitioning one caliper in A (outer) and the other one in C (inner). Although the bone thickness of 3 to 4 mm is related to a third-trimester fetus, it represents 3 to 4 percent of the BPD also during the second trimester

The OFD is obtained by positioning the calipers at both ends of the longest diameter perpendicular to the BPD. The HC measurement is made by tracing around the outer edge of the circumference of the image. Intra- and interobserver errors of 0.57 percent (+/-2.1 SD) and 1.2 percent (+/-4.4 SD), respectively, have been estimated.[21] At least two studies have shown that HC can be determined from BPD and OFD, assuming that the cross-section of the head in the BPD plane is an ellipse, with an accuracy similar to that obtained by direct measurement.[22]

Head changes in shape, such as in dolicocephaly (BPD to OFD ratio <0.75), affecting approximately 8 percent of fetuses, more frequently those in breech presentation, can affect single diameter measurement but they do not significantly affect the HC, which should be used in preference, at least in these cases. Moreover, prenatal and postnatal HC values can be compared directly, since both measurements are made in the same location.

Trunk Size

Among all the possible sections and parameters of the fetal trunk, the abdominal circumference (AC) has been chosen because it reflects changes in liver size which occur early in many fetuses with growth abnormalities (because of the availability and maintenance of blood glucose, for instance) and can be measured in a well-defined plane (Fig. 6.5).

The long axis of the fetus is found by obtaining a longitudinal section through the fetal spine or aorta. The aorta is preferable to the spine, as it is not as wide as the spine, therefore minimizing the degree of obliquity of the true longitudinal plane. The transducer is then rotated through 90° to obtain a transverse image of the fetus at the level of the umbilical vein and of the stomach. The transverse section should be circular in outline as well as the outline of the aorta and the fetus spine.[23] These landmarks will be seen in several sections, but the correct one will show the portion of the umbilical vein situated most centrally as it enters the portal system within the liver. The umbilical vein runs in an anteroposterior and caudocranial direction, on a plane at approximately 40° to the longitudinal axis of the fetus. For this reason a cross-section of the fetal abdomen showing the umbilical vein from its insertion will be at approximately 50° to the correct plane and therefore unsuitable for measurements, which would be overestimated (Fig. 6.6).

When a satisfactory image is obtained, the circumference can be measured by tracing around the outer edge of the image. The intra- and interobserver errors have been reported to be –0.5 percent (+/–2.6 SD) and 2.4 percent (+/–1.6 SD), respectively.[10] As shown for HC, the AC values obtained from perpendicular diameters, assuming an elliptic shape for the cross-section of the fetal abdomen, are similar to those obtained by direct measurement.[24]

Comparison of pre- and postnatal AC measurements are affected by several variables, including the different levels of measurement and changes in liver position due to the initiation of breathing. Since these differences are systematic, they can be reduced by using an appropriate correction factor.[25]

Length

The femur diaphysis length has been utilized as an indirect indicator of fetal length, since this parameter is strongly related with postnatal crown-heel length measurements (Fig. 6.7)[26].

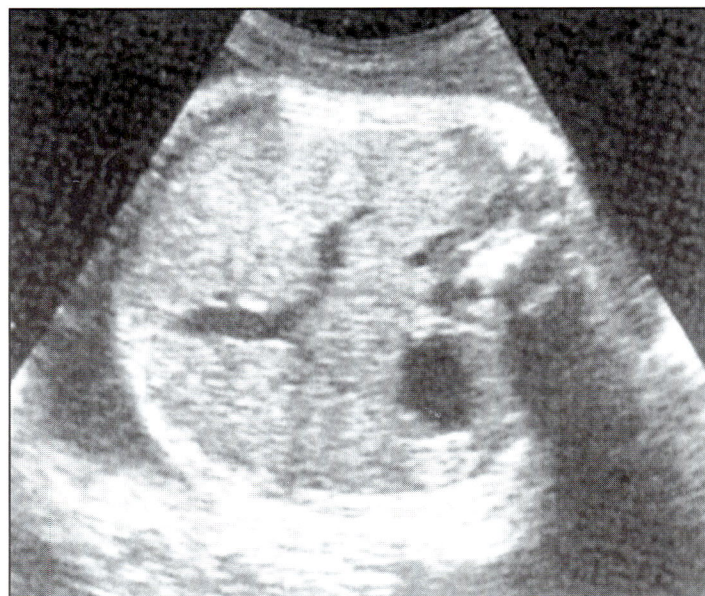

A

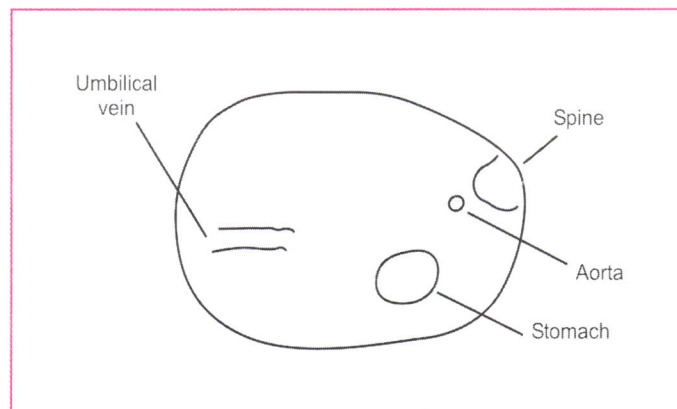

B

Fig. 6.5: (A) Ultrasound image of appropriate section for the measurement of abdominal circumference, (B) Line diagram illustrating anatomical landmarks shown in (A)

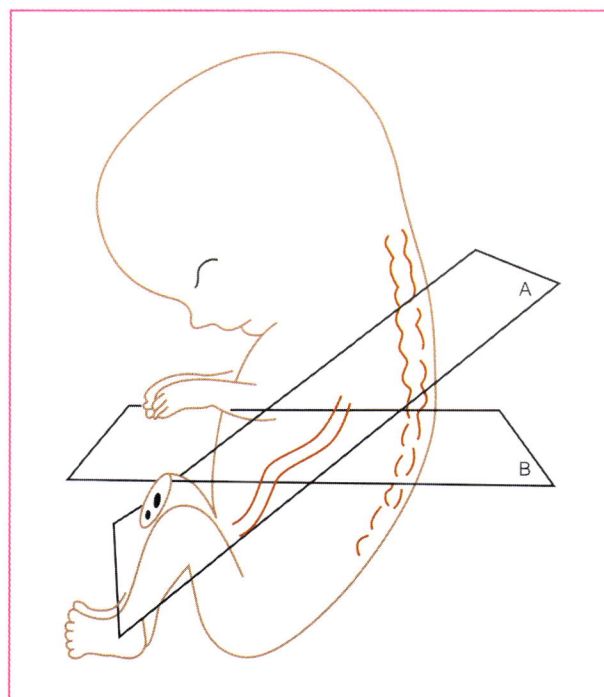

Fig. 6.6: Representation of the umbilical vein course. A is the correct plane for the measurement of abdominal circumference; B is the incorrect plane

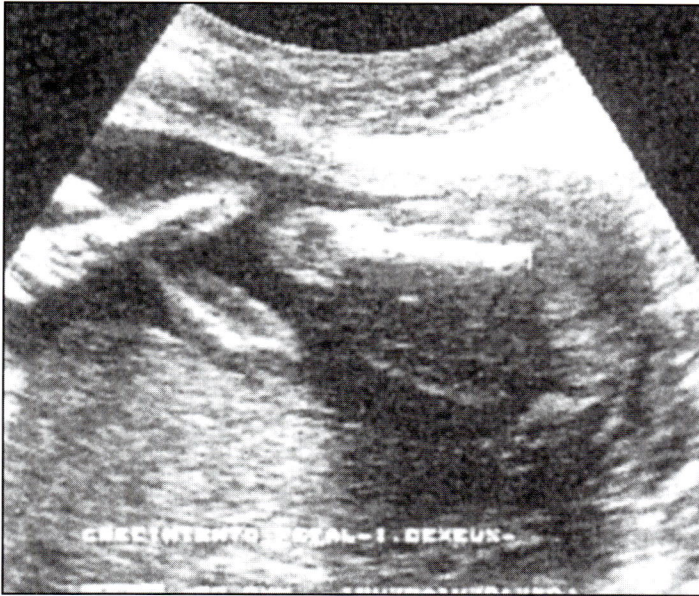

Fig. 6.7: Femur length. The ultrasound image of the femur has clear sharp ends

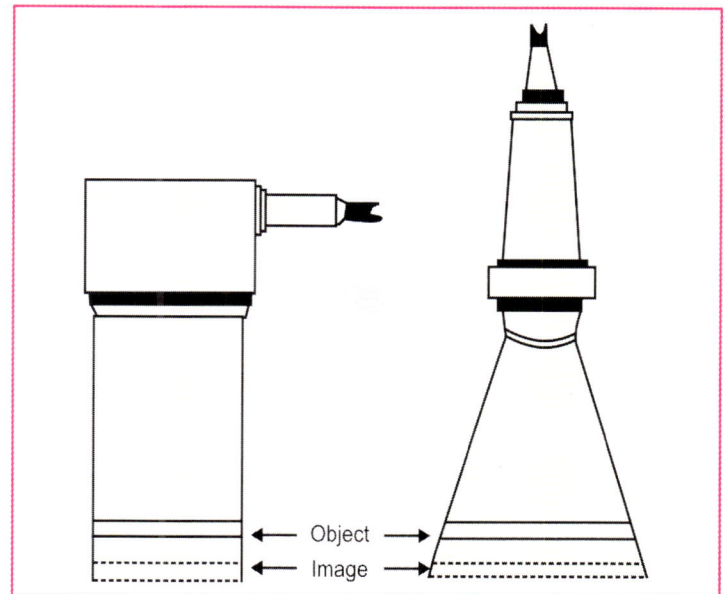

Fig. 6.8: Effect of the difference in sound velocity on ultrasound measurements. By using a linear array probe (A) the apparent object is imaged 3.36 percent deeper than it actually is, but the apparent length is unaffected. By using a sector scanner (B) the apparent object is imaged 3.36 percent deeper than it actually is, but the apparent half-length is also increased by 3.36 percent through the rules of trigonometry

The long axis of the fetus is found and the femora identified as the single long bones at its caudal end. The transducer is rotated until the longest possible image of the femur is obtained and the transducer is along the long axis of the femur. On the frozen image the femur image will have clear blunt ends, if the true long axis is obtained. A straight-line measurement is made between the two ends of the femoral diaphysis (the distal femoral epiphysis should not be included). The measurement is repeated until three values, all within 1 mm of each other, are obtained; the largest of these is considered as the femur length (FL).[23]

It should be noted that difference in orientation can affect this measurement, owing to the differences in axial and lateral resolution.[27] Consequently the femur should be measured when it is parallel or slightly oblique to the transducer.

Linear array scanners and sector scanners give different measurements of femur length, owing to the difference in apparent depth of the image. Although the difference is usually within acceptable limits (approximately 4%), the importance of these variations should be remembered when fetal age or growth is assessed during the third trimester (Fig. 6.8).[28]

Fetal Weight

There are several situations (preterm labor, breech presentation, diabetes, previous cesarean section) when it is of clinical value to have a single estimate of the fetal weight at one point in time. Formulae for using various ultrasonic parameters for estimating fetal weight are numerous, although no procedure is free of problems and errors as high as 15 percent can be expected with even the best methods. All the formulae tend to overestimate the weight of the low-weight fetus (<1550 g) and underestimate the weight of the high-weight fetus (>4000 g).[29]

According to Deter and Harrist,[30] although several methods appear to give similar results, those involving HC, AC and FL seem to be the most appropriate and consistent, since three of the five major body components (brain, trunk, skeleton, muscle and fat) are represented with minimal effects due to shape changes. They recommend the weight estimation function of Hadlock and coworkers:[31]

log 10 weight = 1.326 + 0.107 (HC) + 0.0438 (AC) + 0.158 (FL) – 0.00326 (AC x FL).

Body Proportion

Several ratios of fetal anatomic parameters have been used for evaluation of body proportions. From a general point of view, ratios of head circumference to other body parts gradually decrease with increasing gestational age, which ratios not involving the head remain relatively constant after 20th week of gestation. The most popular are as follows.

1. The HC/AC ratio is commonly used to differentiate symmetric versus asymmetric growth anomalies, although this ratio has been proved to change considerably from one fetus to another in advancing gestational age.[32]
2. The thoracic circumference (TC)/AC ratio is used in detecting pulmonary hypoplasia, although more recently Doppler studies have demonstrated a higher sensitivity.[33]
3. The BPD/FL ratio has been used in screening for Down syndrome, usually in combination with other sonographic markers of chromosomal aberration.[34]

The FL/HC ratio seems to be quite sensitive to both head (microcephaly) and long bone (dwarfism) growth abnormalities, although some skeletal dysplasia not involving head size and/or femur length may require measurement of other parameters (Table 6.2).[35]

Table 6.2: Prenatal growth profile. Variables and sonographic parameters

Variables	Measured parameters
Head size	Head circumference (HC)
Trunk size	Abdominal circumference (AC)
Soft tissue mass	Thigh circumference
Length	Femur length (FL)
Weight	Estimated weight
Body proportionality	HC/AC, FL/HC ratios

REFERENCES

1. Robinson HP. Sonar measurement of fetal crown-rump lenth as means of assessing maturity in first trimester of pregnancy. Br Med J 1973;4:28-31.
2. Nelson LH. Comparison of methods for determining crown-rump measurement by real-time ultrasound. J Clin Ultrasound 1981;9:67-70.
3. Drumm JE, Clinch J, Mackenzie G. The ultrasonic measurement of fetal crown-rump length as a method of assessing gestational age. Br J Obstet Gynaecol 1976;83:417-21.
4. Hadlock FP, Shah YP, Kanon DJ, Lindsay JV. Fetal crown-rump lenth: reevaluation of relation to menstrual age (5-18 weeks) with high-resolution real time US. Radiology 1992;182:501-5.
5. Selbing A, McKay K. Ultrasound in first trimester shows no difference in fetal size between the sexes. Br Med J 1985;290:750.
6. Dubowitz LMS, Goldberg C. Assessment of gestation by ultrasound in various stages of pregnancy in infants differing in size and ethnic origin. Br J Obstet Gynaecol 1981;88:255-9.
7. Pedersen JF. Ultrasound evidence of sexual difference in fetal size in first trimester. Br Med J 1980;281:1253.
8. Gardosi J. Ethnic differences in fetal growth. Ultrasound Obstet Gynecol 1995;6:73-4.
9. Brooke OG, Butters F, Wood C, Bailey P, Tukmachi F. Size at birth from 37-41 weeks gestation: ethnic standard for British infants of both sexes. J Hum Nutr 1981;35:415-30.
10. McFadyen IR, Campbell-Brown M, Abraham A, North WRS, Haines AP. Factors affecting birthweight in Hindus, Moslems and Europeans. Br J Obstet Gynaecol 1984;91:968-72.
11. Chetcuti P, Sinha SH, Levine MI. Birth size in Indian ethnic subgroups born in Britain. Arch Dis Child 1985;60:868-70.
12. Shiono PH, Klebanoff MA, Graubard BI, Berendes HW, Rhoads GG. Birth weight among women of different ethnic groups. JAMA 1986;255:48-52.
13. Overpeck MD, Hediger ML, Zhang J, Trumble AC, Klebanoff MA. Birth weight for gestational age of Mexican American infants born in the United States. Obstet Gynecol1999;93:943-7.
14. Hata T, Deter RL. A review of fetal organ measurements obtained with ultrasound: normal growth. J Clin Ultrasound 1992;20:155-74.
15. Aoki S, Hata T, Kitao M. Ultrasonographic assessment of fetal and neonatal spleen. Am J Perinatology 1992;9:361-7.
16. Hata T, Deter RL, Aoki S, Makihara K, Hata K, Kitao M. Mathematical modeling of fetal splenic growth: Use of the Rossavik Growth Model. J Clin Ultrasound 1992;20:321-7.
17. Hata T, Deter RL, Nagata H, Makihara K, Hata K, Kitao M. Mathematical modeling of fetal organ growth using the Rossavik Growth Model: Adrenal gland. Am J Perinatol 1993;10:97-100.
18. Senoh D, Hata T, Kitao M. Fetal liver length measurement does not provide a superior means for prediction of a small for gestational age fetus. Am J Perinatol 1994;11:344-7.
19. Altman DG, Hytten FE. Assessment of fetal size and fetal growth. In Chalmers Y, Enkin M, Kerse MJNC (eds). Effective Care in Pregnancy and Childbirth. Oxford: Oxford University Press, 1990: 411-18.
20. Hadlock FP, Deter RL, Harrist RB, et al. Fetal biparietal diameter: rational choice of plane of section for sonographic measurement. Am J Roentgenol 1982;138:871-4.
21. Deter RL, Harrist RB, Hadlock FP, et al. Fetal head and abdominal circumferences. 1. Evaluation of measurement errors. J Clin Ultrasound 1982;10:357-63.
22. Shields JR, Medearis AL, Bear MB. Fetal head and abdominal circumferences: ellipse calculations versus planimetry. J Clin Ultrasound 1987;15:237-9.
23. British Medical Ultrasound Society. Fetal Measurement Working Party Report. Clinical Applications of Ultrasonic Fetal Measurements. London: British Institute of Radiology, 1990.
24. Hadlock FP, Kent WR, Loyd JL, et al. An evaluation of two methods of measuring fetal head and body circumferences. J Ultrasound Med 1982;1:359-60.
25. Deter RL, Hill RM, Tennyson LM. Predicting the birth characteristics of normal fetuses 14 weeks before delivery. J Clin Ultrasound 1989;17:89-93.
26. Vintzileos AM, Campbell WA, Keckles S, et al. The ultrasound femur length as a prediction of fetal length. Obstet Gynecol 1984;64:779-82.
27. Pretorius DH, Nelson FR, Manco-Johnson ML. Fetal age estimation by ultrasound: the impact of measurement errors. Radiology 1984;152:763.
28. Jeanty P, Beck GJ, Chervenak FA, et al. A comparison of sector and linear array scanners for the measurement of the fetal femur. J Ultrasound Med 1985;4:525.
29. Miller JM, Kissing GA, Brown HL, et al. Estimated fetal weight: applicability to small- and large-for-gestational-age fetus. J Clin Ultrasound 1988;16:95-7.
30. Deter RL, Harrist BH. Assessment of normal fetal growth. In Chervenak F, Isaacson G, Campbell S, eds. Ultrasound in Obstetrics and Gynecology, Vol. 1. Boston: Little Brown, 1993;1:361-85.
31. Hadlock FP, Harrist RB, Sharman RS, et al. Estimation of fetal weight with the use of the head, body and femur measurements. A prospective study. Am J Obstet Gynecol 1985;151:333-7.
32. Deter RL, Harrist RB, Hadlock FP, et al. The ultrasound in assessment of normal fetal growth. J Clin Ultrasound 1981;9:481-93.
33. Johnson A, Callan NA, Bhutani VK, et al. Ultrasonic ratio of fetal thoracic to abdominal circumference : an association with fetal pulmonary hypoplasia. Am J Obstet Gynecol 1987;157:764-9.
34. Brumfields CG, Hauth JC, Cloud GA, et al. Sonographic measurements and ratios in fetuses with Down syndrome. Obstet Gynecol 1989;73:644-6.
35. Romero R, Pilu GL, Jeanty Ph, et al. Prenatal Diagnosis of Congenital Anomalies. Norwalk, CT : Appleton & Lange, 1988.

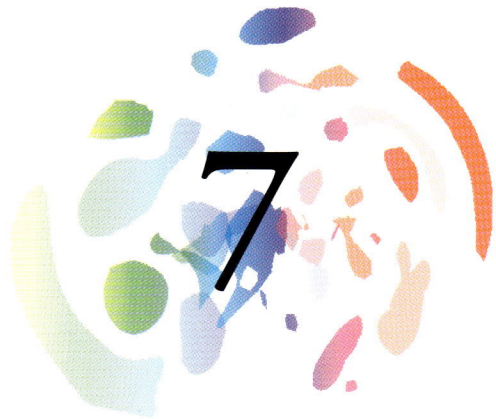

**N Maiz, JM Carrera
MA Rodriguez, M Ruiz**

7

Ultrasonographic Diagnosis of Intrauterine Growth Restriction

INTRODUCTION

Intrauterine growth restriction (IUGR) undoubtedly is one of the most challenging areas of research for obstetricians today.[1,2] Fetuses with IUGR greatly contribute to perinatal mortality and morbidity due to congenital abnormalities, perinatal asphyxia and other neonatal processes (persistent fetal blood flow, hypothermia, hypoglycemia, polycythemia, etc). On the other hand continues to be associated a long-term morbidity: learning problems, abnormal behavior patterns, neurological deficits, etc.[3,4] Even in the adult age, the arterial hypertension and the cardiovascular diseases increase.[5]

DEFINITIONS AND INCIDENCE

Regarding the fetal weight anomalies, a clear distinction should be made between the meaning of three different terms: Low birth weight (LBW), small for gestational age (SGA), and intrauterine growth restriction (IUGR). The LBW refers only to newborn infants weighing less than 2500 g. independently of gestational age. Some of these newborns will be premature, and others will be newborns with a growth restriction. The SGA is a term based on a statistical definition, which includes all newborn infants found below the lower confidence limit of normal weight-weeks of gestation curve. Depending upon the type of curve, the lower confidence limit may be the 3rd, 5th, or 10th percentile or -1 or -2 SD. The IUGR refers to any process that is capable of limiting intrinsic fetal growth potential "*in utero*". It is thus a heterogeneous entity with a variety of possible etiologies.

Unfortunately, in literature, the terms IUGR and SGA are frequently considered as synonymous. This confusion was increased even more the National Institute of Child Health and Human Development in the USA stated that for "both medical and research purposes, intrauterine growth restriction should be defined as a situation which results in a newborn weight that is lower than 10th percentile for its gestational age."

The incidence of IUGR varies greatly in the literature, with reports of figures ranging from 1 percent to 12 percent. The reason for this may be found in different factors, including the social and economic status of the population studied, different criteria used for discrimination (10th percentile, 5th percentile, etc), different ways in which standard curves are drawn, data obtained from transverse or longitudinal studies, etc.[6]

ANTENATAL DIAGNOSIS OF IUGR

It is possible to make several prenatal diagnosis:
a. Screening for IUGR,
b. Ultrasound diagnosis of IUGR,
c. Type of IUGR, and
d. Fetal hemodynamics.

Ultrasound Screening of IUGR

This is perhaps the most important and the most difficult diagnosis to make when we consider that more than 50 percent of pregnancies are free of any associated conditions that would alert obstetricians to the possibility of IUGR.

Serial Measurements of Biparietal Diameter

Initially, and still in many places, the biparietal diameter (BPD) was the only measurement that was routinely taken for the assessment of fetal growth. When pregnancy is normal, this parameter falls within the normal range and can be considered a representative indicator of the growth of other fetal organs and tissues, but when pregnancy is abnormal it may still fall within the normal range (head size is rarely affected in many cases of IUGR) although in this case it is not representative of the growth of other fetal structures.

The substitution of BPD by head circumference or cephalic area does not substantially improve the sensitivity of the method (Fig. 7.1).

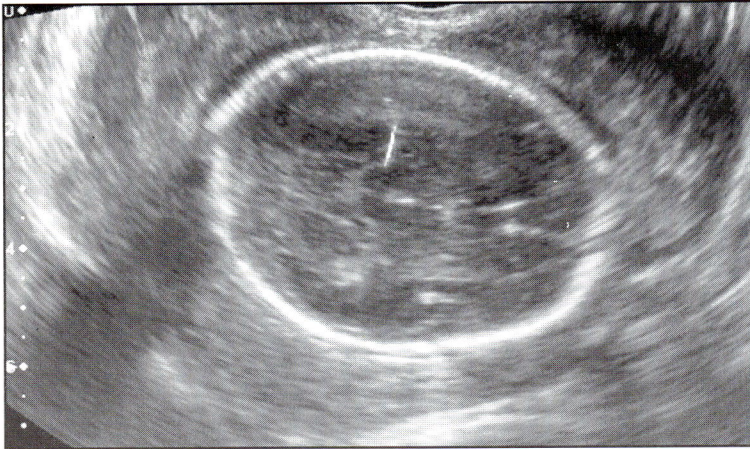

Fig. 7.1: BPD at 20th weeks

Measurement of Biparietal Diameter and Length of the Femur

With the purpose of improving the screening method, measurement of the length of the femur has been introduced (Fig. 7.2). It has the advantage that it measures a component of fetal longitudinal growth and does not suffer the sudden flattening out characteristic of cephalic parameters at term, although it has the disadvantage of not being a useful parameter for establishing the diagnosis of IUGR early stages.

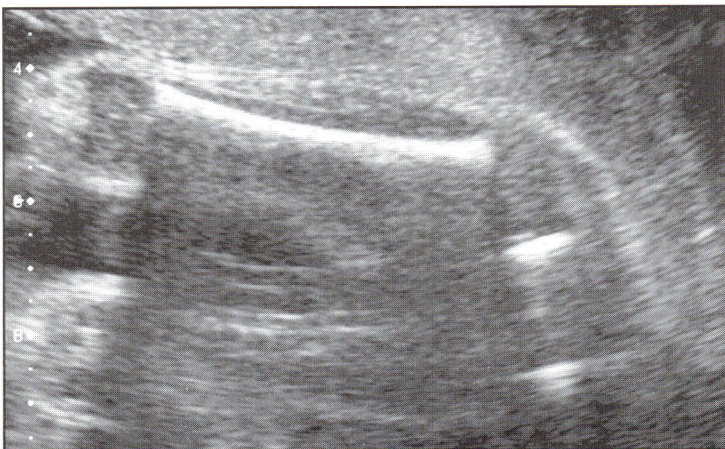

Fig. 7.2: Femur length

Measurement of Biparietal Diameters, Length of the Femur and an Abdominal Parameter

The combination of these three parameters, if they are correctly measured, provides a considerably higher sensitivity than a measurement of BPD alone or in association with the length of the femur. Inclusion of an abdominal parameter (abdominal diameter, abdominal circumference or abdominal area) adds a

measurement that is earlier affected by growth restriction than cephalic or longitudinal development. An important limitation, hower, is the high variability and low reproductibility of these measurements. Values within the normal or abnormal ranges may be found according to the section site (Fig. 7.3).

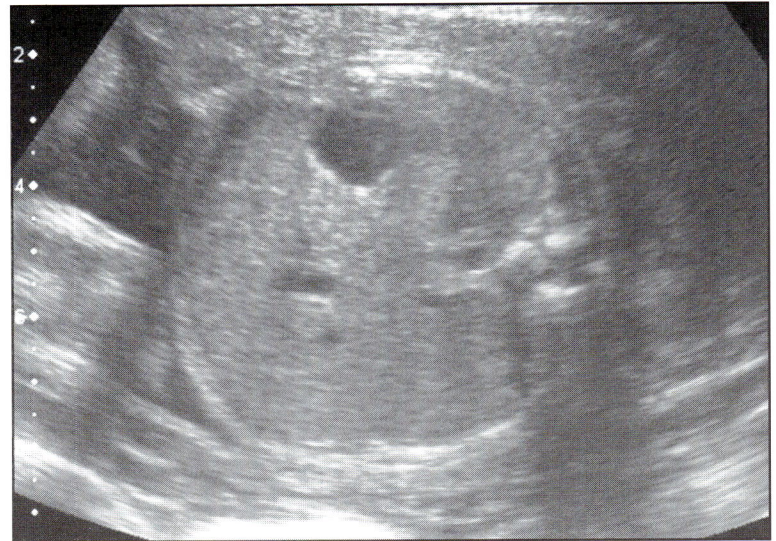

Fig. 7.3: Fetal abdomen

Ultrasound Diagnosis of IUGR

Ultrasound screening of abnormal fetal growth is based on results of the three basic sonographic studies generally recognized as necessary in the control of a supposedly normal pregnancy. That is, at 8 to12, 18 to 22 and 34 to 36 weeks of gestation. Measurement of the crown-rump length (CRL) is obtained in the first examination, so that gestational age is determined with notable accuracy, whereas other biometric parameters are measured on the second and third occasions of echographic study. Comparison of data obtained in both these examinations will permit identification of deviations from normality.

The diagnosis of IUGR is based on biometrics parameters recorded during ultrasound scanning. However, for the correct evaluation of those it is fundamental that a correct gestational age has been previously assigned. If it is not clinically reliable, it must be determined by using measurements of fetal structures that are affected either little or not all by fetal growth retardation, such as transverse cerebellar diameter[7,8] (Fig. 7.4).

Although there are multiple standardized measurements of fetal parameters for which tables or curves showing normal values have been developed, the following parameters are those used in clinical practice.

Crown-rump Length

The greatest value of this parameter is the early confirmation of the gestational age, which, if measured in all gestations, allows for the early diagnosis of IUGR (Figs 7.5 and 7.6).

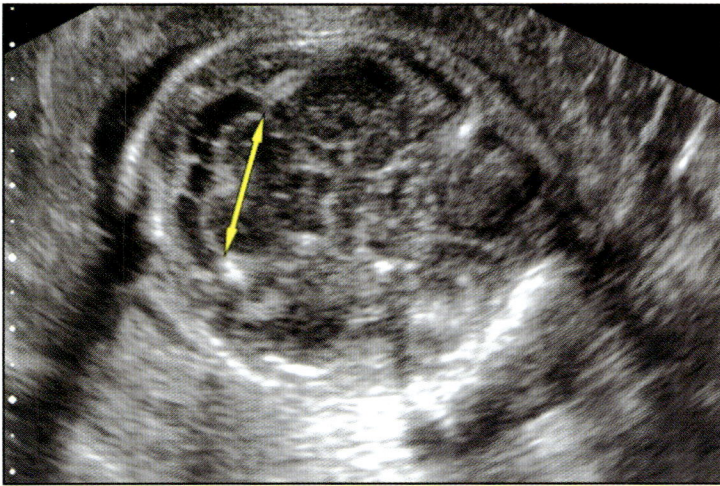

Fig. 7.4: Cerebellar diameter

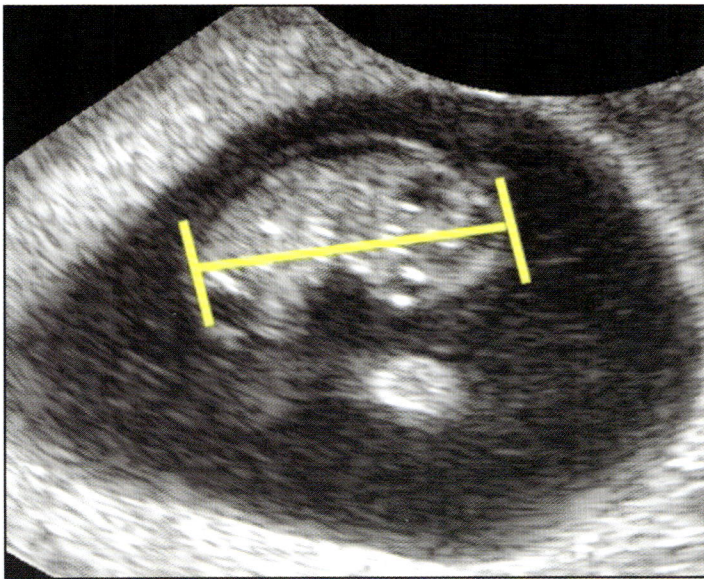

Fig. 7.5: CRL at 8th week

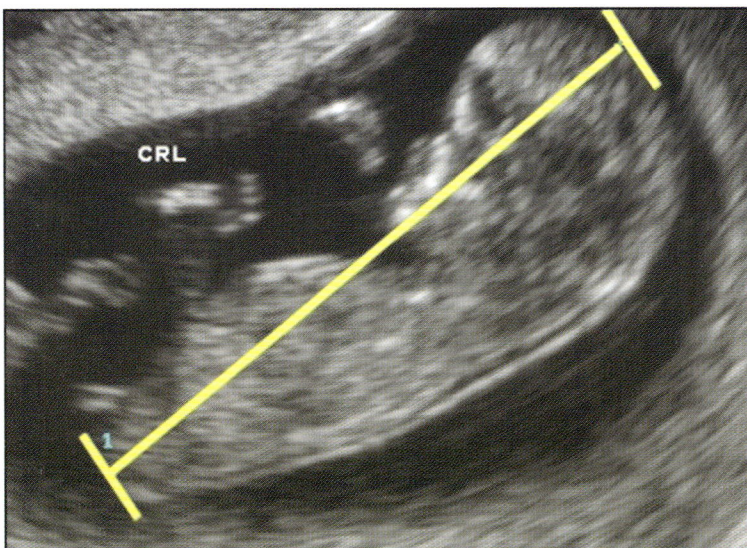

Fig. 7.6: CRL at 11th week

is an exponential increase in CRL although this increase later appears to be linear. The maximum error obtained when calculating this parameter with respect to gestational age is +/– 5 days in 95 percent of cases (between weeks 6 and 14, fetal growth is rapid and the limits of confidence are very narrow). If an embryo falls well outside the normal curve, the presence of chromosome anomalies or dysmorphy should be suspected. Fetal surveillance using ultrasound imaging should be instituted and the karyotype determined.

Biparietal Diameter

This is the most reproducible parameter; it may be determined from weeks 13 to 14 of gestation. Many would consider this biometric parameter to be the most useful, not only to determine gestational age, but also to diagnose IUGR.

The principal advantage of this measurements is the fact that it is relatively little affected by processes of nutritional deprivation or placental insufficiency, which permits it to be used, in spite of these conditions, for the determination of the probable gestational age.

The sonographic section, from front to back includes[9] the most anterior portion of the longitudinal fissure, the cavum of the septum pellucidum, the thick line of the third ventricle and quadrigeminal cisterna with the punctiform echo on the pineal body. Frontal horns of the lateral ventricle and thalami on either side of the third ventricle should be visible[9,10] (Fig. 7.7).

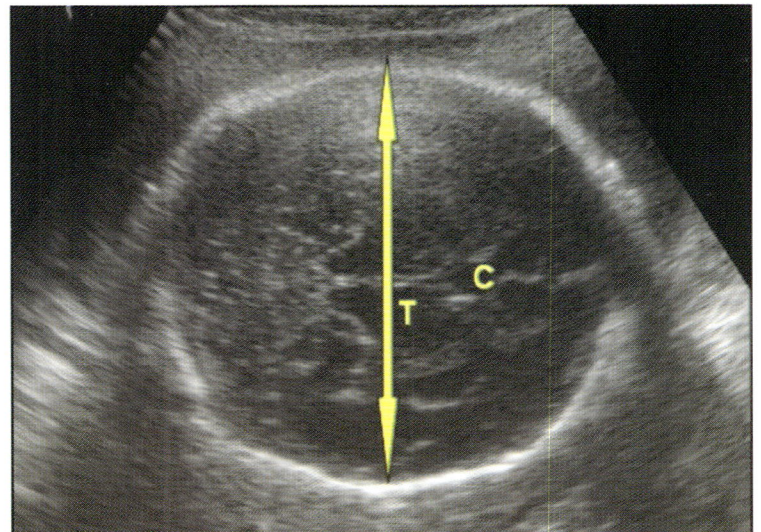

Fig. 7.7: BPD at 29th week. T: Thalami; C: Cavum of the septum pellucidum

Technically the only limitation is the progressive bending of the embryo which makes measurements less reliable after weeks 10 to 12 of gestation. Between weeks 6 to 12 of gestation there

Until week 30th of gestation, increases in BPD are reasonably linear, with weekly increases of 3 mm approximately equal to the standard deviation of mean values for this period.[11,12] From weeks 30 to 38, the rate of change gradually slows, with weekly increases of about 1.5.[12,13] From week 38th to term, weekly increases are 1 mm, and virtually nil as from week 42nd. The sum of the different rates of increase in BPD causes standard deviations to increase as pregnancy reaches term.

The sensitivity of the BPD as the only cephalometric parameter does not exceed 50 percent[14] (varying from 26.9 to 48%).[15-18] In our experience, the sensitivity of the BPD between weeks 34 and 36 of gestation is 45 percent.

Sabbagha and associates[19] proposed determining the so-called growth-adjusted sonar age in order to determine sonar age precisely and to improve the prediction of IUGR. The ideal evolution of the 226 cases in which serial measurements of BPD were made (the first within the 24th week and the last after the 30th) on an original centile curve as is shown in Figure 6.8.

The diagnosis of IUGR is specially consistent when cephalic measurements are initiated early. If the cephalic curve remains parallel to the standard curve throughout the gestation, then we are dealing with a pregnancy with earlier dates. In contrast, if we are dealing with IUGR, the curve will deviate from the theoretical standard curve at a given moment during the gestation (Fig. 7.8).

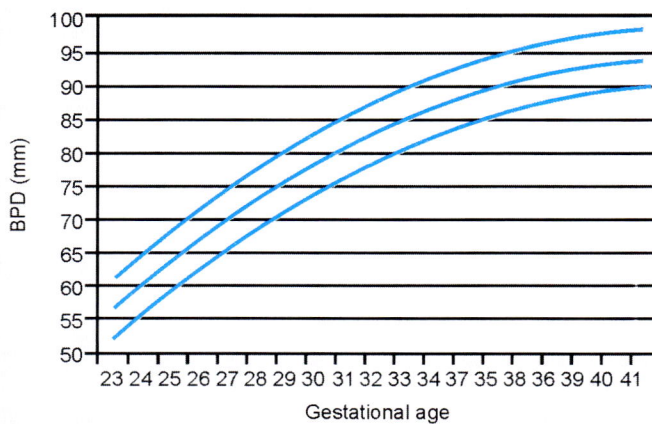

Fig. 7.9: Head circumference or cephalic area

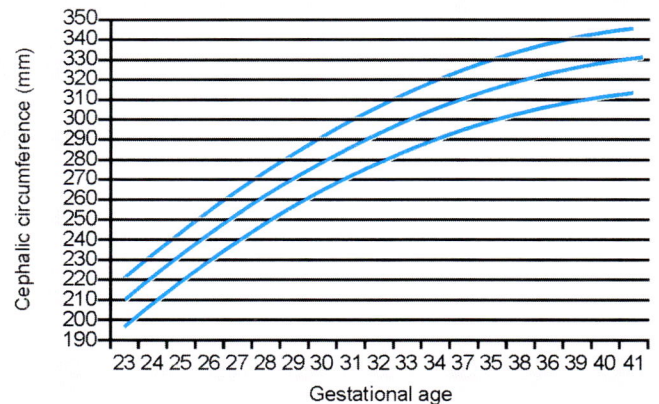

Fig. 7.10: Cephalic circumference curve

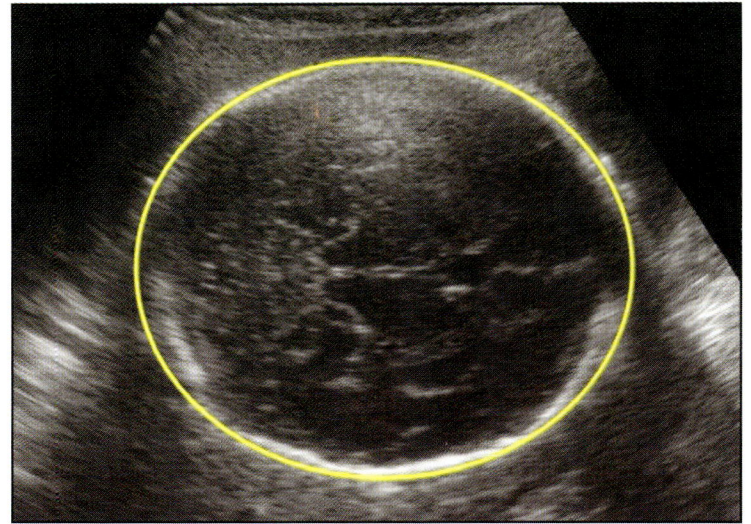

Fig. 7.8: BPD curve

Head Circumference and/or Cephalic Area

Measuring the head circumference of cephalic area is a more complex procedure than measuring BPD since, for measurements to be correct, the sonographic section should include both the biparietal and the fronto-occipital diameters (Figs 7.9 and 7.10).

The sensitivity of head circumference measurements is 52 percent and therefore, somewhat higher than that of BPD. Specificity, however, is similar (80%).

Abdominal Diameters

Both transverse and anteroposterior abdominal diameters have been used to assess fetal development (Fig. 7.11). Some

authors[20,21] consider that measurement of abdominal diameters has the advantage over abdominal circumference or abdominal area of being much simpler and open to fewer errors.

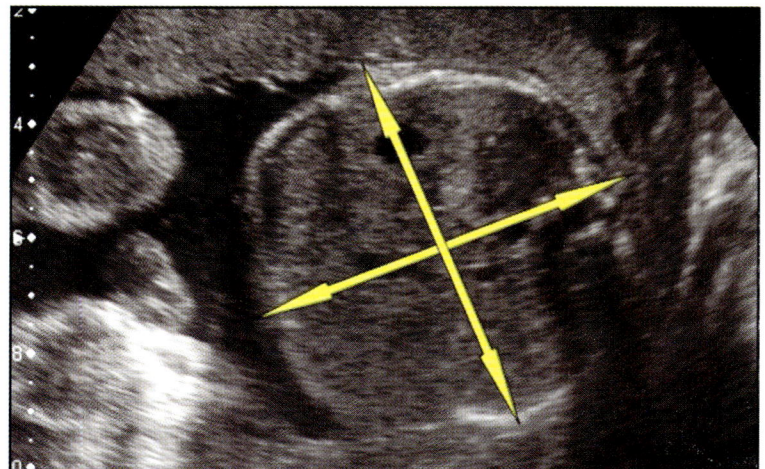

Fig. 7.11: Transverse and anteroposterior abdominal diameters

These parameters are considered to be the best indicators of fetal growth, since they reflect the volume of an important complete organ, such as the fetal liver.

Measurement of the abdominal circumference or abdominal area of the fetus is facilitated by the cylindrical shape if this body segment and the existence of an excellent point of reference (the umbilical vein) (Fig. 7.12). The curve of values for the abdominal circumference during pregnancy shows as almost linear increase until week 36th with a slight decrease from this time onwards (Fig. 7.13).

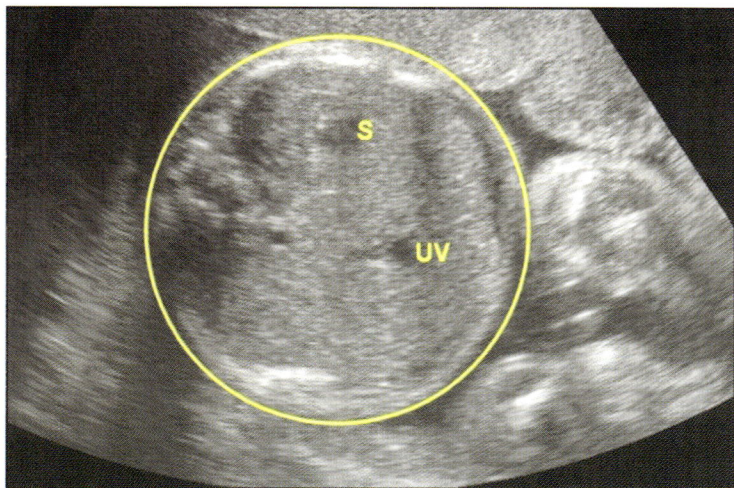

Fig. 7.12: Abdominal circumference or abdominal area. S=Stomach UV=Umbilical vein

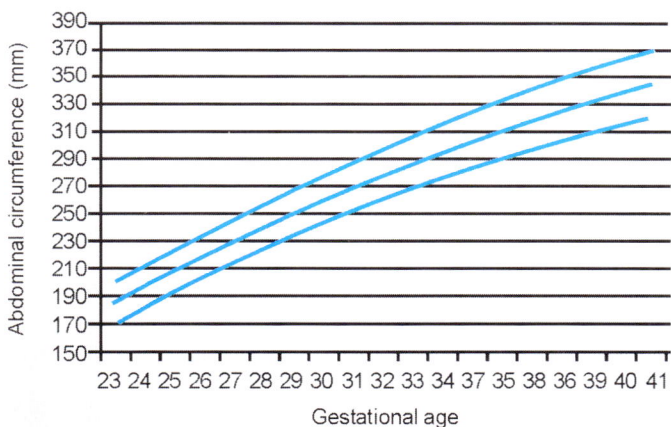

Fig. 7.13: Abdominal circumference curve

Length of Femur

The femur is the easiest long bone to identify and measure (Figs 7.14 and 7.15). On the other hand, it offers an advantage over the BPD since it does not change with morphological changes of the fetal head, and it also permits the evaluation of certain types of skeletal dysplasias. Its typical "golf club"-like appearance and moderate curvature from week 18th are unmistakable. The normal curve for length of femur, similar to that of abdominal parameters, does not suffer the sudden flattening out characteristic of cephalic parameters (Fig. 7.16).

Hadlock and colleagues[22] have emphasised the usefulness if the femur length/abdominal circumference ratio, which not only presents acceptable levels of sensitivity (63%) but also has the advantage of being independent of gestational age. Indeed, this ratio remains constant (22 +/– 2%) as from week 22nd of gestation. Its predictive value, however, is less than 30 percent.[23]

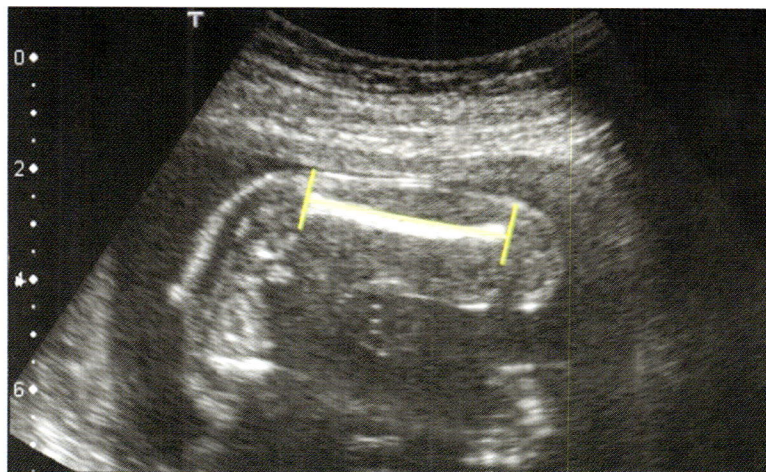

Fig. 7.14: Femur length at 21st week

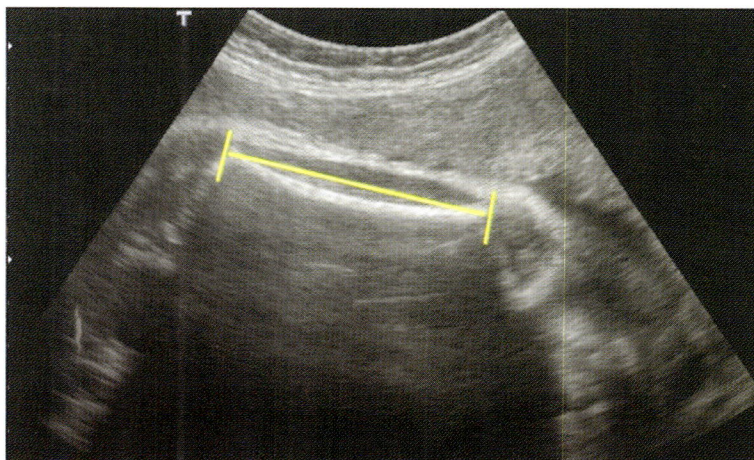

Fig. 7.15: Femur length at 33rd week

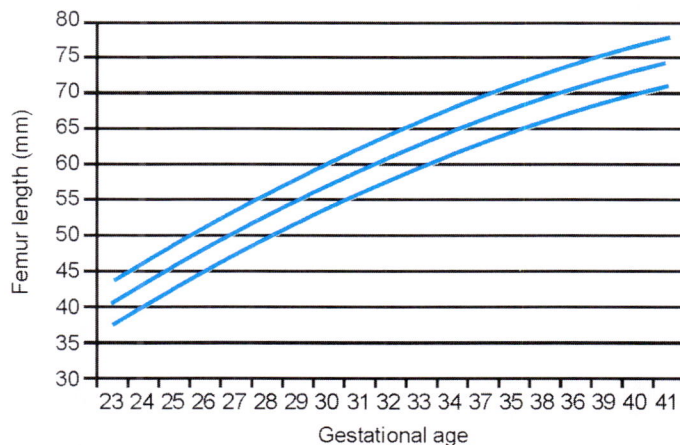

Fig. 7.16: Femur length curve

Diagnosis from the Delay of the Growth of BPD and Femur Length

A computerized technique is to calculate the pregnancy weeks from the values of BPD and/or femur length. The IUGR is suggested, if the pregnancy weeks determined by the computer programs repeatedly delay in the third trimester from the weeks determined by the CRL or correct LMP.

Fetal Organs Biometry

Currently we study the biometry of certain organs (diameters, estimation of volume, etc.) of diverse fetal organs such as the brain, the heart, the lungs, the liver, the spleen, the pancreas, the stomach, the suprarenal glands, the intestine and the bladder.[24] Nevertheless, in general, the use of parameters is not generalized.

Diagnosis of Type of IUGR

Most Anglo-Saxon specialists[25] adopted the classification of symmetrical and asymmetrical IUGR, with some[26] adding a third category known as symmetrical IUGR with "femur sparing", characterized by femur length appropriate for gestational age but out of proportion to all other biometrical parameters.

Integrated Classification of IUGR

This classification has been proposed by our group[27-33] since 1976, and takes into account all the basic aspects of IUGR, such as onset (early or late), etiology (intrinsically abnormal developmental process, etc.), anthropometric data of the newborn infant (weight, length, head circumference), general morphology (proportionate, disproportionate, semiproportionate), trophism (eutrophic, hypotrophic, dystrophic), etc. In accordance with these characteristics, three types of IUGR have been recognized.

Type I implies a decrease in intrinsic fetal growth potential and is also known as intrinsic, harmonious, proportionate, symmetrical or early. In this case, the adverse factor-excerpts its influence from the time of conception, or at least from the embryonic stage (hyperplastic stage). Due to the early onset of the process, the three parameters that are usually assessed to determine IUGR are uniformly affected: fetal weight, length and head circumference (Fig. 7.17). Newborn infants are hypoplastic of microsomic, but their appearance is clearly eutrophic. The incidence of congenital malformations is very high (aneuploidy in 25% of fetuses with severe growth retardation in the early stages of gestation).[34] It is thus advisable to carry out routine studies of fetal karyotype. Approximately 20 to 30 percent of cases of IUGR are of this type.[35-37]

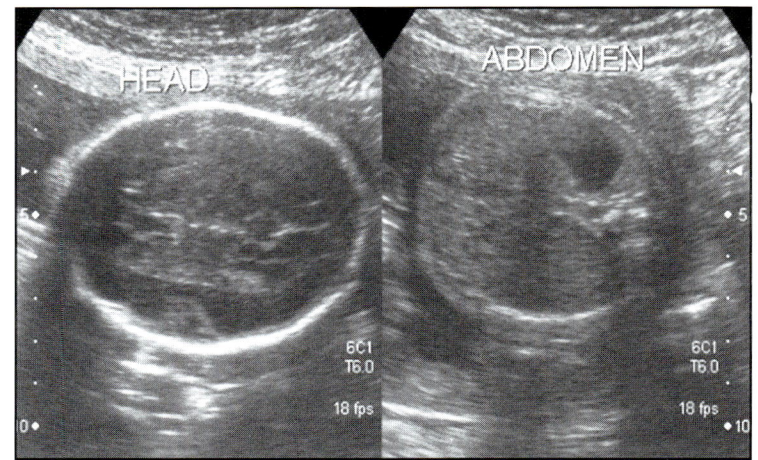

Fig. 7.17: Abdominal and cephalic parameters are uniformly affected

Type II is known as extrinsic, disharmonious, disproportionate, asymmetrical or late, and uteroplacental insufficiency. It has the etiopathogenetic mechanism. Since factors involved in uteroplacental insufficiency are particularly common during the last trimester of pregnancy (hypertrophic stage), only fetal weight is affected, whilst little or no effect is evident in fetal length or head circumference. The physical appearance of the neonate is characteristic, with a disproportionately large head and dystrophic, undernourished body. Cases of in utero fetal death and fetal distress during delivery are most often found in this group. Approximately 70 to 80 percent of cases of IUGR are thought to be of this type.[38,39]

Type III is somewhat mixed in comparison with the other two types. While the factors at work are apparently extrinsic and appear relatively early on in pregnancy (nutrient deficiency), the consequences are more akin to those associated with intrinsic IUGR, where fetal weight and length, in particular, are modified. Neonates in this group are characterized by semiharmonious morphology and a hypotrophic, undernourished appearance.

The ultrasonographic identification of the type of IUGR is based on three evaluations: (i) a profile of the cranial parameters, (ii) calculation of the HC/AC ratio, and (iii) calculation of the diameter of the fetal thigh.

Hemodynamic Study of Fetal Deterioration

The reduction in the number of functional arterioles in the tertially villi, of progressively increases the circulatory resistance in the umbilical artery, and gives rise to a decrease in the PO_2 in the umbilical vein. Both these events set into motion a phenomenon of circulatory redistribution principally characterized by the centralization of blood flow. The better oxygenated blood goes towards the most vital organs (brain, heart, the adrenals), whilst vasoconstriction limits the blood's arrival at the organs considered less indispensable (digestive system, lungs, skin, skeleton, etc.).[40]

The redistribution or centralization of blood flow has been studied in animal experimentation by various researchers[41-43] and the above-mentioned mechanical pattern has been confirmed. However, it should be stressed that when fetal hypoxemia was induced by maternal hypoxemia, not only was there an increase in cardiac and cerebral perfusion, but there was also a significant increase in the umbilical blood flow, and this was not the case when the fetal asphyxia originated from microembolization of the umbilical arteries, thus creating conditions similar to those of a human fetus with a placental lestion.[44-46]

REFERENCES

1. Carrera JM. Fetal growth characteristics. In Kurjak A (Ed): Textbook of Perinatal Medicine. London: The Parthenon Publishing 1998;2:1129-31.
2. Carrera JM. Crecimiento Intrauterino retardado: conceptoy frecuancia. En: J.M. Carrera y col. (Eds). Crecimiento fetal normal y patologico. Barcelona: Editorial Masson 1997;219-22.
3. Spinillo A, Capuzzo E, Piazzi G, Baltaro F, Stranati M, Ornetto A. Significance of low birth weight for gestational age among vey preterm infants. Br J Obstet Gynaecol 1997;104:668-73.
4. Leviton A, Gilles F. Ventriculomegaly, delayed myelination, white matter hypoplasia, and periventricular leukomalacia: how are they related? Pediatr Neurol 1996;15:127-36.
5. Baker DJP. The fetal origins of coronary heart disease. Acta Pediatr 1997; (Suppl). 442:73-7.
6. Carrera JM. Definitions, etiology and clinical implications. In Carrera JM, Mandruzzato GP, Maeda K (Eds): Ultrsound and Fetal Growth, London: Parthenon Publishing 1999;17-34.
7. Goldstein I. Reece Ea, Pilu G, Bovicelli L, Hobbins JC. Cerebellar measurements with ultrasonography in the evaluation of fetal growth and development. Am J Obstet Gynecol 1987;156:1065-9.
8. Reece EA, Goldstein I, Pilu G, Hobbins JC. Fetal cerebellar growth unaffected by intrauterine growth retardation: a new parameter for prenatal diagnosis. Am J Obstet Gynecol 1987;157:632-8.
9. Shepard M, Filly RA. A standardized plane for biparietal diameter measurement. J Ultrasound Med 1982;1:145-54.
10. Johnson ML, Dunne MG, Mack LA, Rashbaum CL. Evaluation of fetal intracranial anatomy by static and real-time ultrasound. J Clin Ultrasound 1980;8:311-8.
11. Campbell S. Ultrasonic fetal cephalometry during the second trimester of pregnancy. J Obstet Gynaecol Br Commonw 1970;77:1057-63.
12. Varma YR. Prediction of delivery date by ultrasound cephalometry. Br J Obstet Gynaecol 1973;80:316-9.
13. Campbell S, Newman GB. Growth of the fetal biparietal diameter during normal pregnancy. J Obstet Gynaecol Br Commonw 1971;78:513-9.
14. Seeds JW. Impaired fetal growth: Ultrasonic evaluation and clinical management. Obstet Gynecol 1984;63:577-82.
15. Rosendahl H, Kivinen S. Routine ultrasound screening for early detection of small for gestational age fetuses. Obstet Gynecol 1988;71:518-21.
16. Arias F. The diagnosis and management of intrauterine growth retardation. Obstet Gynecol 1977;49:293-8.
17. Kurjak A, Kirkinen P, Latin V. Biometric and dynamic ultrasound assessment of small-for-dates infants. Report of 260 cases. Obstet Gynecol 1980;56:281-4.
18. Geirsson RT, Patel NB, Christie AD. Intrauterine volume, fetal abdominal area and biparietal diameter measurements with ultrasound in the prediction of small-for-dates babies in a high-risk obstetric population. Br J Obstet Gynaecol 1985;92:936-40.
19. Sabbagha R, Hughey M, Depp R. Growth adjusted sonographic age. A simplified method. Obstet Gynecol 1978;51:383-6.
20. Macler J, Rosenthal C, Burgun P, Renaud R. The interest of ecotography measurements of the transversal abdominal diameter in the poor intrauterine fetal growth. In Salvadori B, Bacchi-Modena A (Eds). Poor Intrauterine Fetal Growth. Parma: Minerva Medica, 1977.
21. Zoltan I. Poor intrauterine fetal growth: Constitutional factors/weight and size. In Salvadori B, Bacchi-Modena A (Eds): Poor Intrauterine Fetal Growth. Parma: Minerva Medica, 1977; pp 51-5.
22. Hadlock FP, Deter RL,Harrist RB, Roecker E, Park SK. A date independent predictor of intrauterine growth retardation: Femur length/abdominal circumference ratio. AJR Am J Roentgenol 1983;141:797.
23. Benson CB, Doubilet PM, Saltzman DH, Jones TB. FL/AC ratio: poor predictor of intrauterine growth retardation. Invest Radiol 1985;20:727-30.
24. Hata T, Deter RL. A review of fetal organs measurements obtained with ultrasound: normal growth. J Clin Ultrasound 1992;20(3):155-74.
25. Warsof SL, Cooper DJ, Little D, Campbell S. Routine ultrasound screening for antenatal detection of intrauterine growth retardation. Obstet Gynecol 1986;67:33-9.
26. Clark SL. Patterns of intrauterine growth retardation. Clin Obstet Gynecol 1992;35:194-201.
27. Carrera JM. Intrauterine growth retardation.Abstracts of VIII World Congress of Gynecology and Obstetrics (FIGO), Mexico, DF, October 17-22, 1976.
28. Carrera JM, Barri PN. Diagnosis of the intrauterine growth retardation. In: Salvadori B, Bacchi-Modena A (Eds). Poor intrauterine fetal growth. Parma, Italy: Minerva Medica, 1977:277-81.
29. Carrera JM. Concepto, seleccion y clasificacion delos recien nacidos pequenos por retardo de crecimiento intrauterino. Prog Obstet Ginecol 1978;21:197-208.
30. Carrera JM, Mallafre J. Tratamiento "in utero" el retardo de crecimiento fetal. In Esteban Altirriba J, Perinatologia Clinica 3, 1980 (Barcelona: Salvat Editores, S.A.E.).
31. Carrera JM. Regulacion del crecimiento fetal. In Carrera JM (Ed): Biologia Y Ecologia Fetal1981;217. (Barcelona: Salvat Editores, S.A.E.).
32. Carrera JM. Clasificacion del crecimiento intrauterine retardado. Tesisdoctoral, Santiago de Compostela, 1981.
33. Carrera JM. Ecografia Obstetrica, 2nd edition, 1985, Barcelona: Salvat Editores,S.A.E.
34. Weiner CP, Williamson RA. Evaluation of severe retardation using cordocentesis-hematologic and metabolic alterations by etiology. Obstet Gynecol 1989;73:225-9.
35. Carrera JM. Intrauterine Growth Retardation. Abstracts of VIII World Congress of Gynecology and Obstetrics (FIGO), Mexico, DF, October 17-22, 1976.
36. Lockwood CJ, Weiner S. Assessment of fetal growth. Clin Perinatol 1986;13:3-35.
37. Mintz M, Landon M. Sonographic diagnosis of fetal growth disorders. Clin Obstet Gynecol 1988;31:44-52.
38. Carrera JM, Devesa R, Serra B. Classification of intrauterine growth restriction. In Kurjak A (Ed): Textbook of Perinatal Medicine. London. Parthenon Publishing 1998;1192-1200.
39. Brar HS, Rutherford SE. Classification of intrauterine growth retardation. Semin Perinatol 1988;12:2-10.
40. Carrera JM, Devesa R, Torrents M, Munoz A, Comas C, Nortera C, Serra B. Natural history of fetal compromise in intrauterine growth retardation. In Kurjak A (Ed): Textbook of Perinatal Medicine (vol. 2). London, Parthenon Publishing, 1226-43.
41. Rudolph AM, Heymann MA. The circulation of the fetus "in utero". Methods for studying distribution of blood flow, cardiac output and organ blood flow. Circ Res 1967;21:163-7.
42. Johanson GN, Palahniuk RJ, Tweed WA, Jones MV, Wade JG. Regional cerebral blood flow changes during fetal asphyxia produced by slow partial umbilical cord compression. Am J Obstet Gynecol 1979;135:48-52.
43. Behrman RE, Lees MH, Peterson EN, De Lannoy CW, Seeds AE. Distribution of the circulation in the normal and asphyxiated fetal primate. Am J Obstet Gynecol 1970;108:956-69.
44. Morrow RJ, Adamson SL, Bull SB, Ritchie JWK. Ante hypoxemia does not effect umbilical artery waveforms in sheep. Obstet Gynecol 1990;75:590-3.
45. Morrow RJ, Adamson SL, Bull SB, Ritchie JWK. Hypoxia acidaemia, hyperviscosity and maternal hypertension do not affect the umbilical artery velocity waveforms in fetal sheep. Am J Obstet Gynecol 1990;163:1313-20.
46. Hecher K, Bilardo CM, Stigler RH, et al. Monitoring of fetuses with IUGR: A longitudinal study. Ultrasound Obstet Gynecol 2001;18:564-70.

**N Maiz, JM Carrera
MA Rodriguez, P Prats**

8

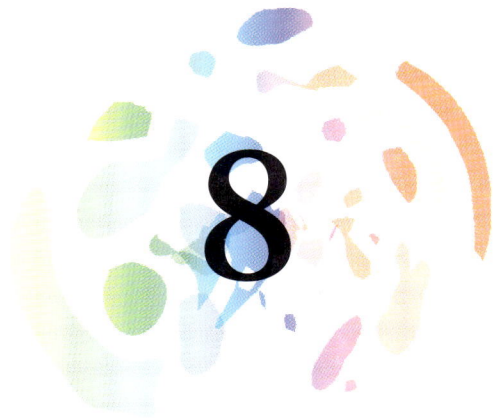

Natural History of Fetal Deterioration

INTRODUCTION

The degree of fetal wellbeing or fetal deterioration can be determined by the evaluation of various biophysical and biochemical proceeding. But, in this moment, the hemodynamic study of fetal deterioration while Doppler, is the best and more used technique.

Nowadays, Doppler enables a hemodynamic profile to be drawn up that includes the functionality of vascular (arterial and venous) and cardiac systems (Table 8.1)[1] (Figs 8.1 to 8.4).

Table 8.1: Hemodynamic profile

	Normal pattern	Pathological pattern
1. Arterial parameters		
• Umbilical artery (PI)	<P-95	>P-95
• Aorta artery (PI)	<P-95	>P-95
• Carotid artery (PI)	>P-5	>P-5
• Middle cerebral artery (PI)	>P-5	>P-5
2. Venous parameters		
• Umbilical vein	Non-pulsating	Pulsating
• Inferior vena cava (VPI)	<P-95	>P-95
• Ductus venosus (VPI)	<P-95	>P-95
3. Intracardiac parameters		
• Diastolic function	>P-5	>P-5
• E/A Transmitral	>P-5	>P-5
• E/A Transtricuspid		
4. Dyastolic function		
• Aorta (PSV Ao)	>P-5	>P-5
• Pulmonary (PSV P)	>P-5	>P-5

Thanks to the Doppler technique it is possible to recognize four periods with relatively well defined hemodynamic, biophysical and biochemical patterns. These are: (i) a silent period of increase in resistance; (ii) a period with reduction in umbilical blood flow; (iii) a period with centralization of the blood flow; and (iv) a period with decentralization of blood flow.

The redistribution or centralization of blood flow has been studied in experimental animals, in particular by Rudolph and Heymann[2] and Johnson and colleagues[3] in sheep, and by

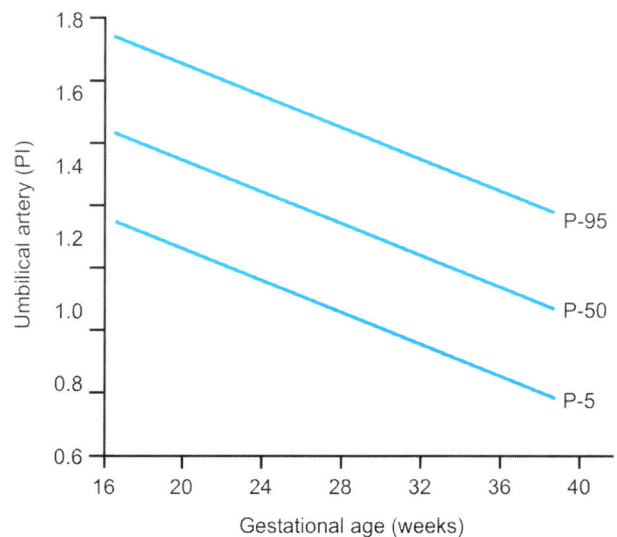

Fig. 8.1: Umbilical artery pulsatility index. 5th, 50th and 95th percentile

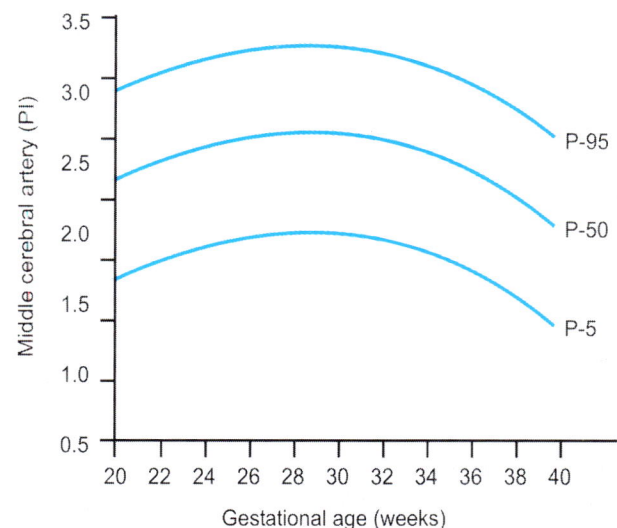

Fig. 8.2: Middle cerebral artery pulsatility index. 5th, 50th and 95th percentile

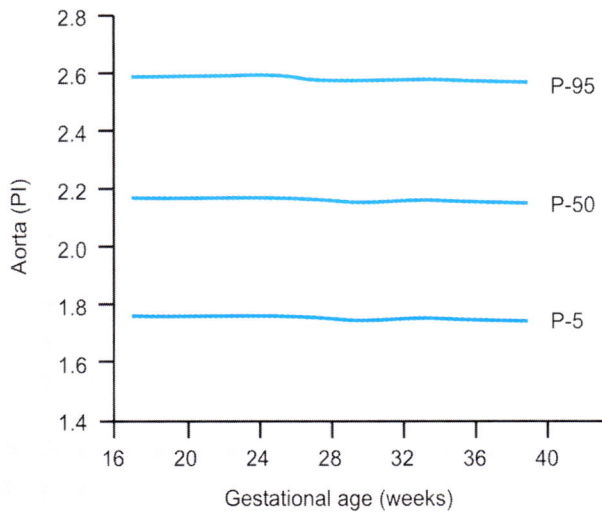

Fig. 8.3: Aortic pulsatility index. 5th, 50th and 95th percentile

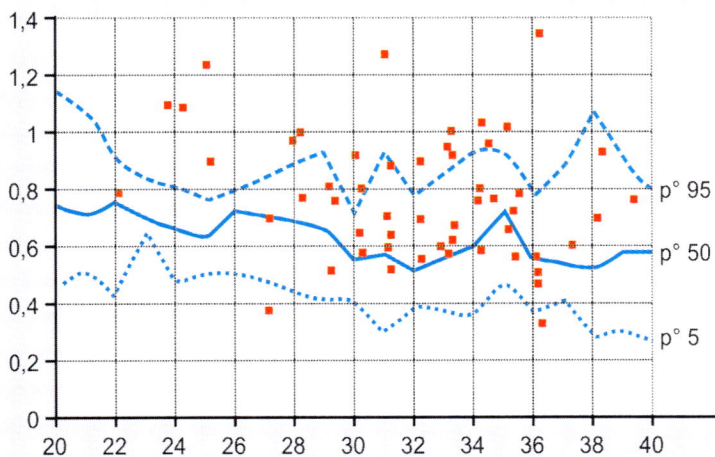

Fig. 8.4: Ductus venosus artery pulsatility index. 5th, 50th and 95th percentile

Berhman and associates[4] in fetal primates. In most cases, blood flow redistribution was assessed by injecting radioactively labeled microspheres, and hypoxemia and acidosis were induced by different procedures, such as maternal breathing of a mixture low in oxygen, hypotension, partial umbilical compression using clamps and microembolization of the umbilical arteries. In all cases the aforementioned pattern of redistribution of blood flow was confirmed. It is worth pointing out, however, that when fetal hypoxemia occurred as a result of maternal hypoxemia, not only did cardiac and cerebral blood perfusion increase but umbilical artery blood flow also increased significantly. This did not occur when fetal asphyxia was induced by microembolization of the umbilical arteries, a condition similar to that encountered in human fetuses with placental lesions.[5,6]

SILENT PERIOD OF INCREASE IN RESISTANCE

Pathophysiological Basis

The progressive deterioration of the villous microcirculation is reflected in the Doppler study of the umbilical artery, when the functional abstruction reaches 50 percent of the villous arteriolar system, and significantly modifies the pulsatility index (PI).[7]

Before this percentage is reached, the capacity of the placental reserves covers the theoretical deficit of gaseous exchange, provided the maternal supply line remains satisfactory.[8]

Doppler Hemodynamic Profile

The hemodynamic profile is completely normal over a certain period (generally 3 to 6 weeks), and there is no pathology of any kind. The flow velocity waveform (FVW) of the umbilical artery is normal (positive blood flow over the whole cardiac cycle, with normal pulsatility indices, resistance or conductancy[9-10] (Fig. 8.5). Doppler studies on the remaining vessels (aorta, common carotid and middle cerebral arteries) also prove normal (Fig. 8.6). We can therefore speak of a "normal hemodynamic pattern."

In a Doppler study we carried out 82 cases of growth retardation confirmed at birth, we demonstrated that 36 of them (43.9%) had a normal umbilical PI; the study of the remaining fetal vessels proved normal in all these cases (Table 8.2). For this reason, we consider it unnecessary in practice to widen the hemodynamic study of the fetus when the umbilical FVW is normal and fetal growth is also apparently normal.

Table 8.2: Cases of intrauterine growth retardation, grouped into four groups according to the pulsatility (PI) results in the umbilical artery and the hemodynamic profile (FHP); thoracic aorta PI, common carotid artery PI and middle cerebral artery. The pH of the umbilical vein was measured at birth

		Cases		Perinatal mortality		pH<7.20	
Group	Association	N	%	N	%	N	%
I	Normal umbilical PI + normal FHP	36	43.9	0	0.0	6	16.6
II	Normal umbilical PI + abnormal FHP	0	0.0	–	–	–	–
III	Abnormal umbilical PI + normal FHP	22	26.8	0	0.0	8	36.3
IV	Abnormal umbilical PI + abnormal FHP	24	29.2	6	25.0	15	62.5
Total		82	100.0	6	7.3	29	35.3

In this period, both the cardiotocography and the remaining parameters of the biophysical profile are normal and the study of fetal blood gases by funicolucentesis is normal. According to the limits of our current experience, such an exploration is therefore not justified when the Doppler study is normal.

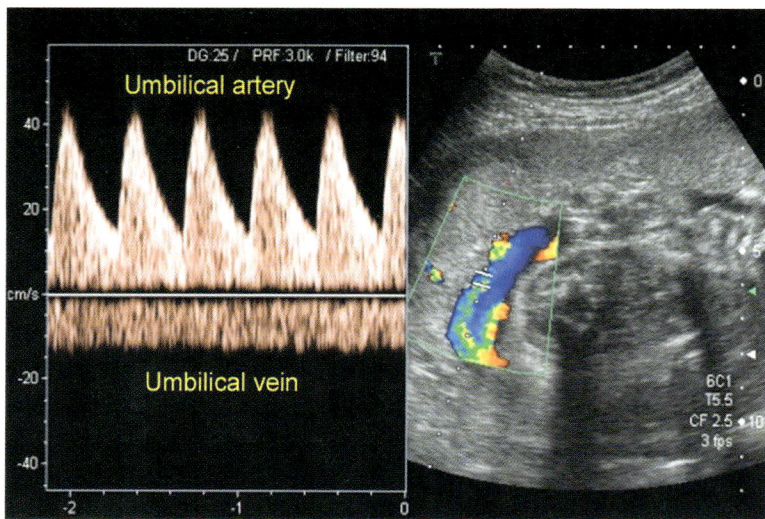

Fig. 8.5: Umbilical artery and umbilical vein: Normal FVW

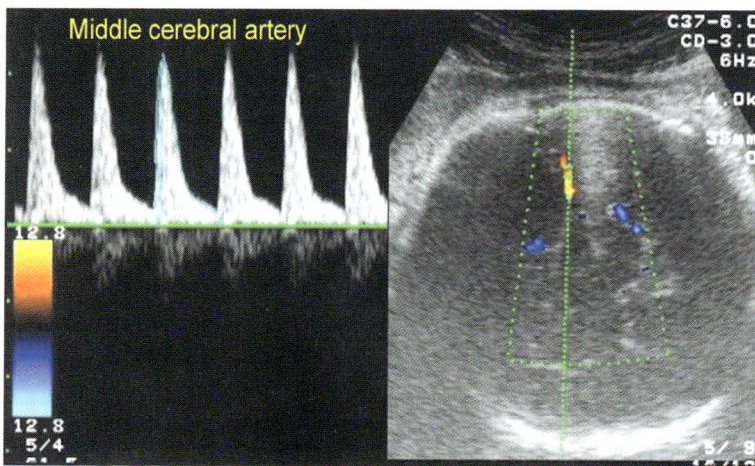

Fig. 8.6: Middle cerebral artery: Normal FVW

For all these reasons, the perinatal mortality rate is not increased.

REDUCTION OF UMBILICAL BLOOD FLOW

This is the first objective sign of the start of chronic fetal distress brought on by the placental lesion.

Pathophysiological Basis

It has been demonstrated that the functional obstruction of over 50 percent of the villous arterioles is translated into a clear deterioration of the umbilical FVW.[11]

Although some studies claim that the umbilical artery is not always the first vessel affected,[12, 13] in our experience and in that of other authors, an increase in umbilical resistance is usually the first observable hemodynamic signal when there is a placental lesion affecting the villous microcirculation. In 15 to 20 percent of fetuses with growth retardation with a placental cause, the abrupt decrease in PO_2 can give rise, through the aortic and carotid chemoreceptors, to an increase in the aortic

and/or cerebral PI, which exceeds and/or precedes those observed in the umbilical artery. On the other hand, it is also possible to observe pathological values of the aortic or cerebral PI before an alteration in umbilical perfusion, when the cause of fetal distress does not reside in the placenta but in a disorder in the mother's internal medium (hypoxemia through maternal cardiorespiratory pathology, an acute deficit of specific nutrients, severe anemia, etc.) or in her hemodynamics (e.g. hypertensive crises with a renal 0 or endocrine origin). Even in these cases, umbilical conductance may be increased. So, brain-sparring may develop independently of the umbilical artery waveform[14-16] (Figs 8.7 and 8.8).

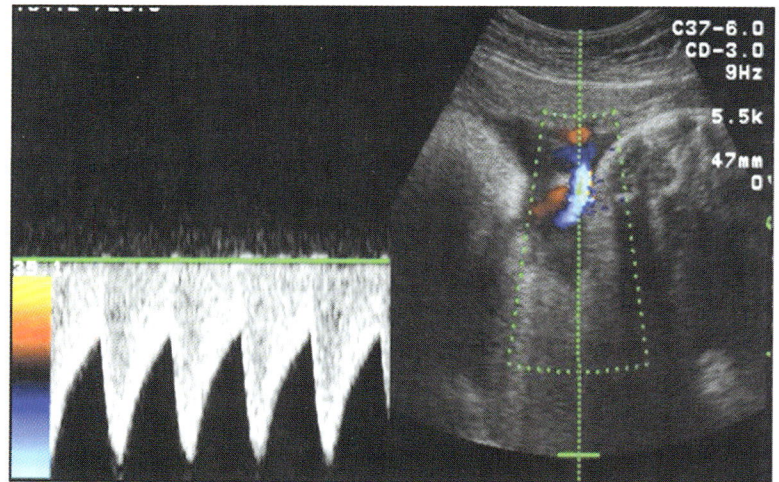

Fig. 8.7: Umbilical artery: Normal FVW

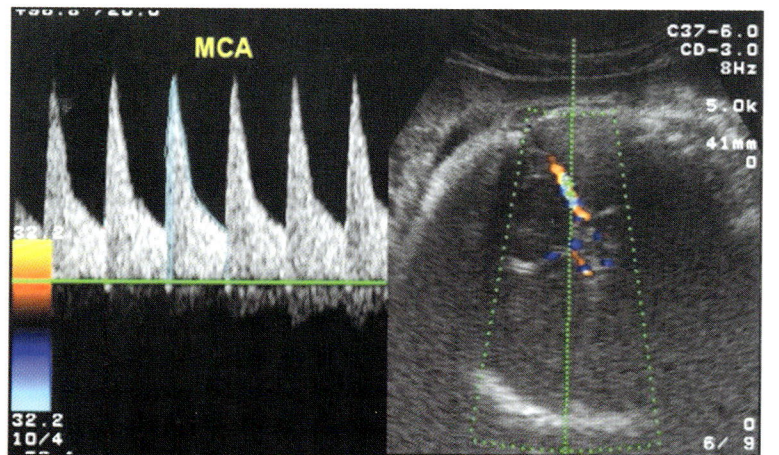

Fig. 8.8: Middle cerebral artery: Brain-sparing

Alternatively, there is experimental evidence that a placental lesion is followed by a decrease in umbilical arterial perfusion. Morrow and coworkers [5,6,17] working with fetal sheep subjected to an embolism of the villous microcirculation (plastic micropistons 50 … in diameter), observed gradual changes in the FVW of the umbilical artery similar to those described in human fetuses subjected to growth retardation through villous pathology (reduction in endodiastolic blood flow, zero diastole and, finally, reserve blood flow). The cause, therefore, of the deterioration of the umbilical FVW lies in the increase in microvillous vascular resistance which, whilst primarily inducing a deficit in the perfusion in the umbilical artery, is also the reason for a progressive decrease in the PO_2 in the umbilical vein. Hypoxemia is thus the result and not the cause of the hemodynamic umbilical-placental alteration. This is why a reduction in PO_2 without any placental lesion does not give rise to any change in the umbilical FVW [18,19] and neither does this change occur through an increase in hematic viscosity or a rise in maternal blood pressure.[18,20]

Doppler Hemodynamic Profile

A moderate increase in umbilical resistance is the only finding capable of revealing the onset of chronic fetal distress for a specific period of time, the duration of which largely depends on how quickly the placental lesion takes effect. During this period the Doppler study of the rest of the fetal circulatory system, including the aorta, is usually normal. In our experience 56 percent of fetuses with growth retardation presented an altered umbilical PI, but of these only 52 percent were accompanied by a pathological hemodynamic pattern.

The umbilical FVW presents positive flow velocities throughout the entire cardiac cycle, but the pulsatility (or conductance) incides reveal values outside the accepted limits for the gestation (Fig. 8.9).

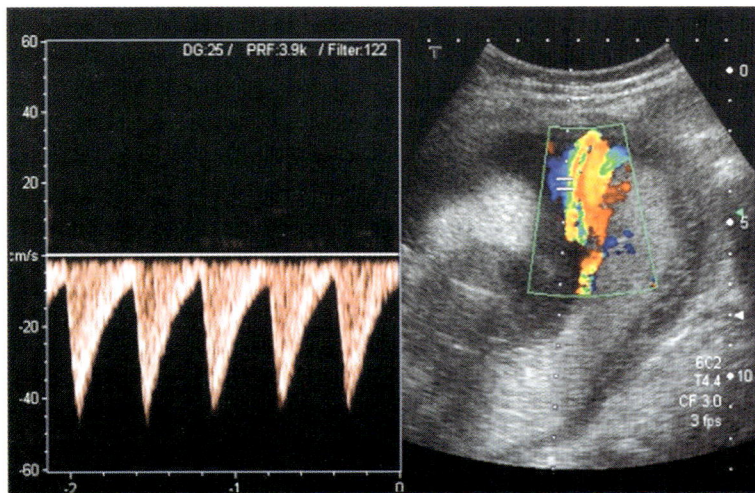

Fig. 8.9: Umbilical artery: Increased resistance or pulsatility

The only compensatory hemodynamic process that can be observed at this time, with the use, in particular, of color Doppler, is the reopening of the ductus venosus, the caliber of which if physiologically reduced at the end of the second trimester (Fig. 8.10). This mechanism makes it possible to extract a significant amount of blood from the fetal liver, and this goes directly to the heart. This "shunt" can delay by some weeks the need for a centralization of the blood flow, but induces the appearance of typical asymmetric growth retardation.[21]

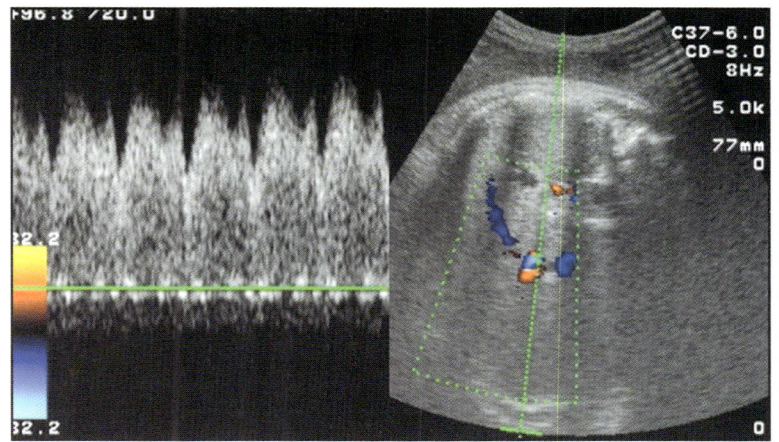

Fig. 8.10: Ductus venosus

In the cerebral circulation, it is also possible to confirm, in some cases, the experience of a decrease in the PI of the M2 sector of the middle cerebral artery, with the M1/M2 index passing from below 1 (normal) to being over 1 (pathological). This occurrence, secondary to the selective vasodilation of that arterial tract, which can be considered as the subcortical sector of the artery, represents a preservation mechanism for specific areas in the brain, and precedes the authentic brain-sparring effect.

The objective of these two compensatory mechanisms is to delay as far as possible the stimulation of the aortic and carotid chemoreceptors which will set in motion the centralization of flow.

In this period the fetus is normally in normoxia. In our experience it is not necessary to carry out diagnostic funiculocentesis in this phase if there is confirmation that centralization of the blood flow has not begun.

There were no fetal deaths in our statistics for this group but there was a significant increase in the percentage of small-for-dates neonates. For this reason the percentage of neonates with pH below 7.20 reached 38 percent. In fact, the percentage of intrapartum fetal distress tripled, proof of a greater fetal vulnerability. The cesarean section rate rose to 30 to 40 percent.[11]

CENTRALIZATION OF BLOOD FLOW

Pathophysiological Basis

As the resistance in the umbilical arterial system increases, there is also a corresponding decrease in the PO_2 in the umbilical vein. This means that the fetus must carry out, in addition to a reopening of the ductus venosus, a redistribution of its blood flow once a specific PO_2 value has been reached, in order to protect its most important structures from hypoxia. As we have already explained, this redistribution consists of a circulatory centralization with selective vasodilatation of certain organs, such as the brain, the heart and the adrenals, and a vasoconstriction of other sites such as the lung, the intestine, the skin, the kidney or the skeleton. This redistribution can be seen with Doppler, which records a successive increase in the PI of the aorta and the renal artery, and a decreased PI in the common carotid artery and the intracranial vessels.

These changes in the perfusion of the various organs are primarily mediated by neuronal stimulation, whether directly by stimulation of the vagal center or through the aortic and carotid chemoreceptors. In 1969 Dawes and colleagues[22] confirmed that the aortic chemoreceptors in sheep respond to small reductions in arterial oxygen levels. However, it is very probable that these vasoconstriction phenomena are modulated by other factors, such as, for example, the direct effect of hypoxemia vasoactive substances, secretion of catecholamines, or an overall increase in the activity of the autonomic nervous system.

Although the chronological pattern is not well established, it seems that the first vessel to be affected after the umbilical artery is the aorta. The increase in resistance in the descending thoracic aorta is the result of the combined action of several factors: an increase in umbilical-placental resistance, arterial vasoconstriction resulting in progressive hypoxemia and, finally, a decrease in myocardial contractility.[23] Lingman and coworkers[24] postulate an inverse relationship between myocardial contractility and the aortic and umbilical PI.

Doppler Hemodynamic Profile

Doppler study reveals an increase in PI, not only in the umbilical artery but also in the descending thoracic aorta and its branches, such as the renal artery.[25-29] There is a progressive loss of end-diastolic velocity in both vessels when the resistance reaches a certain level. At the same time, there is a noticeable decrease in the PI of the cerebral and common carotid arteries, evidence of a further vasodilatation process.

It is often possible to recognize three phases in the centralization of blood flow.

1. *Initial phase:* The PI in the umbilical artery is high, but there are still positive values in the Doppler frequencies throughout the whole cardiac cycle, even in telediastole (Fig. 8.11).

    On the other hand, the FVW of the common carotid artery, which has no end-diastolic frequencies until weeks 32 to 34,[30] recovers its end-diastolic flow shortly after a proven moderate increase in intracranial perfusion. This suggests that the fall in the PI of the common carotid artery is due to the reduction in the resistance of the cerebral vessels. The study of the umbilical PI/middle cerebral PI (U/C) relationship can prove particularly helpful in making a definitive assessment of centralization at this stage. Several

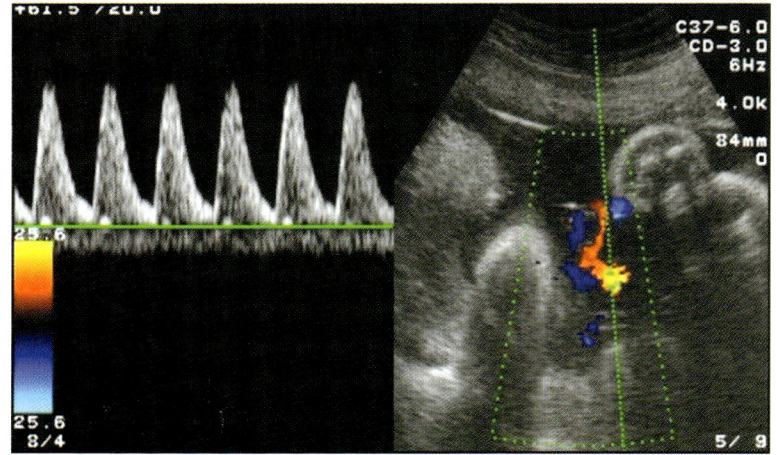

Fig. 8.11: Umbilical artery (38th week), high PI and RI. Positive values in whole cardiac cycle

authors[31-34] maintain that this is the best fluxometric index for tracing IUGR.

2. *Advanced phase:* The umbilical FVW shows zero diastole (Fig. 8.12). The first to disappear were the telediastolic frequencies, but afterwards the lack of blood flow affected the whole diastole (Fig. 8.13). According to Trudinger,[7] the situation occurs when an 80 percent obstruction in the villous arteriolar system has been attained. The FVW of the aorta also loses its end-diastolic values.

    In conjunction with this deterioration in the umbilical blood flow, the vasodilatation of the cerebral vessels arrives at its maximum point, which means that the PI of both the common carotid and the middle cerebral arteries attain their lowest values (Fig. 8.14).

3. *Terminal phase:* In addition to an absence of end-diastolic flow, there is the onset of a reverse flow, both in the umbilical artery and in the aorta, and this obviously aggravates the prognosis (Fig. 8.15). As well as the arterial hemodynamic findings already described, there are signs in this phase of cardiac insufficiency, revealed by Doppler study of the fetal venous circulation through a decrease both in the velocity peaks in the exit tracts and in the ventricular ejection force, and through a possible visualization of the coronary blood flow.[35, 36]

As regards the venous return circulation, there are three signals:

1. Raised reverse blood flow in the inferior vena cava, coinciding with auricular contraction. This finding, which reveals difficulties in the blood flow through the right atrium, can be due both to alterations in the fetal cardiac frequency and to deficient auricular contractility.[37-39] The reverse flow can reach up to 30 percent of the total blood flow (under normal conditions this does not exceed 10%) (Figs 8.16 and 8.17).

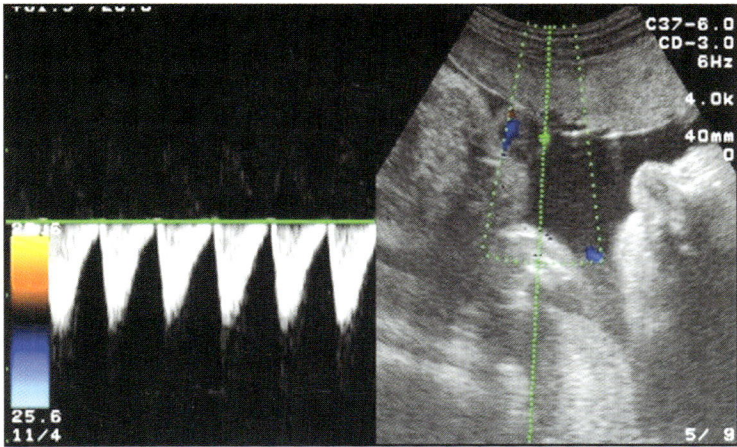

Fig. 8.12: Umbilical artery: Absence of telediastolic flow

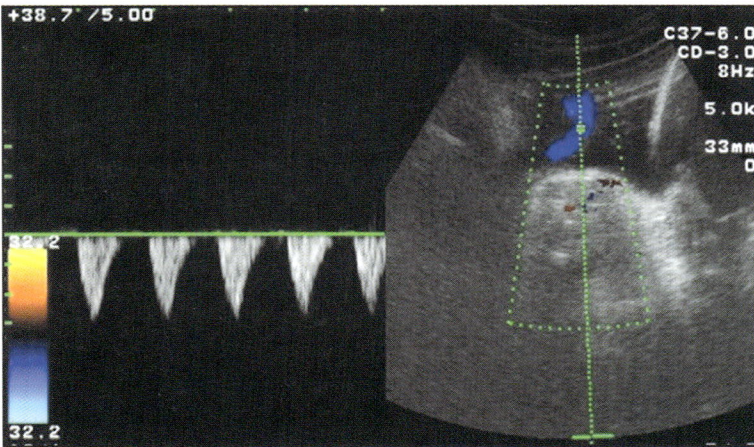

Fig. 8.13: Umbilical artery: Absence of diastolic flow

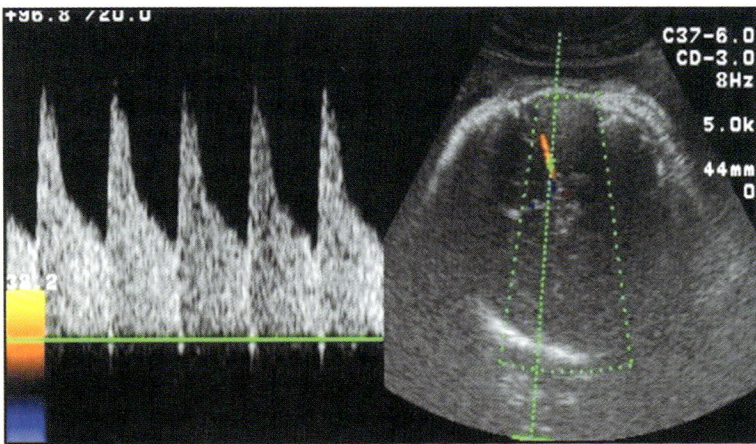

Fig. 8.14: Middle cerebral artery vasodilatation

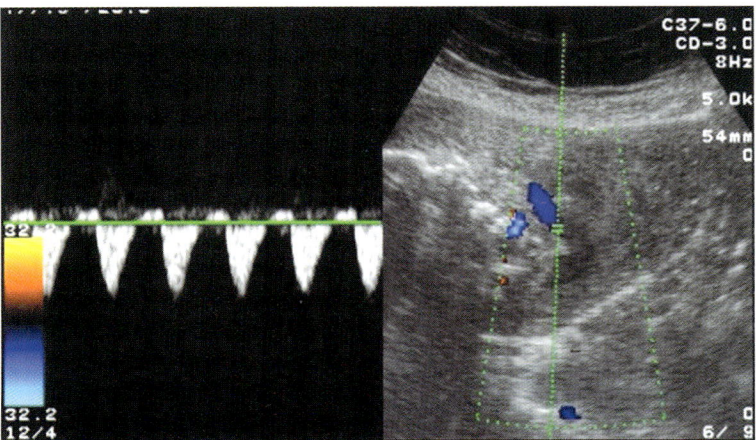

Fig. 8.15: Umbilical artery: Reverse diastolic flow

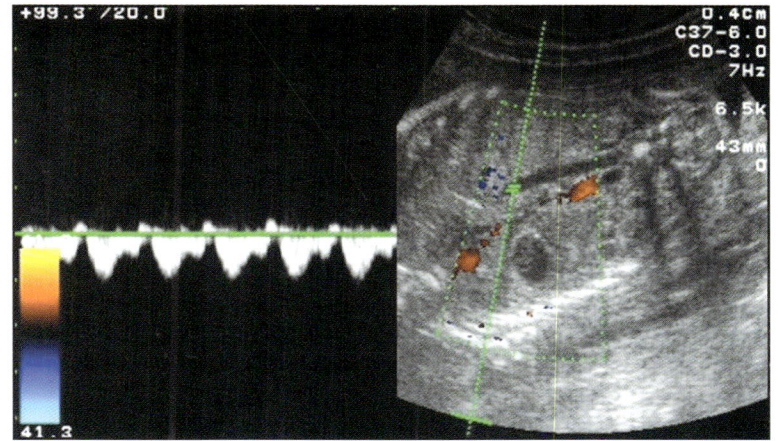

Fig. 8.16: Inferior vena cava: Normal FVW

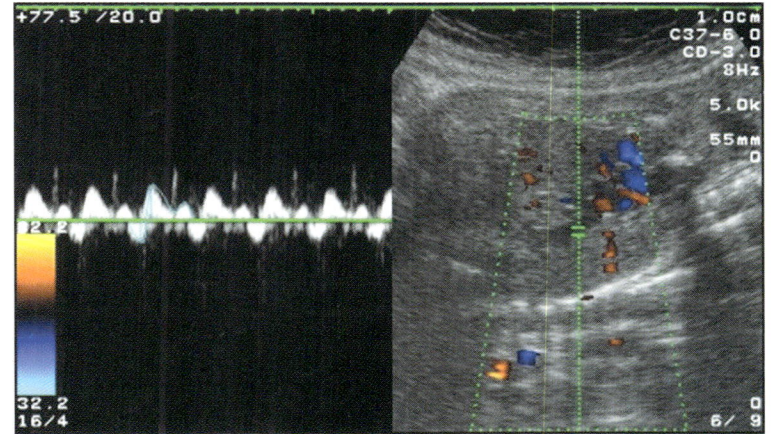

Fig. 8.17: Inferior vena cava: Increased reverse blood flow coinciding with auricular contraction

2. Reduction in the telediastolic velocity values in the ductus venosus(in the notch which reflects the auricular contraction) (Figs 8.18 and 8.19); this reduction can lead to an inversion of the blood flow. This would be secondary not only to the increase in telediastolic; volume determinated by the increase in the peripheral resistance, but also to the reduction in the capacity for myocardial response.[4]

3. "Venous pulsation" in the umbilical vein, with an apparent cyclical decrease in the venous flow coinciding with the zero diastole of the umbilical artery (Figs 8.20 and 8.21).

As regards the exit blood flows, there have been reports of their progressive deterioration in this phase, with a clear reduction in their velocity peaks and decreased cardiac output.[41] The most recent observation in this respect in probably the reduction in the values of the so-called "ventricular ejection force" (VEF).[42]

It has been demonstrated that the VEF values of both the right and the left ventricles are similar and increase throughout gestation in fetuses with normal growth. In contrast, there is a significant decrease in both ventricles, below the 5th centile of the normality curves, in the terminal phase of the centralization of blood flow.[42] Furthermore, there is an excellent correlation between the VEF values and the severity of the acidosis

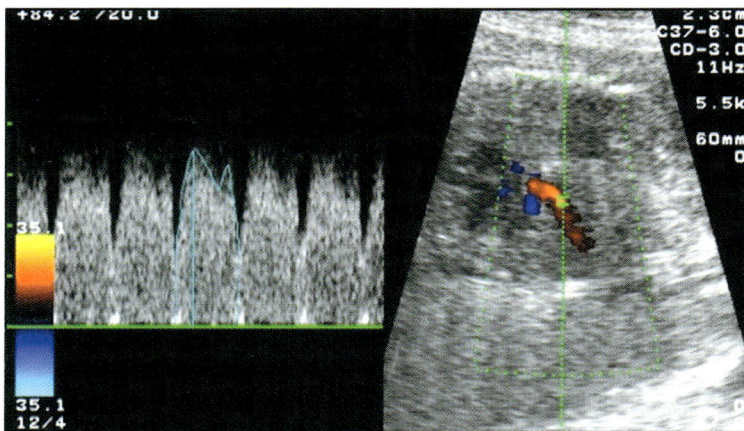

Fig. 8.18: Ductus venosus: Normal FVW

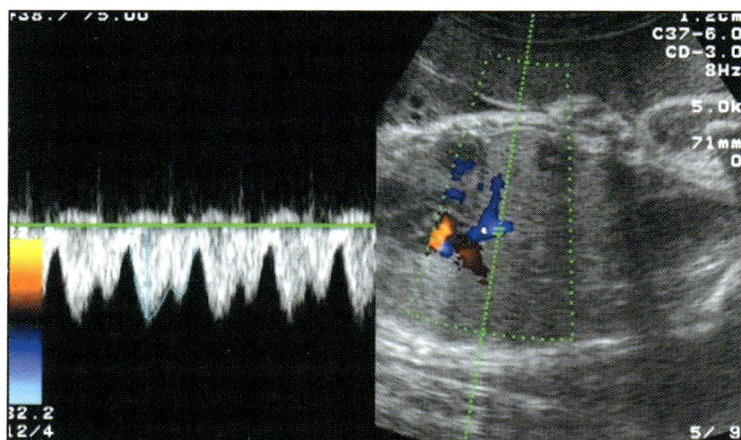

Fig. 8.19: Ductus venosus: Reduction in telediastolic velocity

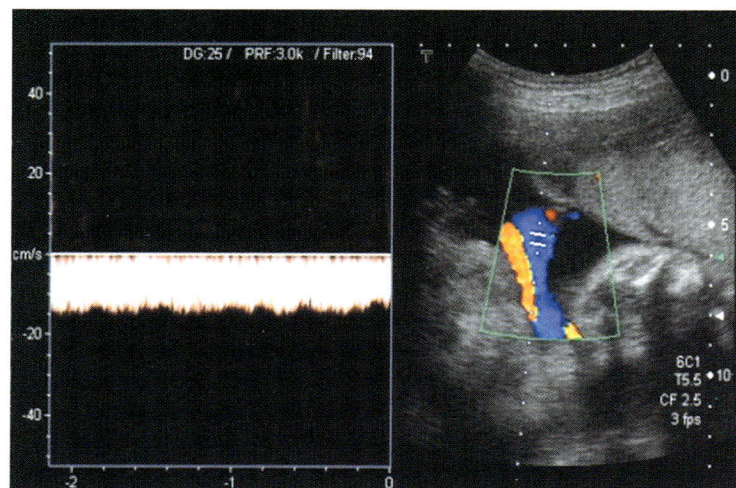

Fig. 8.20: Umbilical vein: Normal FVW

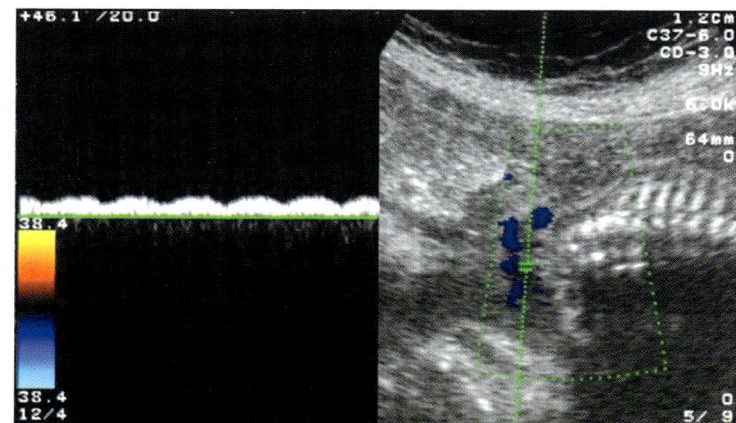

Fig. 8.21: Venous pulsation in umbilical vein

registered by funiculocentesis. It can therefore be stated that this hemodynamic finding is significantly related to a serious fetal compromise.

The visualization of the coronary blood flow, in the context of a severe uteroplacental insufficiency, must be interpreted as a very serious sign of fetal distress, probably premortem. The phenomenon is particularly visible in the diastole.[43]

The coronary vasodilatation which makes it possible can be the result of three different types of mechanism: (a) an attempt at compensation provoked by low myocardial oxygen pressure; (b) loss of myocardial contraction force, which causes a reduction in the pressure on the coronary arteries (especially during the diastole), and (c) decrease in the velocity of the intracardial blood flows, with the same results as in (b) The first autoregulating mechanism described could be called a heart-sparing effect, and this has been studied in detail.[35]

In the initial phase of centralization, the cardiotocographic readings can still apparently be normal and Manning's biophysical profile proves to be unaltered or doubtful.

The biophysical parameters affected most early or are in correlation with behavior. Changes in the cyclical periods of rest/activity[44] and a decrease in multiple rolling movements.

Although there is an increase in the pathological results of the biophysical stress tests with respect to the previous stage, we have not been able to establish whether their comparative percentages are significantly different statistically.

However, in the advanced phase there is a progressive deterioration in the fetal cardiac frequency register and late decelerations appear. The time lapse from the pathological quality of the umbilical PI until the appearance of late decelerations in the register has been evaluated as between 9 and 60 days [45,46] with a mean of 2 to 3 weeks.[47-49] Echographically, on the other hand, there is an evident decrease in fetal movements (somatic and respiratory) and in fetal tone. There can be a marked decrease in amniotic fluid; Phelan and coworkers[50] obtained indices of between 5 and 8. If all these data are marked in accordance with Manning's the biophysical profile usually attains a score of under 7. In the phase the number of positive oxytocin tests is already clearly significant, as are the force tests and the vibroacoustic stimulation. We are then confronted with the decompensation of a chorionic fetal distress which, until then, could be considered as compensated.

Finally, in the late phase, and owing to the loss of cardiac automatism, not only do apparent late decelerations appear in the cardiotocographic reading, but there is also noticeable loss of reactivity.[51] The ominous readings do not appear until 2 to 3 weeks after the minimum values of the cerebral PI have been attained. In fact, this interval depends on the ability of the fetus to compensate for the reduction in the metabolic supply.[7,52,53]

The biophysical profile shows very low values, always under 5, owing to the alteration of all its parameters (severe decrease to the alteration of all its parameters, severe decrease in fetal movements and tone, etc. and an increasingly significant oligohydramnios.

When the velocimetric values are altered not only in the umbilical artery, but also in the remaining fetal vessels (aorta, common carotid and middle cerebral arteries), there is a risk of low pO_2 and pH values in the fetal blood obtained by cordocentesis.[32,44,54,55] In fact, centralization gets underway only when the fetus is already suffering from a degree of hypoxemia and acidosis.

In the initial phase, with end-diastolic frequencies still present in both the umbilical artery and the aorta, the percentage of cases with hypoxemia does not generally exceed 25 to 30 percent.

The situation changes dramatically in the advanced phase, when the to end-diastolic values of the Doppler frequency in those two vessels disappear: in the case 70 to 80 percent of the fetuses present hypoxemia, and 40 to 60 percent present acidosia.[31,32,55,56] The majority of authors[57-59] consider that the absence of end-diastolic flow signifies pathological results in the acid-base study of the fetal blood.[60]

Finally, in the terminal phase, practically all the fetuses have a pO_2 between 2 and 4 SD below the mean.[61]

DECENTRALIZATION OF BLOOD FLOW

Decentralization of blood flow is represented by irreversible hemodynamic changes that follow on from the centralization of blood flow and which precede fetal death.

Pathophysiological Basis

If the hypoxia persists, a phenomenon of generalized fetal vascular paralysis will ultimately occur.

We can probably hypothesize that the situation is similar to those described in the fetuses of monkeys[62] and sheep[63] subjected to severe and sustained hypoxemia. The appearance of cerebral edema and the resulting increase in intracranial pressure hinder the mechanism for cerebral blood perfusion. The cerebral edema is probably brought about by the local accumulation of lactic acid resulting from the sustained anaerobic metabolism, which alters the permeability of the cellular membrane, increases the osmotic intracellular pressure and ultimately leads to the edema and eventual tissue necrosis.

The result of all this is that, in addition to the hypoxemia of the cerebral centers, there is a progressively irreversible interference in the control mechanism of the arterial tone. The situation usually occurs when the hypoxemia is extreme: more than 4 SD below the mean.[61,64,65]

Doppler Hemodynamic Profile

The diagnosis of decentralization of blood flow essentially rests on two findings:
1. Confirmation of resistance in the umbilical and peripheral circulation (aorta, renal…) with the presence of reserve end diastolic flow; and
2. Increase, after a brief period of stabilization, in the PI in the intracranial arteries, the values of which can appear normal; there are even FVW without diastoles or with reverse flow.[66]

It is not known how much time can pass from the onset of this picture until in utero fetal death, but it is probably no more than 2 to 3 days, and in many cases only a few hours; this explains the remote possibility of observing in through Doppler.

Biophysical Correlation

If a cardiotocographic examination is carried out at this point, it is certain that a terminal pattern will be observed, indicating the so-called "intrauterine brain death syndrome".[67-72] The readings invariably show a fixed fetal cardiac frequency, with no variability from one heartbeat to another and a complete absence of accelerations or decelerations, even when contractions are induced by an oxytocin test or an EVA is performed. The biophysical profile, on the other hand, will show an immobile atonic fetus, drawn in on itself and with hardly any amniotic fluid, although some authors[71-73] have described some cases with hydramnios. The score will not exceed 2 points.

Only on very rare occasions will it be possible by echography to confirm the existence of cystic periventricular cerebral lesions (porencephaly) or evident ventriculomegaly[72,74,75] the consequence of the hypoxic necrosis.[67,74,76]

As has already been mentioned above, that a funiculocentesis will confirm extreme hypoxemia (values of $PO_2 - 4$ SD below the mean) and a significant acidosis.

REFERENCES

1. Carrera JM, Torrents M, Muñoz A, Figueras F, Comas C. The role of Doppler in prenatal diagnosis. Ultrasound Rev Obstet Gynecol 2002;2:240-50.
2. Rudolph AM, Heymann MA. The circulation of the fetus "in utero". Methods for studying distribution of blood flow, cardiac output and organ blood flow. Circ Res 1967;21:163-7.

3. Johnson GN, Palahniuk RJ, Tweed WA, Jones MV, Wade JG. Regional cerebral blood flow changes during fetal asphyxia produced by slow partial umbilical cord compression. Am J Obstet Gynecol 1979;135:48-52.

4. Behrman RE, Lees MH, Peterson EN, De Lannoy CW, Seeds AE. Distribution of the circulation in the normal and asphyxiated fetal primate. Am J Obstet Gynecol 1970;108:956-69.

5. Morrow RJ, Adamson SL, Bull SB, Ritchie JWK. Ante hypoxemia does not effect umbilical artery waveforms in sheep. Obstet Gynecol 1990;75:590-3.

6. Morrow RJ, Adamson SL, Bull SB, Ritchie JWK. Hypoxia acidaemia, hyperviscosity and maternal hypertension do not affect the umbilical artery velocity waveforms in fetal sheep. Am J Obstet Gynecol 1990;163:1313-20.

7. Trudinger BJ. Doppler ultrasound study and fetal abnormality. In Drife JO, Donnan D (Eds): Antenatal Diagnosis of Fetal Abnormalities. London: Springer-Verlag, 1991;113.

8. Gruenwald P. The relation of deprivation to perinatal pathology and late sequels. In Grunewald P (Ed): The placenta. Lancaster Gr: Med. Tech. Publish. Co., 1975.

9. Laurin J, Marsal K, Persson PH, Lingman G. Ultrasound measurement of fetal blood in predicting fetal outcome. Br J Obstet Gynaecol 1987;94:940-8.

10. Laurin J, Lingman G, Marsal K, Persons PH. Fetal blood flow in pregnancies complicated by intrauterine growth retardation. Obstet Gynecol 1987;69:895-902.

11. Carrera JM, Devesa R, Torrents M, Muñoz A, Comas C, Nortera C, Serra B. Natural history of fetal compromise in intrauterine growth retardation. In Kurjak A (Ed): Textbook of Perinatal Medicine (Vol. 2). London: Parthenon Publishing, 1998;1226-43

12. Guidetti R, Luzi G, Simonazzi E, Tini M, Chicodi A, Di Renzo GC, Cosmi E. Correlation between cerebral blood flow and umbilical blood flow in the fetus recorded with a pulsed Doppler system. Abstract book of the XI European congress of perinatal medicine. Roma: CIC, 1988:252.

13. Baschat AA, Weiner CP. Umbilical artery Doppler screening for detection of the small fetus in need of antepartum surveillance. Am J Obstet Gynecol 2000;182:154-8.

14. Severi FM, Bocchi C, Viscuti A, et al. Uterine and fetal cerebral Doppler predict the outcome of third trimester small-for-gestational age fetuses with normal umbilical artery Doppler. Ultrasound Obstet Gynecol 2002;19:225-8.

15. Hershkowitz R, Kingdom JC, Geary M, Rodeck CH. Fetal cerebral blood flow distribution in late gestations: identification of compromise in small fetuses with normal umbilical artery Doppler. Ultrasound Obstet Gynecol 2000;15:209-12.

16. Mc Cowan LM, Harding JE, Roberts AB, et al. A pilot randomized controlled trial of two regiments of fetal surveillance for small-for-gestational age fetuses with normal results of umbilical artery Doppler velocimetry. Am J Obstet Gynecol 2000;182:81-6.

17. Morrow RJ, Adamson SL, Ritchie JWK, Pearce JM. The pathophysiological basis of abnormal flow velocity waveforms. In Pearce JM (Ed): Doppler Ultrasound in Perinatal Medicine. Oxford: Oxford University Press, 1992.

18. Arduini D, Valensise H. Fetal hemodynamics in growth retardation. In Kurjak A (Ed): Textbook of Perinatal Medicine. London: Parthenon Publishing 1998:1217-25.

19. De Haan J. Fisiopatologia de los cambios de los indices de flujo Doppler en la circulacion fetal. In Carrera JM (Ed). Doppler en Obstetricia. Barcelona: Masson-Salvat, 1992:89-97.

20. Laurini R, Laurin J, Marsal K. Placental histology and fetal blood in intrauterine retardation. Acta Obst Gynecol Scand 1994;73:529-34.

21. Giorlandino G, Vizzone A. Flussimetria ostetrica materna e fetale. Testo Atlante. Roma: CIC Edizione Inter, 1993.

22. Dawes GS, Duncan SL, Lewis BV, Merlet CL, Owen-Thomas TB, Reeves JT. Cyanide stimulation of the systemic arterial chemoreception in foetal lambs. J Physiol 1969;201:117-28.

23. De Vore GR. Examination of the fetal heart in the fetus with intrauterine growth retardation using M-mode echocardiography. Semin Perinatol 1988;12:66-79.

24. Lingman G, Legarth J, Rahman F, Stangenberg M. Myocardial contractility in the anemia human fetus. Ultrasound Obstet Gynecol 1991;1:266-8.

25. Marsal K, Lingman G, Giles W. Evaluation of the carotid, aortic and umbilical blood velocity waveforms in the human fetus. XI Annual Conference of the Society for the study of fetal physiology, Oxford. Oxford: The Nuffield Institute, 1984:C33.

26. Marsal K, Lindblad A, Lingman G, Eik-Nes SH. Blood flow in the fetal descending aorta: intrinsic factors affecting fetal bllod flow, i.e. fetal breathing movements and fetal cardiac arrhythmia. Ultrasound Med Biol 1984;10:339-48.

27. Wladimiroff JW, Tonge HM, Stewart PA. Doppler ultrasound assessment of cerebral blood flow in the human fetus. Br J Obstet Gynaecol 1986;93:471-5.

28. Arabin B, Bergmann PL, Saling E. Simultaneous assessment of blood flow velocity waveforms in uteroplacental vessels, the umbilical artery, the fetal aorta and the common carotid artery. Fetal Ther 1987;2:17-26.

29. Arabin B, Siebert M, Jimenez E, Saling E. Obstetrical characteristic of a loss of end-diastolic velocities in the fetal aorta and/or umbilical artery using Doppler ultrasound. Gynecol Obstet Invest 1987;25:173-80.

30. Bilardo CM, Campbell S, Nicolaides KH. Mean blood velocity and flow impedance in the fetal descending thoracic aorta and common carotid artery in normal pregnancy. Early Hum Dev 1988;18:213-7.

31. Montenegro CA. Perfil hemodinamico fetal-Diastole-Zero "revisitada". J Brasileiro Ginecol 1992;102(10):375-80.

32. Montenegro CA, Meirelles J, Fonseca AL, Netto MC, Amin Junior J, Rezende-Filho J, Jacyntho C. Cordocentèse et evaluation du bien-être foetal dans une population à très haut risque. Rev Franç Gynecol Obstet 1992 ;87 :467-77.

33. Gramellini P, Folli MC, Raboni S, Vadora E, Merialdi A. Cerebral-umbilical Doppler ratio as a predictor of adverse perinatal outcome. Obstet Gynecol 1992;79:416-20.

34. Ferrazi E, Belloti M, Galan H, Pennati G, Bozzo M, Rigano S, Battaglia FC. Doppler investigation in intrauterine growth restricion – from qualitative indices to flow measurements: a review of the experience of a collaborative group. Ann NY Acad Sci 2001;943:316-25.

35. Grmbruch U, Baschat AA. Demonstration of fetal coronary blood flow by color-coded and pulsed wave Doppler sonography: a possible indicator of severe compromise and impending demise in intrauterine growth retardation. Ultrasound Obstet Gynecol 1996;7:10-6.

36. Rigano S, Bozzo M, Ferrazi E, Belloti M, Battaglia FC, Galan HL. Early and persistent reductionin umbilical vein blood flow in the growth restricted fetus: a longitudinal study.Am J Obstet Gynecol 2001;185:834-8.

37. Indik JH, Chen V, Reed KL. Association of umbilical venous with inferior vena cava blood flow velocities. Obstet Gynecol 1991;77:551-7.

38. Reed KL. Venous flow velocities in the fetus. In: Jaffe R, Warson SL (Eds): Color Doppler Imaging in Obstetrics and Gynecology. New York: McGraw Hill, 1992:179.

39. Rizzo G, Arduini D, Romanini C. Inferior vena cava flow velocity waveforms in appropriate and small-for-gestational-age fetuses. Am J Gynecol 1992;166:1271-80.

40. Antolin E, Carrera JM. Ductus venosus in IUGR. Perinatal outcome. In Carrera JM, Cabero L, Baraibar R (Eds): The Perinatal Medicine of the New Millennium. Bologna: Monduzzi, 2001:691-9.

41. Rizzo G, Arduini D. Fetal cardiac function in intrauterine growth retardation. Am J Obstet Gynecol 1991;165:876-82.

42. Rizzo G, Capponi A, Rinaldo D, Arduini D, Romanini C. Ventricular ejection force in growth retarded fetuses. Ultrasound Obstet Gynecol 1995;5:247-55.

43. Baschat AA, Gembruch U, Gortner L, Reiss I, Weiner CP, Harman CR. Coronary artery blood flow visualization signifies hemodynamic deterioration in growth-restricted fetuses. Ultrasound Obstet Gynecol 2000;16:425-31.

44. Arduini D, Rizzo G, Romanini C, Mancuso S. Are blood flow velocity waveforms related to umbilical cord acid-base status in the human fetus? Gynecol Obstet Invest 1989;27:183-7.

45. Reuwer PJ, Sijmons EA, Rietman GW, Van Tiel MN, Bruinse HW. Intrauterine growth retardation: prediction of perinatal distress by Doppler ultrasound. Lancet 1987;2:415-8.

46. Bekedam DJ, Visser GH, Van Der Zee AG, Snijders RJ, Poelmann Weesjes G. Abnormal velocity waveforms of the umbilical artery in growth retarded fetuses: relationship to antepartum late heart rate decelerations and outcome. Early Hum Dev 1990;24:79-89.

47. Arduini D, Rizzo G, Romanini C. Changes of pulsatility index from fetal vessels preceding the outset of latedecelerations in growth retarded fetuses. Obstet Gynecol 1992;79:605-10.

48. Arduini D, Rizzo G. Color Doppler studies of fetal circulation in intrauterine growth retardation. In Jaffe R, Warson SL (Eds): Color Doppler Imaging in Obstetrics and Gynaecology. New York: McGraw-Hill, 1992:183.

49. Griffin DR, Bilardo K, Diaz-Recasens J, Pearce JM, Wilson K, Campbell S. Doppler blood flow waveforms in the descending thoracic aorta of the human fetus. Br J Obstet Gynaecol 1984;91:997-1002.

50. Phelan JP, Smith CV, Bronssard P, Small M. Amniotic fluid volume assessment with the four-quadrant technique at 36-42 weeks of gestation. J Reprod Med 1987;32:540-2.

51. Nijhuis IJ, Hof J, Mulder EJ, Nijhuis JG, et al. Fetal hear rate in relation to its variation in normal and growth retarded fetuses. Eur J Obstet Gynecol Reprod Biol 2000;89:27-33.

52. Manning FA, Harman CR, Menticoglon S, Dayal A, Xic J. mental retardation: prevalence and etiological factors in a large obstetric population. Am J Obstet Gynecol 2000;182:S110.

53. Baschat AA. Integrated fetal testing in growth restriction: combining multivessel Doppler and biophysical parameters. Ultrasound Obstet Gynecol 2003;21:1-8.

54. Nicolaides KH, Bilardo CM, Soothill PW, Campbell S. Absence of end-diastolic frequencies in the umbilical artery: a sign of fetal hypoxia and acidosis. Br Med J 1988;297:1026-7.

55. Nicolaides KH, Bilardo CM, Campbell S. Prediction of fetal anaemia by measurement of mean blood velocity in the fetal aorta. Am J Obstet Gynecol 1990;162:209-12.

56. Hsieh FJ, Chang FM, Ko TM, Chen HY, Chen YP. Umbilical artery flow velocity waveforms in fetuses dying with congenital anomalies. BrJ Obstet Gynaecol 1988;95:478-82.

57. Ferrazzi E, Pardi G, Bauscaglia M, Marconi AM, Gementi B, Bellotti M et al. The correlation of biochemical monitoring versus umbilical flow velocity measurements of the human fetus. Am J Obstet Gynecol 1988;159:1081-7.

58. Tyrell S, Obais AH, Lilford RJ. Umbilical artery Doppler velocimetry as a predictor of fetal hypoxia and acidosis at birth. Obstet Gynecol 1989;74:332-7.

59. Bilardo CM, Nicolaides KH, Campbell S. Doppler measurements of fetal and uteroplacental circulation: relationship with umbilical venous blood gases measured at cordocentesis. Am J Obstet Gynecol 1990;162:115-9.

60. Ferrazi E, Bozzo M, Rigano S, Belloti M, Morabito A, Pardi G et al. Temporal sequence of abnormal Doppler changes in the peripheral and central circulation systems of the severely growth-restricted fetus. Ultrasound Obstet Gynecol 2002;19:140-6.

61. Vyas S, Nicolaides KH, Bower S, Campbell S. Middle cerebral artery flow velocity waveforms in fetal hypoxemia. Br J Obstet Gynaecol 1990;97:797-803.

62. Myers RE, De Courtney-Myers GM, Wagner KR. Effects of hypoxia on fetal brain. In Beard RW, Nathanielsz PW (Eds): Fetal Physiology and Medicine. London: Butterworth, 1984:419.

63. Richardson BS, Rurak D, Patrick IE, Homan J, Carmichael I. Cerebral oxidative metabolism during sustained hypoxaemia in fetal sheep. J Dev Physiol 1989;2:37-43

64. Vyas S. Pulsed Doppler examination of the normal human fetus. In Pearce JM (Ed). Doppler Ultrasound in Perinatal Medicine. Oxford: Oxford University Press, 1992.

65. Vyas S, Campbell S. Doppler studies of the cerebral and renal circulations in small-for-gestational age fetuses. In Pearce JM (Ed). Doppler Ultrasound in Perinatal Medicine. Oxford: Oxford University Press, 1992:268-78.

66. Mari G, Wasserstrum N. Flow velocity waveforms of the fetal circulation preceding fetal death in a case of lupus anticoagulant. Am J Obstet Gynecol 1991;164:776-78.

67. Adams RD, Prod´Hom LS, Rabinowicz TH. Intrauterine brain death. Acta Neuropathol 1977;40:41-9.

68. Gaziano EP, Freeman DW. Analysis of heart rate patterns preceding fetal death. Obstet Gynecol 1977;50:578-82.

69. van der Moer PE, Gerretsen G, Visser GHA. Fixed fetal heart rate pattern after intrauterine accidental decerebration. Obstet Gynecol 1985;65:125-7.

70. Nijhuis JG, Kruy N, Van Vijck JAM. Fetal brain death. Two case reports. Br J Obstet Gynaecol 1988;85:197-200.

71. Nijhuis JG, Crevels AJ, Van Dongen PWJ. Fetal brain death: The definition of a fetal heart rate pattern and its clinical consequences. Obstet Gynecol Surv 1990;45:229-32.

72. Zimmer EZ, Jakobi P, Goldstein I, Gutterman E. Cardiotocographic and sonographic findings in two cases of antenatally diagnosed intrauterine fetal brain death. Prenatal Diagn 1992;12:271-6.

73. Ellis WG, Goetzman BW, Lindenberg JA. Neuropathologic documentation of prenatal brain damage. Am J Dis Child 1988;142:858-66.

74. Nwaesei CG, Pape KE, Martin DJ, Becker LE, Fitz CR. Periventricular infarction diagnosed by ultrasound: a postmortem correlation. J Pediatr 1984;105:106-10.

75. Hill A. Assessment of the fetus: Relevance to brain injury. Clin Perinatol 1989;16:413-4.

76. Larroche JCL, Droulle P, Delezoide AL, Narey F, Nessmann C. Brain damage in monozygous twins. Biol Neonate 1990;57:261-78.

E Scazzocchio, MA Rodriguez
F Astudillo

9

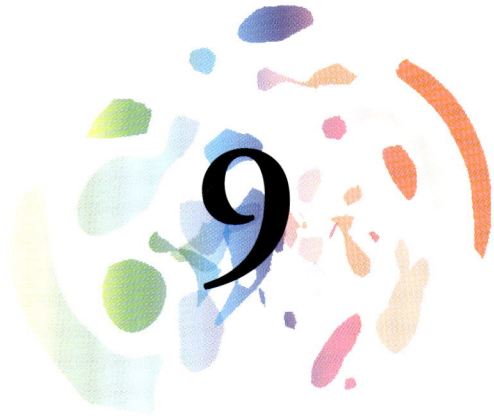

Cervical Incompetence: Ultrasonic Evaluation

INTRODUCTION

In 1658 Riverius and colleagues[1] described for the first time a late spontaneous abortion, whose cause was thought to be the "slackness" of the uterine cervix. Two hundred years later, Gream[2] speculated on the possibility that a "weakness" in the cervical structures prevented them from supporting the weight of the pregnancy to term. It was not until 1947, however, that Danforth[3] correctly described the musculofibrous sphincter mechanism of the internal cervical os of the uterine cervix. The detailed anatomical study enabled Lash and Lash[4], in 1950, to define cervical incompetence, or insufficiency, as "the loss of structural or functional integrity in the sphincter mechanism of the internal cervical os, resulting in the effacement and dilatation of the uterine cervix and the subsequent interruption of the gestation at between 14 and 28 weeks."

DIAGNOSIS

The diagnosis made prior to gestation should be distinguished from that made during pregnancy.

Pregestational Diagnosis

Cervical incompetence should be suspected whenever there is a history of two or more spontaneous abortions in the second trimester (14 to 28 weeks) showing the characteristics typically associated with the condition, namely, rapid, almost painless pregnancy loss with protrusion of the amniotic sac and the expulsion of a living fetus.

Cervical incompetence is unlikely in the case of earlier spontaneous abortions or those which, although occurring during the second trimester, are long and difficult or are preceded by a retained, dead fetus.

The diagnosis may be confirmed by means of various exploratory procedures:

1. The excessive permeability of the internal cervical os.
2. Hysterosalpingography, performed in the second stage of the cycle (if possible with progesterone treatment) and using a cervical suction cannula which does not damage the cervix and enables the whole of it to be visualized. An internal cervical os of greater than 6 mm[5] and the morphology typical of the cervical canal (finger-shaped) usually confirm the existence of cervical incompetence.
3. Transvaginal ultrasound examination of the cervix showing that the width of the internal cervical os is greater than 10 mm.
4. Endocervical hysteroscopy, confirming the incontinence of the internal cervical os.
5. Stress relaxation tests[6] to determine the degree of cervical dilatation under pressure.
6. Uterine rheobase tests[7] aimed at establishing the minimum current required to cause a uterine contraction. These, therefore, measure the degree of uterine irritability.

Gestational Diagnosis

During pregnancy, possible cervical incompetence should be suspected when, regardless of the patient's history, clinical examination reveals:

1. Short and/or dilated cervix (prior to 28th week). This finding is confirmed in around 50 percent of cases of cervical incompetence. The importance of the data obtained from examination depends on whether it is the woman's first pregnancy or not.[8] Some authors consider that these signs are not specific and therefore have a low predictive value. Indeed, various researchers[9,10] have

found significant cervical dilatations (1 to 2 cm) in normal pregnancies at 21st to 28th weeks in 16 percent of primigravidas and 17 to 35 percent of multigravidas.

2. Visualization of the membranes, with or without protrusion of the amniochorionic sac. This finding is practically pathognomonic.

3. Other more indirect signs have also been described, for example, leukorrhea, sensation on the part of the pregnant woman of vaginal pressure or occupation; plaquiuria; and dysuria.

Diagnostic confirmation during pregnancy may be attempted by means of ultrasound, a procedure which should also enable cervical changes to be monitored throughout the first trimester and thus facilitate the decision on which cases would benefit from cervical cerclage when this decision could not be made earlier (owing to the absence of a reliable diagnosis during the pregestational stage).

In 1980 our group[11] published the first ultrasound images consistent with cervical incompetence, showing various stages of the process (isthmic sacculation, isthmic-cervical sacculation, cervical opening, etc.). Currently, a diagnosis of cervical incompetence is considered appropriate when the internal cervical os has a diameter of 23 to 25 mm or more,[12] it being ruled out with lesser diameters. Examination may be either transabdominal or transvaginal. In our service we use a scoring system to try to predict via ultrasound, the likelihood of a preterm birth.[13]

ULTRASONIC EVALUATION OF UTERINE CERVIX

Extensive research has been made so far, in methods of predicting preterm delivery in both asymptomatic and symptomatic patients. During the last few years a clear relationship has been established between decreased cervical length and the risk of spontaneous preterm delivery. Diagnostic ultrasound plays a very important role here. It has been applied mainly in five categories:

   i. women with symptoms of preterm labor,
   ii. asymptomatic women at high risk of preterm delivery,
   iii. asymptomatic women at low risk of preterm delivery,
   iv. women with multiple gestations,
   v. pregnancies complicated by preterm premature rupture of membranes (PPROM).

It is the purpose of this chapter to describe and illustrate the proper use of ultrasound in the accurate and reliable detection of cervical incompetence.

Technique

The cervix can be assessed by transabdominal, transvaginal or transperineal ultrasonography (Figs 9.1A to D). The main disadvantage of the transabdominal route is the need for a full bladder.

When transvaginal sonography is used the bladder is empty and the woman is placed in the dorsal lithotomy position. Then the probe is inserted in the anterior vaginal fornix and a sagittal view of the cervix is obtained. The picture should be magnified to at least 75 percent of the screen (Fig. 9.2).

Transperineal approach is an alternative method of cervical sonographic evaluation. More recently Cicero et al[14] showed that in the vast majority of cases cervical assessment can be performed by the transperineal approach. This method could be the method of choice in patients objecting to transvaginal sonography, or in those with preterm rupture of membranes, where transvaginal ultrasound should be better avoided for fear of infection.

Several other cervical characteristics such as the presence of funneling and the cervical index (funnel length + 1)/cervical length (Fig. 9.3) can be determined by ultrasound. The shape (Y- or U-shaped), the width, the length, and the percentage of funneling have also been evaluated (Figs 9.4 A, B and 9.5 A, B). It seems that a short cervix and funneling usually coexist. Therefore, a single measurement of the cervix is enough, because funneling is not an independent variable for the prediction of preterm birth in most of cases.[15] Several studies proposed transfundal or suprapubic pressure in order to detect cervical shortening. They suggested that this was the earliest sign of cervical incompetence and therefore identification of high-risk cases.[16-18]

Recently, three-dimensional transvaginal sonography has been proposed for the evaluation of cervical morphology. Bega et al[19] showed that three-dimensional ultrasound gave more accurate estimation of the cervical length compared to two-dimensional ultrasound. In a study on multiple gestations Strauss et al[20] failed to show any additional benefit from the use of three-dimensional versus conventional ultrasound for the measurement of the cervical length. Similar findings were observed in a study by Hoesli et al[21] who compared three-dimensional to two-dimensional ultrasound for the measurement of the cervical volume.

The Cervic in Women with Symptoms of Preterm Labor

Transvaginal ultrasound can be used as a screening test for preterm delivery in symptomatic patients. It can be used easily

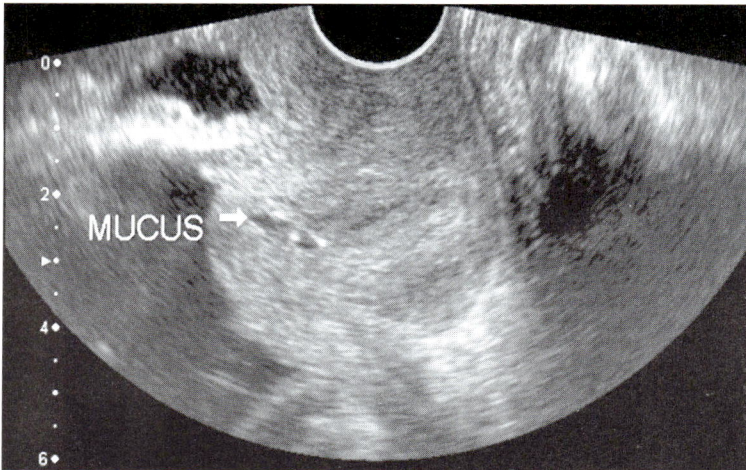

Fig. 9.1A: Transvaginal ultrasound at 20th week. Visualization of bladder, vagina and normal cervix. Visualization of mucus on cervix

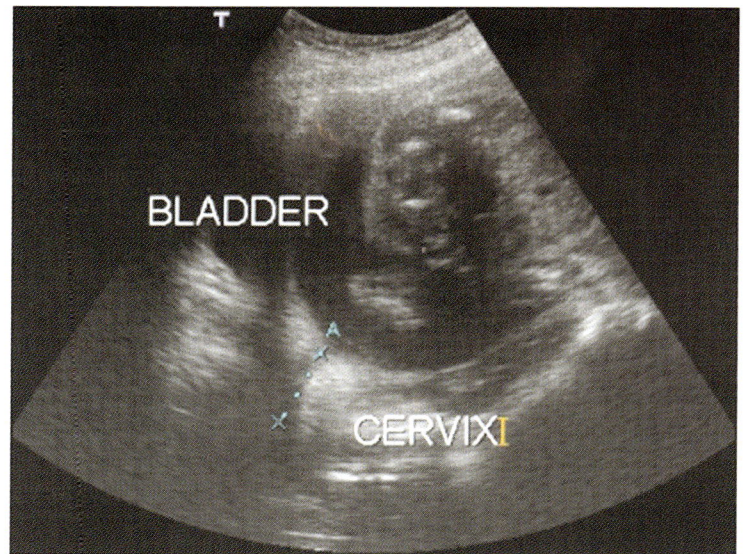

Figs 9.1B$_1$ or B$_2$: Transvaginal ultrasound at 20th week. Visualization of bladder, vagina, cervix and funnel

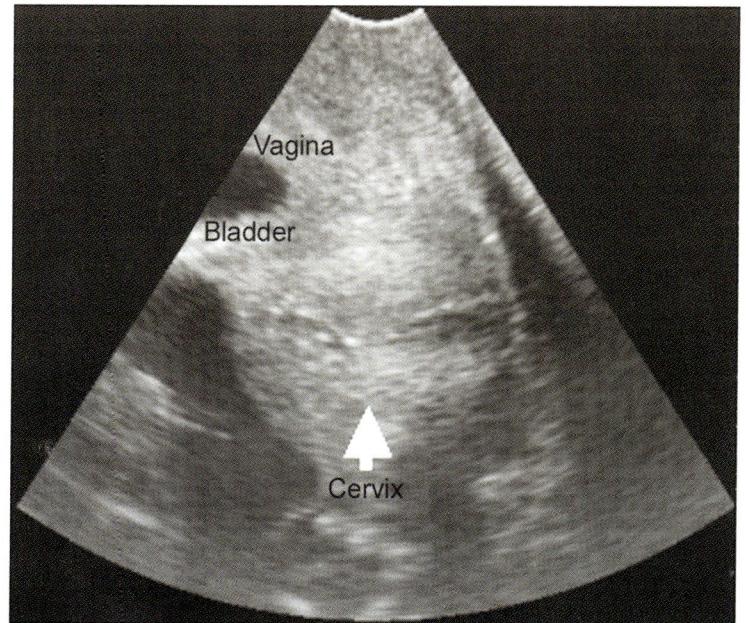

by physicians with the equipment and experience and it can reliably diagnose patients who are in true preterm labor when they present with preterm contractions, reducing the false-positive results. Consequently different management protocols can be used for symptomatic patients, depending on cervical length. A more aggressive tocolytic treatment in combination

Fig. 9.1C: Transabdominal ultrasound at 20th week. Visualization of bladder, vagina, and cervix. Bladder was non-good repletionated so we have image poor quality. When bladder is good repletionated it seems longer cervix that it is

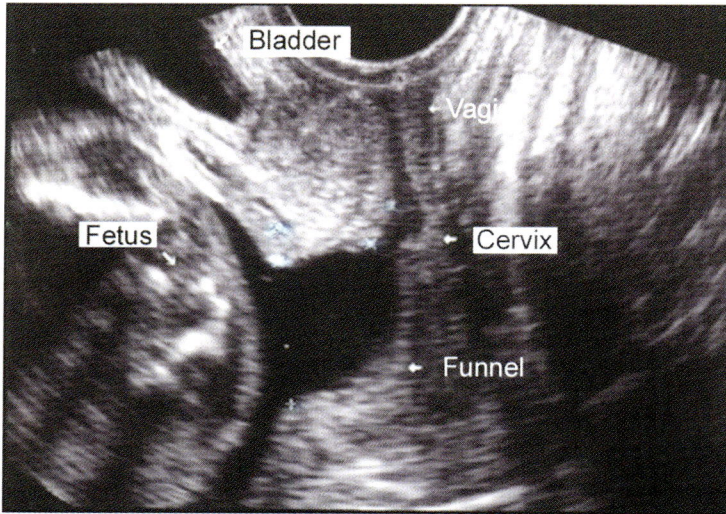

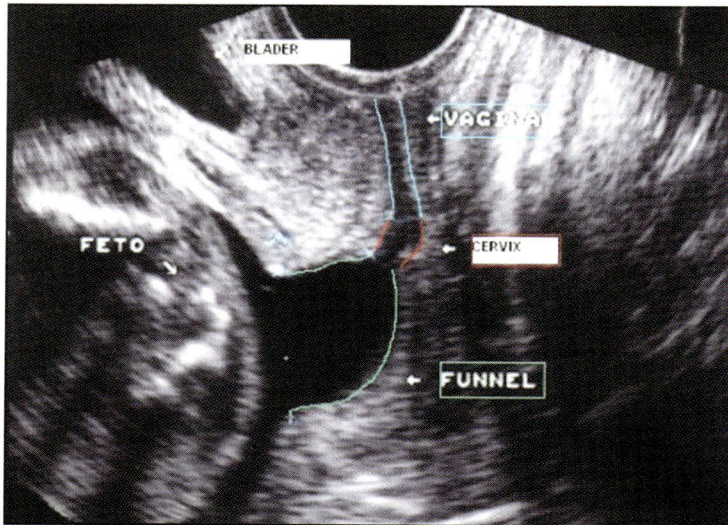

Fig. 9.1D: Transperineal ultrasound at 20th week. Visualization of bladder, vagina, and cervix.

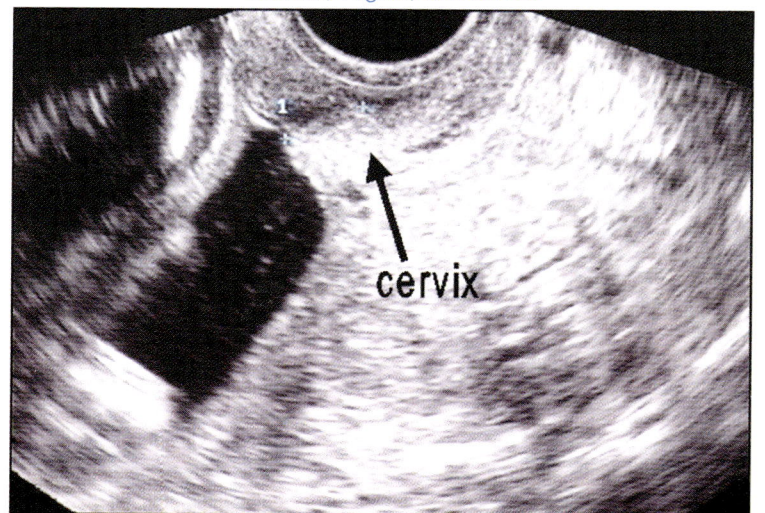

Fig. 9.2:. Incorrect vusualization because minimum magnificance

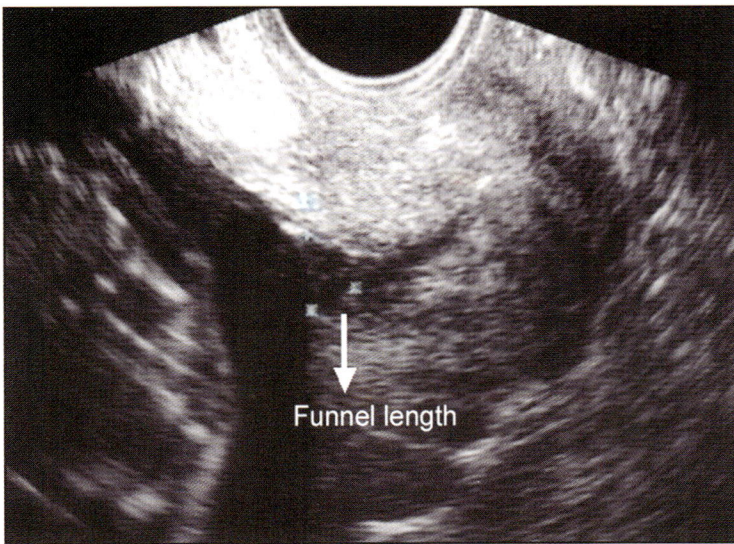

Fig. 9.3: Cervical index [(Funnel length + 1)/cervical length]

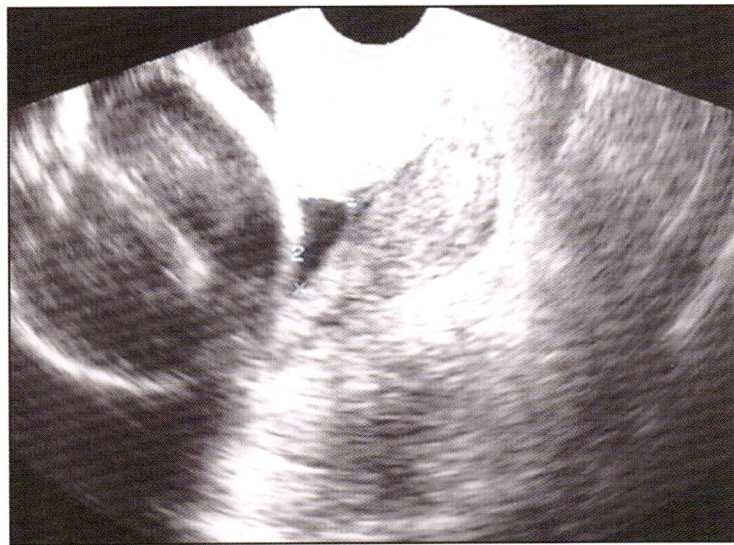

Figs 9.5A and B: U-shaped funneling of cervix

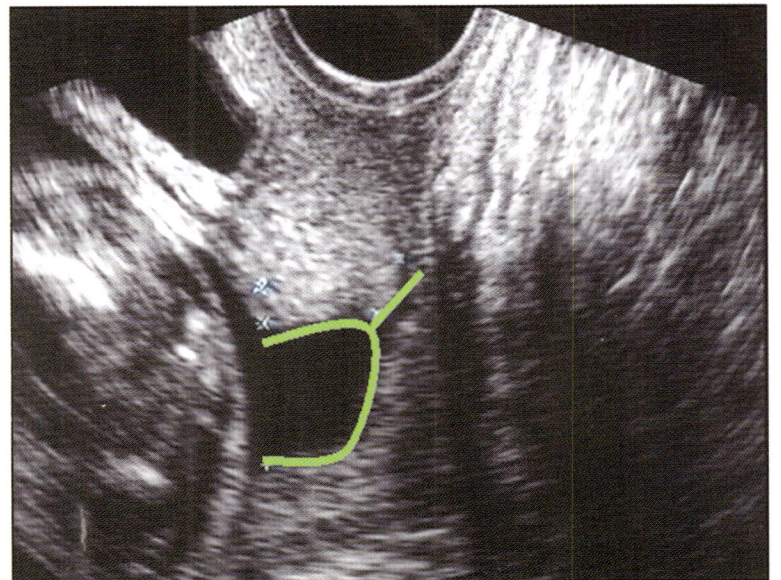

Figs 9.4A and B: Y-shaped funneling of cervix

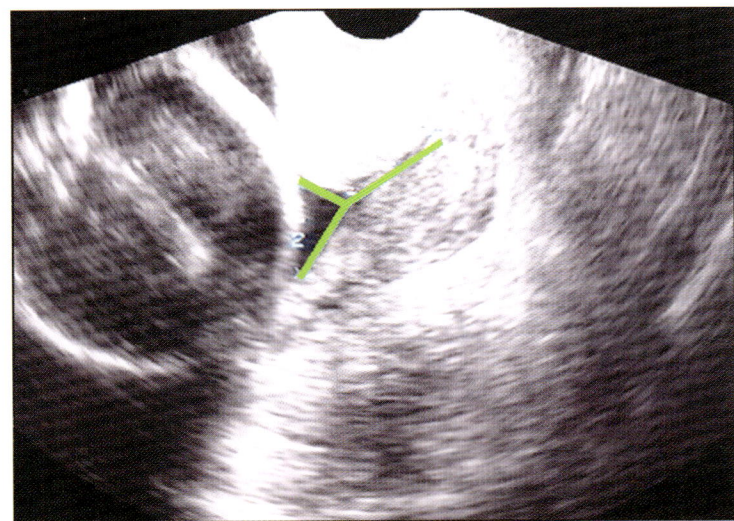

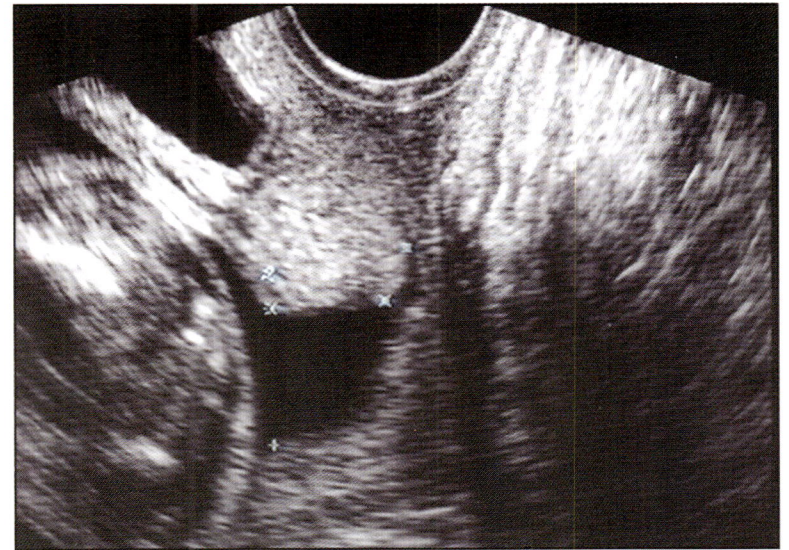

The Cervix in High-risk Asymptomatic Women

The high-risk population for preterm delivery includes women with a previous history of preterm delivery or rupture of the membranes, repeated mid-trimester pregnancy losses, cervical surgery, congenital uterine anomalies, or diethylstilbestrol exposure. Many studies have reported on cervical sonography for the prediction of preterm delivery in this population. The relative risk of preterm delivery using a cervical length cut-off of 25 mm between 16 and 20 weeks was 4.8 (95% CI 2.1-11.1, p=0.0004). Moreover, cervical ultrasonography was a better predictor of preterm delivery, than manual examination of the cervix. Guzman et al[17] examined high-risk women by serial transvaginal cervical ultrasonography with transfundal pressure. Examinations were performed until the cervical length decreased to < 10 mm. They concluded that the shortening of the cervical length, or the prolapse of the membranes into the cervix following transfundal pressure, has a significant predictive value for preterm delivery.

with fetal lung maturation should be considered for those with a short cervix. In contrast, patients with a long cervix should be managed in an outpatient basis, avoiding prolonged hospitalization and potentially dangerous tocolytic treatments.

Vendittelli et al[22] in a prospective study on 200 high-risk women reported that a cervical length of less than 30 mm had a relative risk of preterm delivery of 2.79 (95% CI 1.7-4.59) (Fig. 9.6). The presence of funneling of ≥ 5 mm gave a relative risk of 1.39 (95% CI 0.99-1.95). Obido et al[23] showed that a cervical funneling of more than 75 percent or a cervical shortening of less than 10 mm were predictive of preterm premature rupture of membranes. In a similar study Guzman et al[24] showed that a progressive cervical shortening of ≤ 20 mm before 24 weeks suggested cervical incompetence. Incompetent cervices had significantly greater cervical shortening compared to competent ones (p<0.001). Recently, Berghella et al[25] performed transvaginal cervical sonography in 183 high-risk women having pregnancies between 10th and 14th weeks and concluded that this period was not appropriate for screening for preterm delivery, as in most cases cervical changes develop after this gestational age.

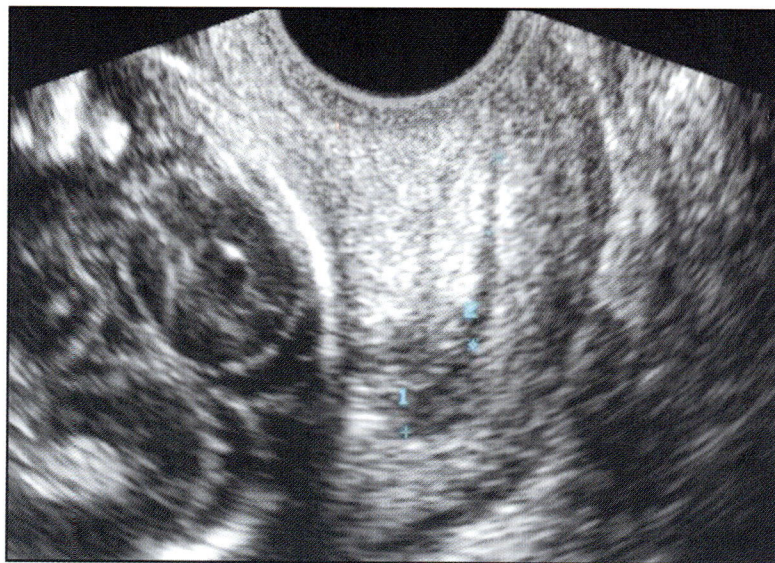

Fig. 9.6: Cervical length less than 30 mm (9.9 + 16.7 = 26.6)

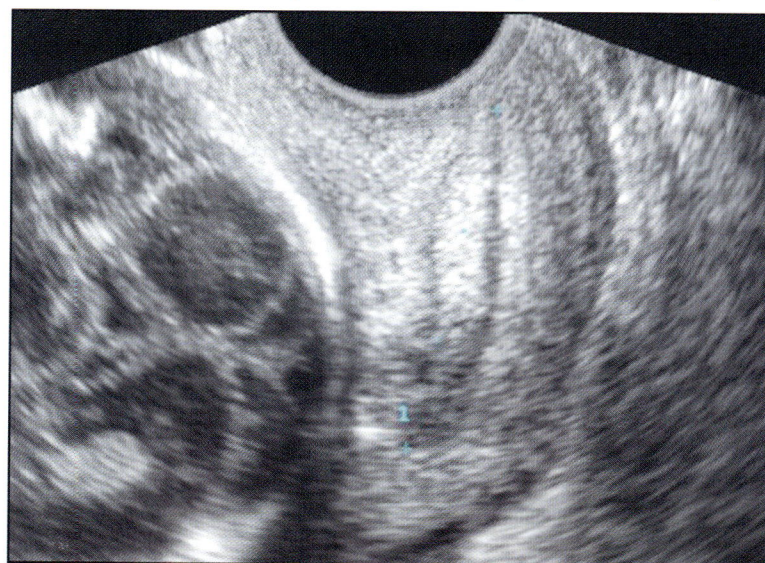

Fig. 9.7: Cervical length less than 35 mm

The Cervix in Low-risk Population

In comparison to women at high-risk of preterm delivery, pregnant women without risk factors have a low prevalence of preterm birth of about 4 to 8 percent. However, more than half of the preterm births occur in these low-risk women. It is therefore of great importance to examine the potential of cervical screening in this population. In 1990 Andersen et al[26] evaluated 178 women with singleton gestations and observed that the majority of preterm deliveries occurred in women with endovaginal ultrasonographic measurements below the median. In a similar study Tongsong et al[27] reported that a cervical length of less than 35 mm between 28th and 30th weeks had a sensitivity for delivery before 37th week of 65.9 percent and a specificity of 62.4 percent (Fig. 9.7).

Antsaklis et al[28] evaluated 1,197 singleton low-risk pregnancies at 23 weeks, with transvaginal sonographic cervical assessment. The preterm delivery rate before 37th week in our population was 8.7 percent, confirming that this was a low-risk population. The distribution of cervical length was normal and the mean cervical length was 38 mm (range: 2 to 70 mm). Less than 20 mm length of the cervix had 17 women (1.4%). Women with a cervical length > 20 mm had 3.31 times increased risk for prematurity (95% CI 10.14-1.08) (p=0.03). The presence of funneling gave a relative risk for preterm delivery of 2.07 (95% CI 0.94-4.54) (p=0.07).

The Cervix in Multiple Pregnancies

Multiple pregnancies are generally considered as high-risk for preterm delivery as the mean gestational age at birth is 35 weeks for twins and 33 weeks for triplets. Although the numbers of published trials in multiples are significantly fewer compared to singletons, sonographic assessment of the cervix appears to be of value in this population. Goldenberg et al[29] prospectively screened 147 twin pregnancies at 24th and 28th weeks for more than 50 potential risk factors for spontaneous preterm birth. They found that at 24th weeks a cervical length ≤ 25 mm was consistently associated with preterm birth.

Ultrasonographic cervical screening has been shown to be also useful in triplet pregnancies. Ramin et al[30] performed transperineal ultrasonographic measurements of the cervix in 32 triplet pregnancies between 10th and 32nd weeks and found that a short cervix and funneling could predict preterm delivery. To et al[31] measured cervical length by transvaginal ultrasound at 23rd week in 43 triplet pregnancies. The rate of preterm delivery increased with decreasing cervical length at 23rd week from 8 percent at 36 to 48 mm, to 11 percent at 26 to 35 mm, 33 percent at 16 to 25 mm and 67 percent at 15 mm or less. Guzman et al[32] evaluated 51 triplet pregnancies between 15th and 28th weeks with transvaginal cervical sonography and transfundal pressure. The cervical parameters evaluated were funnel width and length, cervical length, percentage of funneling and cervical index (Figs. 9.8 A and B). They concluded that cervical lengths of ≤ 25 mm between 15th and 24th weeks and ≤ 20 mm between 25th and 28th weeks were at least as good as other sonographic cervical parameters for the prediction of spontaneous preterm birth.

The Cervix in Preterm Premature Rupture of Membranes

One of the main causes of preterm delivery is preterm premature rupture of membranes (PPROM). Ultrasonographic cervical assessment has been used in this group of patients. Carlan et al[33] studied the use of transvaginal sonography in PPROM and found no relationship between a cervical length cut-off of 30 mm and latency period. Moreover, endovaginal ultrasound in these patients did not appear to increase the incidence of maternal infection.

INTERVENTIONS FOR CERVICAL INCOMPETENCE BASED ON ULTRASONOGRAPHIC FINDINGS

It is obvious that ultrasonographic cervical assessment is extremely useful as a screening method for preterm delivery. However, the usefulness of a screening test depends on our ability to intervene, so that to change the final result. So far, there has not been clear evidence that any treatment is of benefit in a case of short cervix. What seems to be more promising is the placement of a cervical cerclage, which has been shown to lead to an increase in cervical length.

Only two prospective randomized trials have been published so far. In the first of that Rust et al[34,35] examined 113 patients between 16th and 24th weeks. All of them had cervical funneling > 25 percent of the total cervical length, or a shortened distal cervix < 25 mm and were randomly assigned to McDonald cerclage or no cerclage. All women were treated identically before and after randomization. Before randomization they had amniocentesis, multiple urogenital cultures and therapy with indomethacin and clindamycin for 48 to 72 hours. Fifty-five patients were randomly assigned to the cerclage group and 58 were randomly assigned to the no cerclage group. Cerclage did not affect perinatal outcome. In another study Althuisius et al[36] examined 35 patients with risk factors or symptoms of cervical incompetence. Such risk factors included previous preterm delivery before 34th week of gestation that met clinical criteria for the diagnosis of cervical incompetence, previous preterm premature rupture of membranes before 32nd week, history of cold knife

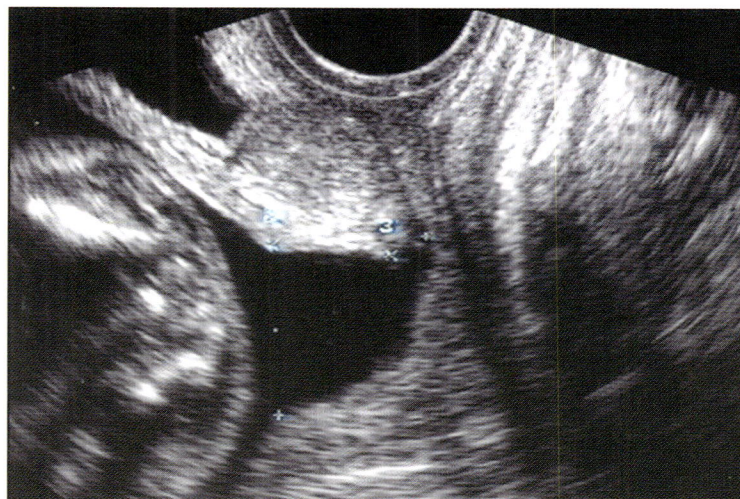

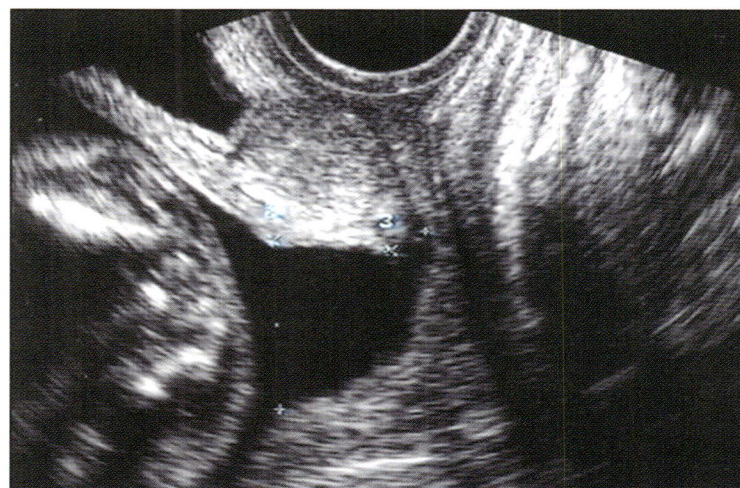

Figs 9.8A and B: Cervical parameters: Funnel width and length, cervical length, percentage of funneling and cervical index

conization, diethylstilbestrol exposure and uterine anomaly. When a cervical length of < 25 mm was found before 27th week, a randomization for cerclage and bedrest or bedrest alone was performed. Nineteen patients were randomly allocated to the cerclage group and 16 to the bedrest group. Preterm delivery before 34th week was significantly more frequent in the bedrest group compared to the cerclage group (7 of 16 vs none, respectively; p=0.002).

In a most recent elegant study by to et al[37] analyzed randomized trials about the use of cervical cerclage. Results of randomized trials have not generally support this practice. A more effective way of identifying the high risk group for early preterm delivery is transvaginal sonographic measurement of cervical length. A multicenter randomized control trial has been undertaken to investigate whether, in women with a short cervix identified by routine transvaginal scanning at 22nd to 24th weeks of gestation, the insertion of Shirodkar suture reduces early preterm delivery. The proportion of preterm delivery before 33rd week was similar in studied and control groups with no significant differences in perinatal or maternal morbidity and mortality. They concluded that although routine transvaginal sonographic measurement of cervical length at 22nd to 24th weeks identifies a group at high risk of early preterm delivery, the insertion of Shirodkar suture in such women with short cervices, does not substantially reduce the risk of prematurity.

CONCLUSIONS

The use of cervical assessment with ultrasound has been well established. It is a widely accepted and well-standardized method which can be easily performed in both high and low-risk patients as a screening test for preterm delivery. All it requires is a well-trained operator and a few minutes to spend on the evaluation of the cervix.

Further improvements are expected with the use of 3D and 4D sonography, in particular in the evaluation of the volume of cervical mucus.

REFERENCES

1. Riverius L, Culperer N, Cole A. On barrenness. In The Practice of Physik, Book 15. London: Peter Cole, 1658:502.
2. Gream GT. Dilatation or division of the cervix uteri. Lancet 1865;1:381.
3. Danforth DN. The fibrous nature of the human cervix and its relation to the isthmic segment in gravid and non gravid uteri. Am J Obstet Gynecol 1947;53:541.
4. Lash AF, Lash SR. Habitual abortion: the incompetent internal os of the cervix. Am J Obstet Gynecol 1950;59:68.
5. Rubovitz FE, Cooperman NR, Lash AF. Habitual abortion. A radiographic technique to demonstrate the incompetent internal os of the cervix. Am J Obstet Gynecol 1953;66:269-80.
6. Van Duyl WA, van der Zon AT, Drogendijk AC. Stress relaxation of the human cervix: a new tool for diagnosis of cervical incompetence. Clin Phys Physiol Meas 1984;5:207.
7. Diener L, Kaden W. Tocometry and rheobase measurement for cervical insufficiency – contribution to pathogenesis of premature birth. Zentralbl Gynakol 1981;103:797.
8. Carrera JM. Protocolos de Obstetricia y Medicina Perinatal, 3rd edn. Barcelona: Masson, 1996.
9. Parikh MN, Mehta AC. Internation cervical os during the second half of pregnancy. J Obstet Gynaecol Br Commonw 1961;68:818.
10. Schaffner F, Schanzer SN. Cervical dilatation in the early third trimester. Obstet Gynecol 1966;27:130.
11. Carrera JM. Ecografia patologica del 1er trimestre. In Carrera JM, ed. Ecografia Obstetrica. Barcelona: Salvat,1980.
12. Brook I, Feingold M, Schwartz A, Zakut H. Ultrasonography in the diagnosis of cervical incompetence in pregnancy. A new diagnostic approach. Br J Obstet Gynaecol 1981;88:640-3.
13. Carrera JM, Mallafre J. Incompetencial cervical y su tratamiento. In Carrera JM, Kurjak A, eds. Medicina del Embrion. Barcelona, Spain: Masson, 1997;47:487-510.
14. Cicero S, Skentou C, Souka A, et al. Cervical length at 22-24 weeks of gestation: comparison of transvaginal and transperineal-translabial ultrasonography. Ultrasound Obstet Gynecol 2001;17:335-40.
15. Bergelin I, Valentin L. Patterns of normal change in cervical length and width during pregnancy in nulliparous women: a prospective, longitudinal ultrasound study. Ultrasound Obstet Gynecol 2001;18:217-22.
16. Guzman Er, Walters C, Anath CV, et al. A comparison of sonographic cervical parameters in predicting spontaneous preterm birth in high-risk singleton gestations. Ultrasound Obstet Gynecol 2001;18:204-10.
17. Guzman ER, Vintzileos AM, McLean DA, et al. The natural history of a positive response to transfundal pressure in women at risk for cervical incompetence. Am J Obstet Gynecol 1997;176:634-38.
18. MacDonald R, Smith P, Vyas S. Cervical incompetence: the use of transvaginal sonography to provide an objective diagnosis. Ultrasound Obstet Gynecol 2001;18:211-6.
19. Bega G, Lev-Toaff A, Kuhlman K, et al. Three-dimensional multiplanar transvaginal ultrasound of the cervix in pregnancy. Ultrasound Obstet Gynecol 2000;16:351-8.
20. Strauss A, Heer I, Fuchshuber S, et al. Sonographic cervical volumetry in higher order multiple gestation. Fetal Diagn Ther 2001;16:634-8.
21. Hoesli J, Surbek DV, Tercanli S, Holzgreve W. Three-dimensional volume measurement of the cervix during pregnancy compared to conventional 2D-sonography. Int J Gynecol Obstet 1999;64:115-9.
22. Vendittelli F, Mamelle N, Munoz F, Janky E. Transvaginal ultrasonography of the uterine cervix in hospitalized women with preterm labor. Int J Gynaecol Obstet 2001;72:117-25.
23. Obido AO, Berghella V, Reddy U, et al. Does transvaginal ultrasound of the cervix predict preterm premature rupture of membranes in high-risk population? Ultrasound Obstet Gynecol 2001;18:223-2227.
24. Guzman ER, Mellon C, Vintzileos AM, Annath CV, Walter C, Gibson K. Longitudinal assessment of endocervical canal length between 15 and 24 weeks' gestation in women at risk for pregnancy loss or preterm birth: transfundal pressure, coughing, and standing in predicting cervical incompetence. Obstet Gynecol 1998;92:31-7.
25. Berghella V, Talucci M, Desai A. Does transvaginal sonographic measurement of cervical length before 14 weeks predict preterm delivery in high-risk pregnancies? Ultrasound Obstet Gynecol 2003;21:140-4.
26. Andersen HF, Nugent CE, Wanty SD, Hayashi RH. Prediction of risk for preterm delivery by ultrasonographic measurement of cervical length. Am J Obstet Gynecol 1990;163:859-67.
27. Tongsong T, Kamprapanth P, Srisomboon J, Wanapirak C, Piyamongkol W, Sirichotiyakul S. Single transvaginal sonographic measurement of cervical length early in the third trimester as a predictor of preterm delivery. Obstet Gynecol 1995;86:184-7.
28. Antsaklis A, Daskalakis G. Cervical measurements and preterm labour. In Transvaginal Sonography: Jaypee Brothers: New Delhi; Parthenon Publishing: London, 2004 (in press).
29. Goldenberg RL, Iams JD, Miodovnik M, et al. The preterm prediction study: risk factors in twin gestations. Am J Obstet Gynecol 1996;175:1047-53.
30. Ramin KD, Ogburn PL, Mulholland TA, Breckle RJ, Ramsey PS. Ultrasonographic assessment of cervical length in triplet pregnancies. Am J Obstet Gynecol 1999;180:1442-5.
31. To MS, Skentou C, Cicero S, Liao AW, Nicolaides KH. Cervical length at 23 weeks in triplets: prediction of spontaneous preterm delivery. Ultrasound Obstet Gynecol 2000;16:515-8.
32. Guzman ER, Walters C, O'Reilly-Green C, et al. Use of cervical ultrasonography in prediction of spontaneous preterm birth in triplet gestations. Am J Obstet Gynecol 2000;183:1108-13.
33. Carlan SJ, Richmond LB, O'Brien WF. Randomized trial of endovaginal ultrasound in preterm premature rupture of membranes. Obstet Gynecol 1997;89:458-61.
34. Rust OA, Atlas RO, Jones KJ, Benham BN, Balducci J. A randomized trial of cerclage versus no cerclage among patients with ultrasonographically detected second-trimester preterm dilatation of the internal os. Am J Obstet Gynecol 2000;183:830-5.
35. Rust OA, Atlas RO, Reed J, Van Gaalen J, Balducci J. Revisiting the short cervix detected by transvaginal ultrasound in the second trimester: why cerclage therapy may not help? Am J Obstet Gynecol 2001;185:1098-1105.
36. Althuisius SM, Dekker GA, Hummel P, Bekedam DJ, Van Geijn HP. Final results of the cervical incompetence prevention randomized cerclage trial (CIPRACT): Therapeutic cerclage with bed rest versus bed rest alone. Am J Obstet Gynecol 2001;185:1106-12.
37. To MS, Alfirevic Z, Heath VCF, et al. Cervical cerclage for prevention of preterm delivery in women with short cervix: randomised controlled trial. The Lancet 2004;363:1849-53.

C Millán, JM Carrera
A Muñoz, N Maiz

10

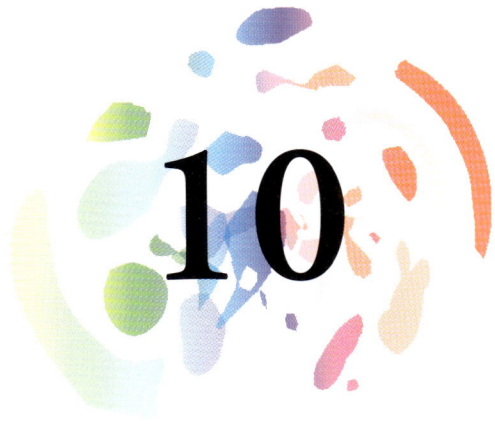

Placenta and Umbilical Cord

INTRODUCTION

The sonographic examination of the placenta and umbilical cord is fundamental in the sonographic assessment of pregnancy.

PLACENTA

From 7 to 8 weeks it is already possible to identify the placing of the placenta.

The thickness of the placenta increases until 36th week reaching the value approximated to gestational age in mm.[1] In normal conditions it cannot surpass 40 mm. In cases of IUGR or pre-eclampsia, the placenta may be thinner than expected. On the contrary, much thicker placenta is associated with intrauterine infection, hydrops, etc.

Placental Grading

The deposition of calcium in the placenta is normal physiologic process in pregnancy.[2] These calcifications primarily appear on the basal plate and septa, but later on can be found in the perivillous and subchorionic spaces.

Grannum et al [3] classified the placenta into four grades: 0, 1, 2 and 3.

- In grade 0, the chorion plate is smooth and well defined, tissue of the placenta is homogenous and the basal plate has no echoes (Fig. 10.1).
- Grade 1 appears after 28th week; the chorion plate is slightly irregular in shape, there are few "dot-like" calcifications without acoustic shadowing and basal plate does not present refringencies (Fig. 10.2).
- After 36th week, the placenta is classified as grade 2. "Notches", which do not reach basal plate and have hyperechogenic echoes, appear in the chorion plate. The tissue presents several notches with calcifications (Fig. 10.3).

Finally, after 38th week, the placenta is classified as grade 3 in which calcification appears on septa up to basal plate. Circular calcifications are observed in placental tissue with or without central anechogenic areas. The basal plate presents larger echoes with shadowing (Fig. 10.4).

The significance of placental grading and "aging" is not clear. However, the presence of grade 3 can help predict fetal maturity.[4]

Morphological Anomalies of the Placenta

By means of sonography it is possible to diagnose the place of insertion of the umbilical cord, which may be central, lateral or marginal (Figs 10.5 to 10.10) and several morphological anomalies, specially placenta succenturiate (or accessory lobes), velamentous insertion (vasa praevia), placenta membranacea, etc.

- In *placenta succenturiate*, the sonographic study has shown a separate mass of placental tissue connected to the rest of the placenta by vessels. The prenatal diagnosis is important since it is possible that the accessory lobe remains retained inside the uterus after delivery.
- In the named *velamentous insertion of placenta*, the umbilical cord is inserted on the chorioamniotic membranes instead on the main portion of the placenta. Fetal vessels from the placenta or umbilical cord cross the internal cervical os (vasa praevia). The fetal mortality is very high in this condition (50 to 90%) which is a result of blood vessel tearing at the time of fetal membranes rupture or in labour. With color Doppler the diagnosis is easy (Figs 10.11 to 10.27).
- *Placenta membranacea*, includes annular or ring-shaped placenta. The ultrasonographic exploration has shown a mass of placental tissue which extends over most of the uterine cavity.[5] It is associated with prenatal or postnatal hemorrhage.

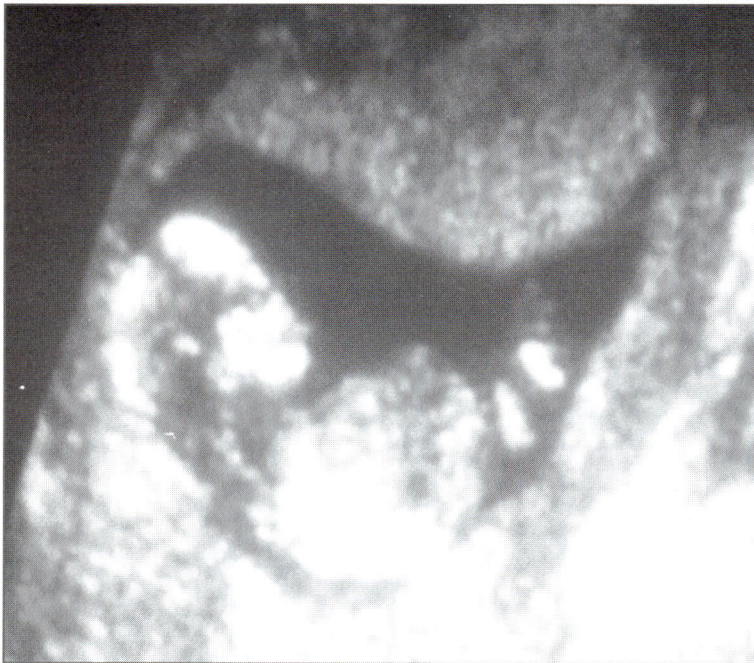

Fig. 10.1: Anterior insertion of the placenta showing grade 0 of Grannum at 14th week

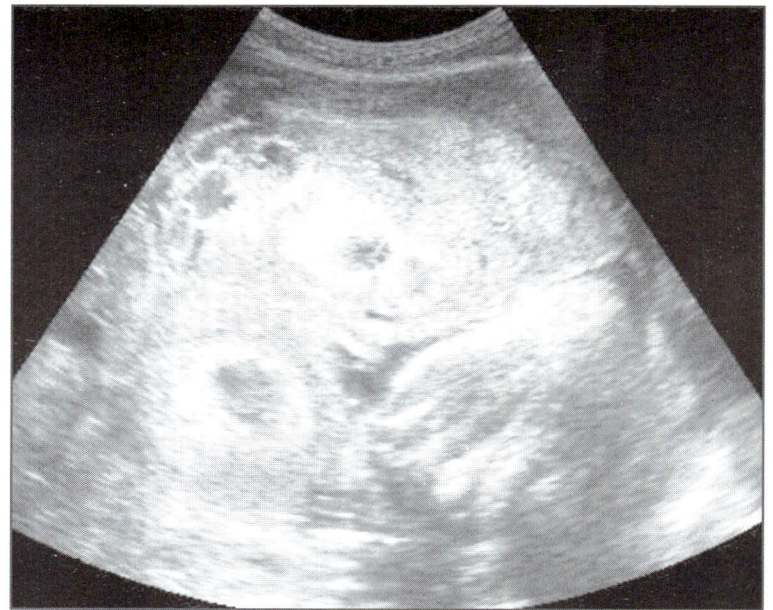

Fig. 10.2: Posterior insertion of the placenta showing grade 1 of Grannum at 30th week

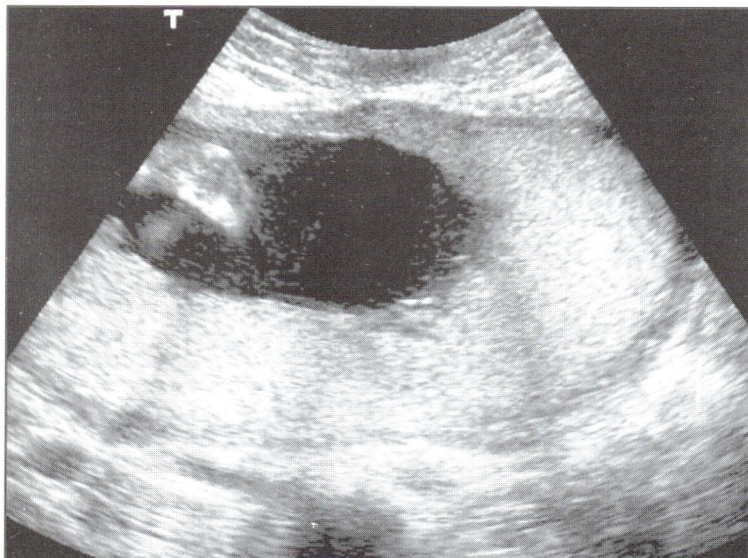

Fig. 10.3: Posterior insertion of the placenta showing grade 2 of Grannum at 32nd week

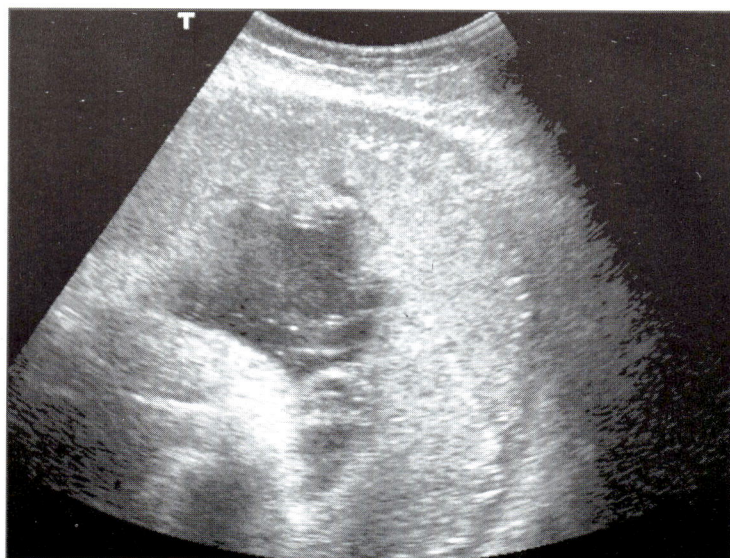

Fig. 10.4: Anterior insertion of the placenta showing grade 3 of Grannum at 37th week

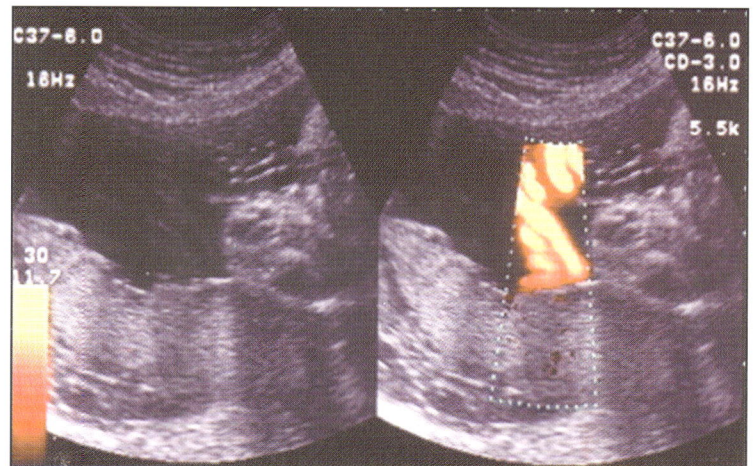

A

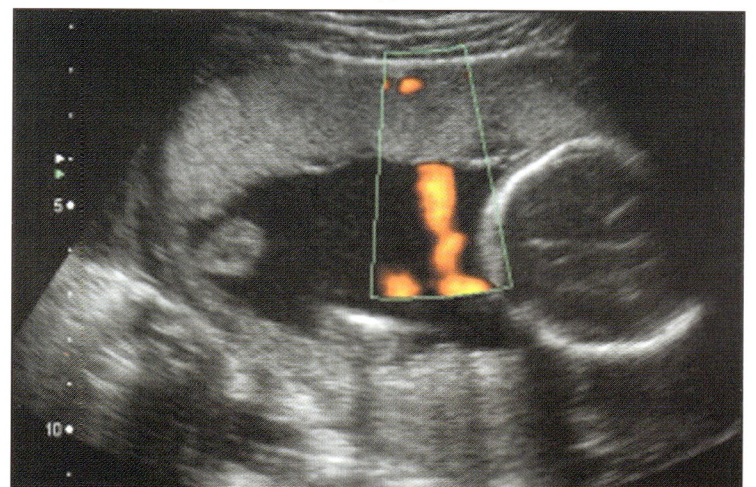

B

Figs 10.5A and B: Sonogram showing a central insertion of the umbilical cord in the placenta in the third term using power Doppler

Retroplacental Space

Under this heading, we included three pathological conditions: retroplacental hematomas, placental abruption, and subamniotic hematoma.[6]

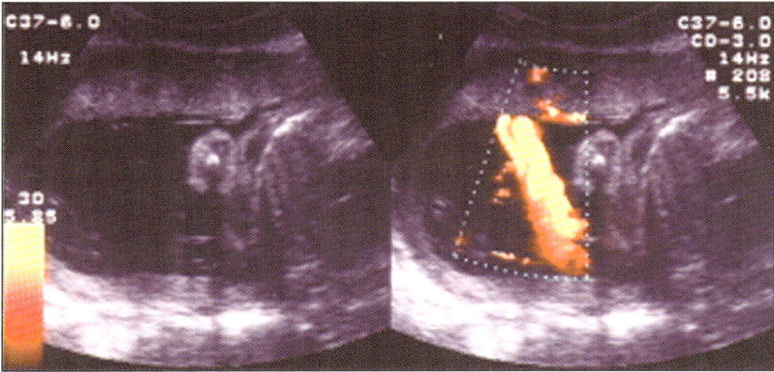

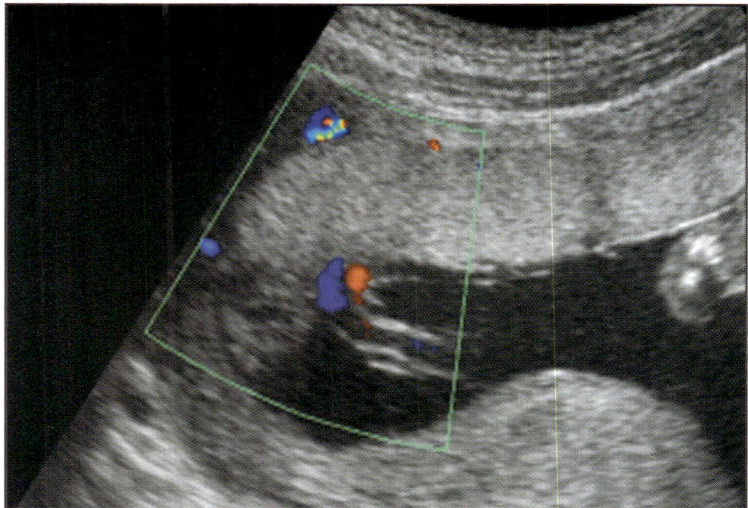

Figs 10.6A and B: Sonogram showing a lateral insertion of the umbilical cord in the placenta in the third term using power Doppler on the left and color Doppler on the right

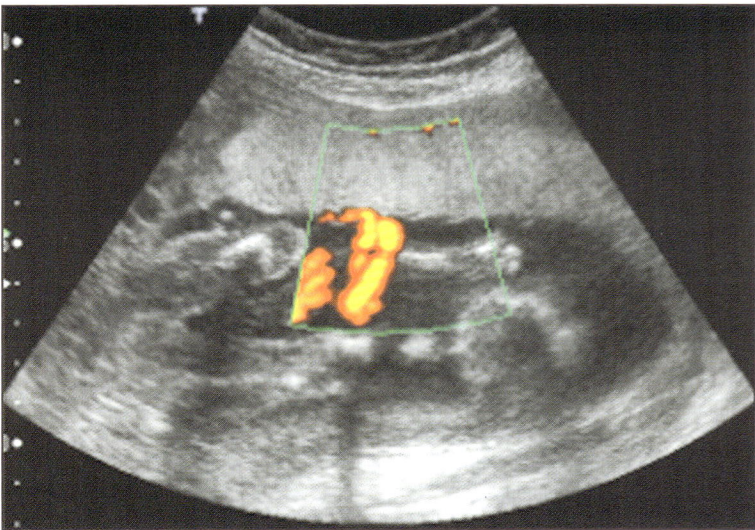

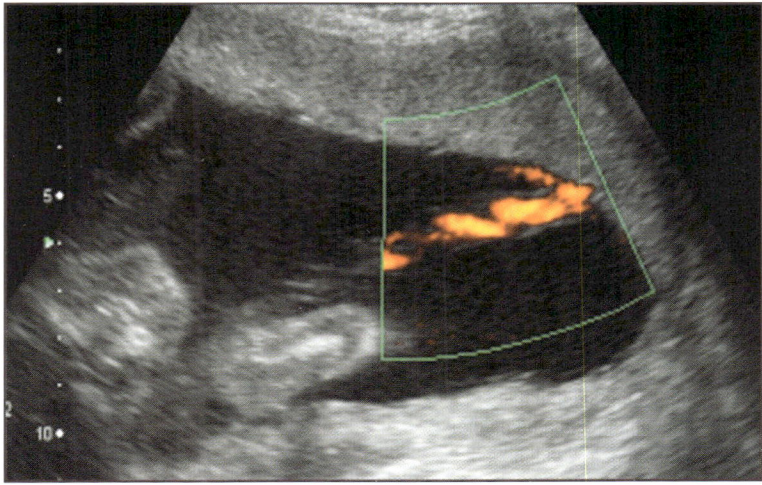

Fig. 10.7: Sonogram showing a lateral insertion of the umbilical cord in the placenta in the third term using power Doppler

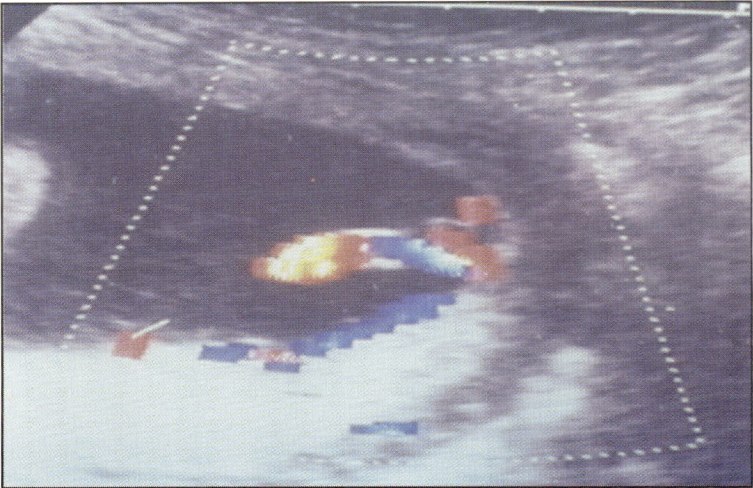

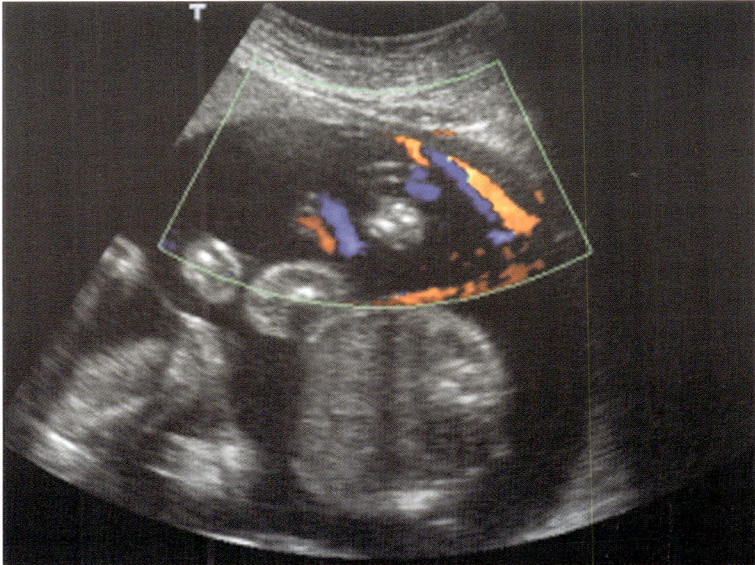

Figs 10.8A and B: Sonogram showing a marginal insertion of the umbilical cord in the placenta at 22nd week using color Doppler

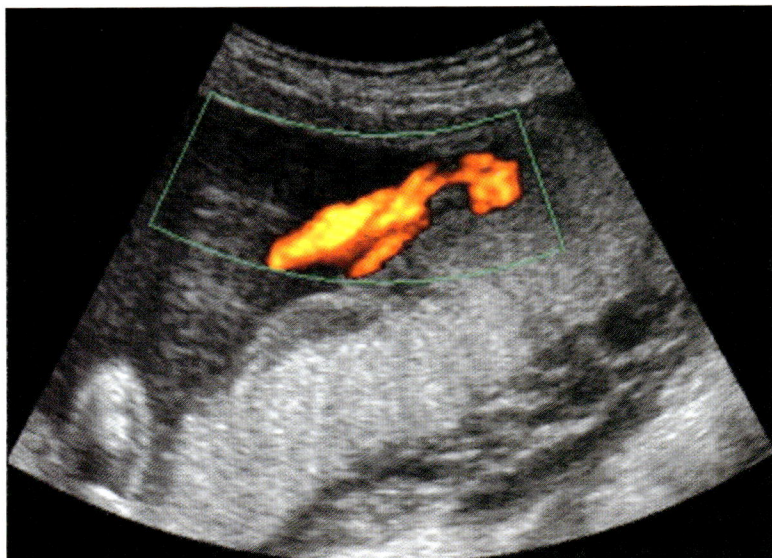

A

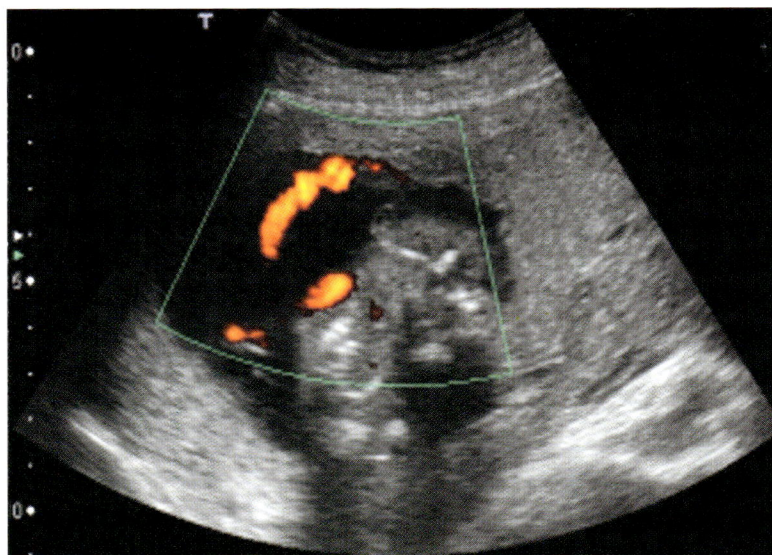

B

Figs 10.9A and B: Sonogram showing a marginal insertion of the umbilical cord in the placenta using power Doppler at 22nd week on the left and at 16th week on the right

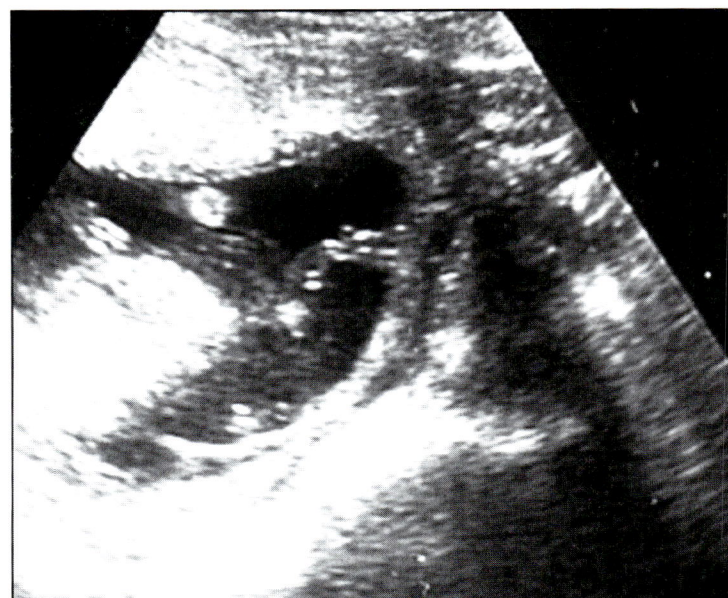

Inbercion marcinal

Fig. 10.10: Marginal umbilical cord insertion at 28th week

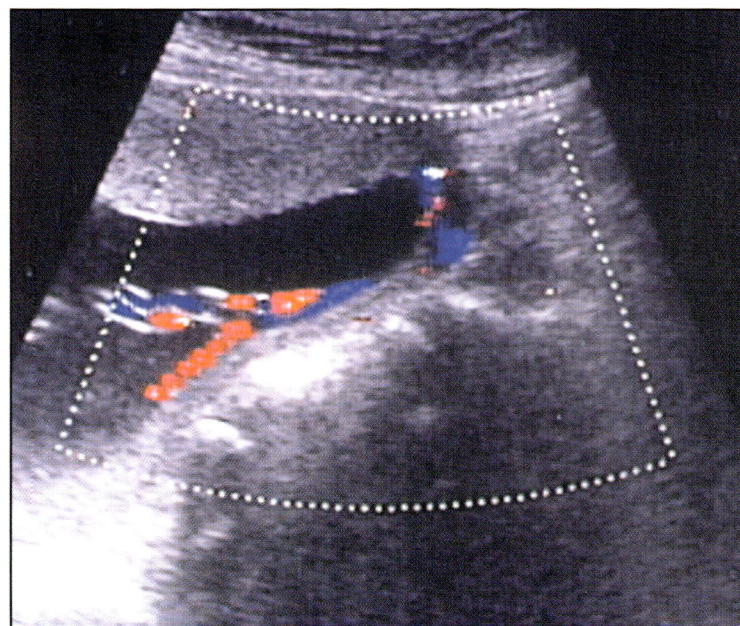

Fig. 10.11: 2D scan showhing a velamentous insertion of placenta at 27th week

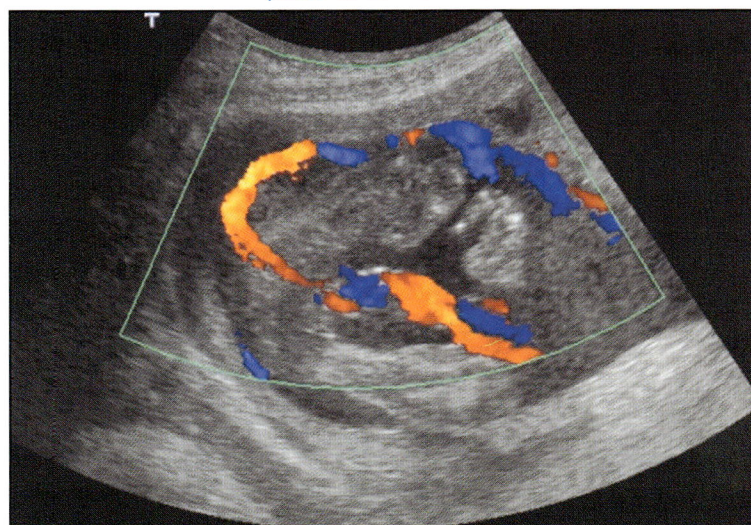

Fig. 10.12: Color Doppler showhing a velamentous insertion of placenta at 26th week

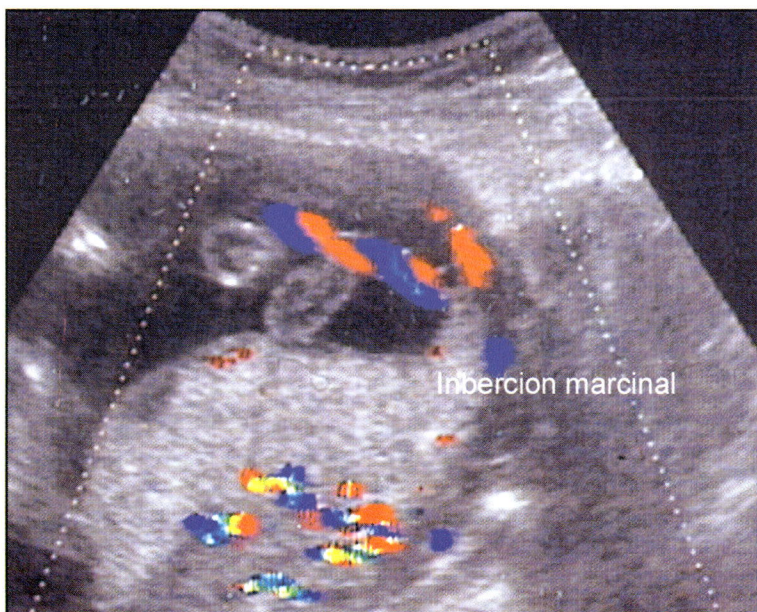

Fig. 10.13: Color Doppler showing a velamentous insertion of placenta at 27th week

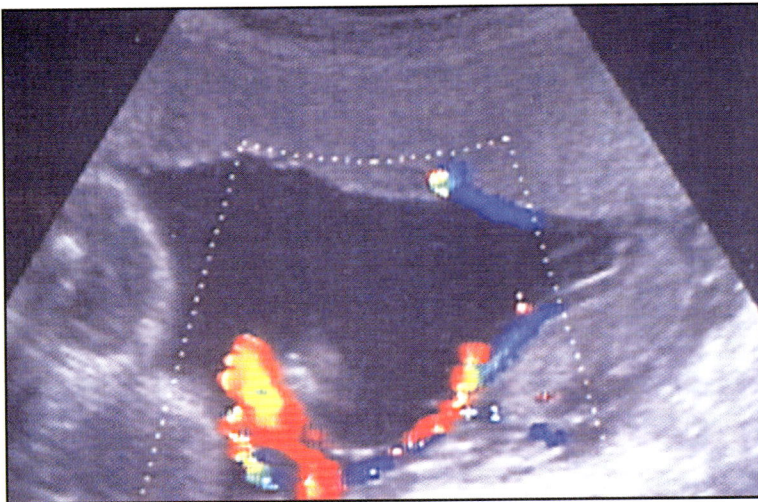

Fig. 10.14: Velamentous insertion of placenta with a long portion of the umbilical vessels along the membranes

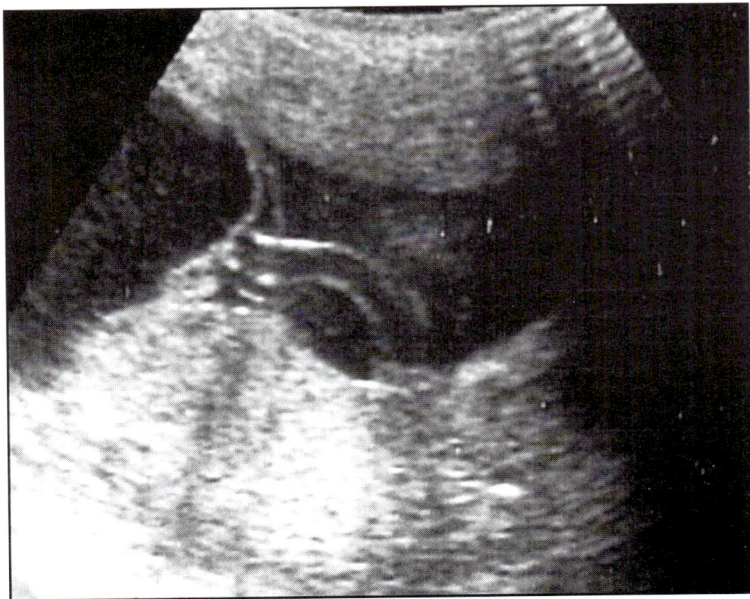

Fig. 10.15: 2D scan showing a velamentous insertion of placenta in a twin gestation at 28th week

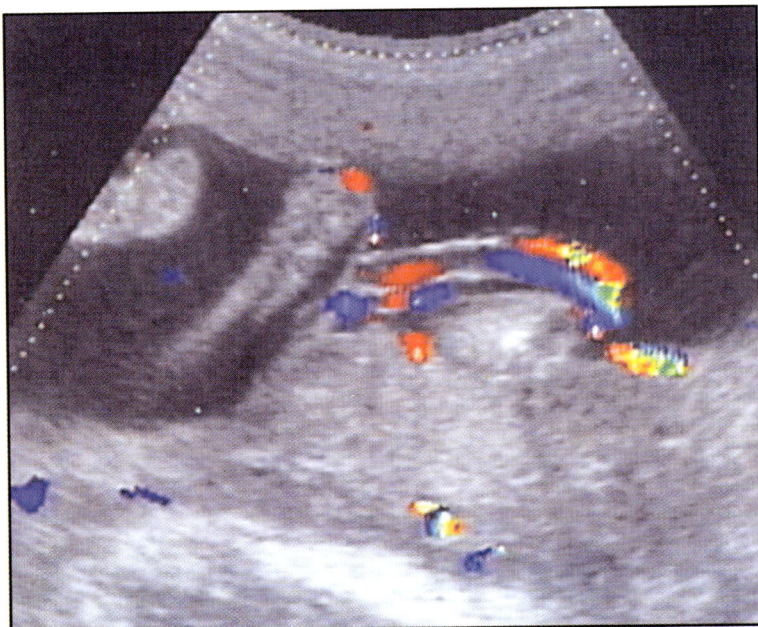

Fig. 10.16: Color Doppler showing velamentous umbilical cord insertion at 28th week in a twin gestation

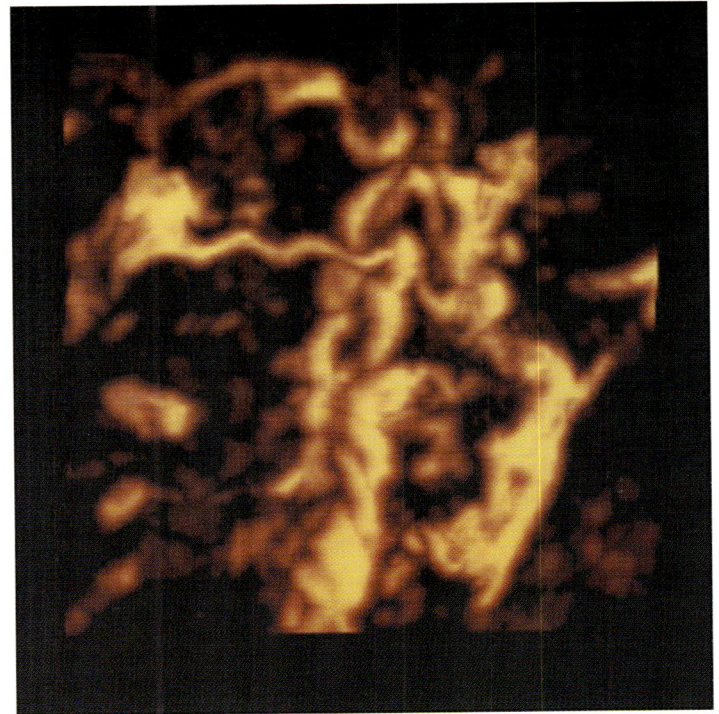

Fig. 10.17: 3D scan with power Doppler showing a velamentous insertion of the placenta

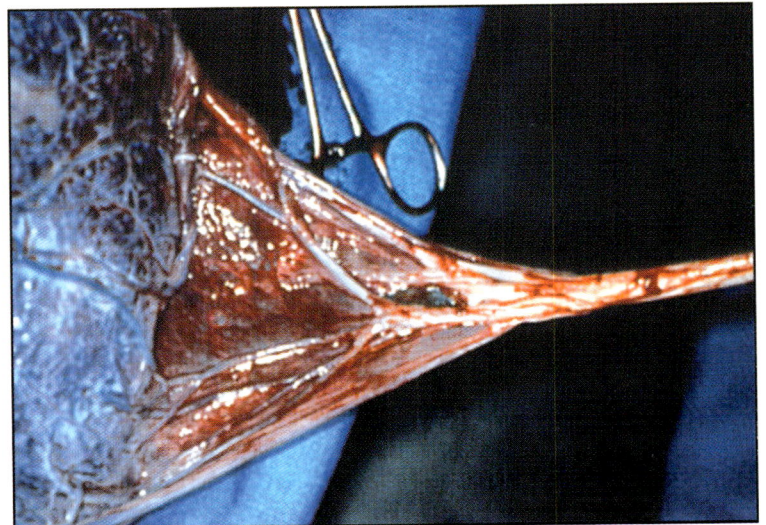

Fig. 10.18: Placenta after delivery showing velamentous insertion of the umbilical cord

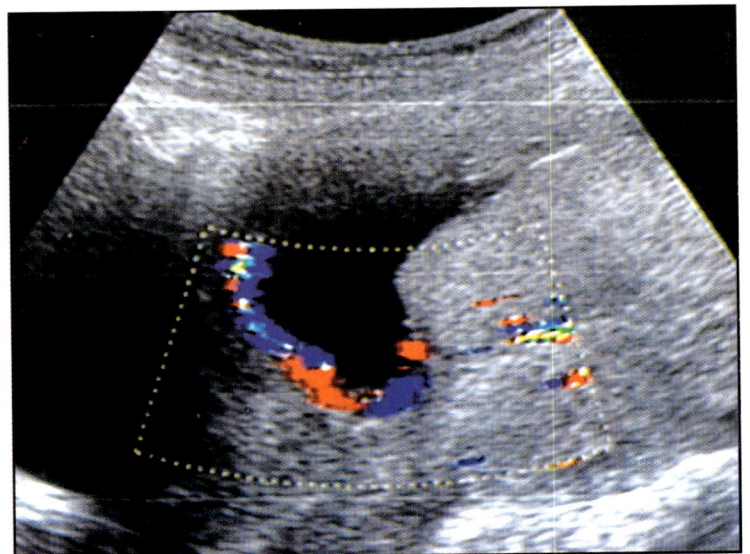

Fig. 10.19: Vasa praevia and velamentous insertion of placenta

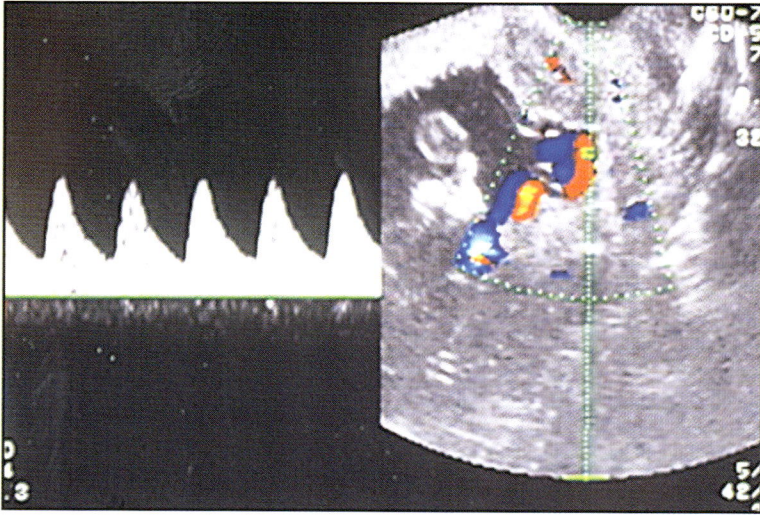

Fig. 10.20: Vasa praevia and velamentous insertion of placenta with color Doppler showing normal arterial flow

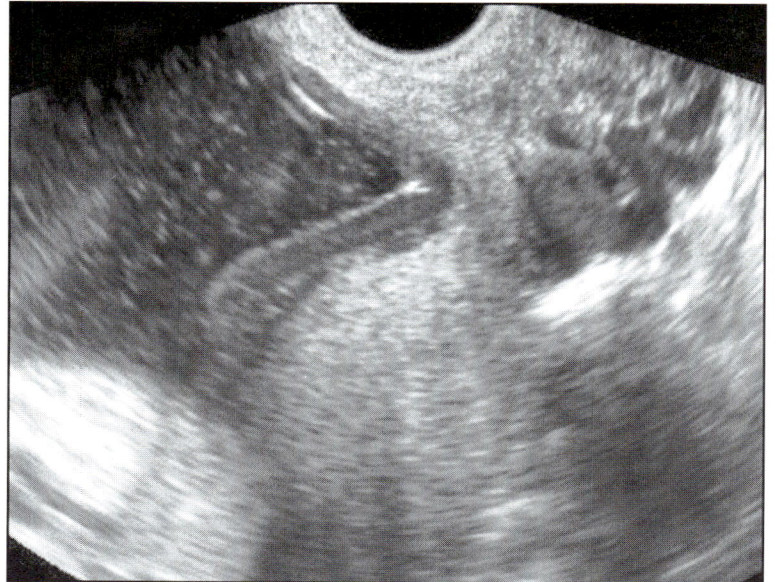

Fig. 10.21: Transvaginal scan at 34th week showing vasa praevia with normal Doppler

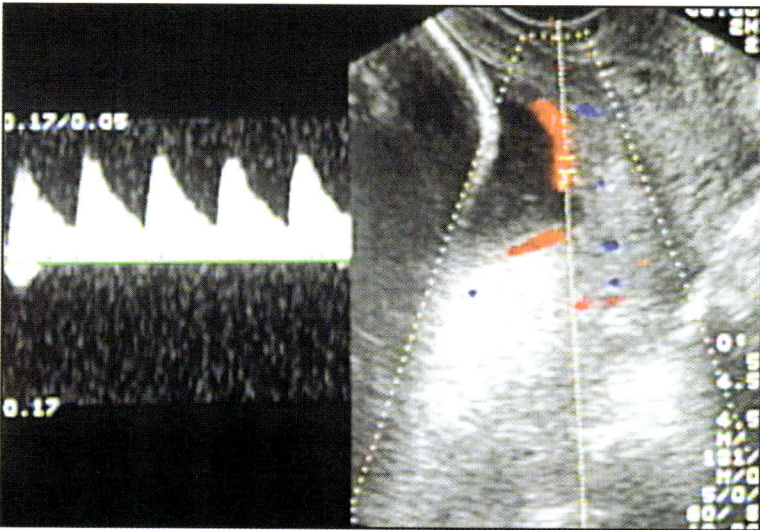

Fig. 10.22: Transvaginal scan at 34th week showing vasa praevia with normal venous flow

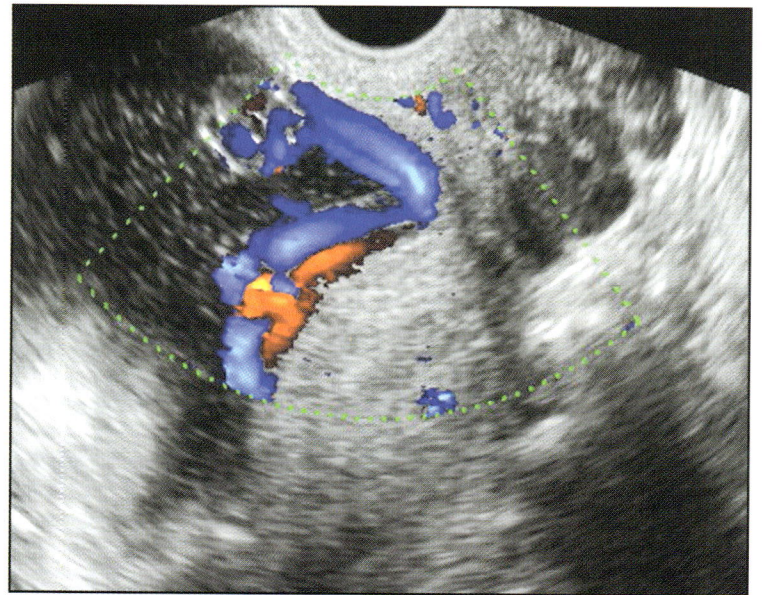

Fig. 10.23: Transvaginal scan showing the umbilical vessels running between the cervix and the fetal head at 36th week (vasa praevia)

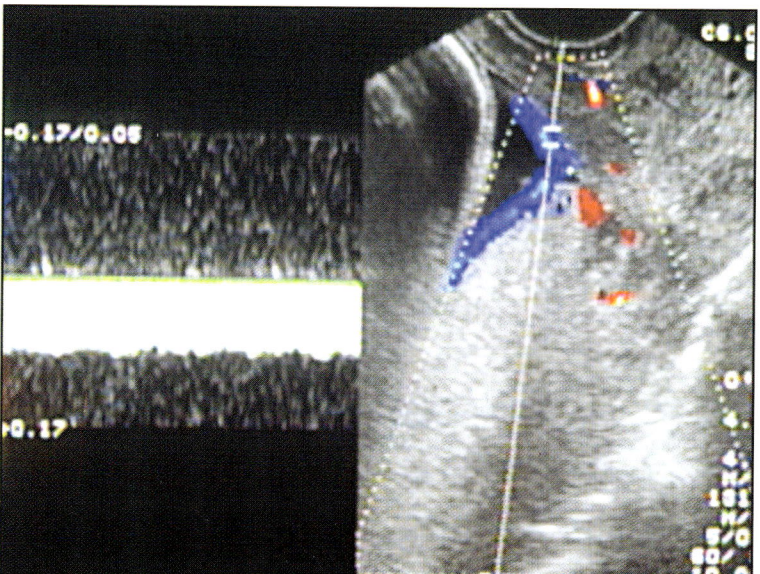

Fig. 10.24: Transvaginal scan with color Doppler showing the umbilical vessels running between the cervix and the fetal head at 36th week (vasa praevia)

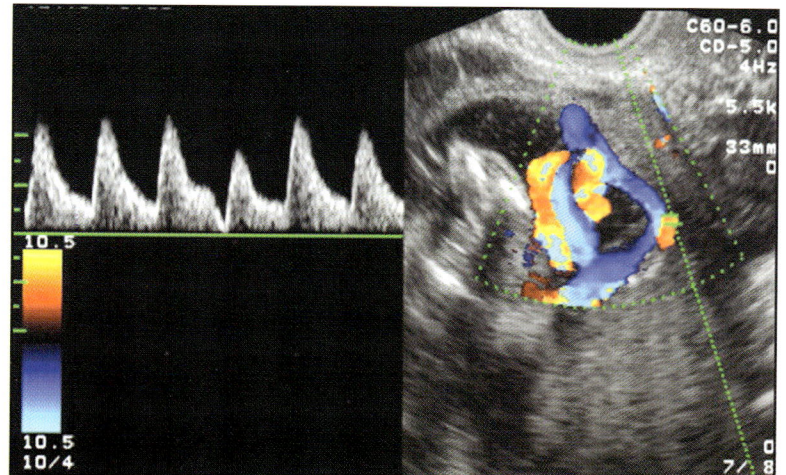

Fig. 10.25: Transvaginal scan with color Doppler showing a normal blood flow through the umbilical vessels at 36th week (vasa praevia)

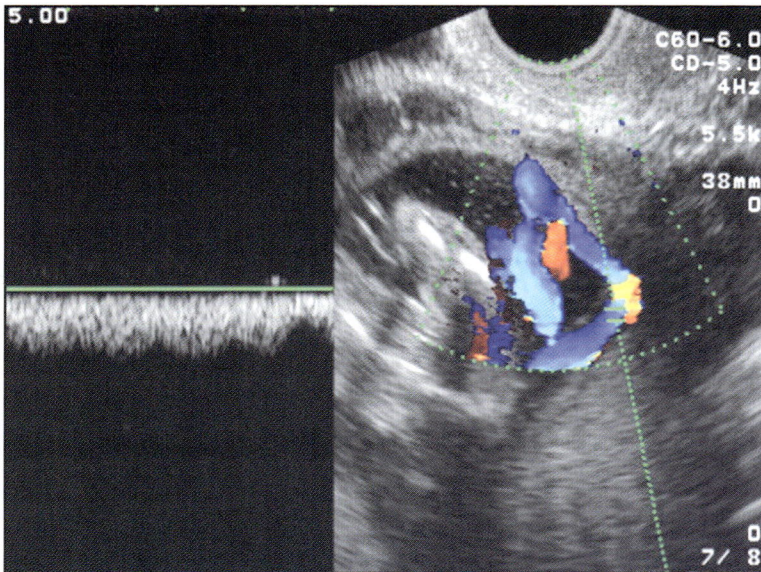

Fig. 10.26: Transvaginal scan with color Doppler showing a normal venous flow through the umbilical vessels at 36th week (vasa praevia)

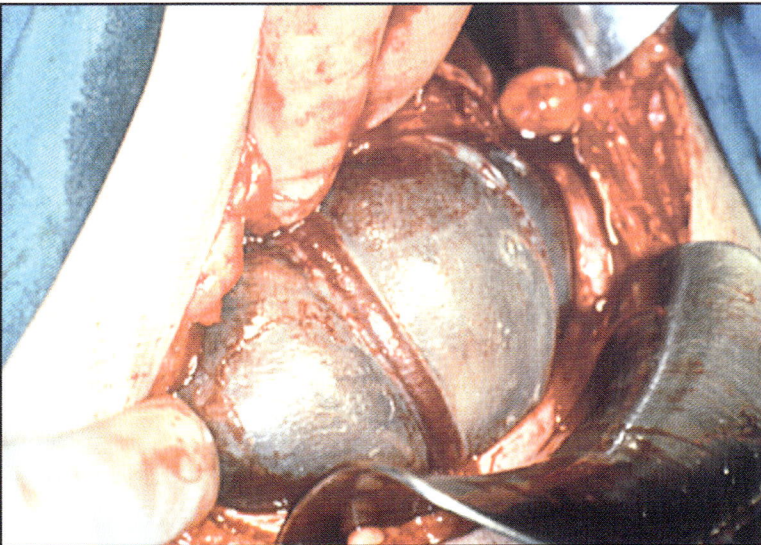

Fig. 10.27: Picture showing the vasa praevia during the cesarean before the fetal presentation

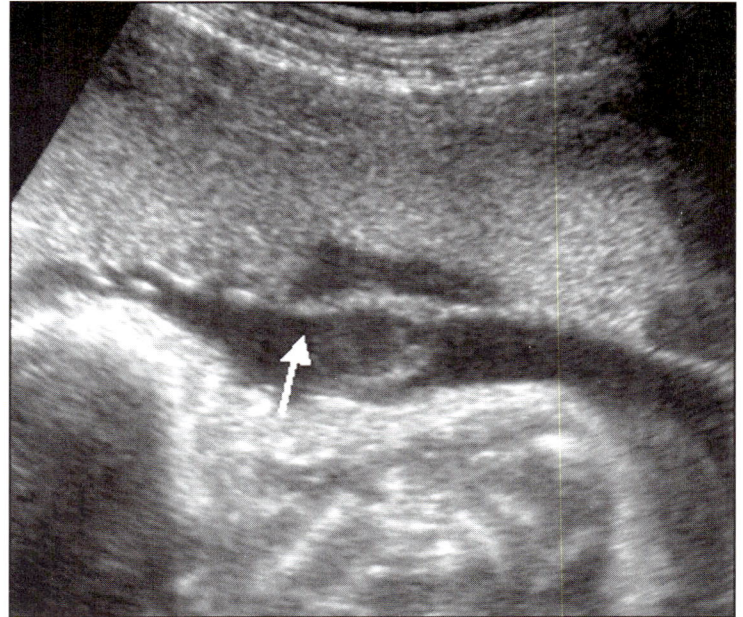

A

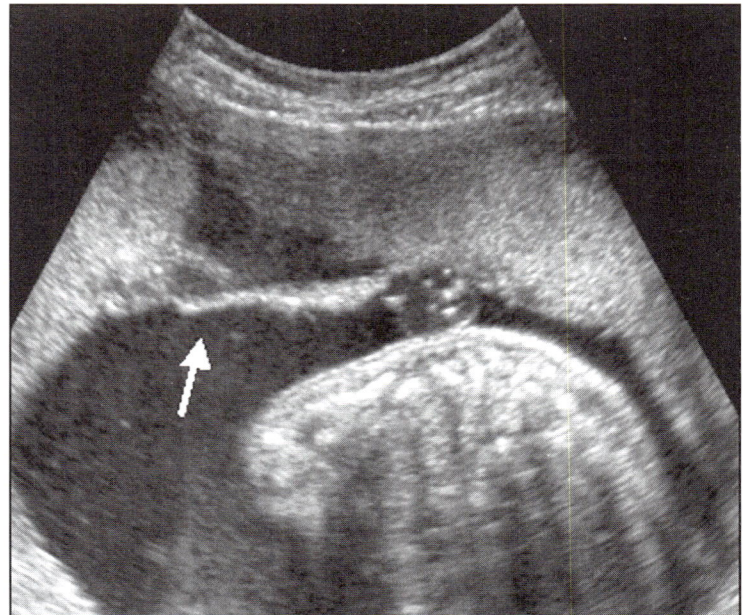

B

Figs 10.28A and B: Sonogram showing different sections of a subamniotic hematoma at 35th week

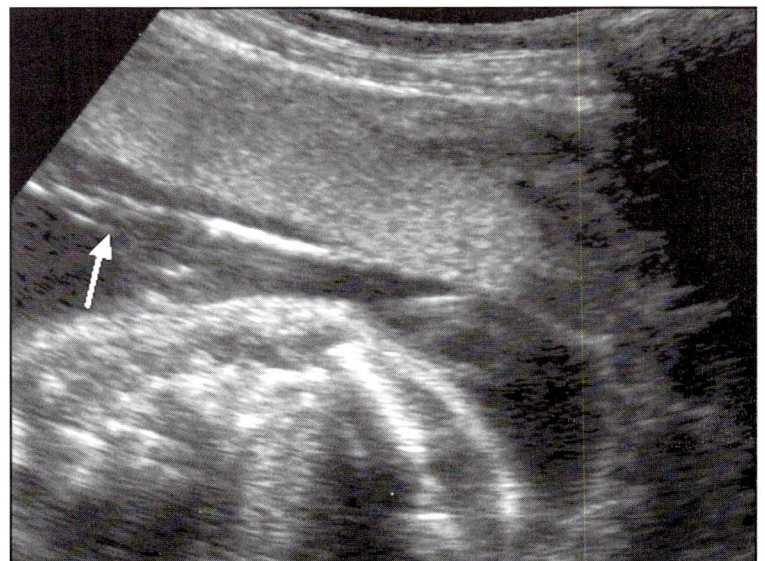

Fig. 10.29: Sonogram showing a subamniotic hematoma at 37th week

- *Retroplacental hematoma* sonographically presents as a complex or hypoechoic mass in the close proximity of the placenta. These hematomas are most common in early pregnancy.

- *Placental abruption* defines acute placental separation of the placenta from the uterus before the delivery of the fetus. Ultrasound appearance of this condition varies. Usually it is characterized by the presence of bizarre echoes between placenta and myometrium with a very variable grade of size and echogenicity.[6] If the abruption is small it might be unrecognized at ultrasonographic examination.

- The *subamniotic hematoma* is a "cystic" structure containing a thrombotic mass arising from the amniotic membrane. The sonographic features were those of a poorly reflective oval-shaped cystic mass overlying the fetal plate of the placenta and covered in a thin membrane[7] (Figs 10.28 and 10.29).

Placental Tumors

Apart from the gestational trophoblastic disease, it is possible to diagnose two types of tumors in the placenta: chorioangioma and teratoma.

- From the aspect of ultrasound, *chorioangioma* is an intraplacental mass, more or less solid, of variable echogenicity, situated usually near the fetal surface. Color and pulsed Doppler may demonstrate vascularity of the tumor. If large, it can be associated with fetal hydrops, cardiomegaly, IUGR and fetal death (Figs 10.30 to 10.33).

- *Placental teratomas* are very rare.[8] Ultrasound appearance is a heterogene mass, with solid and liquid areas (echonegatives). In several cases it is possible to observe hyperechogenic areas that correspond to calcifications. Teratomas may present throughout the variety of fetal lesions, for example, an acardiac fetus.[9]

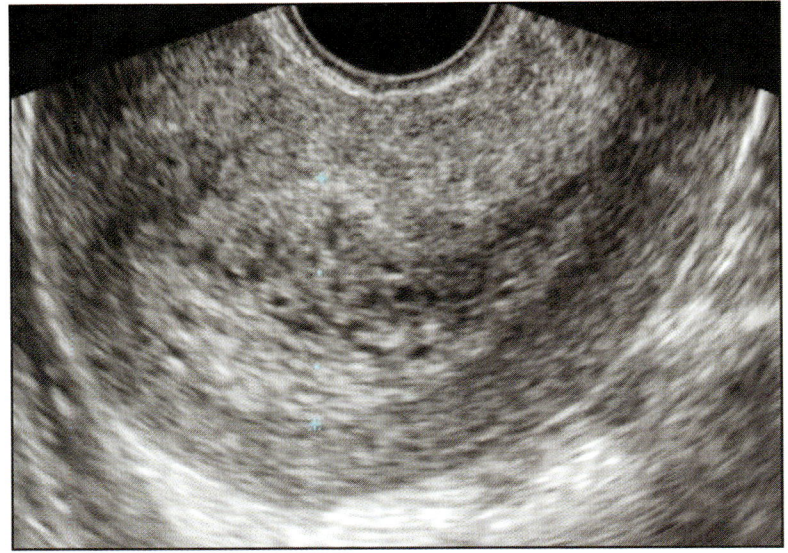

A

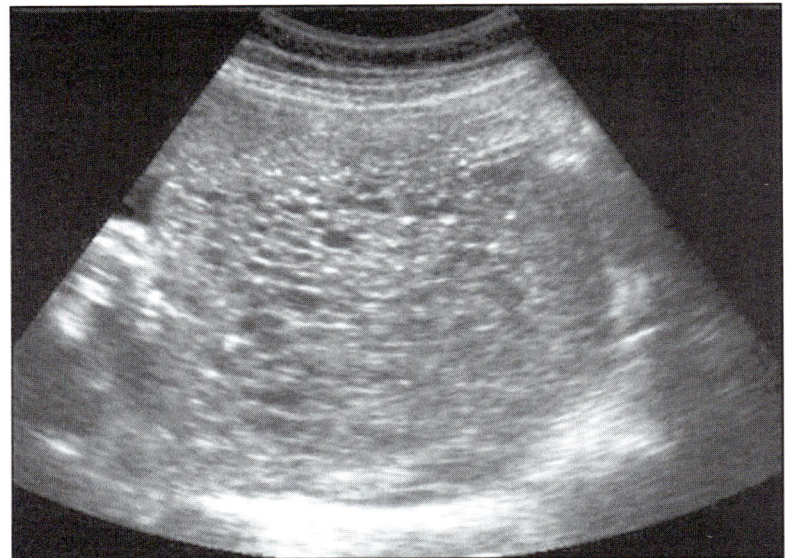

B

Figs 10.30A and B: Sonogram showing a heterogenic mass occupying the uterus and higly vascularized with color Doppler; gestational trophoblastic disease

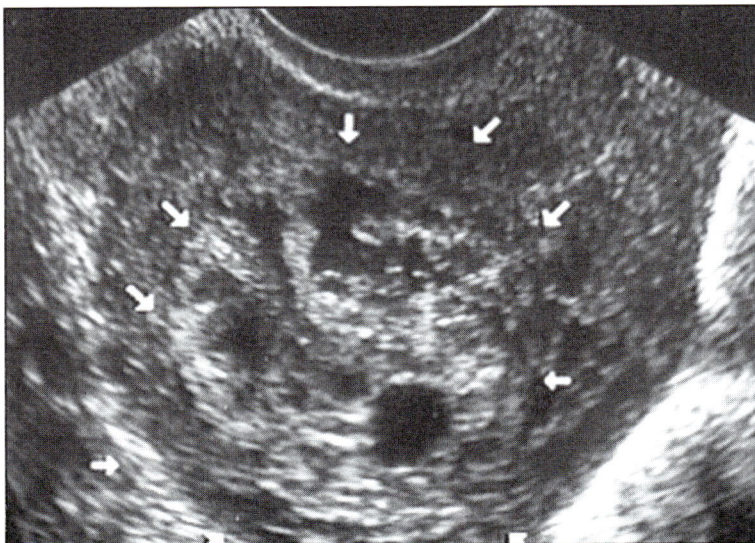

A

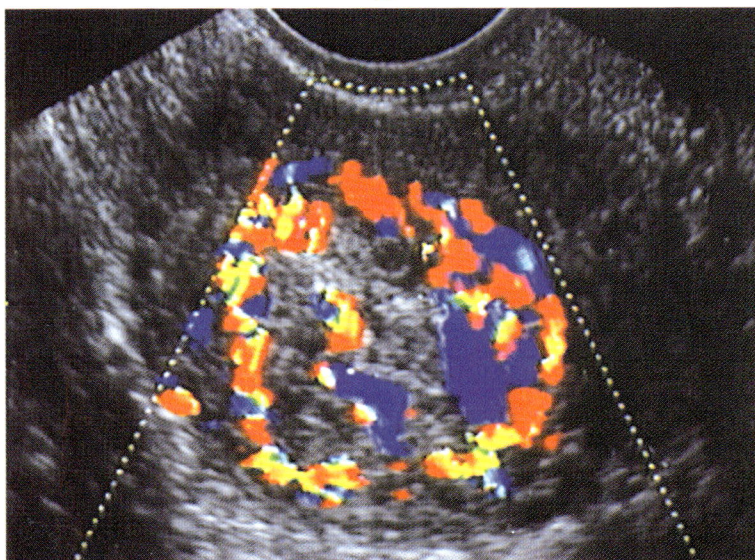

B

Figs 10.31A and B: Sonogram showing a heterogenic mass occupying the uterus; gestational trophoblastic disease

Placental Infarcts

Placental infarction is a consequence of the disruption of blood supply to the placenta. The sonographic diagnosis is not easy. It usually adopts the form of the intraparenchymatous areas, irregular, hyperechogenic in the first moment (acute stage) and hypoechogenic in advanced stages. In many occasions presented a halo very... Usually are present on the placental basis, in the close proximity to the basal plate. The size is very variable.

Placenta Previa

Correct diagnosis of placenta previa cannot be made before 30th to 32nd weeks.[6] Usually this pathologic condition is overdiagnosed (diagnosis before formation of lower uterine segment, and also for full urinary bladder and uterine contractions).

In diagnosing placenta previa, transvaginal approach was found to be much better compared to transabdominal ultrasound examination.[10]

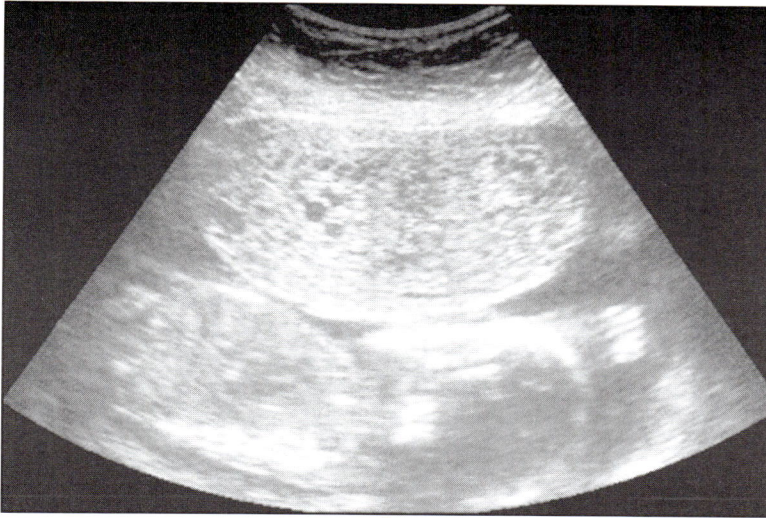

A

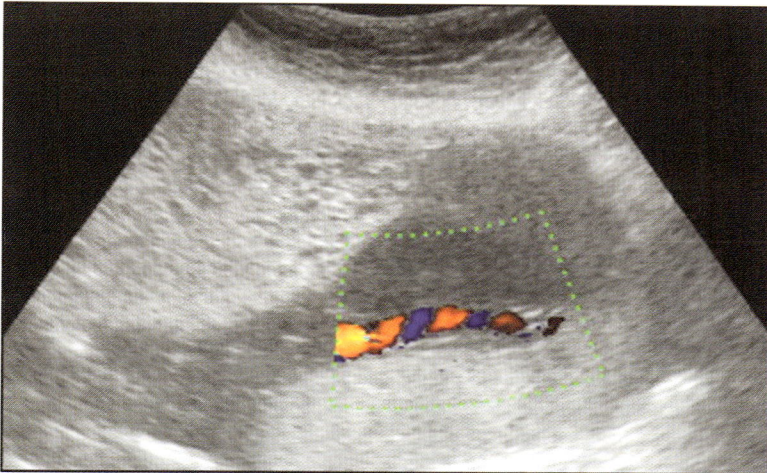

B

Figs 10.32A and B: Twin gestation with gestational trophoblastic disease in one of the sacs and a normal gestation in the other sac

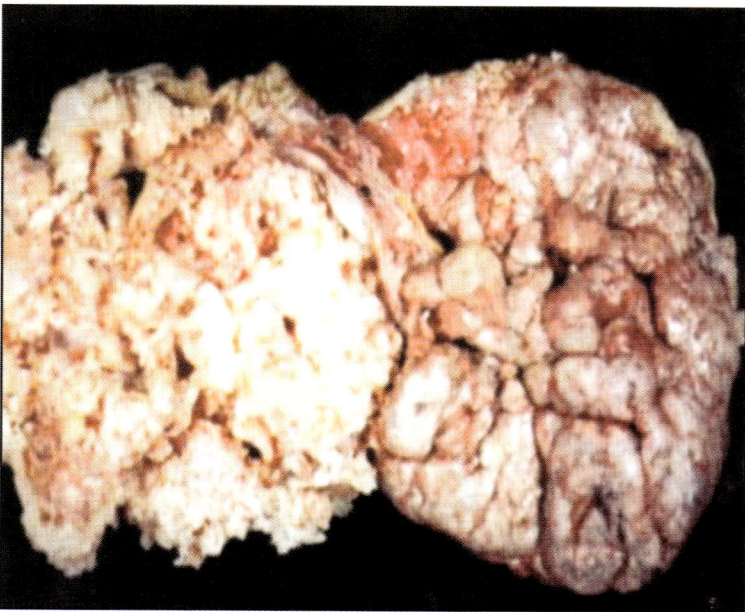

Fig. 10.33: Placenta after delivery, normal placenta and gestational trophoblastic disease

The aim of the sonographic examination is to try to establish the relation between the placenta and internal cervical os, with the purpose that not only establishes the diagnosis of placenta

previa, but also determines the grading of placenta previa. Lamentably, when the placenta is located in posterior wall of the uterus, the presenting part of the fetus can obstruct the clear visualization of internal cervical os making the diagnosis very difficult or impossible.[6] For this reason it is good to use the transvaginal approach (Fig. 10.34).

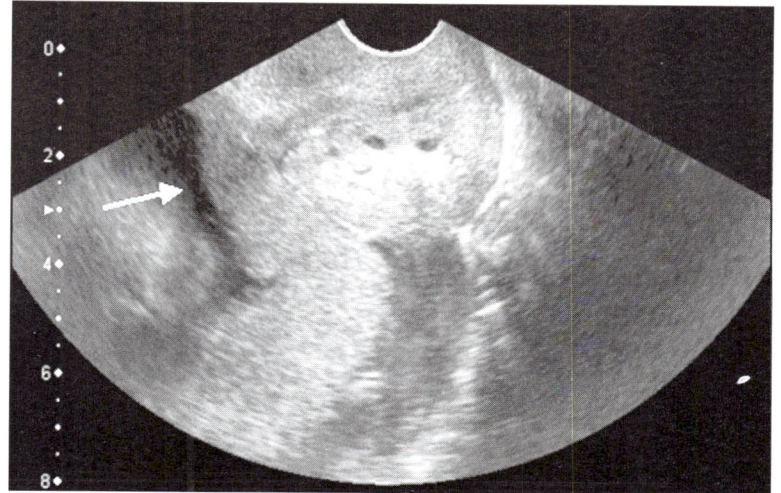

Fig. 10.34: Transvaginal scan at 31st week showing placenta previa obstructing the cervix

Placenta Accreta

Sonographic diagnosis of placenta accreta is not easy, although it can be diagnosed mostly by the absence of retroplacental hypoechogenic zone of the decidua/myometrium.[11] In these cases the subplacental-vascular complex disappears. Color Doppler can help in making this diagnosis.

UMBILICAL CORD

The sonographic aspect of the umbilical cord is well known. In a cross-sectional view, the presence of the two arteries and one vein surrounding for Wharton's jelly that protects the umbilical circulation against compression, stretching and torsion, is evident. And, very early, from the 8th week of pregnancy, umbilical cord develops its characteristic helical structure (Figs 10.35 to 10.42).

Several studies have demonstrated that there is an association between alterations of umbilical cord structure and adverse perinatal outcome. For this reason it is important to integrate the sonographic assessment of the umbilical cord in prenatal screening programs.[12]

Umbilical Cord Measurement

In literature there is a consensus that the morphometry of the umbilical cord might be useful in predicting perinatal outcome.

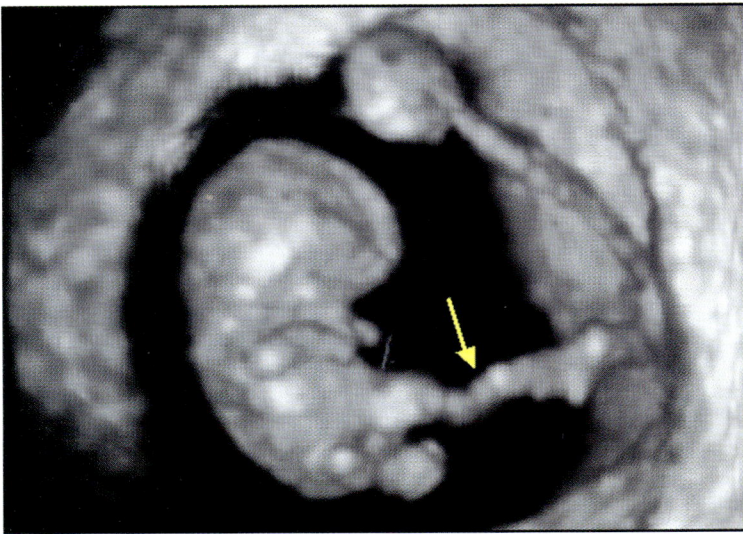

Fig. 10.35: Transvaginal 3D scan at 8th week showing the initial umbilical cord

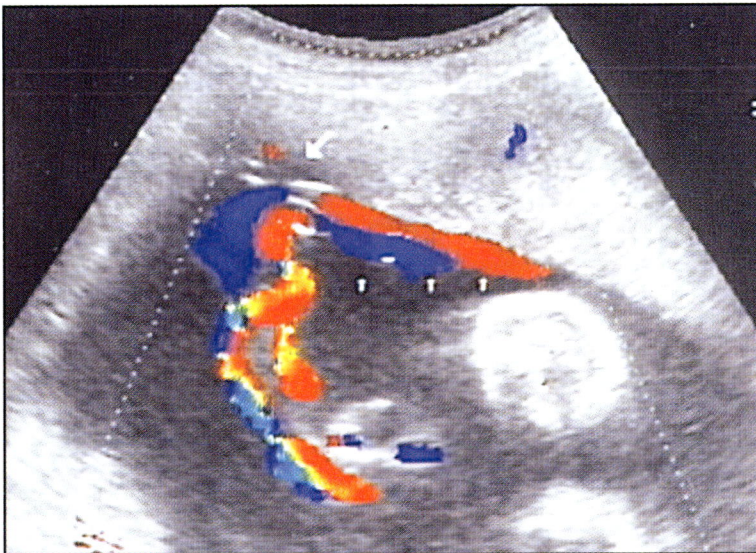

Fig. 10.36: Sonogram showing the number of vessels, the size, and the placental insertion of the umbilical cord

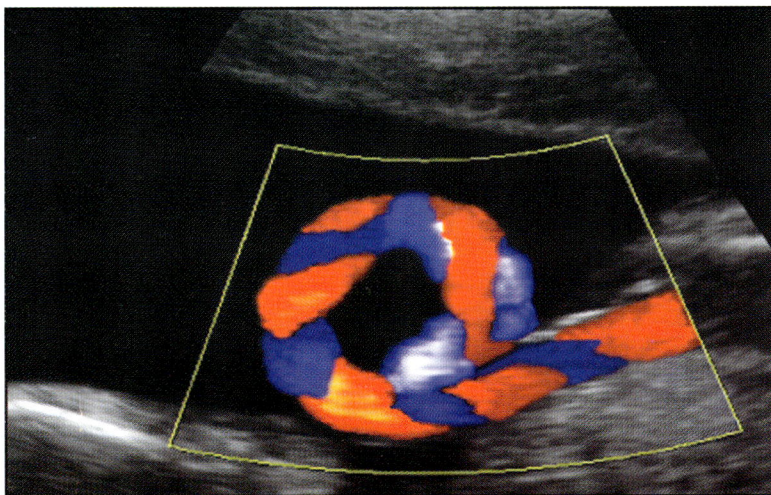

Fig. 10.37: Color Doppler showing a normal umbilical cord at 30th week

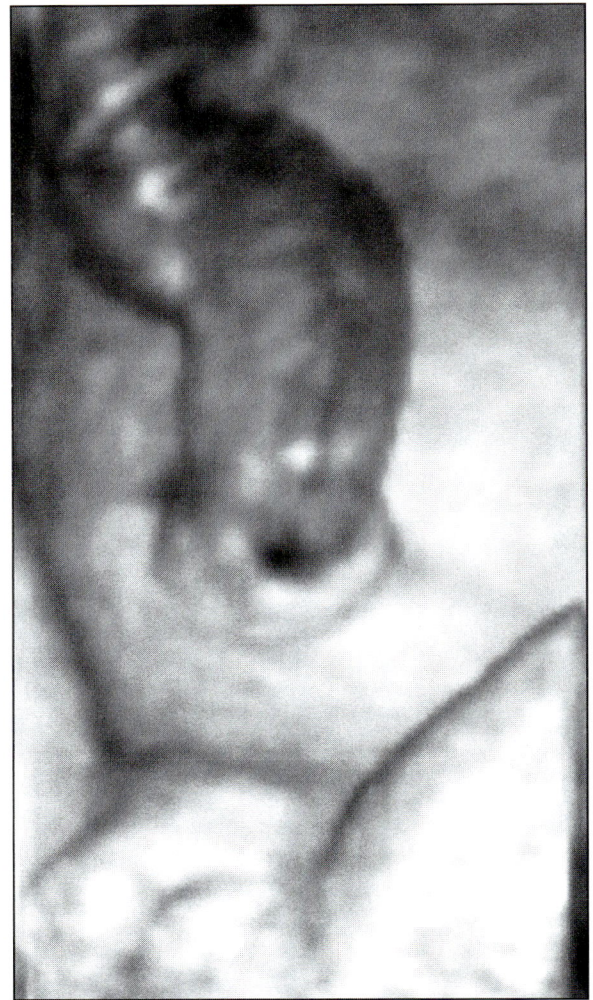

Fig. 10.38: 3D scan showing the insertion of the umbilical cord into the fetus at 31st week

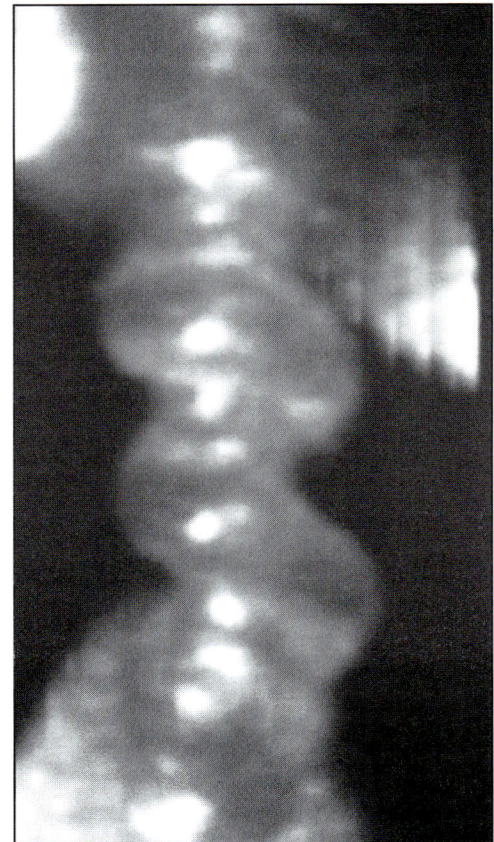

Fig. 10.39: 3D scan showing a normal umbilical cord in the third term

In the first trimester, a significant correlation was observed between umbilical cord diameter and gestational age. Ghezzi et al [13] have verified that umbilical cord diameter increases steadily from 8th to 15th weeks, and they have confirmed

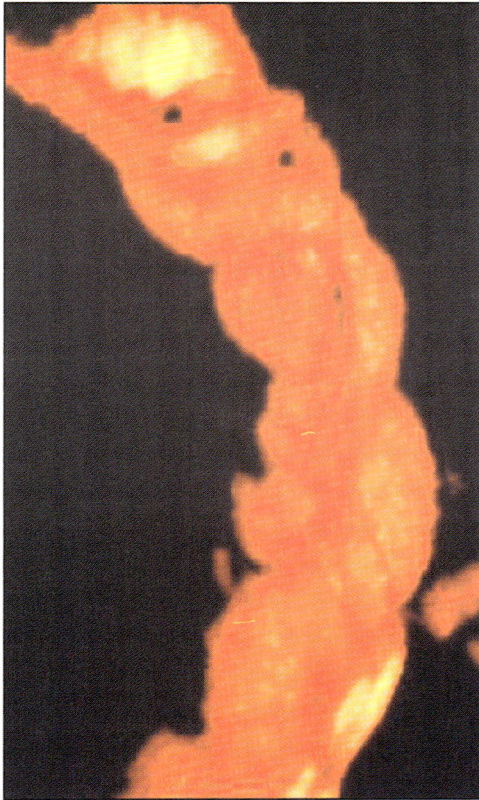

Fig. 10.40: 3D scan with power Doppler showing the umbilical vessels in the third term

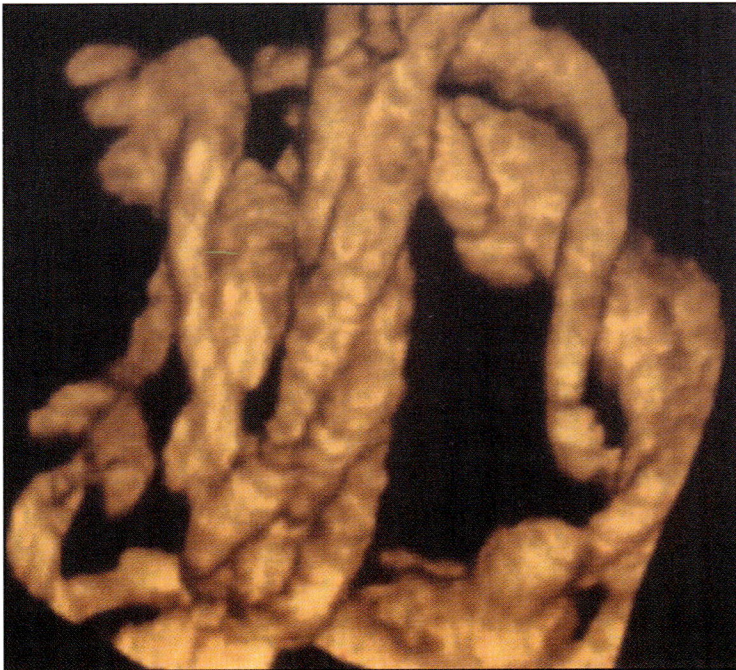

Fig. 10.41: 3D scan with power Doppler showing a normal umbilical cord at 35th week

existence of a significant correlation between umbilical cord diameter, CRL and biparietal diameter. Apparently, the pregnancies with low values of umbilical cord diameter (below the 5th centile or — 2 SD) have a high risk for miscarriage and pre-eclampsia. On the contrary, if the values are above the 95th centile, the incidence of aneuploidies is high.[14]

In the second half of gestation, the cross-sectional area increases as a function of gestational age, reaching a plateau from 32nd week until term, when a progressive reduction occurs.

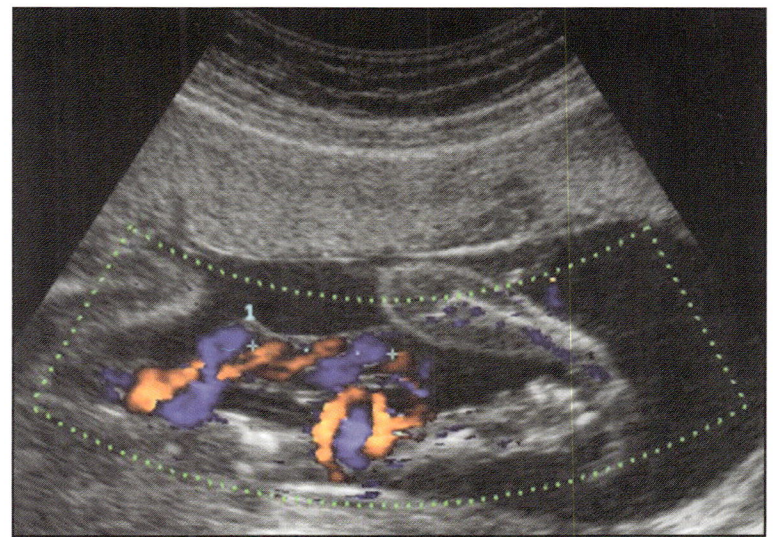

Fig. 10.42: Sonogram showing the number of vessels, the size, and the placental insertion of the umbilical cord

Several studies[6,15] have shown that the umbilical cord cross-sectional area correlated with fetal biometry, and that values situated below the 10th centile for gestational age indicated high risk for IUGR, fetal distress and intrapartum complications[16] (Figs 10.43A to D).

Umbilical Cord Coiling

The spiral structure of umbilical cord is fully developed from 8th to 9th weeks of gestation.

The number of umbilical vascular coils present in the first trimester is very similar at term gestation.

Strong et al[17] introduced a standard method to quantify the degree of umbilical vascular coiling. It is called "umbilical coiling index" (UCI). It is calculated as dividing the total number of complete vascular coils by the umbilical cord length. When the UCI is less than 0.1 coils/cm we speak about hypocoiled cord, and if the value surpasses 0.3 coils/cm, it is considered as hypercoiled cord. Both conditions are associated with increased fetal risk. Particularly, a consistent association between hypocoiled cord and IUGR, unexplained fetal demise, intrapartum complications, and also chromosomal abnormalities, seems evident[18,19] (Figs 10.44 to 10.46).

Single Umbilical Artery

The sonographic diagnosis is very easy since there are only two vessels in umbilical cord. Usually, the single artery is larger. The diameter of the artery can even reach that of the vein.[20]

A huge number of studies published so far have found an association between single umbilical artery and fetal structural and chromosomal abnormalities, but also with IUGR, unexplained fetal death, etc.[21] For this reason, when this abnormality is diagnosed, it is necessary to make an exhaustive study of fetal anatomy as well as to study the fetal karyotype (Figs 10.47 to 10.55).

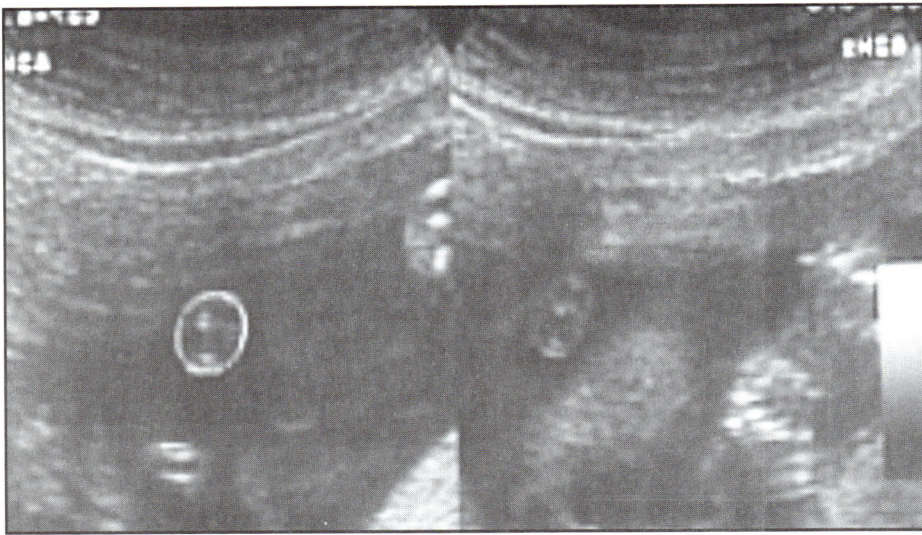

A

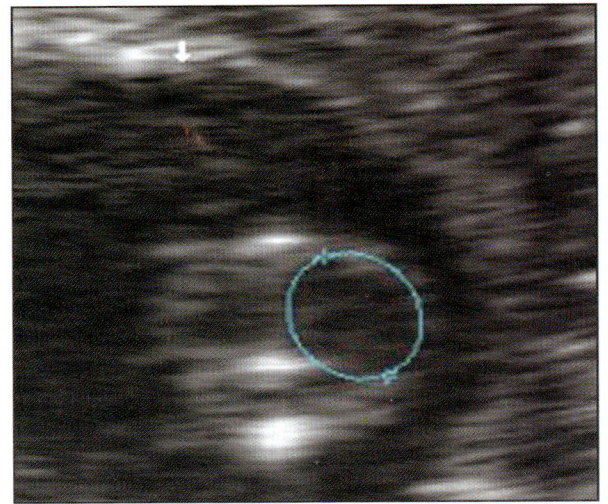

B

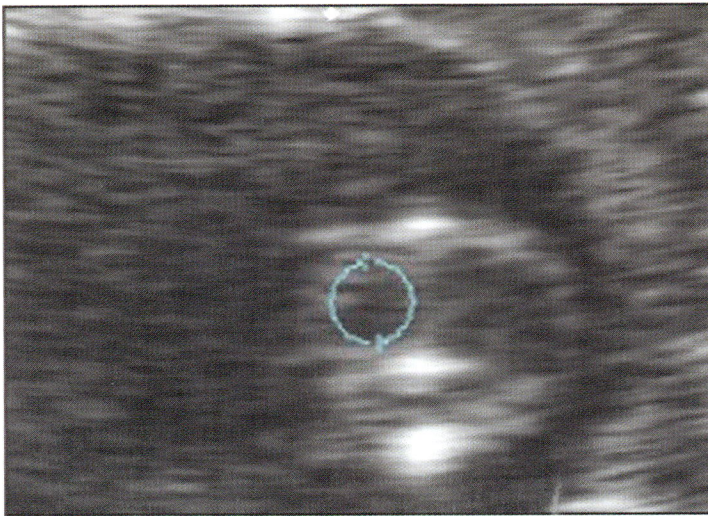

C

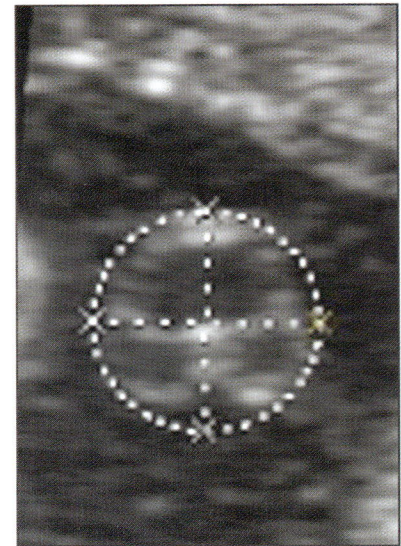

D

Figs 10.43A to D: Estimation of the circumference size of the umbilical cord for comparison using normality tables

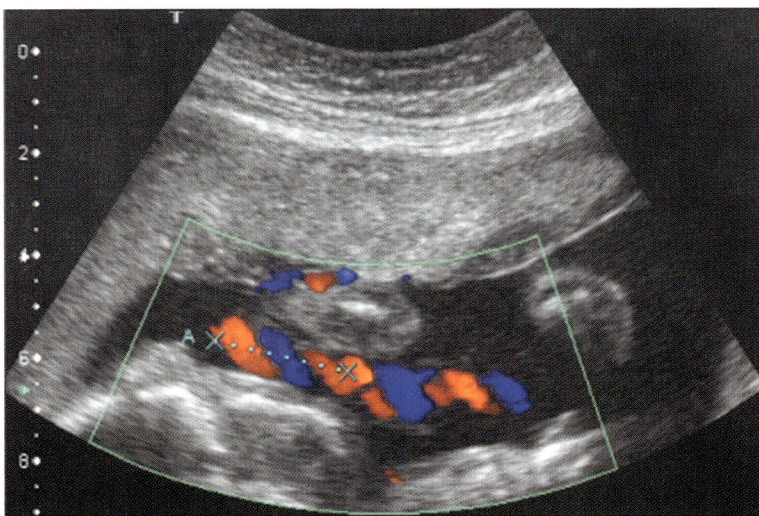

Fig. 10.44: Umbilical cord in the the third term: Measurement shows a normal number of coils "umbilical coiling index" (UCI)

Occasionally, it is possible to observe discordant umbilical arteries that are usually of similar diameter. Apparently, the discordant arteries may be caused by absence or malfunction of the Hyrtl anastomosis.[22] The fact is that this abnormality produces differences in blood flow between both lobes of the placenta which can increase the risk for IUGR and preterm delivery (Figs 10.56 to 10.61).

Umbilical Cord Tumors

The umbilical cord can be the location for several cysts and solid tumors. The most frequent are: omphalomesenteric duct cyst, allantoid cyst, hemangiomas, teratomas, etc. The multiple umbilical cord cysts are highly associated with structural and chromosomal abnormalities.[23] Hemangiomas can cause fetal cardiac dysfunction and polyhydramnios [24] (Figs 10.62 to 10.75).

Miscellaneous Abnormalities

Different pictures showing the umbilical cord during a fetus blood sampling in a twin gestation and showing normality (Figs 10.76 to 10.82).

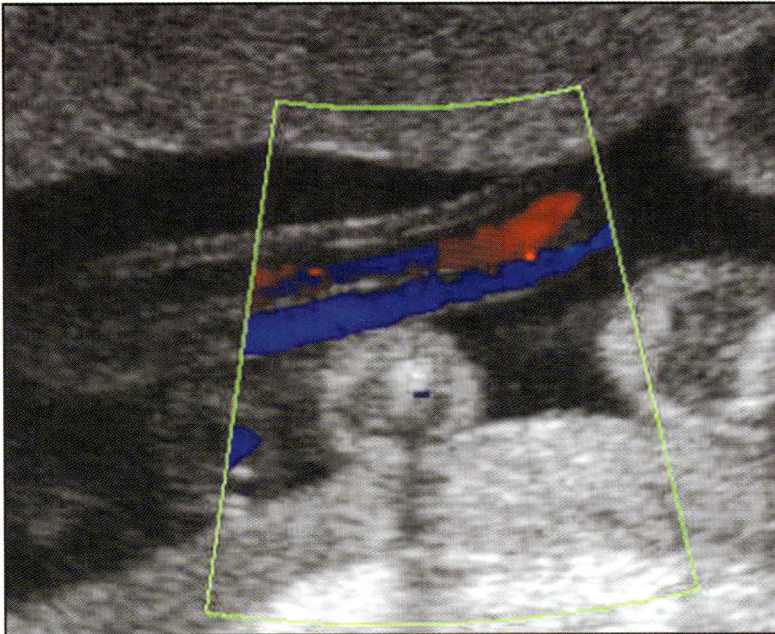
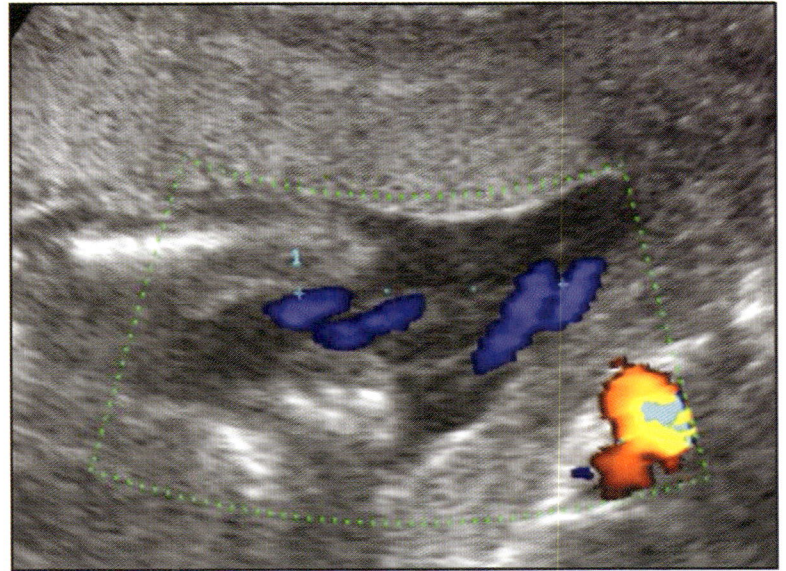

A   B

Fig. 10.45: Sonogram showing the umbilical cord at 33rd week with less than 0.1 coils/cm; hypocoiled cord

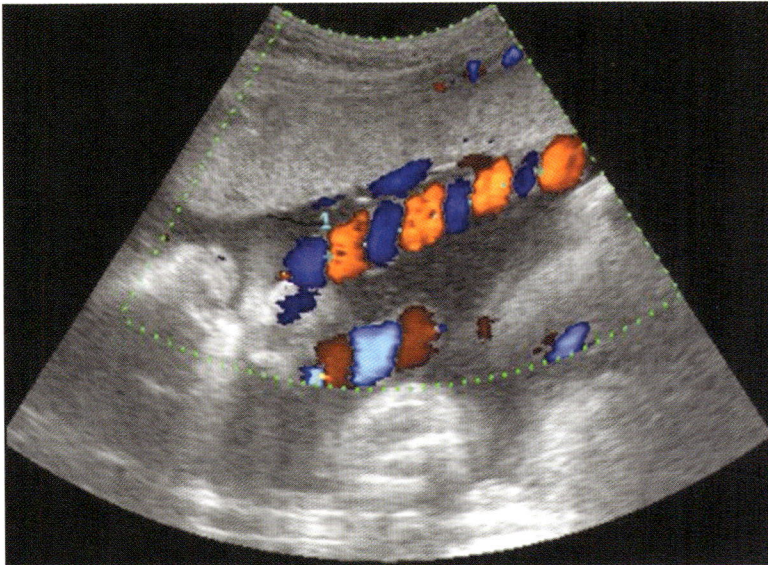

Fig. 10.46: Sonogram showing the umbilical cord at 32nd week with more than 0.3 coils/cm hypercoiled cord

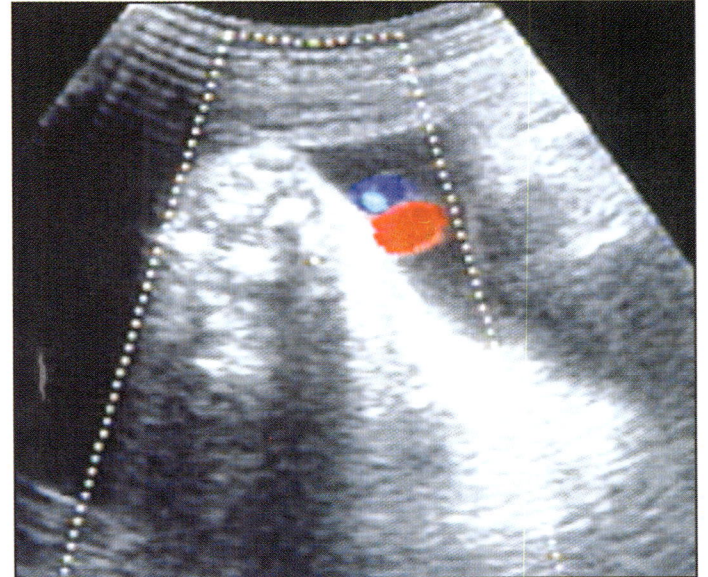

Fig. 10.48: Cross-section of umbilical cord with color Doppler showing two vessels (single umbilical artery)

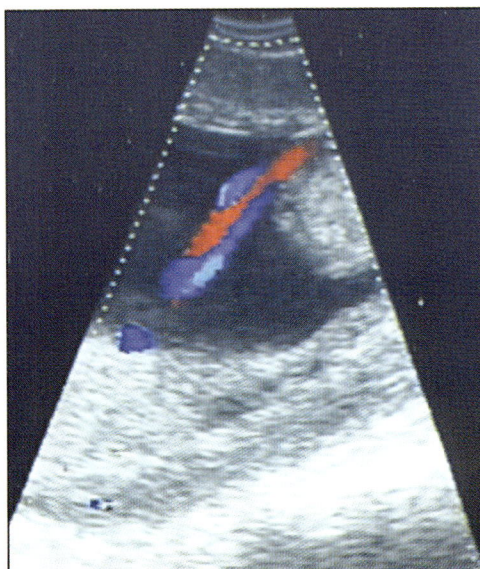

Fig. 10.47: Longitudinal section of umbilical cord showing single umbilical artery

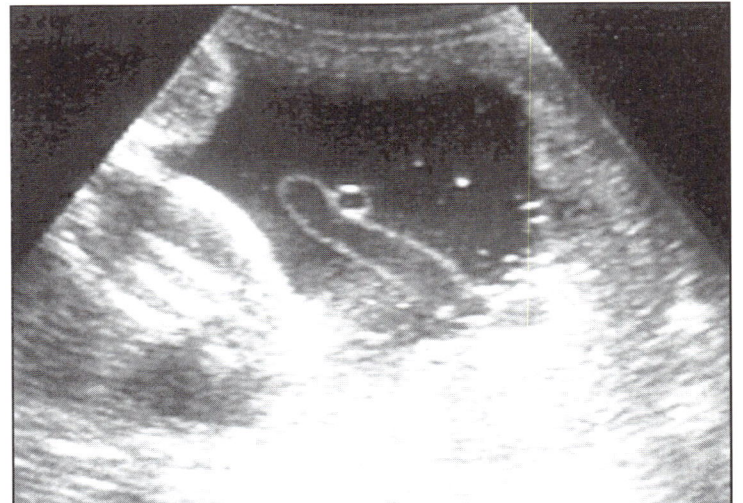

Fig. 10.49: Sonogram showing two vessels (single umbilical artery) at 25th week

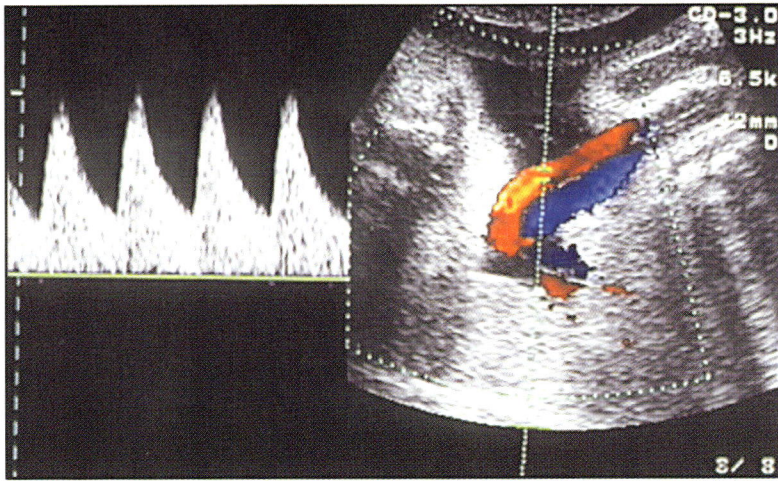

Fig. 10.50: Umbilical single artery Doppler with its normal waveform pattern

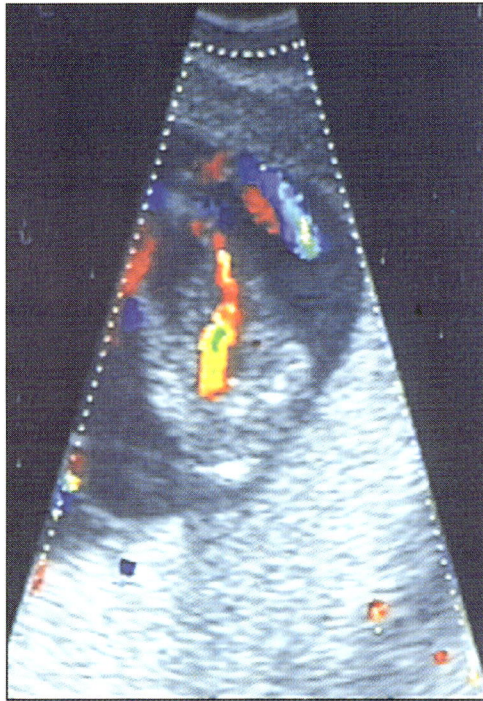

Fig. 10.53: Power Doppler shows a single umbilical artery coursing around the urinary bladder at 13th week

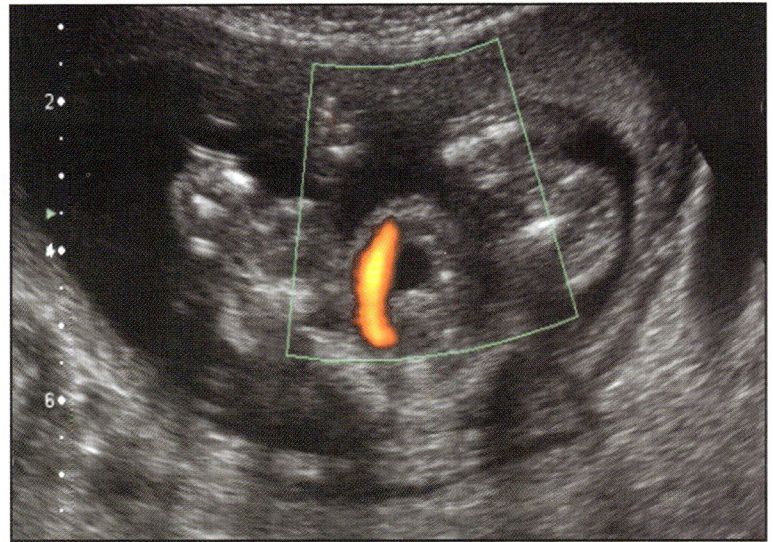

Fig. 10.51: Color Doppler shows a single umbilical artery coursing around the urinary bladder at 13th week

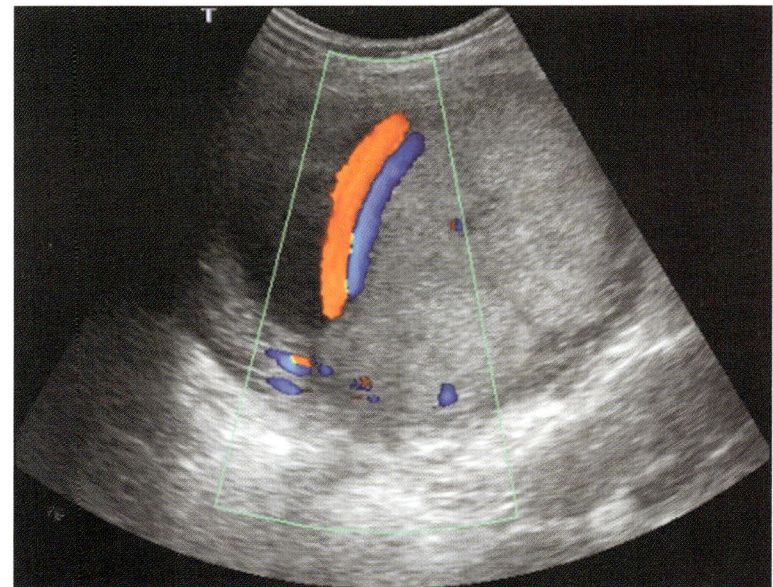

Fig. 10.54: Longitudinal section of umbilical cord showing single umbilical artery at 27th week

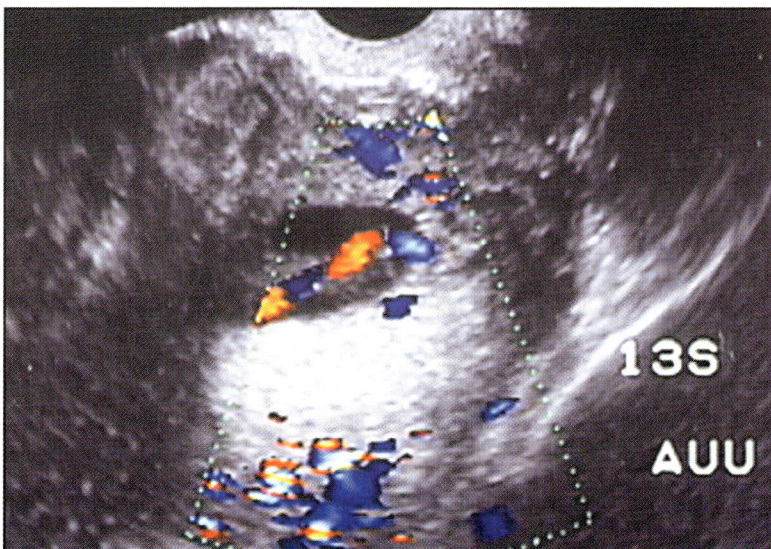

Fig. 10.52: Color Doppler shows a single umbilical artery at 13th week

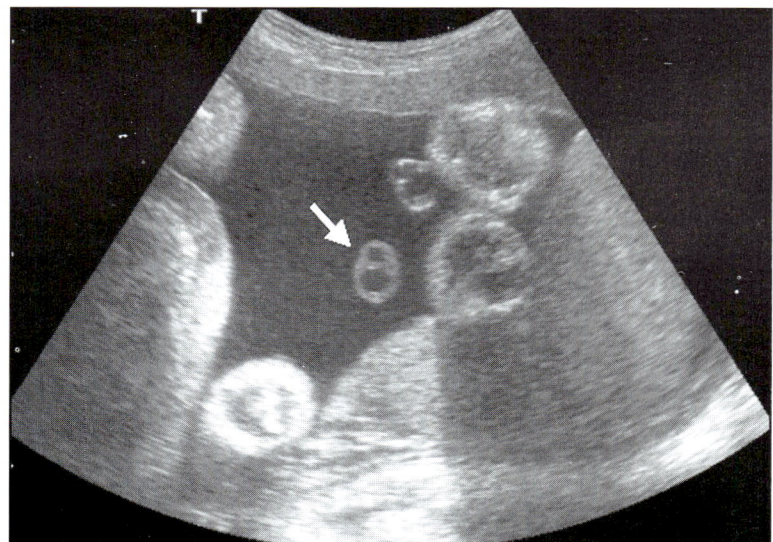

Fig. 10.55: Cross-section of umbilical cord showing single umbilical artery at 27th week

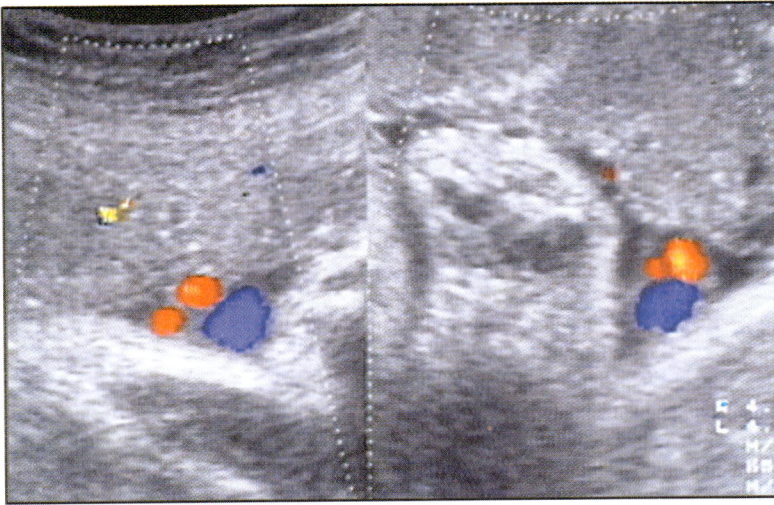

Fig. 10.56: Cross-section showing a normal umbilical cord on the left and on the right showing an hypoplasic umbilical artery at 32nd week

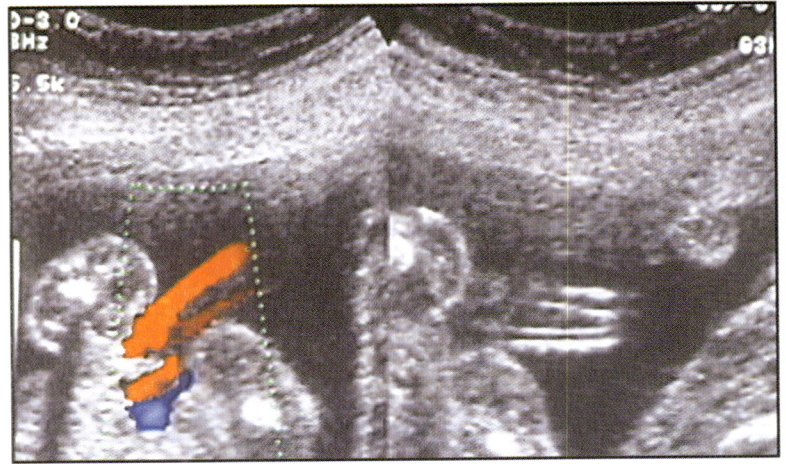

Fig. 10.59: Longitudinal section showing the difference in the diameter of an hypoplasic umbilical artery with color Doppler on the left and without on the right

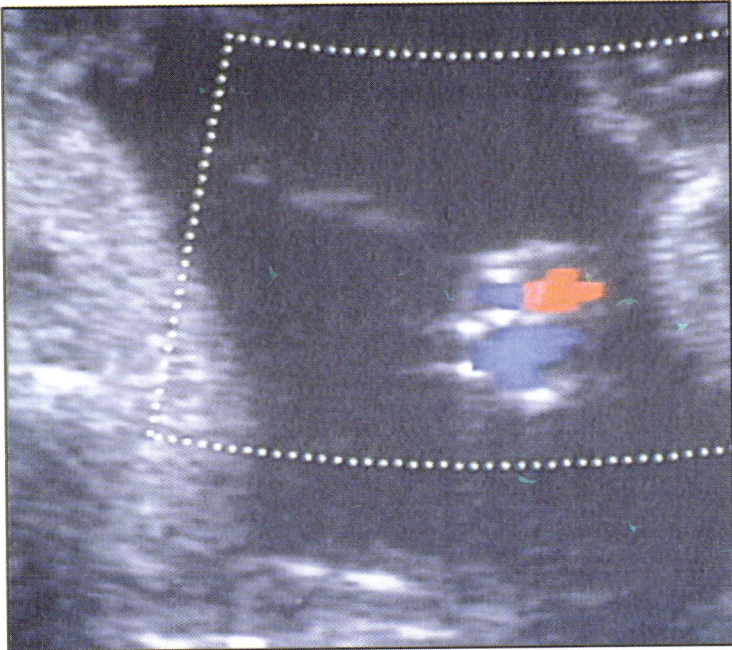

Fig. 10.57: Cross-section showing the difference in the diameter of an hypoplasic umbilical artery

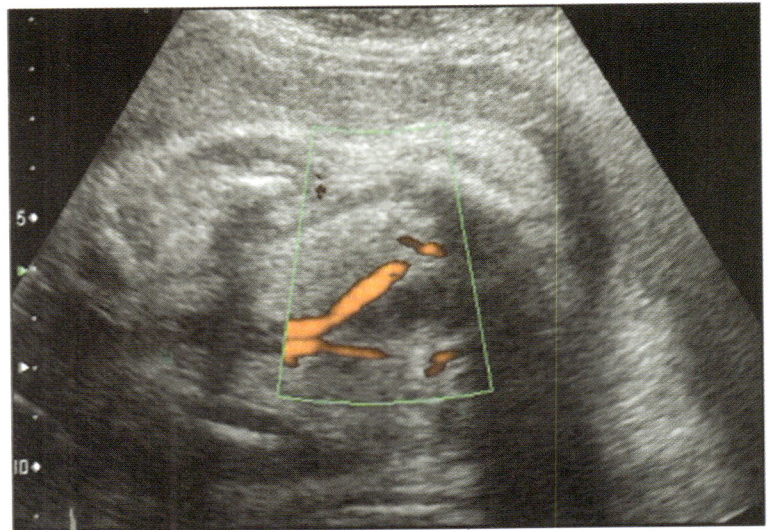

Fig. 10.60: Longitudinal section showing the difference in the diameter of an hypoplasic umbilical artery with power Doppler

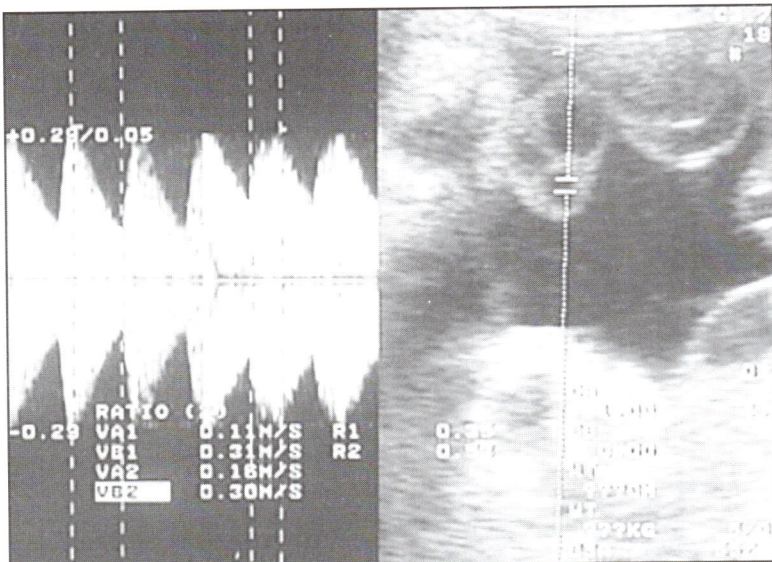

Fig. 10.58: Umbilical artery Doppler with its normal waveform pattern

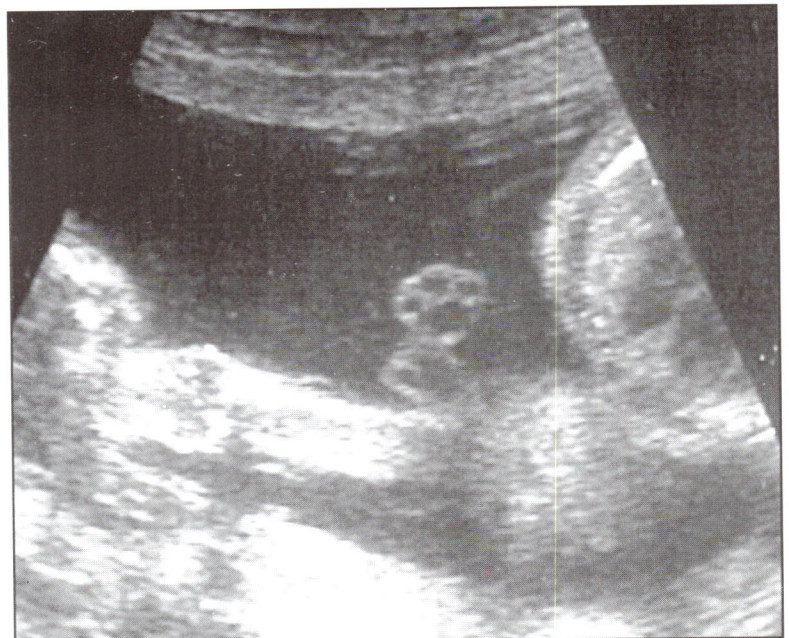

Fig. 10.61: Cross-section of umbilical cord showing four vessels

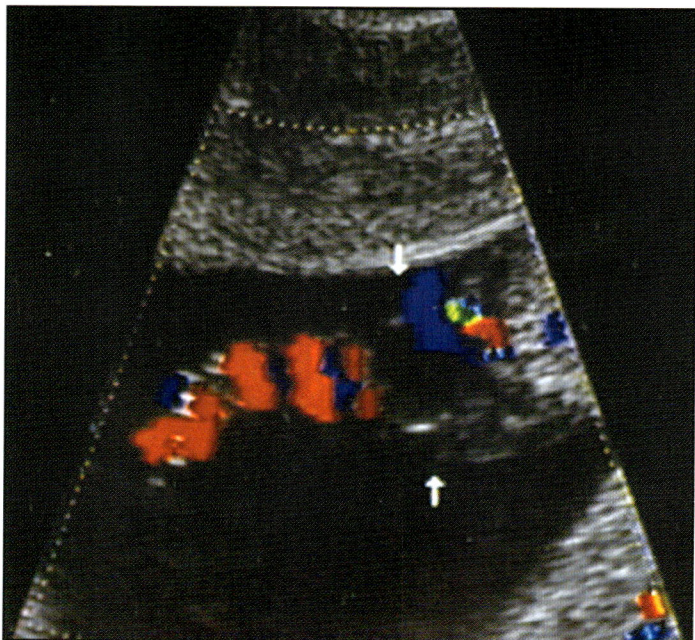

A

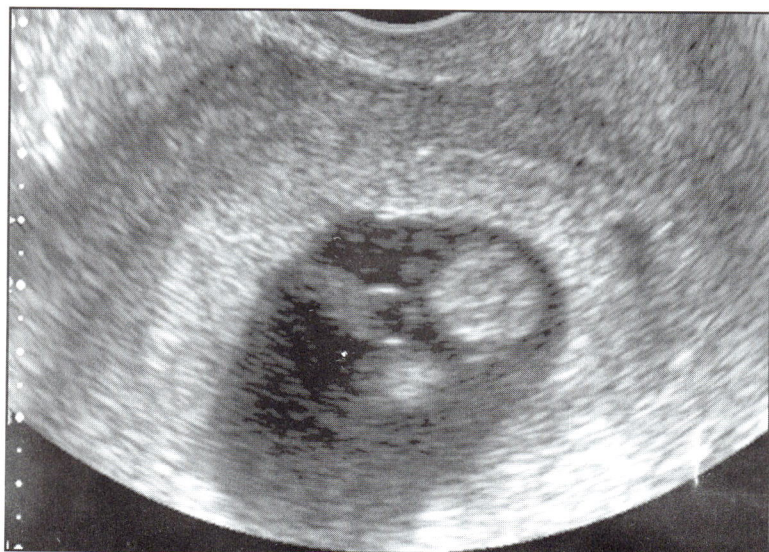

B

Figs 10.62A and B: Umbilical cord cyst in the first term

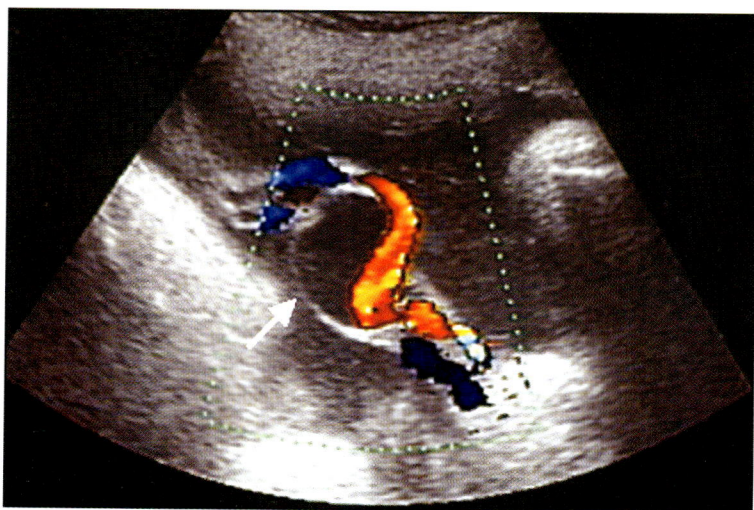

Fig. 10.63: Umbilical cord cyst in the third term, probably pseudocyst

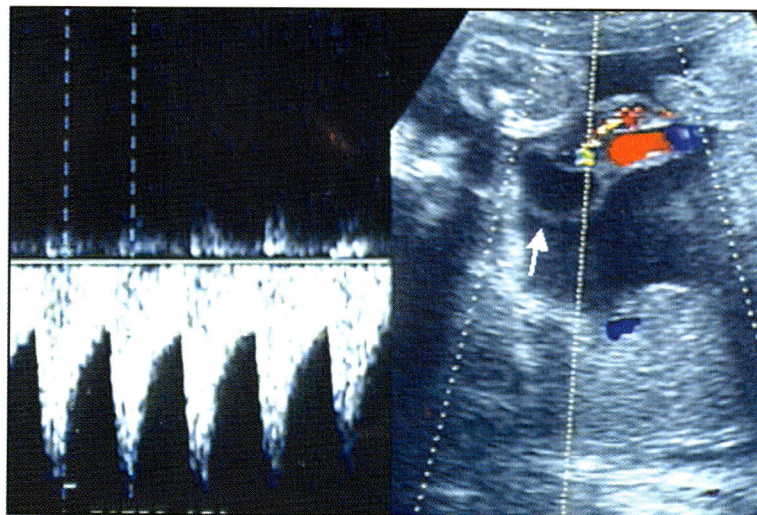

Fig. 10.64: Umbilical cord cyst in the third term with normal Doppler

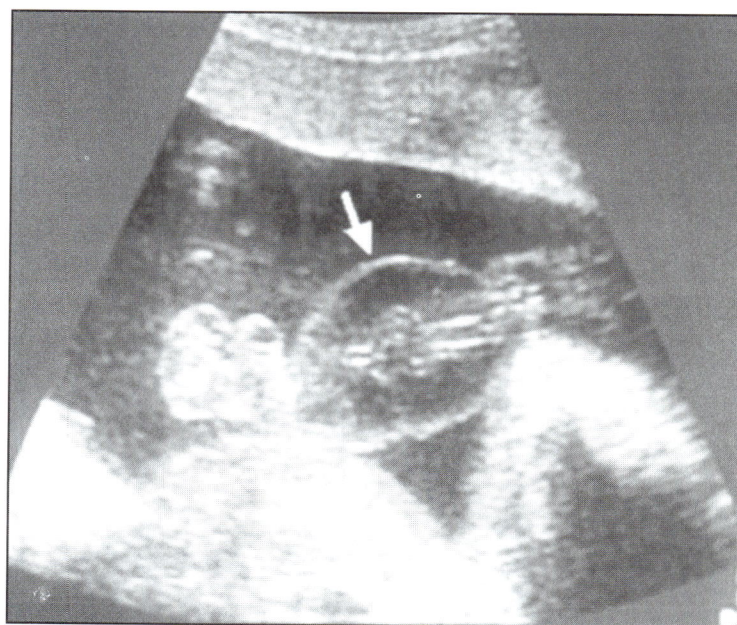

Fig. 10.65: Umbilical cord cyst near of fetal insertion. Fetus with trisomy 18

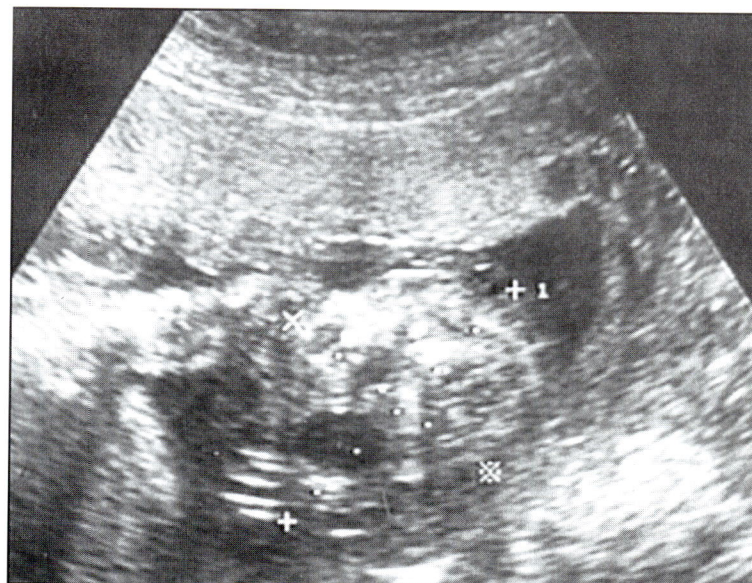

Fig. 10.66: Solid and cystic tumor of the umbilical cord in the third term

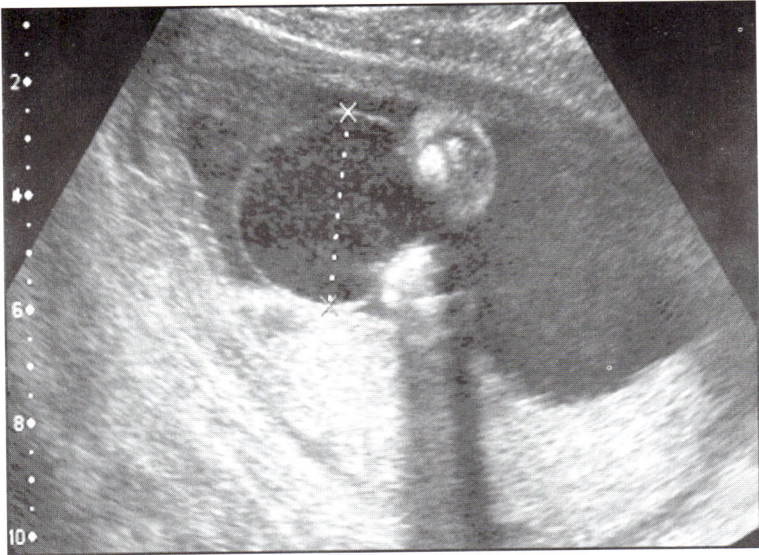

A

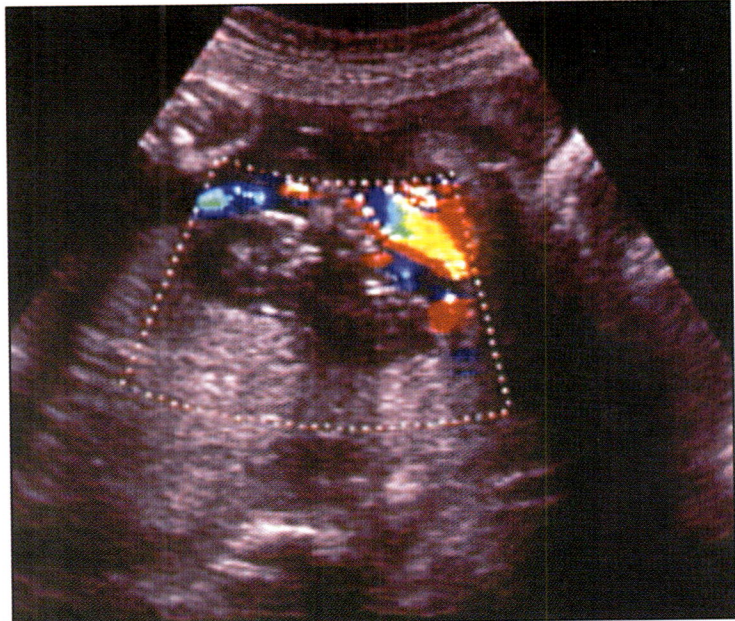

Fig. 10.69: Solid and cystic tumor of the umbilical cord with normal Doppler

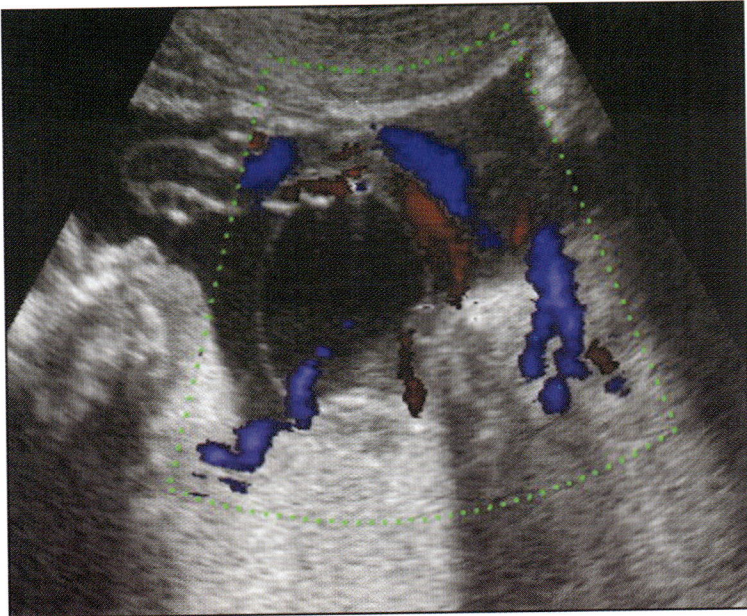

B

Figs 10.67A and B: Umbilical cord cyst in the third term without Doppler on the left and with color Doppler on the right

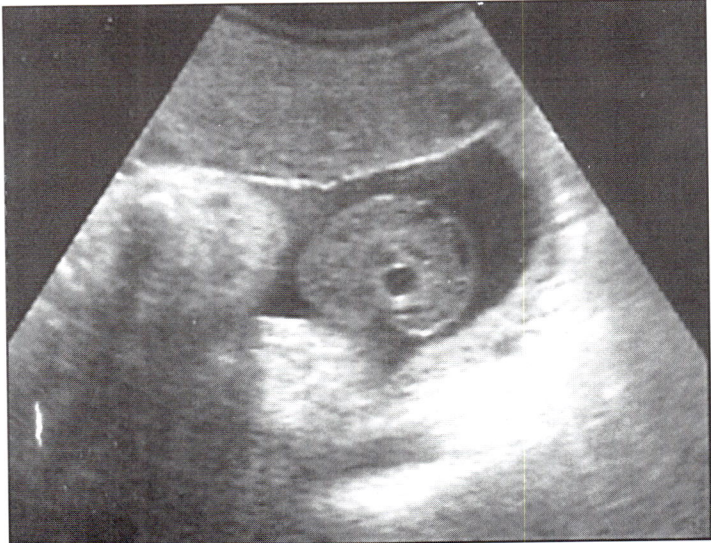

A

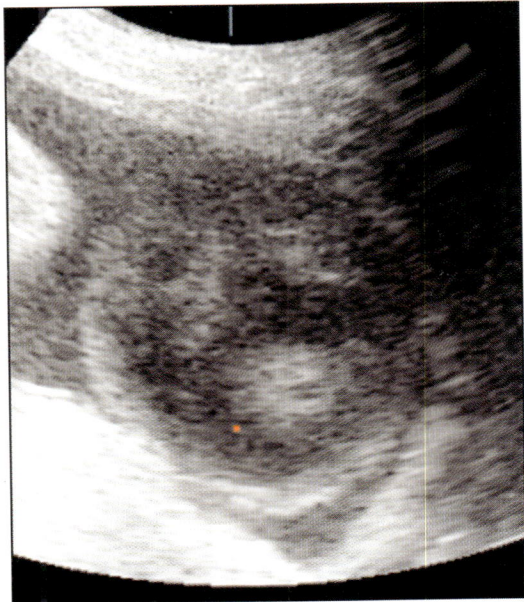

B

Fig. 10.68: Solid and cystic tumor of the umbilical cord with normal Doppler

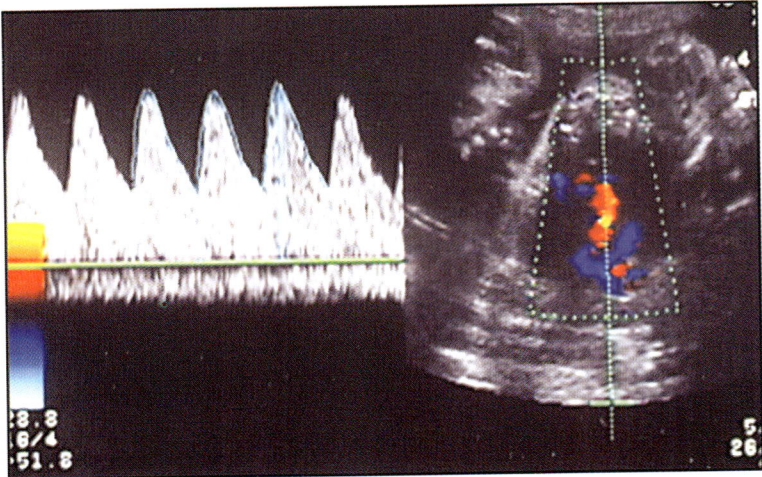

B

Figs 10.70A and B: Cross-section of the umbilical cord in the third term of pregnancy showing an increase in the Wharton's jelly probably due to edema

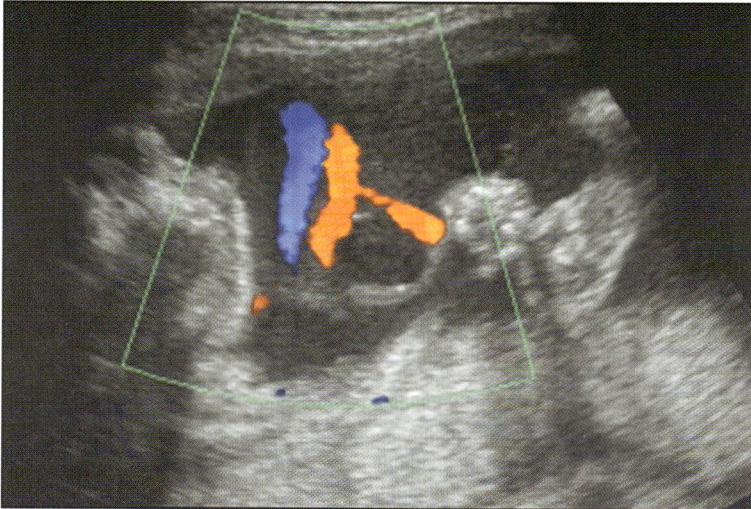

A

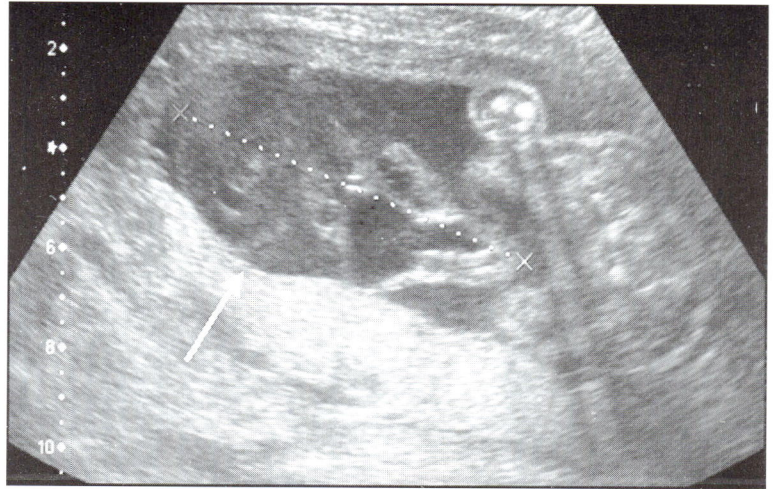

Fig. 10.73: Longitudinal section showing a solid-cystic tumor of the umbilical cord in the third term before its insertion at the fetus

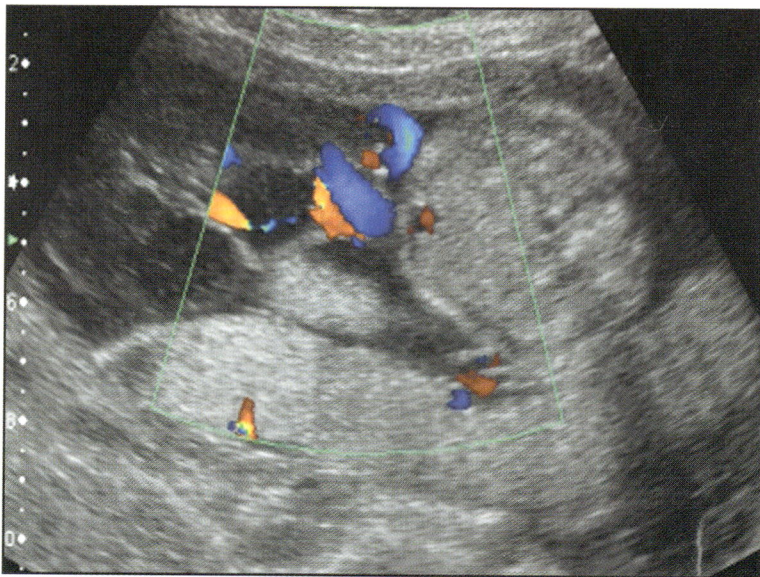

B

Figs 10.71A and B: Cross-section on the left and longitudinal section on the right showing a cyst between the two arteries which have a normal diameter in the third term

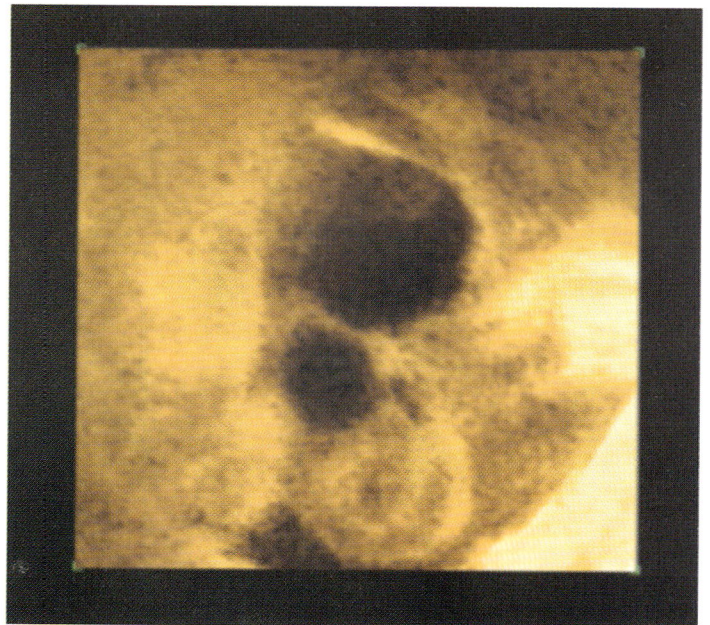

Fig. 10.74: 3D scan showing a cross-section of the umbilical cord in the third term with a cystic tumor

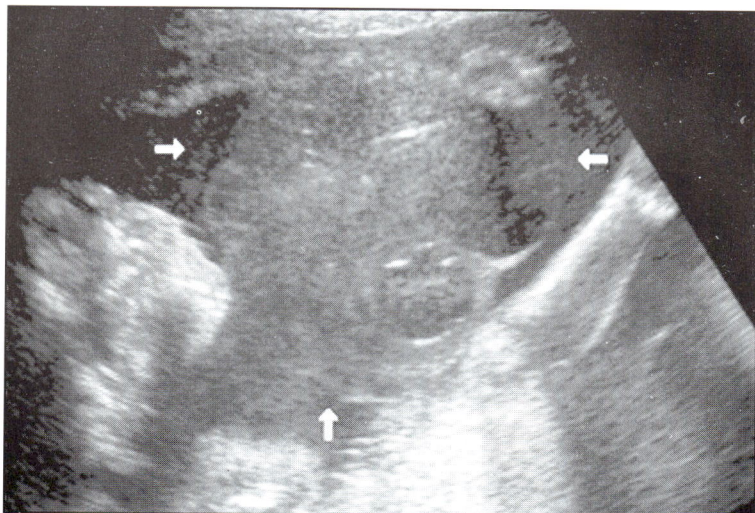

Fig. 10.72: Cross-section of the umbilical cord in the third term of pregnancy showing an increase in the Wharton's jelly probably due to edema

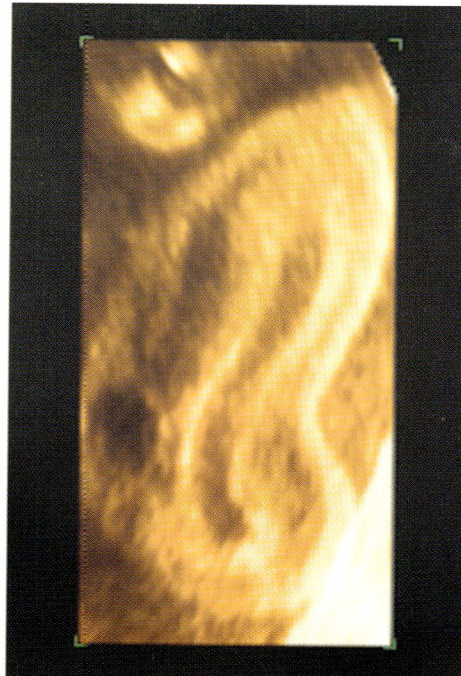

Fig. 10.75: 3D scan showing a longitudinal section of the umbilical cord In the third term with an increase of the wharton's jelly and edema

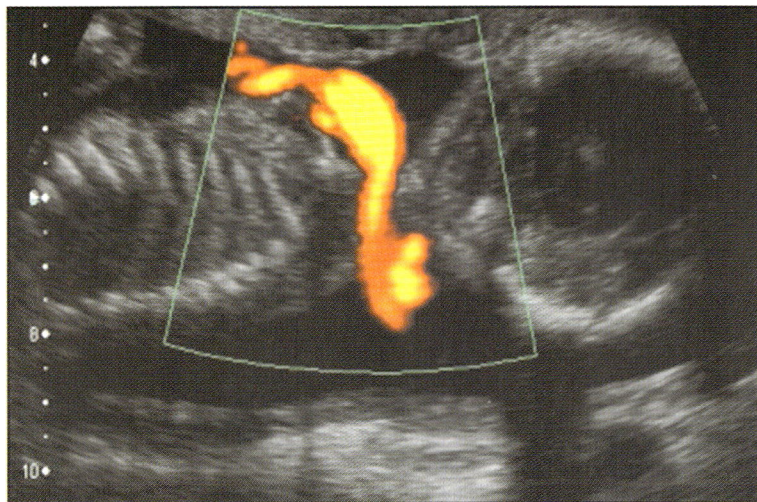

A

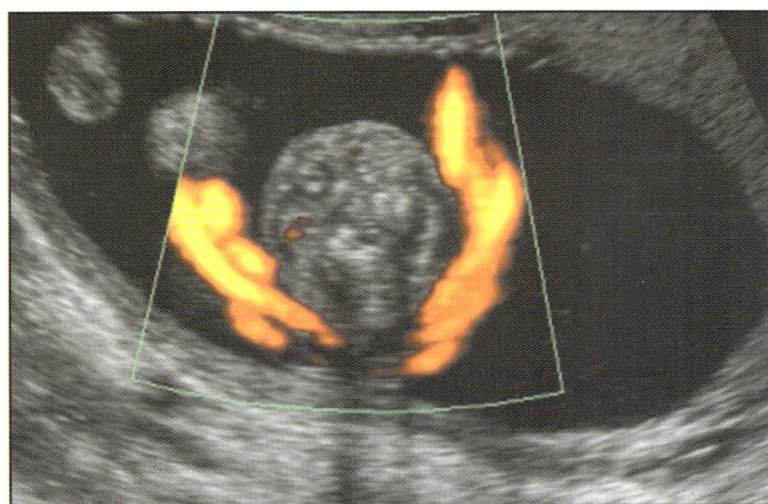

B

Figs 10.76A and B: Power Doppler scan showing the umbilical cord around the fetus neck

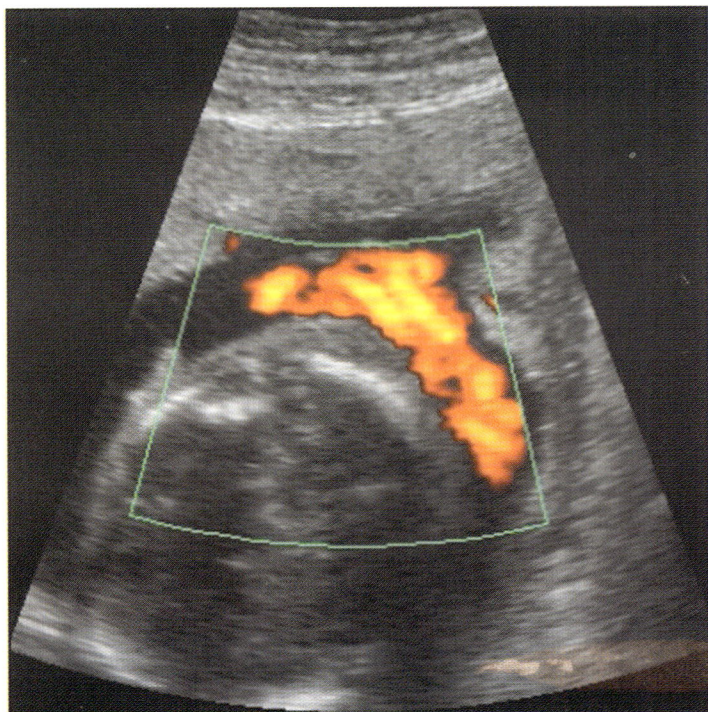

Fig. 10.77: Power Doppler scan showing the umbilical cord around the fetus neck

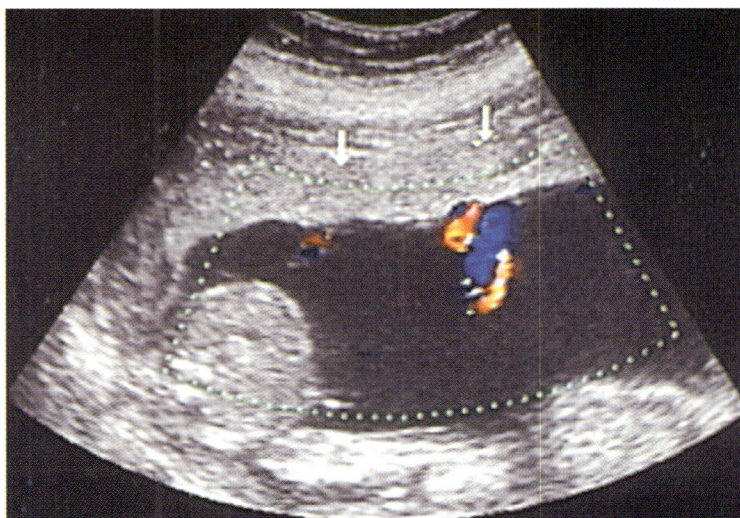

Fig. 10.78: Doppler shows the difference in the size of the umbilical cord in a twin-twin transfusion syndrome in a monochorionic pregnancy during the second term

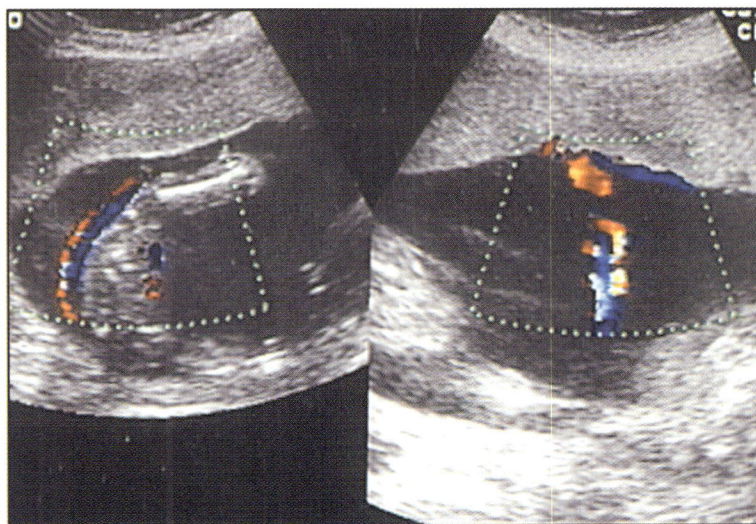

Fig. 10.79: Doppler shows the difference in the size of the umbilical cord in a twin-twin transfusion syndrome in a monochorionic pregnancy during the second term

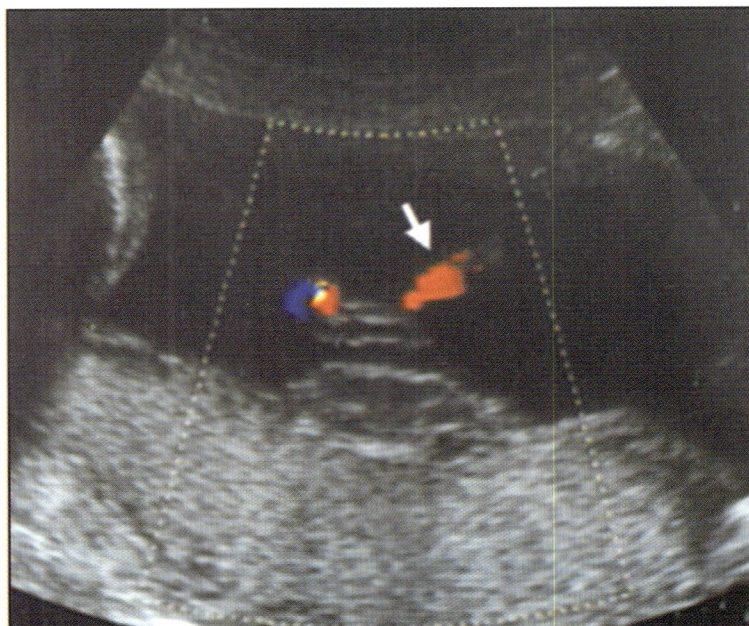

Fig. 10.80: Blood leak following the removal of the needle during a fetal blood sampling in the second term

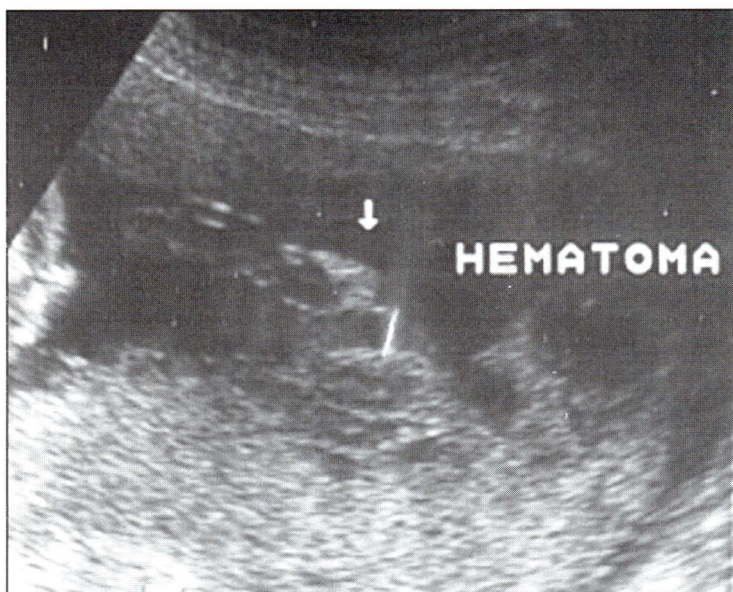

Fig. 10.81: Hematoma at the puncture site following fetal blood sampling in the second term

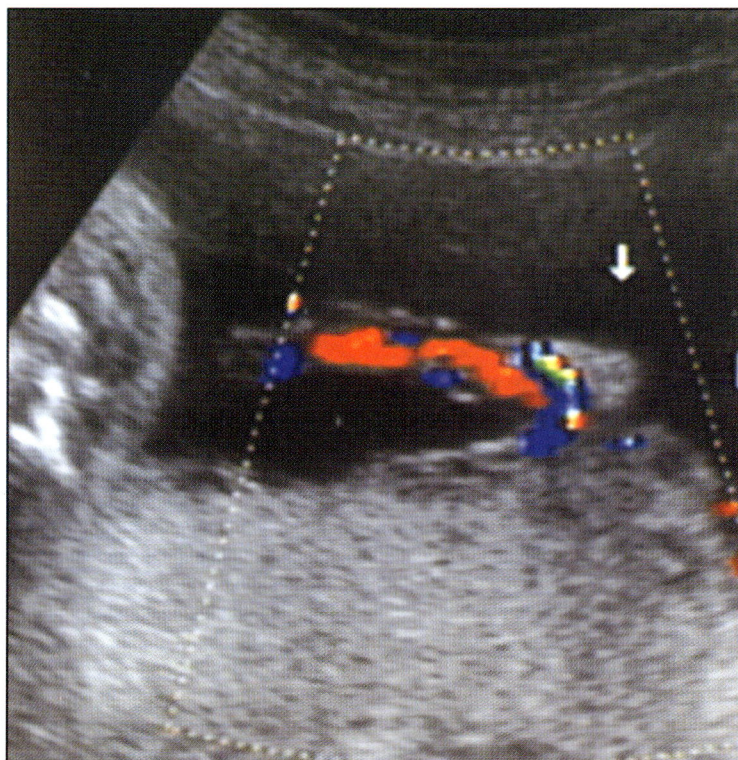

Fig. 10.82: Normal blood flow through the umbilical cord with the hematoma following fetal blood sampling

REFERENCES

1. Spirt BA, Gordon LP. The placenta as indicator of fetal maturity. Facts and fancy. Semin Ultrasound 1984;13:501.
2. Fox H. Pathology of placenta. WB Saunders: Philadelphia, 1978.
3. Grannum PAT, Berkowitz FL, Hobbins JD. The ultrasonic changes in the maturing placenta and their relation to fetal pulmonic maturity. Am J Obstet Gynecol 1979;133:915-22.
4. Loret de Mola JR, Judge N, Entsminger C, De Viney M, Mvise KL, Dudron MA. Indirect prediction of fetal lung maturity. Value of ultrasonographic colonic and placental grading. J Reprod Med 1998;43:898-902.
5. Molloy CE, Mc Dowell W, Armour R. Ultrasonic diagnosis of placenta membranacea in utero. J Ultrasound Med 1983;3:337.
6. Matijevic R. The placenta. In Kurjak A, Chervenak FA (Eds): Donald School Textbook of Ultrasound in Obstetrics and Gynecology. Jaypee Brothers: New Delhi, 2004, pp 326-39.
7. Deans A, Jauniaux E. Prenatal diagnosis and outcome of subamniotic hematomas. Ultrasound Obstet Gynecol 1998;11:319-23.
8. Meinhard K, Dimitrov S, Nicolou A, Dimitrova V, Vassilev N. Placental teratoma – a case report. Pathol Res Pract 1999;195:649-51.
9. Gillet N, Hustin J, Magritte JP, Givron O, Longueville E. Placental teratoma: differential diagnosis with fetal acardia. Gynecol Obstet Biol Reprod (Paris) 2001:30:789-92.
10. Smith RS, Lauria MR, Comstock CH, Treadwell MC, Kirk JS, Lee W, Bottoms SF. Transvaginal ultrasonography for all placentas that appear to be low-lying or over the internal cervical os. Ultrasound Obstet Gynecol 1997;9:22-4.
11. Finberg HJ, Williams JW. Placenta accreta. Prospective sonographic diagnosis in patients with placenta previa and prior cesarean section. J Ultrasound Med 1992;11:333.
12. Di Naro E, Raio L, D'Addario V. The umbilical cord: sonographic assessment. In Kurjak A, Chervenak, FA (Eds): Donald School Textbook of Ultrasound in Obstetrics and Gynecology. Jaypee Brothers: New Delhi, 2004, pp 320-5.
13. Ghezzi F, Raio L, Di Naro E. First trimester sonographic umbilical cord diameter and the growth of the human embryo. Ultrasound Obstet Gynecol 2001;18:348-51.
14. Ghezzi F, Raio L, Di Naro E. First trimester umbilical cord diameter: a novel marker of fetal aneuploidy. Ultrasoun Obstet Gynecol 2002;19:235-9.
15. Raio L, Ghezzi F, Di Naro E. Sonographic measurement of the umbilical cord and fetal anthropometric parameters. Eur J Obstet Gynec Reprod Biol 1999;83:131-5.
16. Bruds JF, Sibony O, Benali K. Computerized microscope morphometry of umbilical vessels from pregnancies with IUGR and abnormal umbilical artery Doppler. Hum Pathol 1997;28:1139-45.
17. Strong TA Jr, Jarles DL, Vega FS, Feldman DB. The umbilical coiling index. Am J Obstet Gynecol 1994;170:29-32.
18. Degani S, Leibovich Z, Shapiro I. Early second-trimester low umbilical coiling index predicts small-for-gestational age fetuses. J Ultrasound Med 2001;20:1183-8.
19. Georgiou HM, Rice GE, Walker SP. The effect of vascular coiling of venous perfusion during experimental umbilical cord encirclement. Am J Obstet Gynecol 2001;184:673-8.
20. Persutte WH, Lenke RR. Transverse umbilical arterial diameter: a new technique for the prenatal diagnosis of singled umbilical artery. J Ultrasound Med 1994;13:763-6.
21. Heifetz SA. Single umbilical artery: a statistical analysis of 237 autopsy cases and review of the literature. Perspect Pediatr Pathol 1994;8:345-78.
22. Raio L, Ghezzi F, Di Naro E. In-utero characterization of the blood flow in the Hyrtl anastomosis. Placenta 2001;22:597-601.
23. Sepulveda W, Leible S, Ulloa A. Clinical significance of first trimester umbilical cord cyst. J Ultrasound Med 1999;18:95-9.
24. Tennstedt C, Chaoui R, Bollmann R. Angiomyxoma of the umbilical cord in one twin with cystic degeneration of Wharton's jelly. A case report. Pathol Res Pract 1998;194:55-8.

11

Fetal Pathology

A Muñoz, JM Carrera,
P Prats, M Ruiz

FETAL INFECTIONS

Certain ultrasonographic signs, even though they are nonspecific, can alert on the presence of a fetal infection. These signs include oligohydramnios, an enlarged placenta (Fig. 11.1), hepatosplenomegaly (Fig. 11.2) and fetal ascites.[1] In addition, if the fetus also demonstrates pattern of IUGR, then one can be assured that one is heading with a fetal infection.

Ultrasonography, in addition, gives us information about the possible specific embryonic pathologies, especially in the case of cytomegalovirus, rubella and toxoplasmosis.

In the case of *cytomegalovirus*, in addition to the nonspecific abnormalities, it is possible to find intracerebral calcifications (Figs 11.3A to C) (punctiform and periventricular), moderate hydrocephaly (Fig. 11.4) (frequently associated with an expansion of the subarachnoid space), microcephaly, intra-abdominal echogenic images, pleural effusions and anasarca (Figs 11.5A and B).

If the fetal infection is obvious by serological analysis, the ultrasonographic evaluation will permit one to define the prognosis by classifying the causes as: (i) asymptomatic fetal infection; (ii) discrete or moderate infection (few ultrasonographic findings), and (iii) fetal infection of the pleura and viscera. In this case, which is common in primary infections in the first half of gestation, the perinatal mortality is very high (30 to 40%) and also the risk for perinatal sequela.

In the case of *rubella* it is possible to observe various malformations by ultrasonography: cardiovascular malformations (ductus arteriosus, interventricular defects), anomalies of the central nervous system (microcephaly, cerebral microcalcifications) and hepatosplenomegaly. However, some of the expected anomalies that have no echographic manifestation (ophthalmic malformations, deafness, mental

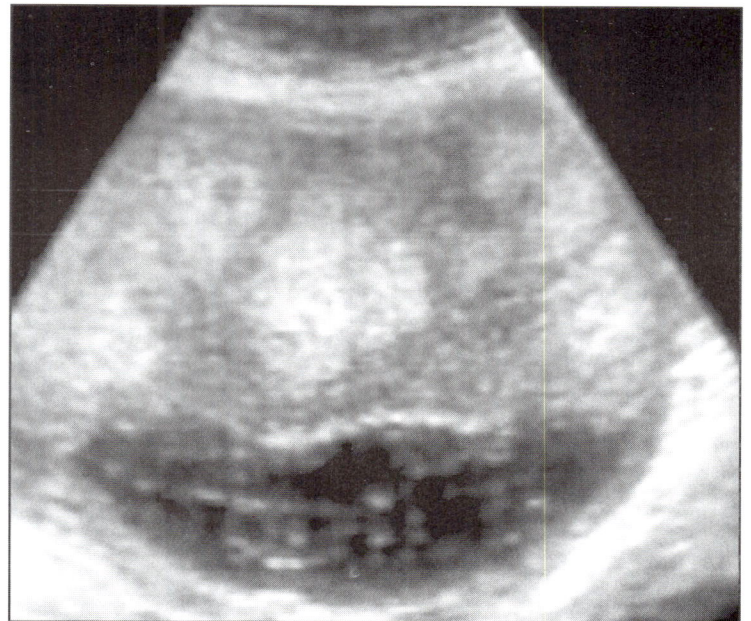

Fig. 11.1: Congenital infection: Placentomegaly

retardation, immunological defects, behavioral abnormalities, etc.) should make us cautious in predicting the prognosis. It should be taken into account that serious abnormalities are the rule before 11th week of gestation; in contrast, important abnormalities are rarely found after 18th week of gestation.

With respect to *toxoplasmosis*, the usual case is that the embryonic infections provoke an abortion or "intrauterine death." In the fetus, the lesions are essentially cerebral. The ventricular enlargements are usually bilateral and symmetrical and often originate in the occipital horns. The intracranial calcifications are the consequence of zones of necrotic cerebrum. Other anomalies such as intrahepatic densities, ascites and pericardial effusions are also possible.

The prognosis depends on the gestational age in which the fetal infection occurs and the cerebral lesions that are diagnosed echographically. Infections that occur before 10th week of

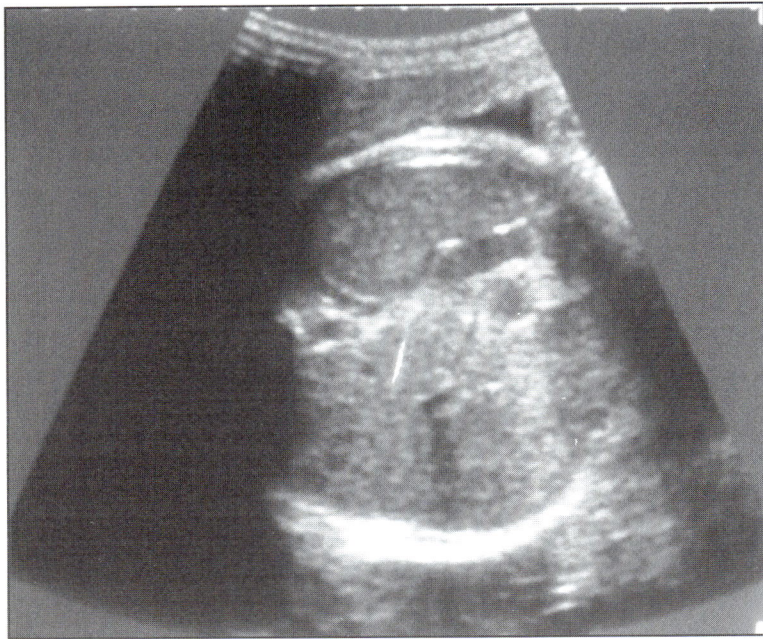

A

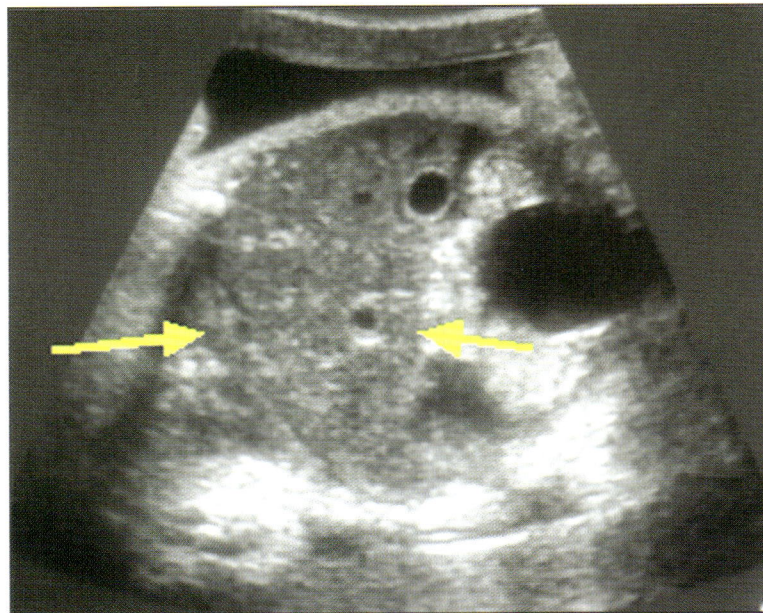

B

Figs 11.2A and B: *Lysteria* infection: Hepatosplenomegaly, with heterogeneous appearance of the liver

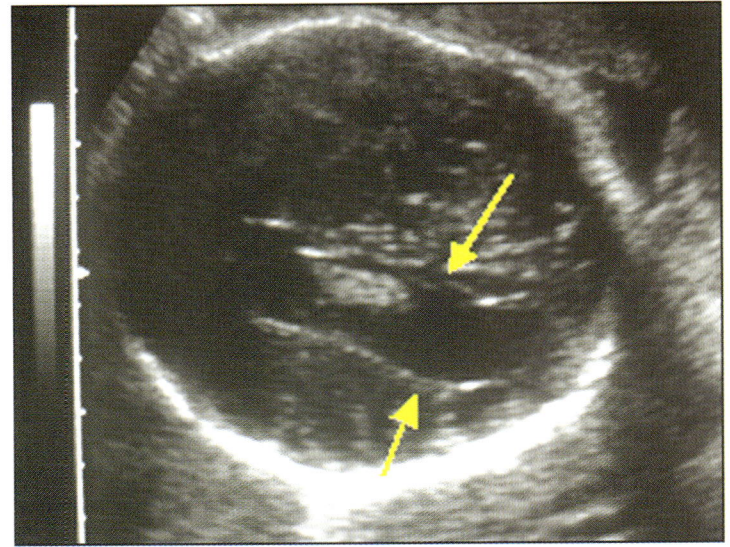

A

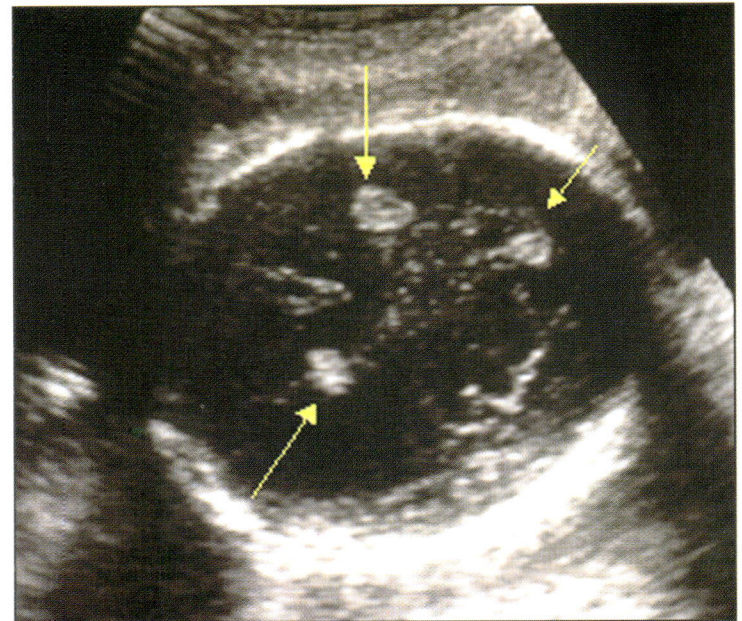

B

Figs 11.3A and B: Fetal infections: Cytomegalovirus ventriculomegaly, coronal view of the brain shows bright echogenic area consistent with calcification

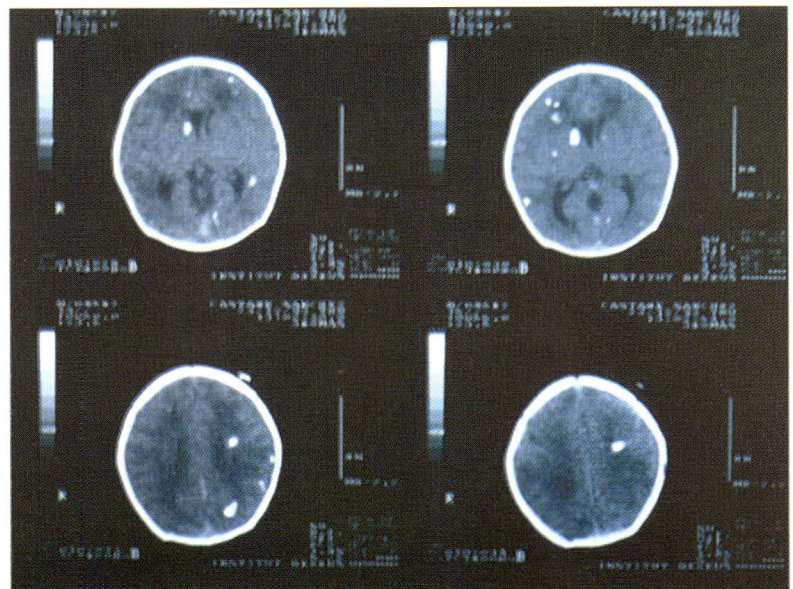

Fig. 11.3C: A postnatal computed tomogram shows calcification of the basal ganglia

gestation and that have cerebral necrotic lesions should be considered to have a very poor neurological prognosis. In contrast, fetuses that are infected in or beyond the second trimester and that have only isolated calcifications may suffer only from epilepsy and not necessarily from mental retardation. The rapid evolution of the lesions (ventricular dilatation, for example) should also signal a poor prognosis.[2]

ALLOIMMUNIZED PREGNANCY

Traditionally, the ultrasound has been used in the management of alloimmunized pregnancy, as an adjunct for diagnosis and treatment. Thanks to ultrasonography, the invasive methods of diagnosis (amniocentesis and cordocentesis) and also of

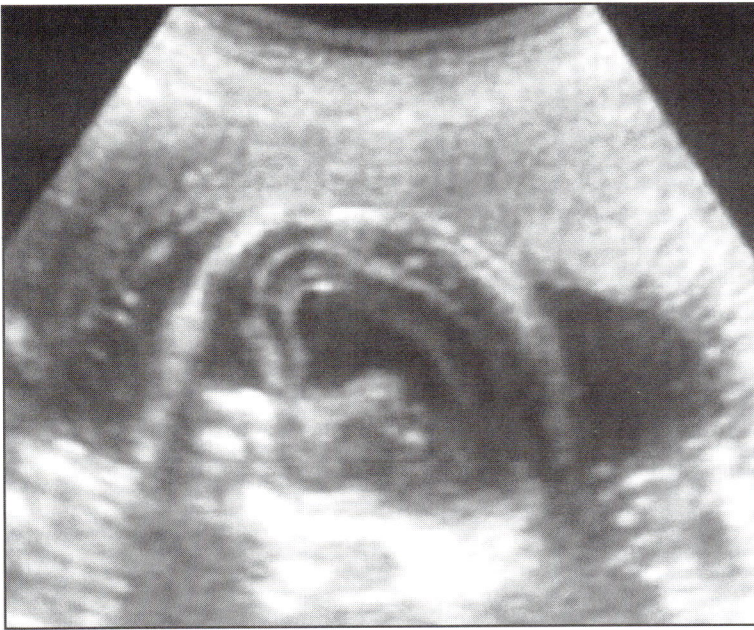

Fig. 11.4: Congenital cytomegalovirus infection. Sagittal scan shows ventriculomegaly

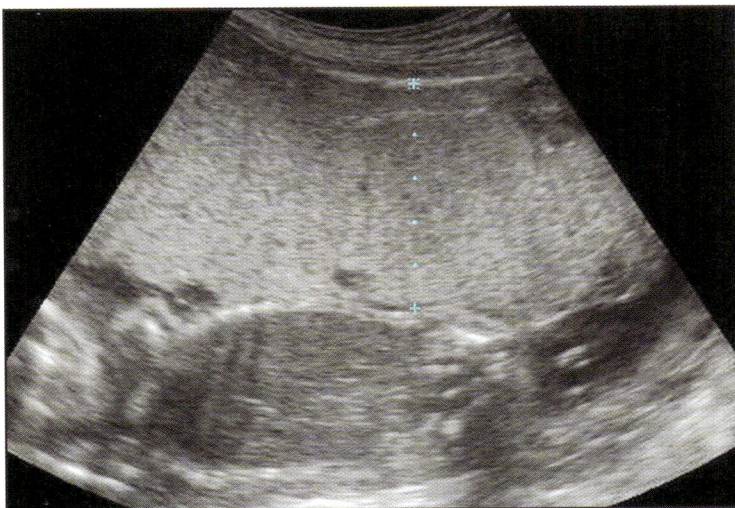

Fig. 11.5A: Congenital cytomegalovirus infection: Placentomegaly

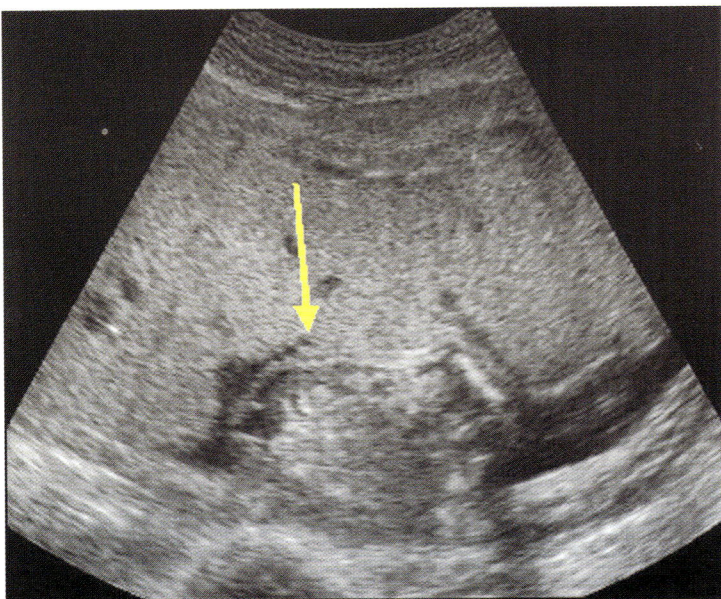

Fig. 11.5B: Congenital cytomegalovirus infection: Hyperechoic bowel

treatment (percutaneous intraperitoneal fetal transfusion (IPT) or intravascular intrauterine transfusion (IUT), were realized with notable safety. Effectively, ultrasound has been commonly used to guide the needle, through the maternal abdomen into the amniotic cavity, peritoneal space or fetal umbilical vein.[3]

But in this moment, the role of the amniocentesis in the diagnosis of alloimmunized pregnancy is null and void. The reason is that the early diagnosis of fetal anemia is possible with the use of ultrasonography and Doppler.

The conventional ultrasonographic examinations have discovered the signs that indicated fetal anemia in moderate grade: incipient ascites, thickened placenta, incipient pleural or pericardial effusions, etc. But, the Doppler technique is the method that permits the early diagnosis of fetal anemia, prior to the development of hydrops fetalis. This fact is fundamental for avoiding fetal mortality.

The Doppler measurement of the peak systolic velocity of the middle cerebral artery (MCA-PSV) allows prediction of fetal anemia. The reason is that viscosity of blood flow is inversely correlated with the speed of blood flow. When fetal anemia is severe, the viscosity of blood is markedly decreased, and for this reason peak systolic velocity is increased.[3,4]

The measurements should be taken using color Doppler, magnifying the image of the screen, with a zero degree angle of incidence, and in absence of marked fetal body and breathing movements.[4,5]

Usually, when the alloimmunization is diagnosed, it is necessary to permute ultrasonography and Doppler study each week. The proceeding minimizes fetal complications associated with invasive testing.[6]

HYDROPS FETALIS

The hydrops fetalis is a condition characterized by abnormal accumulation of fluid and edema in the fetus.

Usually, hydrops fetalis has been described in cases of Rhesus alloimmunization. It is the so-called "isoimmune" fetal hydrops. On the contrary, if there is no evidence of fetal-maternal group incompatibility, hydrops is considered "nonimmune." Traditionally, isoimmune fetal hydrops has been considered the primary cause. However, the implementation of preventive measures for this condition, has decreased its incidence. For this reason, at present, the ratio between isoimmune and nonimmune hydrops is 9 to 1.

Literature recognizes five pathophysiological mechanisms for nonimmune fetal hydrops; (i) fetal anemia (probably the most frequent cause of hydrops); (ii) venous return obstruction for thoracic masses or pleural effusions; (iii) increased capillary permeability for congenital infections, umbilical cord pathology or placental pathology; (vi) increased capillary pressure for cardiac malformation, structural or functional; and (v) decreased plasma oncotic pressure for increased albumin excretion (or, on the contrary, for decrease albumin formation).

The most used sonographic criteria for diagnosis are: (i) generalized skin thickening (more than =5 mm); (ii) accumulation of serous fluids in serous cavities: ascites, pleural effusion (Figs 11.6A to D), pericardial effusion, etc.; (iii) placental enlargement; and iv) hemodynamics features (Figs 11.7A to D).[7]

After the ultrasound diagnosis of the fetal hydrops, it is necessary to investigate: maternal conditions, possibility of fetal chromosomopathies, of fetal malformations (especially congenital heart diseases), and to study the fetal venous return by means of Doppler.

The list of malformations associated to non-immune fetal hydrops is very extensive, but the most important are: (i) lymphatic defects, as a cystic hygroma (Figs 11.8 A to D); (ii) cranial abnormalities, as an absent corpus callosum; (iii) thorax mass, as a mediastin teratoma; (iv) vascular malformations as a hepatic angioma or umbilical vein thrombosis; (v) gastrointestinal abnormalities, as a meconium peritonitis; (vi) neoplasm, as a sacrococcygeal teratoma; (vii) skeletal dysplasias, as an imperfectostogenesis; (viii) renal dysplasia, or congenital nephrosis; and (ix) very specially structural and functional cardiac defects.[8]

Advances in ultrasound (pulsed Doppler, color Doppler, power Doppler, etc.) have made the diagnosis of these defects possible early in gestation. For this reason, in all cases of fetal hydrops, an echocardiographic study of the good level is necessary.

The investigation of fetal venous return is very important in this field. Today it is possible to investigate the fetal venous return and preload by means of umbilical pressure measurement, or by means of measurement of preload conditions with Doppler. Thanks to the Doppler, one can define the preload conditions, with the help of two indexes: venous pulsatility index and pre-load index, calculated in accordance with the aforesaid three parameters: velocity in ventricular sistole, ventricular diastole and atrial contraction.

Therefore, pathological patterns of the venous return assures the presence of cardiac failure. And this is a very important knowledge to make a realistic prognosis.

But the most important progress in this field is the noninvasive diagnosis of anemia with the use of middle cerebral artery Doppler velocity.[8,9]

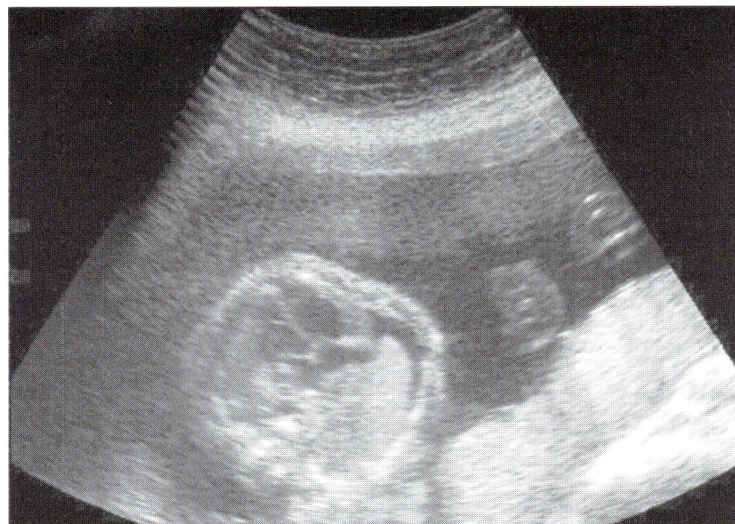
Fig. 11.6A: Idiopathic hydrothorax. The pleural effusions are unilateral

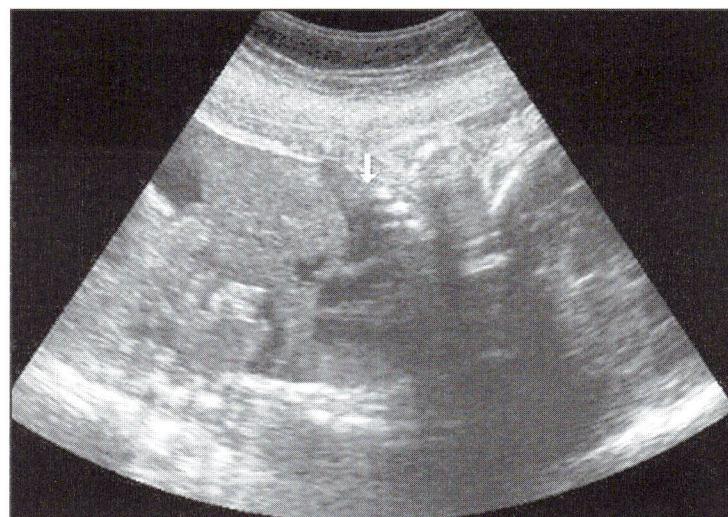
B

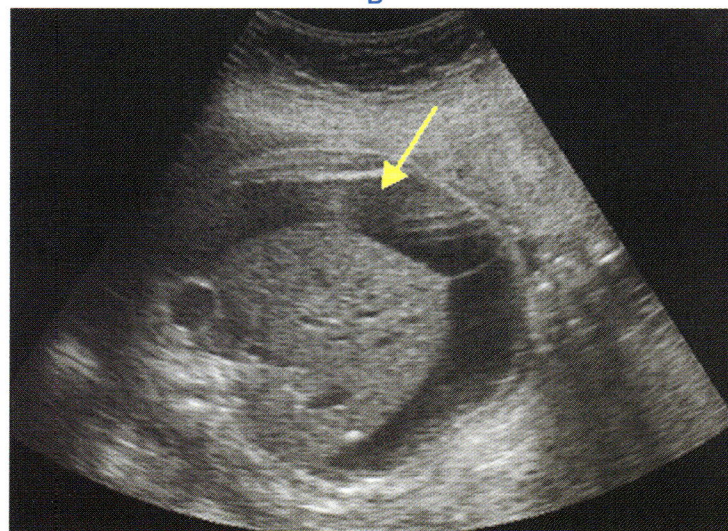
C

Figs 11.6B and C: Hydrops: Ascites hydrothorax

REFERENCES

1. Jacquemard F, Capella-Panlovsky M, Mac Aleere J, Mirlesse V, Daffos F. Aport de l'établissement du pronostic des principales infections foetales. Med Fœtal Echogr Gynecol 1994 ;18 :16-23.
2. Carrera JM, Maeda K, Comas C, Torents M. Diagnosis of intrauterine growth restriction: diagnosis of fetal anomalies. In Carrera JM, Mandruzzato GP, Maeda K (Eds): Ultrasound and fetal growth. Parthenon Publishing: London, 2001, p 35-70.

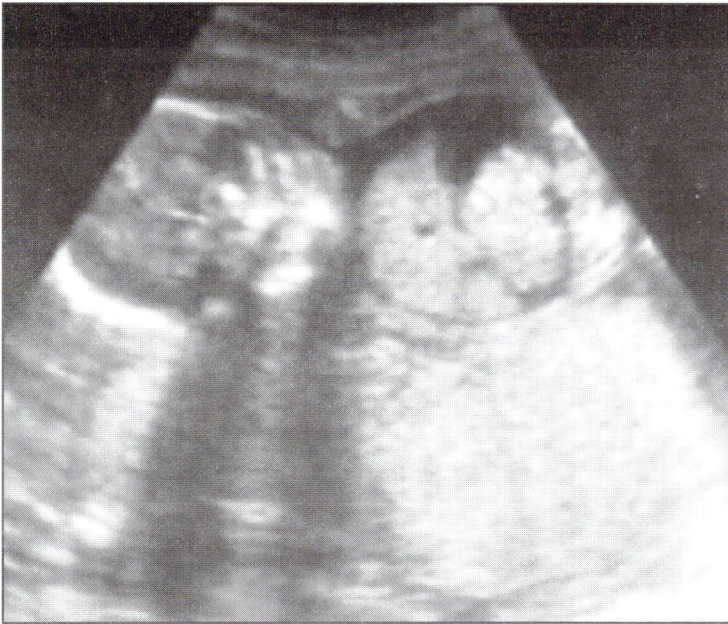

Fig. 11.6D: Hydrops: Congenital parvovirus infection. Longitudinal view shows pleural effusions and ascites

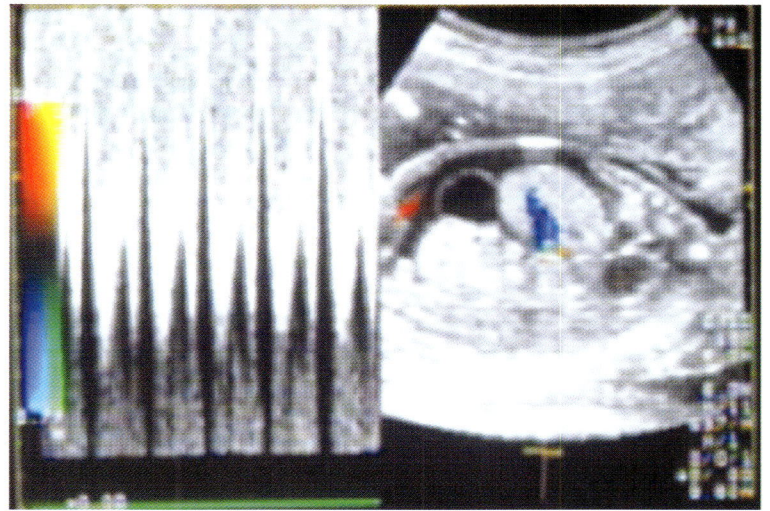

Fig. 11.7C: Nonimmune hydrops. Longitudinal view shows ascites. Doppler shows abnormal ductus venosus wave

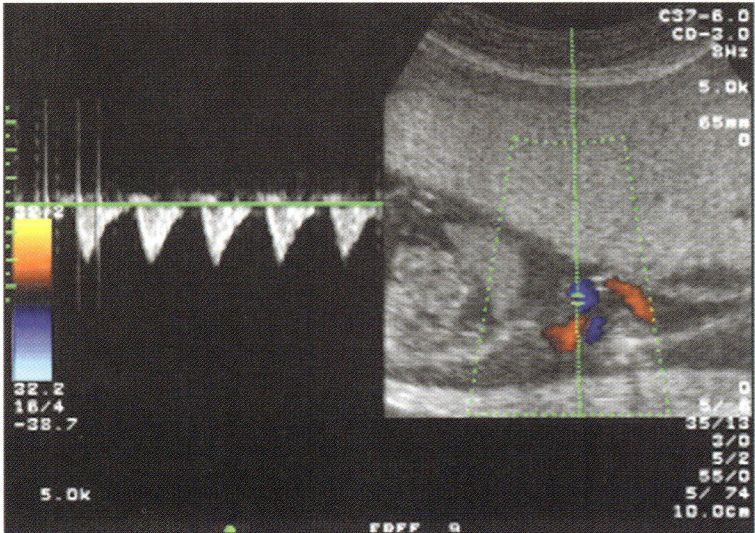

Fig. 11.7A: Hydrops immune (antibody Kell). Umbilical artery, Doppler shows abnormal waveform pattern with reversal wave

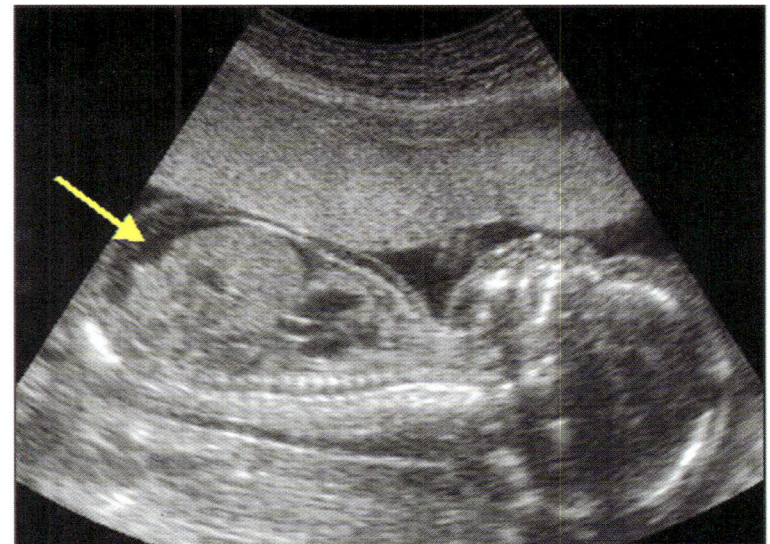

Fig. 11.7D: Hydrops immune (antibody Kell). Longitudinal view shows ascites

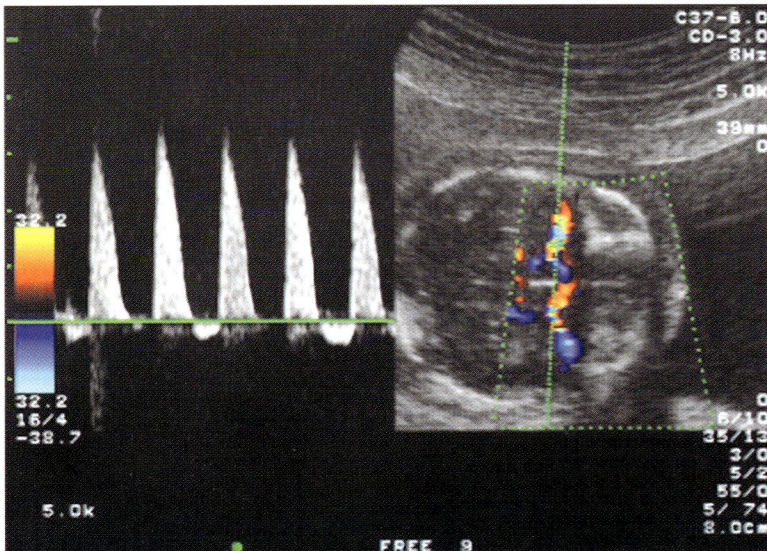

Fig. 11.7B: Hydrops (antibody Kell). Midline cerebral artery. Doppler shows abnormal waveform pattern with reversal wave

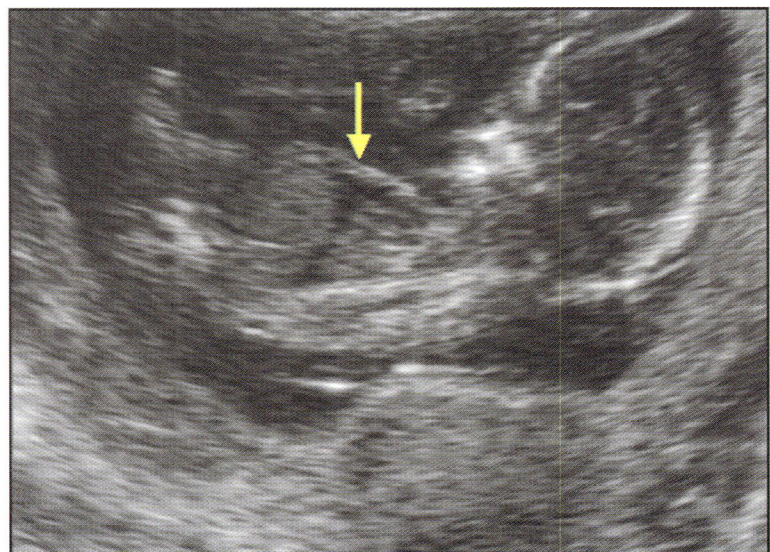

Fig. 11.8A: Cystic hygroma: View for hydrothorax

3. Skupski DW. Ultrasound in the management of the alloimmunized pregnancy. In Kurjak A, Chervenak FA (Eds): Donald School Textbook of Ultrasound in Obstetrics and Gynecology. Jaypee Brothers: New Delhi, 2004; pp 379-85.
4. Whitecar PW, Poise KJ. Sonographic methods to detect fetal anemia in red blood cell alloimmunization. Obst Gynecol Survey 2000;55:240-50.

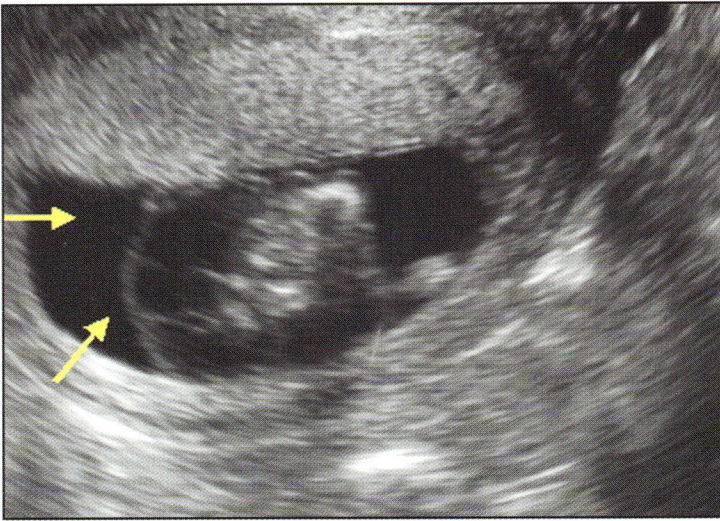

B

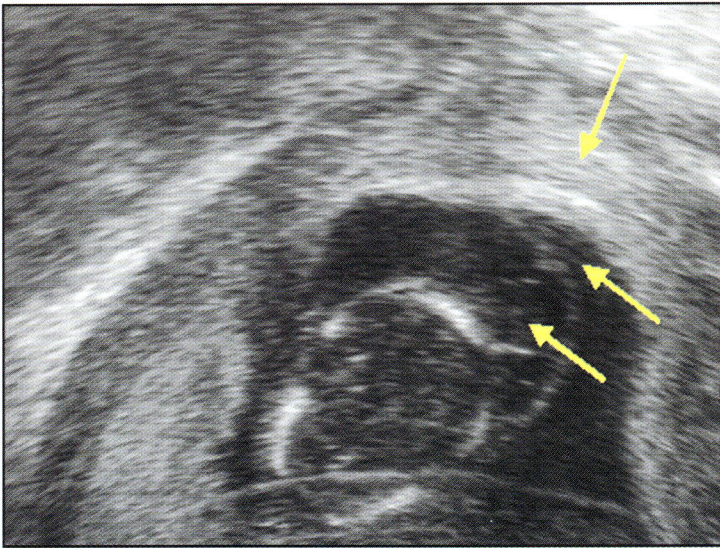

Figs 11.8B and C: Cystic hygroma

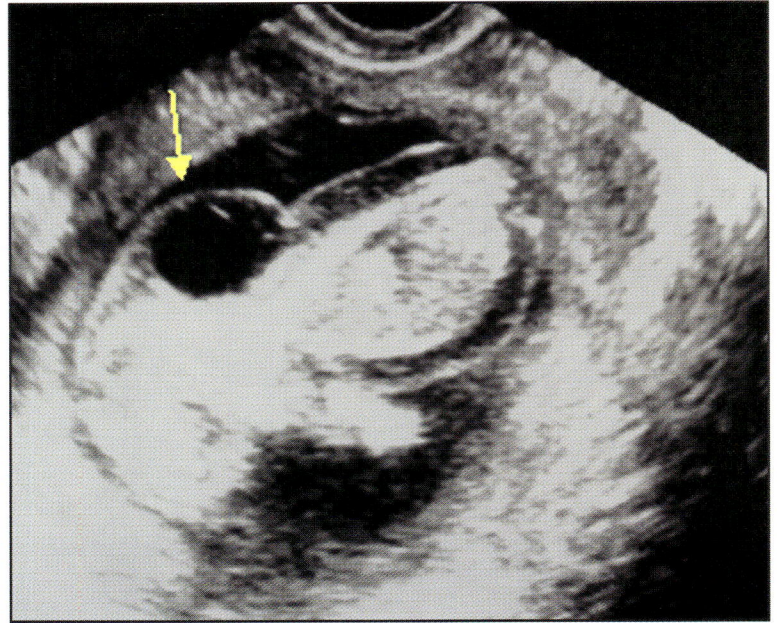

Fig. 11.8D: Longitudinal section of the fetus, showing loculated cystic lesions posteriorly. Lymphedema in the body

5. Divakaran TG, Wangh J, Clark TJ, Khan KS, Whittle MJ, Kilby MD. Noninvasive technique to detect fetal anemia due to red blood cell alloimmunization: a systematic review. Obstet Gynecol 2001;98:509-11.
6. Moise KJ. Management of rhesus alloimmunizationin pregnancy. Obstet Gynecol 2002;100:600-11.
7. Bruner JP, Fleischer AC, Leanty P, Bohem FH. Sonography of nonimmune hydrops fetalis. In Fleischer AC, Manning FA, Jeanty P, Romero R (Eds): Sonography in Obstetrics and Gynecology: Principles and Practice. Appleton and Lange, 1996; p. 565.
8. Abdel-Fattah SA, Soothill PW, Carroll SC, Kyle PM. Noninvasive diagnosis of anemia in hydrops fetalis with the use of middle cerebral artery Doppler velocity. Am J Obstet Gynecol 2001;185:1411-5.
9. Matijevic R. Fetal hydrops. In Kurjak A, Chervenak FA (Eds): Donald School Textbook of Ultrasound in Obstetrics and Gynecology. Jaypee Brothers: New Delhi, 2004; pp 372-78.

P Prats, N Vecek, W Andonotopo, JM Carrera, A Kurjak

12

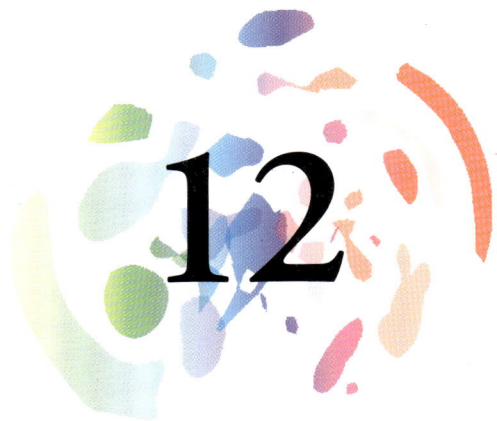

Assessment of Multifetal Pregnancies

INTRODUCTION

The use of Assisted Reproduction Techniques (ART) has resulted in significant increase in the incidence of multiple pregnancies throughout the world. The triplet birth rate in the Netherlands increased from 10/100.000 in 1970 up to 60/100.000 in 1994.[1] Seoud et al reported an incidence of 2.6 percent triplet gestations from ART. Multiple pregnancies are associated with a higher risk of perinatal and neonatal morbidity and mortality. Borlum reported a fetal mortality rate of 64 per 1000 in triplet pregnancies in Denmark.[3]

Two-dimensional sonography (2D) is still the primary modality for diagnosing and evaluating multiple pregnancy. However, 2D sonography can be soon overcome by three-dimensional (3D) sonography. This technique is complementary to 2D sonography and additional information that assists in the clinical management could sometimes be provided. The main disadvantage of 3D sonography is time-consuming procedure and the need for absence of fetal activity what is the precondition for good 3D imaging.[4]

Rapid improvements in the capacity of data processing due to technological breakthroughs in processor engineering is the basis of spatial imaging.[4] Spatial imaging is the main benefit of 3D sonography and it is used for visualization of fetal anatomy in three dimensions. Modern machines are capable of performing spatial imaging in near realtime, called four-dimensional (4D) sonography. 4D in multifetal pregnancies can be used for detection and evaluation of intertwin contacts, because it allows simultaneous visualization of both fetuses and assessment of their motor activity. The main benefits of 4D sonography include: accurate recognition of an isolated motor activity of a single fetus; distinguishing between spontaneous and stimulated motor activity; and spatial visualization of the intertwin area.[4]

Fetal activity such as kicking has been used as a sign of fetal viability from ancient times. It was found that fetal motor activity is present for some period before the mother feels it. Reinold was one of the first to describe fetal activity using ultrasound, stressing the spontaneous character of early prenatal movements.[5] Furthermore, de Vries and colleagues described types of fetal activity according to their onset in singleton pregnancy.[6] These authors were analyzing spontaneous motor activity. Hooker showed that the embryo responds to a stimulus.[7] The embryos used for this purpose originated from pregnancies terminated by hysterectomy. They were maintained in an isotonic bath. The discovery that the fetus responds to a tactile stimulus created a hypothesis that the motor activity of a twin could be either spontaneous or induced by the co-twin. Endogenous activity is the dominant behavioral pattern in singleton pregnancy. Sometimes, the mother's movements such as walking or running can initiate fetal motor activity. On the other hand, in multiples two types of fetal activity are present: endogenous–spontaneous motor activity and motor activity that is a reaction to an exogenous stimulus. This hypothesis was confirmed in vivo by Arabin and colleagues, who reported an embryonic reaction to a tactile stimulus between 8th and 9th weeks of gestation.[8] In more advanced pregnancy, with the use of realtime 2D sonography, according to the part of body, four types of intertwin contacts were recognized (contact with the head, contact with the body, contact with the hand and contact with the leg).[8] According to the speed of initiation and reaction, four combinations of interactions were recognized: slow or fast initiations and slow or fast reactions. Slow initiation was equal to a tactile stimulus, and fast initiation to a kick stimulus.

DIAGNOSIS OF MULTIPLE PREGNANCY BY 2D SONOGRAPHY

The diagnosis of multiple pregnancy (triplets, quadruplets, quintuplets, etc.) with 2D sonography usually requires a long examination period and an experienced ultrasonographer. If one uses transvaginal sonography (TVS), multifetal pregnancies can be diagnosed as early as 5th to 6th weeks of gestation (Figs 12.1 to 12.6). An early diagnosis can be associated with numerous pitfalls. One embryo arises usually from a single gestational sac. However, two embryos arise from a single gestational sac in monozygotic twins. The number of gestational sacs always correlates to the numbers of placentas, and very often to the number of embryos, but not always. Therefore, reliable prediction of the number of embryos on the basis of the number of gestational sacs is not accurate. Even a finding of a gestational sac with a single yolk sac does not exclude monoamniotic (MA) twins. Only one (large or irregular) yolk sac can be seen in MA twin pregnancies.[9] Therefore, until 7th week of gestation when the embryo is recognizable sonographically, reliable counting of the embryos is not possible. Only number of the embryos is important for final diagnosis of the number of multiples.

Three gestational sacs have to be recognized in the case of trichorionic-triamniotic triplets (Fig. 12.5). However, even when two gestational sacs are seen, the diagnosis of triplets is not yet excluded, and the possibility of dichorionic triamniotic triplets (complex chorionicity) should be taken in consideration. Only counting the number of embryos is essential for diagnosis of triplets.

Determination of cardiac activities is another important prognostic factor (Figs 12.7 to 12.19). The chance of delivering twins when two chorionic sacs are seen is 57 percent, but when two cardiac activities (two viable embryos) are present, the chance increases to 87 percent. Similarly the chance of delivering triplets after visualization of three gestational sacs is 20 percent, but with three viable embryos the chance increases to 68 percent.[5] The viability of each embryo can be confirmed using color Doppler imaging of the corresponding fetal circulation (Figs 12.7 to 12.19).

Determination of the Number of Gestational Sacs

Pregnancy number before the 6th week is determined by counting the number of gestational sacs. Using this method, the examiner must aware of what has been characterized as the late-appearing twin phenomenon "undercounting". The late appearance of twins is recognized on the basis of the discrepancy between two sonograms, in which comparison of an initial sonogram, usually obtained at 5.0 to 5.9 weeks, and a subsequent sonogram 6 or more weeks demonstrates more embryos or fetuses than the previously counted gestational sacs. There are two types of undercounting: polyzygotic and monozygotic.

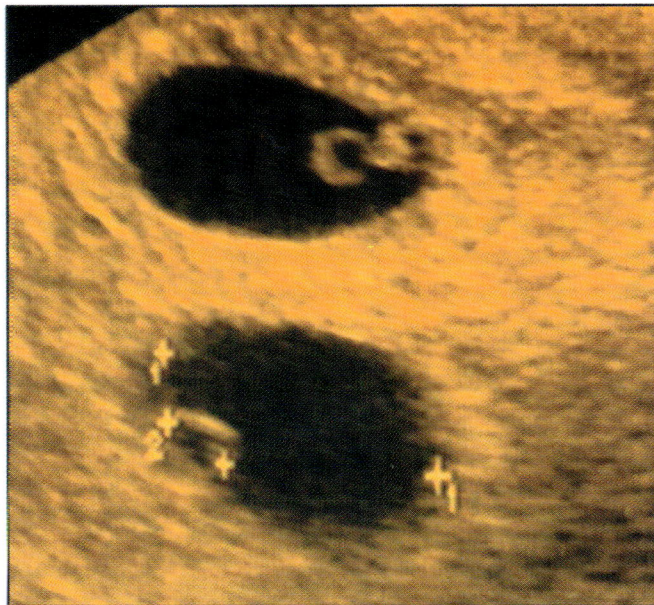

Fig. 12.1: The first visible structure of dizygotic and diamniotic twins. Note the number of gestational sac and the yolk sac

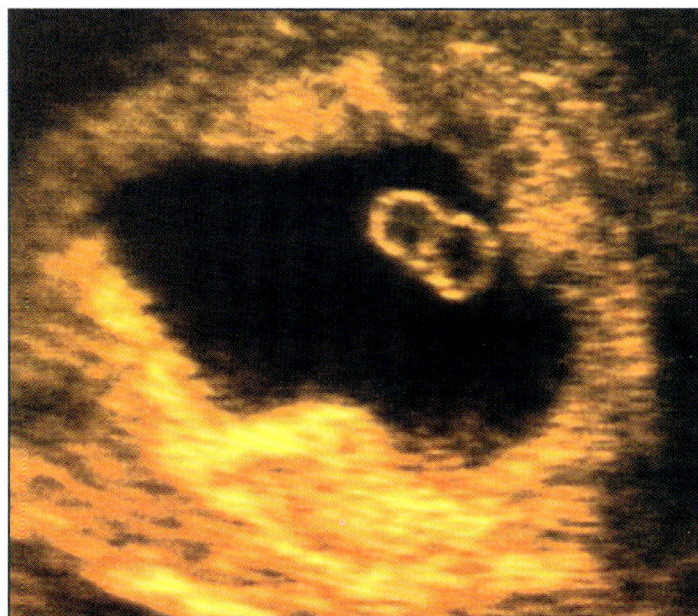

Fig. 12.2: One gestational sac and two yolk sacs fused together are visible in this image

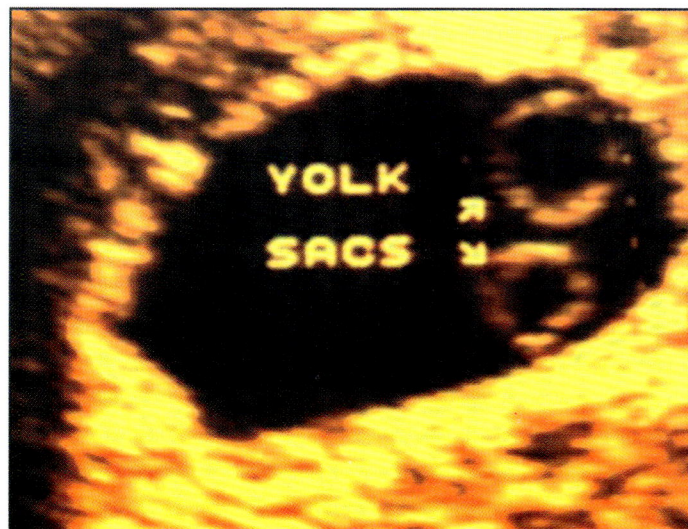

Fig. 12.3: Note the separated yolk sac is demonstrated in early diagnosis of monozygotic twins

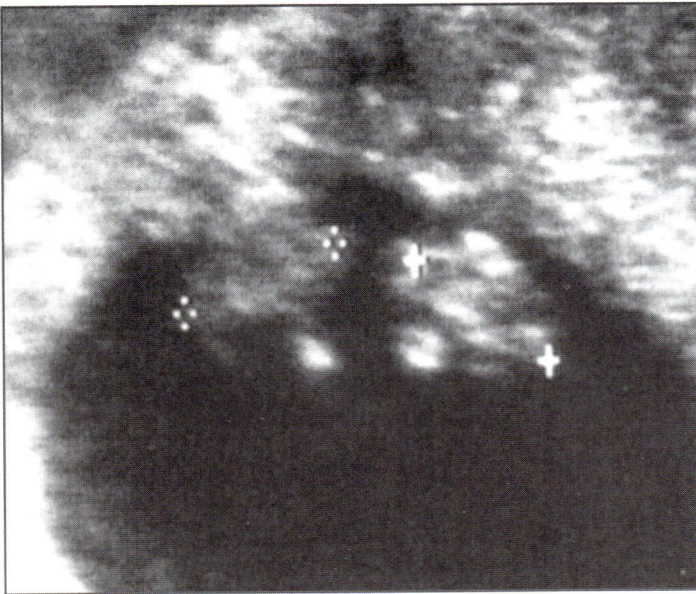

Fig. 12.4: Two embryos are visible in the monozygotic twins pregnancy

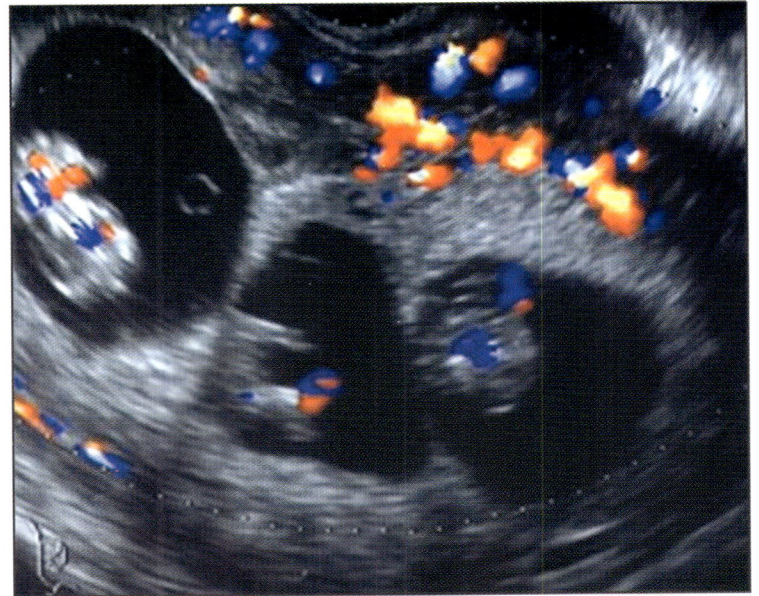

Fig. 12.7: 2D Color Doppler demonstrated live embryos in triplet pregnancy

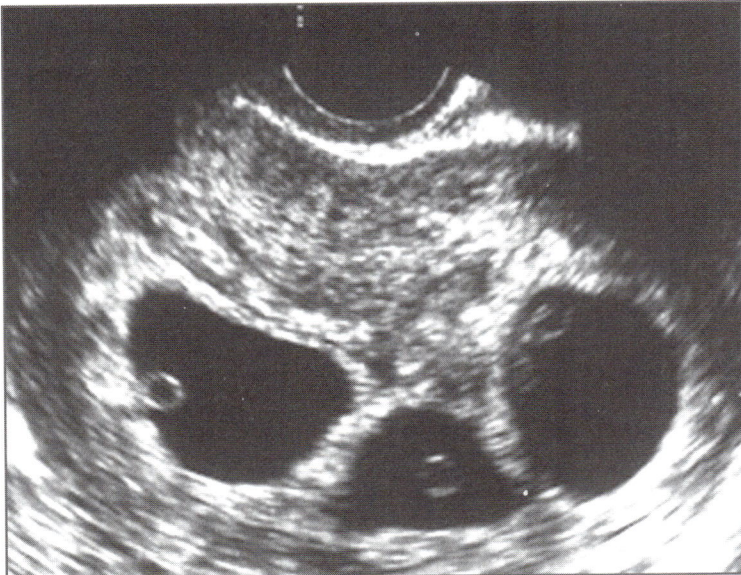

Fig. 12.5: Transvaginal ultrasound of triplets at 6th week of gestation

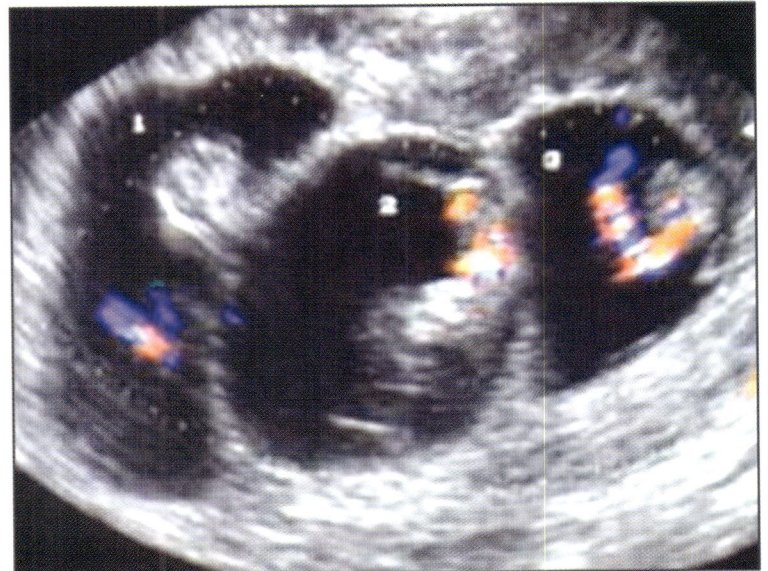

Fig. 12.8: 2D color Doppler demonstrated blood flow depicted from triplet pregnancy

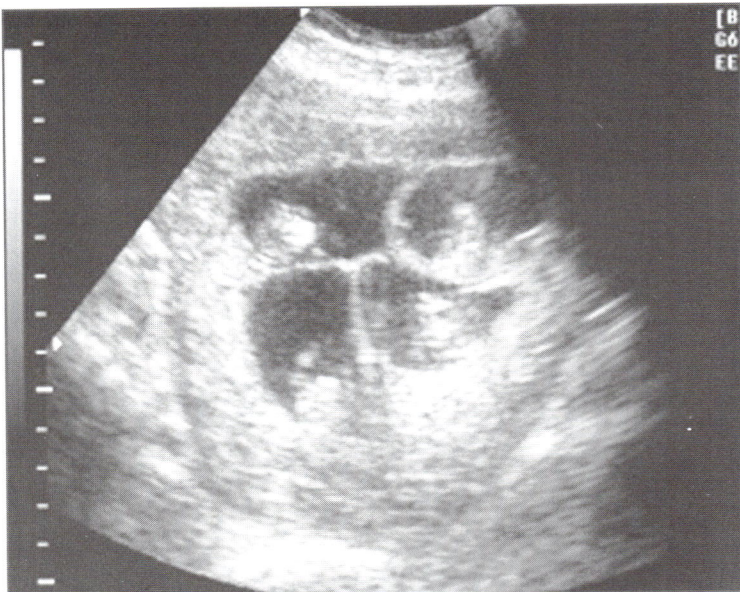

Fig. 12.6: Transvaginal ultrasound of quadruplets at 6th week of gestation. There is a high probability for quadruplets as each gestational sac contains a single yolk sac

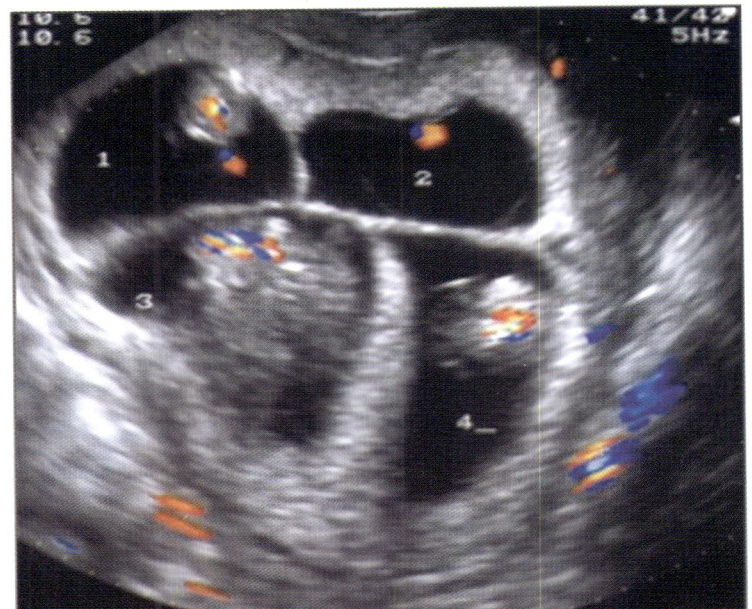

Fig. 12.9: 2D color Doppler imaging of quadruplet pregnancy

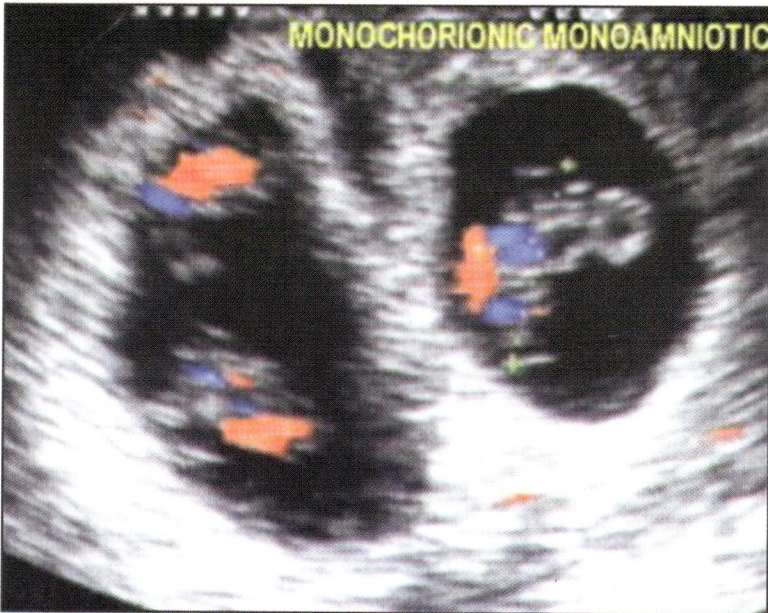

Fig. 12.10: 2D color Doppler scan of a dichorionic triplet pregnancy at 7th week of gestation. Monochorionic twins are visualized on the left side of the scan and show regular cardiac activity. The third embryo is contained within its own chorionic and amnion

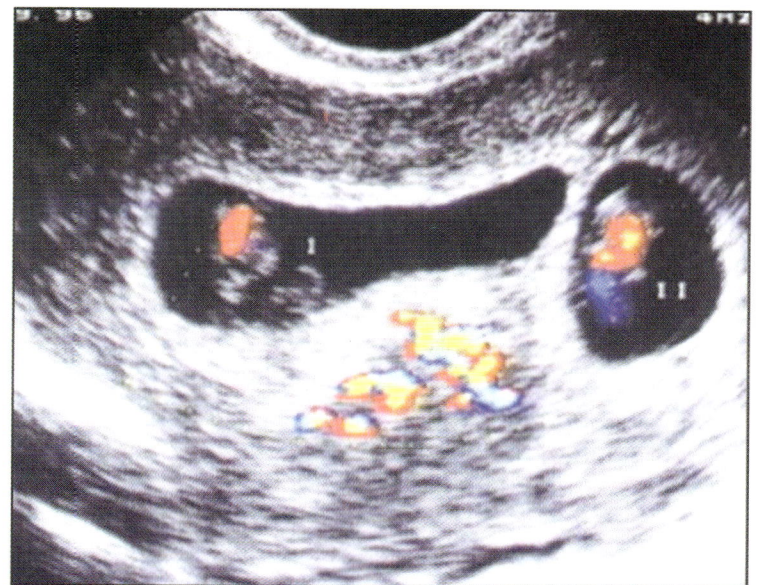

Fig. 12.13: Transvaginal color Doppler scan of dichorionic twins at 7th week of gestation. Each gestational sac contains a single fetus

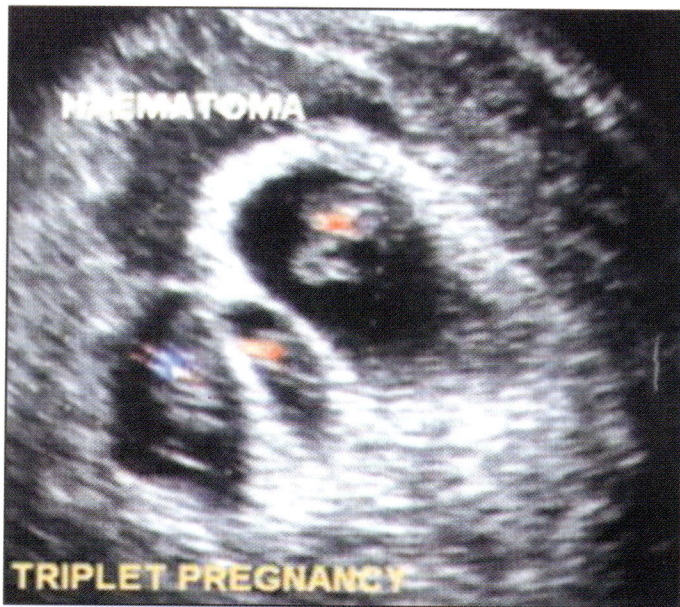

Fig. 12.11: Transvaginal color Doppler scan of triplet prenancy at 7th week of gestation complicated by intrauterine hematoma

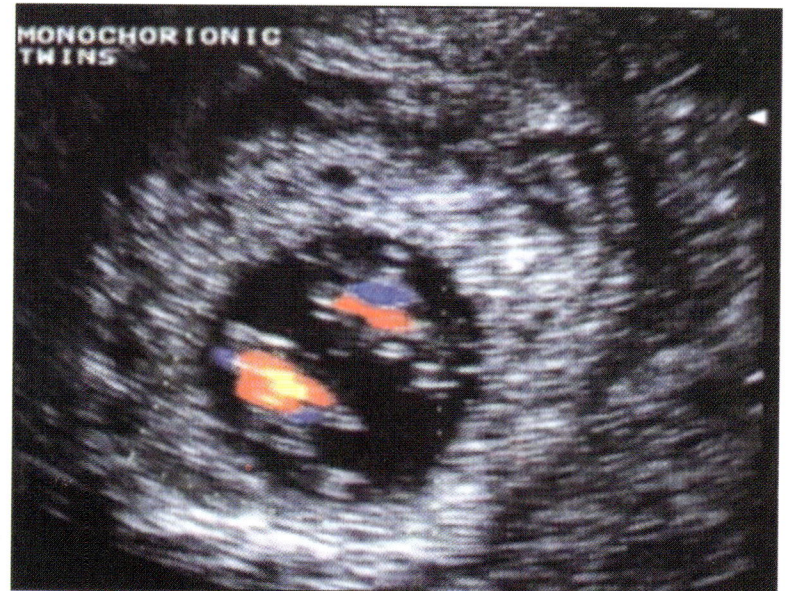

Fig. 12.14: Another case of monochorionic twins at 7th week of gestation demonstrated regular heart activity

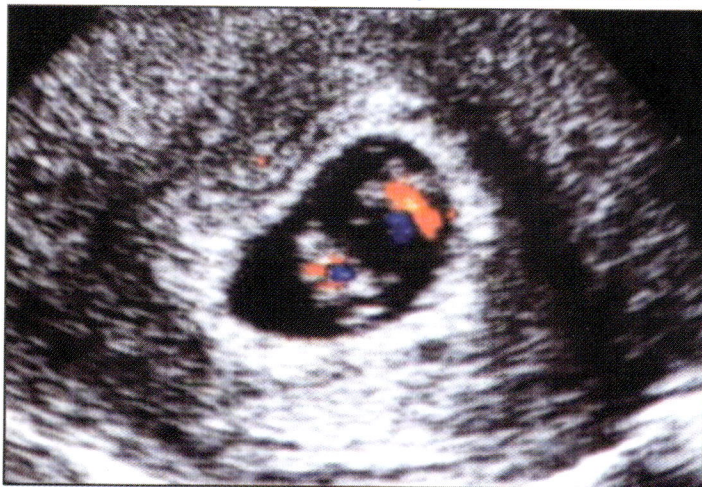

Fig. 12.12: Monochorionic twins at 7th week of gestation. Color signal indicate regular heart activity of both embryos

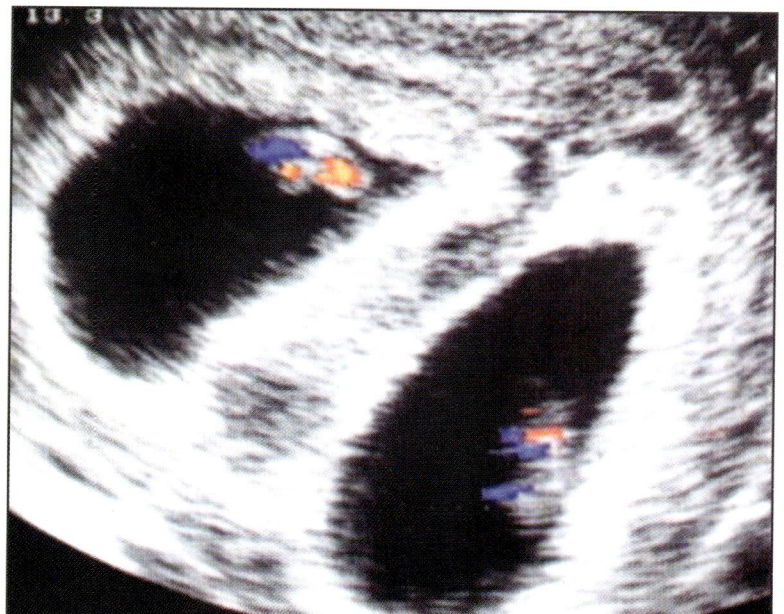

Fig. 12.15: Transvaginal color Doppler scan of dichorionic twins

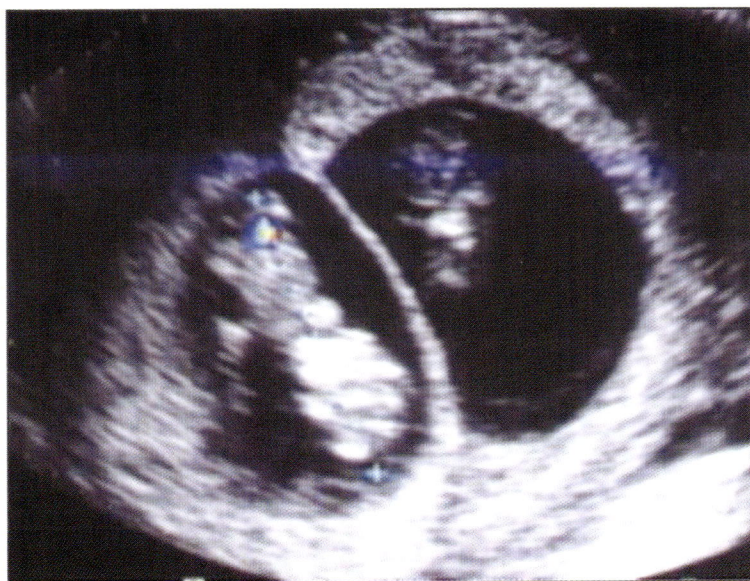

Fig. 12.16: Transvaginal color Doppler scan of dichorionic twins. Color Doppler reveals heart action in only one twin

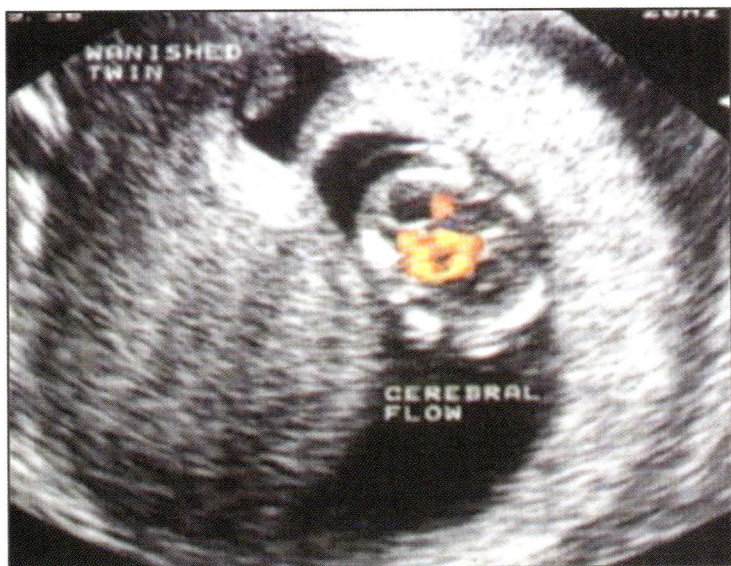

Fig. 12.17: Transvaginal color Doppler scan of a gestational sac at 9th week of gestation. A vanished twin is visualized on the left image

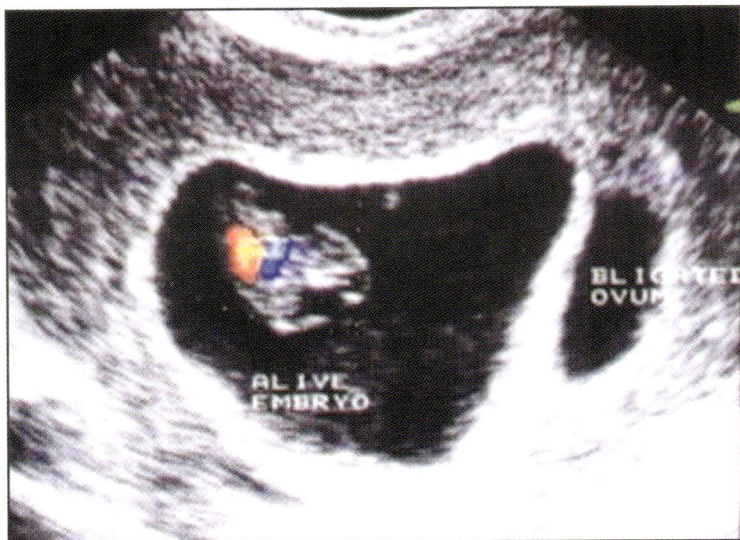

Fig. 12.18: Transvaginal color Doppler scan of twin pregnancy at 8th week of gestation. Note the cardiac activity of the living embryo (left), while the blighted ovum is detected on the right

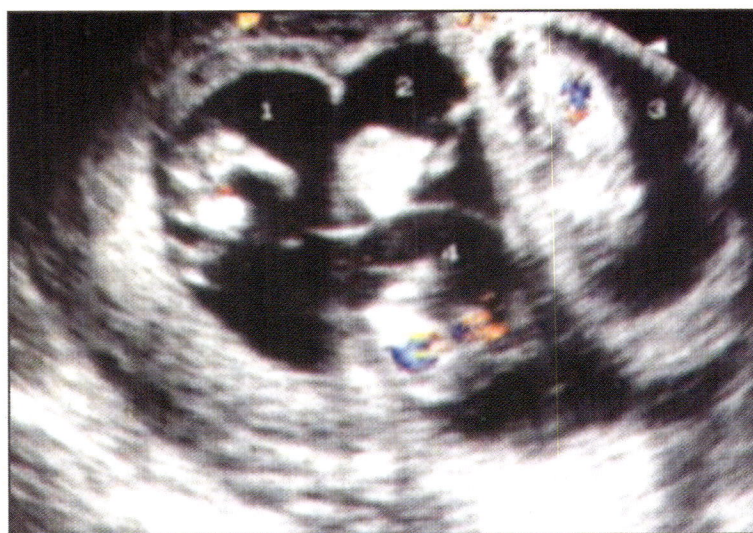

Fig. 12.19: Quadruplet pregnancy at 9th week of gestation. Color Doppler facilitates detection of heart action

Polyzygotic undercounting is a result of the limitations of 2D TVS. The anatomy of the female reproductive tract as well as contemporary probe design limits the number of examination planes to the sagittal and transverse. Because the uterus can only be examined in these two planes, it is possible that an examiner fails to visualize the total number of gestational sacs on a single screen. Stated in other way, one or more gestational sacs may be overlooked. This problem is enhanced in high-order multiple pregnancy in which it is impossible to visualize all gestational sacs on a single screen (Figs 12.20 to 12.29). Therefore, the risk of undercounting is correlated to the number of embryos. Undercounting of the number of gestational sacs is the most common pitfall during the first trimester. This pitfall can be avoided either by conventional or by three-dimensional sonography. How the undercounting phenomenon can be avoided by 2D sonography is illustrated in Figures 12.20 and 12.24. Sometimes detailed 2D examination characterized by slight probe movement can reveal an additional gestational sac.

Chorionicity and Amnionicity Determination

During the first and second trimesters chorionicity can be determined directly and indirectly (Figs 12.30 to 12.41). Direct determination of chorionicity is based on the counting of placentas. This method is easy to perform when the placentas are separated. Unfortunately, in multichorionic pregnancies, fusion of different placentas occurs during the second trimester. Distinguishing between single and fused placenta accomplished by considering of the so-called "twin peak" sign (Figs 12.35 and 12.36). "Twin peak" sign (lambda sign) is a triangular projection of a placental tissue beyond the chorionic surface, extending between the two chorionic layers of the intertwin

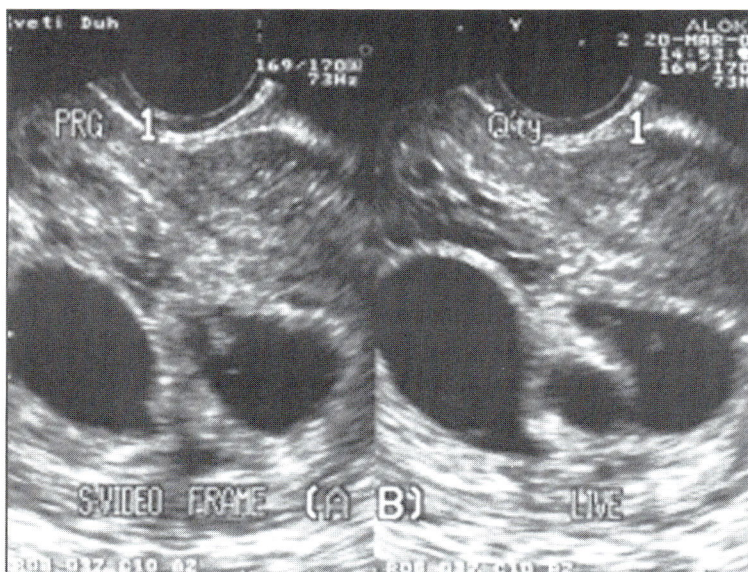

Fig. 12.20: Demonstration of detailed examination of the number of gestational sac using 2D sonography. Note in the left image only two gestational sacs are seen. In the right image, between two gestational sacs, the third appears

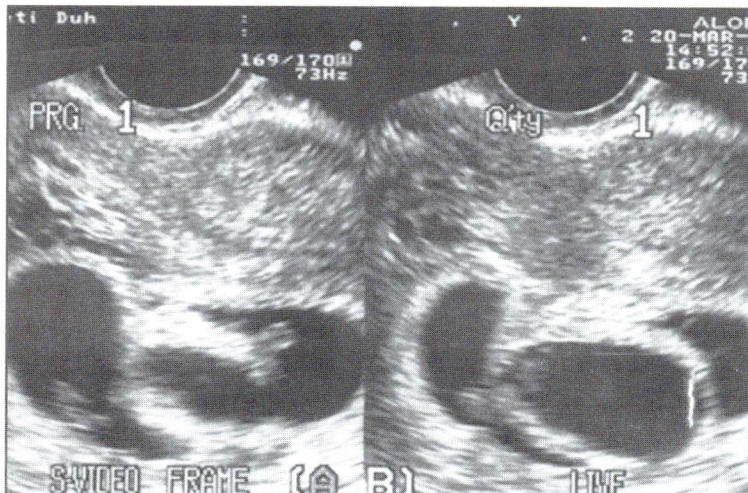

Fig. 12.21: Demonstration of detailed examination of the number of gestational sac. Note in the left image ovoid shape undoubtfully confirms third gestational sac. In the right image, the dimension of third gestational sac is similar to the other two

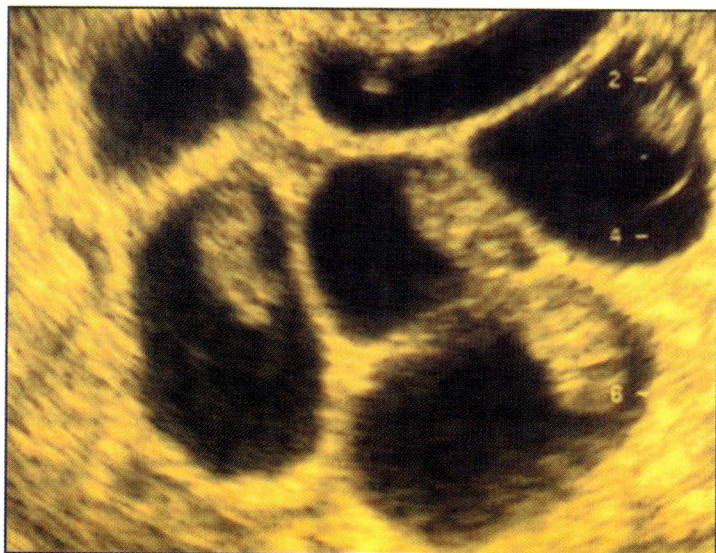

Fig. 12.22: Demonstration of septuplet pregnancy after ovulation induction and in vitro fertilization

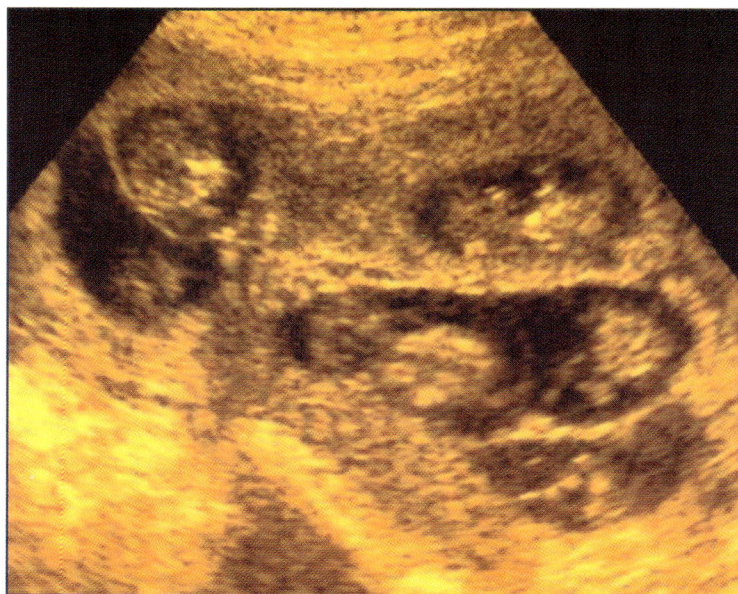

Fig. 12.23: This image demonstrated multiple pregnancy after in vitro fertilization

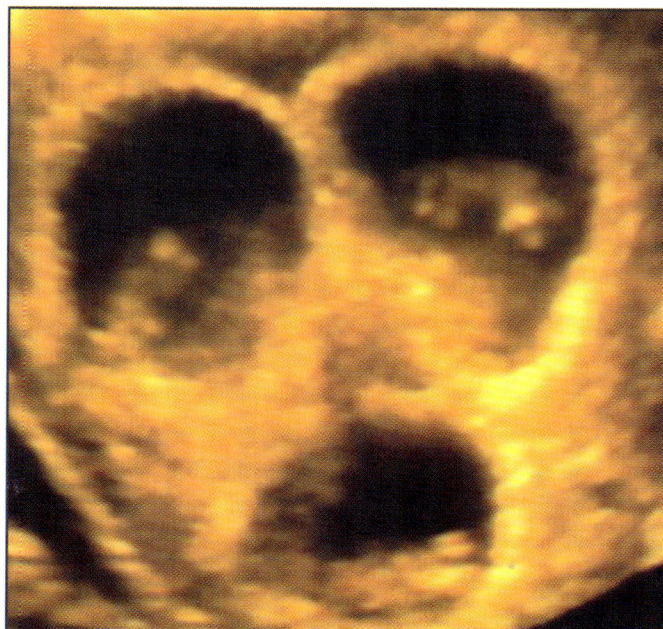

Fig. 12.24: 2D image of triplet pregnancy

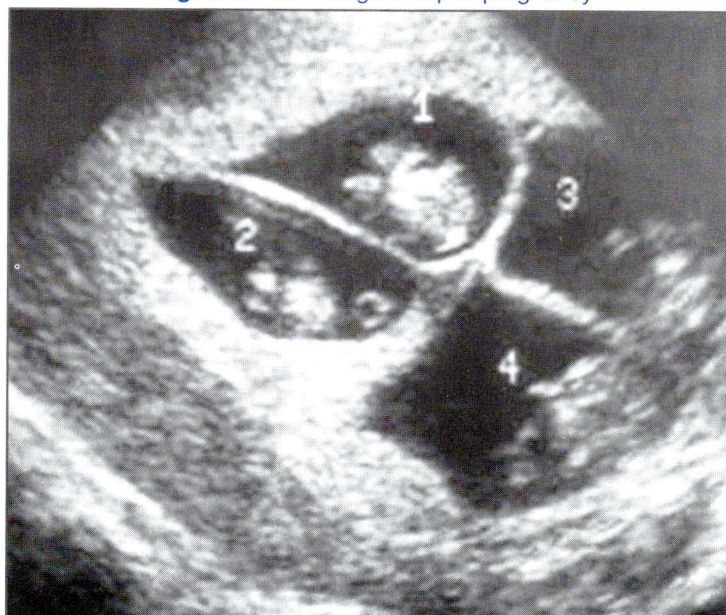

Fig. 12.25: 2D image of quadruplet pregnancy

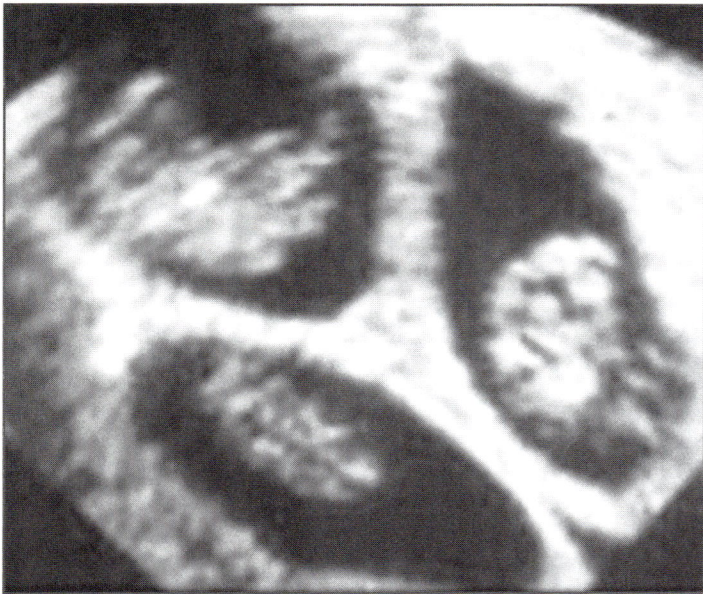
Fig. 12.26: 2D image of triplet pregnancy

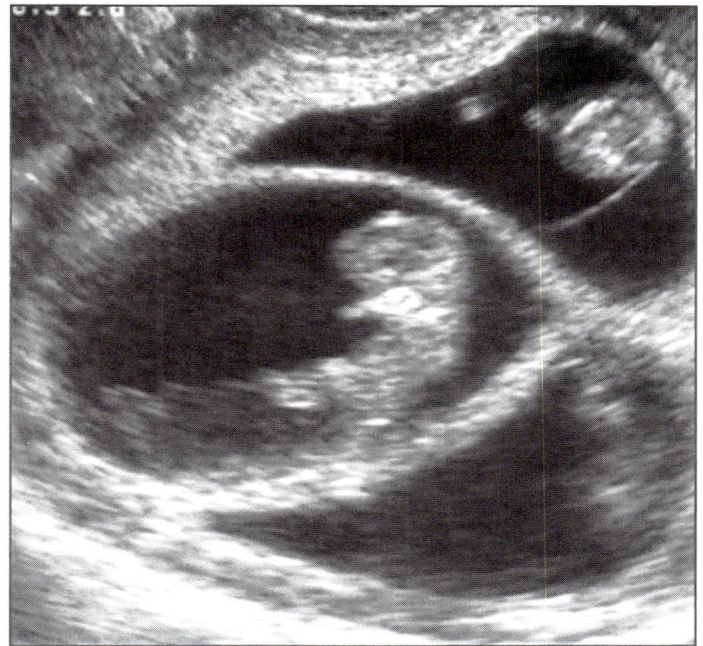
Fig. 12.27: 2D image of quintuplet pregnancy

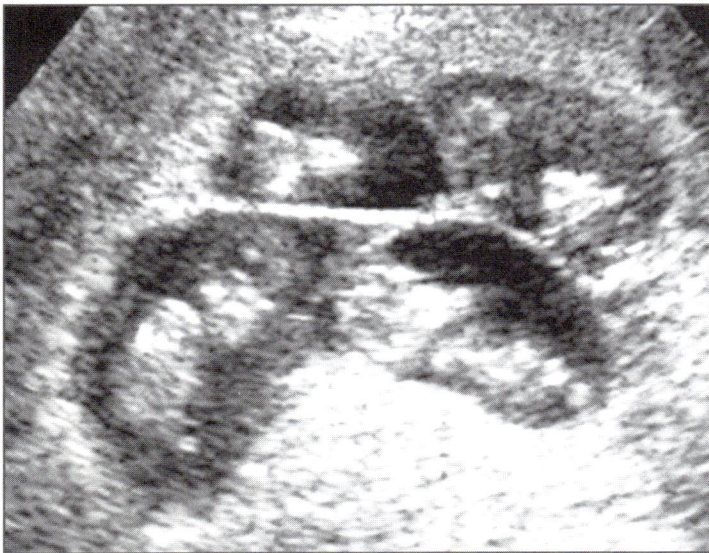
Fig. 12.28: Transvaginal ultrasound of triplets at 8th week of gestation: 3 embryos in three gestational sacs (TCTA-trichorionic-triamniotic triplets)

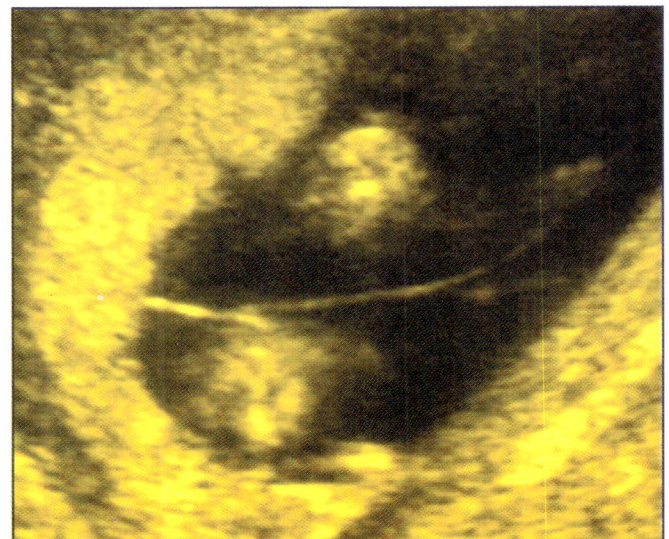
Fig. 12.29: Another case of triplet pregnancy

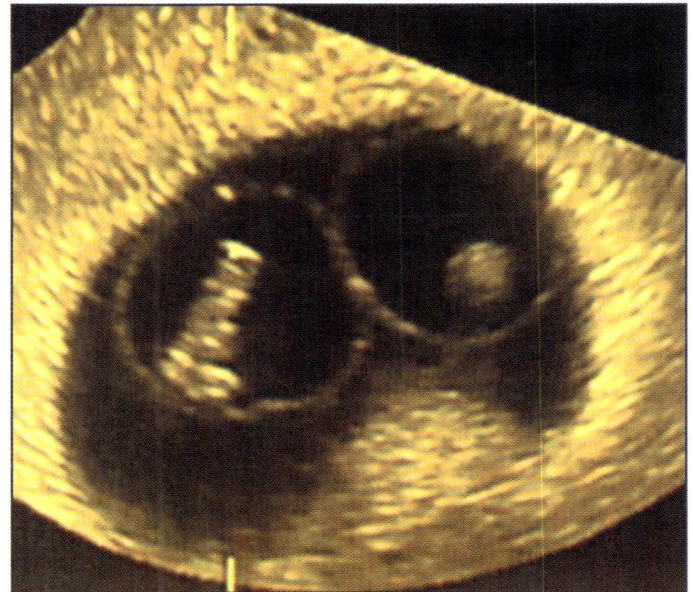
Fig. 12.30: Early diagnosis of the twins demonstrated embryos and amniotic membranes at 7th week of gestation

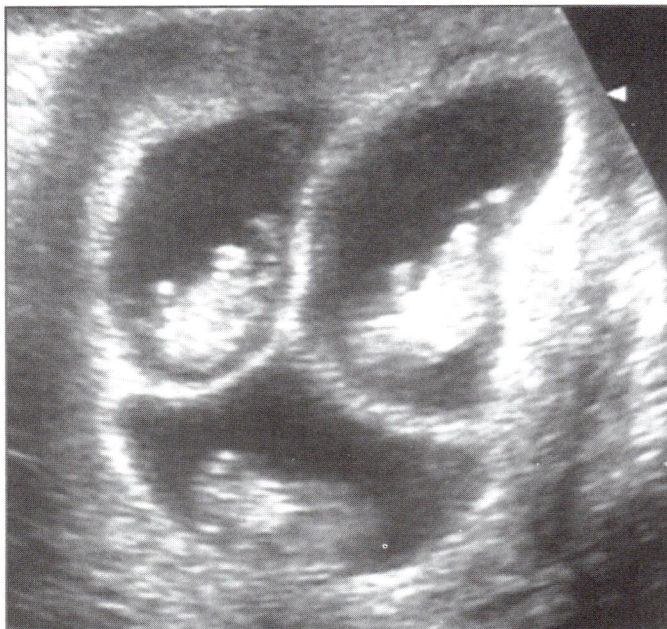
Fig. 12.31: Early diagnosis of the monochorionic-diamniotic twins by 2D transvaginal sonography at 7th week of gestation

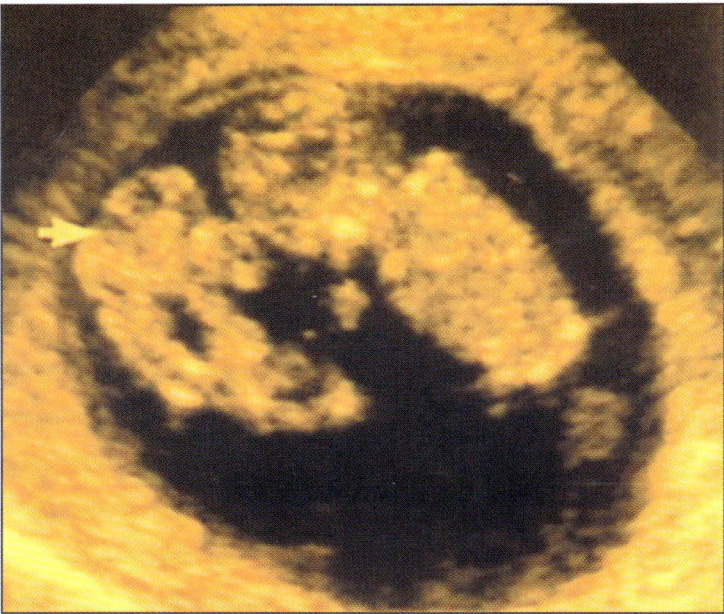

Fig. 12.32: This figure demonstrated early diagnosis of amnionicity. Note the monoamniotic and monochorionic twins pregnancy

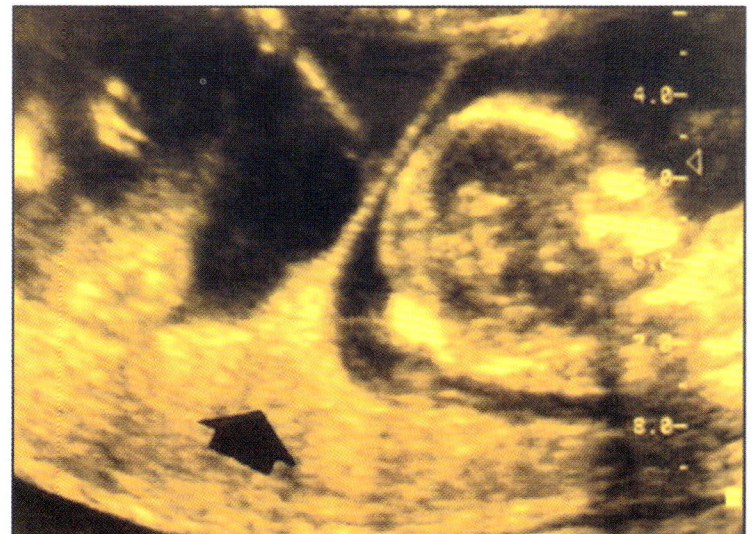

Fig. 12.35: Demonstration of chorionicity and amnionicity in early gestational period

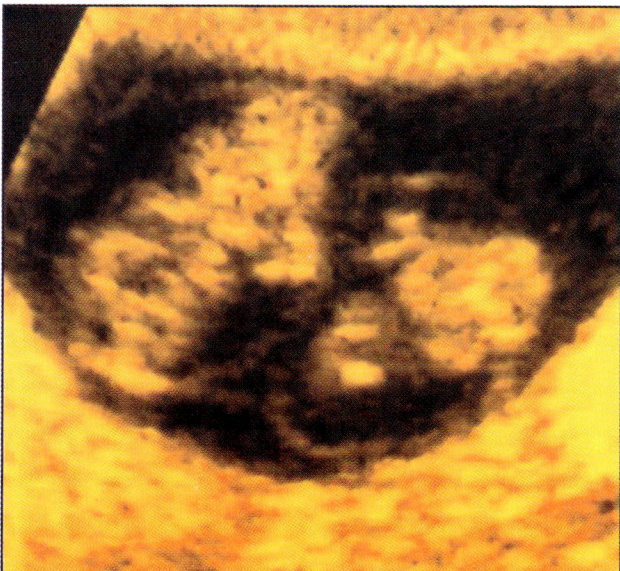

Fig. 12.33: A firm diagnosis of the number of embryos and amniotic membranes demonstrated in this image at 7th week of gestation

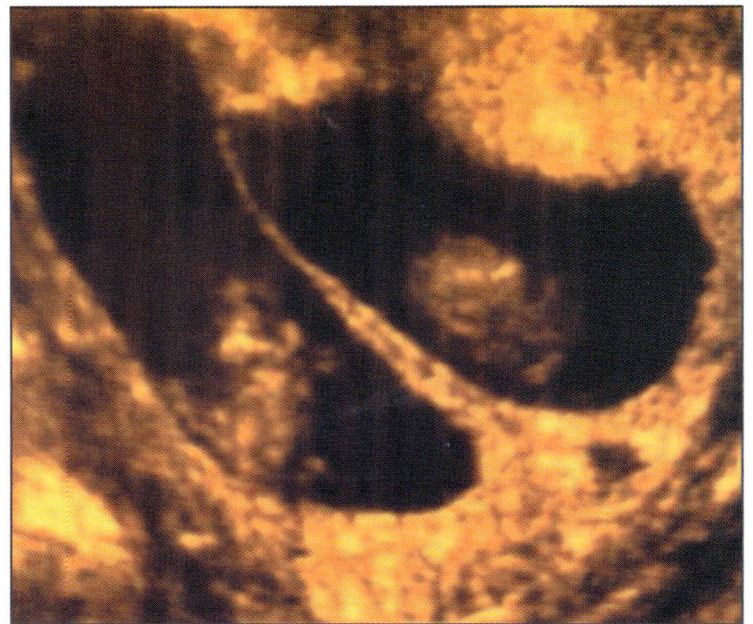

Fig. 12.36: 2D image demonstrated determination of chorionicity and amnionicity. Note the characteristic of the Lambda sign in dichorionic-diamniotic pregnancy

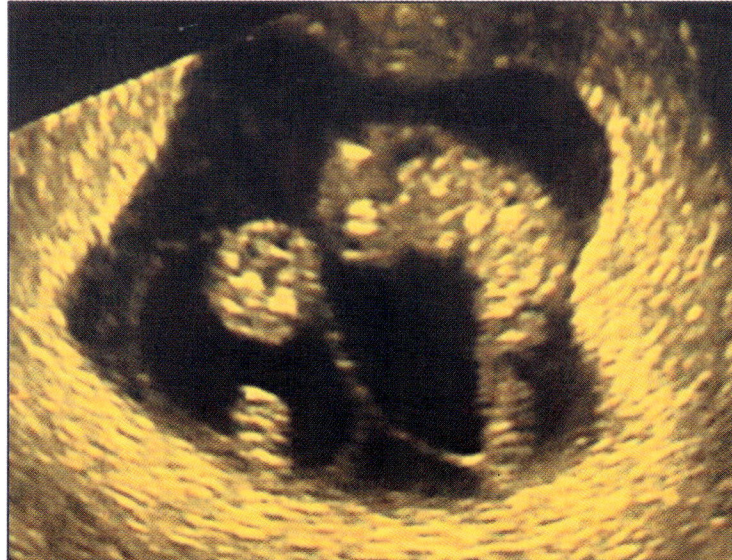

Fig. 12.34: Simultaneous visualization of two embryos and amniotic membranes at 7th week of gestation

membrane. It provides reliable evidence that there are two fused placentas (dichorionic, diamniotic) rather than a single shared placenta (monochorionic, diamniotic) (Fig. 12.37).[10]

The junction of two placentas can be visualized in the early second trimester using high-resolution 2D ultrasonography. When lambda sign is seen, dichorionic pregnancy is diagnosed.

Assessment of the Junction of Interfetal Membranes

The junction of three interfetal membranes represents "Y" zone (Fig. 12.38). Sepulveda and coworkers reported about a complete correlation between the findings at the "Y" zone and transvaginal ultrasonography at 6th and 7th weeks.[11] However, in advanced pregnancy when placentas cannot be seen, then examiner should examine junction between the membranes. The

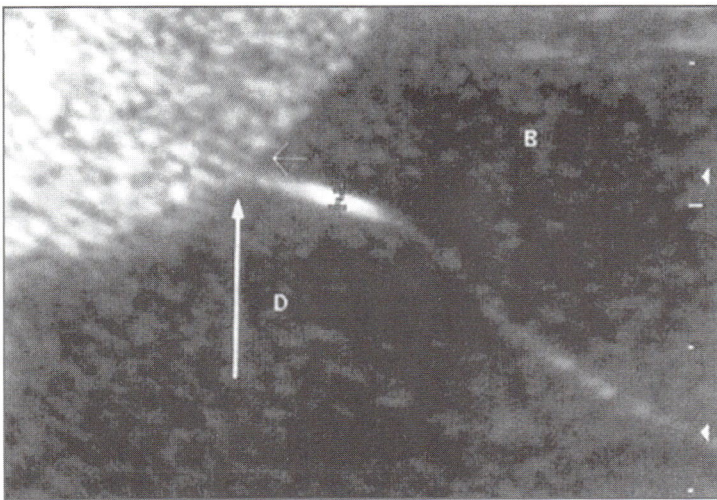

Fig. 12.37: 2D image demonstrated T sign in monochorionic-diamniotic pregnancy

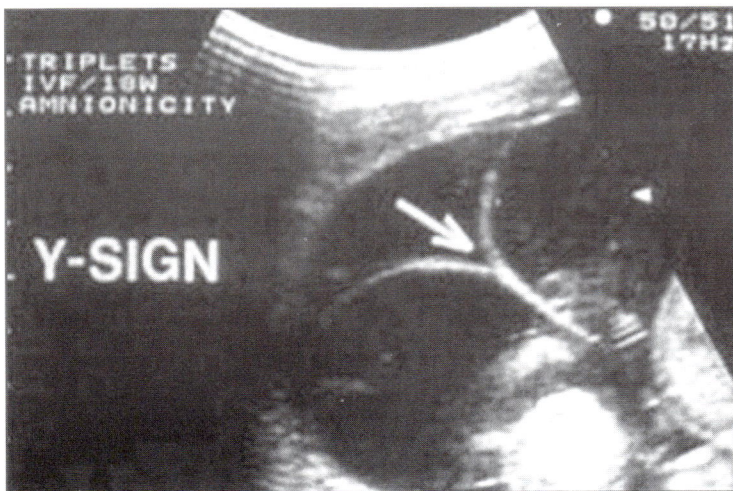

Fig. 12.40: This image demonstrated monoamniotic-monochorionic twins pregnancy at 14th week of gestation

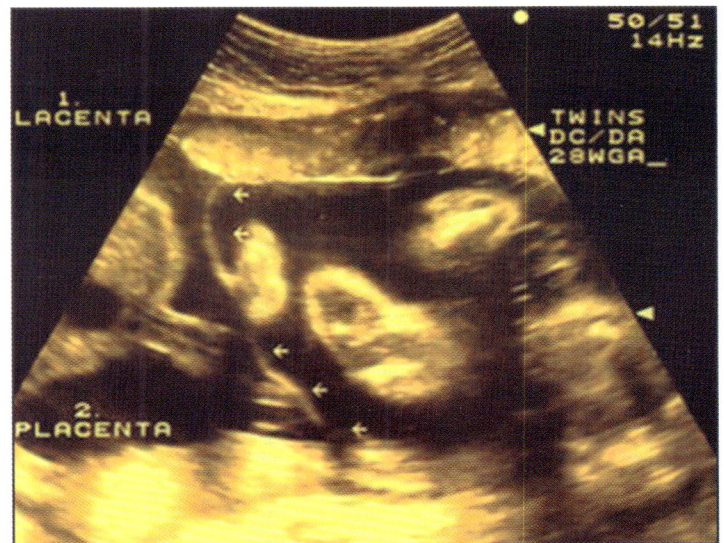

Fig. 12.38: 2D image demonstrated determination of chorionicity and amnionicity. Note the characteristic of the Y sign in triplet pregnancy

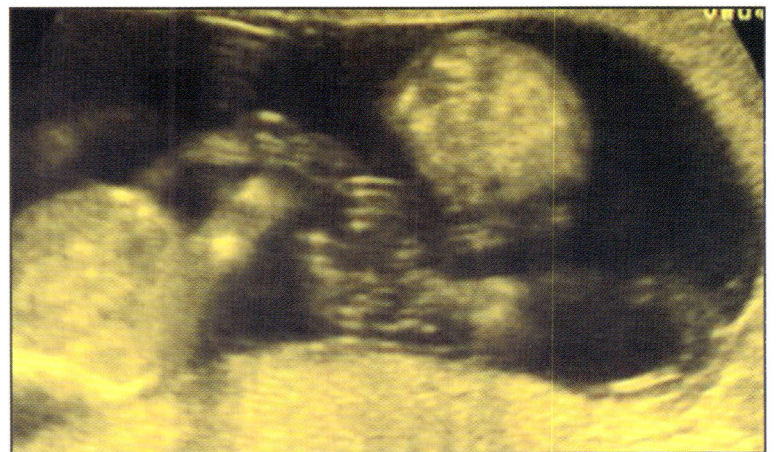

Fig. 12.41: Determination of chorionicity in second trimester. Note two separated placentas and one amniotic membrane

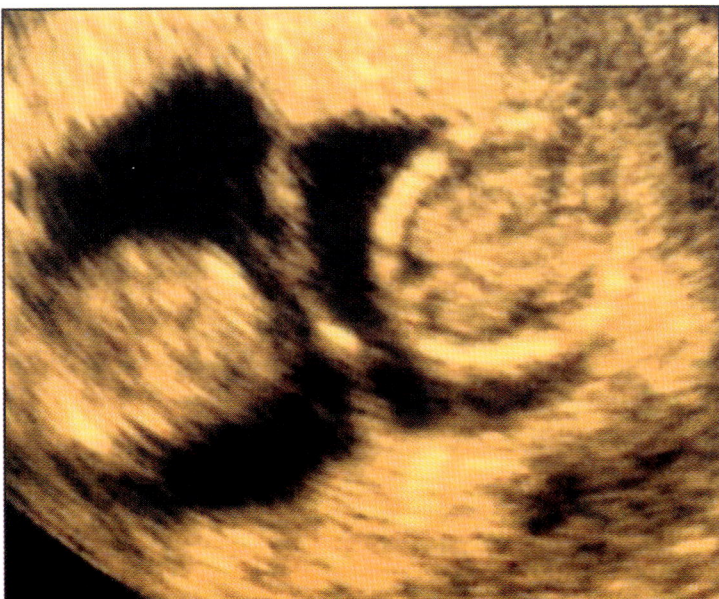

Fig. 12.39: Demonstration of corresponding body parts of two fetuses in dizygotic twins

absence of the "Y" zone does not exclude trichorionic triplets. In second trimester, the "Y" zone can be absent in cases in which the interfetal membranes do not intersect. Therefore, "Y"

zone assessment should be combined with other parameters for determination of chorionicity.[3]

Embryo is recognizable sonographically at 7th week of gestation. Therefore, reliable confirmation of the presence or absence of embryo or embryos within each gestational sac should be then performed (Figs 12.42 to 12.44). An empty gestational sac in high-order pregnancy should be recognized as vanishing phenomenon. The viability of each embryo can be confirmed using color Doppler imaging of circulation (Figs 12.7 to12.19).

Genetic Defects in Multiple Pregnancy

A recent meta-analysis showed that more than 50 percent pregnancies with 3 or more gestational sacs have spontaneous reduction before 12th week. The surviving fetuses weigh less and are born earlier than unreduced pregnancies with the same initial number of fetuses.[12] Whenever spontaneous reduction is suspected in high-order multiple pregnancy on conventional sonographic exam, the additional use of surface rendering mode

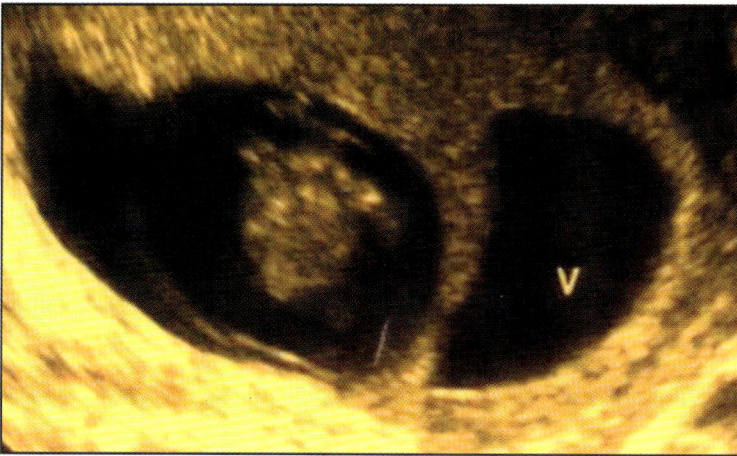

Fig. 12.42: Transvaginal scan of dichorionic twin complicated by a vanished twin (right image)

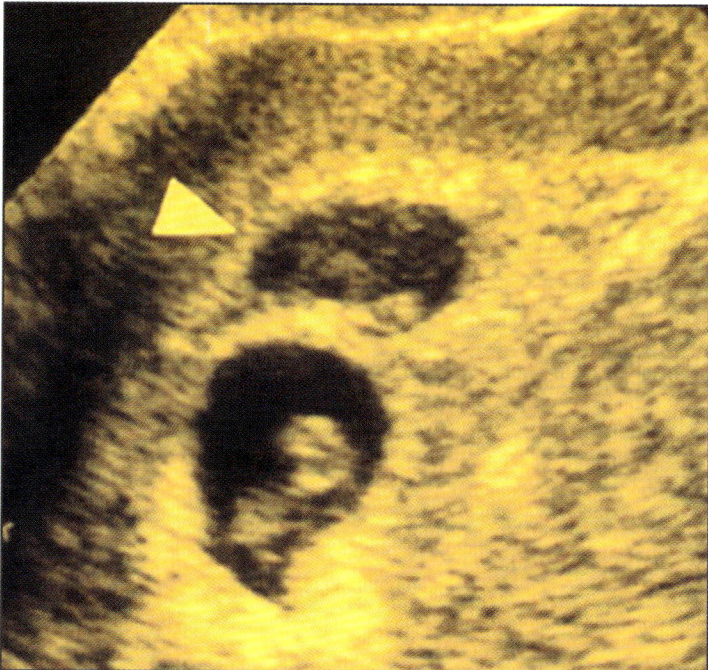

Fig. 12.43: Transvaginal scan of dichorionic twin demonstrated a vanished twin on the upper image

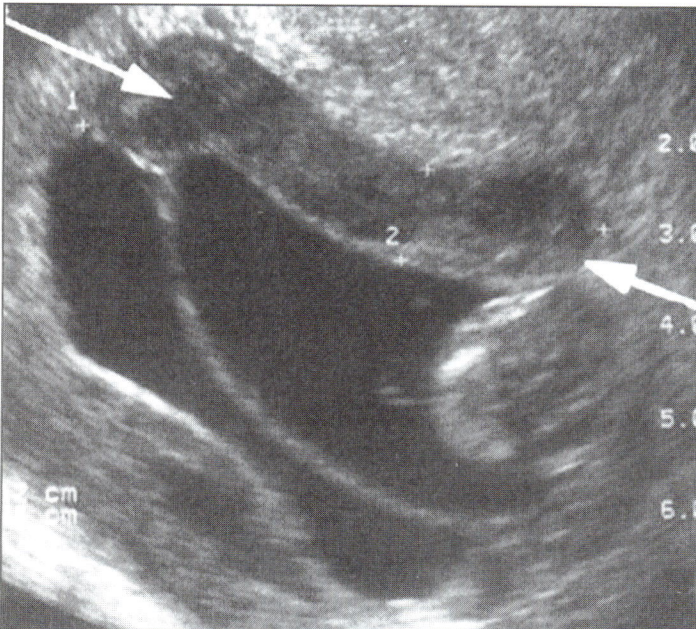

Fig. 12.44: Transvaginal scan of dichorionic-monoamniotic pregnancy complicated by intrauterine hematoma

is recommended. If one uses surface rendering mode, distinguishing between the spontaneous reduction and normal pregnancy in high-order pregnancy can be easily done.

Congenital defects are classified into two main groups:

1. Those unique to twinning such as twin to twin transfusion syndrome, conjoined twins, acardia and fetus in fetu (Figs 12.45 to 12.54).
2. Those not unique to twinning but more common in twins, such as anencephalus, hydrocephalus and congenital heart disease.

The knowledge of sonoembryology enables diagnosis of fetal anomalies in the first trimester. Three-dimensional sonography is useful to recognize the surface morphology of embryos and early fetuses.[13] Maggio and colleagues reported about the first-trimester ultrasonic diagnosis of conjoined twins.[14] Since then several cases confirmed useness of proposed diagnostic criteria.[15-17] The great progress concerning the time of diagnosis-embryonic and early fetal period is achieved, however it seems that delineating of organ sharing cannot be properly done before the second trimester. Moreover, examiner must be aware that following criteria proposed by Maggio are sometimes problematic because two cases of false-positive diagnosis of conjoined twins are reported.[18,19]

Unfortunately, two-dimensional transvaginal sonography limits the number of examination planes to sagittal and transverse. Because the uterus can only be examined in these two planes, it is possible that examiner fails to visualize the coronal section through fetus. Stated another way, a conjoined twin are overlooked.

This problem can be solved using both modalities of the 3D sonography, multiplanar view and surface rendering view. Using the multiplanar imaging the visualization rate of coronal section through fetus is 100 percent, due to unlimited number of section which can be generated by data manipulation.

Maymon and colleagues reported that in a case of conjoined twins at 10th week of gestation, the exact area could be successfully identified by transvaginal 3D ultrasound.[20] We diagnosed this anomaly at 11th weeks of amenorrhea in a fetus of 27 mm in maximum length, showing two separated heads with twins joined at level of the thorax (Figs 12.46 to 12.50). The fetal orientation remained unchanged despite manipulation of with transvaginal probe and prolonged scanning by multiple sonographers.

3D SONOGRAPHY IN THE ASSESSMENT OF MULTIPLE PREGNANCIES

Three-dimensional sonography provides completely new modality of sonographic scanning including coronal section imaging (Figs 12.55 and 12.56), 3D reconstruction and

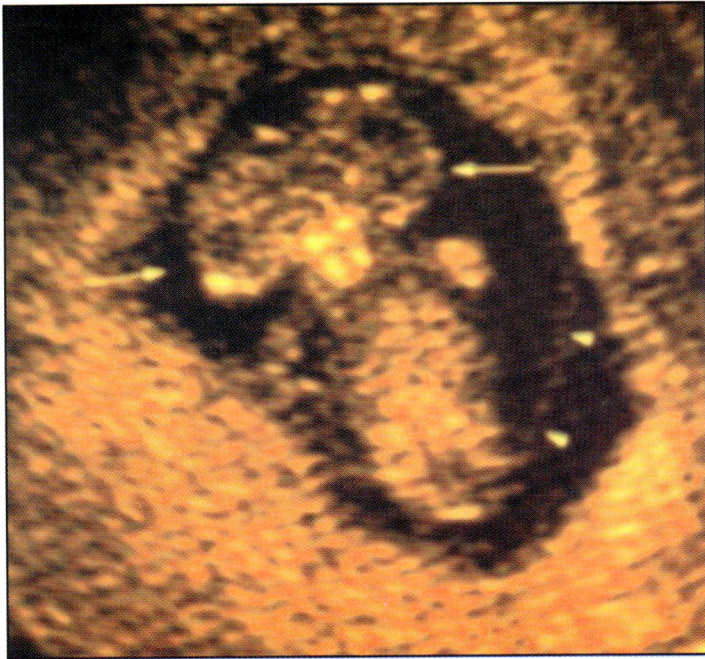

Fig. 12.45: Early detection using 2D ultrasound in diagnosing conjoined twin

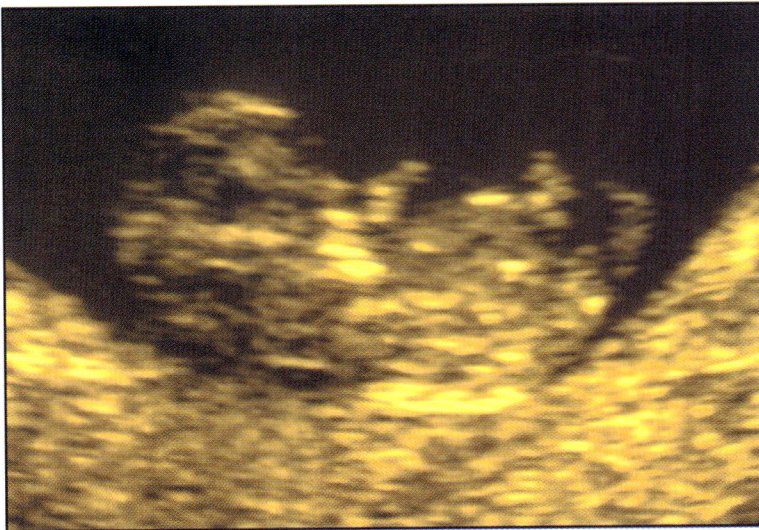

Fig. 12.46: 2D longitudinal sectional imaging demonstrated thoracophagus fetus

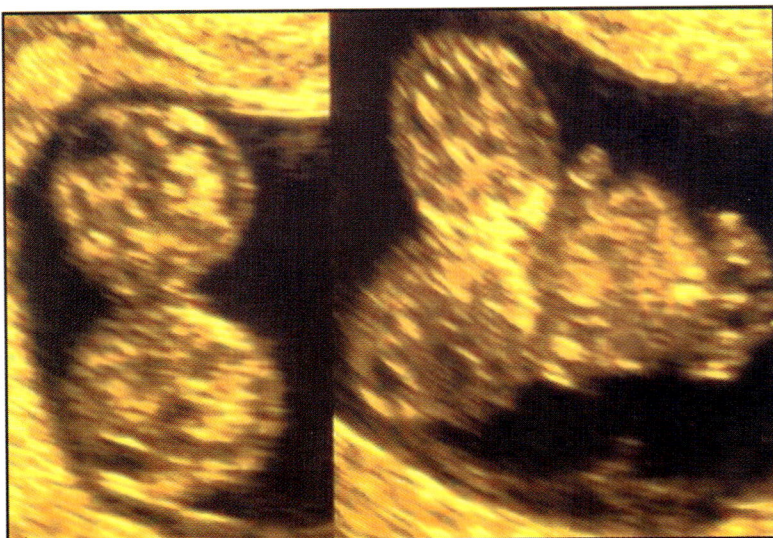

Fig. 12.47: 2D images illustrate thoracophagus fetus with double head in conjoined twin

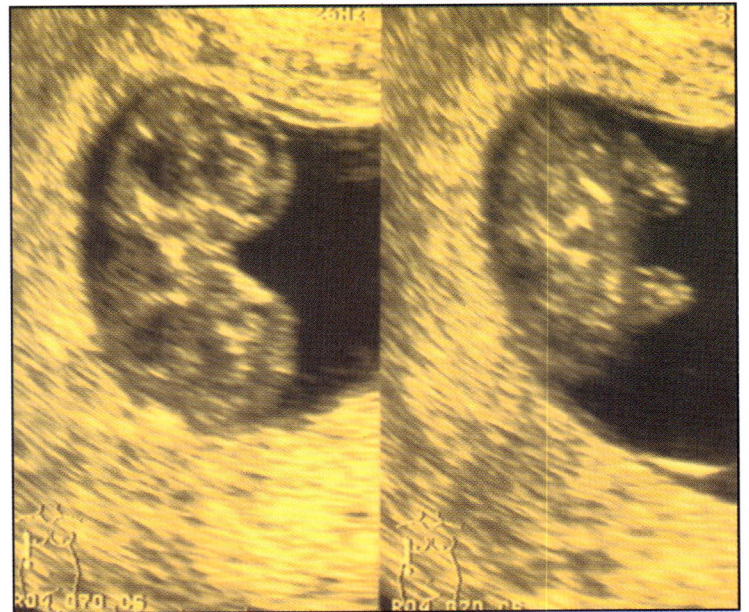

Fig. 12.48: Another 2D images illustrated conjoined twin

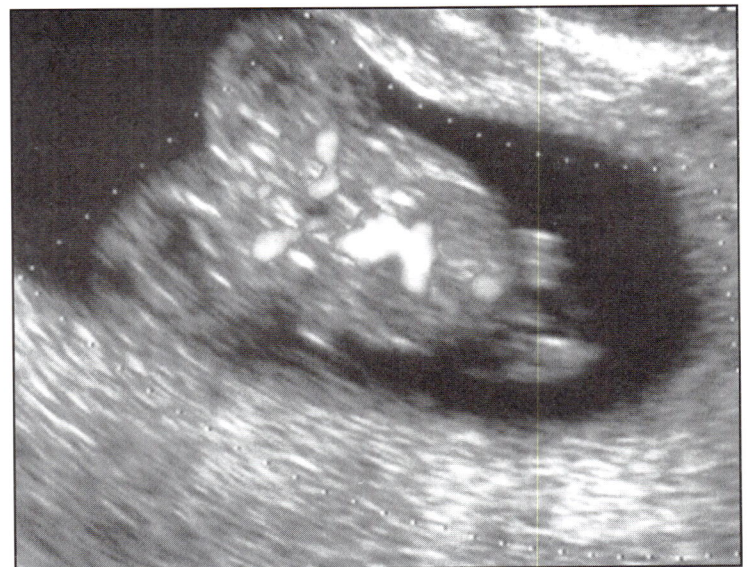

Fig. 12.49: 2D power Doppler image demonstrated single shared circulation in conjoined twin

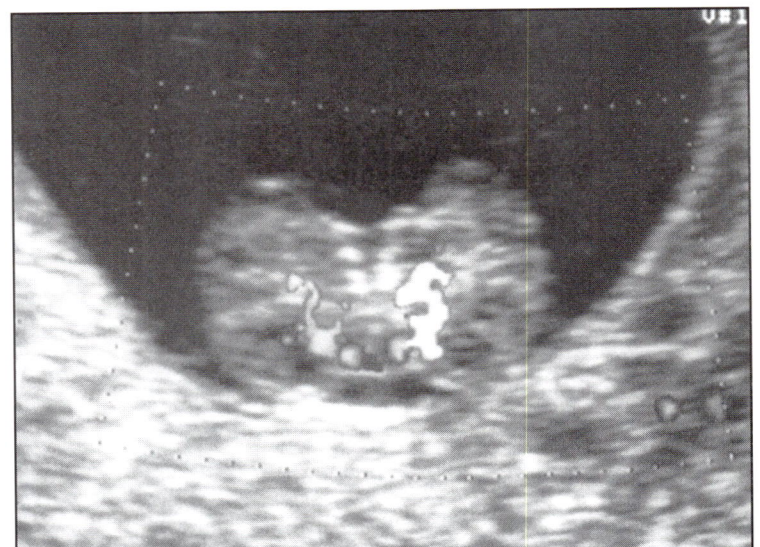

Fig. 12.50: 2D power Doppler image demonstrated circulation in thoracophagus fetus

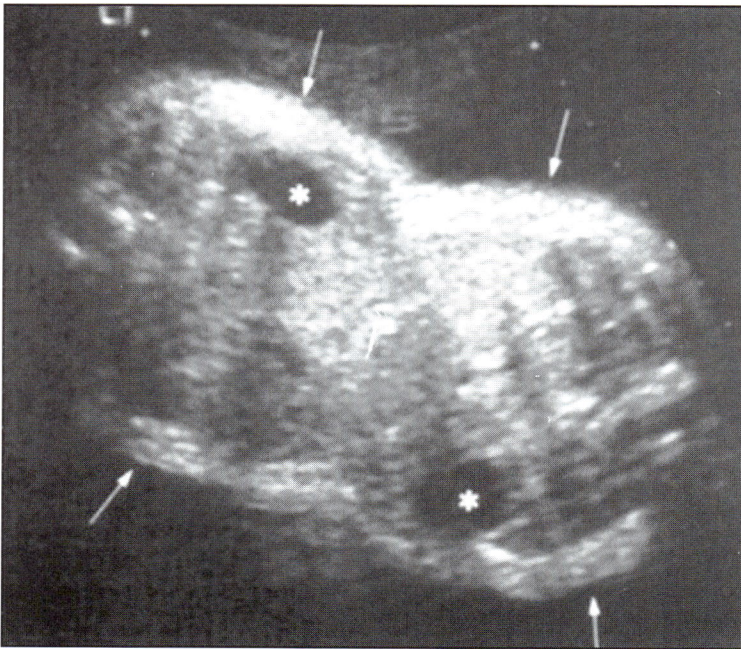

Fig. 12.51: Another case of conjoined twins demonstrated thoraco-omphalophagus

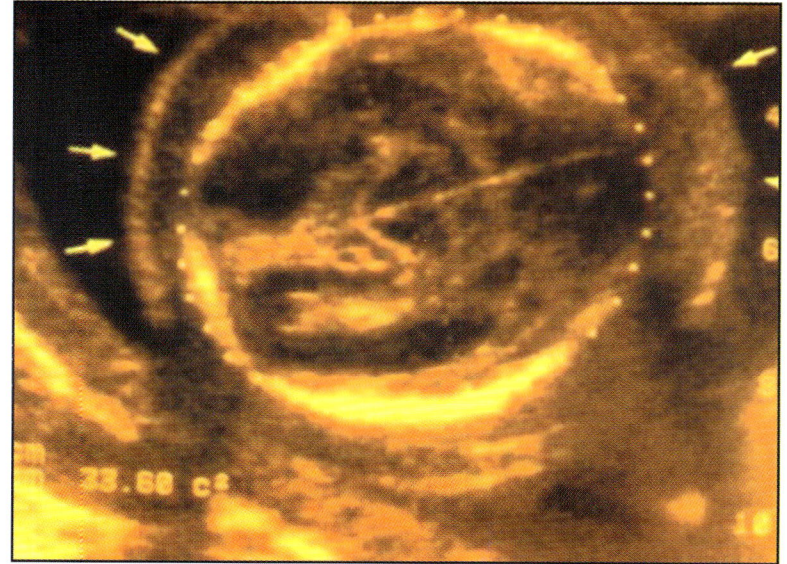

Fig. 12.52: Color Doppler demonstrated blood flow from single shared umbilical cord in thoraco-omphalophagus fetus

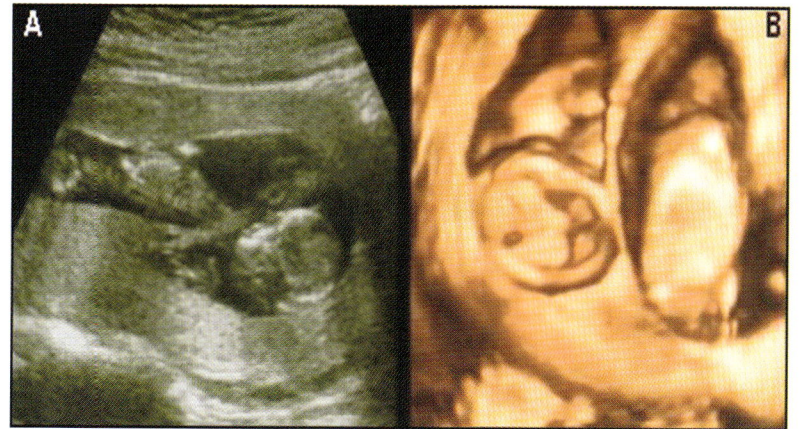

Fig. 12.53: 2D image demonstrated ascites in twin-to-twin transfusion syndrome

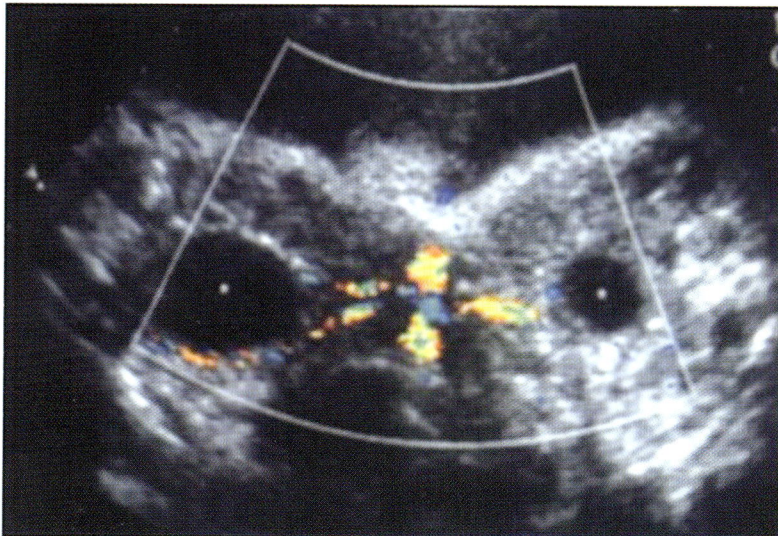

Fig. 12.54: 2D ultrasound image demonstrated scalp edema in twin to twin transfusion syndrome

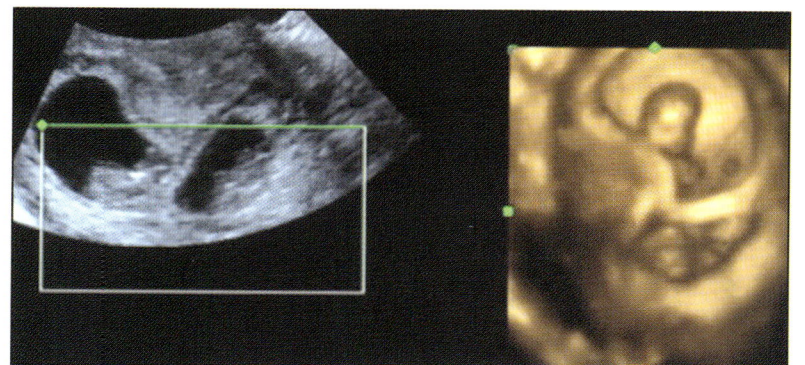

Fig. 12.55: Comparison between sectional 2D image (A) and 3D spatial imaging (B). The advantage of 3D spatial visualization in early pregnancy includes improved visualization of both fetuses and their gestational sacs

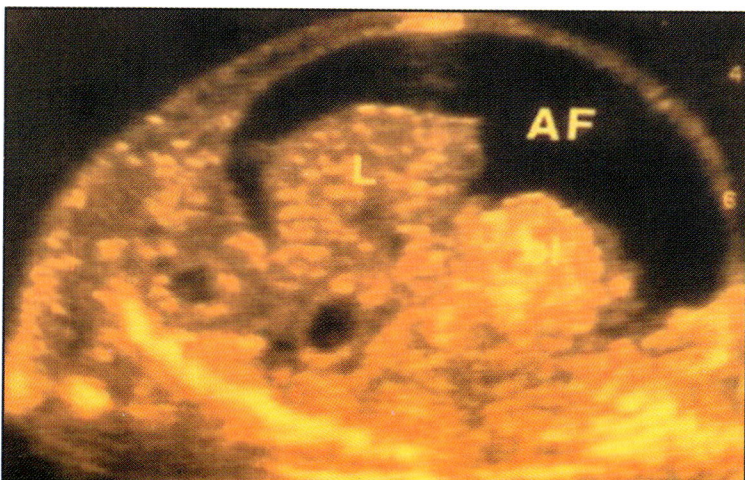

Fig. 12.56: Comparison between 2D and 3D sonography. Both modalities provide an examiner with essential information concerning the management of twin pregnancy including number of fetuses and chorionic status

volumetric calculations. Improved visualization rate, depiction of the spatial relationship, "sculpture like" plastic imaging (Fig. 12.57) and volume measurement are the main benefits of this new technology.

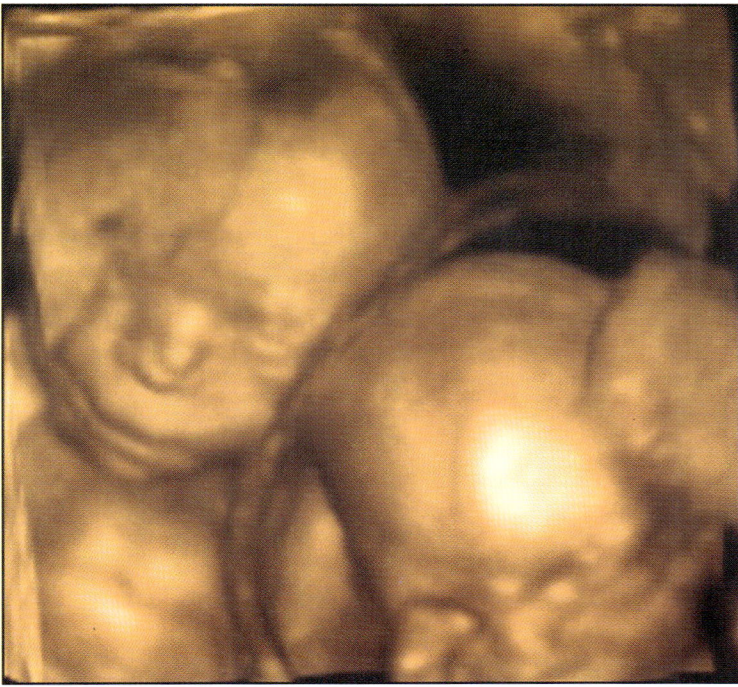

Fig. 12.57: 3D surface imaging demonstrated facial expression of both twins

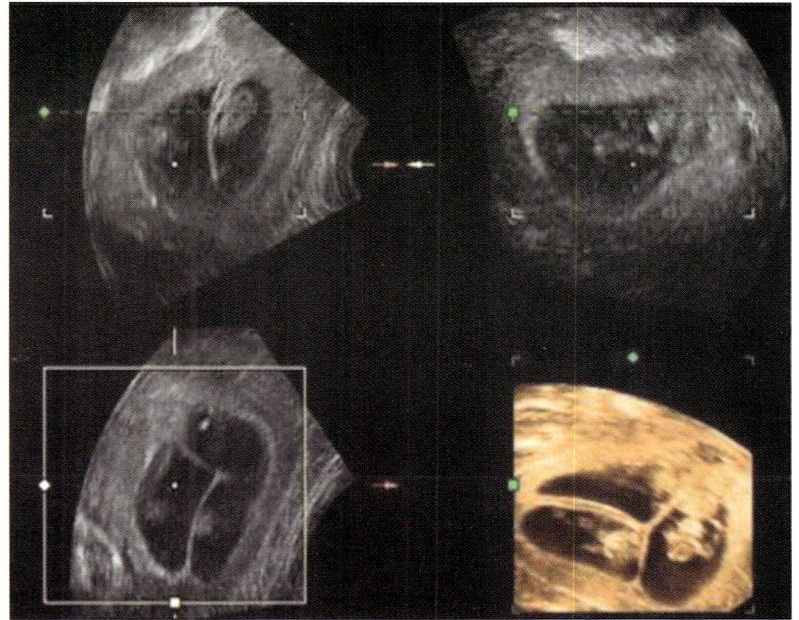

Fig. 12.58: 3D multiplanar view in determination of accurate number of gestational sac of triplet pregnancy at 12th week

3D Multiplanar Imaging

Multiplanar imaging offers an option of synchronous scanning in three orthogonal sections, including even coronal section (Fig. 12.58). Computer data processing provides numerous sections unobtainable by 2D sonography. Multiplanar view will result in simultaneous depiction of three sections orthogonal one to the others. Two of them (transverse and longitudinal) are dependent on angle of insonation, whereas the third one (coronal) is not. This section is orthogonal to the insonation beam.

Elimination of Undercounting Phenomenon

Three-dimensional volume acquisition provides the possibility of simultaneous depiction of three orthogonal planes of examinations. Moreover, it is possible to perform systematic examinations of acquired volumes with three different directions of scanning. For example, frontal (coronal) plane enables examination of the uterine cavity in sections which are unobtainable with conventional 2D sonography. Further, 3D sonography enables the appropriate counting of gestational sacs without any risk of undercounting even for less experienced ultrasonographers (Figs 12.59 to 12.66). Therefore, interobserver variability in detecting the number of gestational sacs is significantly lower. Even quadruplet is recognizable without any difficulties (Fig. 12.65). This advantage strongly suggests that 3D sonography should become the new standard in the early management of high order multiple pregnancies. Before introduction of 3D ultrasound, 11 percent of dichorionic twins

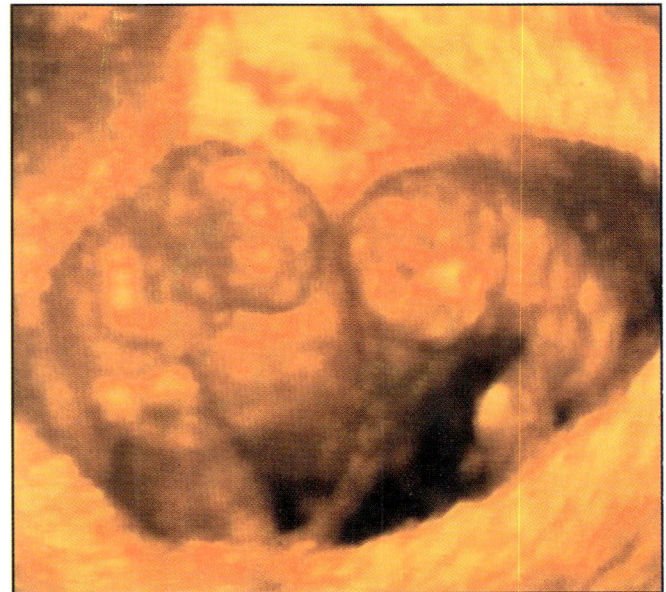

Fig. 12.59: 3D surface rendering of monochorionic-monoamniotic pregnancy

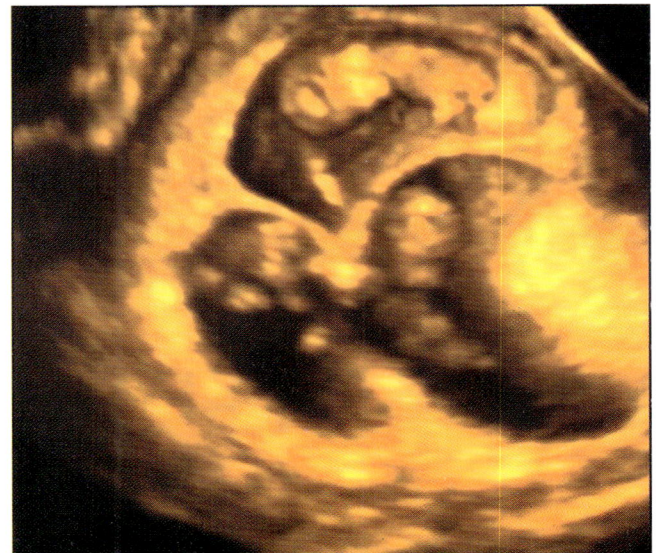

Fig. 12.60: 3D surface rendering of trichorionic-triamniotic triplet pregnancy

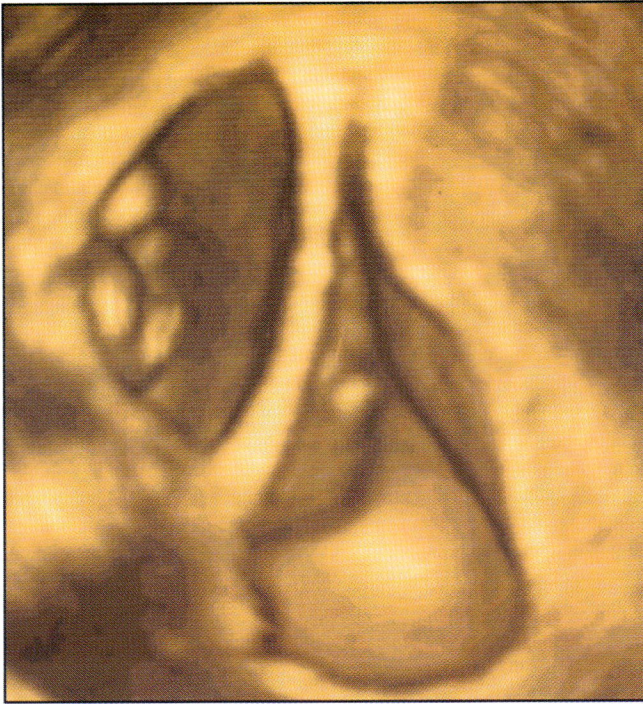

Fig. 12.61: 3D surface rendering illustrated dichorionic-diamniotic pregnancy

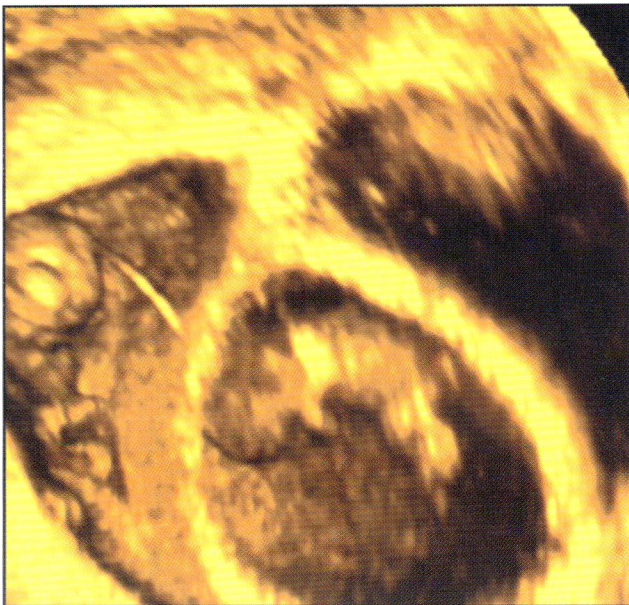

Fig. 12.62: 3D surface rendering demonstrated trichorionic-triamniotic triplet pregnancy

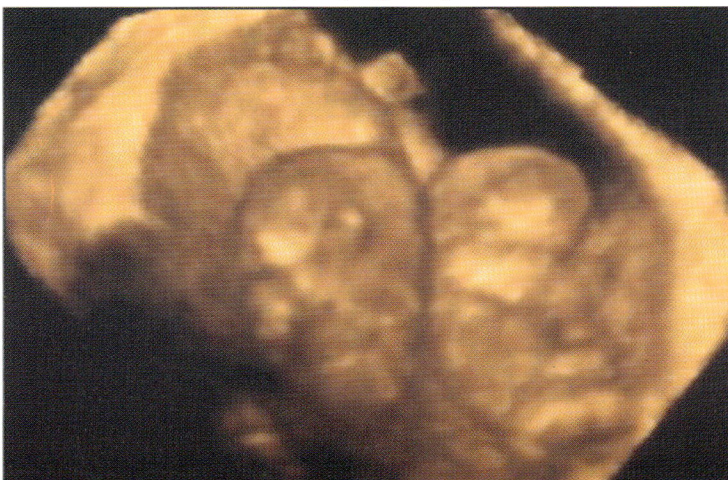

Fig. 12.63: 3D surface rendering demonstrated embryos in monochorionic-monoamniotic pregnancy

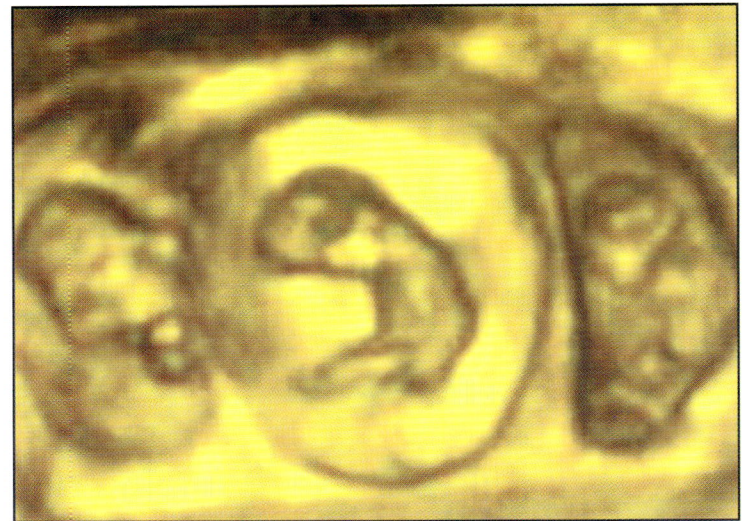

Fig. 12.64: This Figure shows surface features of fetuses including yolk sacs. The spatial relationship of fetuses toward each other can be easily assessed. Simultaneous visualization of three fetuses enables differentiation between active and passive twin

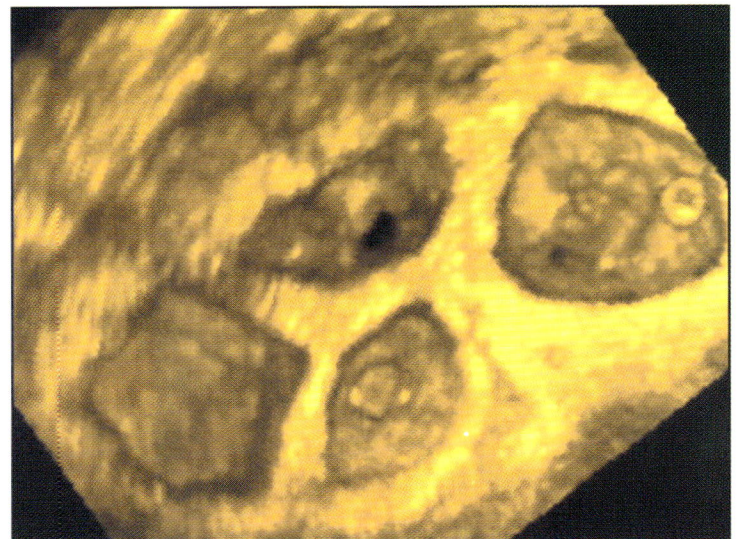

Fig. 12.65: 3D scan of an accurate number of gestational sac. Final diagnosis of quadruplets with 3D surface rendering mode. In contrast to 2D manual slicing, an analysis of 3D volugrams reveals the accurate number of gestational sacs

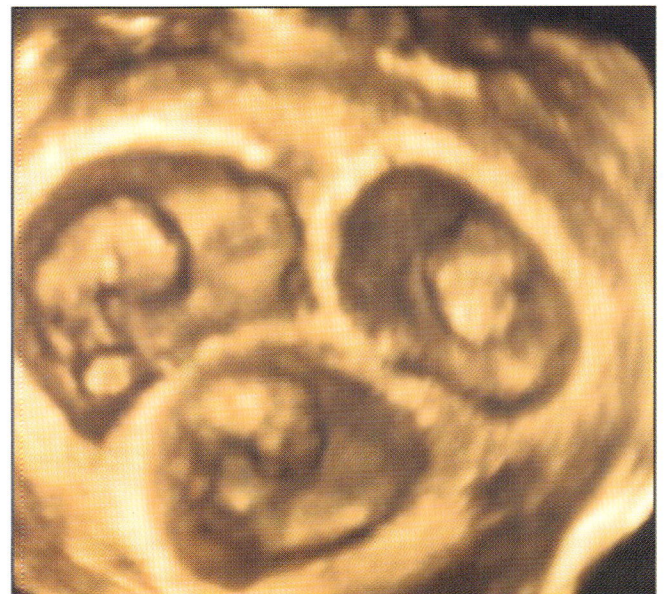

Fig. 12.66: Transvaginal 3D ultrasound of triplets at 8th week of gestation: 3 embryos in three gestational sacs (TCTA-trichorionic triamniotic triplets)

were initially undercounted as singletons, and 16 percent of high order multiple gestations were also undercounted.[21]

Prediction of Spontaneous Abortion

First-trimester spontaneous abortions can be predicted from alterations in the gestational sac size. For this purpose nomograms relating the ratio of mean sac diameter to crown-rump length (S/CR) to the gestational age (last menstrual period [LMP]) were constructed.[22] Using this method a sensitivity of 78.3 percent, a specificity of 97.8 percent and a false-positive rate of 2.2 percent can be achieved. Therefore, S/CR measurement in early pregnancy is a simple and reliable method of predicting first-trimester abortions. However, because of limitations regarding probe manipulations due to the anatomy of female reproductive tract and contemporary probe design some sections are unobtainable by 2D sonography. Using this method, the examiner should be aware that sometimes all gestational sacs are impossible visualized in sections referent for measurement of the gestational sac diameter. This method was often useless before the introduction of multiplanar imaging.

Detection of Fetal Anomalies

Three-dimensional sonography improves the diagnostic capability by offering more diagnostic information in evaluating fetal malformation than fetal growth (Figs 12.67 to 12.69), particularly in displaying the fetal malformations of the cranium, face, spine and extremities and body surface.[23]

The ideal visualization rate of a desired structure regardless of its anatomical limitations is the major advance of 3D sonography. This advantage can be used when the finding of 2D sonography is incomplete in terms of either fetal anatomy or placentation, due to incovenient anatomical relations.

In a singleton pregnancy, the empiric risk for major fetal malformations is approximately 3 percent. In trichorionic triplets the empiric risk for major fetal malformations within each fetus is independent of the others, so that probability of having at least one malformed fetus is approximately 9 percent.[24] According to the Eurofetus study sensitivity of a routine 2D sonography for detecting malformation is 61.4 percent.[25] The sensitivity is lower in multiple pregnancies as a consequence of overcrowding. As 3D sonography offers an ideal visualization rate of the desired structure, achieved by the manipulation within the volugram data, it is reasonable to expect that usage of this technology will increase sensitivity of the detection of malformations in multifetal pregnancies. There are varieties of anomalies involving the multifetal pregnancy. They can be divided in those unique to twins, especially monochorionic twins, such as conjoined twins (Fig. 12.67) or acardiac twins, and those not unique to twins such as neural tube defects, teratomas and congenital heart defects.

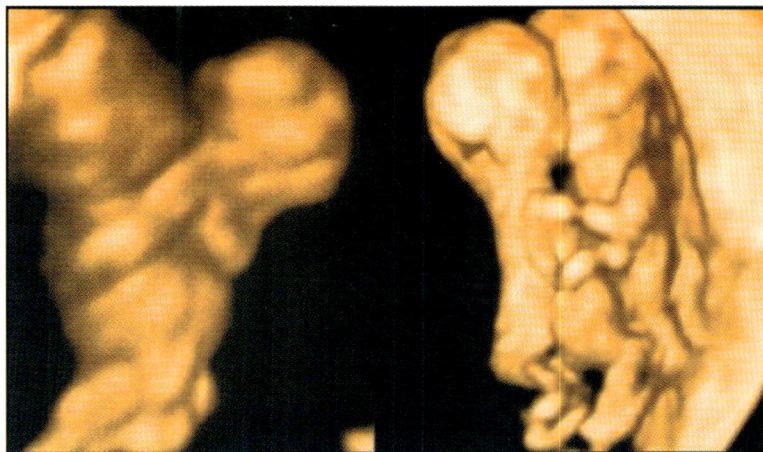

Fig. 12.67: Another case of conjoined twins demonstrated thoracophagus

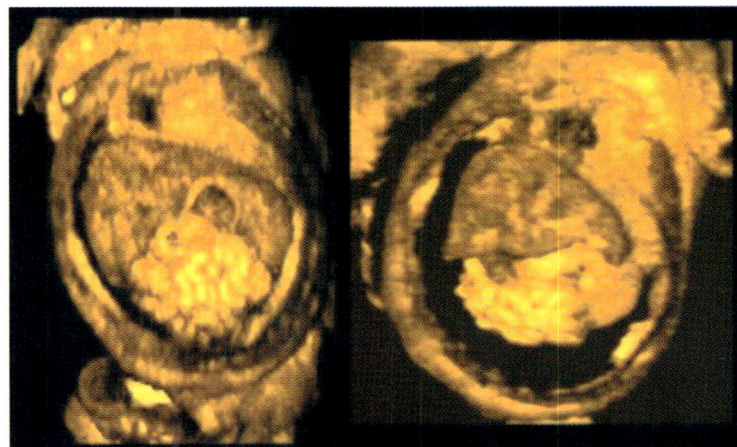

Fig. 12.68: 3D surface rendering demonstrated ascites in twin-to-twin transfusion syndrome fetus

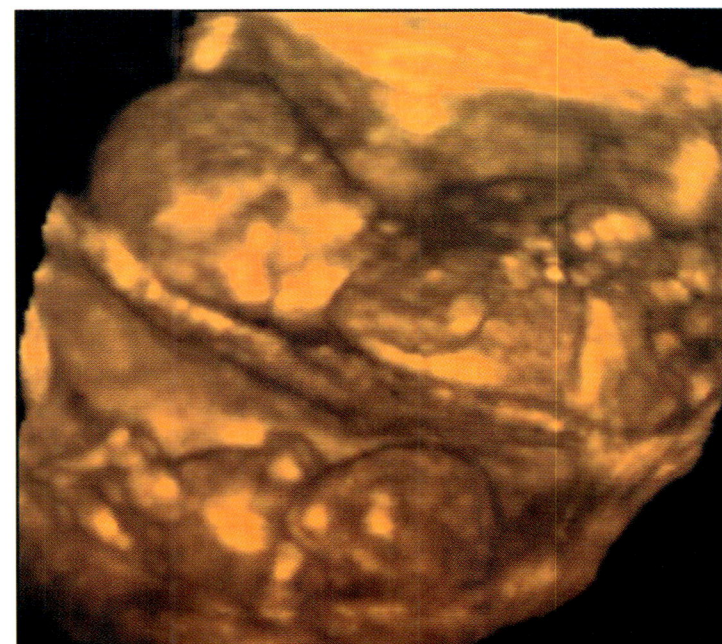

Fig. 12.69: Another case of discordant twins demonstrated using 3D surface rendering mode

Determination of Placentation

Using 2D ultrasound, membranes can be evaluated, counted and measured only when they are at 90°. In other words, the orientation of the membranes studied should be positioned parallel with the transducer cristal array. Clearly, 3D ultrasound enables us to achieve a "perfectly" oriented picture. The rate of appropriate chorionicity determinations should be ideal (100 percent) in the second and third trimesters.

The most revealing area in which to study the chorionicity and amnionicity of the multifetal pregnancy is the location within the uterine cavity in which the membranes change the orientation of their surfaces from covering the placenta or the uterine wall to meet each other and to form the interfetal or intertwin membrane. Using 2D ultrasound this area should be studied by placing the scanning plane at 90° to the plane of the intertwin membrane. This fact explains the potential role of 3D ultrasound in the examination of the origin of the intertwin membranes. The most important step in management of the triplet pregnancy is determination of the number of placentas. When placentas are separate, this is not a problem. Unfortunately, the placentas are usually fused.

In the case of dichorionic-triamniotic triplets (complex placentation), the placenta is represented by the T-sign and lambda sign with one thin and one thick membrane (Figs 12.70 to 12.74). Using conventional sonography it is difficult to distinguish between a single placenta and fused placentas of the twins and this is especially so in triplet pregnancy. Such a complex placentation types can be examined more easily using 3D ultrasound regardless of the gestational age.

3D Spatial Reconstruction

Integration of data obtained by volume scanning can be used to depict 3D plastic (sculpture-like) reconstruction of the region of interest (ROI) (Fig. 12.75). Three-dimensional reconstruction can be presented in surface mode. In the surface mode, only the signals from the surface of ROI are extracted and displayed in plastic appearance. Surface rendering provides an examiner with additional information confirming the normal anatomy either evaluation of the extent of lesion. Surface rendering provides spatial reconstruction of intertwin area, which may be useful in distinguishing between conjoined twins from monoamniotic twins positioned next to each other. At present, it is the safest means to accomplish this distinction.

With 3D ultrasound conjoined twins (Fig. 12.67) can be demonstrated in three perpendicular 2D planes (i.e. sagittal, coronal and transverse) which are simultaneously displayed on the monitor, allowing access to an almost infinite array of sections

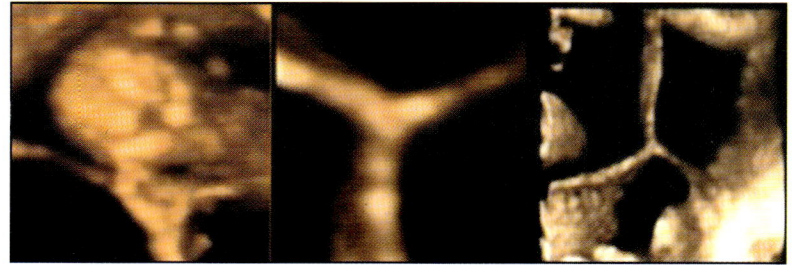

Fig. 12.70: 3D ultrasound determination of the chorionicity in the late second trimester. "Mercedes" or Y sign represents the junction of fetal membranes in triplet pregnancy

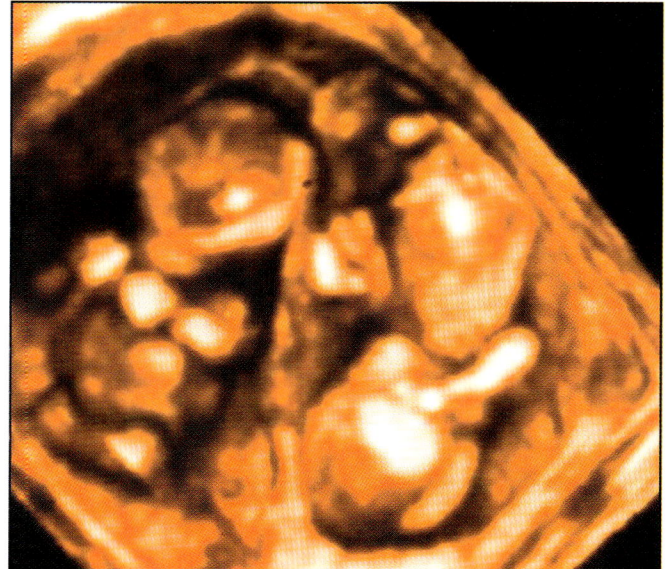

Fig. 12.71: This 3D image shows that on single image chorionicity and external frontal anatomy can be evaluated

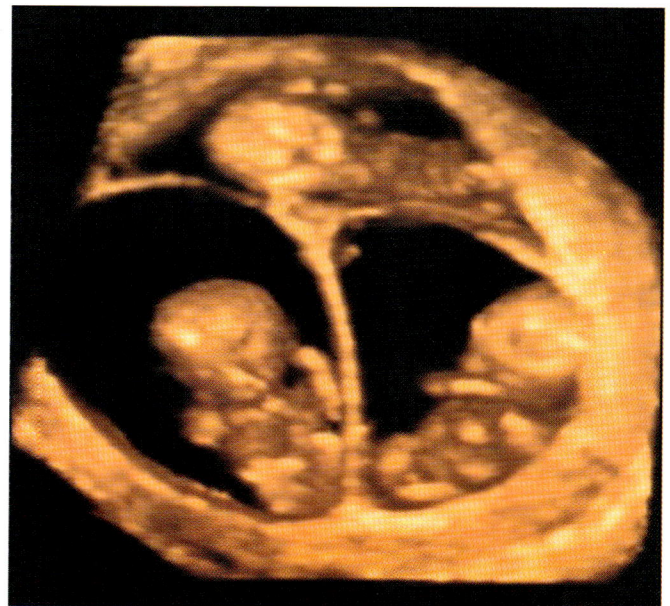

Fig. 12.72: 3D image of triplet pregnancy and external frontal anatomy. Further more orientation of one twin toward other can be simultaneously assessed

in any desired plane. On the other hand, surface rendering enables assessment of their topographic orientation to each other. From these acquired 3D volumes, the exact area of conjunction can be analyzed to assist in planning the postnatal management.

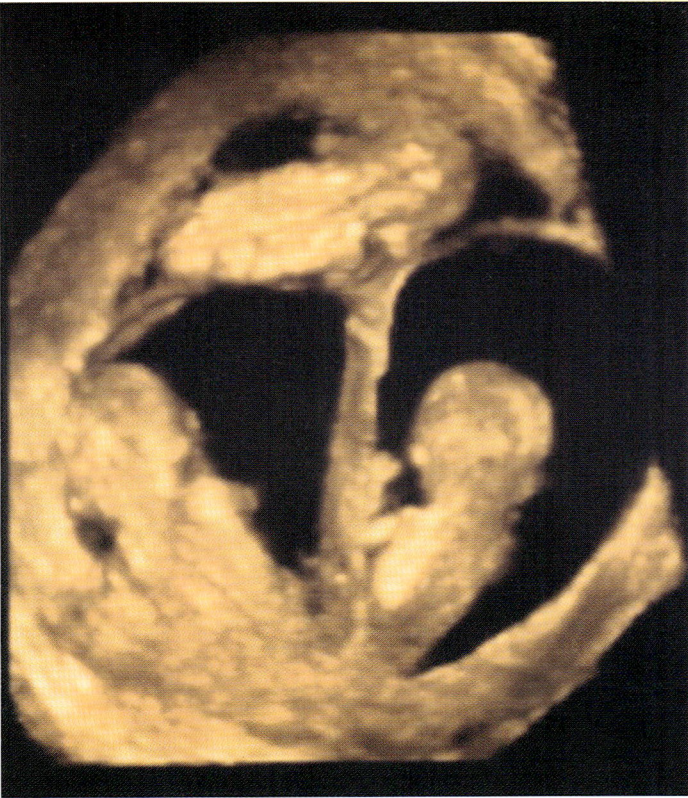

Fig. 12.73: 3D scan of dichorionic-diamniotic twins in the second trimester of gestation. Further more orientation of one twin toward other can be simultaneously assessed. This image illustrates twins seen from back. Interwin membrane and back surface anatomy are seen

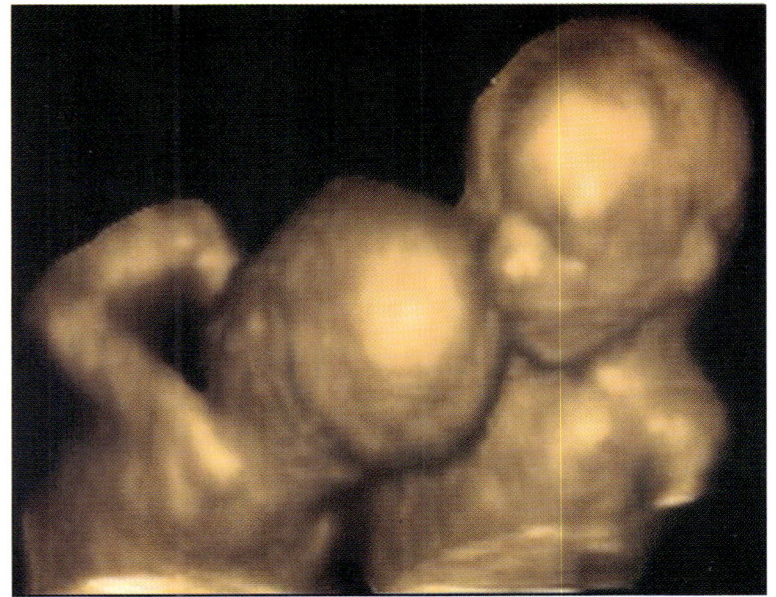

Fig. 12.75: 3D surface rendering shows first fetus (left) lay down in the shoulder of the other twin (right)

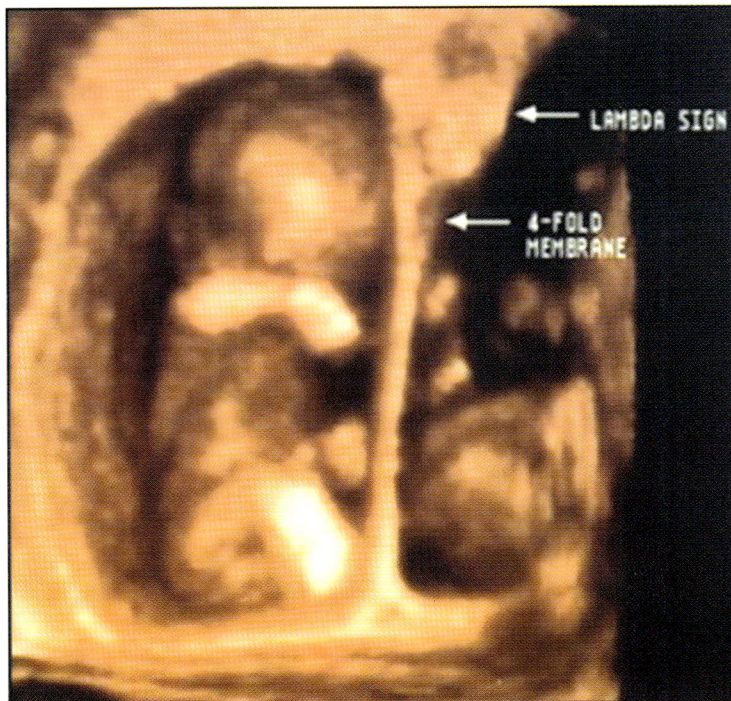

Fig. 12.74: Spatial reconstruction of membrane take-off site provides easier differentiation between dichorionic and monochorionic placentation. Furthermore, membrane thickness can be simultaneously evaluated. Therefore, 3D US is more comprehensive tool for understanding of accurate placentation

Volumetric Calculations

Three-dimensional measurement of the organ volume (volumetric) is obtainable using sequential slice-stepping measurements of areas through the volugram of the targeted organ. The volume assessment by 2D sonography includes the approximation of volume based on assumption that fetal organs have an ideal geometric shape, however it could be erroneous.

The prognostic meaning of early discordant growth in multiple pregnancy is still matter of scientific controversy. Some authors report about association of early discordant growth with major anomalies and poor pregnancy outcome.[26,27] In contrast, Vecek and coworkers reported early discordant growth with normal pregnancy outcomes.[28] All cases were after IVF-ET was performed.

Gassner and coworkers proposed the role of sonographic placental volumetry as a mean of early detection of chromosomal anomaly in multiple pregnancy.[29] They described a dichorionic twin pregnancy discordant in growth with distinctly small placental volume of a growth restricted fetus at 12th week of gestation. These two markers were present before a severe heart defect and bilateral cleft lip and palate were sonographically recognizable.

According to Gassner, volume of the placenta should be recommended criteria distinguishing between pregnancy at risk and without risk for major anomalies and poor outcome in multiple pregnancy.[29] Small placental volume in addition to growth restriction of one fetus early in the course of a twin pregnancy could be an important early marker influencing the decision for chorionic villous sampling at 12th week instead of amniocentesis at 16th week and it could lead to an earlier selective pregnancy termination of a triploid twin.

Placental volumetry is easy to perform when the placentas are separated. Unfortunatelly, in multichorionic pregnancies fusion of different placentas occurs during the second trimester.

Therefore, volumetric measurement should be perfomed at the end of the first trimester or at the beginning of the second trimester.

3D Angio Mode

Three-dimensional angio mode operates on technological basis of high-energy powered Doppler. Its greater sensitivity is related to direction independent scanning and better detection of smaller vessels. This mode provides optimal visualization and selective 3D reconstruction even of tortuous parts of vessels and blood flow arborization. More recently, 3D reconstruction of the vascular channels has been accomplished utilising the Doppler amplitude mode.[30,31] The implementation of 3D power Doppler imaging permits the physician to investigate the anatomy and topography of hemodynamics within the particular organ or ROI.

The diagnosis of cord entanglement with 2D realtime sonography (Figs 12.76 to 12.78) usually requires long examination period. Due to limitations of sectional imaging, examination is informative only to the quality and number of loops and final diagnosis is postponed. The main problem is distinguishing between adjacent and entangled cord. Cords positioned close to each other without torsion around one over the another umbilical cord is defined as adjacent umbilical cords, whereas, cords torquired one over another is called cord entanglement.

Much more information about umbilical cord can be obtained by 3D sonography (Fig. 12.79). Three-dimensional power Doppler permits imaging of curvatures of the umbilical cord and the number of involved loops in entanglement can be easily determied. Counting the number of the loops involved in entanglement is useful method for longitudinal evaluation of entanglement.

There are two types of the umbilical cord knots: true and false. A focal redundancy of the vessels, which sonographically appear as a vascular protuberance that does not persist in all scanning planes is called false-umbilical cord knot.[32] This condition should be differentiated between true umbilical cord knot which is a life-treatening condition.

NEUROLOGICAL DEVELOPMENT IN MULTIPLE GESTATIONS

Reinold was one of the first to describe fetal activity using ultrasound, and he stressed the spontaneous character of early prenatal movements.[33] There are two types of motor activity in multiple gestation: spontaneous and stimulated. Spontaneous motoric activity is defined as each embryonic or fetal activity which is not evoked by internal or external stimuli. On the other

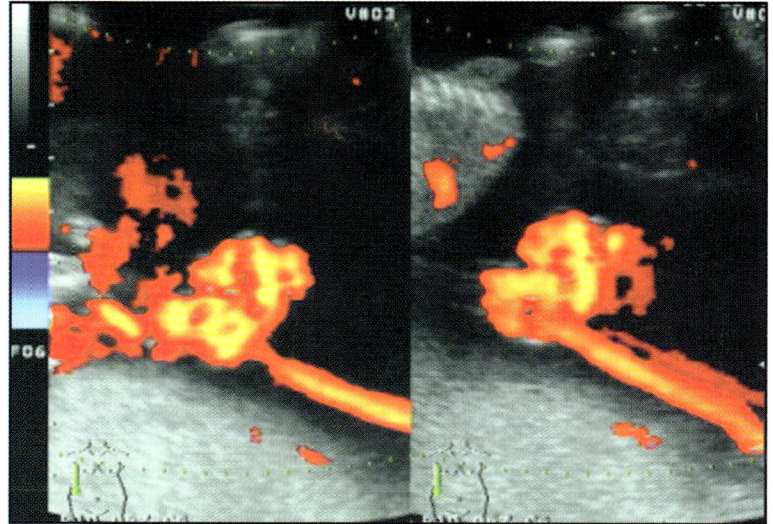

Fig. 12.76: Power Doppler imaging demonstrated cord entanglement in monochorionic-monoamniotic pregnancy

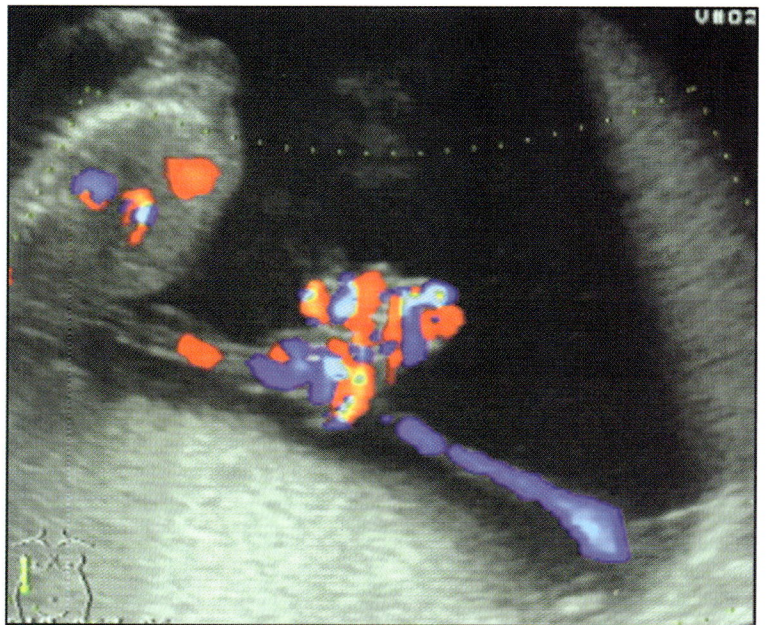

Fig. 12.77: Color Doppler imaging improved visualization of cord entaglement in monochorionic-monoamniotic pregnancy

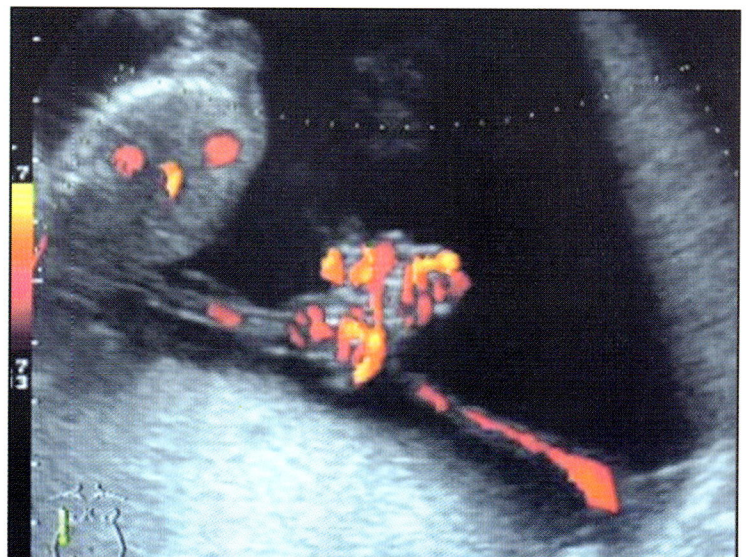

Fig. 12.78: Another imaging of cord entanglement using power Doppler technique

hand, activity evoked by intertwin contacts is called stimulated activity. Spontaneous motoric activity precedes to the stimulated motoric. The effect of prenatal reactions evoked by internal stimulus in twinning phenomenon due to intertwin contacts on the neurologic maturation was in the focus of interest of the systematic research initiated by Arabin.[8] They used realtime 2D sonography for detection and evaluation of the intertwin contacts. Due to sectional imaging, simultaneous visualization of both fetuses and assessment of their motor activity was impossible. Therefore, motor activity of a single fetus was possible to assess and unfortunately only to a limited extent. Similarly the intertwin area is tomogramically visualized and some of intertwin contacts are overlooked. Therefore, using this method distinguishing between spontaneous and stimulated motor activity is very difficult and sometimes impossible. If one perfomes 3D sonography complete anatomy of more fetuses and embryos can be visualized simultaneously. Inspite achieved progress this technology is not suitable for behavioral research because the images are static. Moreover, fetal movements which are in the focus of interest for behavioral studies cause significant artifacts in visualization.

We found that movement activity of each fetus in twin or multiple pregnancy can be easily determined by 4D sonography in the first and early second trimesters.[34] For the first time we can see that one twin is active whereas cotwin or cotriplets are active or not. Simultaneous visualization of motoric activity of each fetus enables study of their isolated motoric activity.

Arabin defined for the first time intertwin contacts.[8] Among them, complex interactions are recognized but complete definition of this phenomenon could not be achieved due to limitations of realtime 2D sonography. According to this group of authors those movement patterns are consisted of initiations and reactions of both twins which are sometimes difficult to distinguish and last longer than a few seconds. Using 4D sonography complex parts of these interactions could be analyzed for the first time. Furthermore, 4D sonography could be useful in evaluation of the altered motoric development such as in pathologic pregnancy.

Sadovsky concluded, " The possibility that movements of one twin stimulate the other to move".[35] However, Ferrari and co-workers came to different conclusion. According to their observations intertwin contacts have been supposed to cause increased rates of simultaneous twin activities in early pregnancy.[36] Arabin and coworkers used video documentation for continuous observation of intertwin activity.[8] The first interhuman contacts were determined (action and reaction within a second of interaction). Using the speed of initiations

this group found slow initiations followed by slow or fast reactions and fast initiations followed by slow or fast reactions.[8]

SONOGRAPHIC METHODS FOR PRENATAL ASSESSMENT OF FETAL BEHAVIOR

Total fetal activity is called fetal behavior. Some activities can be seen by ultrasound. Modern sonography uses two types of imaging: planar and spatial. Planar imaging provides a 2D image. 2D sonography is capable only of sectional imaging enabling sectional reconstruction of internal anatomy with clear visualization of organs and bones (Fig. 12.110). On the other hand, spatial imaging provides a 3D image (Fig. 12.80). Three-dimensional sonography is capable of spatial imaging providing more height, width and depth. Such imaging provides more perceptible surface reconstruction of the defined fetal region of interest. The amount of information obtainable from a single image is called image informativity. Informativity depends on the image type and the quality of the section. In general, planar images taken from referent sections are less informative than spatial images. Although informativity of surface-rendered images surpasses that of sectional 2D images, this view is limited to the visualization of fetal external anatomy. Therefore, sectional imaging is an important part of the sonographic examination. If one uses 3D sonography, the machine instead of the examiner perfoms matching and construction of the sectional images into a single 3D image. The finding is less dependent on the sonographer's experience in analyzing the sectional images and constructing a complete 3D image, and more dependent on the sonographer's technical experience in how to obtain a quality spatial image (Figs 12.81 to 12.104).

ASSESSMENT OF FETAL BEHAVIOR IN MULTIPLE PREGNANCY BY 4D SONOGRAPHY

Four-dimensional sonography provides spatial visualization of the fetal anatomy and movements almost simultaneous with their appearance. Simultaneous visualization of the entire anatomy (head, body and extremities) of two or more fetuses with their movements can be achieved by 4D sonography. Therefore, the type of movements, isolated movement of each twin or high order multiplet, intertwin contacts and interactions can be recognized without difficulties (Figs 12.105 to 12.121).

3D images presented in such a way to create a three-dimensional 'movie'. In contrast to 3D sonograpy, 4D sonography is characterized by continuous volume scanning with creation of a surface-rendered image, whereas 3D ultrasound is characterized by single volume scanning.[37] Rapid

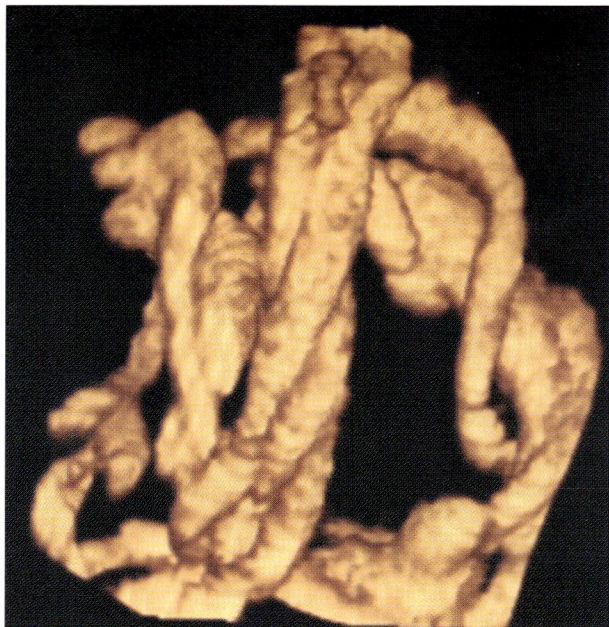

Fig. 12.79: 3D power Doppler reconstruction of umbilical cord with possibility to differentiate between false and true knots in multiamniotic or umbilical cord entanglement and adjacent cords in monoamniotic pregnancies

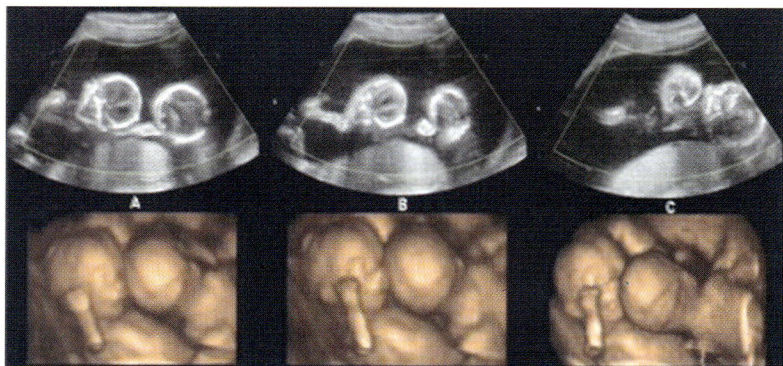

Fig. 12.80: Comparison between two techniques for evaluation of fetal behavior using realtime 2D sonography (upper) and 4D (below). Note hand to head contact together with head to head intertwin contact can be recognized

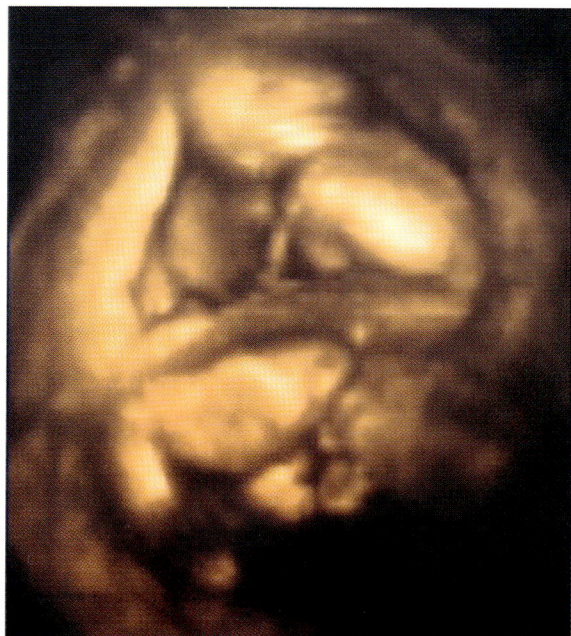

Fig. 12.81: 3D surface rendering illustrated reconstruction of intertwin contact activity at 13th week of pregnancy

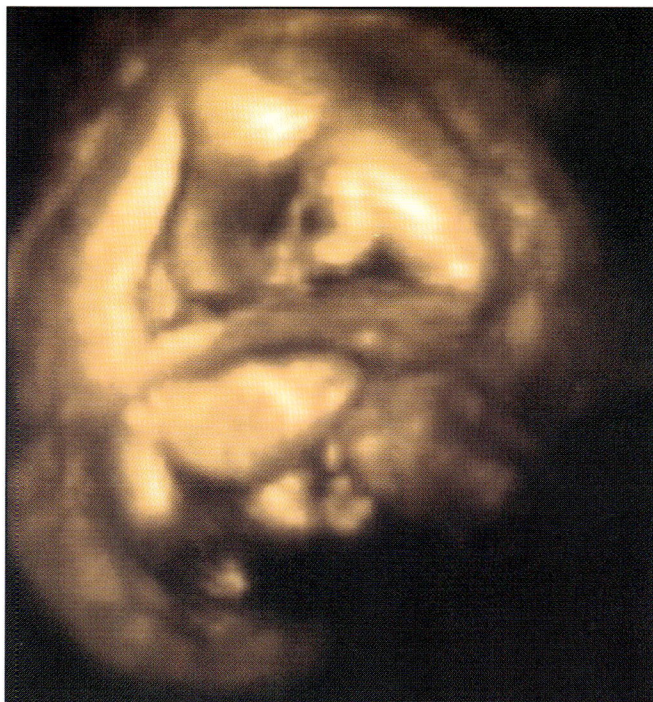

Fig. 12.82: 3D surface rendering demonstrated position of one twin to another due stretching movement pattern. It causes the change of postures

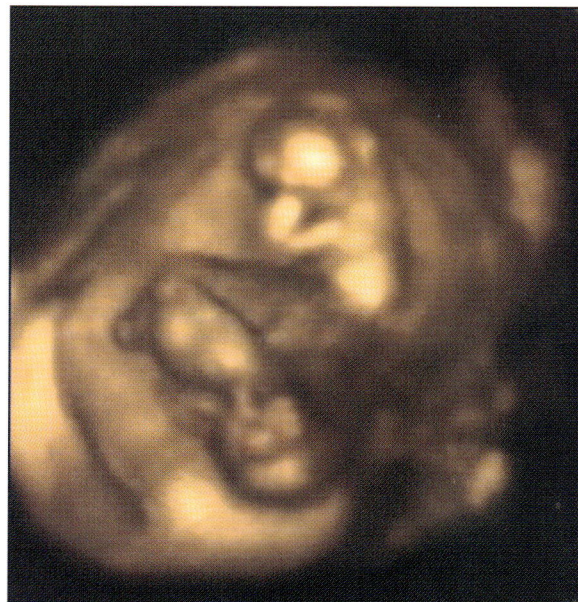

Fig. 12.83: 3D surface rendering of intertwin contact and motoric activity in twins at 13th week of pregnancy. In this image fetal hand is positioned in front of the fetal face in the first twin

development of computer technology has provided more and more capable processors that have reduced the time necessary for image construction. The duration of data acquisition and processing should be several times faster than the duration of fetal movements. When this condition is fulfilled, reliable fetal movements can be observed.

Two types of motor activity are possible in multiple gestation: spontaneous and stimulated. Spontaneous motor activity is defined as embryonic or fetal activity that is not evoked by internal or external stimuli. Activity evoked by intertwin contacts is

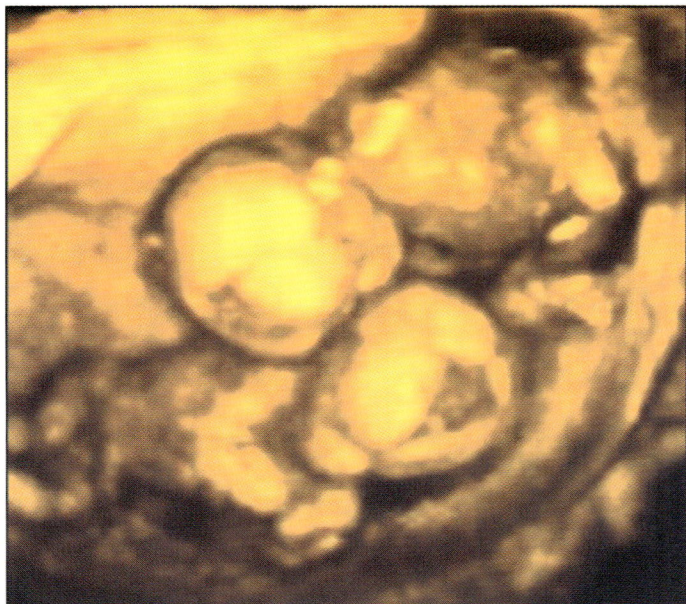

Fig. 12.84: 3D surface rendering showed intertwin contact in monochorionic-monoamniotic twins pregnancy

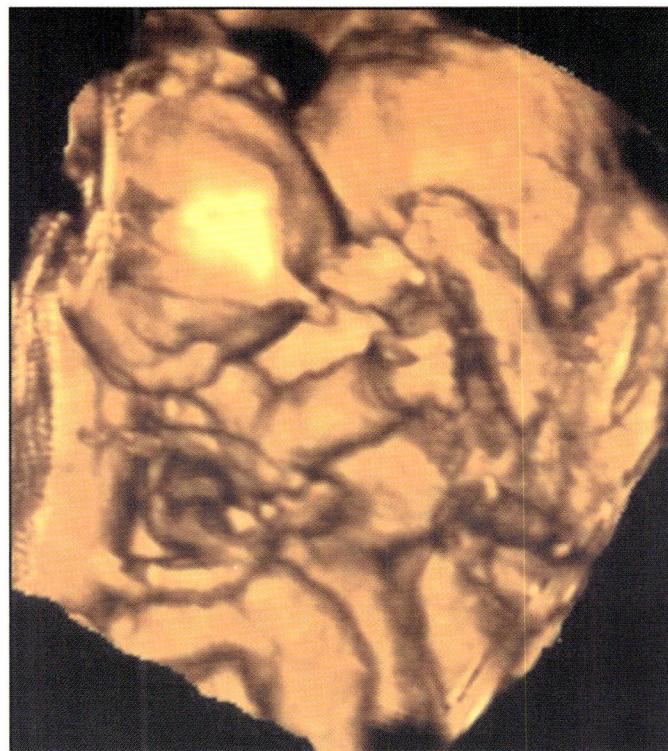

Fig. 12.85: 3D surface rendering demonstrated intertwin contact in another case of monochorionic-monoamniotic twins pregnancy

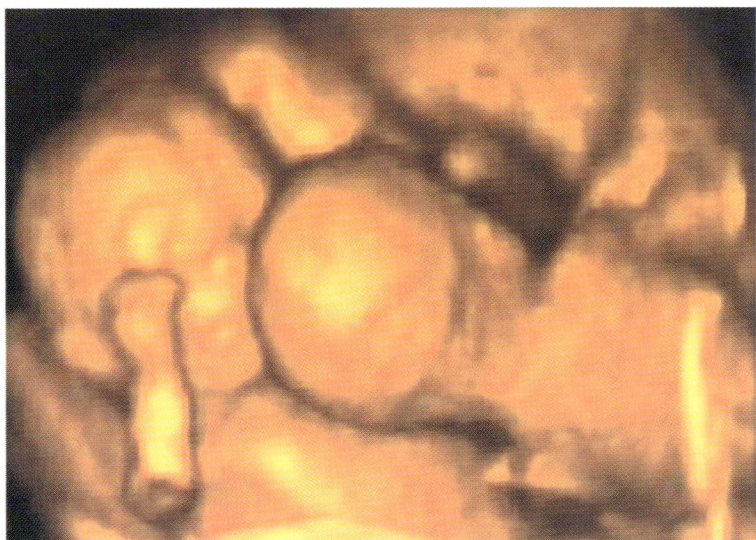

Fig. 12.86: 3D surface rendering demonstrated the first fetus lay down in another fetus behind

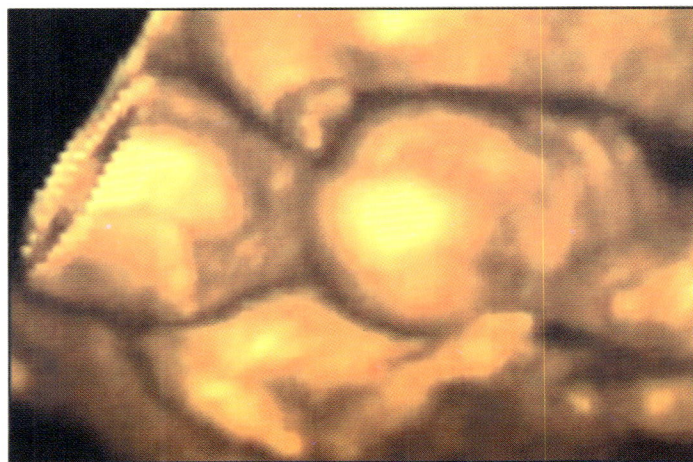

Fig. 12.87: 3D surface rendering showing intertwin contact in monochorionic-monoamniotic pregnancy. Both of fetuses in this image seem to be fighting

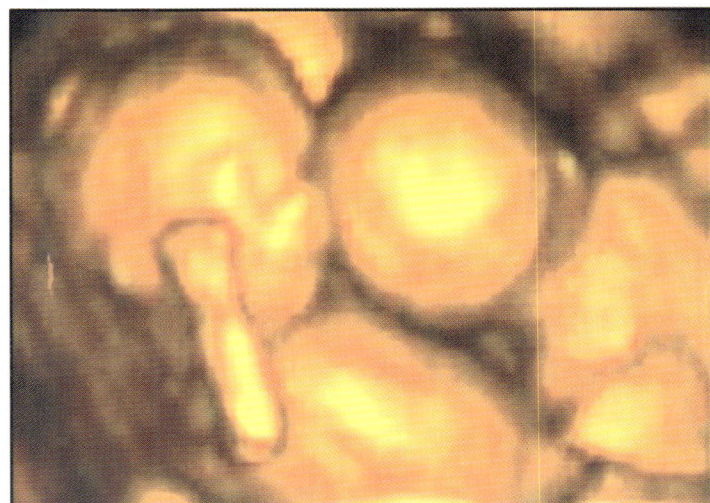

Fig. 12.88: This image showing intertwin contact and fetal motoric activity of both fetuses. Note the fetal hand movement (left) in the direction to the fetal head is depicted

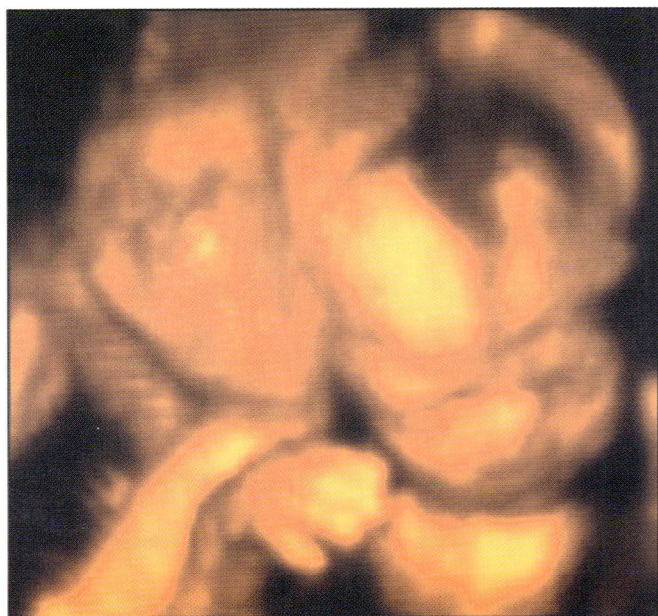

Fig. 12.89: 3D surface rendering of intertwin contact shows first fetus (left) seems try to grasp the second fetus

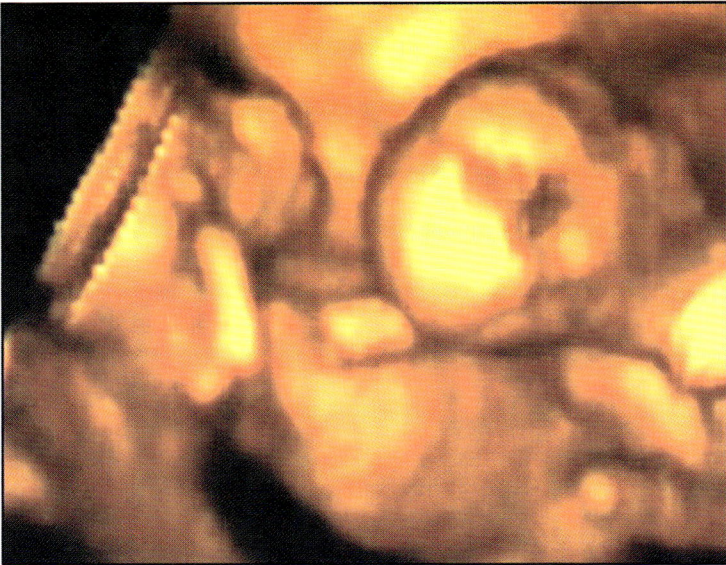

Fig. 12.90: 3D imaging of fetal motoric activity of the monochorionic-monoamniotic twin demonstrated hand to head movement of the first fetus

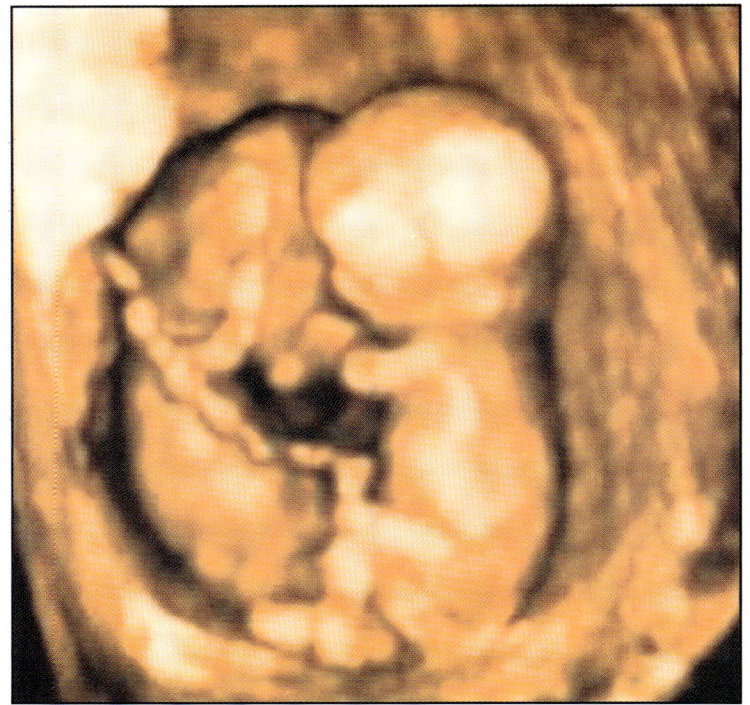

Fig. 12.91: 3D scan shows motoric activity of both fetuses

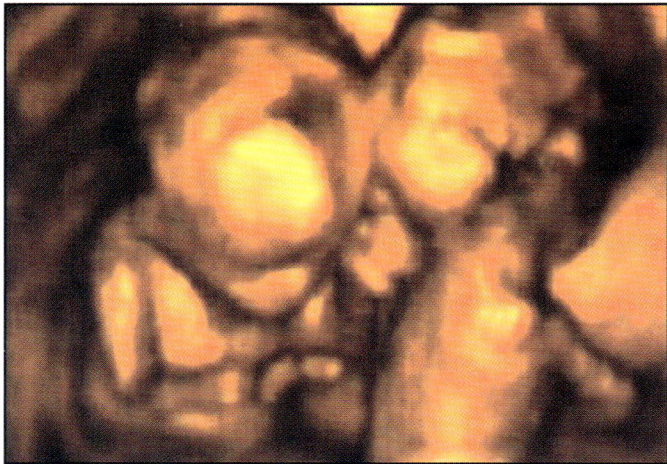

Fig. 12.92: 3D surface scan shows both fetuses are in the same position

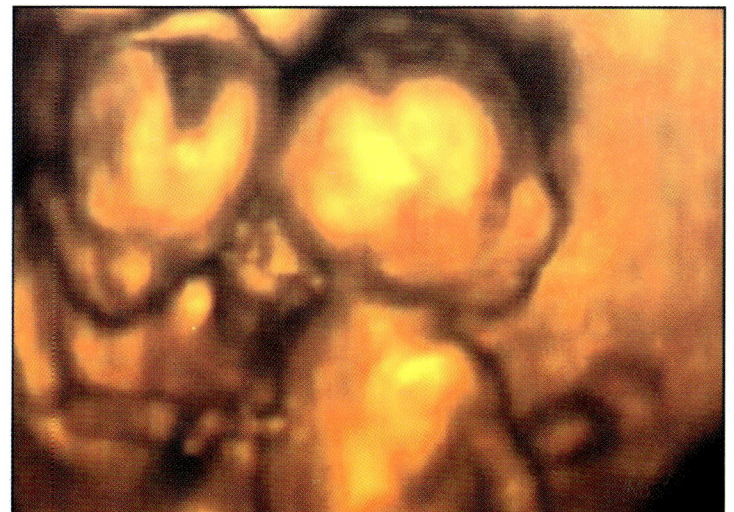

Fig. 12.93: 3D surface rendering shows front-to-front position of both fetuses

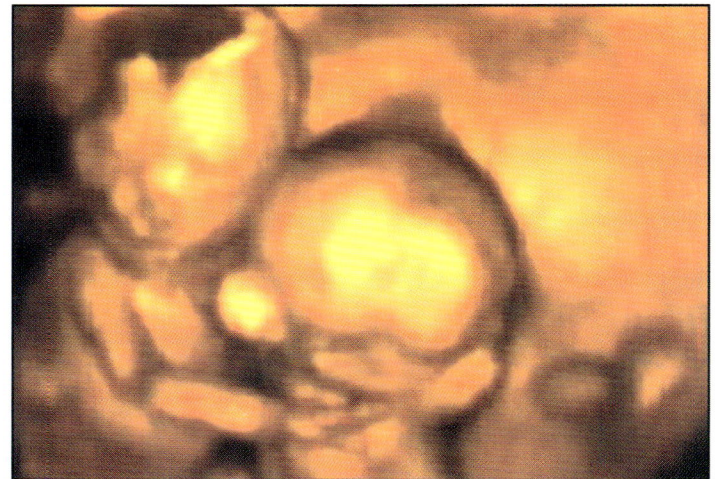

Fig. 12.94: 3D surface imaging demonstrated hand movement of the first twin (left image) in direction to the second twins' shoulder (right)

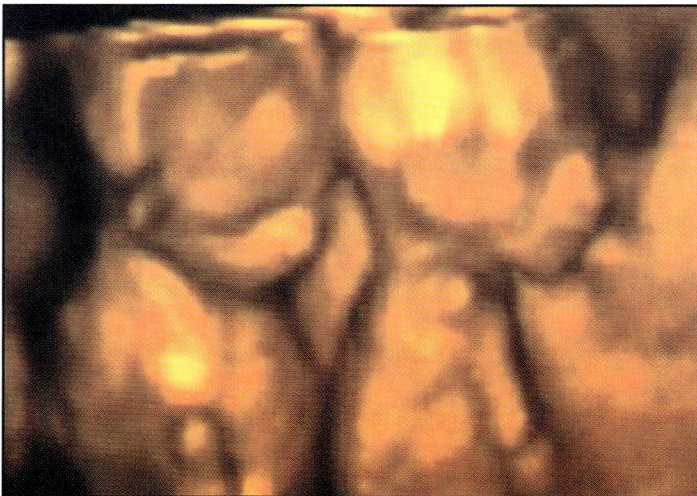

Fig. 12.95: 3D imaging demonstrated hand movement from the first twins in direction to the second twin's back. Note head rotation from the second twin (right) immediately after the first twin touch the fetal back

characterized as stimulated activity (Figs 12.108 to 12.116). Spontaneous motor activity precedes stimulated activity in terms of gestational age of onset.

The effect of prenatal reactions evoked by internal stimuli was the focus of interest of the systematic research initiated by

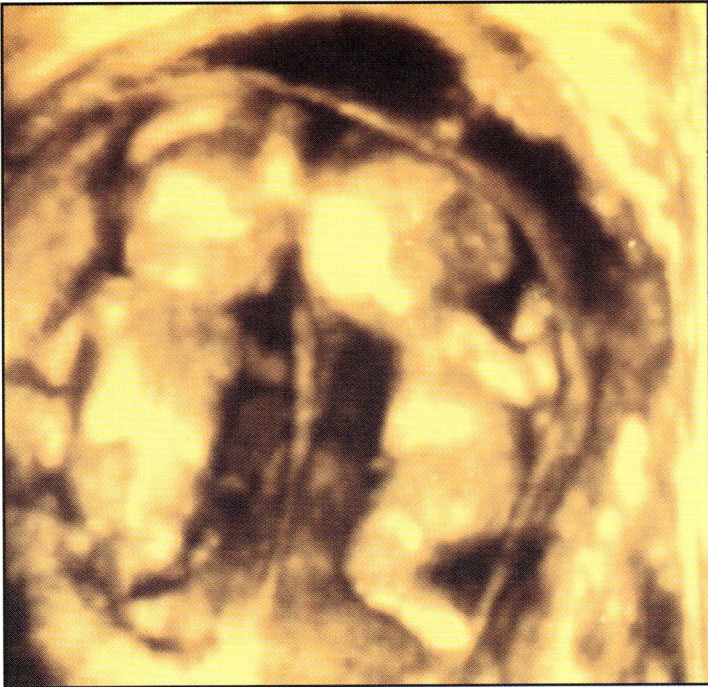

Fig. 12.96: 3D scan illustrated both of twins seen from back. Interwin membrane and back surface anatomy are seen

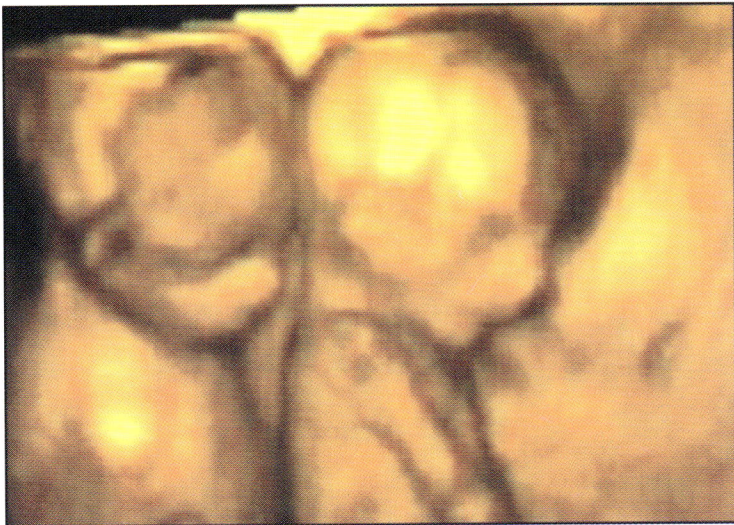

Fig. 12.99: Another 3D image demonstrated intertwin contact. Note the second fetus seems to lean againts the first fetus (left)

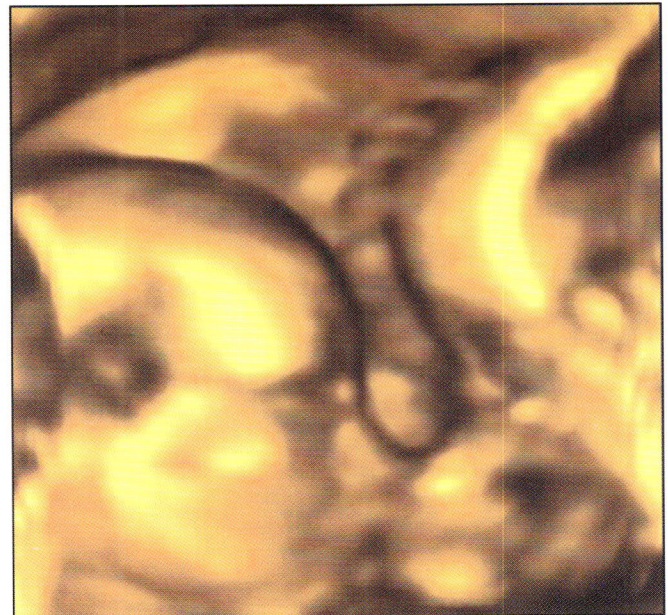

Fig. 12.97: 3D surface rendering illustrated front-to-back position in intertwin contact. Both of the fetuses seem to be passive at this image

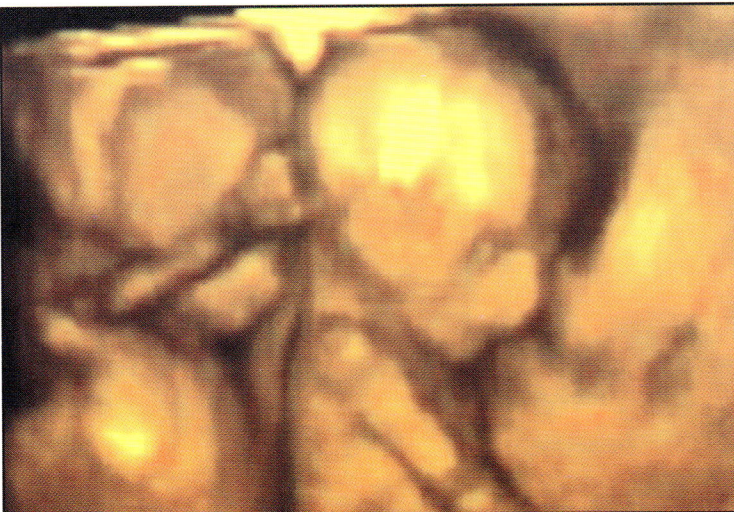

Fig. 12.100: Face-to-face intertwin contact is demonstrated in this image using 3D surface rendering

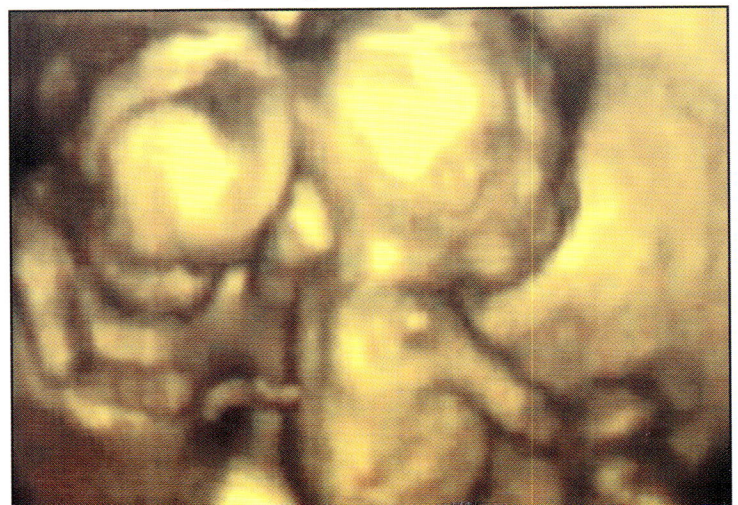

Fig. 12.98: Another 3D image shows hand movement from the first twins to the head of the second twin (right image)

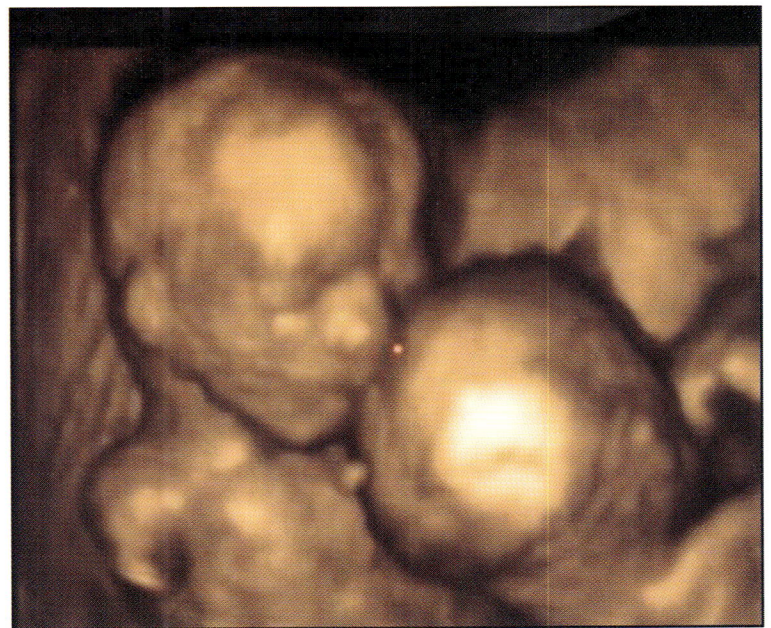

Fig. 12.101: 3D surface rendering demonstrated hand movement of the first twin

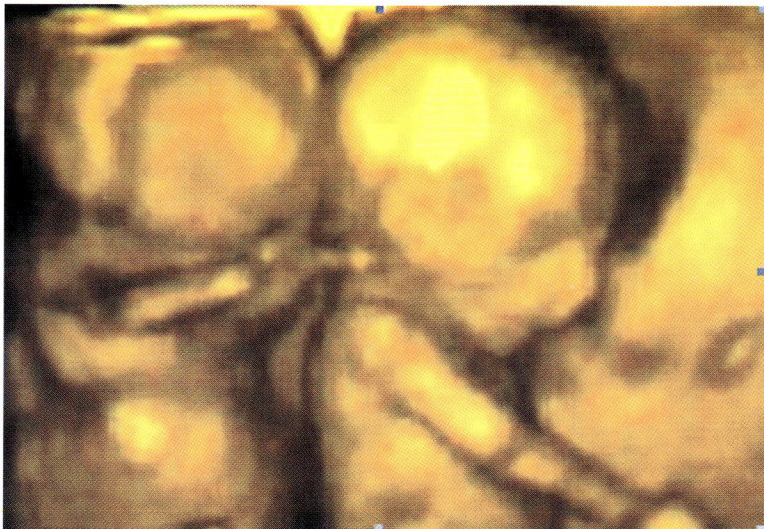

Fig. 12.102: 3D scan shows hand movement from the first fetus (left) to the right ear of the second twin (right)

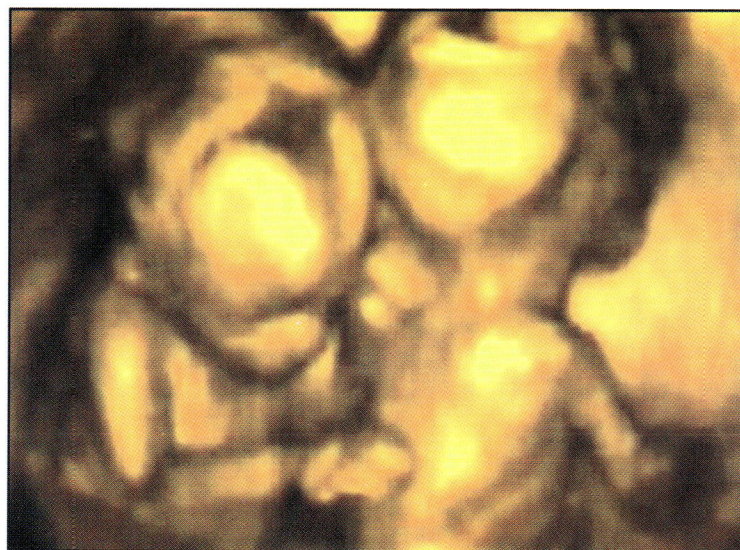

Fig. 12.104: 3D surface rendering illustrated intertwin contact. Note the movement of the second fetus (right), while the first fetus (left) try to grasp the second fetus' shoulder

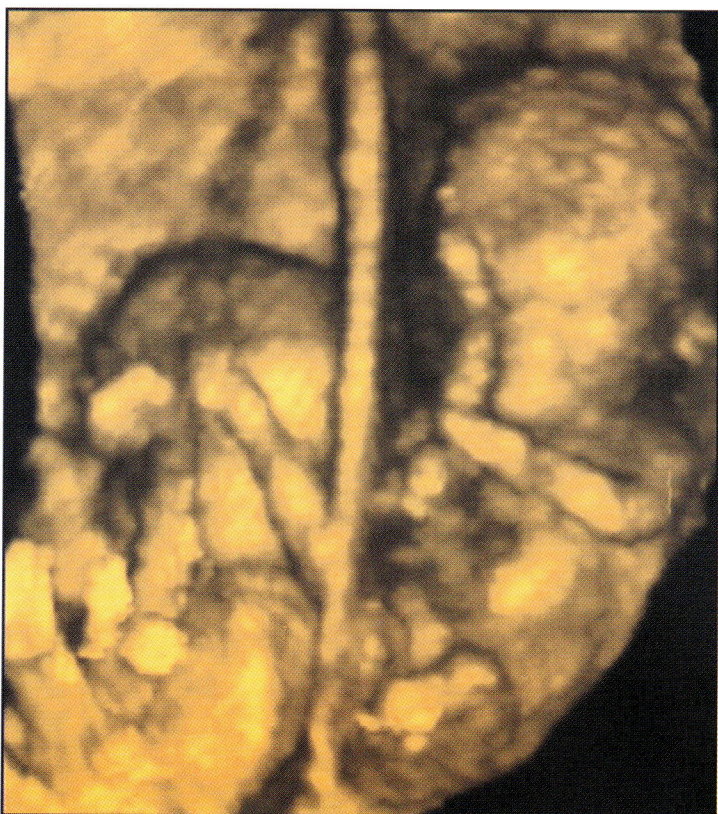

Fig. 12.103: 3D surface rendering illustrated both of the fetus not in the direct contact

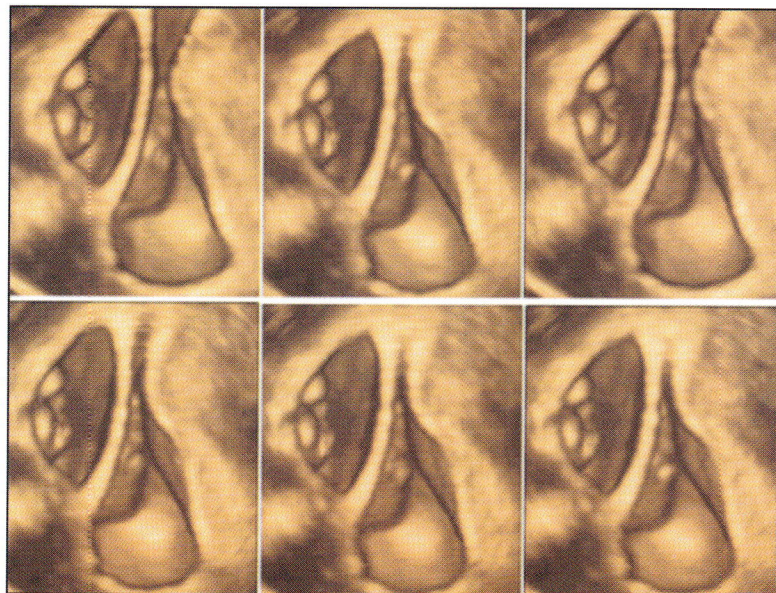

Fig. 12.105: 4D image demonstrated movements of the embryos in diamniotic-dichorionic pregnancy

the group of Arabin and colleagues.[8] These investigators used realtime 2D sonography for detection and evaluation of intertwin contacts. However, owing to sectional imaging, simultaneous visualization of both fetuses and assessment of their motor activity was impossible. Therefore, the motor activity of a single fetus only provided limited information. The same limitation applies to the intertwin area when it is tomographically visualized. Therefore, using this method to distinguish between spontaneous and stimulated motor activity is not only difficult, but sometimes impossible. If, on the other hand, one performs 3D sonography, the complete anatomy of both fetuses can be visualized simultaneously. In spite of this progress, the technology is not suitable for behavioral research because the images are static. Moreover, fetal movements, the focus of interest for behavioral studies, cause significant artifacts in visualization.

All these problems are resolved by 4D sonography, which provides spatial visualization of the fetal anatomy and movements almost simultaneously with their appearance. Simultaneous visualization of the entire anatomy (head, body and extremities) of two or more fetuses along with their movements allows the characterization of the type of movement, isolated movements of

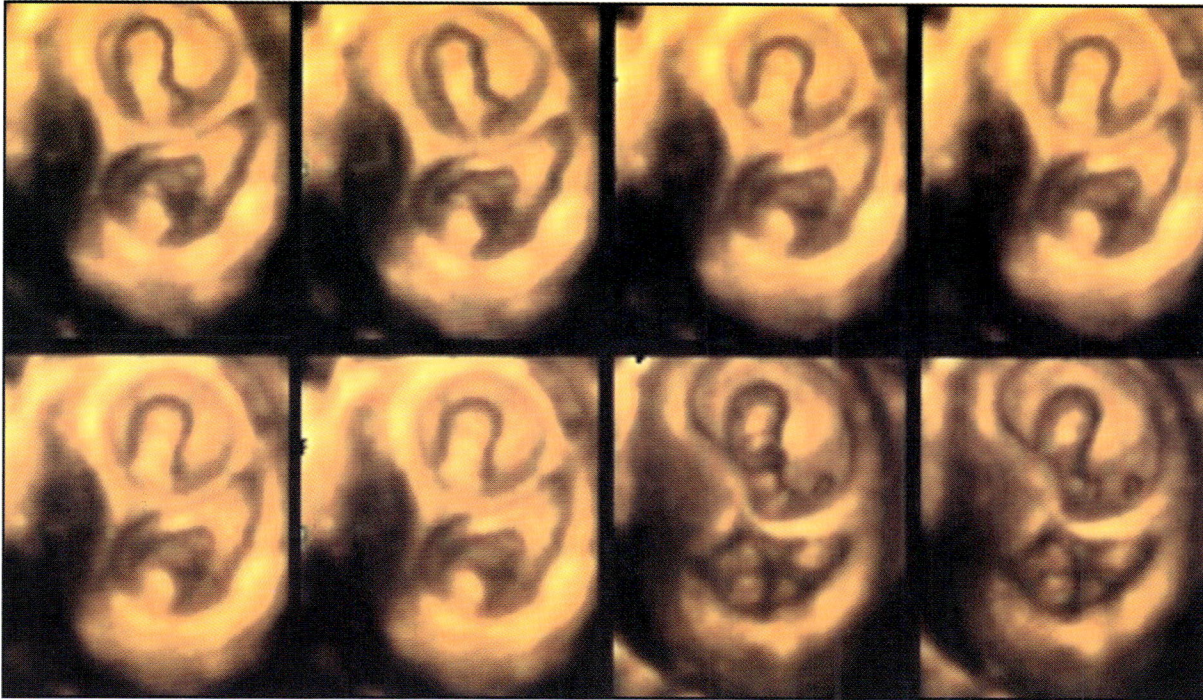

Fig. 12.106: 4D sequence demonstrated embryonic movements in dichorionic-diamniotic pregnancy

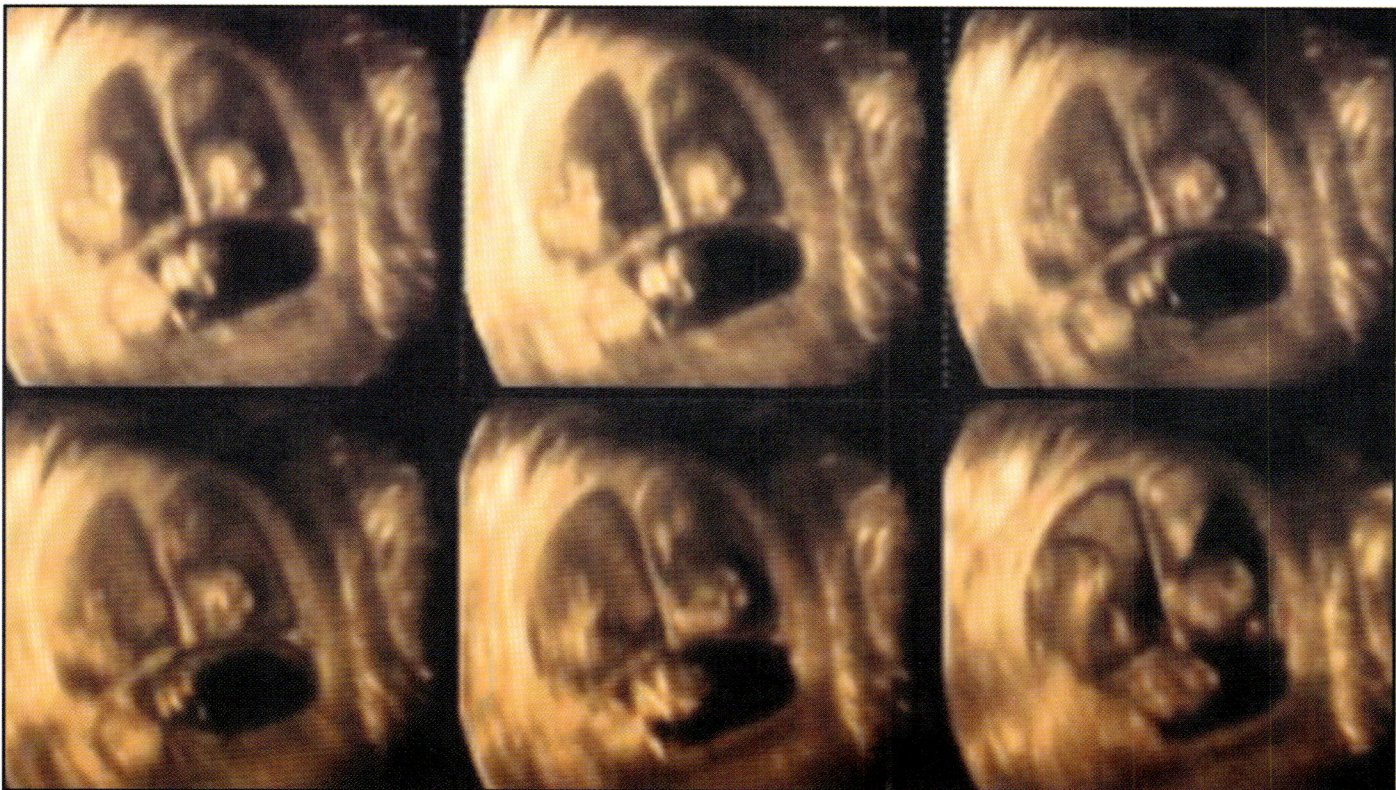

Fig. 12.107: 4D sequence illustrated embryonic movements in triplet pregnancy

each fetus, as well as intertwin contacts and interactions. Movement activity of each fetus can be easily determined in the first and early second trimesters.[35] Simultaneous visualization of motor activity of each fetus enables study of their isolated motor activity. It is possible to determine that one twin is active when the cotwin or cotriplets are either active or not. 4D sonography could be used for further analysis of the quality of interhuman contacts. The initiation and reaction movements are visualized in three dimensions allowing more detailed study of this subject.

CONCLUSIONS

Despite the great progress achieved in management of multiple pregnancy, due to limitations of 2D sonography an additional

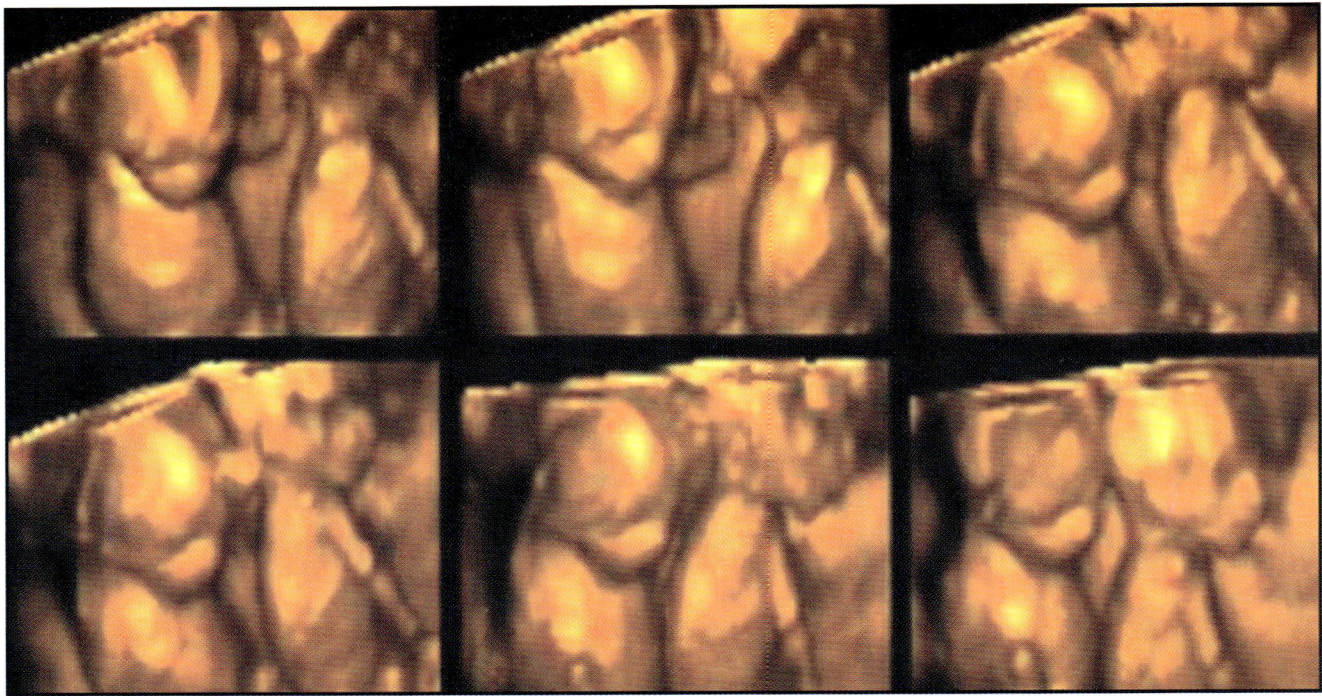

Fig. 12.108: 4D sequence showing intertwin contact and motoric activity. Note the actively hand movement of the first twin (left), while the second fetus seems to be passive

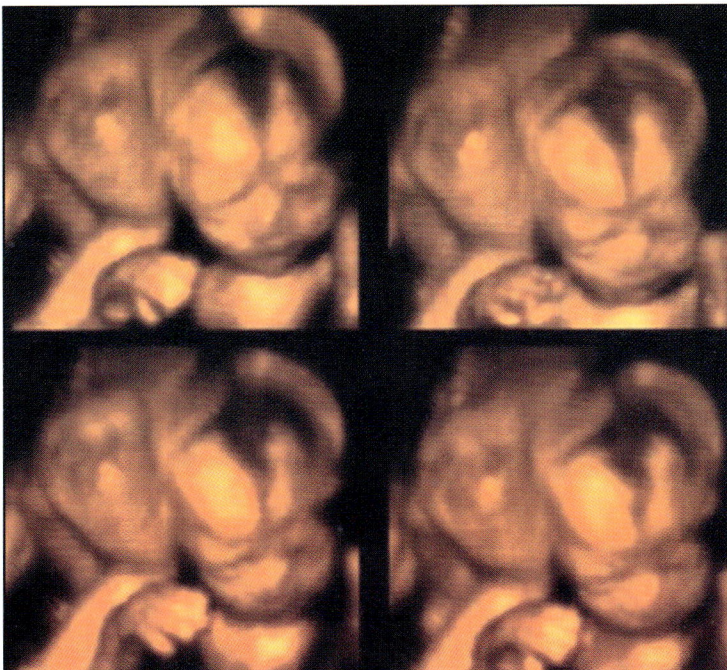

Fig. 12.109: 4D sequence shows intertwin contact. The first fetus (in front) lay down in second fetus (behind), while the right hand of the second fetus is positioned in the right shoulder of the first fetus

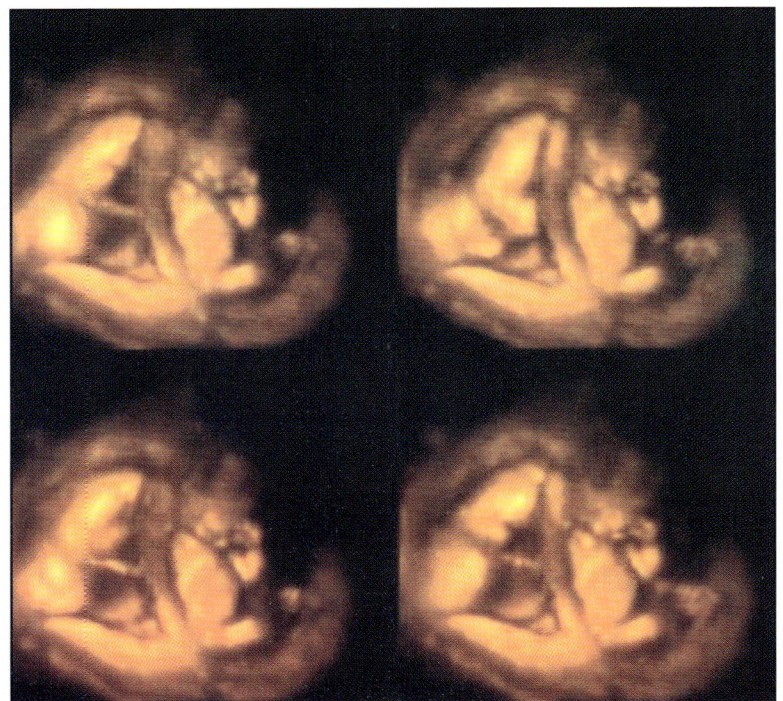

Fig. 12.110: 4D sonography provides us with an option of separated evaluation of fetal activity of each twin. First twin (left) is active, whereas second twin (right) is passive.

three-dimensional scan is recommended, because it provides more reliable or additional information important for management of multiple pregnancy. Four-dimensional sonography has several advantages over realtime 2D sonography in the assessment of twin behavior. These include the capability of simultaneous visualization of both fetuses and assessment of their motor activity. The same advantage applies to the intertwin area. Therefore, it should be considered as a method of choice for accurate diagnosis of isolated motor activity of single twins. 4D sonography is undoubtedly a powerful new imaging tool whose scientific and clinical potential should be established in the coming decade.

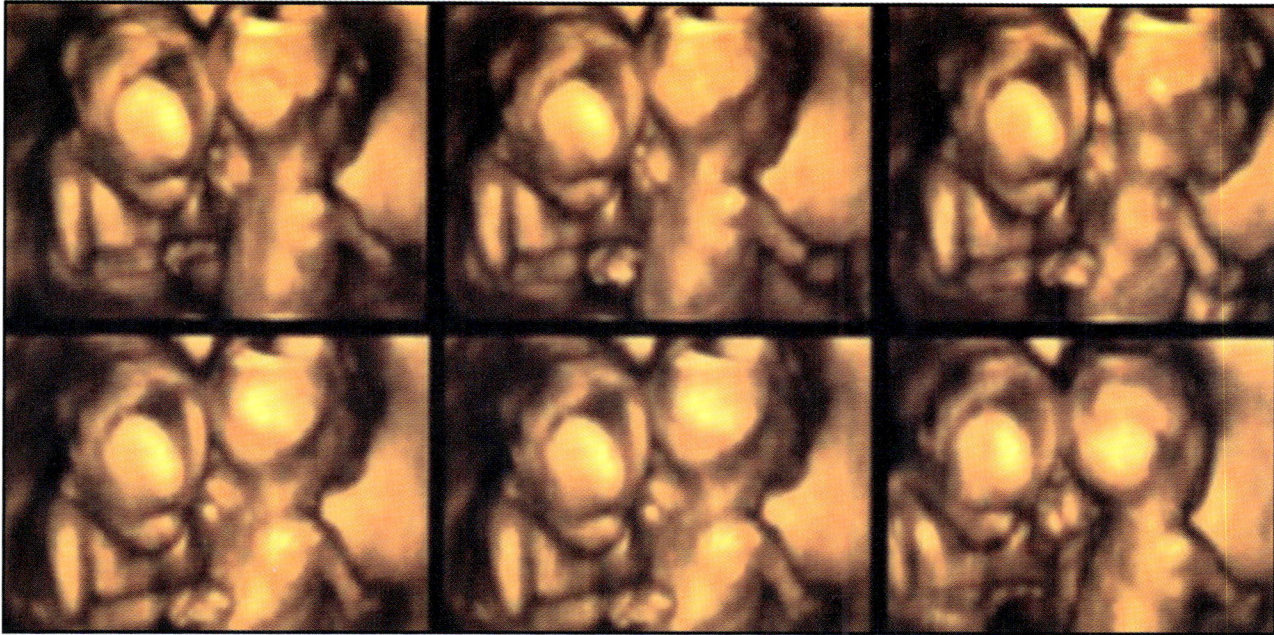

Fig. 12.111: 4D sequence demonstrated intertwin contact. Note lateral head rotation from the second twin (right) when the first twin seems try to touch the second twin's back

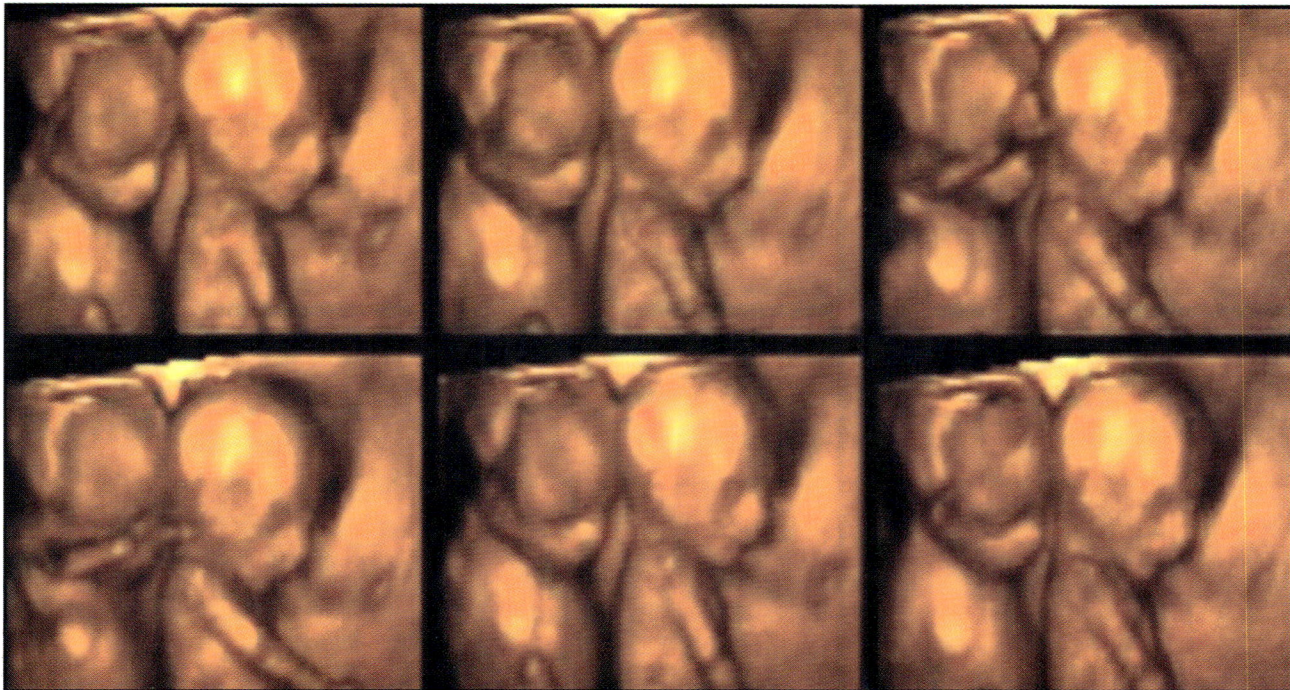

Fig. 12.112: 4D sequence demonstrated intertwin contact. Note active hand movement of the first twin (left image)

REFERENCES

1. Steegers-Theunissen RP, Zwertbroek WM, Huisjes AJ, et.al. Multiple birth prevalence in The Netherlands. Impact of maternal age and assisted reproductive techniques. J Reprod Med. 1998; 43: 173-9.
2. Seoud MA, Kruithoff C, Muasher SJ.Outcome of triplet and quadruplet pregnancies resulting from in vitro fertilization. Eur J Obstet Gynecol Reprod Biol 1991;41:79-85.
3. Borlum KG. Third trimester fetal death in triplet pregnancies. Obstet Gynecol 1991;77:6-9.
4. Vecek N, Kurjak A, Azumendi G. Fetal behaviour in multifetal pregnancies studied by 4D sonography. Ultrasound Rev Obstet Gynecol 2004;4:52-8.
5. Reinold E. Clinical value of fetal spontaneous movements in early pregnancy. J Perinat Med 1973;1:65-72.
6. de Vries JI, Visser GH, Prechtl HF. The emergence of fetal behaviour. I. Qualitative aspects. Early Hum Dev 1982;7:301-22.
7. Hooker D. The Prenatal Origin of Behavior. Kansas: University of Kansas Press, 1952.
8. Arabin B, Bos R, Rijlardsdam R, et al. The onset of inter-human contacts. Longitudinal ultrasound observations in twin pregnancies. Ultrasound Obstet Gynecol 1996;8:166-73.
9. Bromley B, Benacerraf B. Using the number of yolk sacs to determine amnionicity in early first trimester monochorionic twins. J Ultrasound Med 1995;14:415-9.
10. Finberg HJ. The "twin peak" sign: reliable evidence of dichorionic twinning. J Ultrasound Med 1992;11:571-7.
11. Sepulveda W, Sebire NJ, Odibo A, et.al. Prenatal determination of chorionicity in triplet pregnancy by ultrasonographic examination of the ipsilon zone. Obstet Gynecol 1996;88:855-8.
12. Dickey R, Taylor S, Peter YL, et.al. Spoontaneous reduction of multiple pregnancy: Incidence and effect on outcome. Am J Obstet Gynecol 2002;186:77-83.
13. Yonemoto H, Yoshida K, Kinoshita K, et.al. Embryological evaluation of surface features of human embryos and early fetuses by 3-D ultrasound. J Obstet Gynaecol Res. 2002;28:211-6.

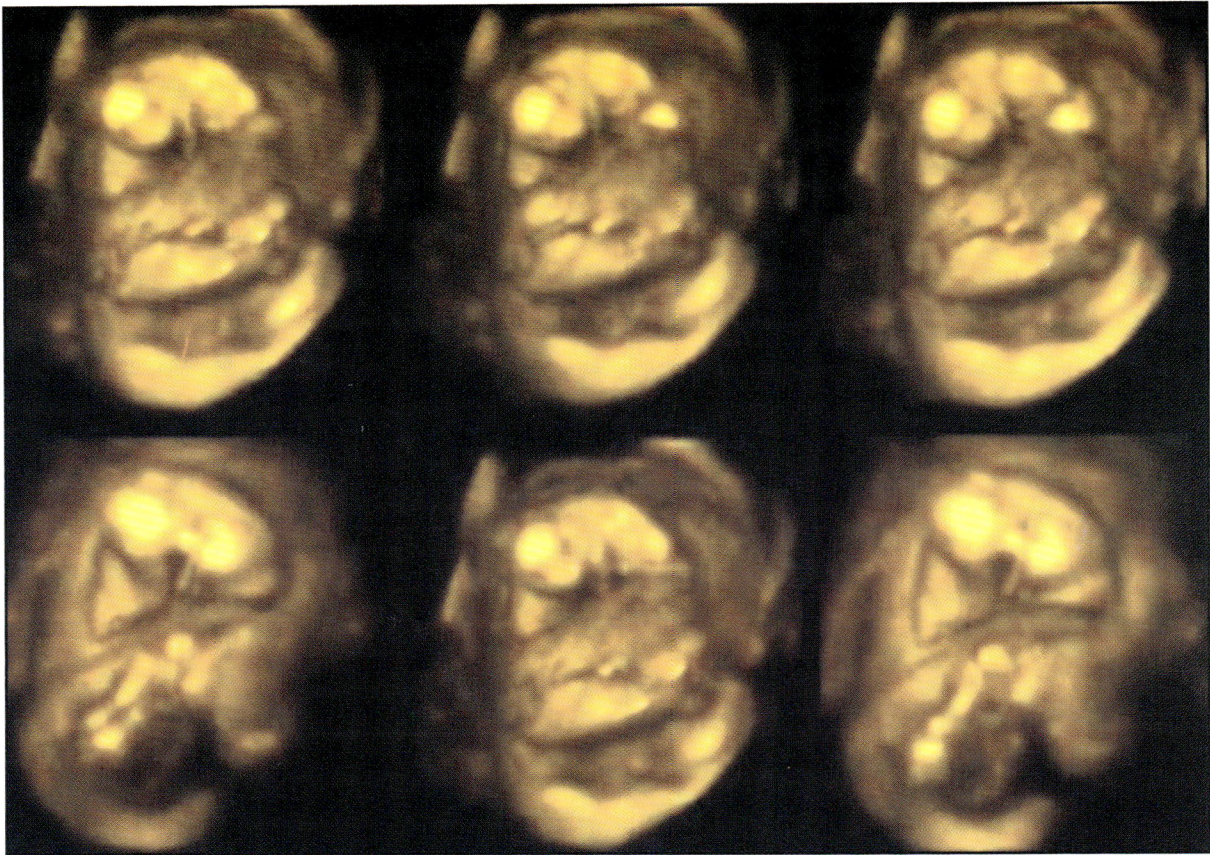

Fig. 12.113: 4D sequence of twins demonstrated active stretching movement of the second twin (below), while the first twin (upper) seems to be passive

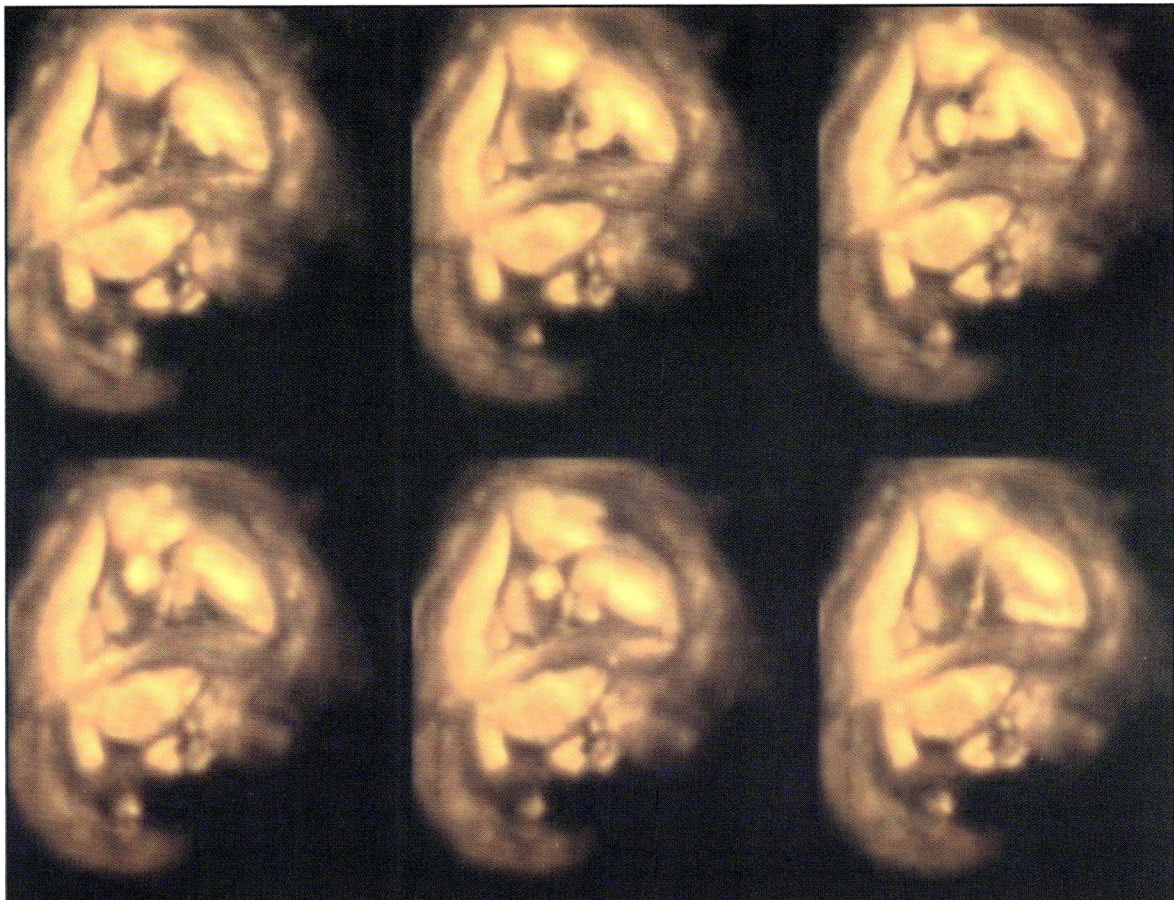

Fig. 12.114: 4D imaging illustrated active fetal hand movement from the first twin (upper), while the second twin (below) is passive

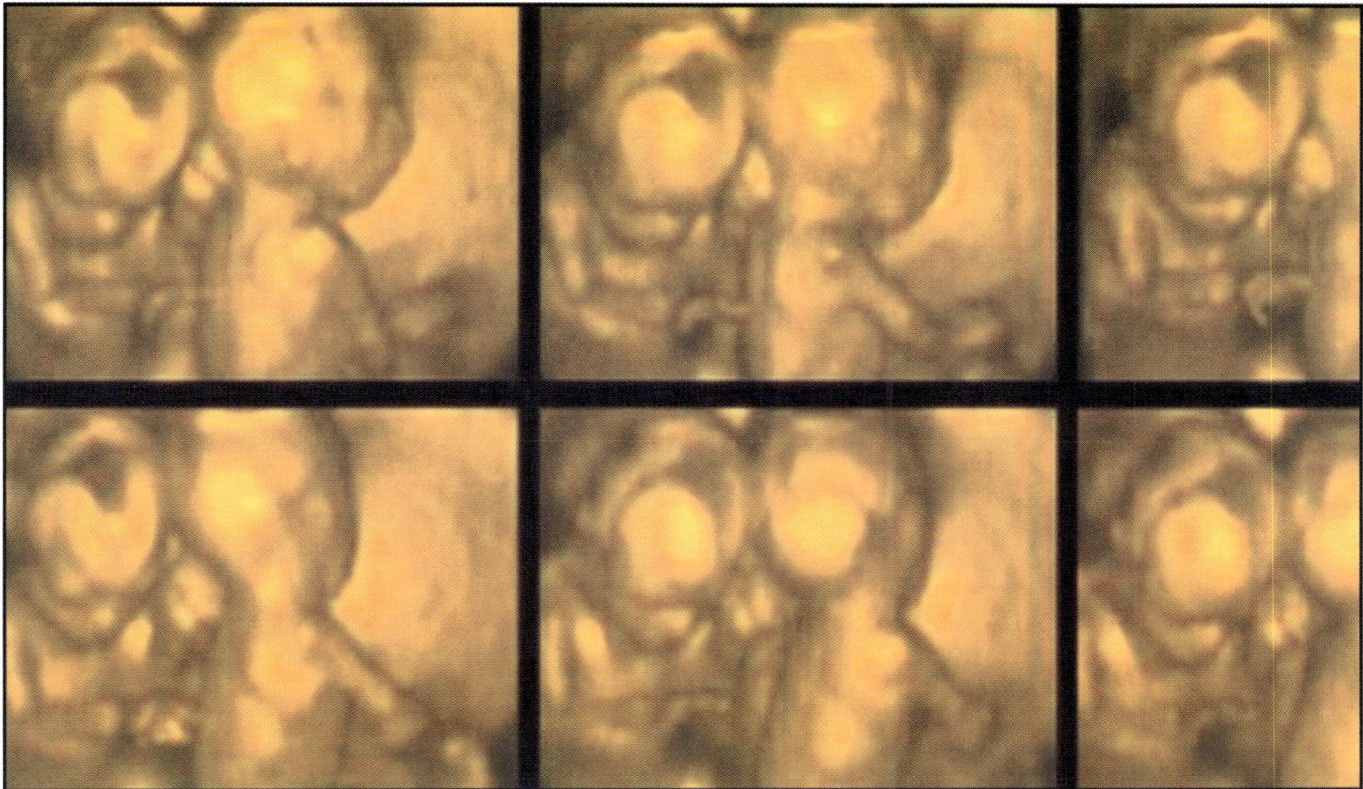

Fig. 12.115: 4D sequence of fetal motoric activity in both fetuses. Note the intertwin contact from the first fetus (left)

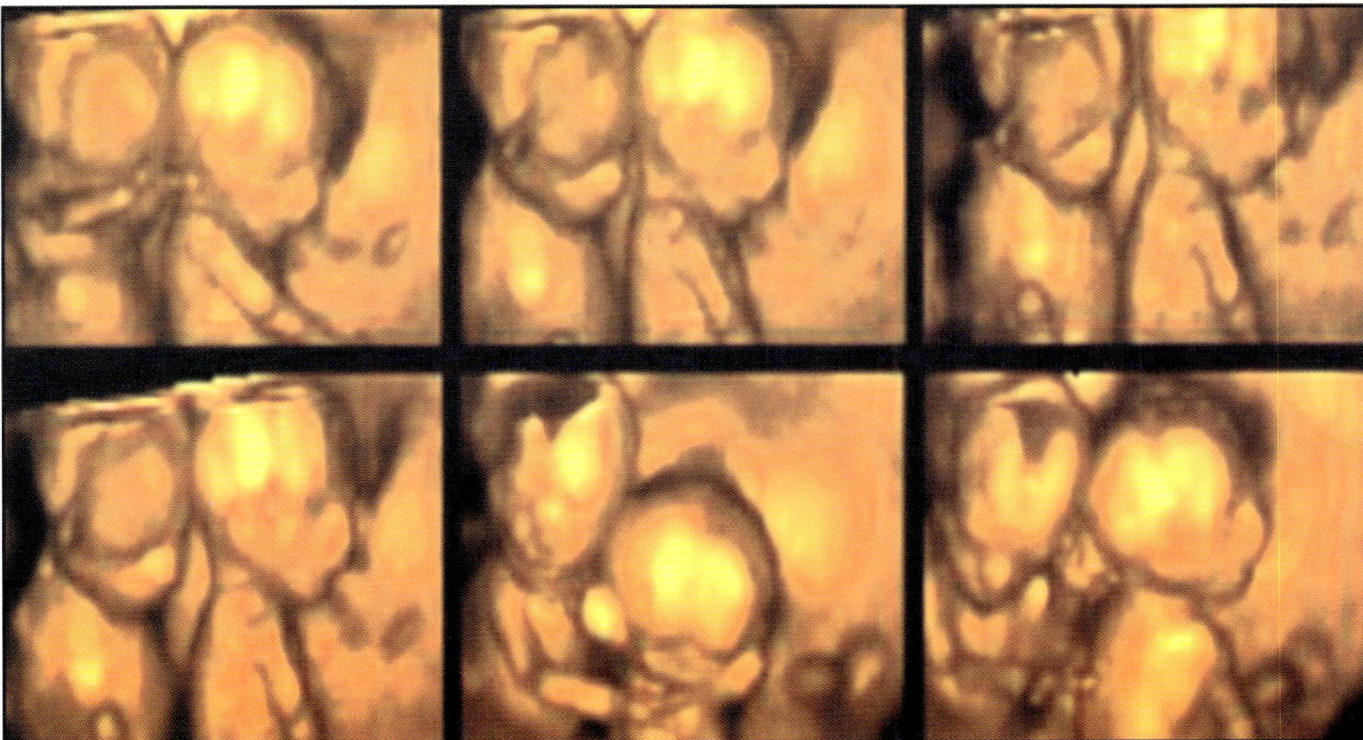

Fig. 12.116: 4D scan demonstrated separated evaluation of fetal activity of each twin. The first twin (left) demonstrated active body movements, while the second twin (right) is passive

14. Maggio M, Callan NA, Hamod KA, et.al. The first-trimester ultrasonographic diagnosis of conjoined twins. Am J Obstet Gynecol. 1985;152:833-5.

15. Lam YH, Sin SY, Lam C, et.al. Prenatal sonographic diagnosis of conjoined twins in the first trimester: two case reports. Ultrasound Obstet Gynecol 1998;11:289-91.

16. Meizner I, Levy A, Katz M, et.al. Early ultrasonic diagnosis of conjoined twins. Harefuah 1993;124:741-4, 796.

17. Tongsong T, Chanprapaph P, Pongsatha S. First-trimester diagnosis of conjoined twins: a report of three cases. Ultrasound Obstet Gynecol. 1999;14:434-7.

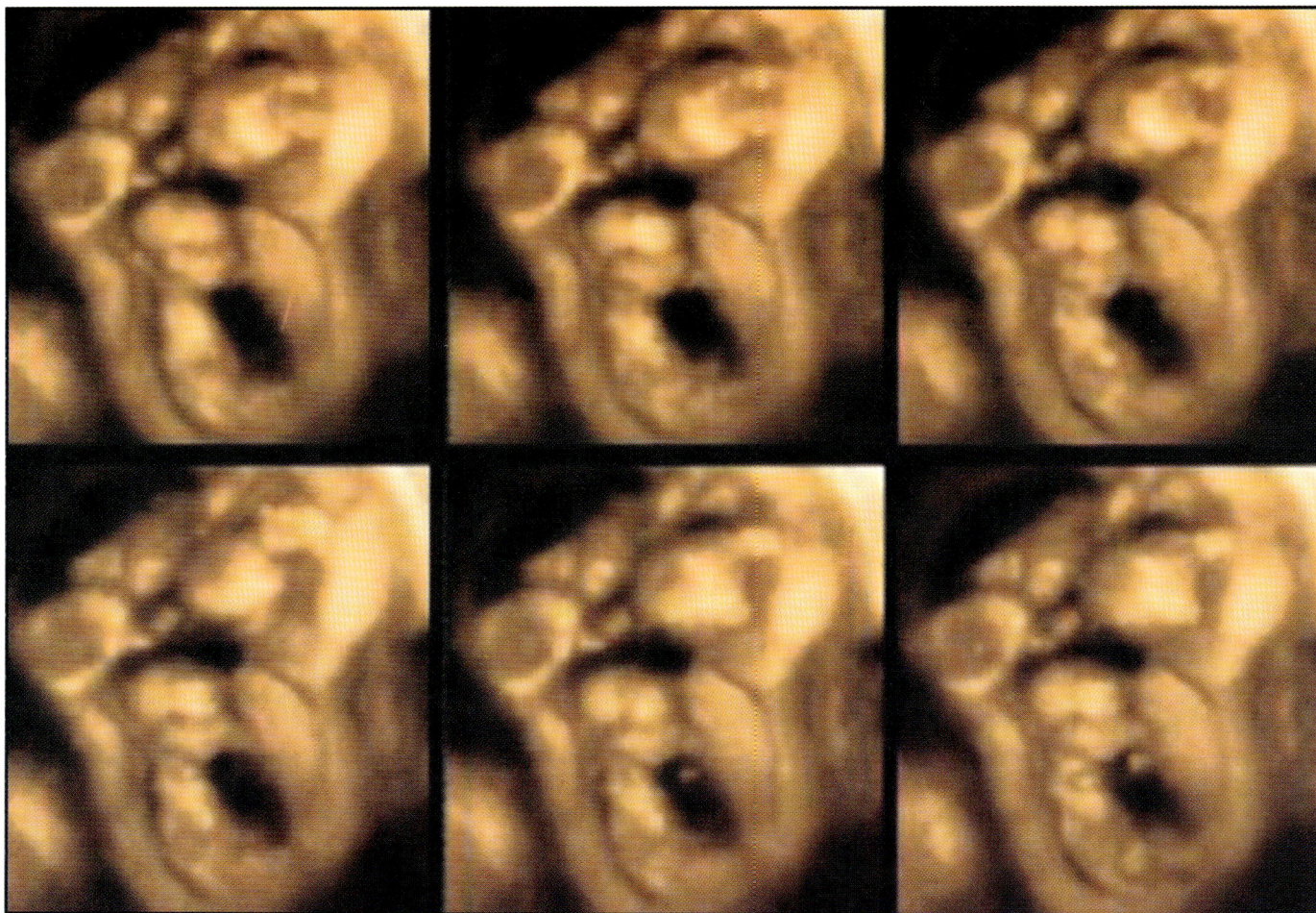

Fig. 12.117: 4D sequence demonstrated separated evaluation of fetal activity of each twin in triplet pregnancy

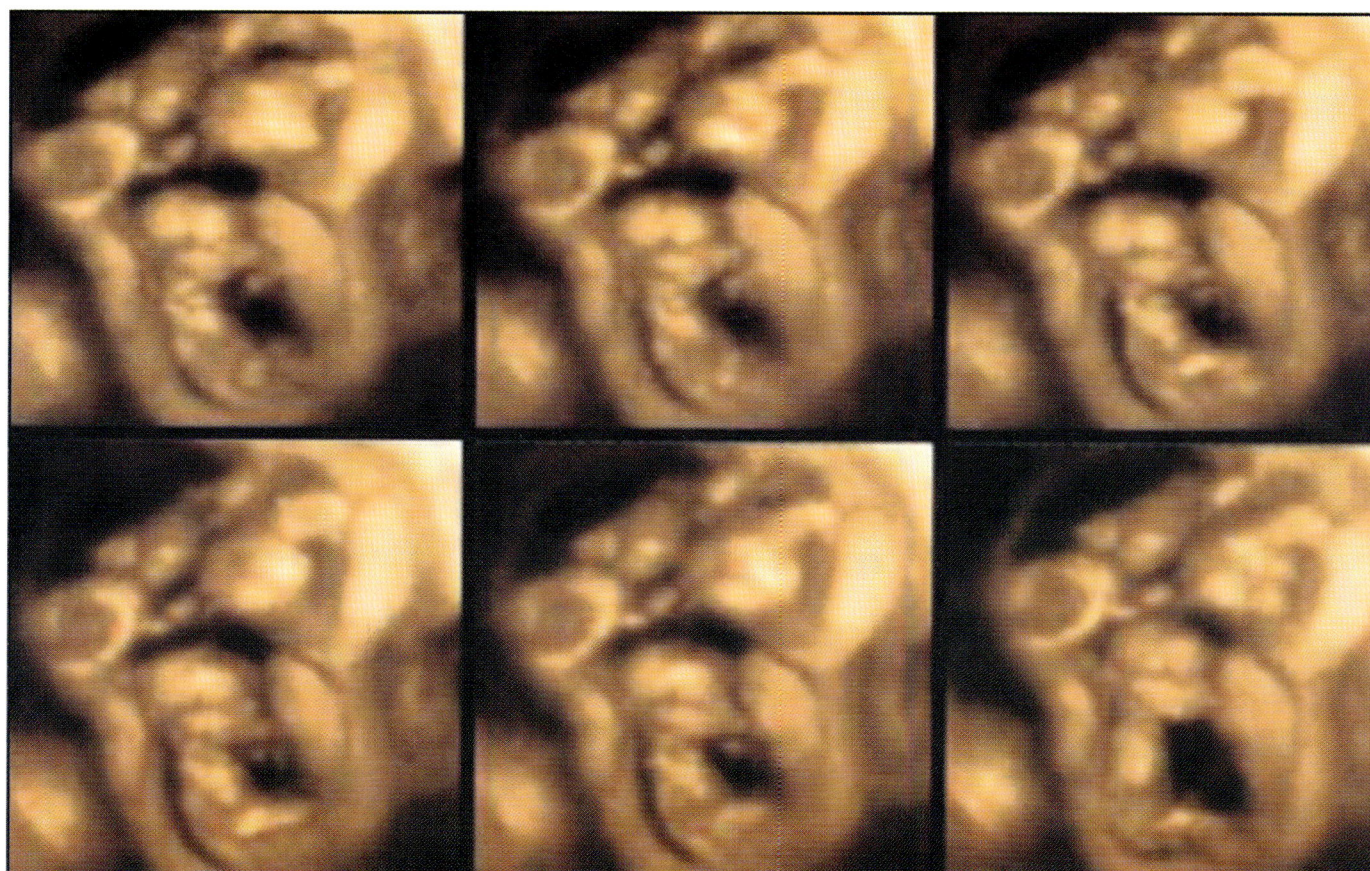

Fig. 12.118: 4D image demonstrated change of position of each twin in triplet pregnancy

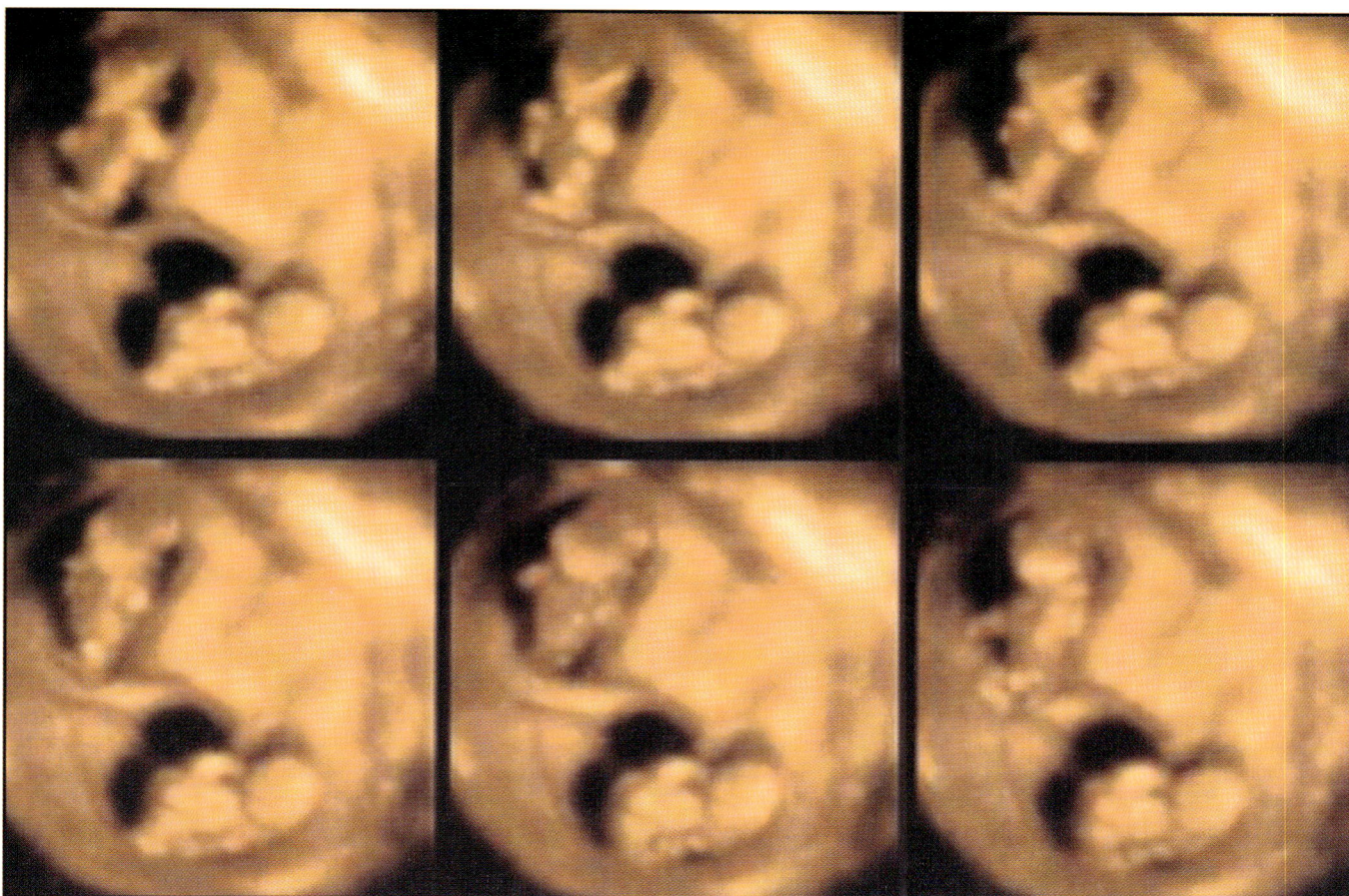

Fig. 12.119: Missed triplet at 13th week of pregnancy by 4D sonography. On the figure sequence the activity of only one twin can be recognized

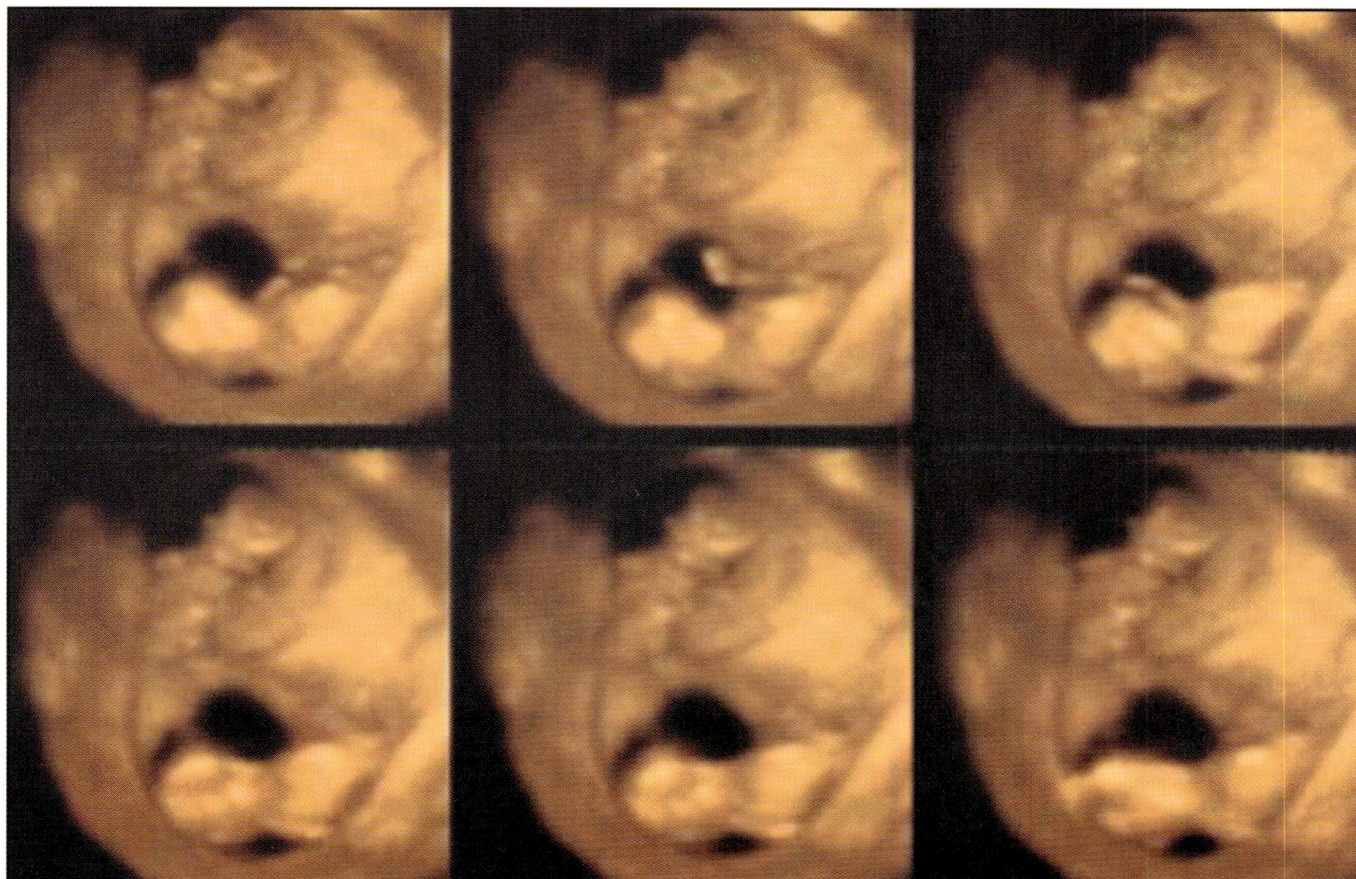

Fig. 12.120: Missed triplet and isolated motoric activity of only one fetus. On this 4D sequence the activity of only one twin can be recognized. Moreover, because of spatial imaging even type of movement can be recognized. It is isolated hand to fluid movement of the first triplet

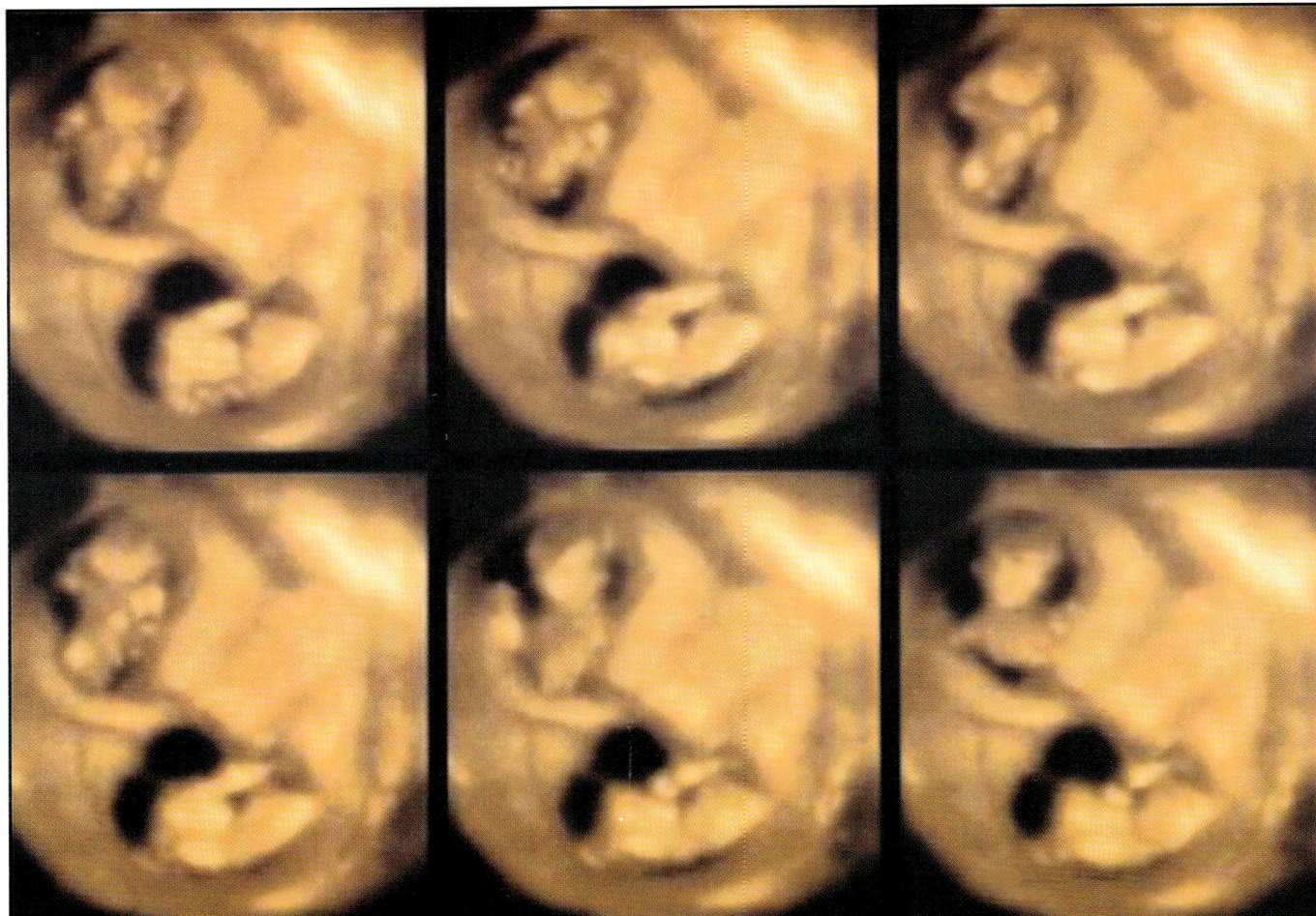

Fig. 12.121: Missed triplet at 13th week of pregnancy diagnosed by 4D sonography. Simultaneous asssessment of complete motoric activity of each fetus can be performed because of simultaneous visualization of two fetuses

18. Usta IM, Awwad JT. A false-positive diagnosis of conjoined twins in a triplet pregnancy: pitfalls of first trimester ultrasonographic prenatal diagnosis. Prenat Diagn. 2000 ;20:169-70.

19. Weiss JL, Devine PC. False-positive diagnosis of conjoined twins in the first trimester. Ultrasound Obstet Gynecol. 2002;20:516-8.

20. Maymon R, Halperin R, Weinraub Z, et.al.Three-dimensional transvaginal sonography of conjoined twins at 10 weeks: a case report. Ultrasound Obstet Gynecol. 1998 ;11:292-4.

21. Doubilet PM, Benson CB. "Appearing twin": undercounting of multiple gestations on early first trimeseter sonograms. Journal of Ultrasound in Medicine. 1998;17:199-203.

22. Tadmor OP, Achiron R, Rabinowiz R, et al. Predicting first-trimester spontaneous abortion. Ratio of mean sac diameter to crown-rump length compared to embryonic heart rate. J Reprod Med. 1994 ;39:459-62.

23. Xu HX, Zhang QP, Lu MD, et.al. Comparison of two-dimensional and three-dimensional sonography in evaluating fetal malformations. J Clin Ultrasound. 2002 ;30:515-25.

24. Kurjak A, Kos M, Veèek N. Pitfalls and caveates in ultrasound assessment of triplet pregnancies. In Keith LG, Blickstein I, Eds. Triplet pregnancies and their consequences. Canforth, UK: Parthenon Publishing 2002:85-105.

25. Grandjean H, Larroque D, Levi S. The performance of routine ultrasonographic screening of pregnancies in the Eurofetus Study. Am J Obstet Gynecol 1999 ;181:446-54.

26. Dickey RP, Olar TT, Taylor SN, et.al. Incidence and significance of unequal gestational sac diameter or embryo crown-rump length in twin pregnancy. Hum Reprod 1992;7:1170-2.

27. Weissman A, Achiron R, Lipitz S, et.al.The first-trimester growth-discordant twin: an ominous prenatal finding. Obstet Gynecol 1994;84:110-4.

28. Vecek N, Rijlarsdam R, Arabin B.Diskordantes Wachstum in Mehrlingsschwangerschaften. 2o. Kongress für Perinatale Medizin Berlin. 2001;29.11-1.12.

29. Gassner R, Metzenbauer M, Hafner E, et.al. Triploidy in a twin pregnancy: small placenta volume as an early sonographical marker. Prenat Diagn. 2003;23:16-20.

30. Downey DB, Fenster A, Williams JC. Clinical utility of three-dimensional US. Radiographics 2000;20:559-71.

31. Downey DB, Fenster A. Vascular imaging with a three-dimensional power Doppler system. Am J Roentgenol 1995;165:665-8.

32. Dudiak CM, Salomon CG, Posniak HV, et al. Sonography of the umbilical cord. Radiographist. 1995;15:1035-42.

33. Reinold E.Clinical value of fetal spontaneous movements in early pregnancy. J Perinat Med 1973;1:65-72.

34. Vecek N, Solak M, Erceg-Ivkosic I. Four-dimensional sonography in multiple pregnancy. Gynecol Perinatol 2003;12:157.

35. Sadovsky E, Ohel G, Simon A. Ultrasonographical evaluation of the incidence of simultaneous and independent movements of twin fetuses. Gynecol Obstet Invest 1987;23:5-9.

36. Ferrari F, Cioni G, Prechtl HFR. Quantitative changes of general movements in preterm infants with brain lesions. Early Hum Dev 1990;23:193-7.

37. Kurjak A, Vecek N, Kupesic S, et.al. Four dimensional ultrasound: how much does it improve perinatal practice? In Carrera JM, Chervenak FA, Kurjak A, (Eds): Controversies in Perinatal Medicine, Studies on the Fetus as a Patient. New York: Parthenon Publishing, 2003:222–34.

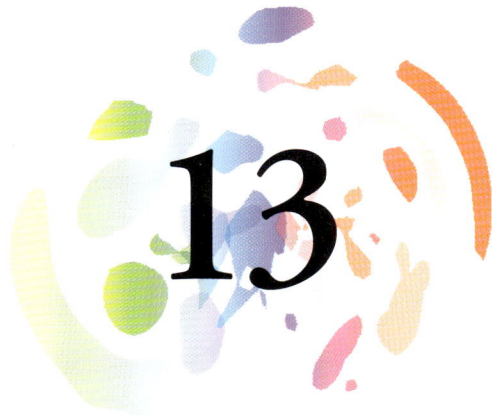

**JM Carrera, M. Torrents, A Muñog,
N Maiz, C. Millán, E Scazzochio,
M Ruiz, MA Rodriguez**

13

Prenatal Diagnosis of Congenital Defects

ULTRASONOGRAPHIC PRENATAL DIAGNOSIS OF MALFORMATIONS

JM Carrera

INTRODUCTION

The principal types of congenital defects (CDs) and their frequency, relative to the number of births and total defects, are indicated in Table 13.1.

Table 13.1: Congenital defects: Types and frequencies

Types	% over births	% over all CD
• Morphological defects	3	60
• Monogenic defects	1.4	28
• Chromosomal disorders	0.6	12
Total	5	100

As it can be observed the malformations constitute, in order of frequency, the CDs numerically higher (3% of all births), followed by monogenic disorders (1.4% of all births) and chromosomal syndromes (0.6% of all births).

The CDs are originated during prenatal development through perturbation of the mechanisms that act during maturation of the gametes and/or during embryonic or fetal development, causing various alterations or patterns (Table 13.2) depending on the pathogeny.

The referred figures vary notably depending on geographical area, ethnic factors, socioeconomic conditions, and, especially, on the methodology utilized in the gathering of information. On the other side, about 30 to 40 percent of CDs studied are finally considered to be of unknown cause. This proportion is especially high in the case of structural defects (Table 13.3).

The index of specific prevalence of various CDs also varies largely depending on the consulted literature.

Ultrasound will be able to detect only morphological anomalies, that have a sufficient anatomical expressiveness, or

Table 13.2: Terminology and pathogenetic classification of morphological defects

Congenital defect:	Anomaly of the morphological, structural, functional or molecular development, which is present at birth (even if it can show later), external or internal, familiar or sporadic, hereditary or non-hereditary, single or multiple. In practice, "congenital defect," "conatal defect" and "birth defect" are considered synonymous.
Malformation:	Structural defect in an organ, part of an organ, or a region of the organism that results from a process of intrinsically abnormal development.
Deformation:	Anomalies of the form or the position of a part of the organism caused by strong intrauterine mechanics that distort the normal structures.
Disruption:	Morphological or structural defect of an organ, part of an organ, or a region of the organism resulting from interference in a process of the development that originally was normal.
Dysplasia:	Abnormal cellular organization (or function) within a specific tissue.
Sequence:	Combination of functional changes or structural defects derived from a unique, known or suspected malformation, disruption, or mechanical factor.
Syndrome:	Pattern of multiple anomalies (malformations, disruptions, deformities, or dysplasia) that affect multiple areas of development, and that are related etiopathogenetically.

Table 13.3: Proportion of cases with known and unknown etiology

	All congenital defects (%)	Structural defects (%)
1. Known etiology	70	40
• Chromosomal abnormalities	2	6
• Monogenic inheritance	4	8
• Multifactorial	56	21
• Chronic maternal disease	1	2
• Maternal infection (TORCH)	4	2
• Chemical (Alcohol-Drugs)	3	1
2. Unknown etiology	30	60

that are accompanied by signs, features, stigmas or markers that can be detected by means of conventional ultrasound and associated techniques. There are several tables or lists, with the grade or percentage of diagnosticability of each anomaly. But the figures change according to the ultrasonographic technology used, and especially the experience of the operator.

Diagnostic Capacity of Ultrasound

Progressive improvements in ultrasound equipment have permitted its diagnostic capacity within the field of prenatal diagnosis of structural fetal anomalies to obtain a sensitivity range of 90 to 95 percent and a specificity range of 95 to 100 percent.[1]

However, these results are only obtained when three basic prerequisites occur: (a) sufficient preparation of the echographist, who should be an expert in fetal dismorphology, (b) utilization of the appropriate instrumentation (high definition equipment, with additional features offered), (c) correct management of prenatal diagnosis allowing the echographist sufficient time, and access to acceptable ultrasound tests for all gestations at the appropriate period.

Appropriate management must include a system of rational levels.

Ultrasonographic Levels

There exists a notable consensus in classifying ultrasound into three levels that take into consideration the preparation and ability of the echographist, and the contents of the exploration.

1. *Level I:* "Obstetrics echography" is performed at this level (State I). It is a simple and brief examination, due to the limitations of equipment and personnel. It consists of the inspection of general fetal anatomy accompanied by a elemental biometry (to verify the gestational age on the basis of CRL), and provides necessary information as to the volume of amniotic fluid, number of fetuses, and viability.

    This level is insufficient if the objective is, with certainty, prenatal diagnosis for the majority of malformations. The reason being that the majority of these examinations are performed by doctors who dedicate only a small part of their time to the practice of echography, and have relatively little experience in prenatal diagnosis.

2. *Level II:* Responsible for the "echography of fetal anatomy" (State II). It consists in an expert and particular study of fetal anatomy, that permits diagnosis of the majority of major malformations.

    This level is performed by doctors with several years of experience in ultrasound diagnosis, and that have familiarity with fetal dismorphology.

    Furthermore, it includes stringent demands on equipment and facilities. It is advisable that it should be located within a hospital and belong to a regional organization.

3. *Level III:* The standard examination at this level is classified as "echography of special fetal anatomy" (State III). It consists of the anatomic, biometric, and functional study of the fetus, utilizing high resolution technology, and it is adept in revealing those problems not detected by levels I and II.

    Echographists, at this level, have a high level of expertise in prenatal diagnostic echography of congenital defects

(specially in the fields of echocardiography and echoneurography), operate within an integrated prenatal diagnostic center, and have at their disposal the support of specialists in other areas (geneticists, cardiologists, dismorphologists, pathologists, pediatricians, neonatal surgeons, etc).

Of course, the rate of PD of fetal malformations has a close relation with the level of the examiner: 22 percent in level I, 40 percent in level II, and 90 percent in level III.

Diagnostic Strategy

In the actuality a majority of countries have adopted the following diagnostic strategy:

1. All gestations must be echographically tested, in accordance with the protocols commonly recommended, to establish a minimum of three-four echographies. These echographic examinations should be performed in level I.

2. The echography done at 18 to 20 weeks, as it is known to be fundamental for diagnosing prenatal malformations, must always be performed in level II.

3. High risk gestations of malformations are to be selected in the first level of screening, and refered to the level II for further study.

4. Level III receives all those with doubtful results from lower levels, specially cardiologic and encephalic pathologies that, due to their complexity, present diagnostic and assistantial problems.

Screening of Malformations

From an epidemiological point of view, there are three possible types of screening:

1. The *population screening* of a given geographical area (several hospitals and doctors taking part, and the diagnosis capacity of several operators is very different).

2. *Multicentric screening*, with patients of two or more centers (working with similar protocols), and

3. Hospital-based screening, whose results are referred to a single hospital, with its particular features. Obviously the results are very different.

The majority of reports of population screening show a detection rate from 20 to 40 percent. In the multicentric screening, results are much better: 60 to 70 percent of detection rate, and finally, the best results are got in some hospital-based screening (level 3 hospital) 80 to 90 percent of detection rate (Table 13.4).

Table 13.4: Topography of fetal abnormalities detected by the ultrasound screening program at Institut Universitari Dexeus (1970-2001)

Topography (single or main anomalies	n	%	n	%	n	%
Renal and urinary tract	508	25.4	484	95.3	227	54.5
Head and neck	348	17.4	296	85.1	226	64.9
Skeleton/muscles	194	9.7	161	83.0	114	58.8
Heart	260	13.0	229	88.1	157	60.4
Gastrointestinal tract	90	4.5	69	76.7	36	40.0
Spinal defects	80	4.0	61	76.3	49	61.3
Ascites/hydrops	86	4.3	82	95.3	55	64.0
Thoracoabdominal wall	63	3.1	59	93.7	30	79.4
Genital tract	69	3.4	45	65.2	23	33.3
Lung	57	2.8	53	93.0	38	66.7
Diaphragm	41	2.0	38	92.7	28	68.3
Polymalformed/ misclellaneous	206	10.3	169	82.0	142	68.9
Total	2002	100.0	1746	87.2	1125	59.6

NORMAL ANATOMY AND MALFORMATIONS OF THE FETAL CENTRAL NERVOUS SYSTEM

M Torrents, C Millán, A Muñoz

INTRODUCTION

Prenatal assessment of the fetal central nervous system (CNS) plays an important role in the field of perinatology. The brain rapidly develops in utero and remarkably changes its appearance from the primitive brain structure in early stage to the well-developed brain in the late pregnancy.[2]

Anomalies in this region are of considerable importance, as they often determine survival, physical appearance and function in society. Some advantages are obtained with the recent introduction of 3D and 4D sonography. They are reviewed in the separate chapters of this book.

NORMAL ANATOMY

A systematic approach to sonographic examination of the fetal neural axis is necessary to reveal the numerous possible abnormalities in this complex region. This topic is important to each person performing obstetric ultrasound, as a careful evaluation of the fetal neural axis should be considered to be an integral part of all second and third trimesters ultrasound examinations.

Neuroimaging of Normal Brain Structure

Following figures will show normal brain imaging in each cutting section of axial, sagittal, parasagittal and coronal sections. Axial section is used to evaluate cerebellar structure, midline, symmetry of both hemispheres (Figs 13.1 and 13.2). In median sagittal section, the corpus callosum (from 18th weeks of gestation),

septum pellucidum, fourth ventricle and sagittal section of cerebellum are demonstrated (Figs 13.3 and 13.4). In parasagittal section, lateral ventricle and choroid plexus, subarachnoid space and insula are visualized (Figs 13.5 and 13.6). In anterior coronal section, anterior horns of lateral ventricle, corpus callosum and sylvian fissure, and in posterior coronal section, posterior horns and cerebellum are demonstrated (Figs 13.7 and 13.8). In late pregnancy, gyral formation is clearly demonstrated (Figs 13.9 and 13.10).

Assessment of Enlarged Ventricles

Hydrocephalus and ventriculomegaly are often used interchangeably to describe dilatation of the fetal lateral ventricles. However, they should be distinguished from each other to assess the enlargement of ventricles. Hydrocephalus is a dilatation of the lateral venticles resulted from increased amount of cerebrospinal fluid and intracranial pressure, while ventriculomegaly is a dilatation of lateral ventricles without increased intracranial pressure due to hypoplastic cerebrum or other intracerebral abnormalities such as agenesis of corpus callosum (Table 13.5). In sonographic imaging, these two intracranial conditions can be differentiated by visualization of subarachnoid space and appearance of choroids plexus (Figs 13.11 and 13.12). The transvaginal oblique and coronal images demonstrate the obliterated subarachnoid space and the dangling choroid plexus in the case of hydrocephalus. In contrast, the subarachnoid space and choroid plexus are well preserved in the case of ventriculomegaly (Fig. 13.13).[3] It is difficult to evaluate obliterated subarachnoid space in the axial section. Therefore, it is suggested that the evaluation of fetuses with enlarged ventricles may be evaluated by parasagittal and coronal views taken by transvaginal way.

Table 13.5: Causes of ventriculomegaly

Hydrocephalus	Atrophy or encephalic destruction	Colpocephalus
↓	↓	↓
Obstruction or overproduction of cephalochoroideus liquid	Encephalic development and posterior destruction	Insufficient encephalic development

Head

Historically, serial transverse sonograms have proved very helpful in evaluating fetal intracranial anatomy.

When accessible to ultrasound examinations, the fetal head is most often in an occiput-transverse position (i.e. the side of the head lies parallel to the mother's abdominal wall). Also, the membranous bones of the fetal cranium do not reflect sound

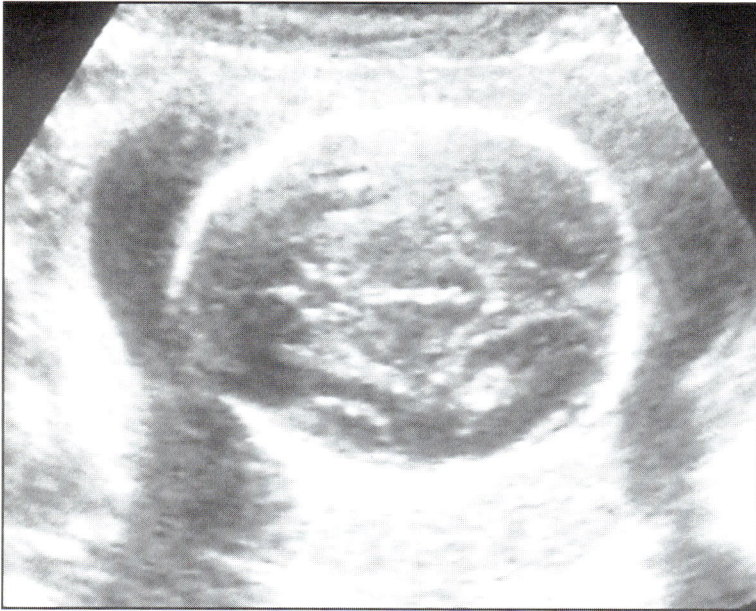

Fig. 13.1: Normal lateral ventricles and cavum septum pellucidum

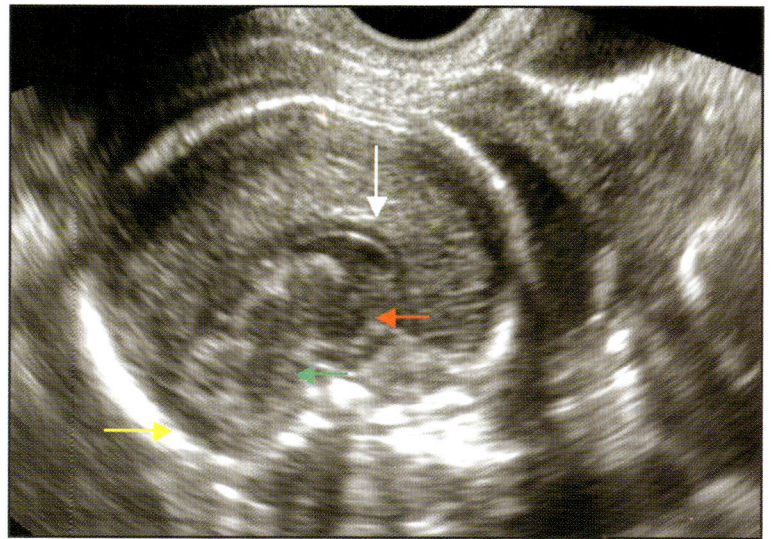

Fig. 13.2: Normal posterior fossa, (oblique views): Cisterna magna, cerebellar hemispheres, mid cerebellar vermis and fourth ventricle

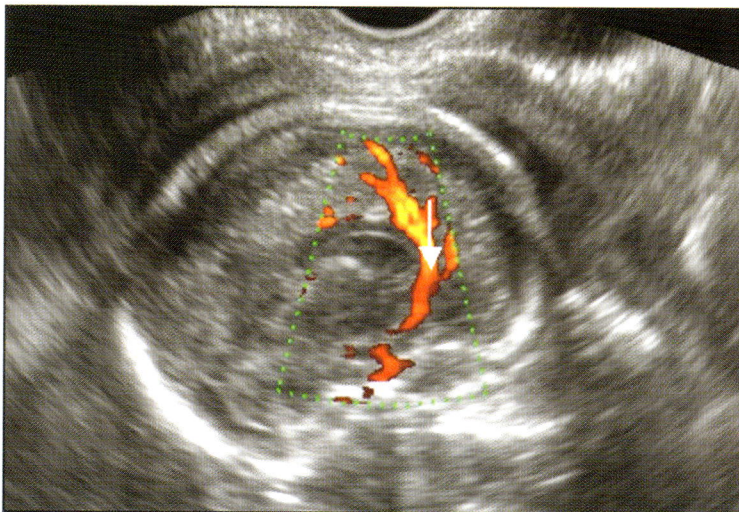

Fig. 13.3: Parasagittal view shows the corpus calosum as an hypoechoic semicircular image (white arrow). Color Doppler shows the pericallosal artery. Under the corpus callosum the cavum of the septum pellucidum is observed and below the red arrow indicates the third ventricle

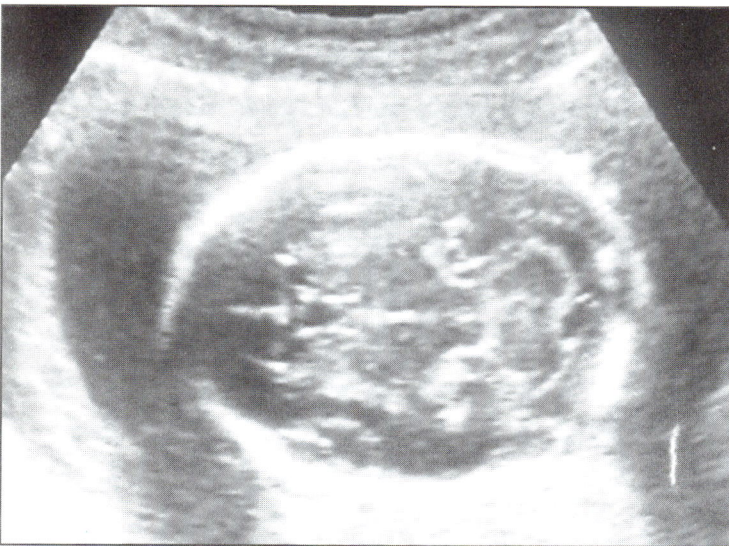

Fig. 13.4: At the posterior fossa the yellow arrow indicates the cisterna magna and the green arrow the fourth ventricle

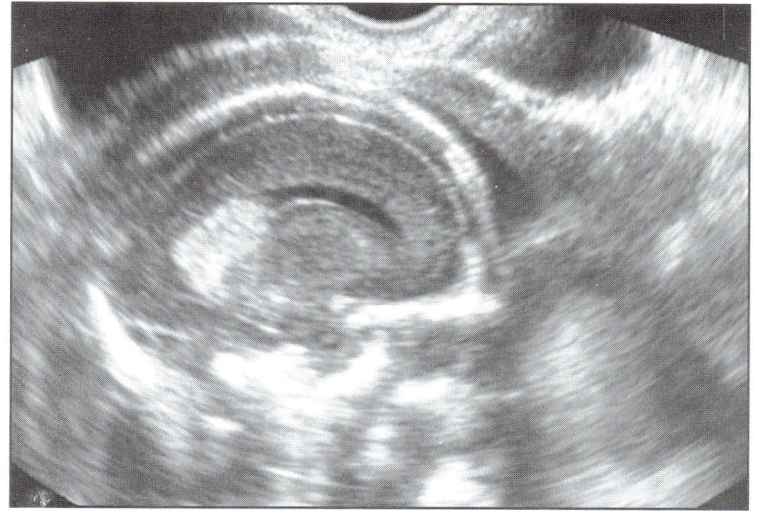

Fig. 13.5: Sagittal scan that shows both lateral ventricles. The dense image of the choroid plexus is observed at the posterior side of the lateral ventricles

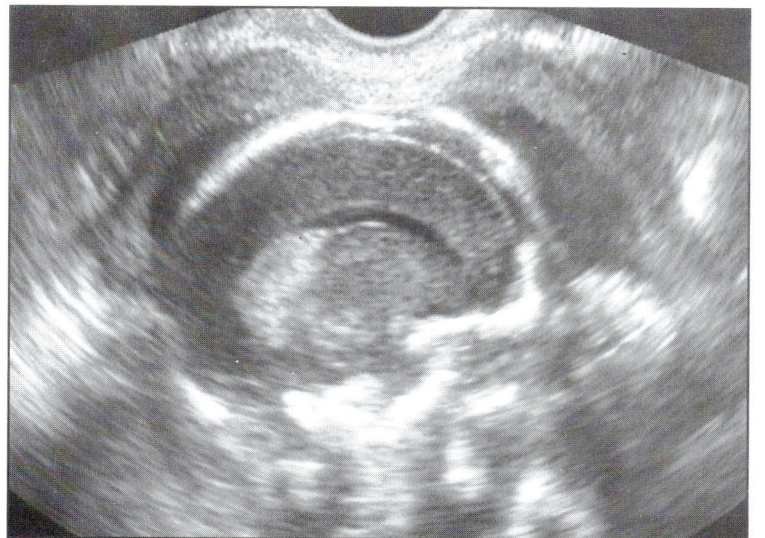

Fig. 13.6: Sagittal scan that shows both lateral ventricles. The dense image of the choroid plexus is observed at the posterior side of the lateral ventricles

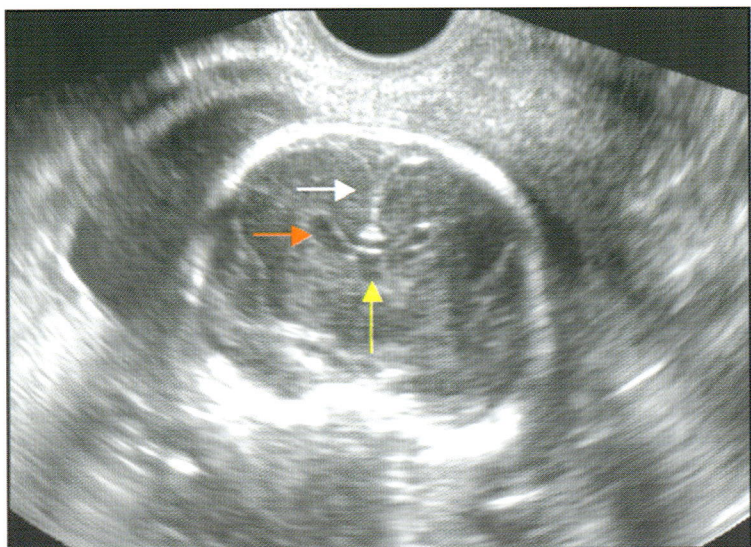

Fig. 13.7: Coronal scan: White arrow shows the echogenic falx, surrounding the subarachnoid spaces. The red arrow indicates the lateral ventricle and the yellow arrow shows the cavum of the septum pellucidum

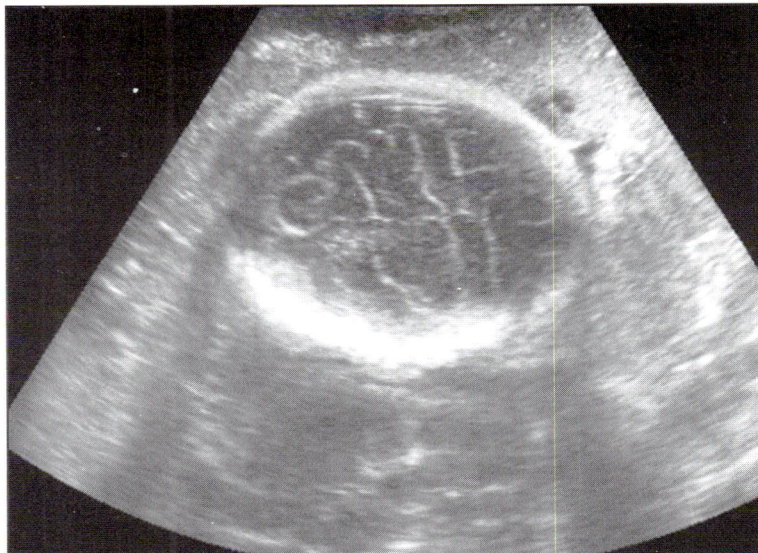

Fig. 13.10: High coronal scan in the third term of pregnancy showing the cerebral convolutions

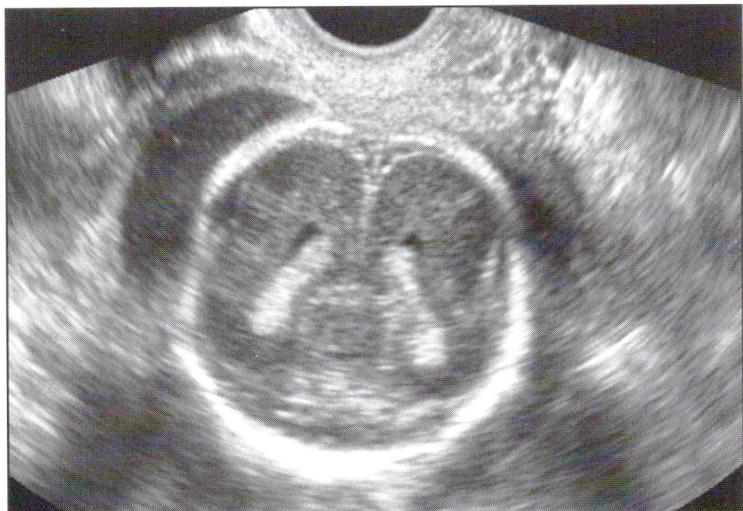

Fig. 13.8: High axial scan that shows the lateral ventricles with the choroid plexus inside (dense image)

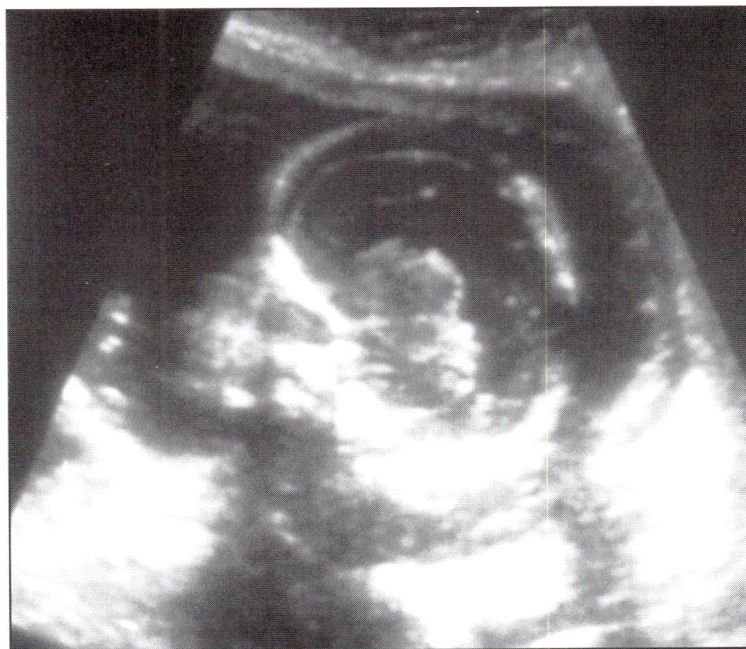

Fig. 13.11: Communicant hydrocephalus

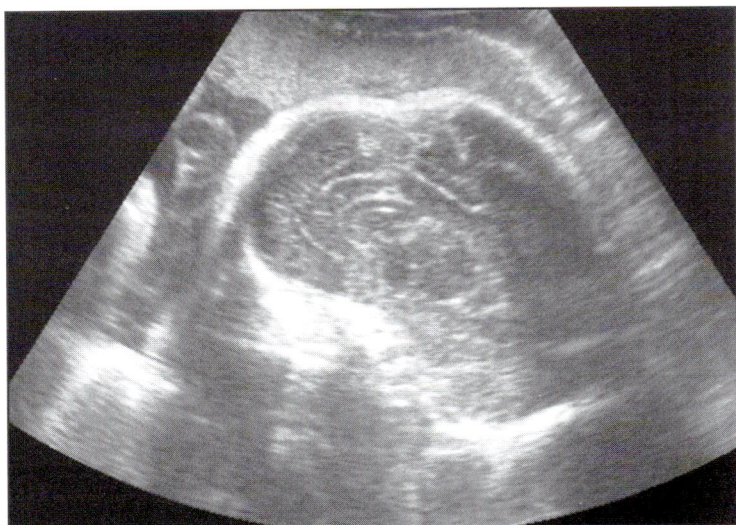

Fig. 13.9: Mid sagittal scan in the third term of pregnancy. The corpus callosum is clearly seen

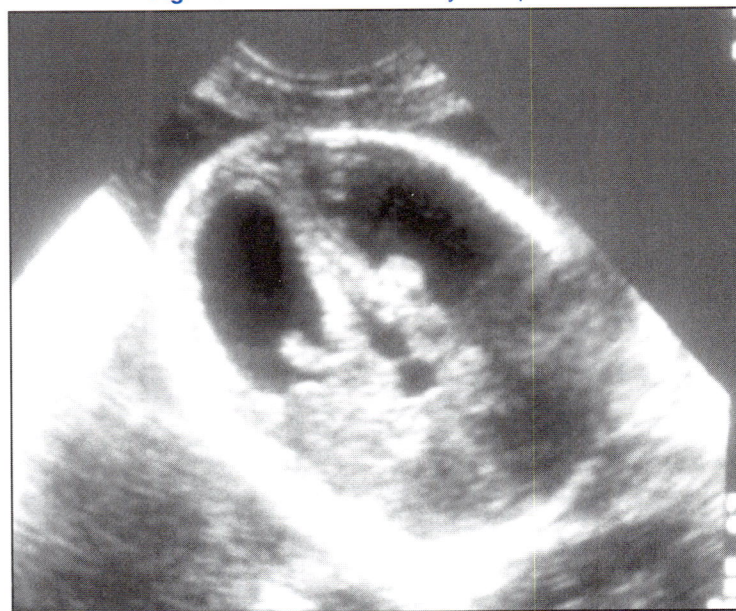

Fig. 13.12: Non-communicant hydrocephalus

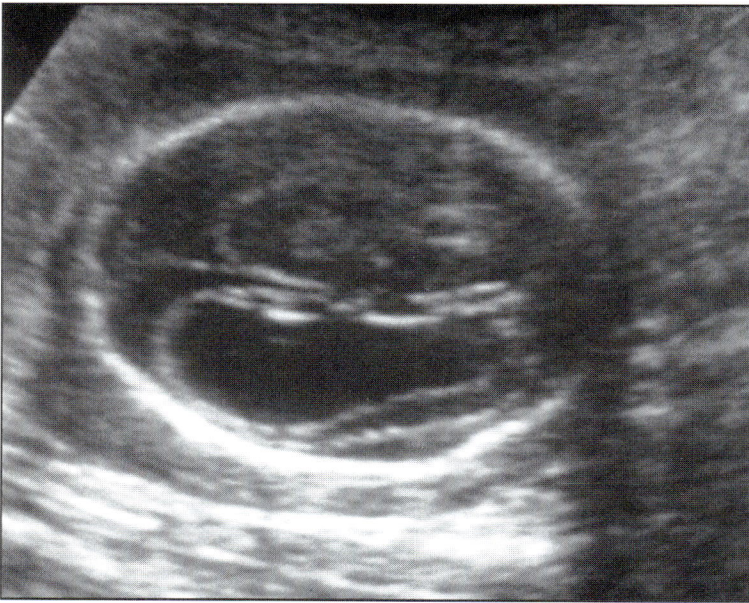

Fig. 13.13: Brain atrophy

waves to the extent that they do when they are more heavily calcified and rigid, in postnatal life. Finally, a transverse plane produces a large cross-section of the brain, in which multiple landmarks may be visualized at one time for orientation. The distal ventricle (i.e. the one farthest from the ultrasound transducer) is chosen for study, as reverberation artifacts often obscure the anatomy of the proximal hemisphere. A prominent echogenic area is often seen within the lateral ventricle, which represents the choroid plexus.

In early fetal life, the ventricular system fills a large portion of the developing brain and has the form of two smooth, curved tubes joined above the third ventricle. As gestation progresses, the ventricular system develops a confirmation that increasingly resembles that in adult life and occupies a decreasing proportion of the brain's volume. Sonographically, this change is manifested by a decrease in the proportion of the brain's cross-section occupied by the lateral ventricles. This evolution has been documented and nomograms generated that compare the width of the lateral ventricle to the width of the cerebral hemisphere at various gestational ages. [4-6]

Biparietal Diameter

Perhaps the most intensely studied transverse section of the fetus is at the level of the biparietal diameter (BPD).

The two landmarks most consistently found are the roughly triangular, paired, non-echogenic thalami and two short anterior lines paralleling the midline, designated the cavum septum pellucidum (see Fig. 13.1).

Cerebellum

The cerebellum may be visualized in a place parallel to the BPD plane. Once located, the cerebellar structures are best studied by rotating the ultrasound transducer farther from the

canthomedial line. In this plane, the cerebellum (with its brightly echogenic, centrally-placed vermis, and two relatively non-echogenic hemispheres) may be evaluated and measured. Frond-like folia are suggested at the borders of the hemispheres and the midbrain may be seen in front of the vermis. The cisterna magna is seen and can be measured between the vermis and the inner table of the occipital bone (see Fig. 13.2).[7,8]

Base of the Skull

The base of the skull level may be identified by an echogenic "X" formed by the lesser wings of the sphenoid bone and the petrous pyramid. These bone ridges demark the anterior, middle and posterior fossae.

Sagittal and Coronal Views

Sagittal views of the fetal brain are sometimes helpful to delineate anatomy. The relationship of midline to cranial structures can be seen in Figure 13.4. Coronal views may also be of value (see Fig. 13.7) (see the heading Agenesis of the Corpus Callosum).

Spine

By 16th week of gestation, individual vertebra may be identified by the observation of three echogenic ossification centers in the transverse plane. Two of these are posterior to the spinal canal in the lamina and one is anterior, representing the vertebral body. If the spine is scanned sagittally, a line of vertebral bodies and a line of posterior elements may be seen on either side of the non-echogenic spinal canal (Fig. 13.14). In the coronal plane, the two echogenic posterior ossification centers are seen to diverge progressively in the cervical region as one moves closer to the base of the skull (Fig. 13.15).[9]

During the third trimester, more detail may be seen. The vertebral body, pedicles, transverse processes, posterior laminae and the spinous process may all be identified as echogenic structures in transverse scans. In addition, the spinal canal and intervertebral foramina may be seen as non-echogenic areas. In the sagittal plane, a line of vertebral bodies is still seen, but the posterior echoes are more complex with spinous processes seen jutting from the line of other elements.[9]

MALFORMATIONS OF THE FETAL NEURAL AXIS

Anencephaly

Anencephaly was the first malformation diagnosed with sufficient certainty for which physicians were willing to perform elective abortion based on sonographic findings.[10]

The diagnosis of anencephaly is made when the upper portion of the cranial vault cannot be visualized. This bony structure can be seen normally after 14th week when the head is not hidden in the pelvis. The area of the cerebrovasculosa, a vascular malformation seen in this disorder, may appear as an ill-defended mass of heterogeneous density above the level of the orbits. Hydramnios may complicate these pregnancies due to poor fetal swallowing (Figs 13.16 to 13.20).

This diagnosis can be made with accuracy. In the combined experiences of six centers, over 130 cases have been detected with no false-positive diagnoses.[11,12]

Anencephaly is a lethal anomaly. The recurrence rate increases with previously affected children as with all neural tube defects.

Hydrocephalus

Hydrocephalus is characterized by a relative enlargement of the cerebroventricular system with an accompanying increase of pressure of the cerebrospinal fluid within the fetal head. Hydrocephalus has been successfully diagnosed by a lateral ventricular atrial width greater than 1 cm an abnormally increased lateral ventricle-to-hemispheric width ratio[13,14] a dangling choroid plexus,[15] and an asymmetric appearance of the choroid plexus.[16,17] Serial measurements are probably the most useful tool to define hydrocephalus in borderline cases. The location of the obstruction may be determined by observing which portions of the ventricular system are enlarged.

Once fetal hydrocephalus is diagnosed, it is essential to search for associated anomalies which have been reported to occur in 83 percent of cases. While spina bifida is the most common associated anomaly, associated structural anomalies may affect any organ system. In addition to meticulous sonographic evaluation, determination of fetal karyotype should be performed.[13, 14]

The prognosis for hydrocephaly is not dependent upon the severity of the hydrocephalus. Associated anomalies may, themselves, determine a poor prognosis (e.g. holoprosencephaly, thanatophoric dwarf with cloverleaf skull). For isolated hydrocephalus there is an outcome range from normal to severe retardation (Figs 13.21 to 13.23).

Microcephaly

Microcephaly means small head.

While different biometric standards have been described to define microcephaly in the neonate, a head perimeter 3 or more standard deviations below the mean for age seems workable, and the correlation with mental retardation is very high.

The BPD (the biometric parameter most commonly measured by sonography) is unreliable in the prediction of microcephaly, with a 44 percent false-positive rate in one study.[18]

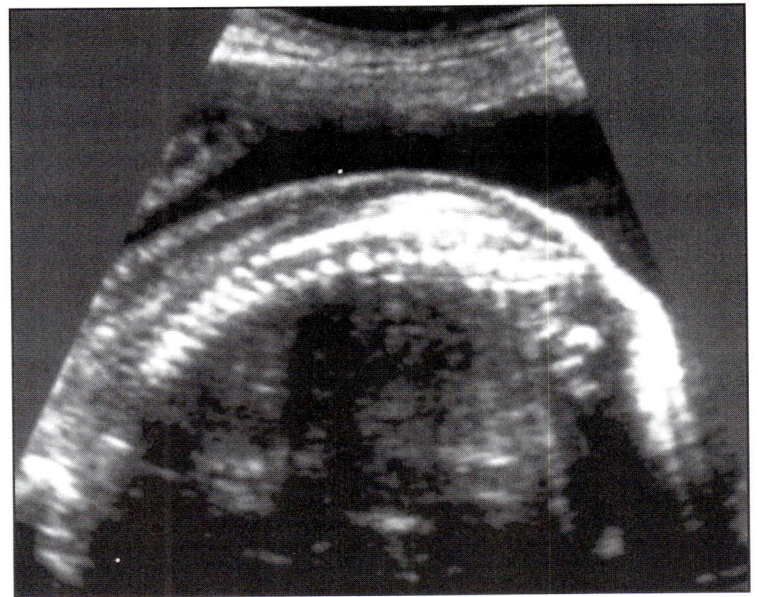

Fig. 13.14: Sagittal section through the lumbosacral vertebrae of a normal fetus

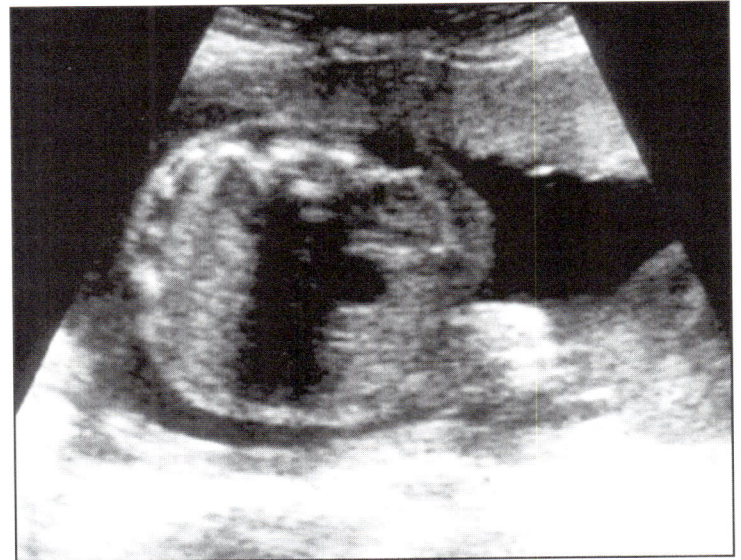

Fig. 13.15: Transverse section through the lumbosacral vertebrae of a normal fetus

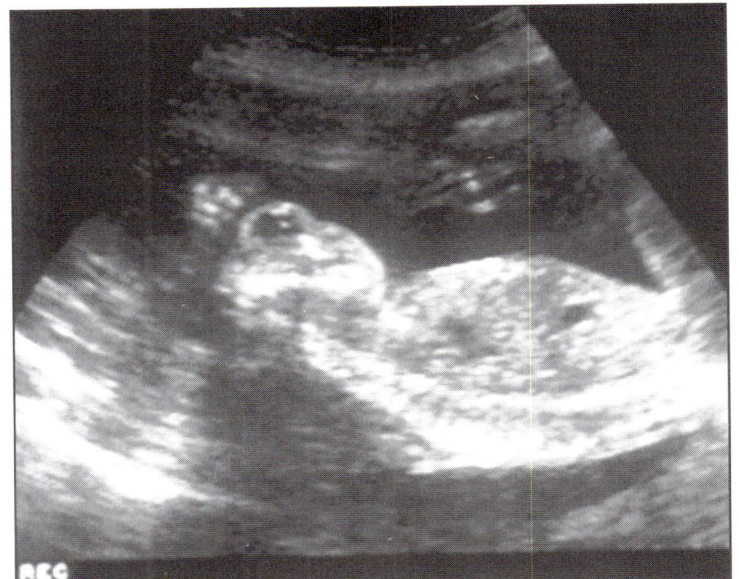

Fig. 13.16: Sagittal section of a second trimester fetus depicting the typical absence of the cranial vault above the orbits, characteristic of anencephaly

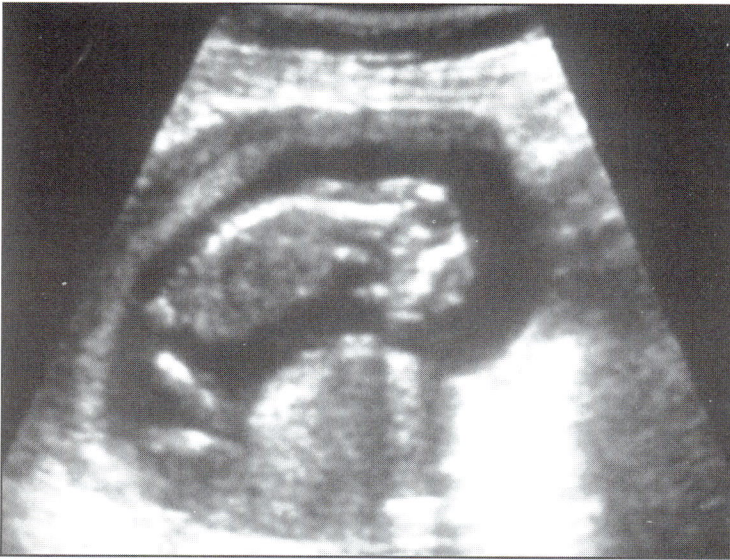

Fig. 13.17: Sagittal scan show an anencephaly with absence of brain and calvaria cephalad to the orbits

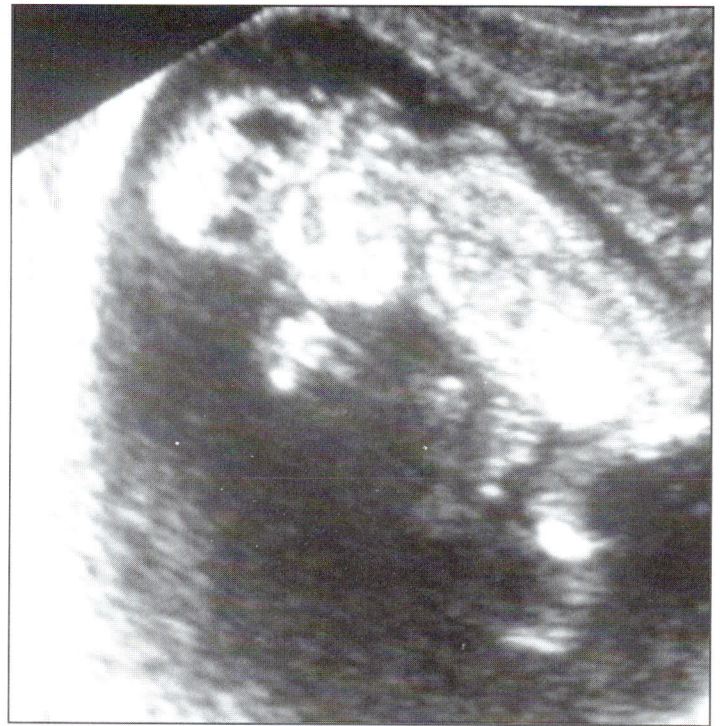

Fig. 13.19: Brain tissue surrounded by amniotic fluid

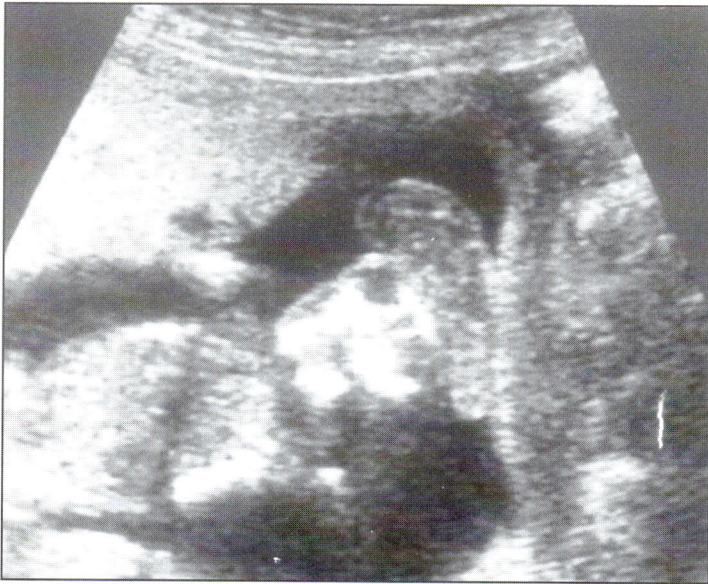

Fig. 13.18: Note the large amount of brain matter that distinguishes this condition from anencephaly. Note also that these images confirm the notion occasionally reported in the literature that acrania is a precursor stage of anencephaly

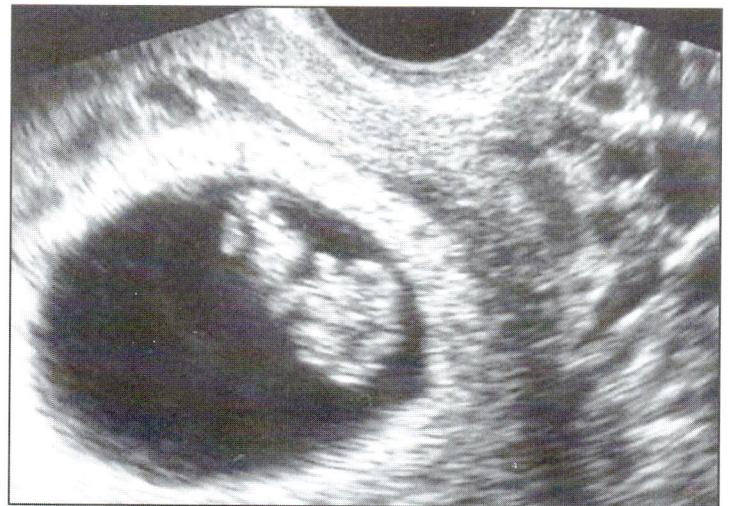

Fig. 13.20: Sagittal section of a 10-week embryo showing absence of the cranial vault

Compression of the fetal head with resultant dolichocephaly in normal pregnancies accounts for many of these errors. A nomogram of head circumference as a function of gestational age, which corrects for such compressive changes, has proved of greater predictive value. Further aids to diagnosis include nomograms of head circumference to abdominal perimeter and of femur length to head circumference ratios. At the present time, it appears that multiple fetal measurements should be utilized for greater accuracy (Figs 13.24 to 13.26).[19]

As with other malformations, the association with other anomalies increases the likelihood of a poor outcome. Risk of recurrence depends on underlying causes.

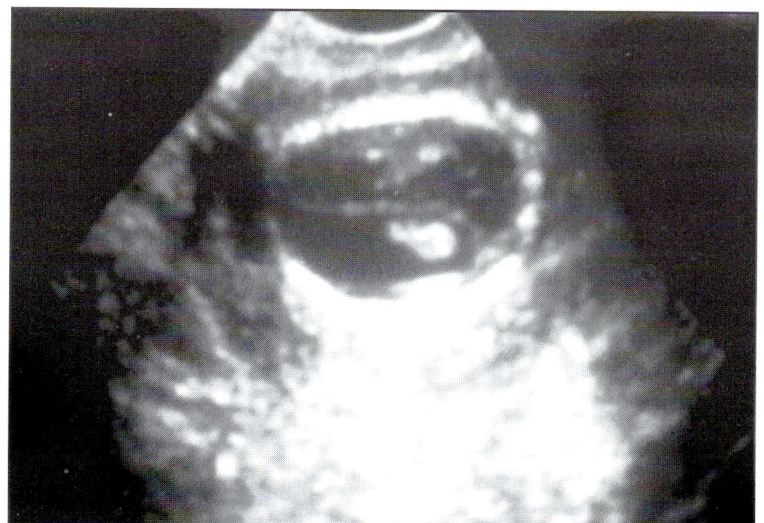

Fig. 13.21: Ventriculomegaly at 14th week

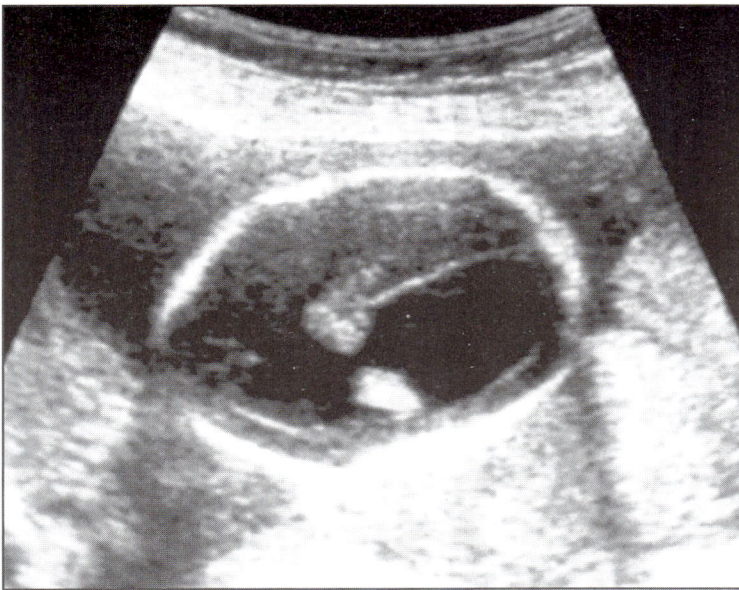

Fig. 13.22: Severe ventriculomegaly

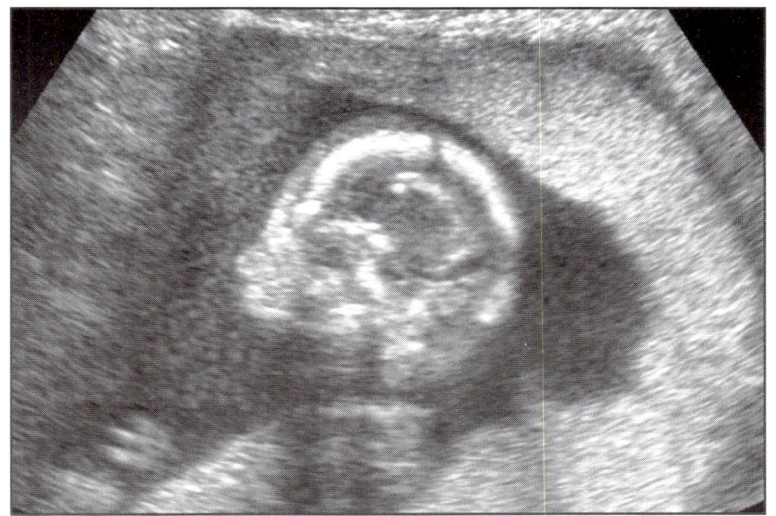

Fig. 13.25

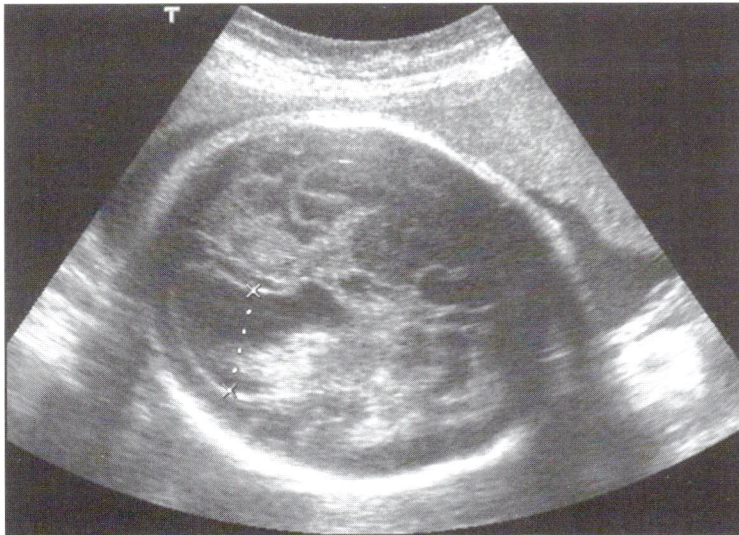

Fig. 13.23: Quadriventricular hydrocephalus secondary to hemorrhage

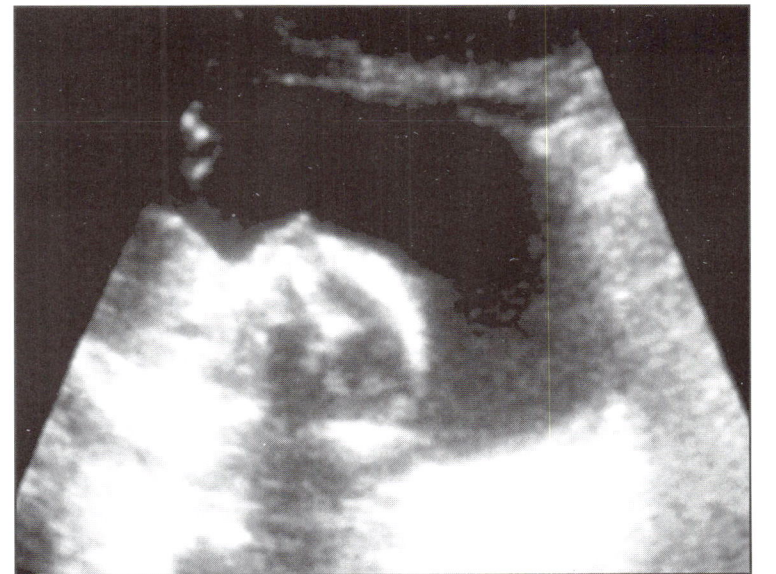

Figs 13.25 and 13.26: A sloping forehead in the fetal profile view with diminished size of the frontal lobe and abnormal shape of the head

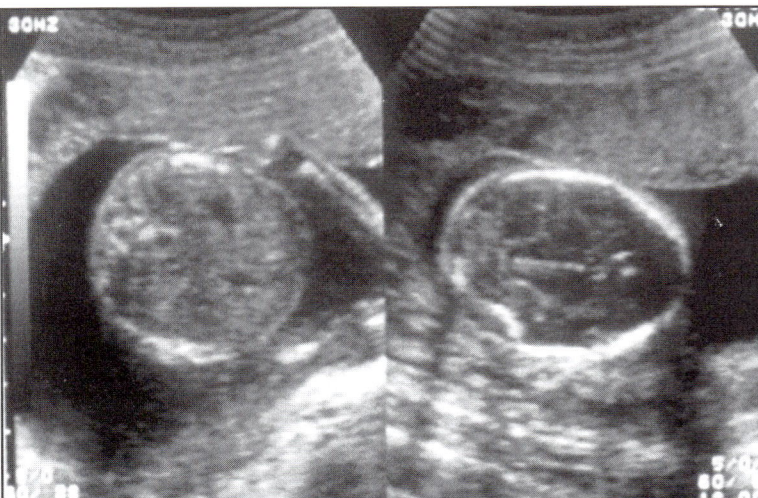

Fig. 13.24: 20 weeks and exposure to teratogens (valproic acid) smaller size of the head in comparison to the abdomen

Holoprosencephaly

Holoprosencephaly is divided into alobar, semilobar and lobar categories, all determined by the degree of separation of the cerebral hemisphere. The alobar variety shows no evidence of division of cerebral cortex. Thus, the falx cerebri and interhemispheric fissures are absent, and there is a single common ventricle. The semilobar and lobar varieties represent a higher degree of brain development with the semilobar having a partial separation and the lobar having a complete separation of the hemispheres. Microcephaly is usually present because of decreased cortical mass, but macrocephaly may be seen if hydrocephalus develops.

The prosencephalon develops from the most rostral part of the neural tube, and gives rise to the cerebral hemispheres, thalamus and hypothalamus. Failure of its sagittal division can result in a common ventricle, a fused thalamus, and a cortex with neither lobes nor an interhemispheric fissure.

In holoprosencephaly, a spectrum of midline facial anomalies may be seen. Indeed, certain facies predict the presence of the alobar type. Cyclopia, the presence of a single median bony orbit with a fleshy proboscis above it, is the most severe of malformations. In cebocephaly, hypotelorism is associated with a normally placed nose and a single nostril. Hypotelorism with a midline facial cleft also predicts the presence of alobar holoprosencephaly.

Alobar holoprosencephaly may be diagnosed before birth if two criteria are met. The midline echo, generated by the interhemispheric fissure should be absent. Hypotelorism can be detected by measuring inner and outer orbital distances. The alobar form of holoprosencephaly carries a dismal prognosis. More subtle forms of them may be associated with minimal neurologic deficits (Figs 13.27 to 13.33).[20, 21]

Cephalocele

Cephaloceles are protrusions of the meninges and frequently of brain substance through a defect in the cranium. The term includes encephaloceles which contain brain tissue, and cranial meningoceles which do not. In the western world, 75 percent of these lesions are occipital, but cephaloceles may be parietal, frontal, or nasopharyngeal.

Hydrocephalus is commonly associated with cephaloceles.[22,23]

Encephaloceles, in general, carry a poor prognosis. Pure meningoceles may have a favorable prognosis and develop normally after surgery (Figs 13.34 to 13.40).

Spina Bifida/Meningomyelocele

Spina bifida refers to a deficit in the spine resulting from a failure of the two halves of the vertebral arch to fuse. These lesions usually occur in the lumbosacral and cervical regions. If the meninges protrude through this defect, the lesion is designated a meningocele; if neural tissue is included, it is a meningomyelocele.

Sonographically, spina bifida is seen as a splaying of the posterior ossification centers of the spine giving the vertebral segment a U-shaped appearance. The posterior ossification centers should be more widely spaced than those in vertebral segments above and below the defect. It should be noted that there is a normal progressive widening of the spinal canal in the cervical region. Although the defect may be visualized on longitudinal scanning, meticulous transverse examinations of the entire vertebral column are necessary to detect smaller defects. When a meningocele or a meningomyelocele is present and intact, a protruding sac may be detected. While detection of small spina bifida defects, especially in the sacral area, remains a challenge, sonographic signs of Arnold-Chiari malformation are of adjunctive value (Figs 13.41 to 13.49).[24, 25]

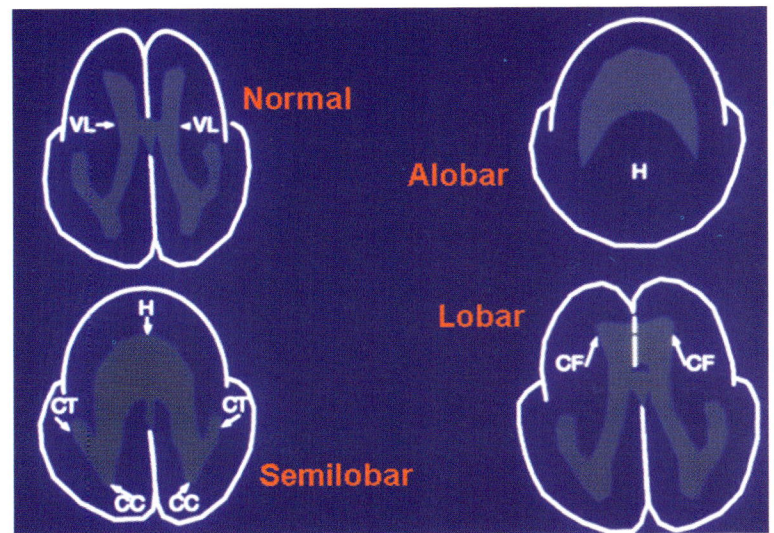

Fig. 13.27: Types of holoprosencephaly: Normal, alobar, semilobar and lobar

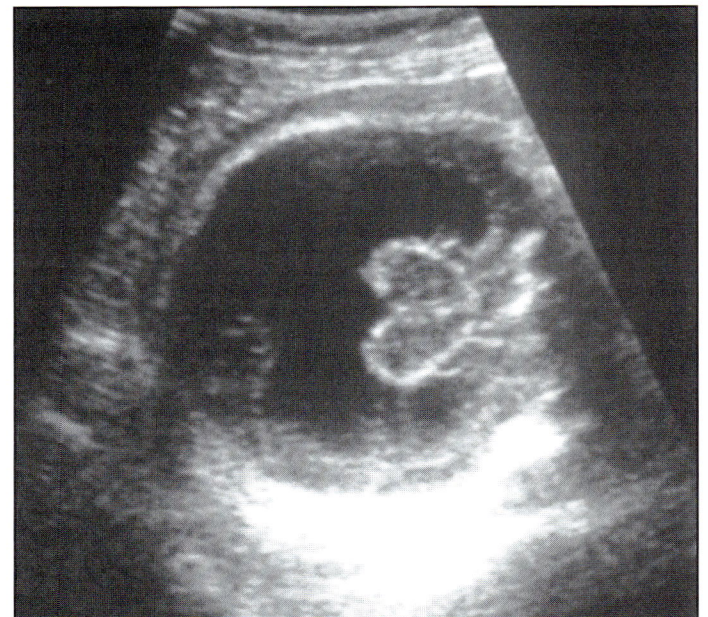

Fig. 13.28: Axial scan at the level of the thalamus, demonstrating the crescent-shaped single ventricle, absence of midline structure in the anterior cortex and fused thalamus

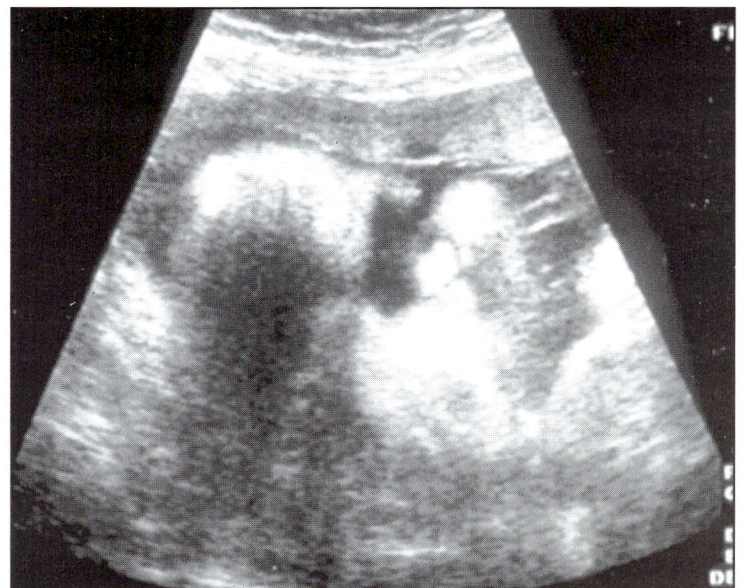

Fig. 13.29: Holoprosencephaly with facial anomalies

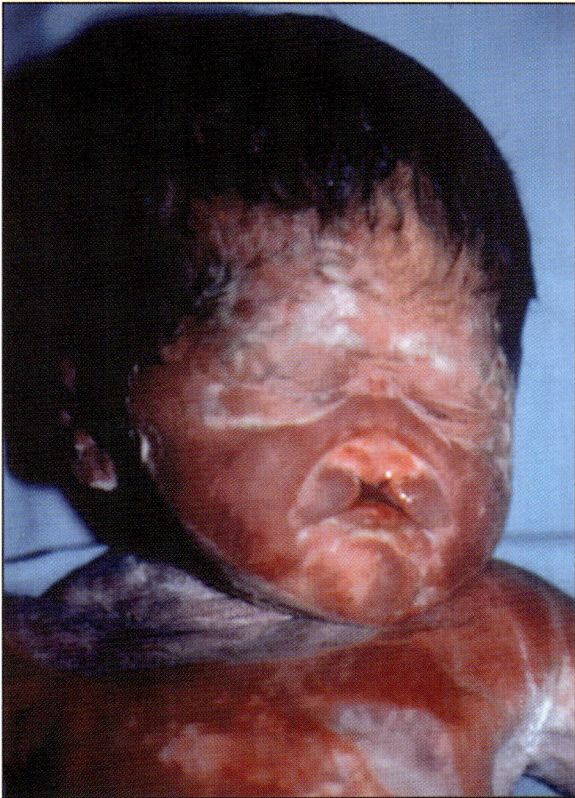

Fig. 13.30: Neonate with holosencephally; A facial anomaly

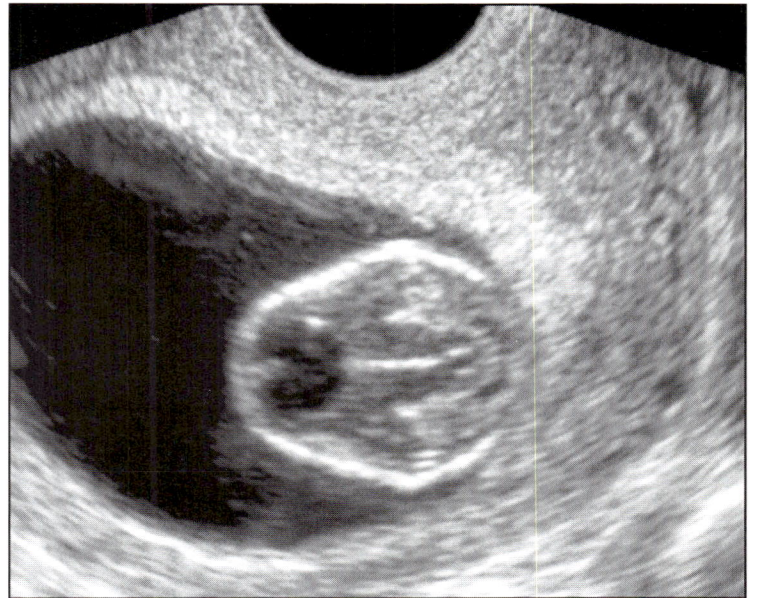

Figs 13.32 and 13.33: Semilobar holoprosencephaly: Transverse image shows partial separation of monoventricle

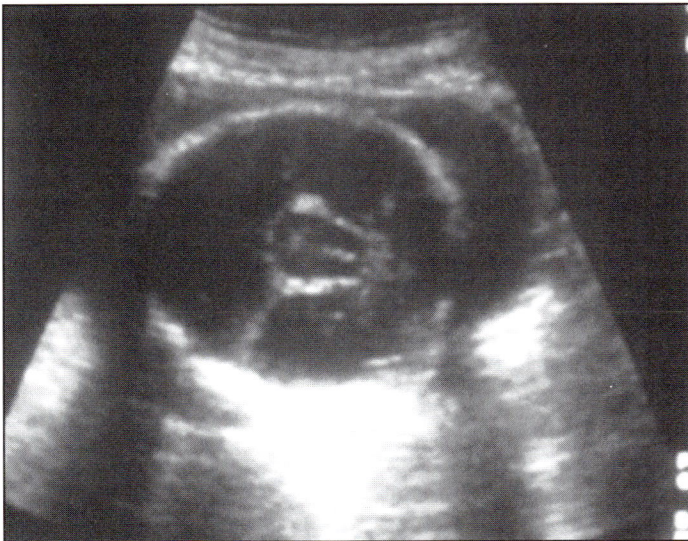

Fig. 13.31: Alobar holoprosencephaly: Transverse view of head shows prominent cerebral fused thalami

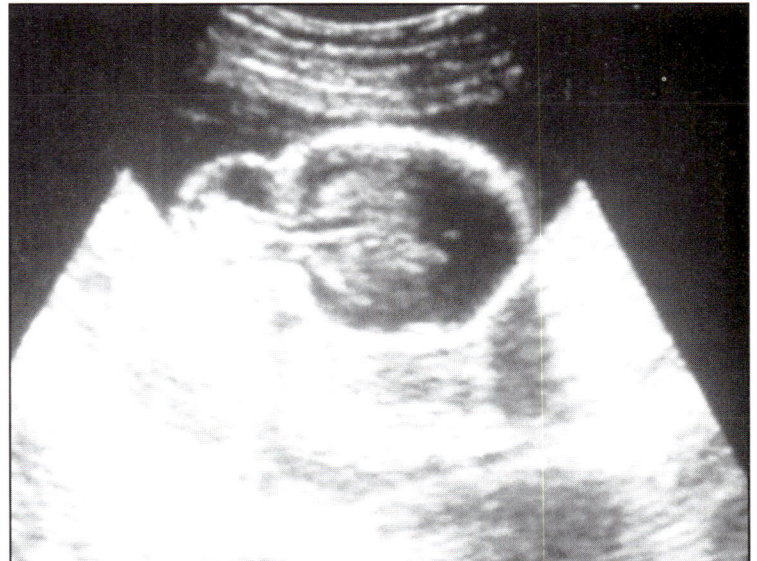

Fig. 13.34: Occipital encephalocele in a second trimester fetus. Transverse view shows defect of posterior calvaria with protrusion of brain

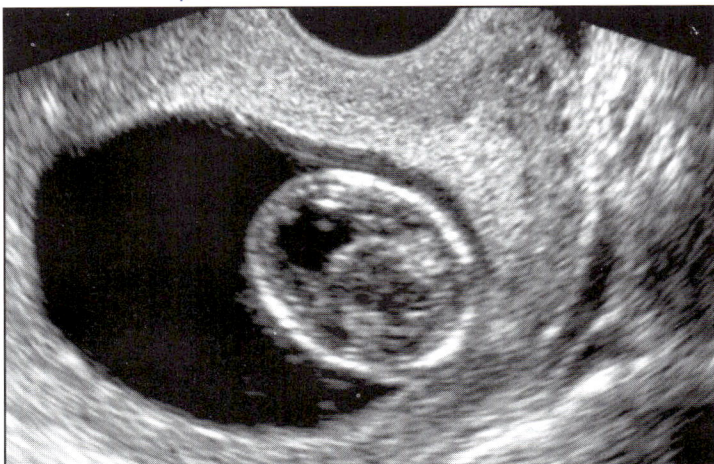

Fig. 13.32

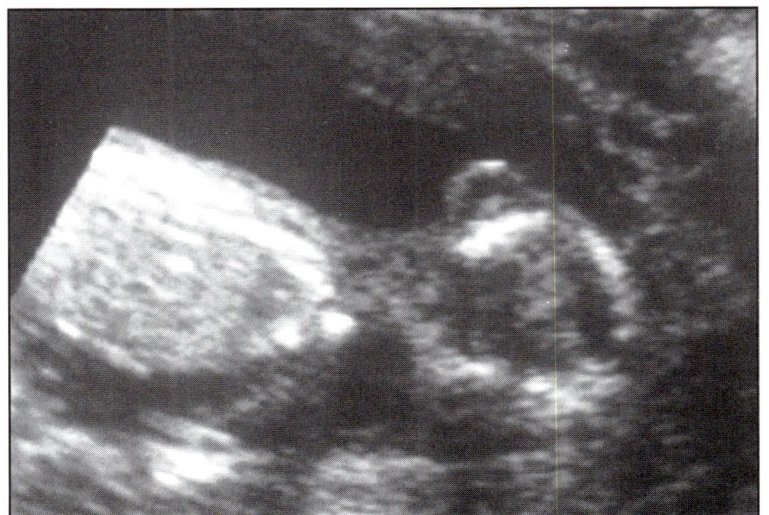

Fig. 13.35

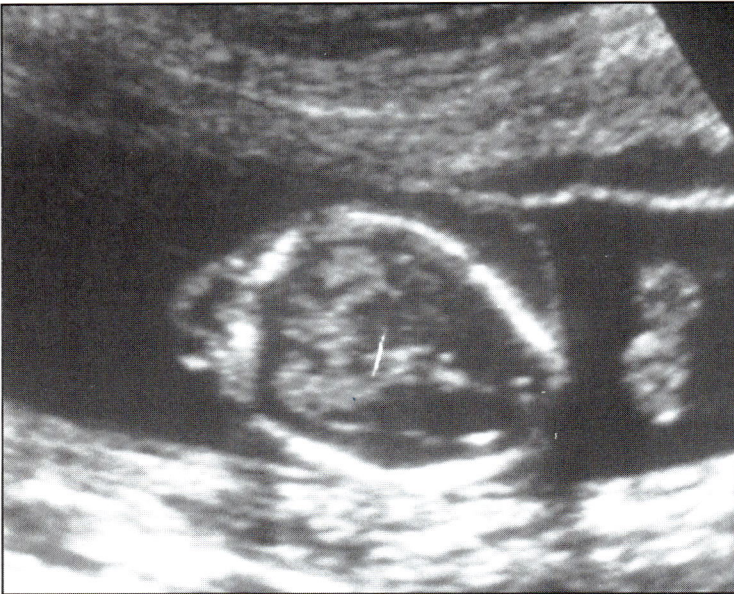

Figs 13.35 and 13.36: Small encephalocele. Small calvarian defect. It appears to contain fluid suggesting a meningocele

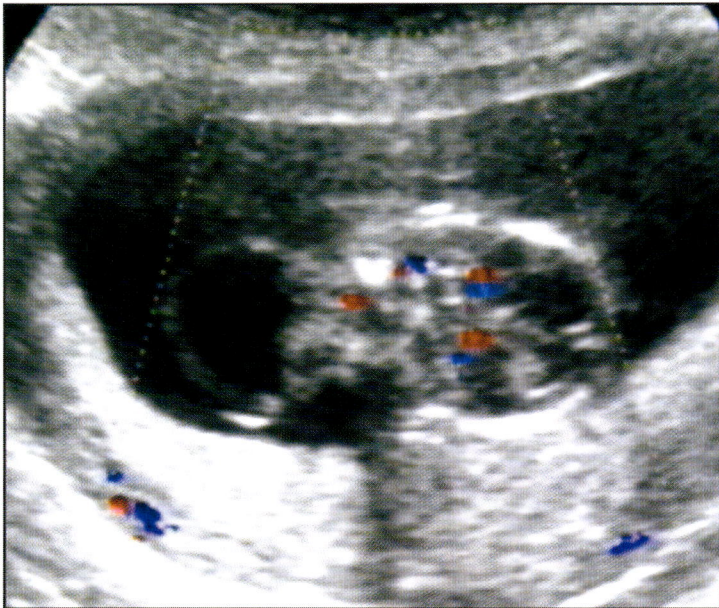

Fig. 13.37: Large encephalocele. Transverse view shows defect of posterior calvaria with protrusion of brain

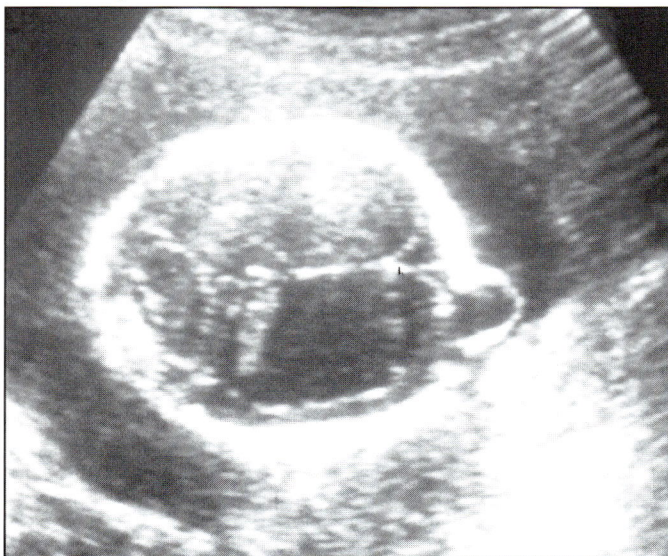

Fig. 13.38: A mass protruding from the top of the head was identified. Ultrasound evaluation confirmed a parietal encephalocele

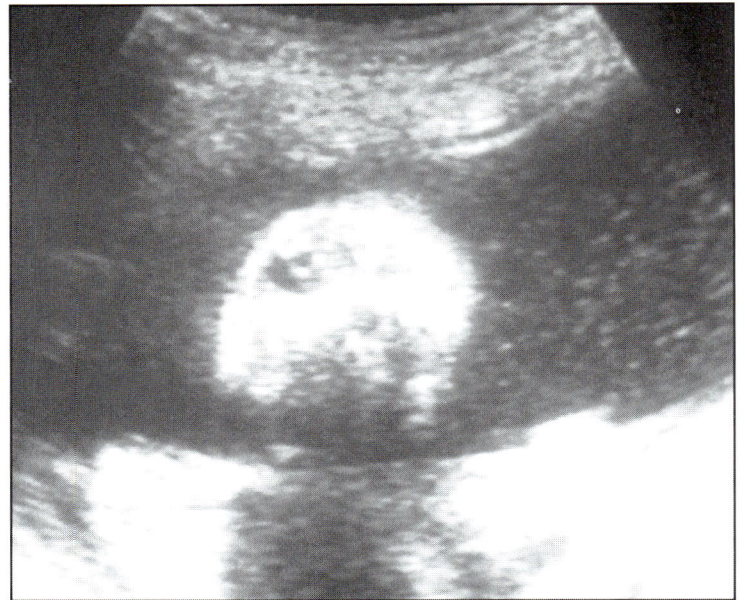

Fig. 13.39: Facial anomalies suggesting amniotic band syndrome

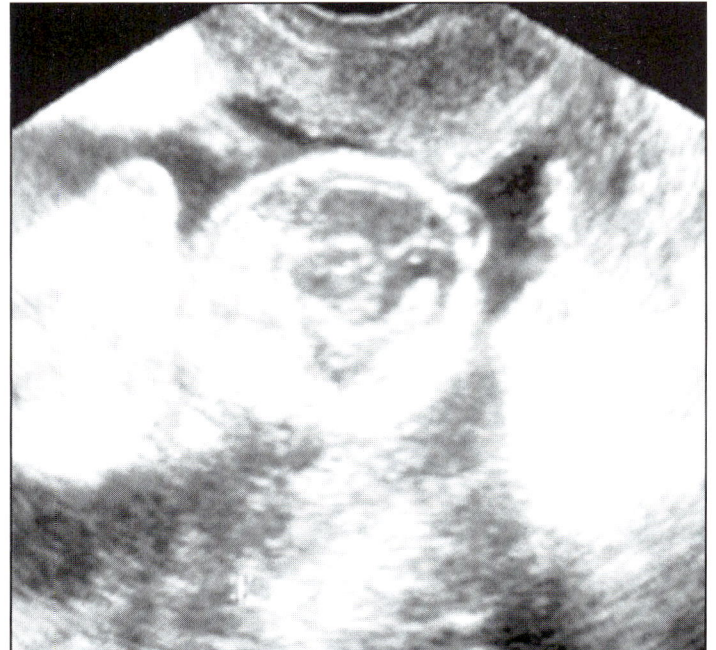

Fig. 13.40: A cystic extracranial mass was noted over the fontanelle. A thin echogenic membrane was seen at the base of the mass thought to represent the periosteum of soft tissue under the mass. There was no intracranial extension of the mass. No defect was seen in the calvarium, and the intracranial anatomy was unremarkable. The diagnosis of an epidermal cyst was therefore suspected

Prognosis with spina bifida is dependent upon the level of the lesion. Bowel and bladder dysfunction, inability to ambulate and complications due to associated hydrocephalus may occur.

Arnold-Chiari Malformation

The Arnold-Chiari malformation is an anomaly of the hindbrain that has two components. The first is a variable displacement of a tongue of tissue derived from the inferior cerebellar vermis into the upper cervical spinal canal. The second is a similar caudal dislocation of the medulla and fourth ventricle. It has

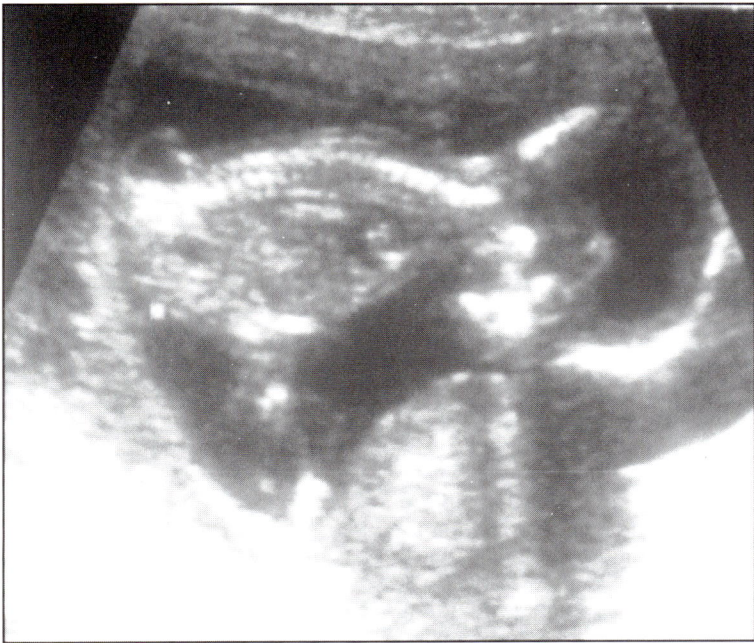

Fig. 13.41: Spina bifida: Sagittal section of the lumbosacral spine of a fetus with spina bifida

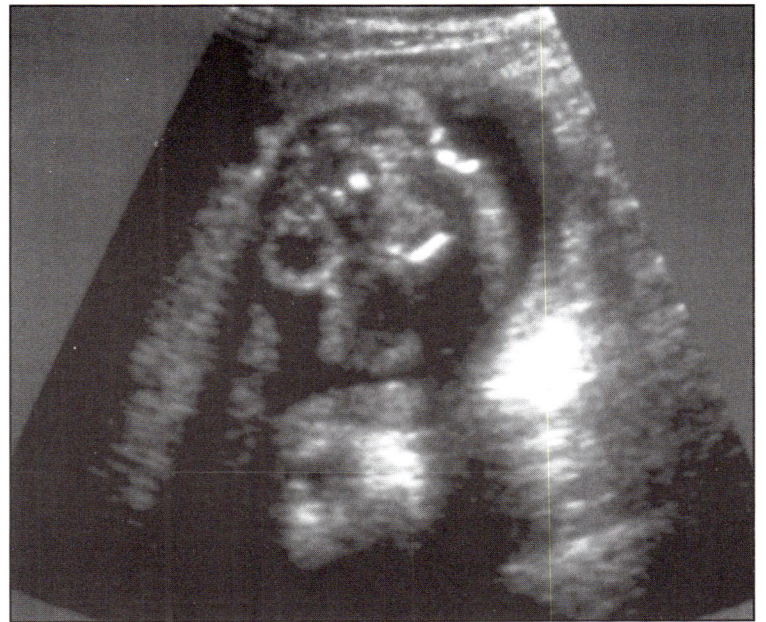

Fig. 13.42

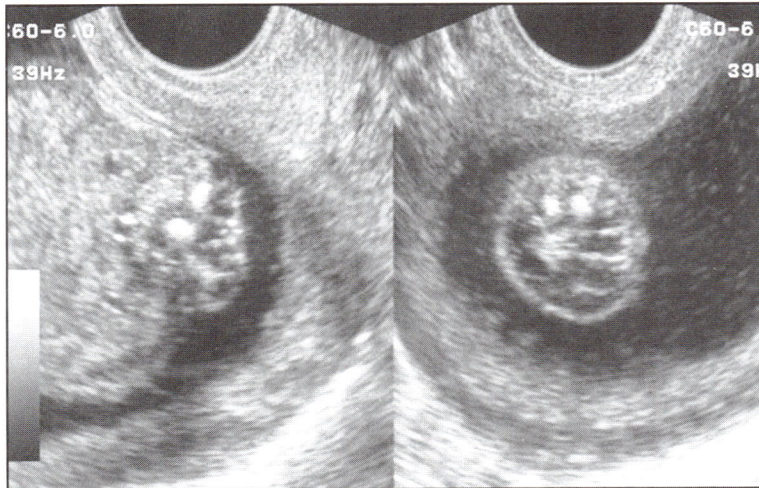

Figs 13.42 and 13.43: Lumbosacral spina bifida: Axial and sagittal planes demonstrating a full thickness defect of the soft tissue overlying spine. U-shaped vertebra with lateral splaying of the lateral process (arrows)

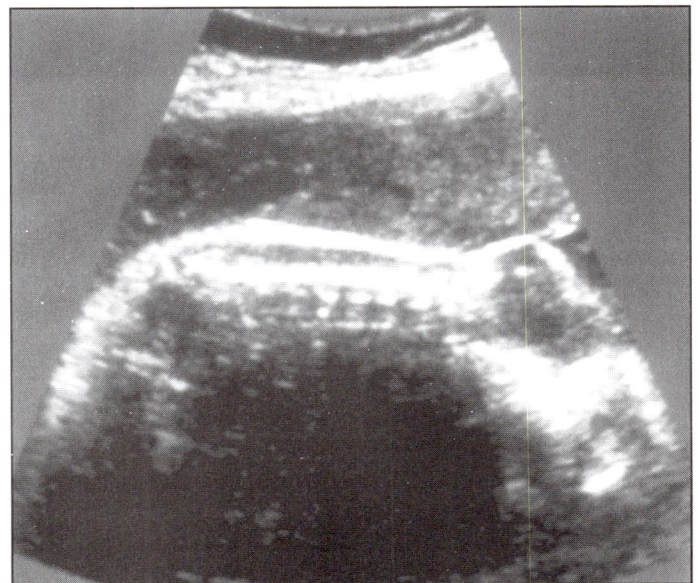

Fig. 13.44

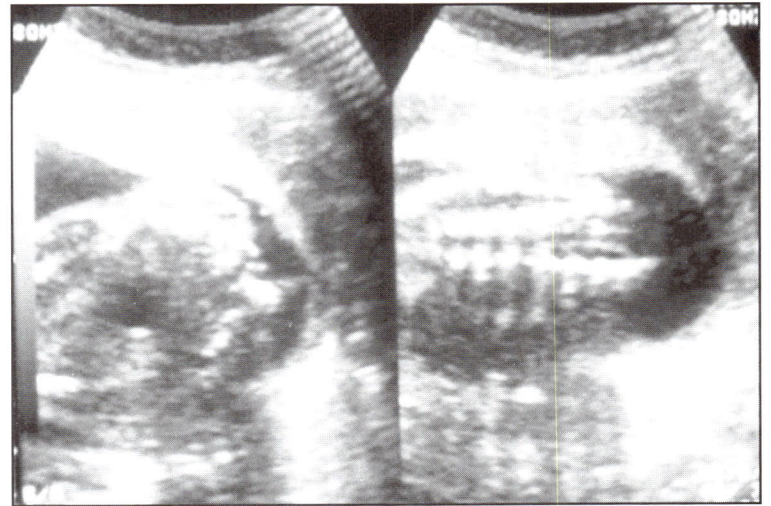

Figs 13.44 and 13.45: Myelomeningocele

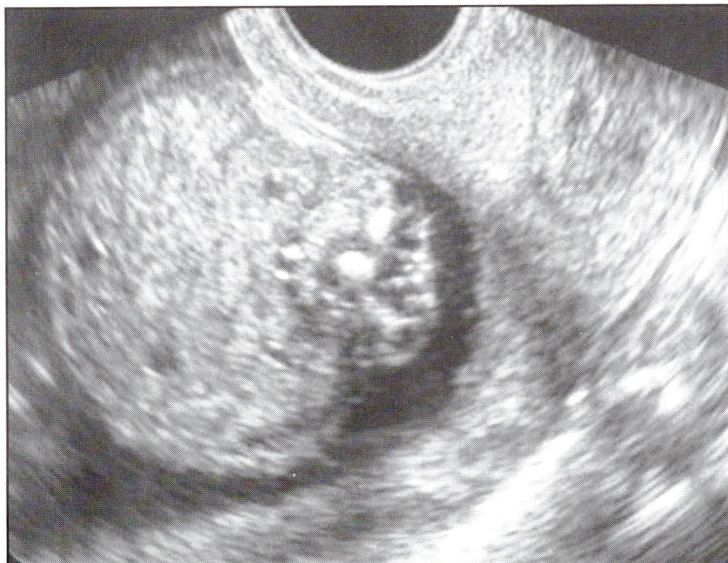

Fig. 13.46

been stated that most, if not all, cases of spina bifida are complicated by the Arnold-Chiari malformation and that 90 to 95 percent of these patients show hydrocephalus.

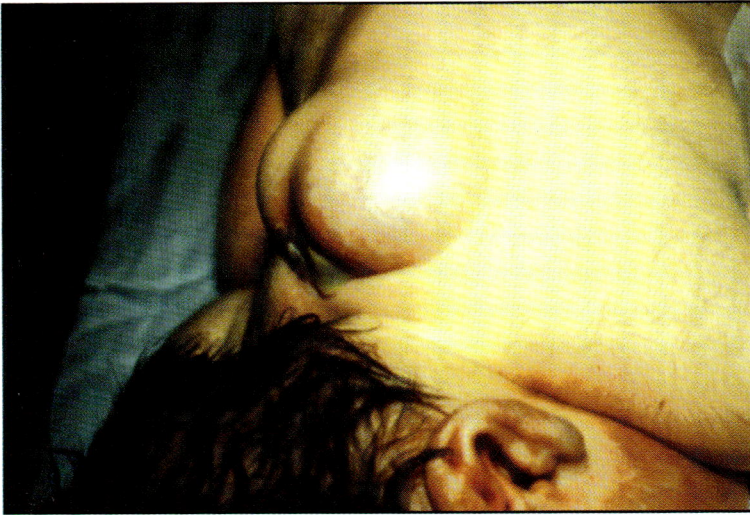

Figs 13.46 and 13.47: Thoracic myelomeningocele

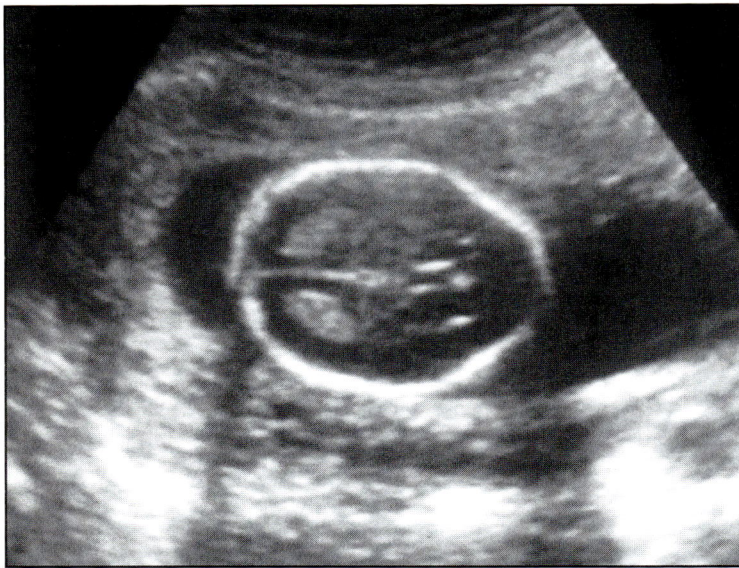

Fig. 13.48: 20 weeks and exposure to teratogens (valproic acid) smaller size of the head

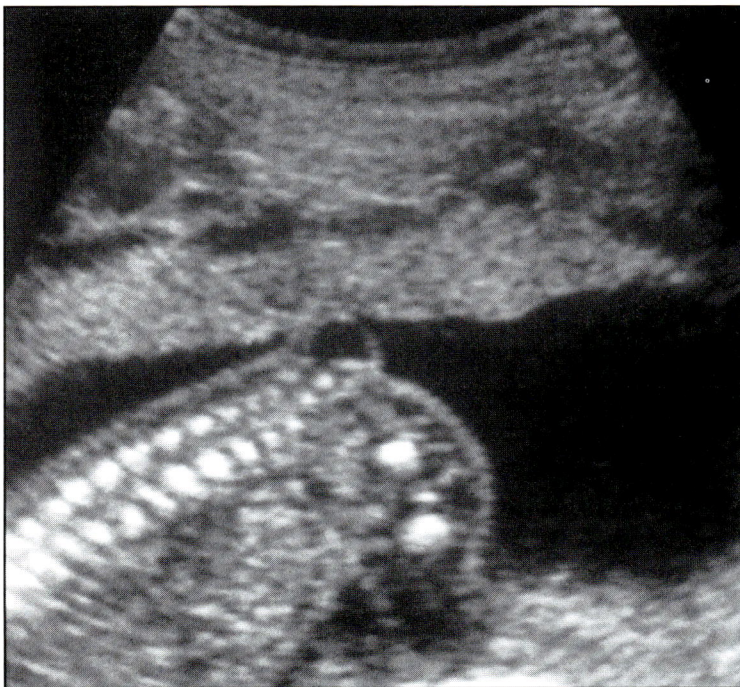

Fig. 13.49: Small sacral meningocele

The Arnold-Chiari malformation can serve, therefore, as an important marker for spina bifida. Two characteristic sonographic signs (the "lemon" and the "banana") of the Arnold-Chiari malformation have been described. A scalloping of the frontal bones can give a lemon-like configuration to the skull of an affected fetus in axial section during the second trimester. The caudal displacement of the cranial contents within a pliable skull is thought to produce this scalloping effect. Similarly, as the cerebellar hemispheres are displaced into the cervical canal, they are flattened anteroposteriorly and the cisterna magna is obliterated, thereby producing a flattened, centrally curved, banana-like sonographic appearance. In extreme cases, the cerebellar hemispheres may be absent from view during fetal head scanning. This characteristic cranial appearance should alert the sonographer to search for spina bifida and has let to its diagnosis in a fetus not previously suspected of having the disorder (Figs 13.50 to 13.53).[26]

Teratomas

Teratomas are neoplasms composed of wide diversity of tissues foreign to the anatomic site in which they arise.

Sacrococcygeal teratomas comprise over 50 percent of these lesions at birth. Those in other locations include intracranial, palatal, cervical, mediastinal, retroperitoneal and gonadal teratomas. The diagnosis of these lesions is of particular importance as they may be resected after birth and the infant cured.

By ultrasound, teratomas characteristically appear both cystic and solid but the solid components may not be observable. The solid components may not be homogeneous in density and may contain calcifications. The cysts frequently have irregular and angulated borders (Figs 13.54 to 13.58).

Choroid Plexus Cyst

Small areas of cystic dilatation may be noted in the choroid plexus of the lateral ventricles of the normal, developing fetus. Generally they resolve before the end of the second trimester without sequelae.

These lesions are usually transient and without clinical significance but warrant a meticulous ultrasound examination to look for anomalies, especially in larger or bilateral lesions (Fig. 13.59).[27, 28]

Agenesis of the Corpus Callosum

The corpus callosum is a bundle of fibers which forms the roof of the third and lateral ventricles. In complete agenesis of the

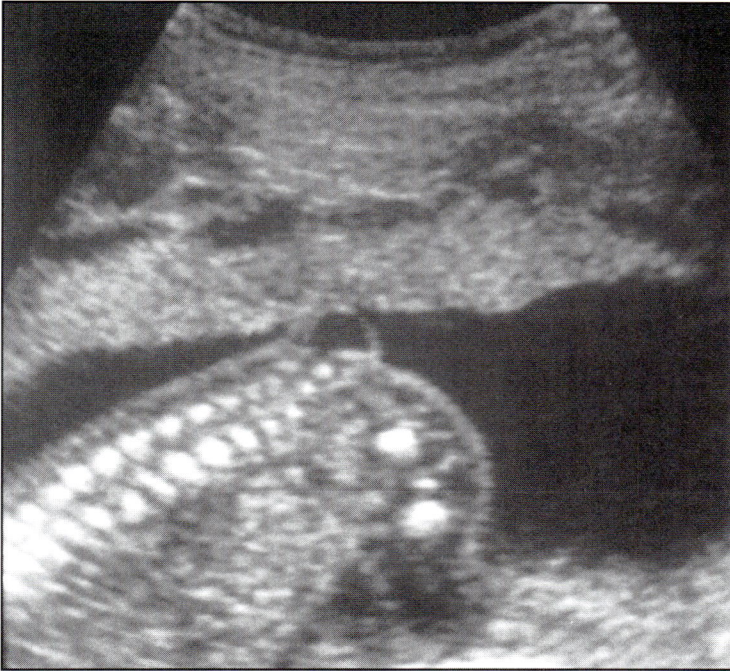

Fig. 13.50

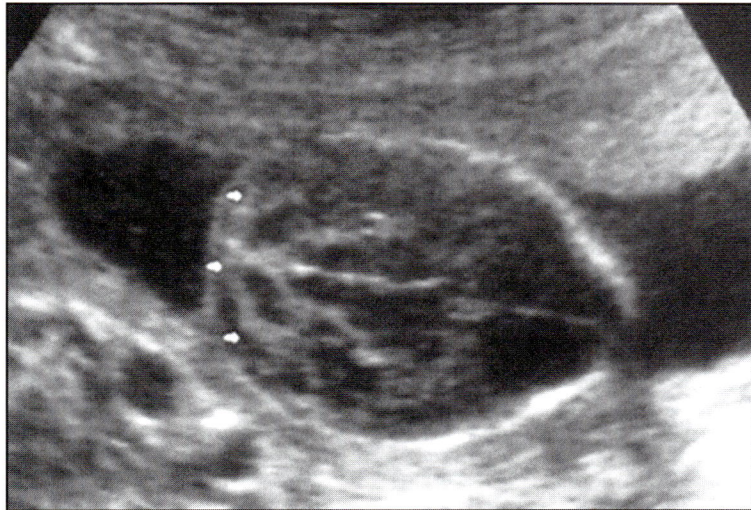

Figs 13.50 and 13.51: Lemon-shaped skull and a banana sign

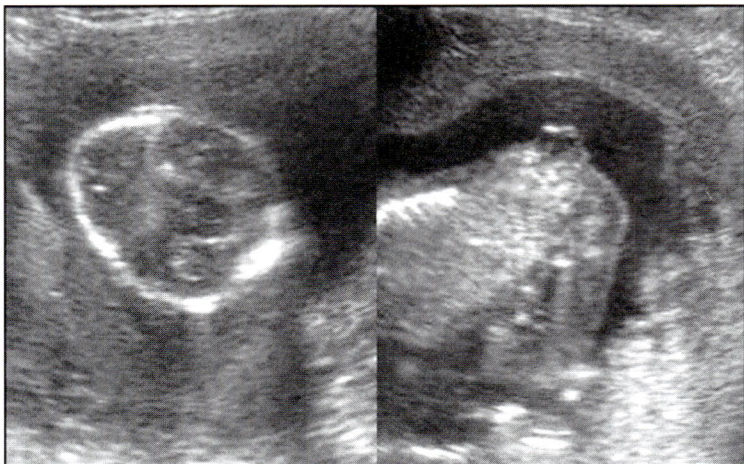

Fig. 13.52: Lemon-shaped skull with cystic meningocele

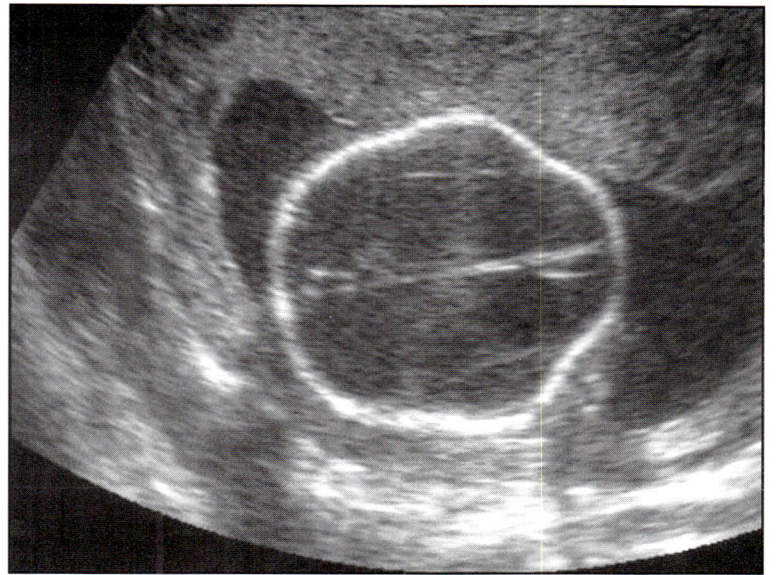

Fig. 13.53: Lemon-shaped skull

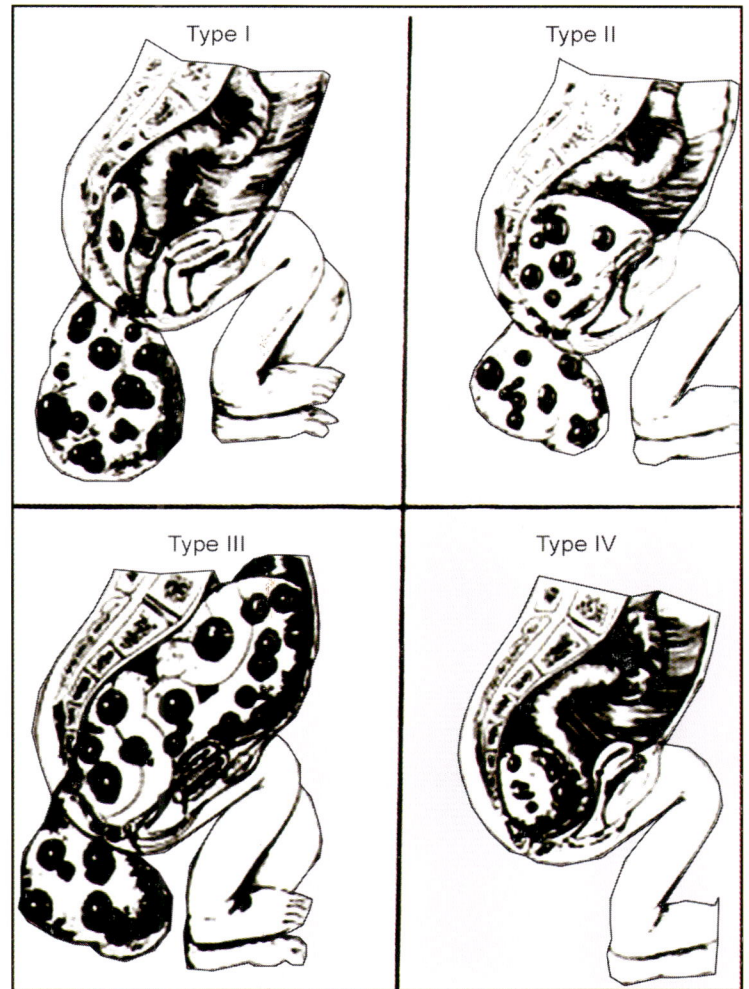

Fig. 13.54: Sacrococcygeal teratoma

corpus callosum the fibers are still present but they lie in bundles medial to the lateral wall of the ventricles. Their presence pushes those walls laterally and makes them concave in appearance with their tip pointing upward instead of laterally. In the coronal sonogram, the widened interhemispheric fissure connected directly with the lateral ventricle.

In a transverse sonogram, the medial walls of the anterior horns of the lateral wall lie close to the falx. Although the anterior

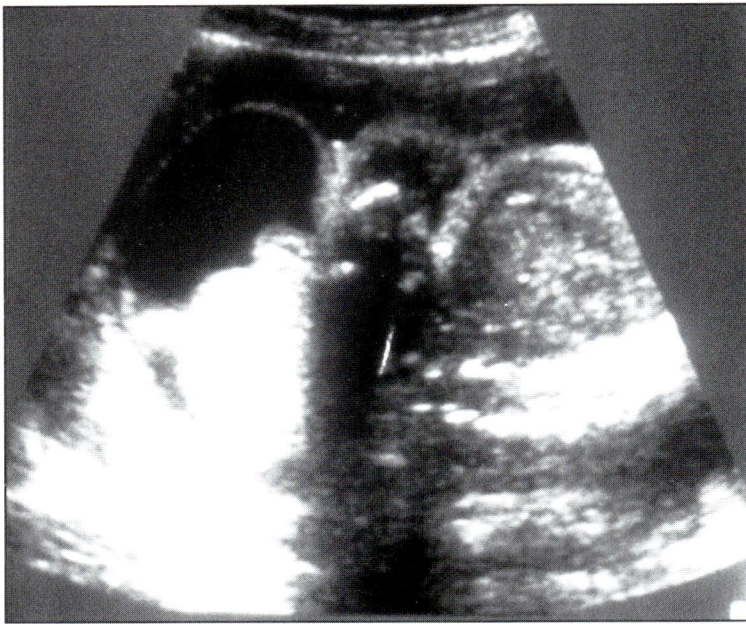

Fig. 13.55

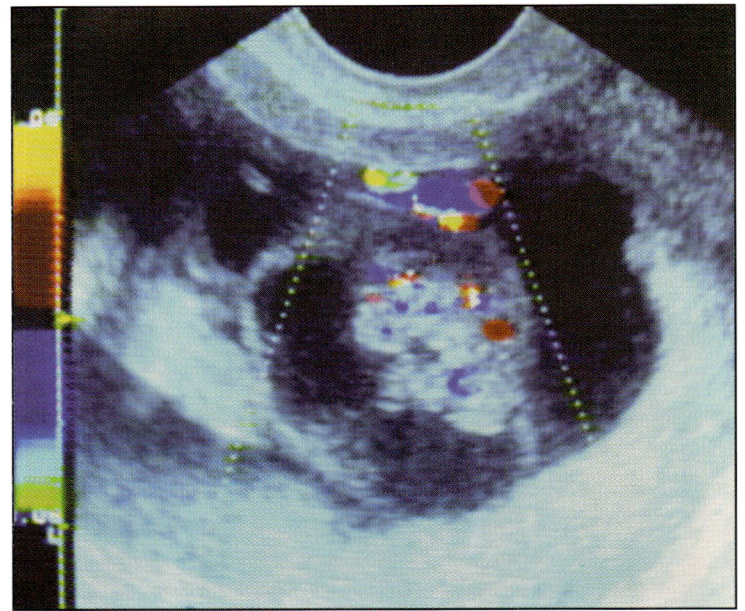

Figs 13.57 and 13.58: Sacrococcygeal teratoma. Low-level venous Doppler signal within the solid component

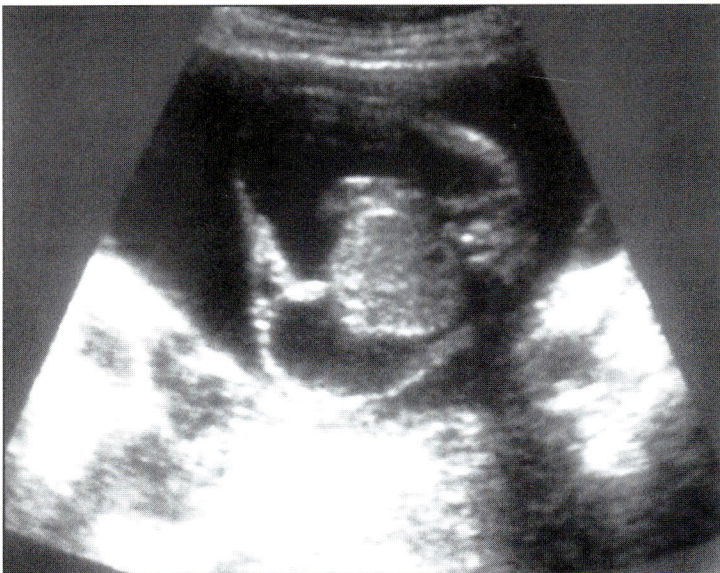

Figs 13.55 and 13.56: Sacrococcygeal teratoma. Note the huge cystic and solid mass originating from the fetal sacrum

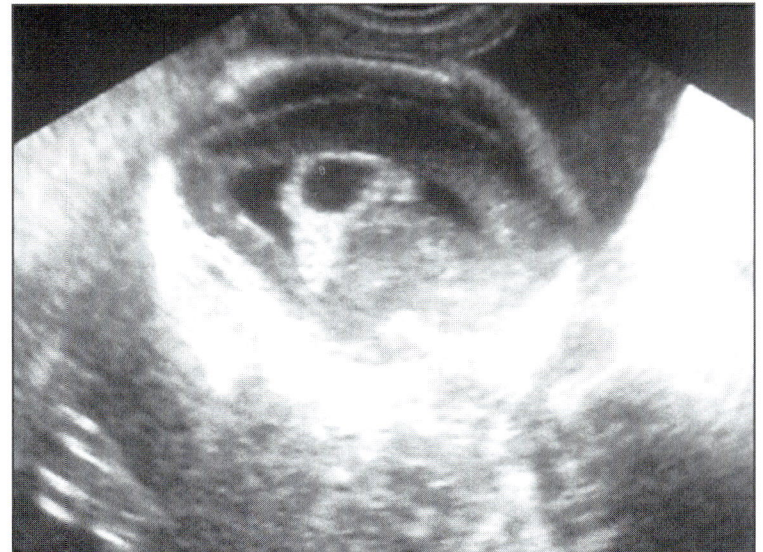

Fig. 13.59: Choroid plexus cysts

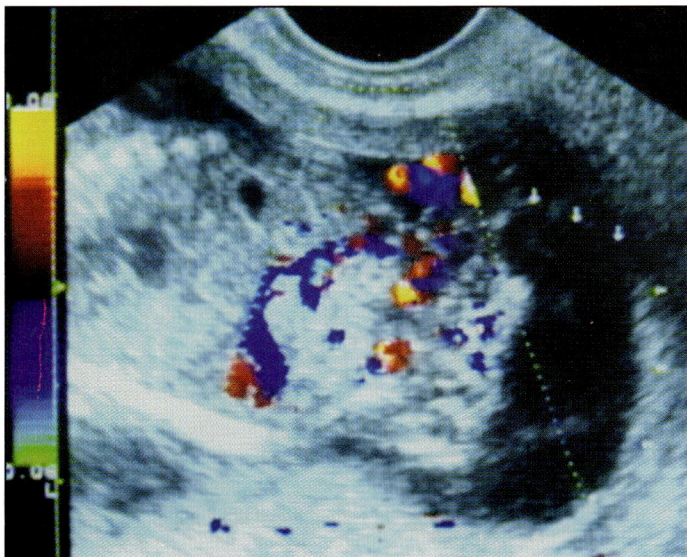

Fig. 13.57

horns are not dilated in agenesis of the corpus callosum, the medial walls are pushed away from their usual midline location. The posterior horns are dilated and, together with the anterior horns, give a tear-drop appearance. The third ventricle is elevated and sometimes dilated.[29, 30]

It is possible to be entirely normal with agenesis of the corpus callosum but, with undetermined frequency in a fetal population, agenesis of the corpus callosum may reflect a more generalized disorder (Figs 13.60A and B to 13.62).

Other Malformations of the Fetal Neural Axis

As experience with ultrasound increases and the resolution of the equipment improves, the list of malformations of the fetal neural axis, detected before birth, continues to grow. Several "cystic" lesions have been detected. Hydranencephaly, appearing as a large, echo-spared area within the head, is distinguished from hydrocephalus by the absence of frontal, temporal and parietal cerebral cortex. Dandy-Walker cyst, prosencephalic cyst, arachnoid cyst and cerebral atrophy all display echo-spared areas as well. Craniofacial duplication, vein of Galen malformation, intracranial hemorrhage, fetal goiter and cloverleaf skull add to the list of malformations detected by antenatal ultrasound (Figs 13.63 to 13.75).[31]

FUTURE ASPECTS

The assessment of the fetal central nervous system plays an important role for the rest of infant's life. As described in this article, advanced sonography combined with methodology of approaching the fetal brain has improved the assessment of fetal intracranial structure and diagnosis of the prenatal brain abnormalities. Recent remarkable development of three-dimensional/four-dimensional ultrasound[32, 33] and advanced MRI technology will produce more accurate evaluation of the brain morphology. A functional evaluation of the intracranial condition and a prenatal prediction of neurological development after birth are also important points in a proper management for fetuses with intracranial abnormalities, but many uncertain and unknown facts still exist. Further studies on the assessment of cerebral function may be expected.

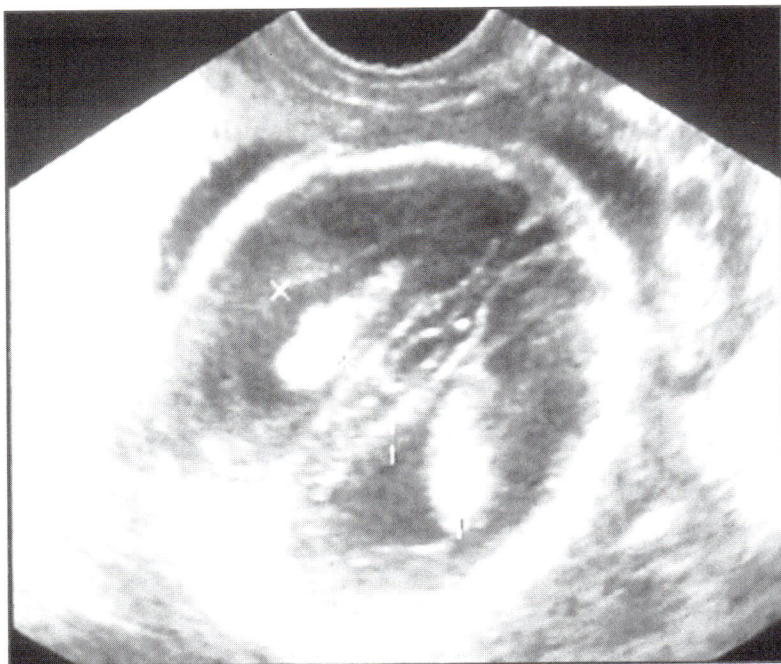

Figs 13.60A and B: Separation of ventricles from midline and upward displacement of the third ventricle. Absence of cavum. Tear drop shape of ventricles

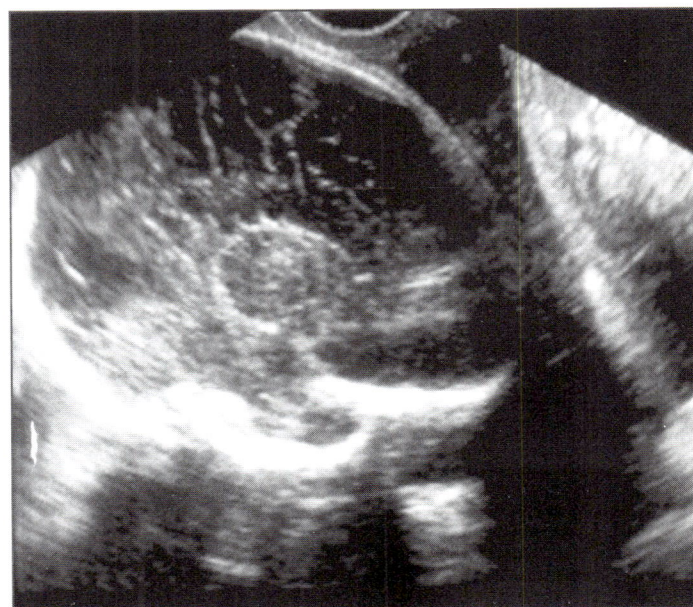

Fig. 13.61: Sigittal view: Absence of the image corpus callosum

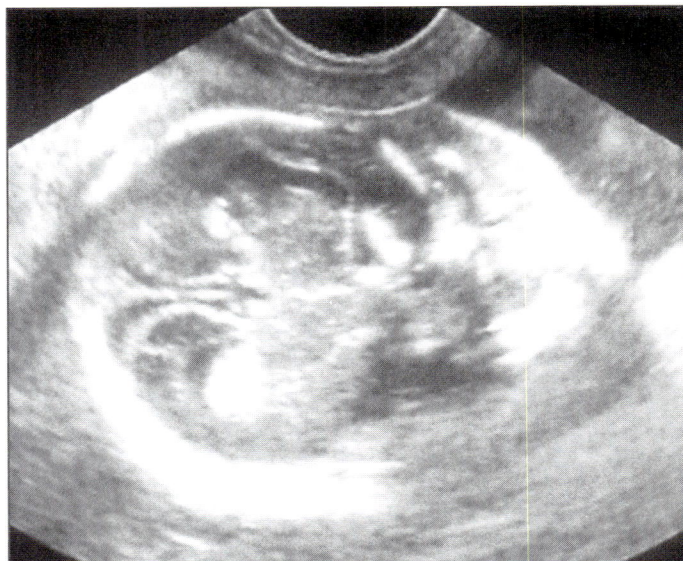

Fig. 13.60A

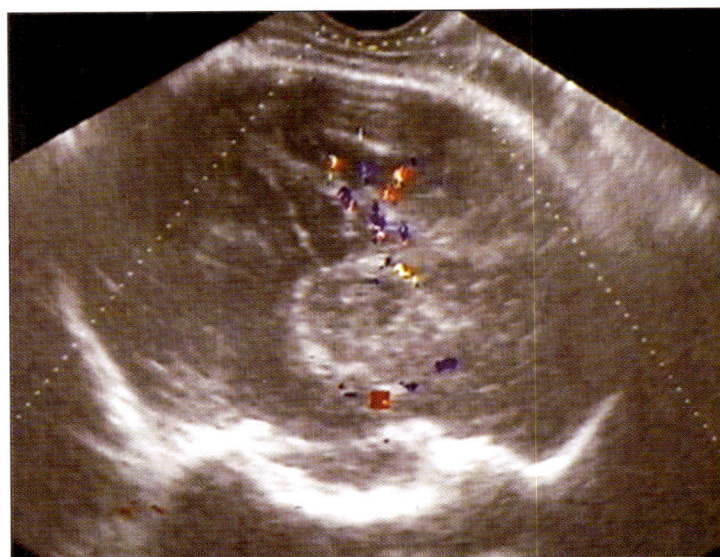

Fig. 13.62: Color Doppler view: Absence of pericallosal artery

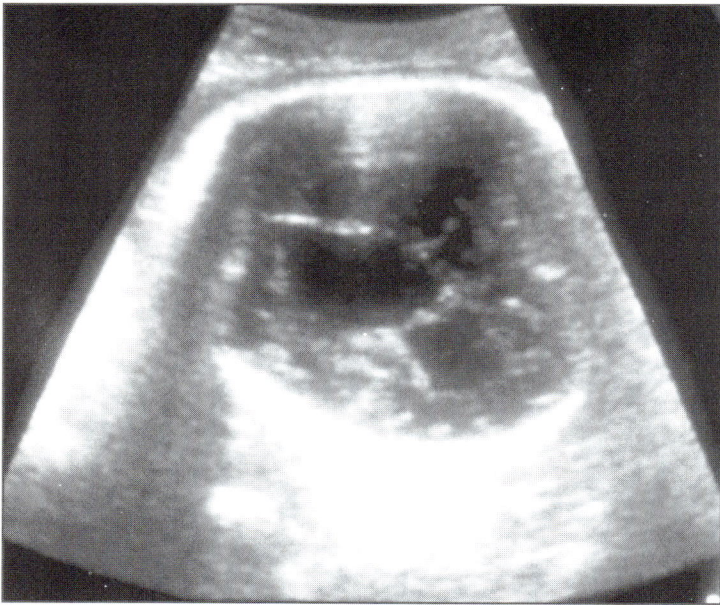

Fig. 13.63: Arachnoid cyst. Axial scan shows a well-defined cyst (arrow) in the temporal fossa

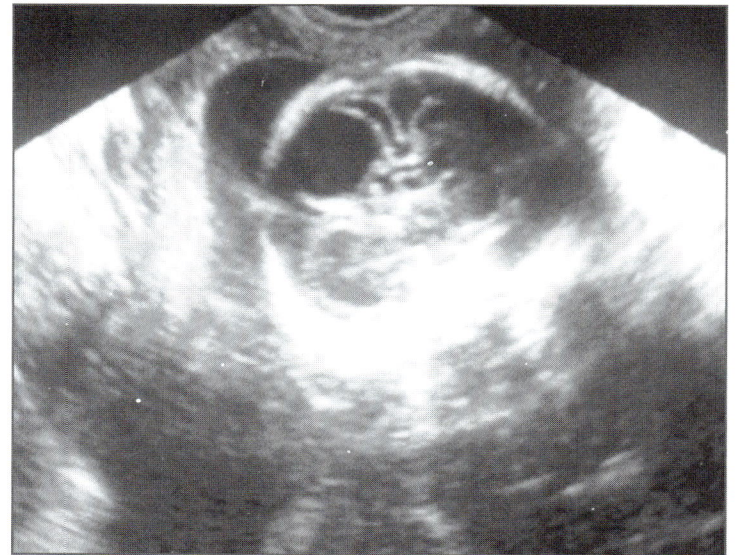

Fig. 12.66

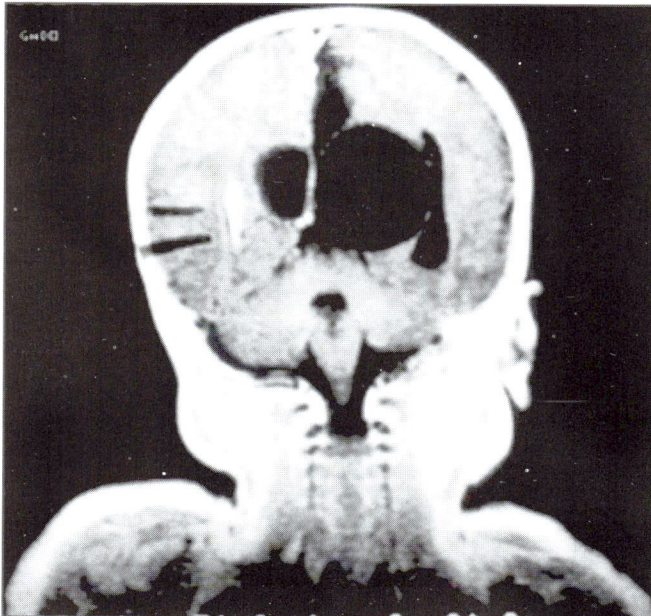

Fig. 13.64: The radiologist images the same case

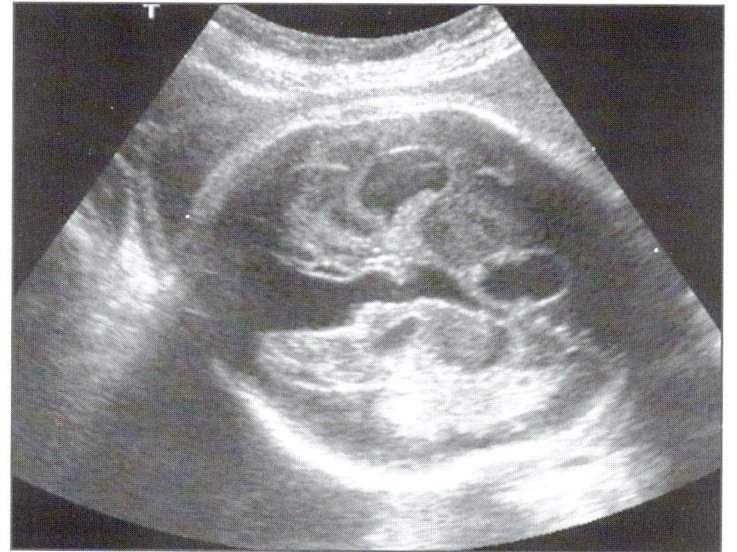

Figs 13.66 and 13.67: Intraparenchymal hemorrhage. A large echogenic image in the lateral hemisphere (arrow)

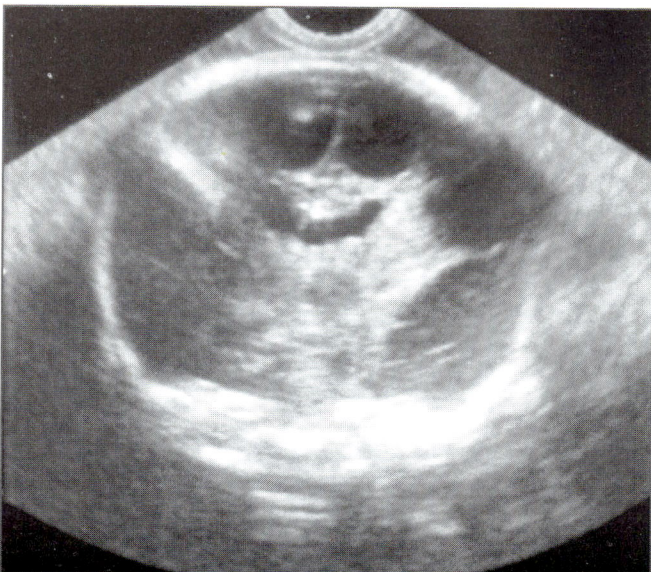

Fig. 13.65: Porencephaly. Coronal scan at 30th week shows bilateral fluid collection (arrow)

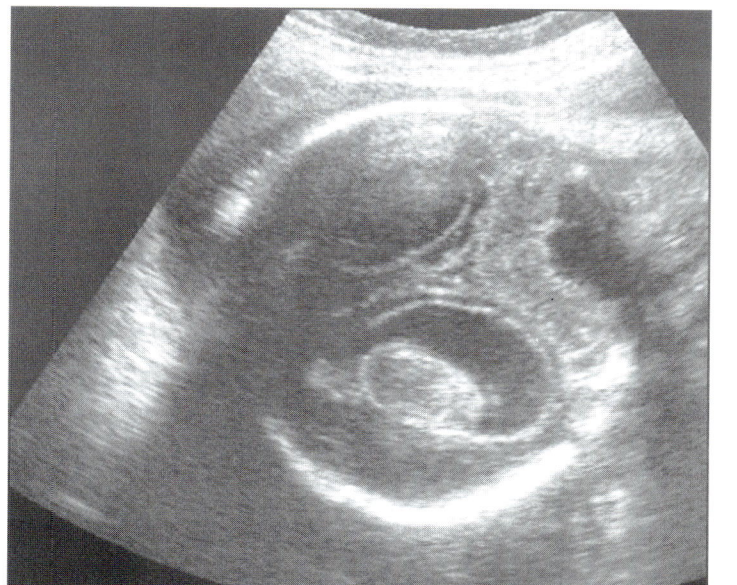

Fig. 13.68: Axial scan shows a large hypoechoic clot extending into the ventricle. The ventricles are dilated

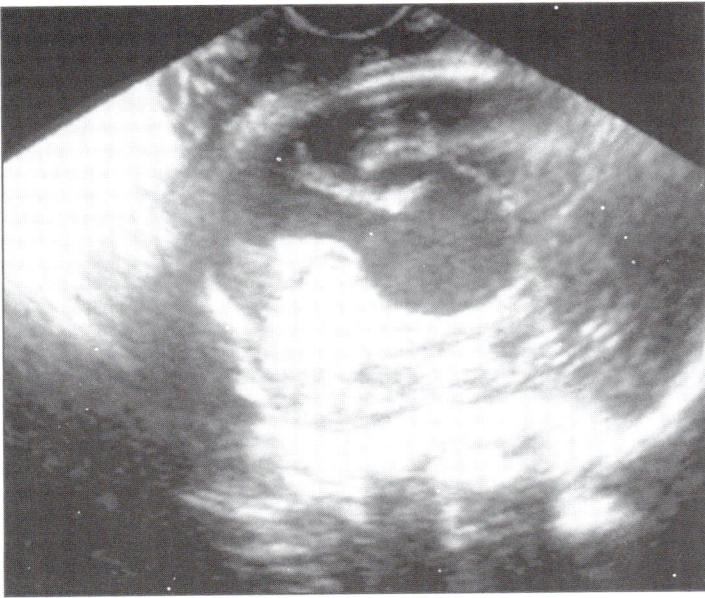

Fig. 13.69: Galen vein aneurysm. A midline supratentorial cystic lesion with draining vessel that extends posteriorly in the direction of the straight sinus is visible

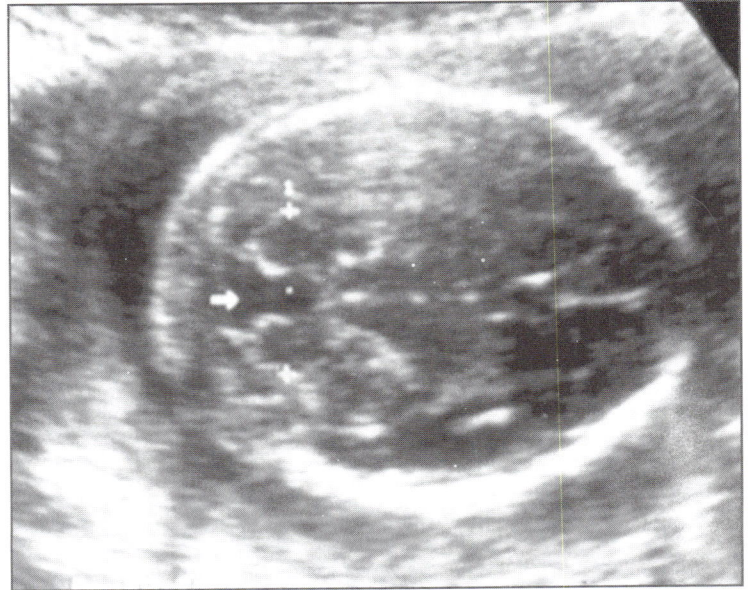

Fig. 13.70: Color and power Doppler demonstrated the high amount of flow and turbulence and exquisitely demonstrates the feeder vessels

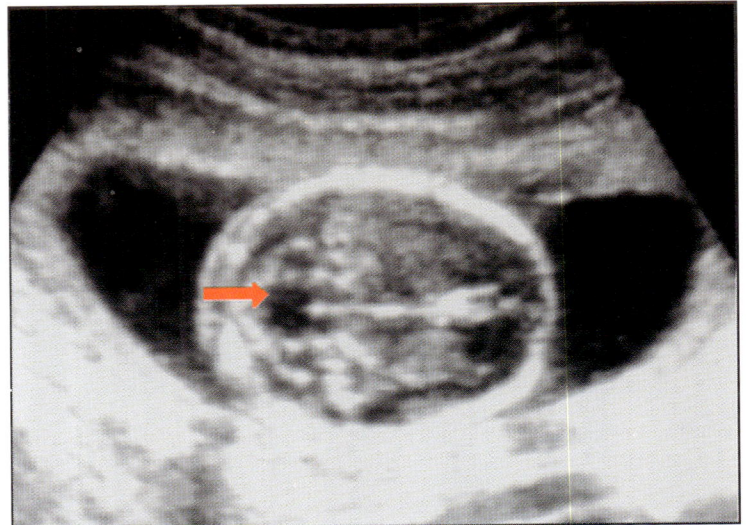

Fig. 13.71: Pulsed Doppler in draining vessel documents continuous venous flow

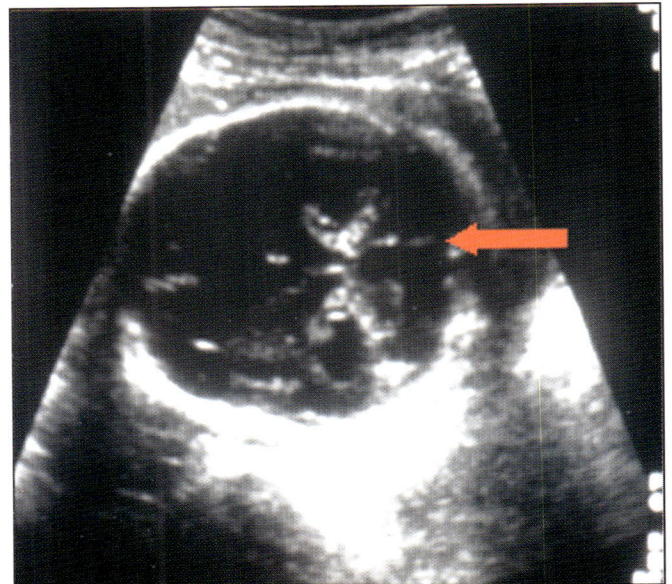

Fig. 13.72: Intratentorial anomalies do not demonstrate the vermis. Instead there is a great big cleft inbetween lateral lobes of the cerebellum

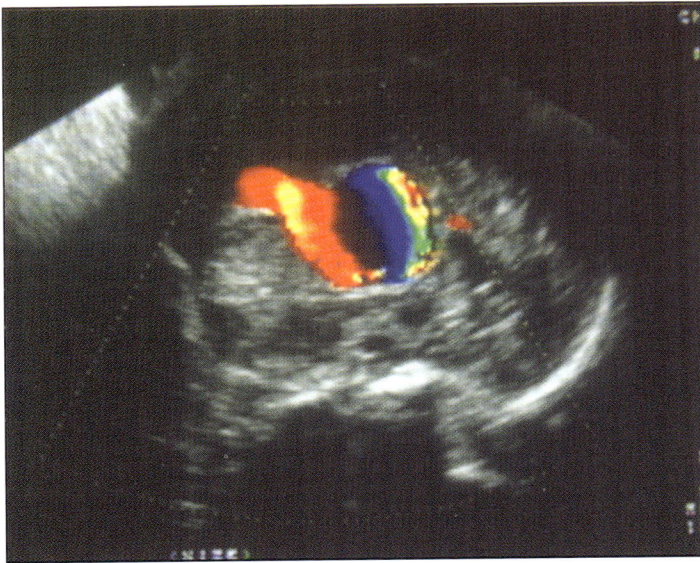

Fig. 13.73: Dandy-Walker malformation. The cerebellar hemispheres are smaller. Absence of the vermis

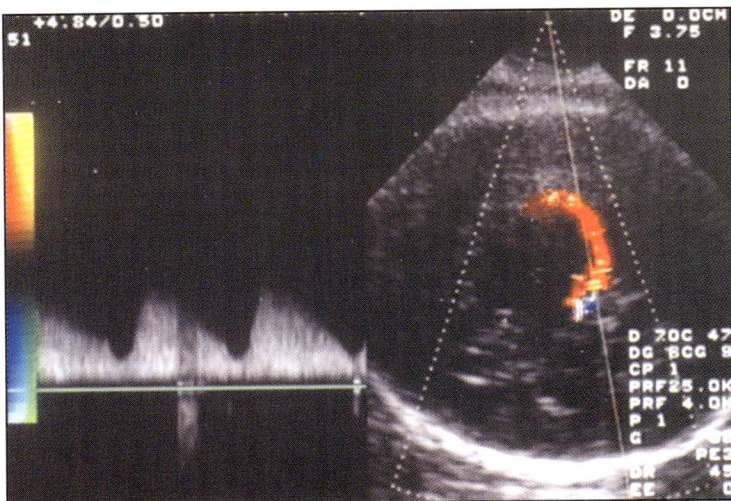

Fig. 13.74: In the axial plane, the cisterna magna is increased in size and the cerebellum is V-shaped because of a large defect in the inferior vermis connecting the cisterna magna to the area of the fourth ventricle

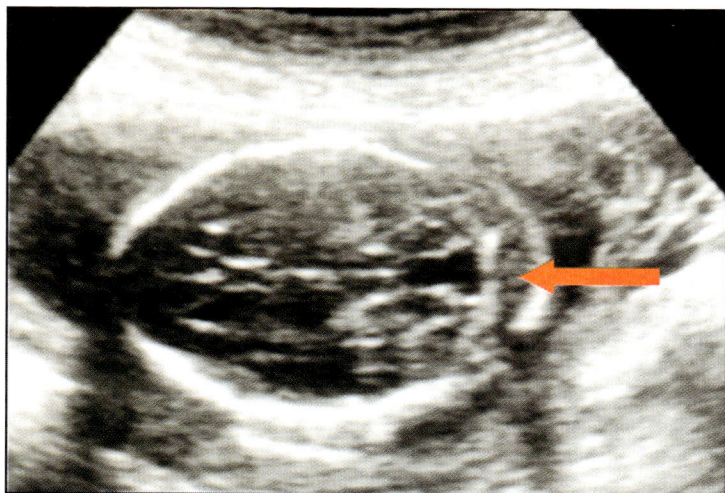

Fig. 13.75: Dandy-Walker variant. Oblique plane through posterior fossa shows partial vermian agenesis with cisterna magna contiguous with posterior aspect of midbrain

FACE AND NECK

M Torrents, JM Carrera, E Scazzocchio, A Muñoz

INTRODUCTION

With the use of ultrasonography it is possible to make prenatal identification of fetal face and neck with great precision. This is particularly obvious in the case of fetal face since, thanks to 3D and 4D technology, the images of fetal face are very realistic.

By means of 2D it is possible to study fetal face in four ultrasonographic sections: lambdoorbitary section, chin-frontal section, vertex-nose section and nose-chin section. Through these sections it is possible to identify all facial structures.

The readers should also study relevant chapters on 3D and 4D sonography.

FACIAL ANOMALIES

At present it is possible to diagnose the majority of facial anomalies by means of different ultrasonographic proceedings: 2D, 3D or 4D.

Cleft Lip

Using transvaginal 2D sonography this anomaly can be diagnosed as early as the end of the first trimester. Fetal lips should be scanned in two perpendicular planes, a tangential coronal plane in a caudorostral direction, and in sagittal paramedian sections.[34,35] But, by means of 3D and 4D, the diagnosis is now very easy.

The defect can be central or bilateral. In the last case it is necessary to make para-medials sections with 2D.

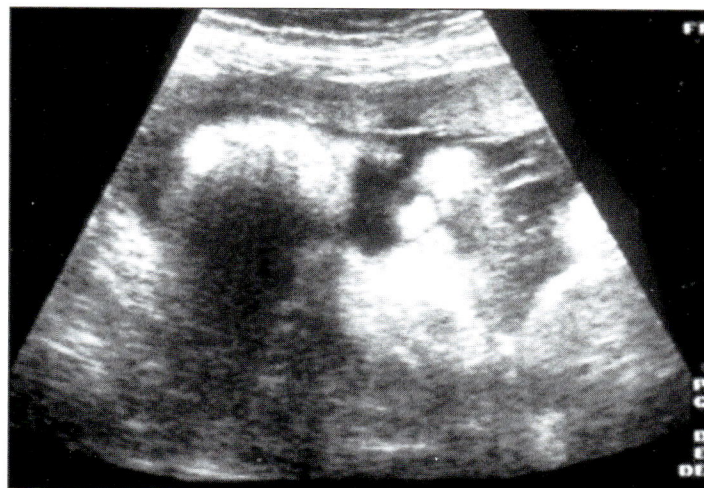

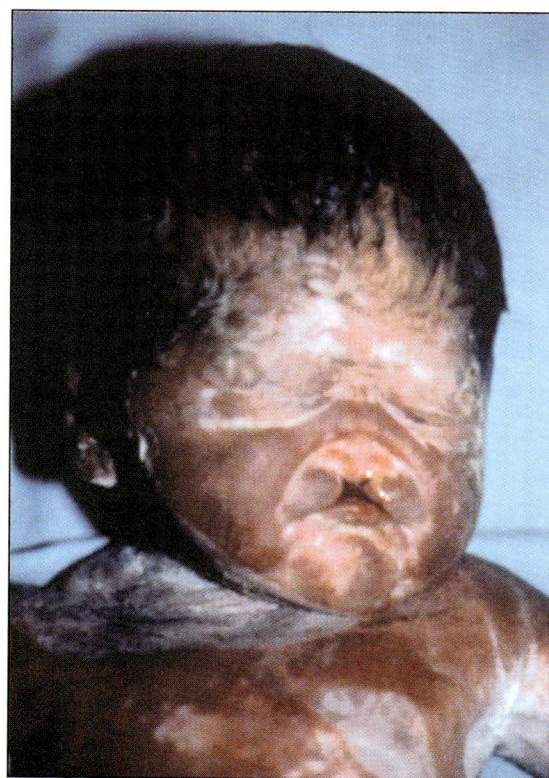

Fig. 13.76A and B: Fetus with T13 presenting hypotelorism, holoprosencephaly, absent nose and midline cleft lip

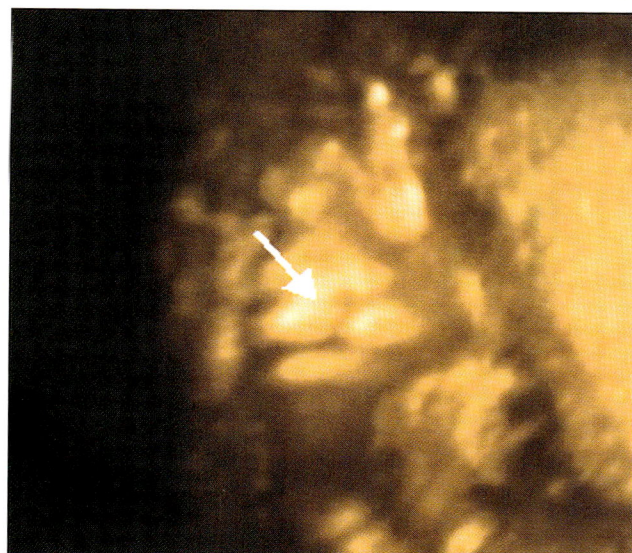

Fig. 13.77: The arrow shows a facial cleft

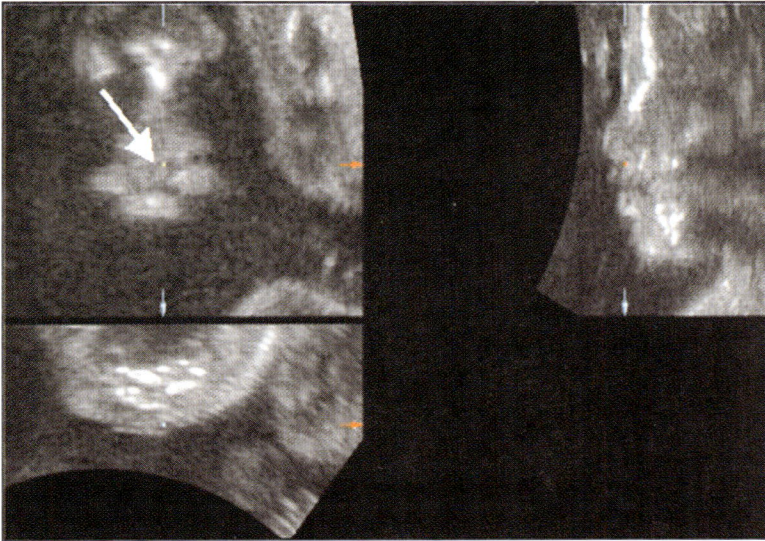

Fig. 13.78: Multiplanar image shows facial cleft in axial, sagittal and coronal planes

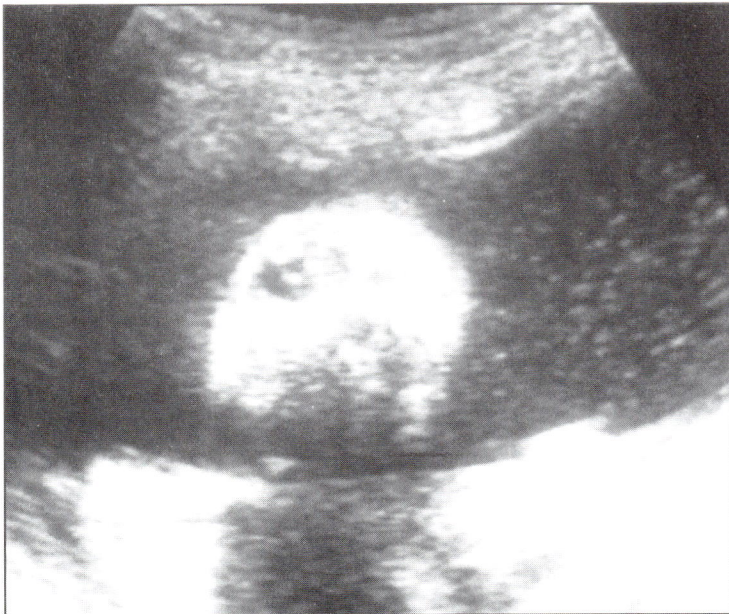

Fig. 13.79: Facial anomalies (only one eye) suggesting amniotic band syndrome

The cleft lip and palate may be associated with other anomalies and syndromes (Figs 13.76A and B to 13.78).

Ocular Abnormalities

The diagnosis of hypertelorism, hypotelorism, anophtalmia-microphthalmia and macroglobus is possible, using the available nomograms.[36] There is a frequent association of these anomalies with several syndromes (Fraser syndrome, Opitz syndrome, etc) and chromosomal abnormalities.[37] The cyclopia, almost always in cases with holoprosencephaly, is easily diagnosed (Fig. 13.79).

At present several cases of *cataract* have been reported in the literature.[38,39] In this situation, the image of the lens is abnormal: thick, irregular, with hyperechogenic borders, opaque, clusters of hyperechogenic material, etc.[34] In some (or any?) cases the hyaloid artery could not be seen.

Nose Malformations

The most frequent anomaly is the absent nose. The presence of the other anomalies, i.e. facial dysmorphs or syndromes is the rule. Therefore, the identification of this anomaly should be target for fetal malformations "work-up" in the ultrasonographic screening (see Figs 13.76A and B).

Ear Malformations

Although the diagnosis of isolated anomalies (anotia, micronotia, etc) is possible, usually they are associated to several syndromes such as Treacher-Collins syndrome, Goldenhar-Gorlin syndrome, etc.

Micrognathia and Retrognathia

These anomalies form part of the multiples syndromes: Robin syndrome, Mohr syndrome, etc. The morphological detection, or the simple suspicion of the fetal facial anomalies, or the constatation of biometrical anomalies, are indication that an exhaustive study of the fetal body, especially intracranial structures, is necessary (Figs 13.80A to D).

NECK ABNORMALITIES

Apart from the "nuchal fold" and "nuchal translucency" that will be studied in another place, various types of cystic lesions and tumors have been diagnosed in the neck. The most frequent are: cystic hygromas (septated and not septated), teratomas, hemangiomas, fetal goiter, etc. Other tumors are only sporadically observed, as a parotid tumor, maxillar tumor, cervical sarcoma or the pterygium syndrome (Figs 13.81 to 13.83).

The hygromas may be associated with other anomalies (ascites, cardiac anomalies, etc) constituting syndromes such as Bonnevie-Ullrich syndrome and Verich-Turner syndrome.

THORAX

A Muñoz, JM Carrera, M Torrents, F Astudillo

INTRODUCTION

The most frequent thoracic anomalies (excluding cardiac anomalies) are: the diaphragmatic hernia, congenital cystic adenomatoid malformation, pleural effusions and sequestration of the lungs.

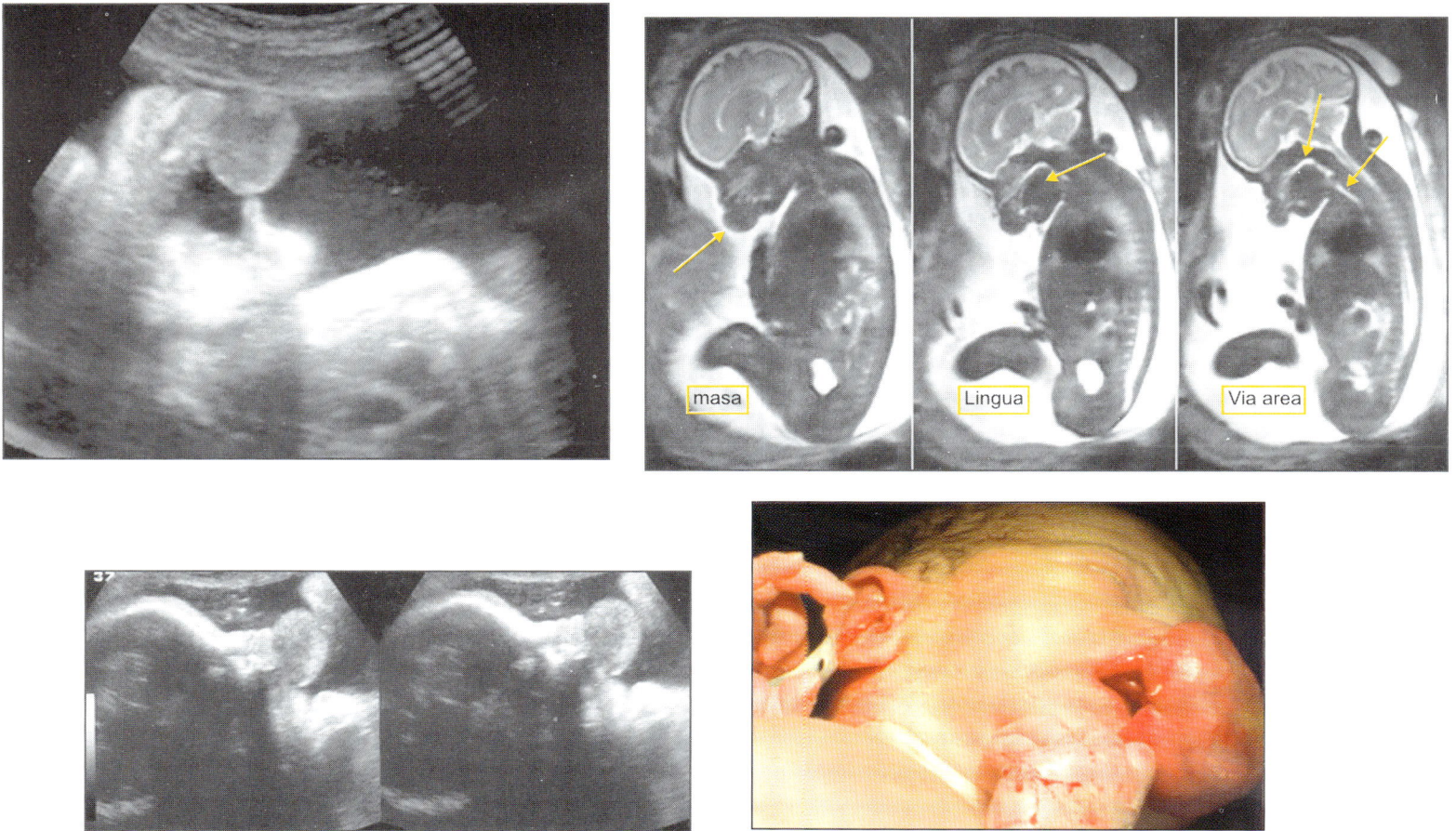

Fig. 13.80A to D: Epulis (congenital)

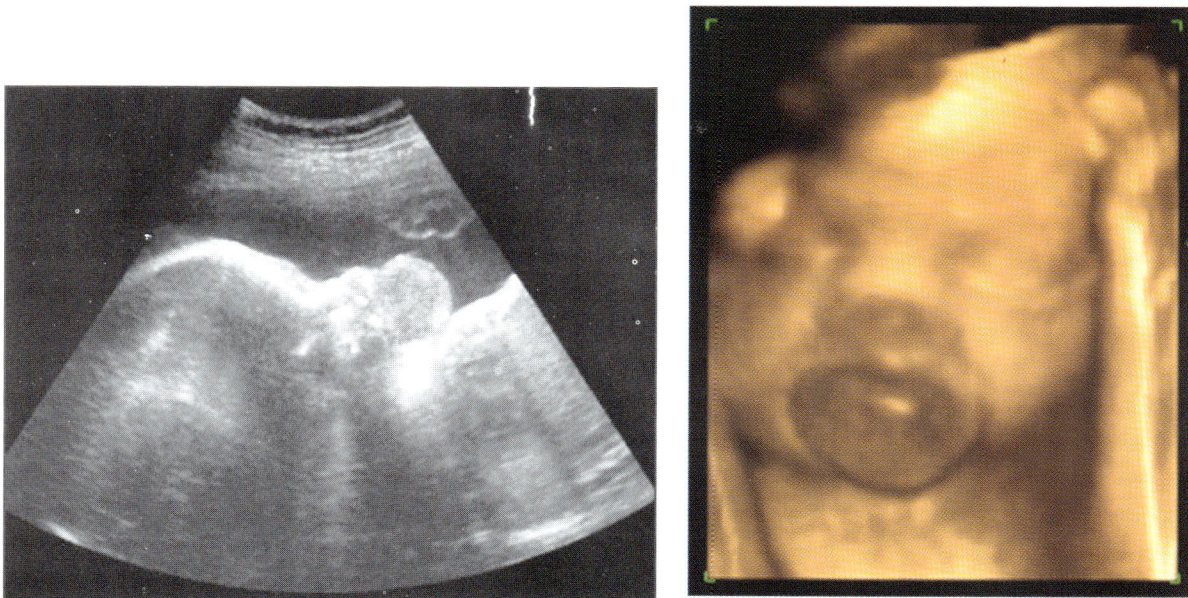

Fig. 13.81A to B: Sagittal scan shows a tumor protruding from the mouth

DIAPHRAGMATIC HERNIA

This anomaly consists of a protrusion of the abdominal organs into the thoracic cavity through a diaphragmatic defect.

The diaphragm is a dome-shaped septum dividing the thoracic and abdominal cavities. The diaphragm closes by the 9th gestational week, and incomplete closure of the diaphragm at 10th week allows the protrusion of abdominal visceral content into the thoracic cavity.

The diaphragm may be imaged as an echogenic line when scanned in a perpendicular section. The spectrum of defects is

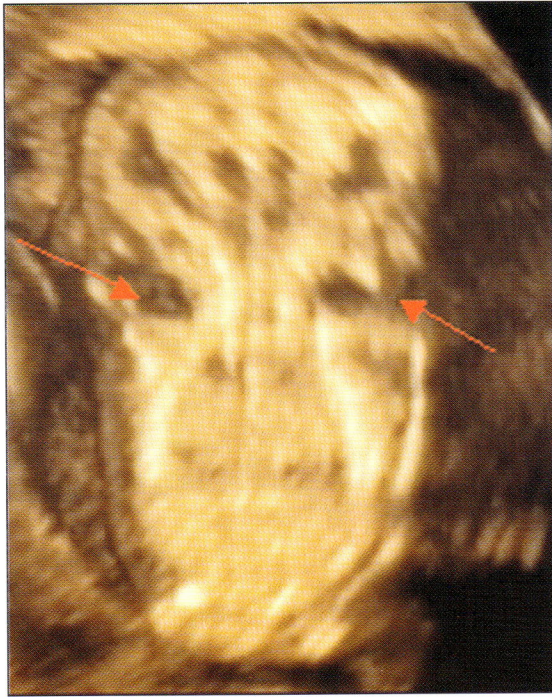

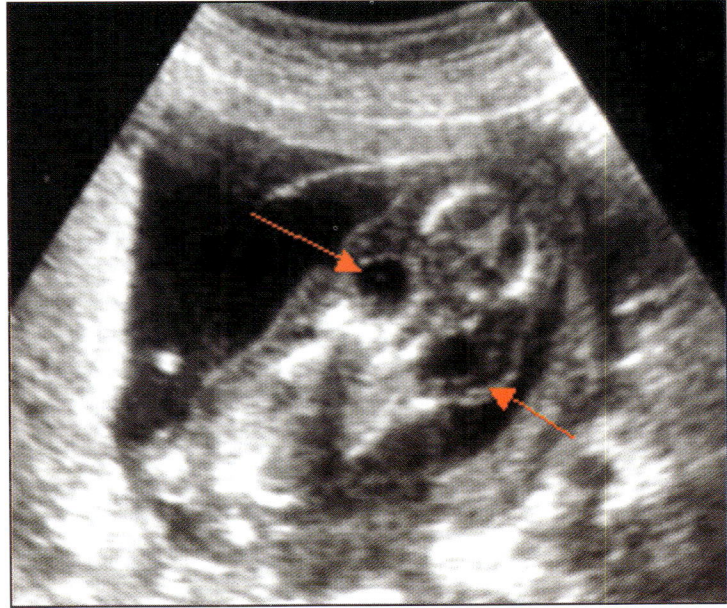

Fig. 13.82A and B: 3D scan. A: Cystic hygroma, B: Cystic hygroma, diffuse edema

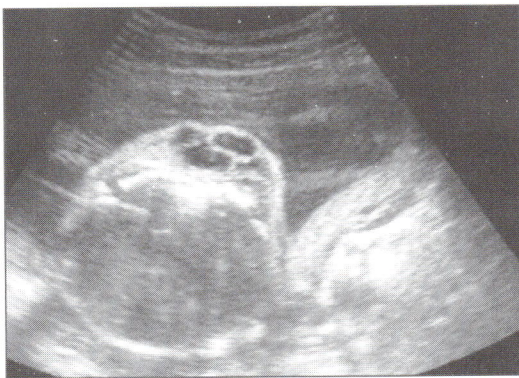

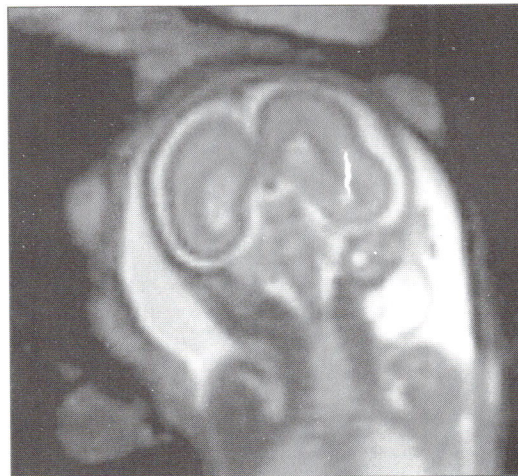

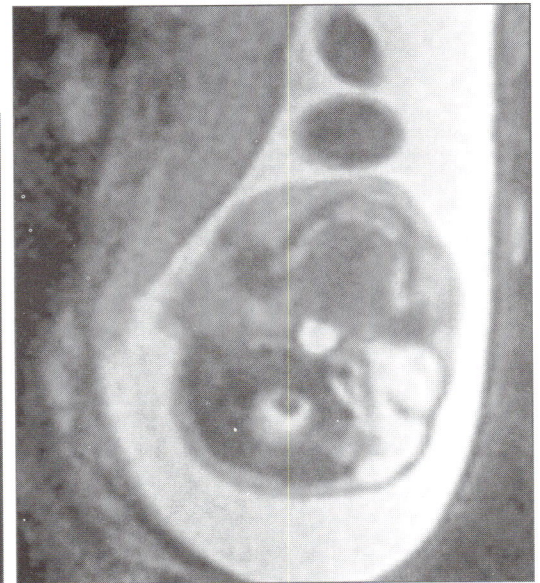

Fig. 13.83A to C: Axial scan shows cystic tumor lateral to the neck

wide, ranging from complete absence of the diaphragm through pathological orifices to congenital hiatal hernia.

The diagnosis of a diaphragmatic hernia is made by imaging the transverse section of the chest, with both the heart and herniated bowel on the same scanning plane.[40] The stomach and intestinal loops displace the heart.

The diagnosis of right diaphragmatic hernia is more difficult because of the similar echogenicity of the liver and lungs (Figs 13.84A and B to 13.91).

The fetal prognosis is bad, due to the hypoplastic lungs and the association with several fetal abnormalities.[41]

CONGENITAL CYSTIC ADENOMATOID MALFORMATION

The most common of the isolated lung malformations is congenital cyst adenomatoid malformation (Figs 13.92 to 13.96). In this condition a large part of the lung is occupied by cyst of variable size and aspect (cystic or solid consistence). It is often large enough to cause a shift of the mediastinal structures and to compress the contralateral lung.[42,43] The cardiac silhouette may be displaced.

Usually, this condition is classified into three subtypes: (i) type I has large cysts, (ii) type II has multiple small cysts (less

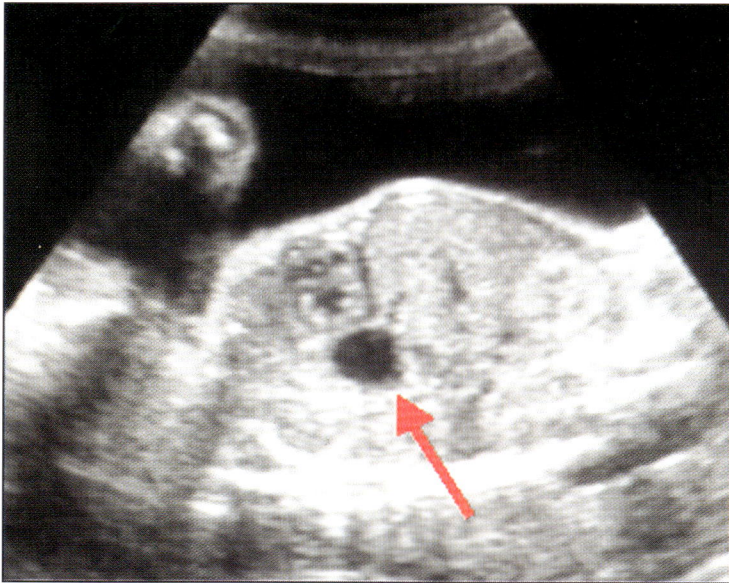

A

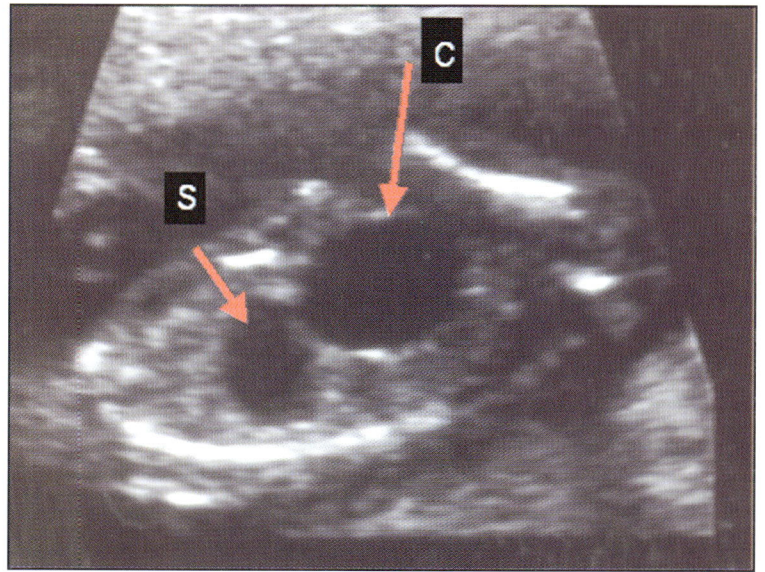

B

Figs 13.84A and B: Left diaphragmatic hernia. Transverse view of the thorax: A . The stomach was herniated into the chest behind the heart. B. The stomach was herniated into the chest

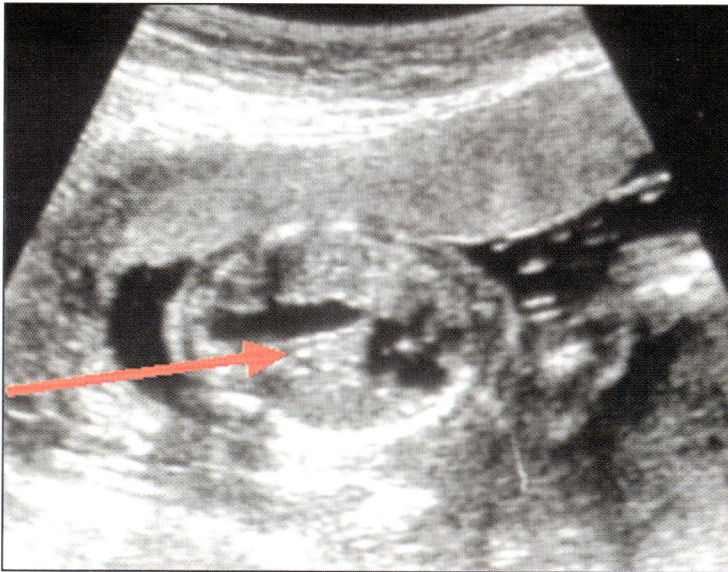

Fig. 13.85: Left diaphragmatic hernia: 13 weeks transverse view of the thorax. The stomach was hermiated in the chest

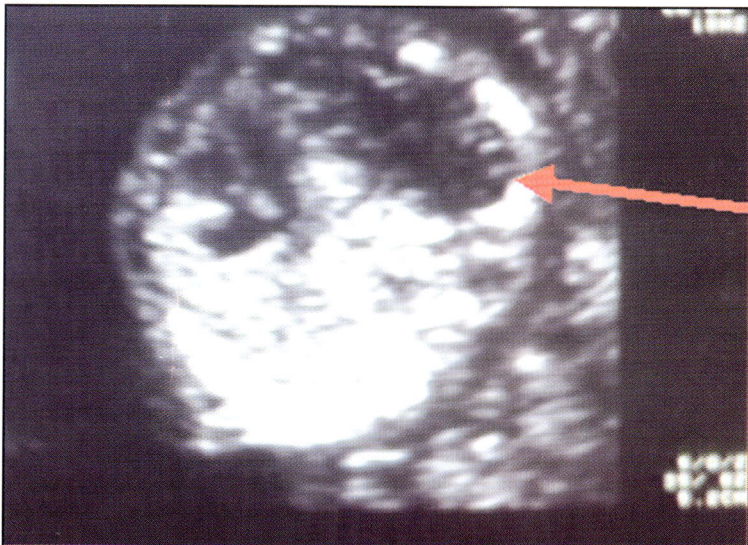

Fig. 13.86: Left diaphragmatic hernia: 13 weeks oblique view of the thorax. The stomach (S) was herniated into the chest. See large abdominal cyst (C)

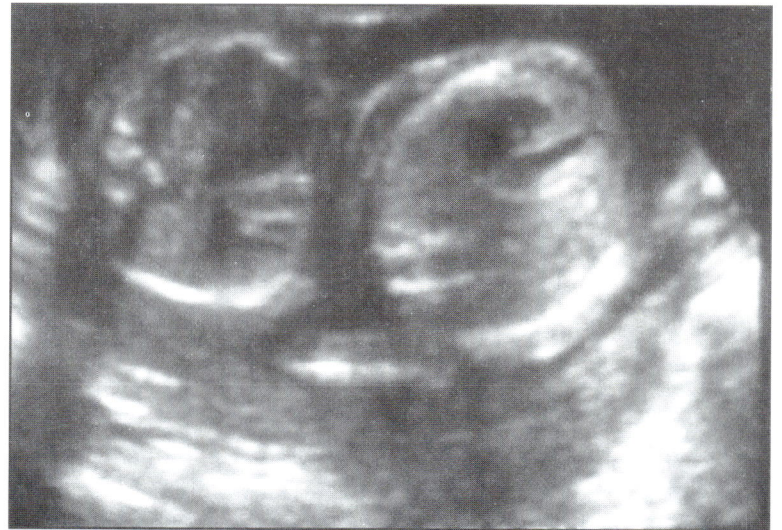

Fig. 13.87: Left diaphragmatic hernia: Twin gestation. Diaphragmatic hernia in both fetuses

than 1, 2 cm in diameter), and (iii) type III consists of a non-cystic or microcystic lesion producing mediastinal shift. The worst prognosis is seen in type III.[44]

Polyhydramnios is consistently present, and the fetus may be hydropic in which case survival is most unlikely.

PLEURAL EFFUSIONS

Fetal pleural effusions consist in the presence of fluid (usually lymph) in pleural cavity. May be unilateral or bilateral, isolated or associated with generalized edema and ascites.

The sonographic diagnosis is easy, but a specific and etiologic diagnosis on the basis of a gross appearance of the effusion is not possible (Figs 13.97 A and B).[43]

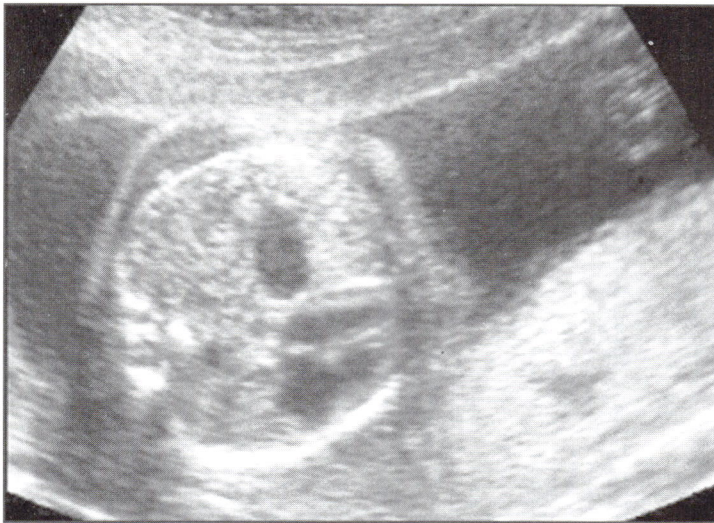

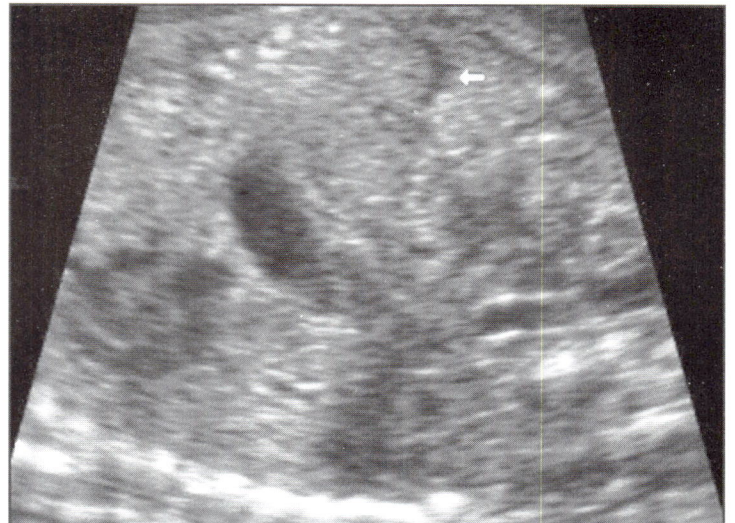

Figs 13.88A and B: Left diaphragmatic hernia: A. Transverse and B. Oblique views of the thorax. The stomach was herniated into the chest

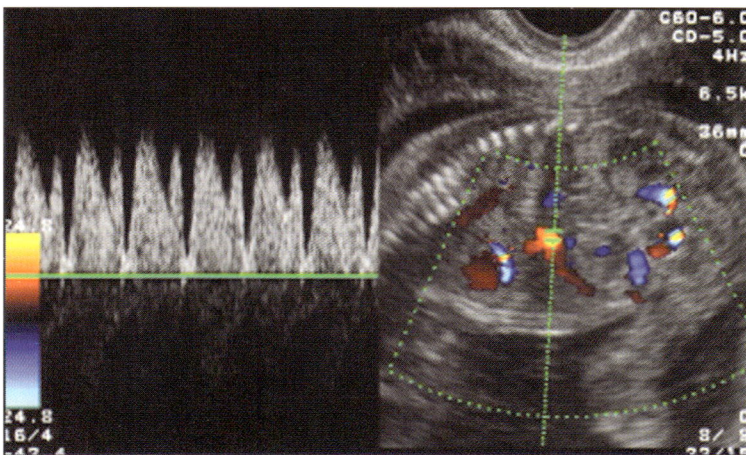

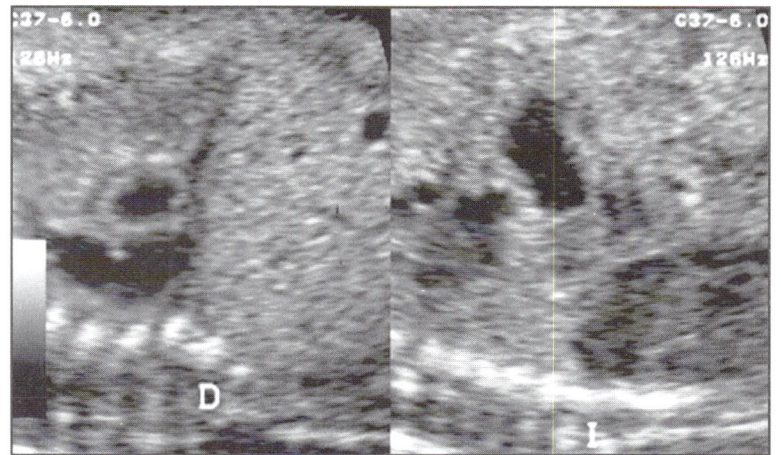

Figs 13.89A and B: Left diaphragmatic hernia: A. Color Doppler shows an abdominal pattern of ductus venosus flow. B. Dual image of right and left side views of the thorax. The stomach was herniated into the chest

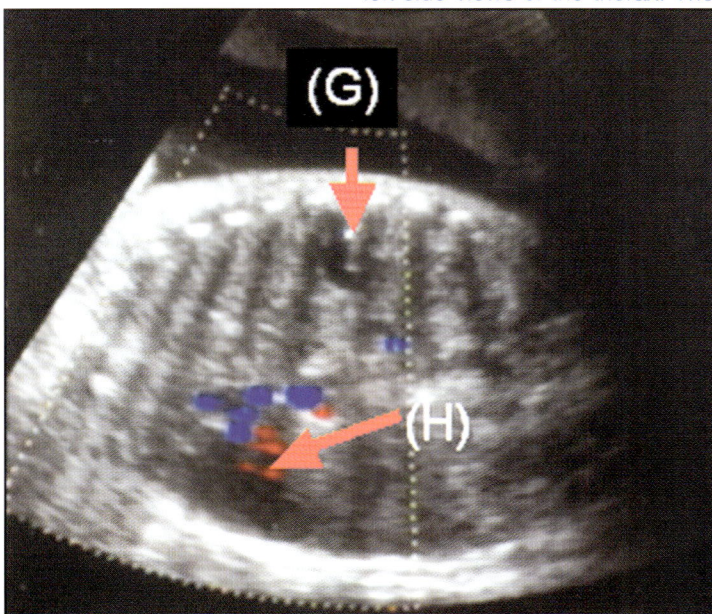

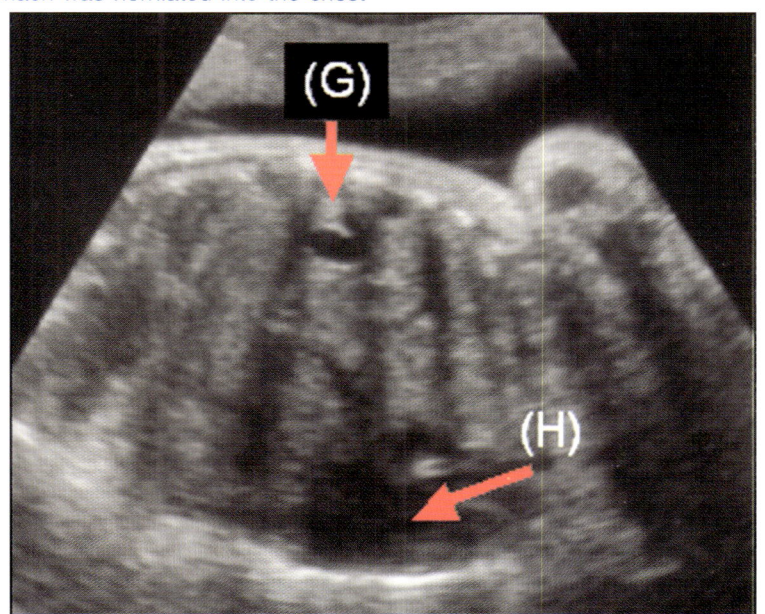

Figs 13.90A and B: Right diaphragmatic hernia: An oblique-coronal view of thorax. Case of right diaphragmatic hernia. Color Doppler shows: A. Heart (H) near gallbladder (G). B. Gallbladder (G) near the heart (H)

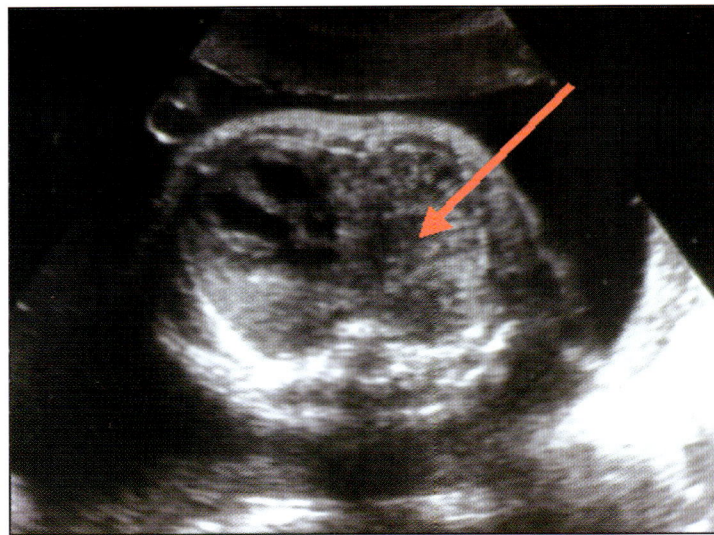

Fig. 13.91: Right diaphragmatic hernia: Case of right diaphragmatic hernia. Transverse image of thorax shows a heart deviation

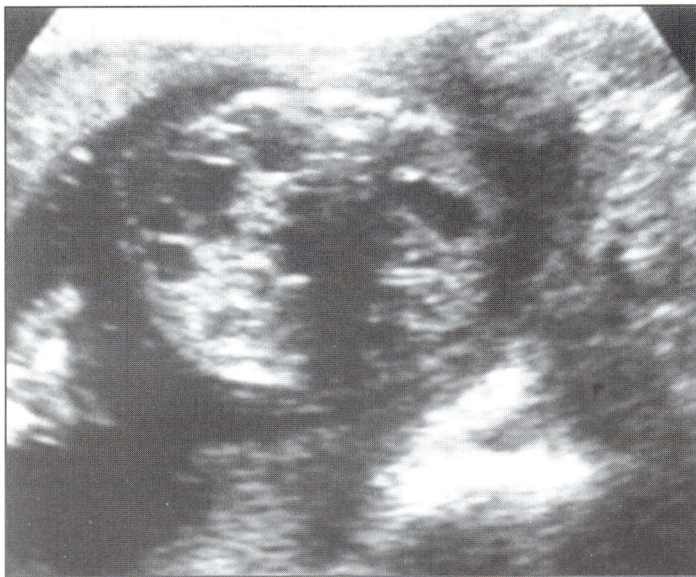

A

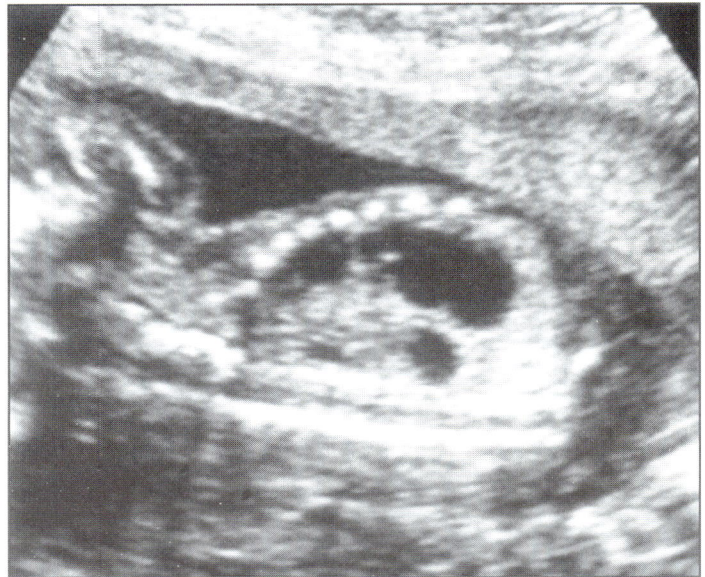

B

Figs 13.92A and B: Congenital cystic adenomatoid malformation. A.Transverse view: This is a case of bilateral cystic adenomatoid malformation of the lungs, macrocyst type. B. Oblique view: Bilateral cystic adenomatoid malformation. See a multiple large cysts surrounded by echogenic tissue

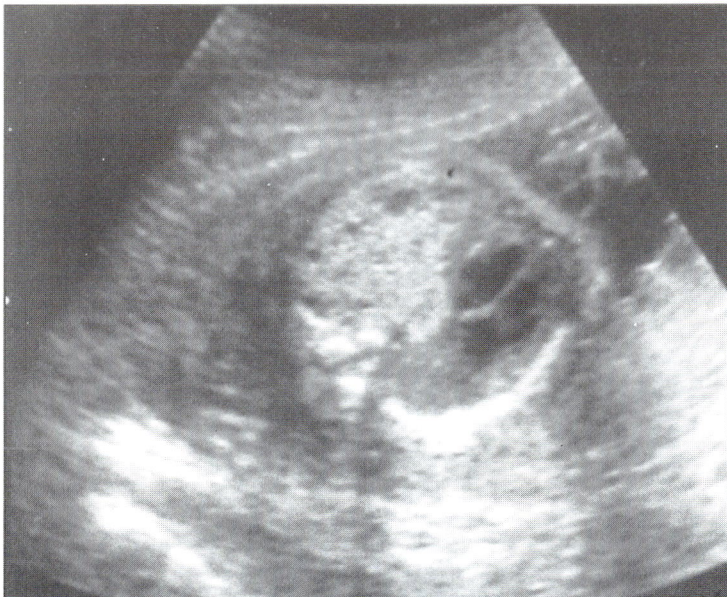

A

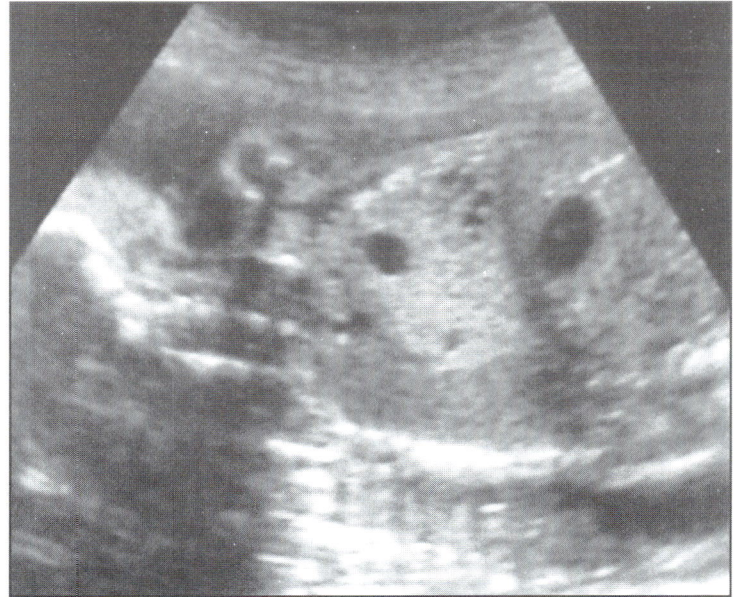

B

Figs 13.93A and B: Congenital cystic adenomatoid malformation. A. Transverse scan. Left cystic adenomatoid malformation of the lung, macrocyst type. B. Oblique view: A case of cystic adenomatoid malformation of the lung, macrocyst type

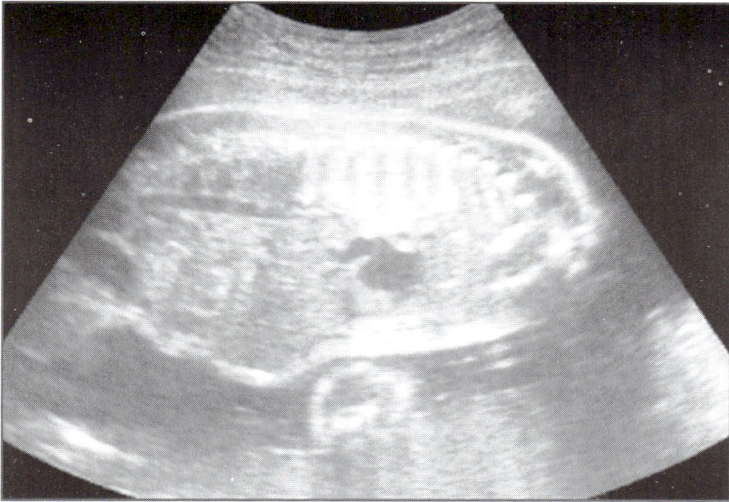
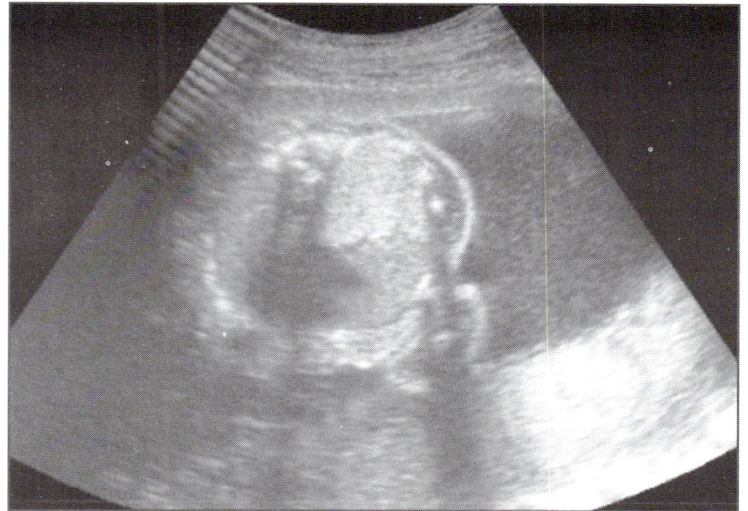

A   **B**

Figs 13.94A and B: Congenital cystic adenomatoid malformation. A. Oblique view demonstrating mass effect of the adenomatoid malformation, microcyst type, with bowing of the diaphragm. B. Transverse image demonstrating a cyst adenomatoid malformation microcyst type, with, displacing the heart

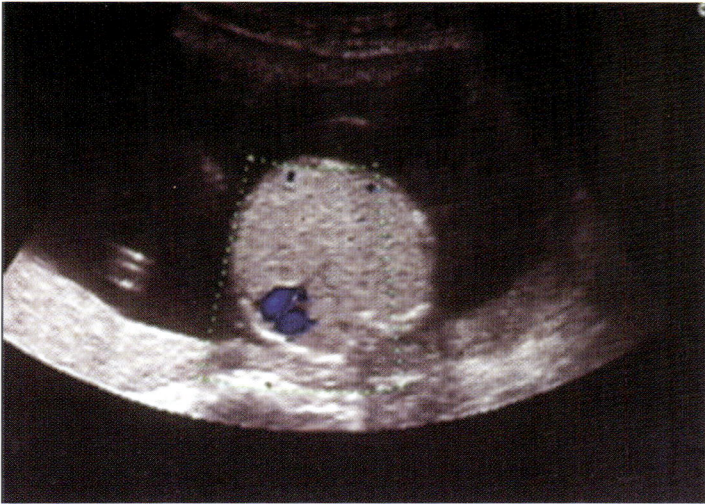
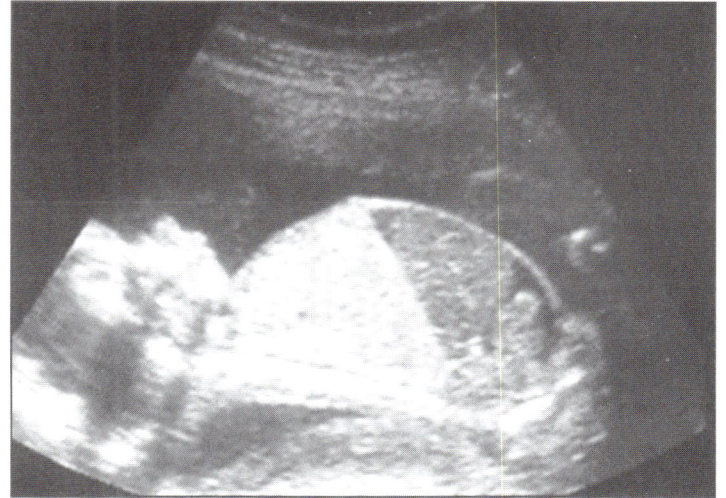

A   **B**

Figs 13.95A and B: Congenital cystic adenomatoid malformation. A. Transverse scan: Bilateral cystic adenomatoid malformation, microcyst type. A hyperechoic mass in the left and right sides. B. Oblique image: Bilateral cystic adenomatoid malformation, large echogenic lungs and ascites

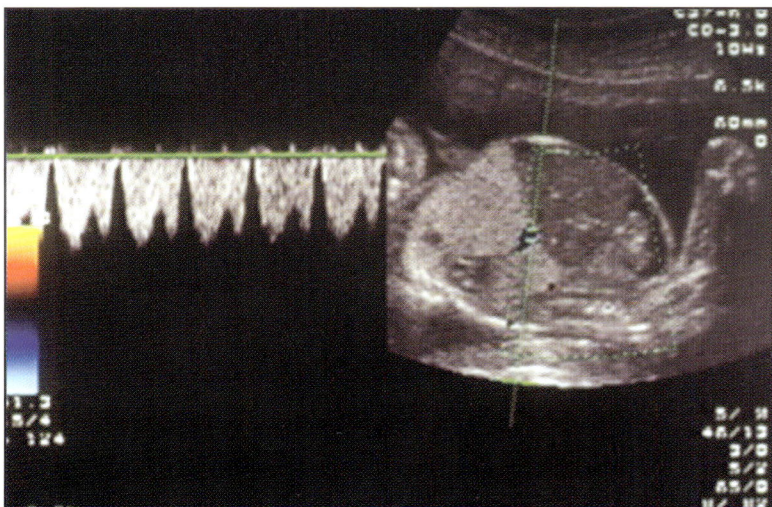
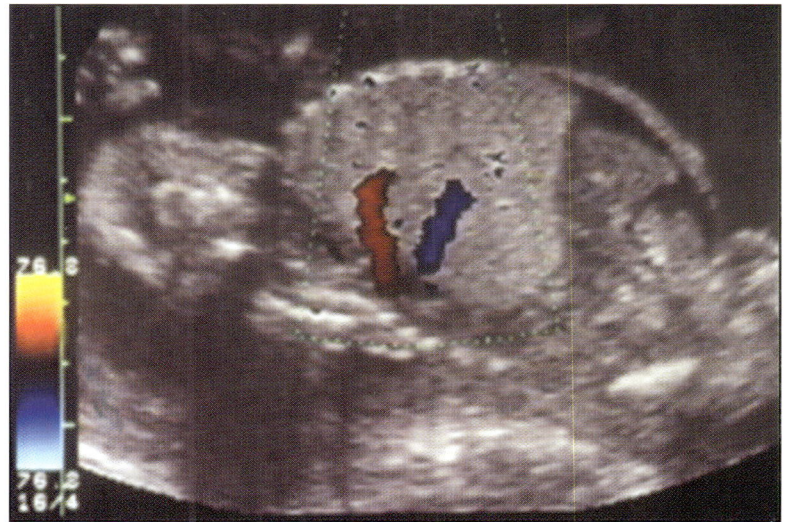

A   **B**

Figs 13.96A and B: Congenital cystic adenomatoid malformation. A. Bilateral cystic adenomatoid malformation, microcyst type color Doppler scan shows a abnormal pattern flow of ductus venosus. B. Bilateral cystic adenomatoid malformation, microcyst type, large echogenic lungs and ascites

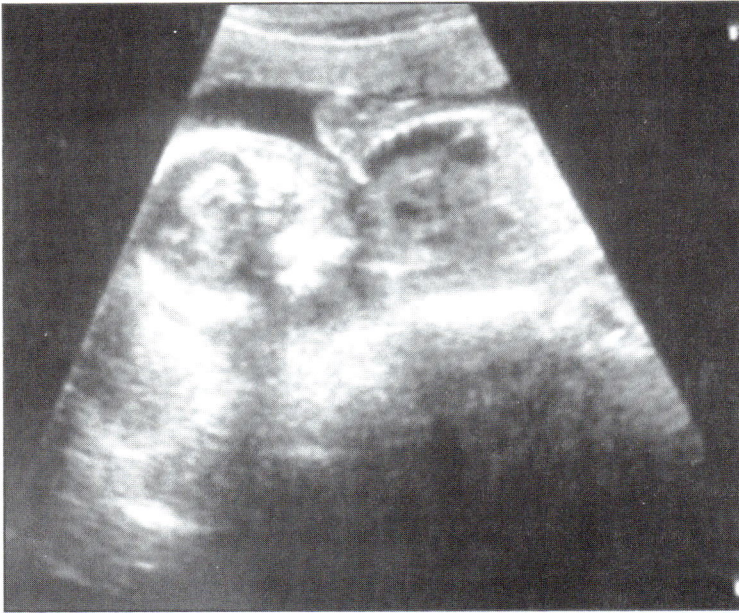

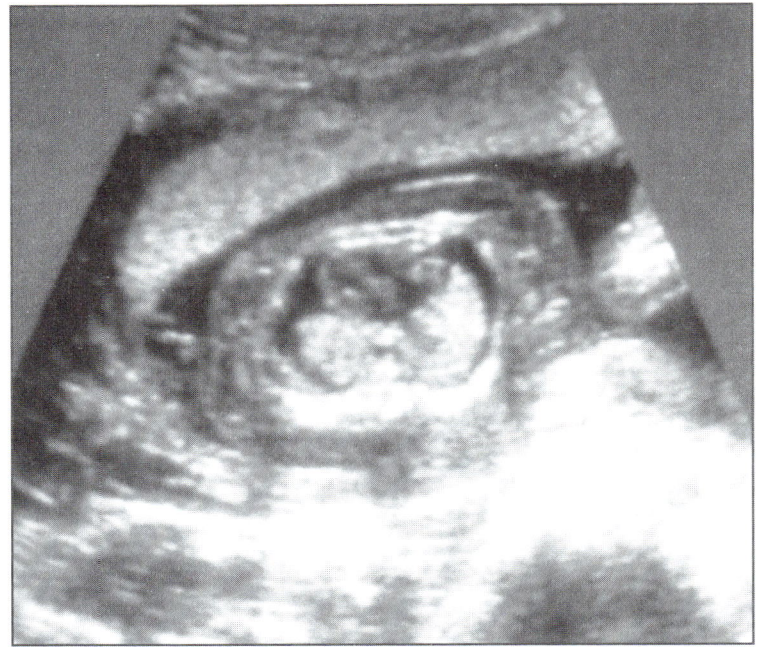

A

B

Figs 13.97A and B: Pleural effusion: A. Oblique image of fetal thorax, Bilateral effusion.
B. Transverse image of the fetal thorax. Bilateral effusion and hydrops.

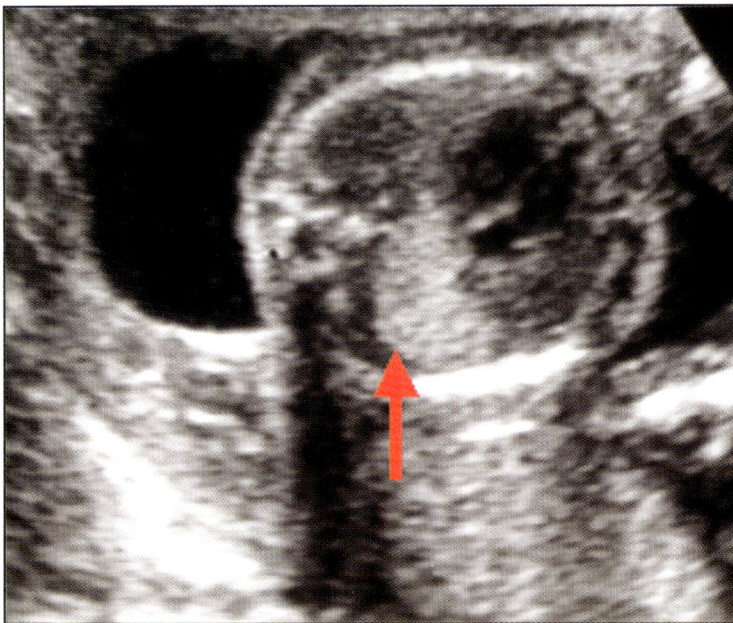

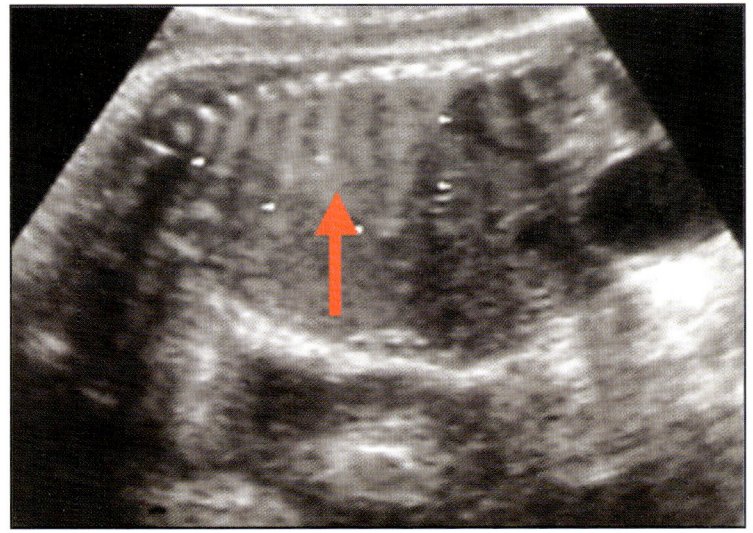

A

B

Figs 13.98A and B: Lung sequestration (intrathoracic). A. Transverse view. A right sided echogenic intrathoracic mass was noted which was a lung sequestration. B. Coronal image: An echogenic intrathoracic mass was noted (lung sequestration)

SEQUESTRATION OF THE LUNGS

This condition appears as a homogeneous and brightly echogenic mass (accessory lung) situated in the lower lobes of the lungs or in the upper abdomen. The diagnosis may be confirmed by color Doppler that shows that vascular supply of the sequestered lobe arises from the abdominal aorta(Figs 13.98 A and B to 13.100A and B).

There are two types of the sequestration of the lungs: intralobar and extralobar sequestration. In the first type, the accessory lung arises before the formation of the pleura and this sequestrated lung will be adjacent to the normal lung and surrounded by the same pleura. On the contrary, when the accessory lung bud arises after formation of pleura, the sequestrated lung will have its own pleura. This is why it is called extralobar.

Large lung sequestration may act as an arteriovenous fistula and cause high-output heart failure and hydrops.[45]

Other lesions that may be diagnosed by ultrasonography are: the *bronchogenic cyst* (Fig. 13.101), and *laryngeal atresia* (Figs 13.102A and B).

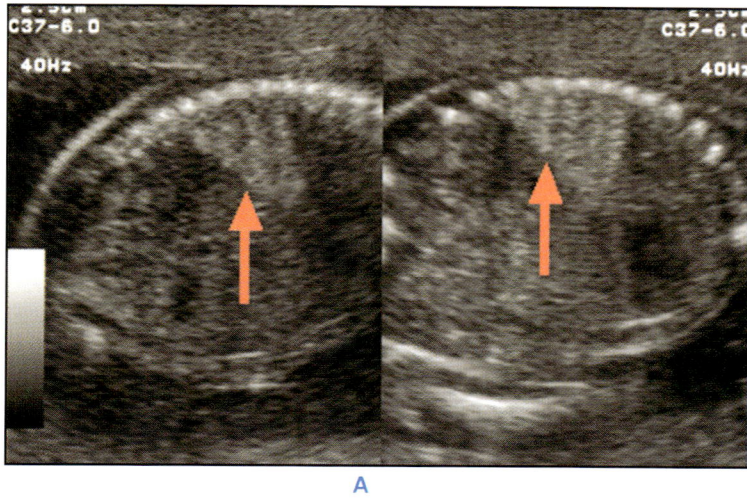

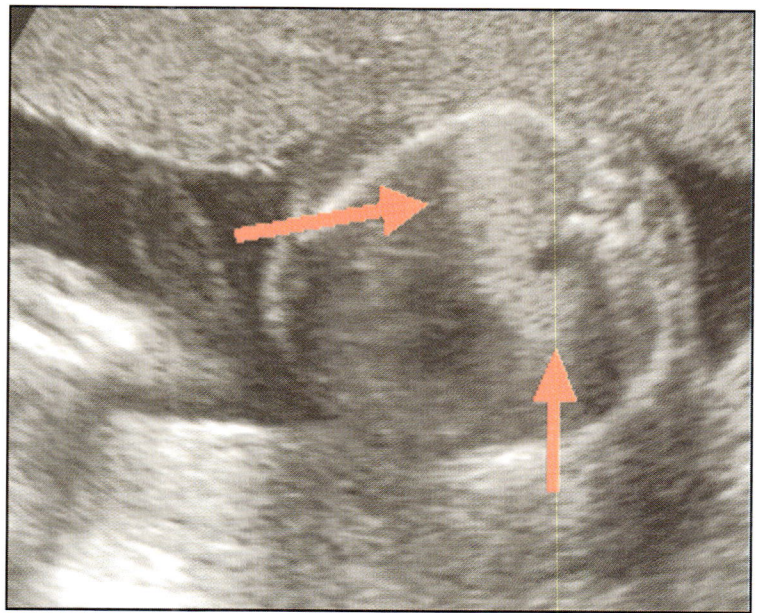

Figs 13.99A and B: Lung sequestration (intrathoracic). A. Dual image of lower pulmonary lobe. A hyperechoic mass in the left and right sides (Bilateral sequestration). B. Transverse view: A hyperechoic mass, located in front of the aorta, extends towards the left and right sides (Bilateral sequestration)

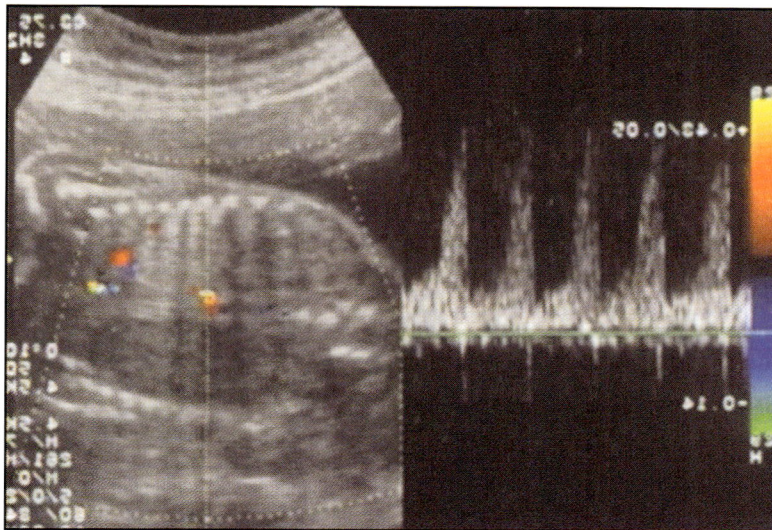

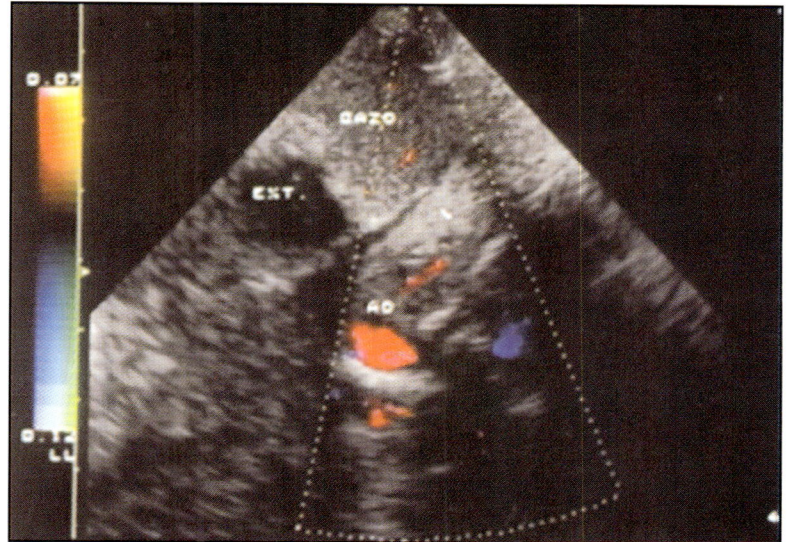

Figs 13.100A and B: Lung sequestration (intrathoracic). A. Thorax view: Color Doppler shows a ectopic vascular supply to a fetal pulmonary sequestration. B. Postnatal scan shows an ectopic vascular supply, confirming the diagnosis of pulmonary sequestration

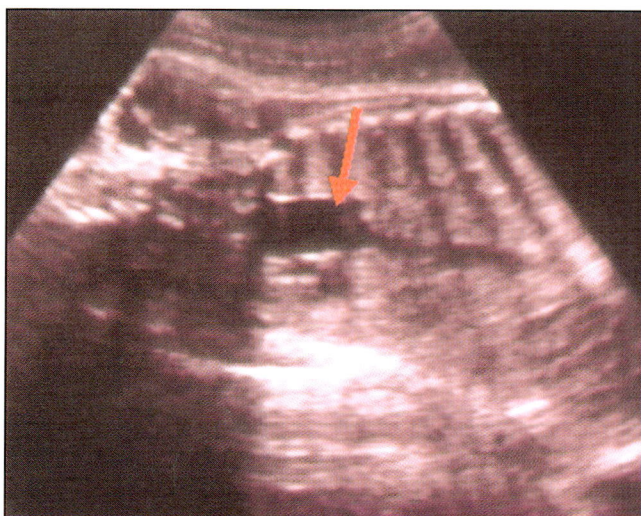

Fig. 13.101: Bronchogenic cyst: Thorax view shows a mediastinal cyst

ANTERIOR ABDOMINAL WALL DEFECTS

A Muñoz, JM Carrera, C Millán, MA Rodriguez

INTRODUCTION

In this section we describe three wall defects: omphalocele, gastroschisis and limb body wall complex.

OMPHALOCELE

Omphalocele is a ventral wall defect in which the abdominal cavity (bowel loops, stomach, liver, etc.) is herniated into a sac

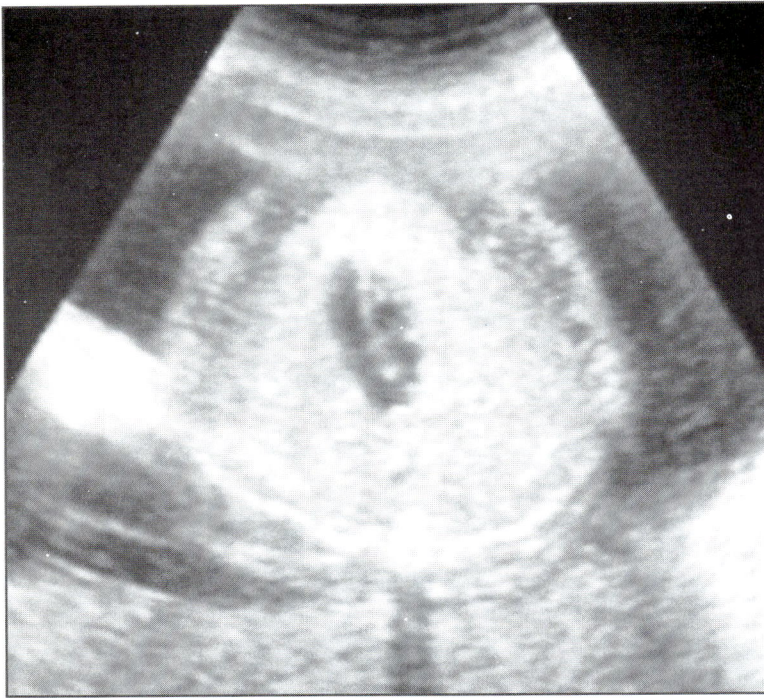

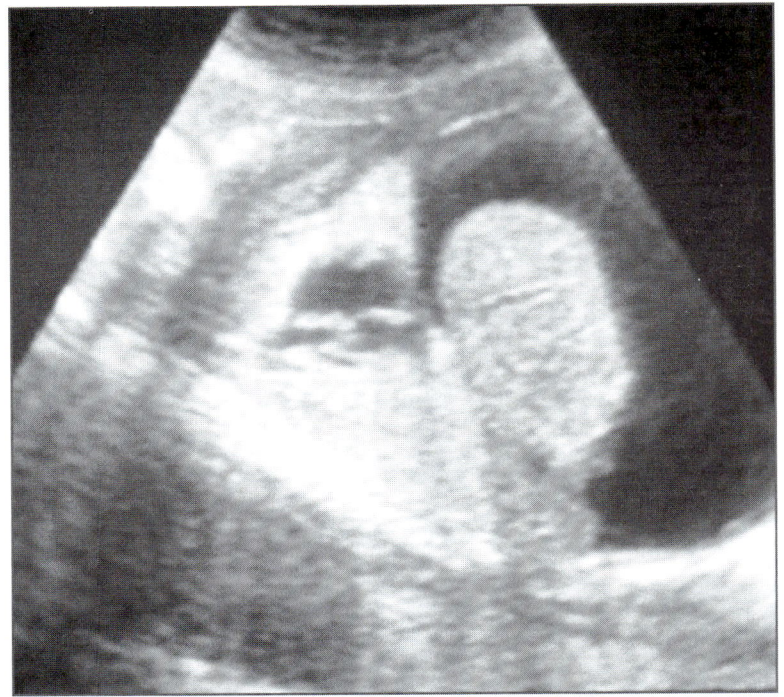

A   B

Figs 13.102A and B: Laryngeal atresia. A .Transverse scan: This is a case of laryngeal atresia with the typical cardiac compression. B. Case of laryngeal atresia. Ascites and edema, large echogenic lung investing the diaphragm

in close proximity to the umbilical cord, and covered with an amnioperitoneal membrane.

The sonographic appearance varies according to the type of defect, the presence of ascites and the organs herniated. The main features are: the umbilical cord insertion into the membrane covering the abdominal wall defect, the confirmation of intrahepatic portion of the umbilical vein in the central portion of the defect, and the presence of a limiting membrane. If the omphalocele does not contain the liver it is difficult to make an early diagnosis (Figs 13.103 to 13.115).

A high incidence of aneuploidy, anomalies of the other organs and different syndromes, especially pentalogy of Cantrell (abdominal defects, deficiency of diaphragmatic periocardium, anterior diaphragm defect, cardiac anomaly) and Beckwitz-Wiedeman syndrome (macroglossia, visceromegaly and omphalocele) are associated with this defect.

It is very important not to confuse the omphalocele with the physiological midgut herniation which subsides at 11 to 12 weeks.[46,47] Therefore, the early diagnosis of omphalocele must be considered after this week.

GASTROSCHISIS

This malformation consists in a paraumbilical defect of the abdominal wall, probably as a consequence of a very early occlusion on the right umbilical or omphalomesenteric vessel.[48,49] Through this defect the abdominal organs protrude into the amniotic fluid, without a covering membrane. For this reason, the sonographic examination shows as "cauliflower-shaped" mass or free-floating loops of bowel.[50] The liver rarely found herniating in this defect (Figs 13.116 and 13.117).

In contrast to omphalocele, gastroschisis is not usually associated with chromosomal abnormalities or other malformations.

LIMB BODY STALK ANOMALY

This defect is caused by the failure of formation of the body stalk. The main features are: absence of umbilical cord and umbilicus, and the fusion of the placenta to the herniated viscera.[51,52]

The sonographic diagnosis is a consequence of the vision of a large anterior wall defect attaching the fetus to the placenta or uterine wall. At the same time pay attention to the absence of umbilical cord, and the visualization of abdominal organs in a sac outside the abdominal cavity (Figs 13.118 to 13.123).

Multiple malformations may be associated. The fetus exhibits a great scoliosis and kyphosis.

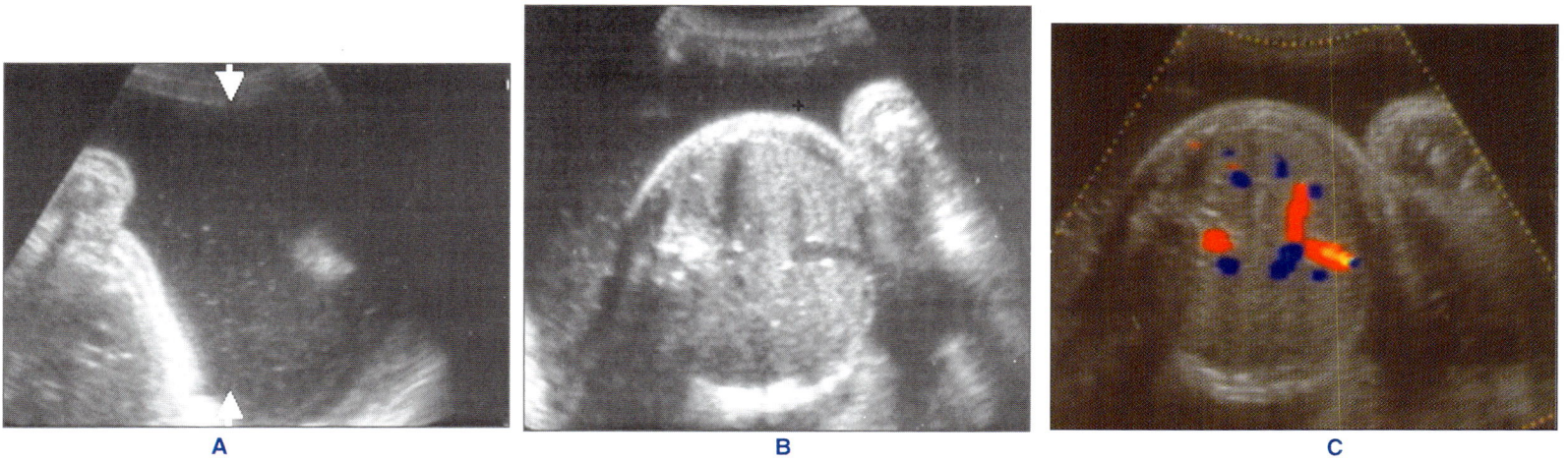

Figs 13.103 A to C: Esophageal atresia: A. Polyhydramnios. B. Transverse view of abdomen shows nonvisualization of stomach. C. Color Doppler shows the umbilical vein and an absent stomach

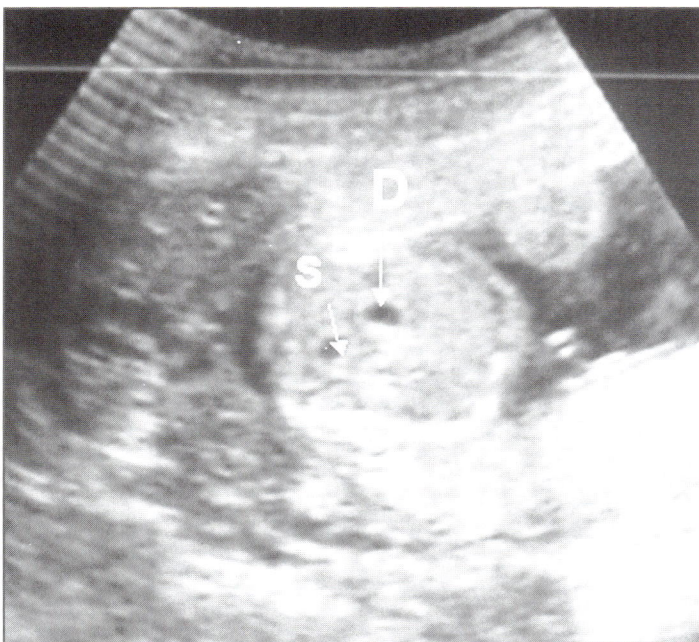
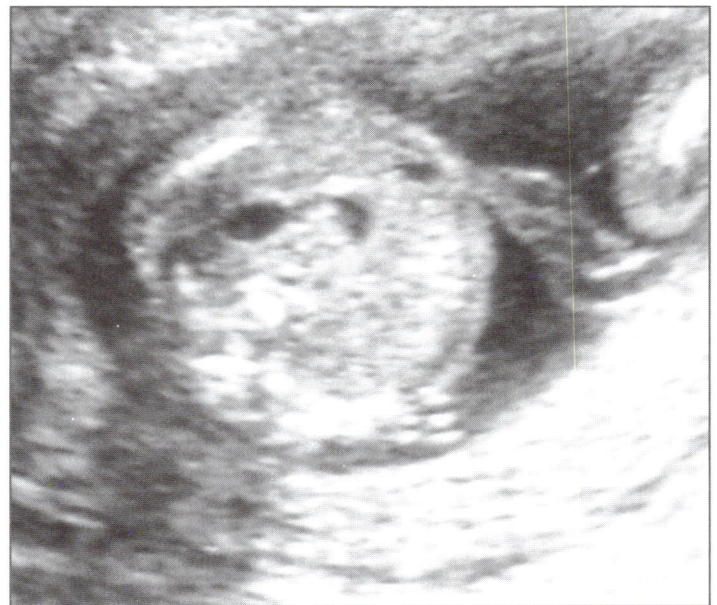

Fig. 13.104

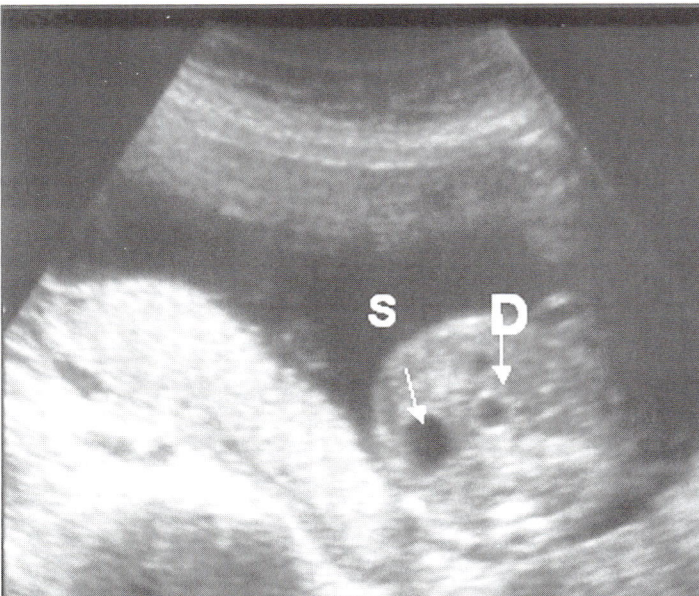
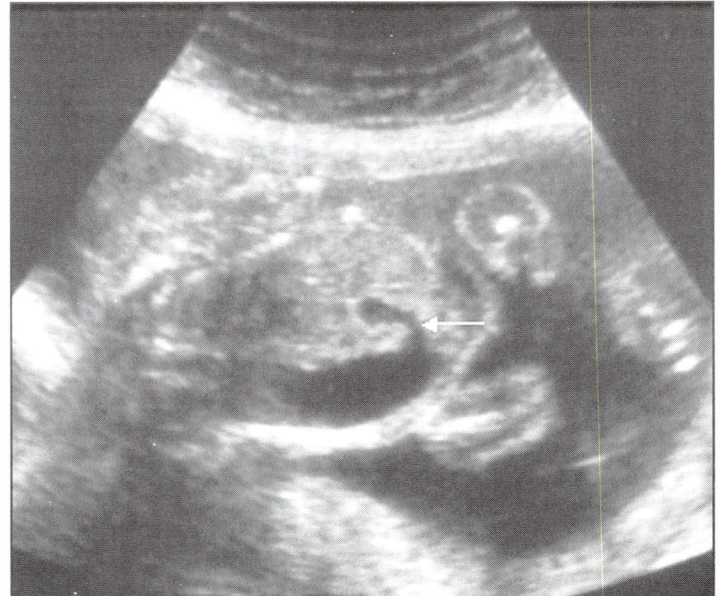

Fig. 13.105

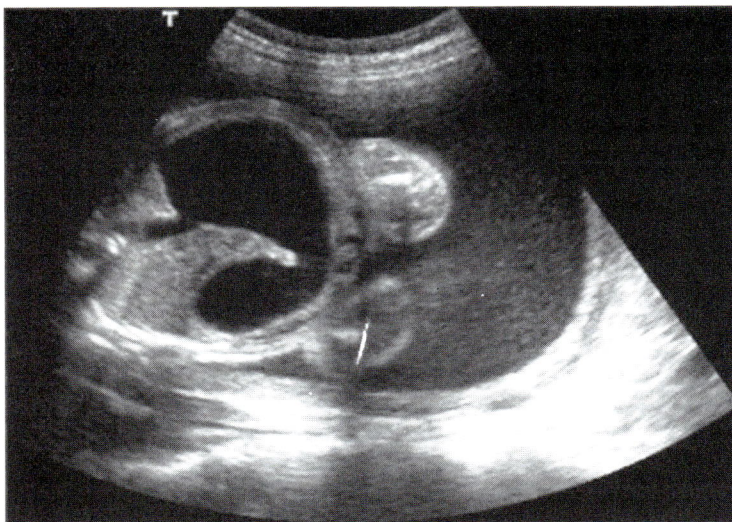

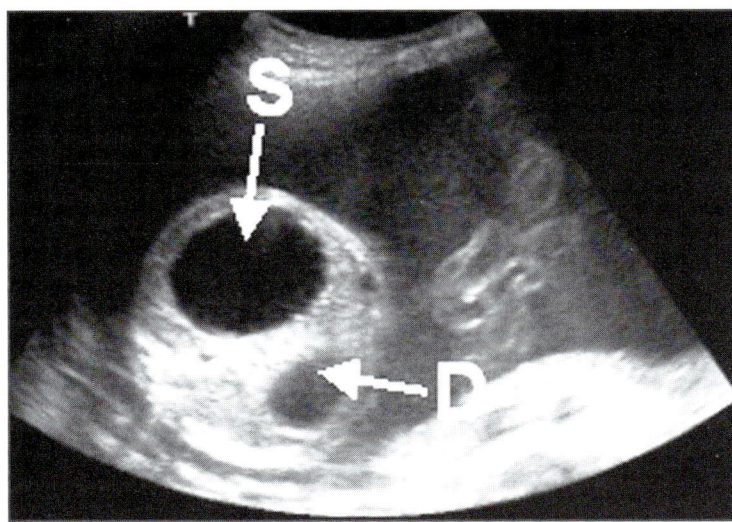

Figs 13.104 to 13.106: Duodenal atresia: Left: The images show the communication between both cystic images which correspond to the stomach and the dilated duodenum. Right: Transverse scans demonstrate the double-bubble representing the fluid-filled stomach and the duodenum

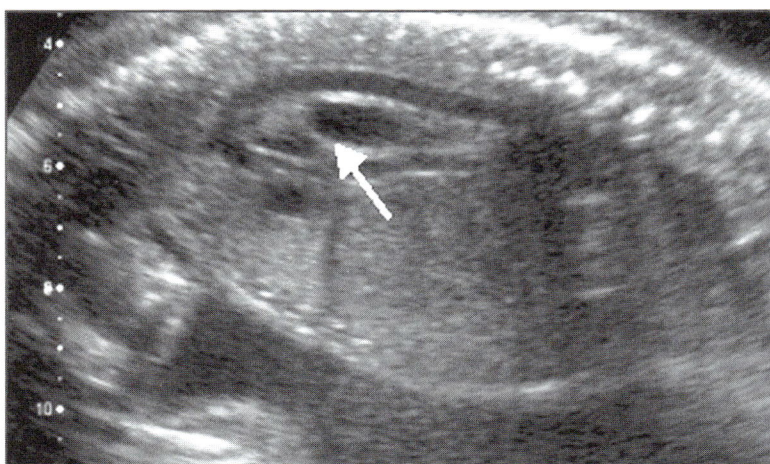

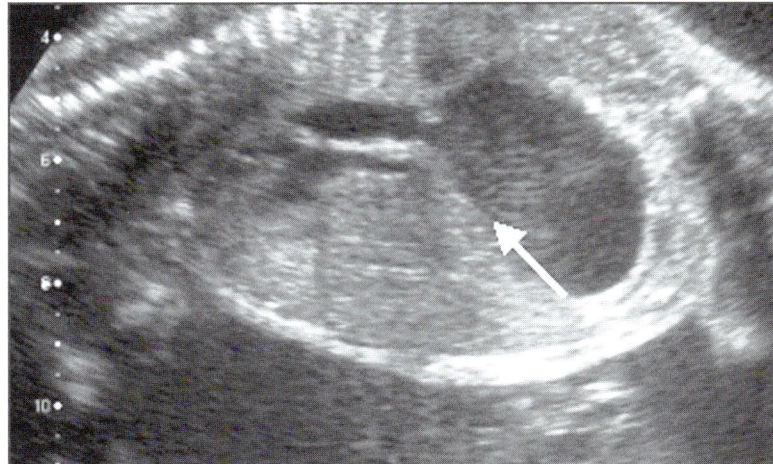

Fig. 13.107: Esophageal and duodenal atresia. Longitudinal scan with a combined esophageal and duodenal atresia. The left cystic image shows the dilated esophage and the right cystic image shows to the dilated stomach

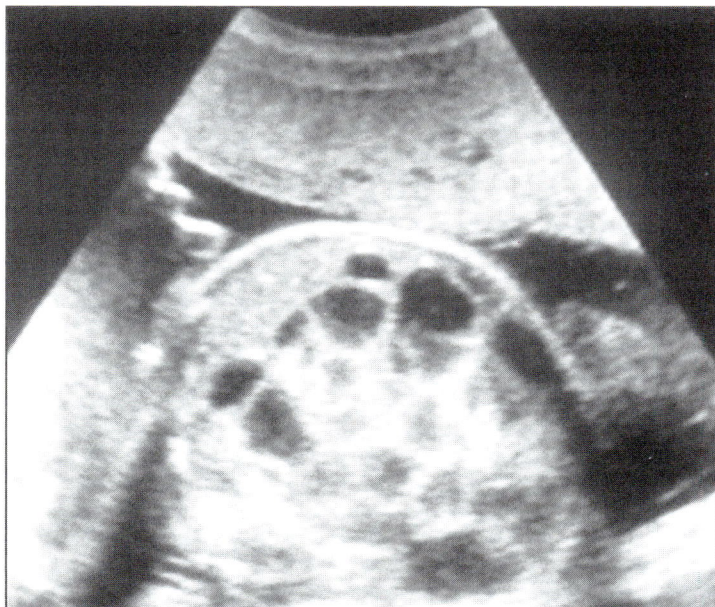

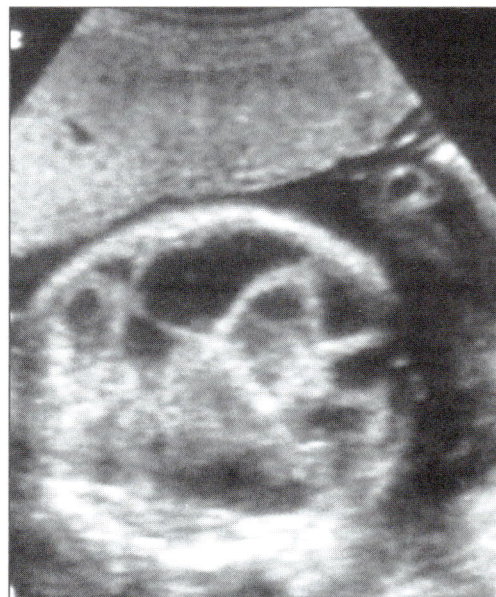

Figs 13.108A and B: Intestinal artresia: A. Transverse of the abdomen. B. Jejunal atresia shows dilated loops of the small bowel

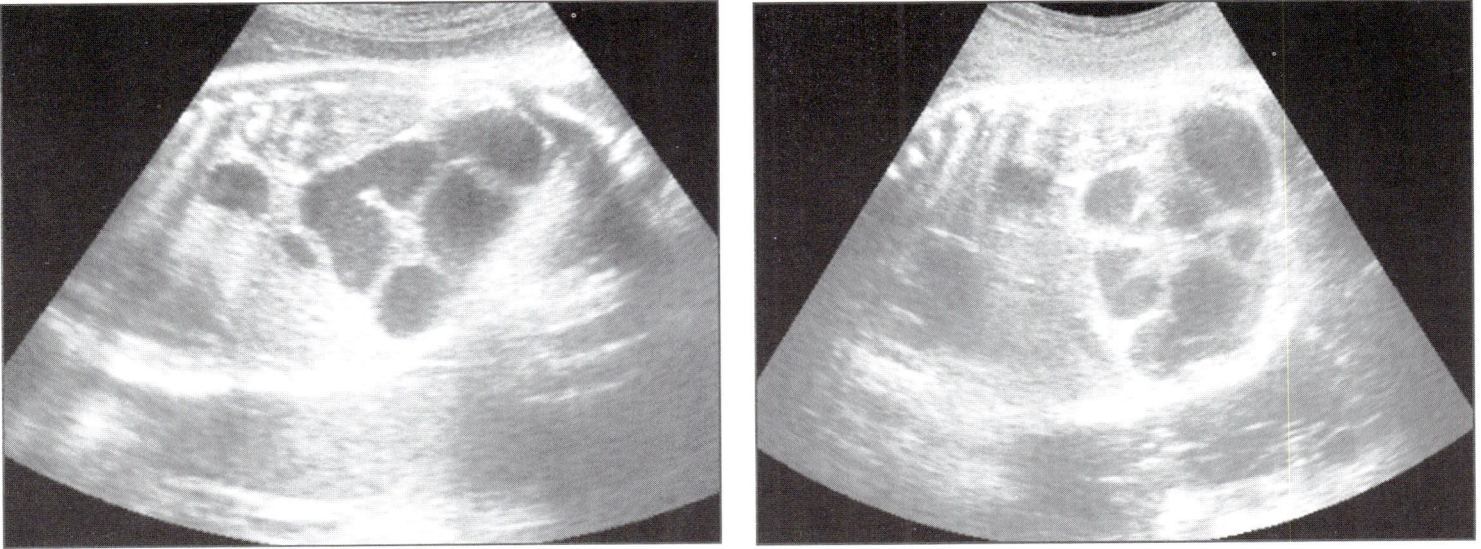

Fig. 13.109: Intestinal atresia: Longitudinal scan shows dilated loops corresponding to a bowel obstruction

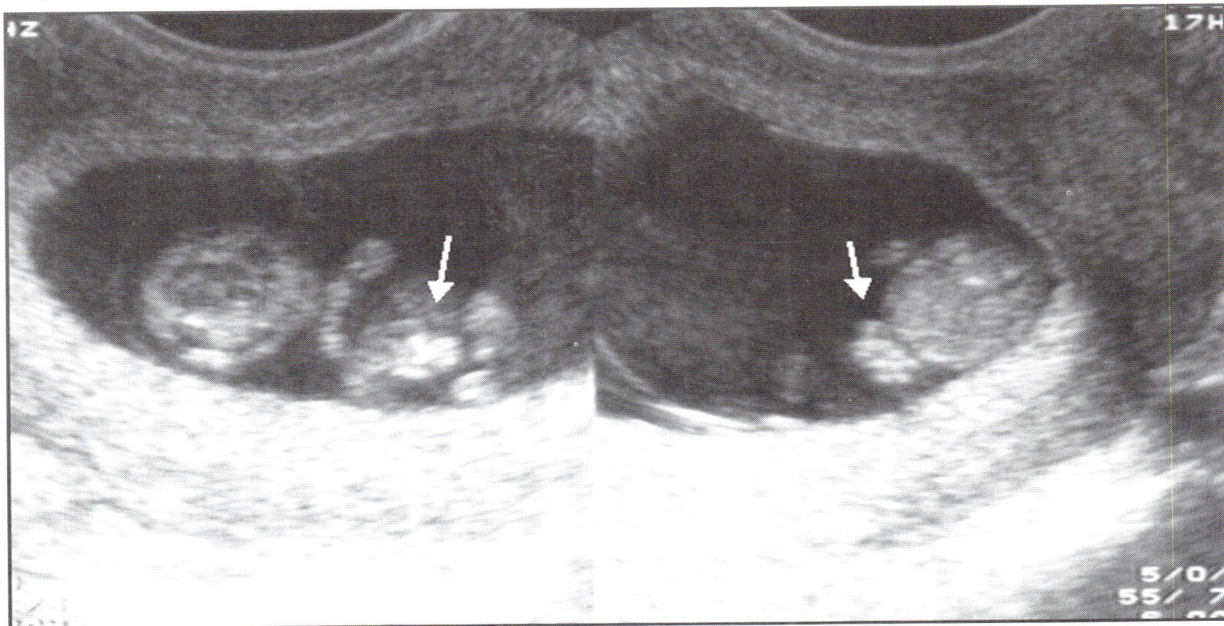

Fig. 13.110: Physiologic bowel herniation: Ninth menstrual week.Longitudinal and transverse view of the physiologic bowel herniation

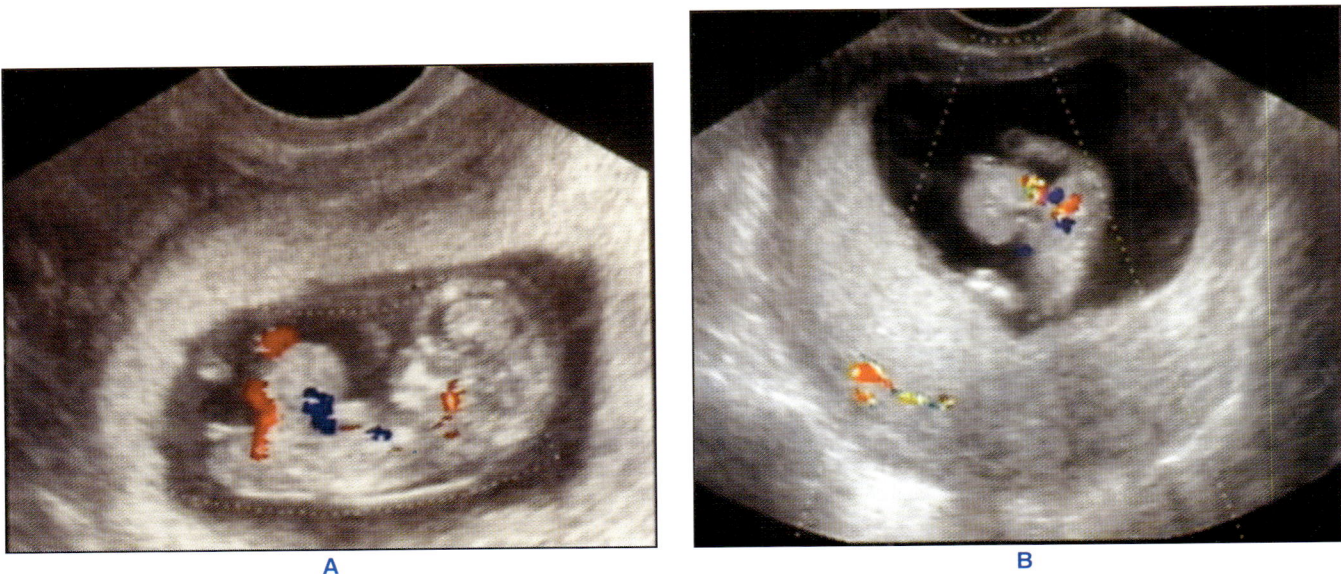

Figs 13.111A and B: Omphalocele: 11 menstrual weeks. A. Longitudinal section through the fetal body shows a solid mass in the cord insertion. B. Color Doppler identifies the umbilical vessels

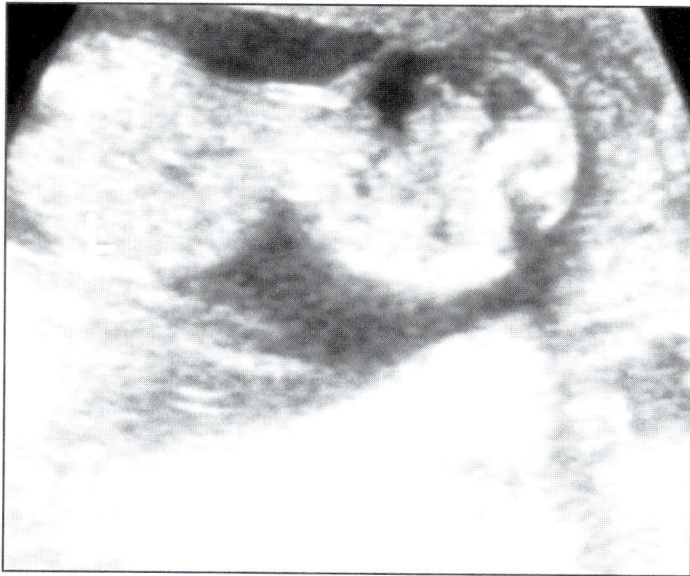

A

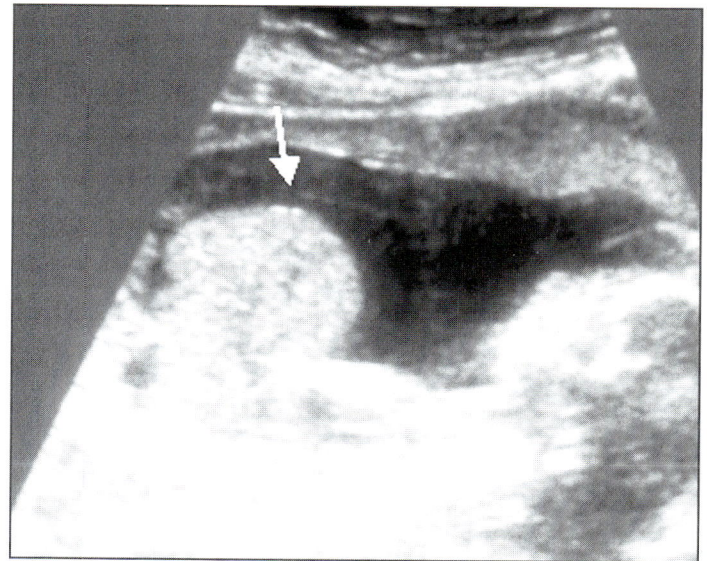

B

Figs 13.112A and B: Omphalocele: 20th menstrual week. A. Transverse section through the fetal body shows a solid mass in the cord insertion. (L) Liver. B. Longitudinal section through the fetal body shows a solid mass

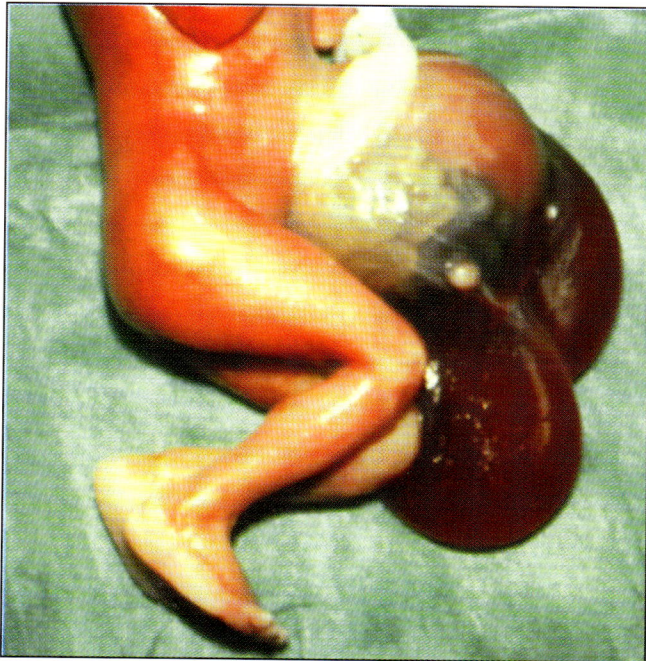

Fig. 13.113: Omphalocele: 20th menstrual week. Omphalocele, extracorporeal liver and bowel surrounded by the membrane

GENITOURINARY TRACT MALFORMATIONS

V Latin, M Kos, U Marton, M Torrents, JM Carrera, F Astudillo, A Muñoz

INTRODUCTION TO URINARY TRACK ANOMALY

Abnormalities of the urinary tract are a group of fetal anomalies which present challenges in prenatal diagnosis. They are easily recognized because they are invariably accompanied by fluid-filled masses in the fetal abdomen. Fetal urine is the major source

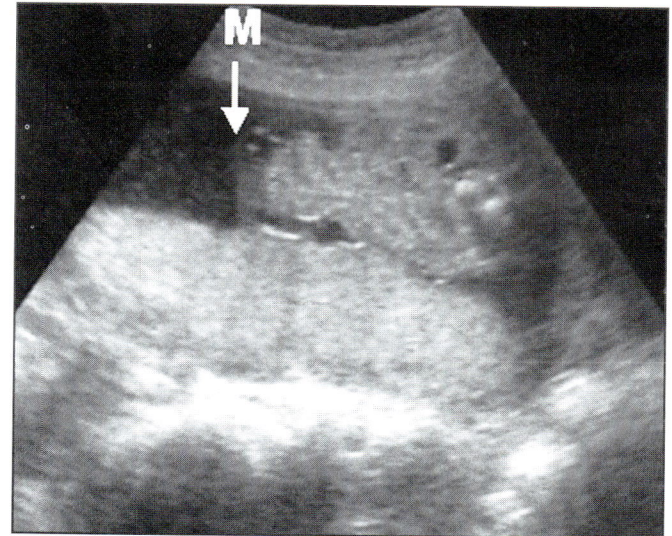

A

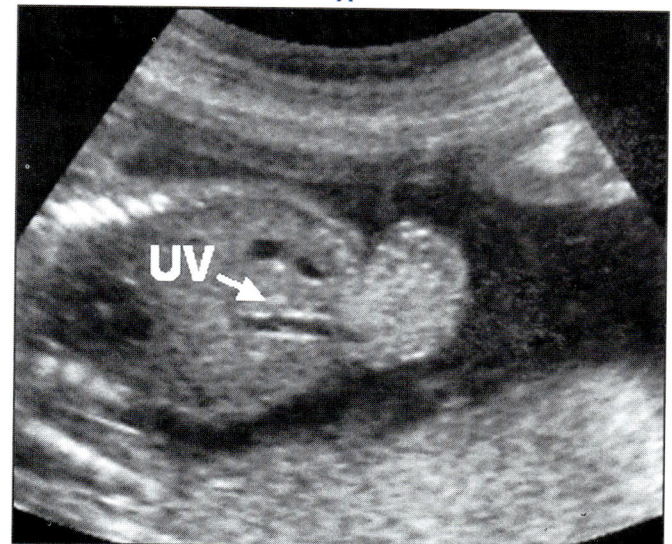

B

Figs 13.114A and B: Omphalocele: 19th menstrual week. A. Transverse view shows the extracorporeal bowel surrounded by the membrane (M). B. Extracorporeal bowel. Umbilical vein (UV)

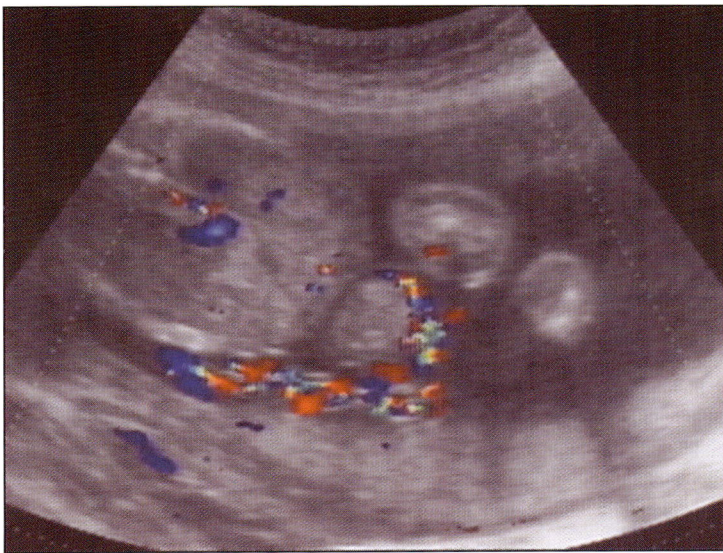
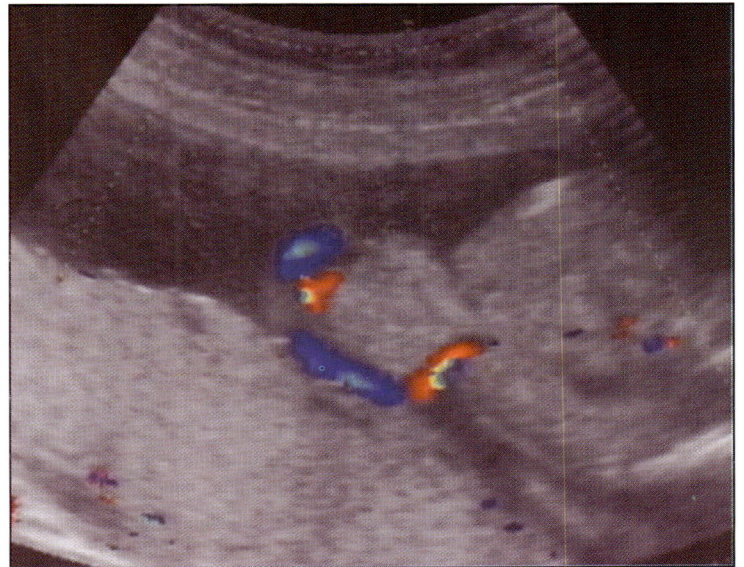

Figs 13.115A and B: Omphalocele: 19th menstrual week. A: Transverse view shows a solid mass (bowel). Color Doppler identifies the cord insertion. B. Transverse view shows a solid mass (bowel). Color Doppler identifies the umbilical vessels

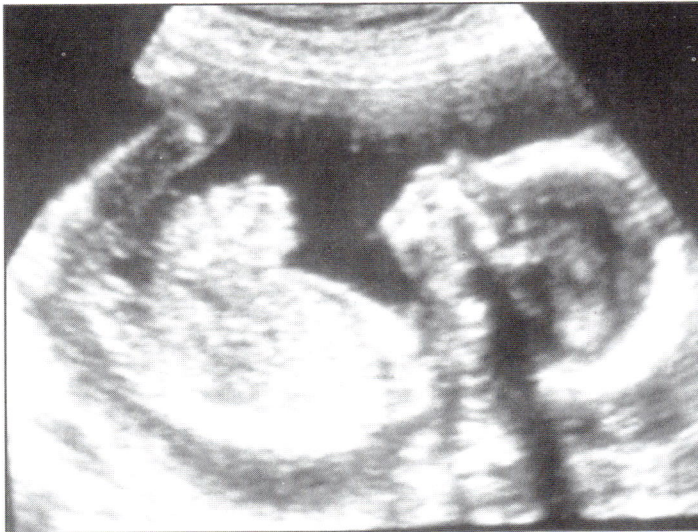
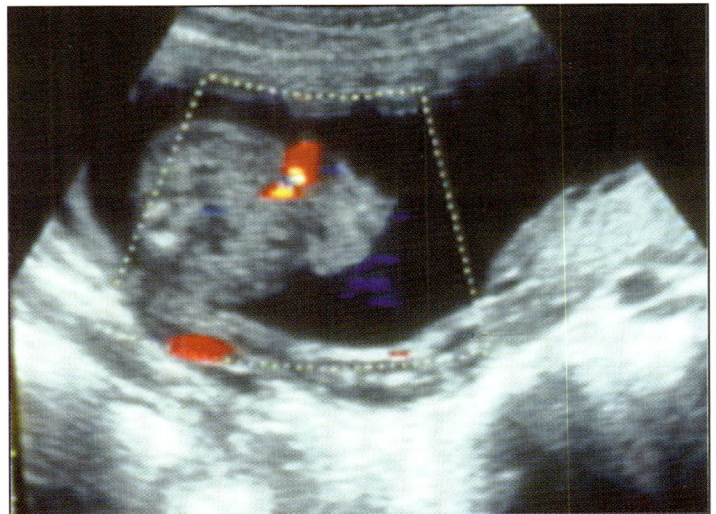

Figs 13.116A and B: Gastroschisis: 19th menstrual week. A. Longitudinal scan shows the loops of bowel protruding through a defect in the abdominal wall, not covered by a membrane. B. Transverse scan: Color Doppler demonstrates clearly that the defect is at the right side of the umbilical insertion. No membrane can be visualized

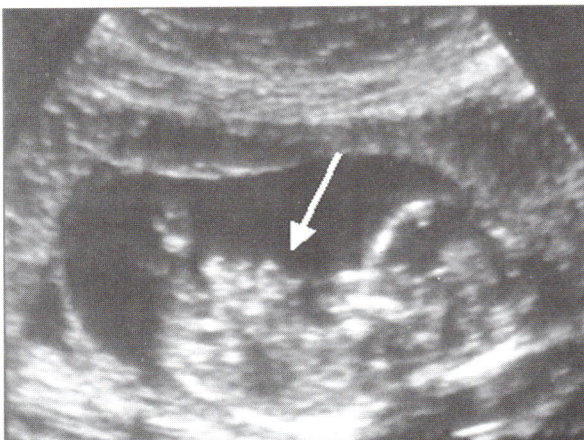
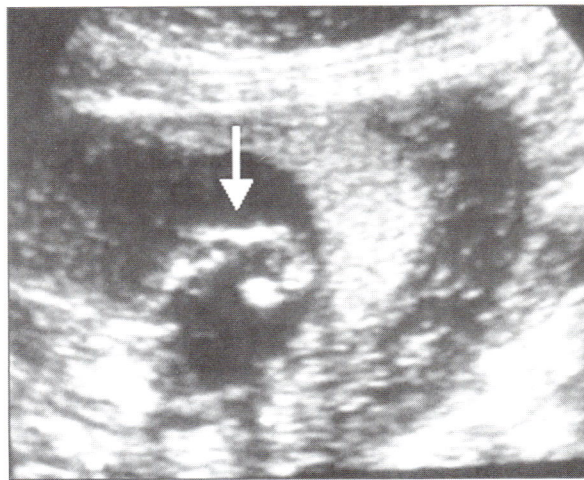
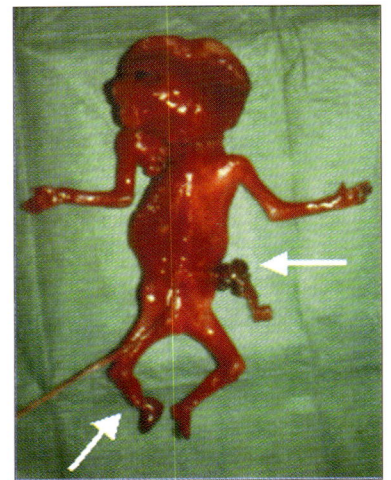

Figs 13.117A to C: Gastroschisis: 12th menstrual week. A. Longitudinal view: Loops of bowel protruding through a defect in the abdominal wall, not covered by a membrane. B. Leg anomalies. C. The pathological examination demostrates the amniotic band syndrome

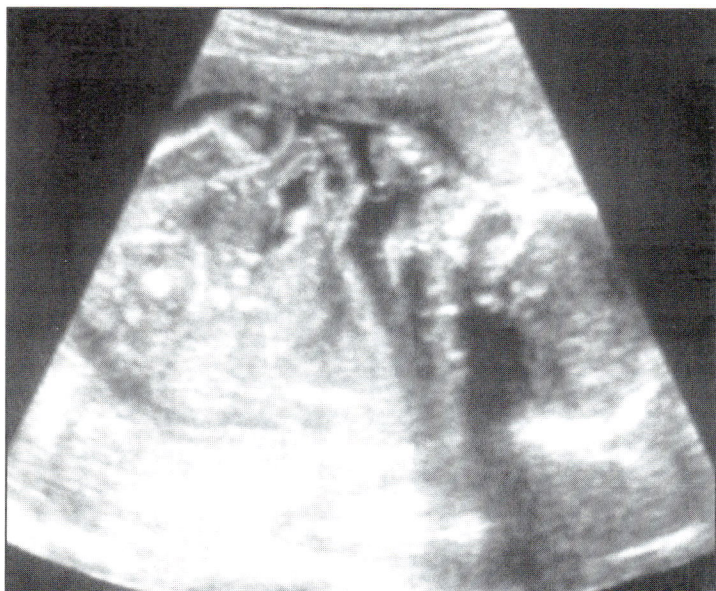

Fig. 13.118: Limb body wall complex: A huge abdominal wall defect extending from the distal part of the sternum to the suprapubic region, caused the evisceration of the fetal liver, stomach and intestines. A rather short umbilical cord connected the fetus tightly to the placenta

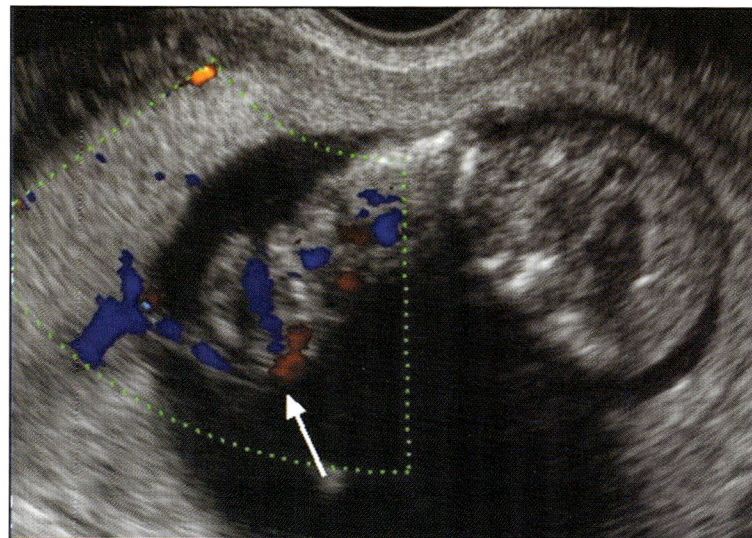

Fig. 13.119: Limb body wall complex: 12th menstrual week. Transverse section through the lower part of the thorax demostrates a large abdominal wall defect. Color Doppler identifies the heart and umbilical vein

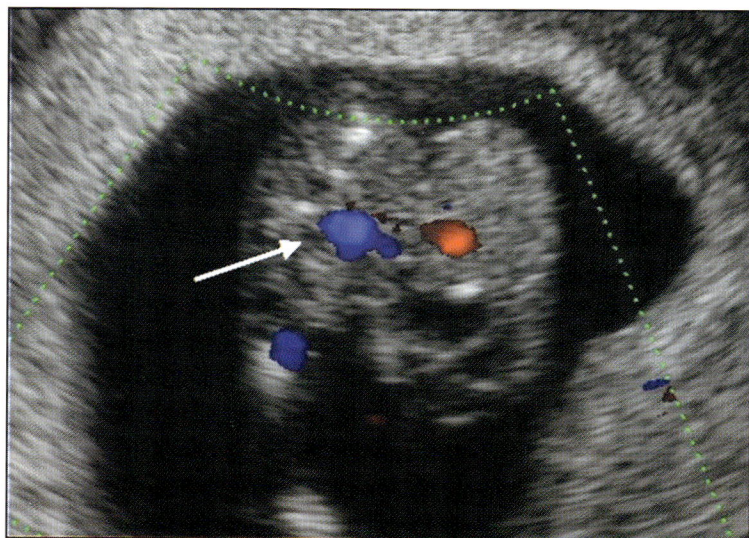

Fig. 13.120: Limb body wall complex: 12th menstrual week. Longitudinal view shows a kyphoscoliosis of the spine

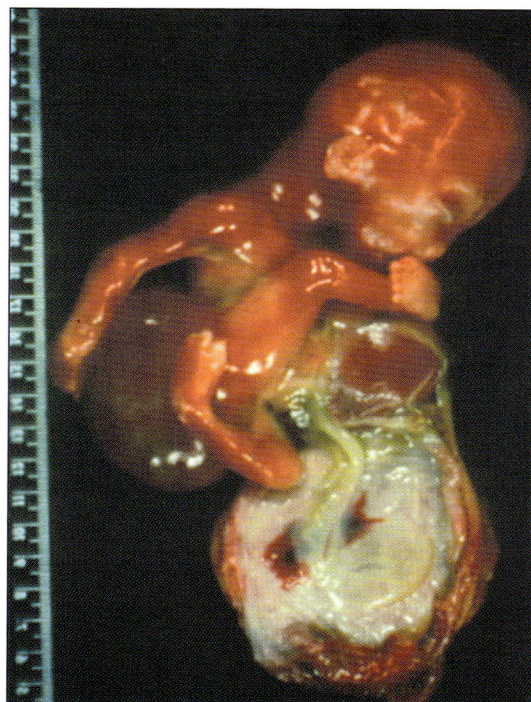

Fig. 13.121: Limb body wall complex: 13th menstrual week. Longitudinal scan of the fetus, the color Doppler shows a short umbilical cord

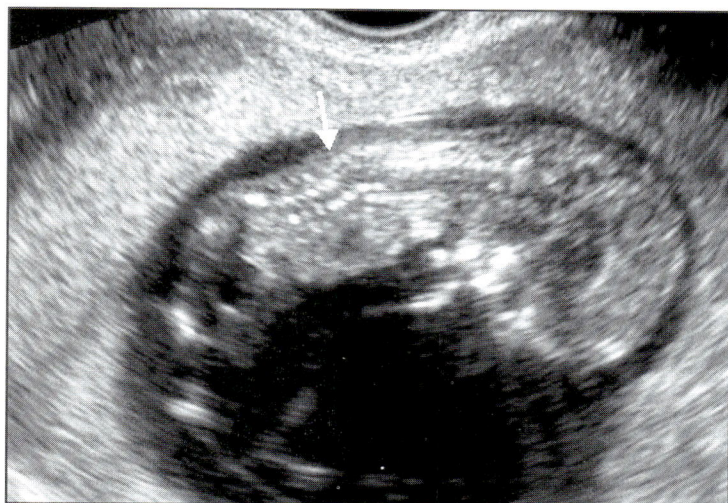

Fig. 13.122: Limb body wall complex: The pathological examination demostrates the large abdominal wall defect, the close relationship of the fetus to the placenta, and the abnormal position of the legs

of amniotic fluid and its decreased excretion or absence will result in oligohydramnios, another common marker of urinary malformations. Correct ultrasound diagnosis significantly influences obstetric management. Diagnosis of renal agenesis is likely to result in conservative management even in the presence of acute fetal distress. Some types of obstructive uropathy may warrant very aggressive management in order to save fetal life. Prenatal diagnosis of congenital hydronephrosis allows early postnatal intervention and preservation of renal function. This compares favorably with cases without antenatal diagnosis in whom the condition is recognized too late, years after delivery.

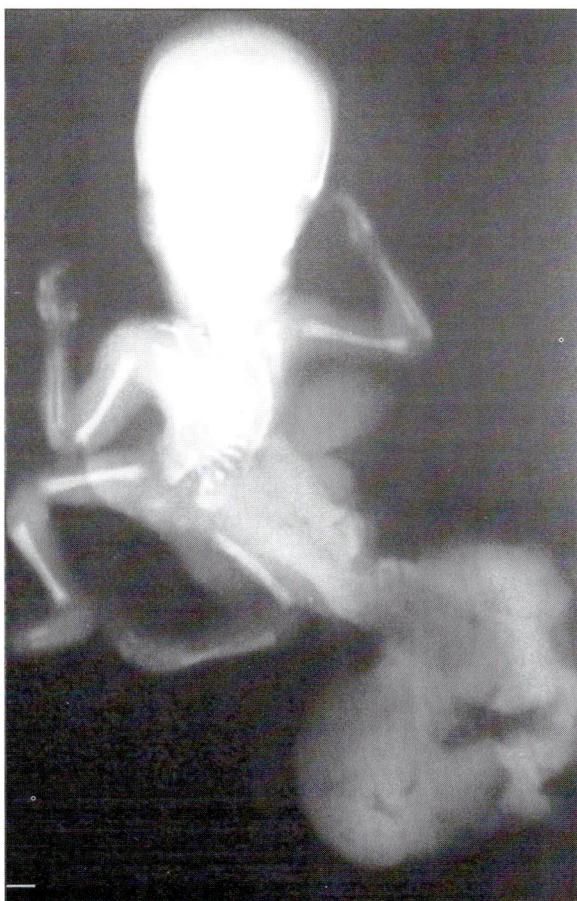

Fig. 13.123: Limb body wall complex: The X-ray examination demonstrates the large abdominal wall defect, the kyphoscoliosis of the spine and the abnormal position of the legs

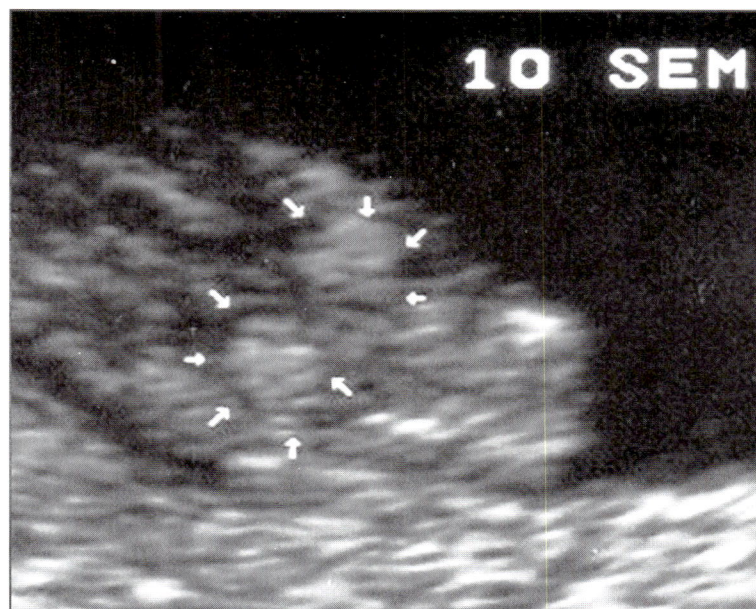

Fig. 13.124: Normal fetal kidney at 10th week. At this stage of gestation, the fetal kidneys have an increased echogenicity

Urinary malformations are relatively common. A prospective antenatal ultrasound study estimated the incidence to be around 0.65 percent.[53] The recurrence risk for genitourinary anomalies is 8 to 10 percent.[54]

NORMAL DEVELOPMENT AND ANATOMY OF THE FETAL URINARY SYSTEM

The fetal kidney can be visualized ultrasonically as early as 9.5 weeks in optimal circumstances.[55] Kidneys are readily seen at the 12th gestational week by abdominal sonography, and between 10th and 11th weeks by transvaginal sonography (Fig. 13.124).[56] At this gestational age, the kidneys can be seen as bilateral echogenic masses with an echogenicity similar to the fetal lungs. It is very easy to differentiate these structures from the hypoechogenic adrenal glands.[57] The visualization rate increases with gestational age from 79.6 percent in the 11th week to 100 percent in the 16th week of pregnancy.[56] In the second part of pregnancy, the kidneys have a typical shape and position with a central echo from the intrarenal part of the collecting system. In transverse section, they appear as two circular structures on either side of the spine and in longitudinal section, they have a typical bean-shaped appearance. Visualization difficulties can arise during the second trimester of pregnancy because the acoustic properties of renal tissue are similar to those of surrounding bowel (Figs 13.125 and 13.126). In the beginning of the second trimester, the fetal kidneys and adrenal glands are of similar size, which may cause confusion. Adrenal glands are seen in the same plane as the fetal stomach, and lie immediately adjacent to the spine, while fetal kidneys lie below the level of the stomach and are found in a transverse plane when viewed axially. Later on, the renal pyramids become evident during the third trimester and the adrenal glands are half the size of the normal kidney. A small fluid collection within the renal pelvis is a normal finding.

The longitudinal, anteroposterior and transverse diameters of the fetal kidney increase linearly throughout pregnancy, the longitudinal from 4.23 ± 0.5 mm at the 11th week to 45.9 ± 5.0 mm at term, the anteroposterior diameter from 3.81 ± 0.53 mm at the 11th week to 28.9 ± 2.4 mm at term, and the transverse from 3.78 ± 0.6 mm to 27.6 ± 2.5 mm.[56,58] The ratio of renal circumference to abdominal circumference in the second and third trimesters is constant.[58]

The fetal urinary bladder can be identified at the 11th week of pregnancy, with a visualization rate of 77.5 percent, and 100 percent at the 16th week using a transvaginal probe (Figs 13.127 and 13.128).[56] The volume of the fetal bladder may vary from 2.2 ml/h at 22nd week to 26.3 ml/h at term. The maximal volume is 50 ml.[59]

Fetal urine in early pregnancy consists of an ultrafiltrate of the fetal serum, with subsequent selective tubular reabsorption

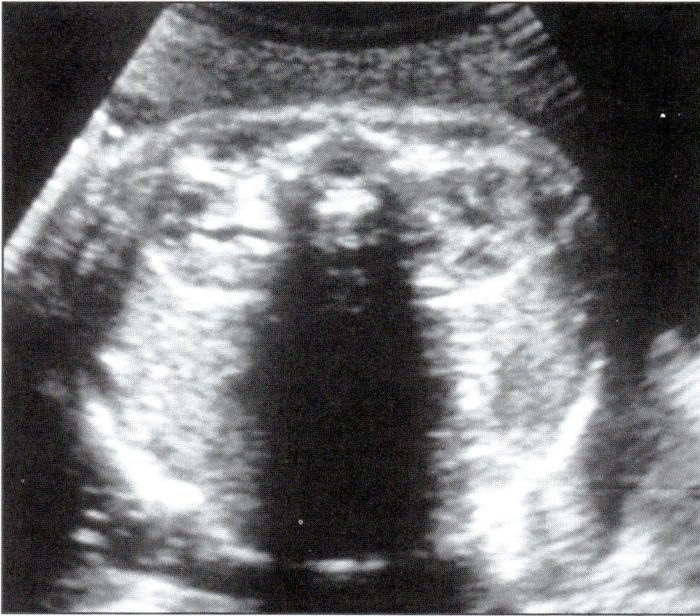

Fig. 13.125

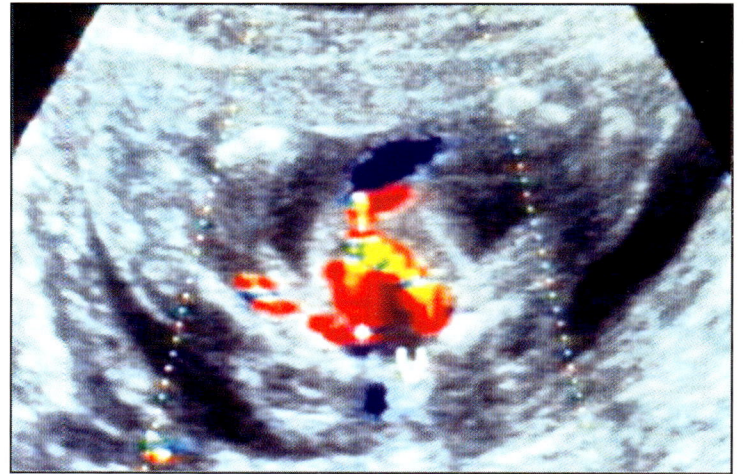

Fig. 13.125 and 13.126: TVS shows fetal kidney at 11th week of pregnancy

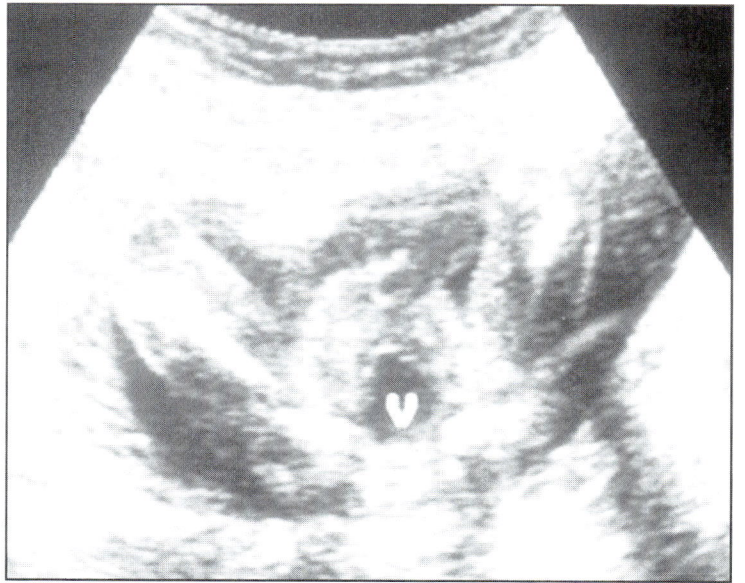

Fig. 13.127

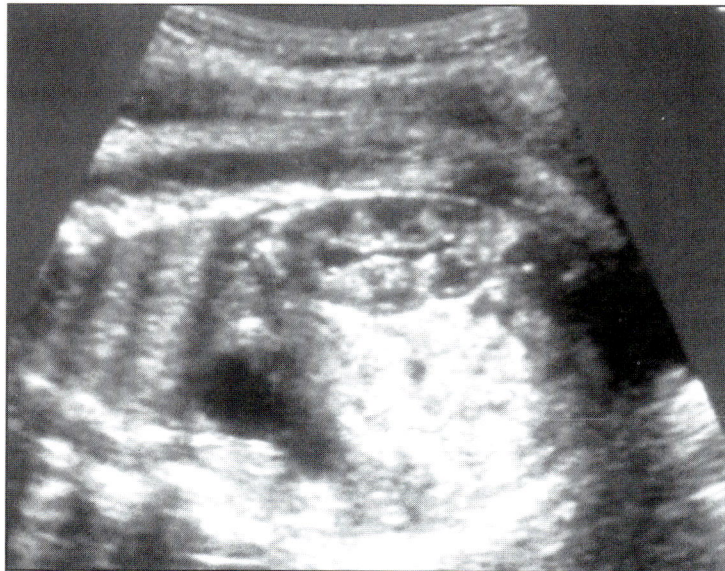

Fig. 13.127 and 13.128: Fetal urinary bladder at 11th week of gestation

of sodium and chloride. The levels of both electrolytes normally fall progressively throughout gestation, and are used in the estimation of tubular reabsorption and kidney damage in utero.[60]

URINARY TRACT MALFORMATIONS

Evaluation of the fetal bladder and kidneys is routine practice in obstetric sonography. Urinary malformations are suspected if there are the following features:

1. Decreased amniotic fluid volume.
2. Dilatation of the urinary tract.
3. Presence of a renal cyst.
4. Change in the size, shape and echogenicity of the kidney.
5. Absence of the bladder.
6. Associated malformations.

Ultrasonically recognizable urinary tract malformations are as follows:

1. Renal agenesis.
2. Renal dysgenesis: Multicystic, polycystic infantile and adult kidney disease, congenital hydro-nephrosis.
3. Bladder outlet obstruction: Posterior urethral valves, urethral stenosis and agenesis, cloacal persistence, megaureter.

Renal Agenesis

The ureteric bud arises from the mesonephric duct during the 5th week of embryonic development and migrates to the metanephros to induce formation of the definitive kidney.[61] Absence of migration will result in renal agenesis, which can be an isolated finding. The frequency of renal agenesis is 1:4000 births. In most cases, it is presumed to be associated with a polygenic inheritance, with the possibility of X-linked recessive, autosomal recessive and autosomal dominant inheritance.

Unilateral renal agenesis is common, occurring in 1 of every 600 individuals. In 40 percent of females and 12 percent of males, it is associated with anomalies of the prostate, testes, epididymis and seminal vesicles.[62] The recurrence risk is 3 percent.[63]

Bilateral agenesis is incompatible with postnatal survival. Typical features include severe oligohydramnios, pulmonary hypoplasia, limb deformities and Potter's face (old man face). The ultrasound image is usually very poor because of oligohydramnios, which can be present as early as 14th weeks, but usually at 16th to 18th weeks of pregnancy. Apart from the absence of the kidneys, the bladder is persistently small or absent, the thorax is hypoplastic and limb deformities may be present if visualization is not too bad. It could be said that the sensitivity of prenatal diagnosis by ultrasound is relatively poor because of oligohydramnios and inadequate visualization. Enlarged adrenal glands which fill the renal fossa can mimic renal appearance. Color Doppler can increase the sensitivity and help in diagnosis, because the presence of the renal artery is very clear and can confirm renal presence.

Approximately 15 percent of fetuses with bilateral renal agenesis have associated anomalies.

Differential diagnosis includes severe intrauterine growth retardation (IUGR) and premature rupture of membranes. In the presence of the latter, normal filling of the fetal bladder will be documented. In IUGR fetuses, urine production is reduced because of the brain sparing effect with diminished renal perfusion. Intravenous administration of 40 mg of furosemide will increase urine production in IUGR fetuses. However, there is doubt about the validity of the furosemide test before 32nd week of gestation.[64]

Bilateral renal agenesis is lethal and termination of the pregnancy should be offered. Isolated unilateral renal agenesis has a very good prognosis and its presence does not alter obstetric management (Figs 13.129 to 13.131).

Renal Dysgenesis

Four types of developmental anomalies are well documented [65-67] and can be diagnosed using ultrasound:
1. Autosomal recessive (infantile) polycystic kidney disease (ARPKD): Potter type I.
2. Multicystic dysplastic kidney disease (MDKD): Potter type II.
3. Autosomal dominant (adult) polycystic kidney disease (ADPKD): Potter type III.
4. Cystic renal dysplasia (CRD): Potter type IV.

Potter Type I

This form of cystic kidney disease is also known as 'infantile polycystic kidney disease' or 'microcystic kidney disease.' It is characterized by abnormal proliferation and cystic dilatation of the renal tubules. The incidence is estimated to be 1:50 000 births.[67] It is transmitted as an autosomal trait.

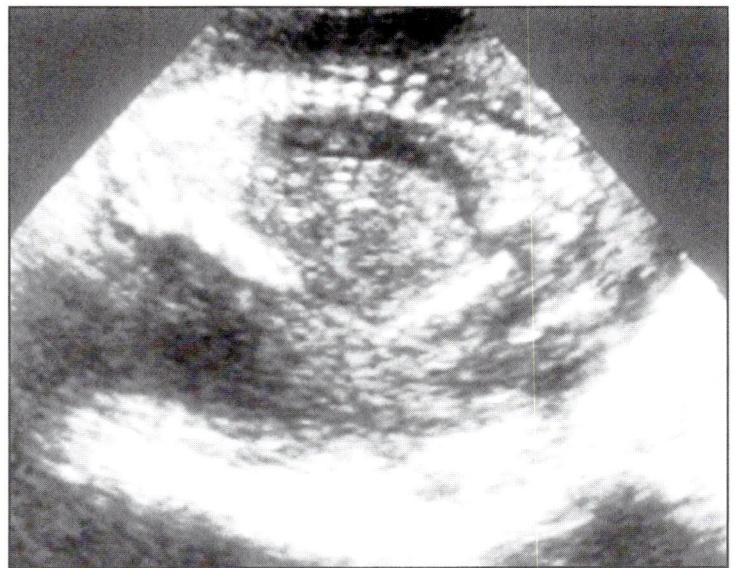
Fig. 13.129: Renal agenesis bilateral. Note the enlarged adrenal gland

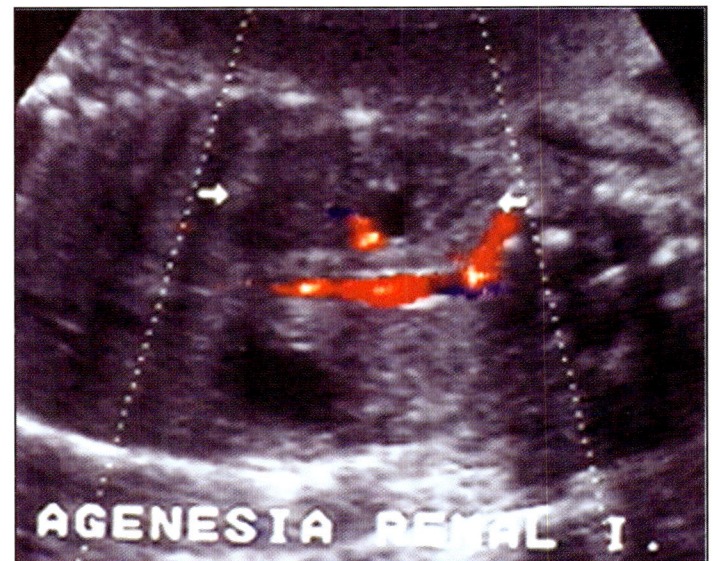
Fig. 13.130: Unilateral renal agenesis. Renal arteries in color Doppler. Notice the absence of the renal arteries

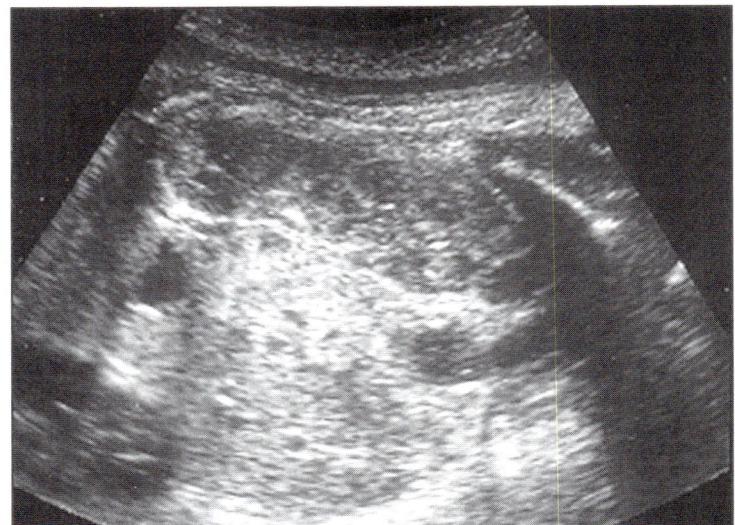
Fig. 13.131: Unilateral renal agenesis . Notice the large kidney

The sonographic picture of a large fetal kidney with hyperechogenic renal structure is very dominant. The kidney parenchyma is replaced by multiple small cysts up to 2 mm in diameter. A 'typical pattern' can be easily recognized. A hyperechogenic structure of the affected kidneys is due to the sound enhancement by the microscopic cysts present in the renal parenchyma. The involvement in ARPKD is invariably bilateral and symmetrical. Other criteria for the diagnosis are absence of the fetal bladder and oligohydramnios. Most of the reported cases were diagnosed after the 24th gestational week.

Affected fetuses with ARPKD may have generalized portal and interlobular fibrosis of the liver, accompanied by biliary duct hyperplasia and small distal vein branches. It should be stressed that ARPKD is not usually associated with other malformations. However, it has been described with Meckel-Gruber syndrome, posterior encephalocele and polydactyly. If the family history is positive, screening for 'silent' disease is advisable.

The prognosis depends on the clinical variety of ARPKD. Subclassification into perinatal, neonatal, infantile and juvenile, according to the patient's age at the time of clinical presentation, is not universally accepted despite good correlation with long-term survival. In the presence of an early prenatal appearance, coupled with severe oligohydramnios and anhydramnios, survival is rare. The perinatal type is a serious condition because 90 percent of the kidney is involved. These changes, with secondary pulmonary hypoplasia, cause rapid neonatal death. Therefore, when the diagnosis is made before fetal viability, termination of the pregnancy should be offered to the parents (Fig. 13.132).

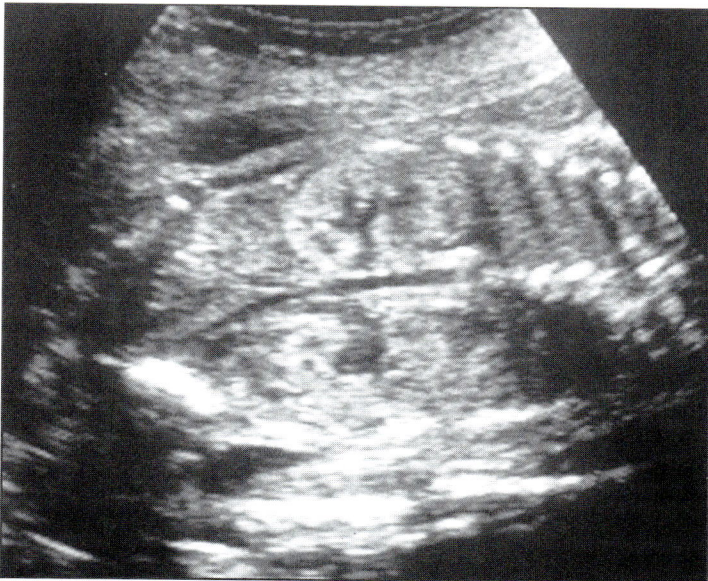

Fig. 13.132: Autosomal recessive polycystic kidney disease: The image shows enlarged kidneys with echogenic parenchyma and the oligohydramnios. The bladder is not visible

Potter Type II

Multicystic dysplastic kidney disease (MDKD) is characterized by cystic lesions which correspond primarily to dilated collecting tubules. The dilatation is a result of ureteric bud system atresia during embryogenesis. The etiology may be secondary to a chromosomal abnormality or mutant gene.[68] It can be unilateral, bilateral and segmental. The incidence of bilateral MDKD is estimated at 1: 10 000, but the real incidence of all MDKD is almost certainly under-estimated, since a certain number of cases are never detected.[68]

The MDKD is characterized by very different pathoanatomic and ultrasound findings, probably as a result of two types of insult: (i) developmental failure of the mesonephric blastema to form the nephrons, and (ii) early obstructive uropathy.

The Potter type IIA is characterized by enlarged or normal, often segmental multicystic kidneys, in contrast to type IIB, which has rudimentary kidneys and a few cysts or only microscopically visible cysts.[67] Sonographic findings of type IIA show one or more non-communicating cysts with no apparent renal pelvis or renal parenchyma. Bilateral changes are accompanied by oligohydramnios. If only one kidney is affected, polyhydramnios may be present. A Potter IIA kidney diagnosed early in the second trimester of pregnancy may change into a Potter IIB in the latter part of pregnancy (Figs 13.133 to 13. 137).[54]

The MDKD can be associated with autosomal recessive syndromes (Meckel, Dandy-Walker, Saldino-Noonan, etc.), autosomal dominant (Apert syndrome) and chromosomal defects (trisomy, del(15)(q22)(q24)), but in the majority of cases the condition is isolated and non-genetic.

The prognosis of bilateral MDKD is fatal and termination of the pregnancy should be offered. Unilateral disease has a good prognosis, particularly if the contralateral kidney is normal and detailed evaluation of the fetal anatomy rules out other anomalies.

Potter Type III

In contrast to Potter type I, adult polycystic kidney disease is rarely detected in utero. It seems that the defect is at the level of the ampulla (distal end of the ureter bud), but the involvement is not universal. The cysts correspond to either dilated collecting ducts or the tubular portion of the nephron. The mode of inheritance is by an autosomal dominant gene with variable expression in adult life. The most common presentation is between the third and fifth decades of life, ranging from a severe form that results in neonatal death, to an asymptomatic form detected only at autopsy. The mutation is located on the short arm of chromosome 16,[69] and antenatal diagnosis in early pregnancy using a highly polymorphic DNA probe genetically linked to the locus of the mutant gene is possible.[70]

The incidence is 1:1000, so adult polycystic kidney disease is one of the most common genetic disorders and the third most prevalent cause of chronic renal failure.[71]

The Potter type III kidney can be associated with cystic lesions in the other organs (liver, spleen, pancreas, etc.) and can be a

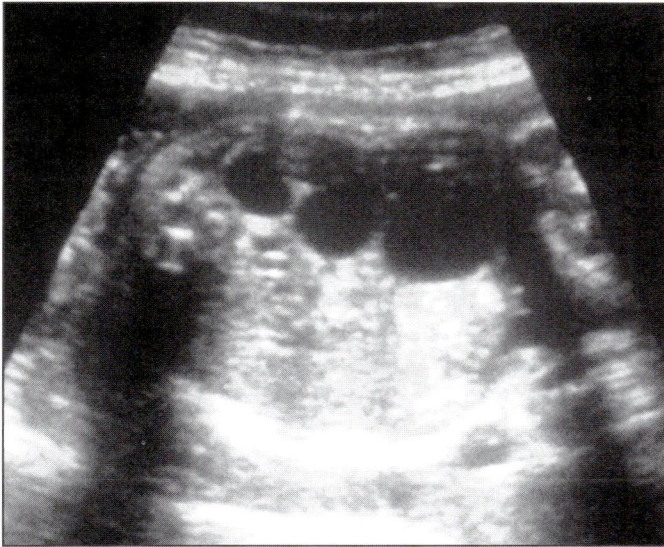

Fig: 13.133

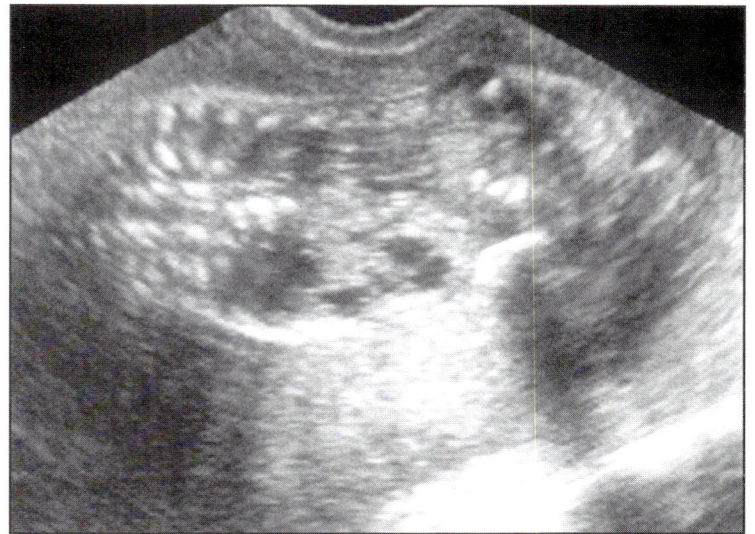

Figs 13.133 and 13.134: Multicystic dysplastic kidney disease. The kidney(s) appear(s) enlarged with multiple cysts which are:

• Mostly randomly positioned, but sometimes peripheral
• Variable in size and
• Non-communicating although artifacts may make non-communicating cysts appear as they communicate
• The parenchyma is seen in small islands between the cysts and the outline of the kidney tends to be lost
• The size of the kidney is proportional to the size and the number of visible cysts[56]

part of various syndromes (Meckel, tuberous sclerosis, von Hippel).

Ultrasound findings are similar to those of IPKD, i.e. renal enlargement with increased echogenicity of the renal parenchyma, or multiple cysts with normal or decreased amniotic fluid volume. The presentation varies and may include involvement of one kidney, ascites or even universal nonimmune hydrops.

If the diagnosis is made before viability, termination of the pregnancy can be offered. If made later on, the diagnosis will not change the obstetric management. Parents should be counseled by experts, because outcomes vary from early neonatal

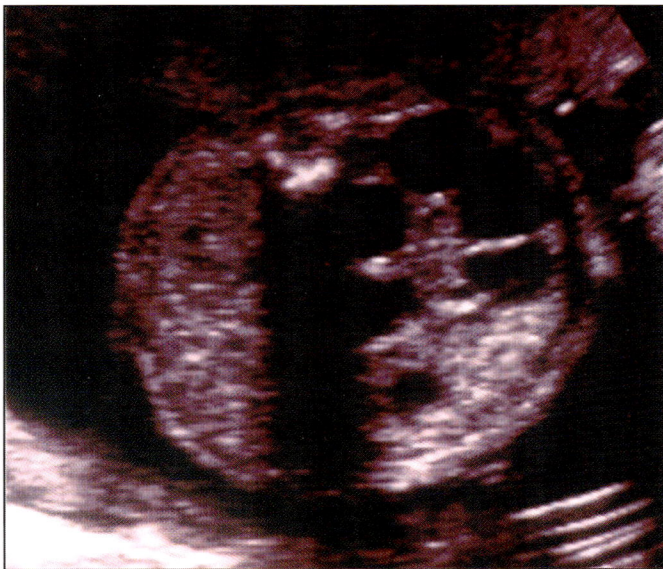

Fig. 13.135

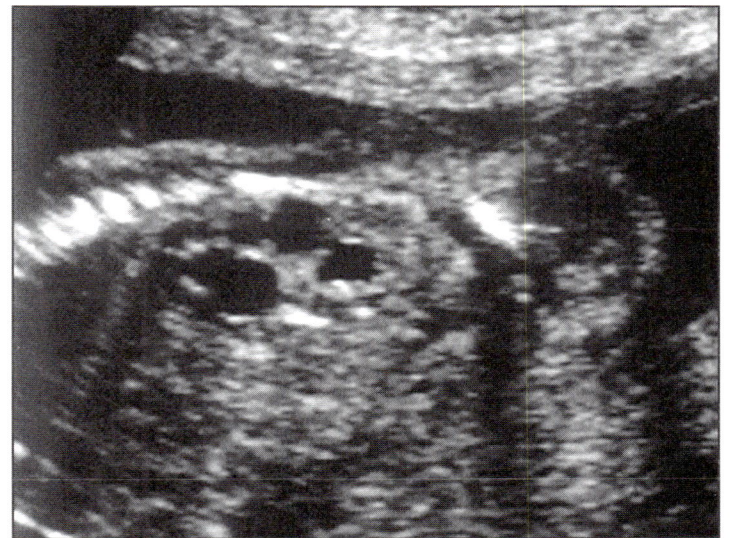

Figs 13.135 and 13.136: Most of the cysts are peripheral; variable in size and noncommunicating

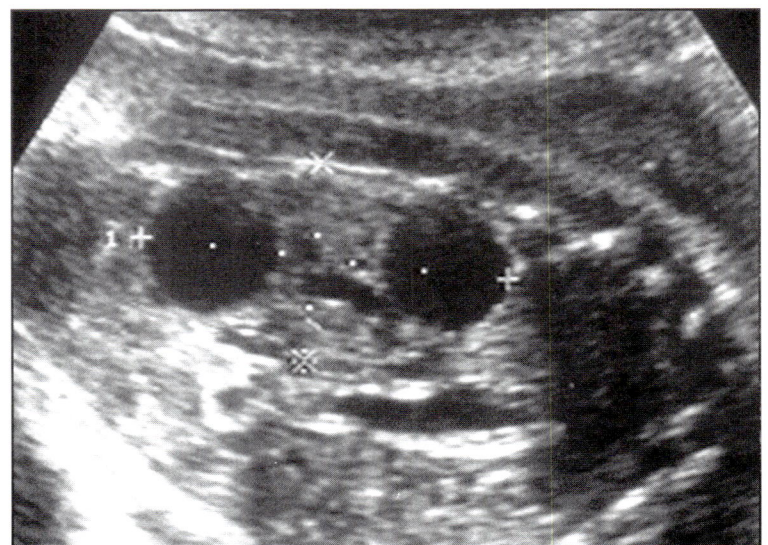

Fig. 13.137: The parenchyma is seen in small islands between the cysts and the outline of the kidney tends to be lost

death, hypertension (present in 50 to 70 percent of patients), and Berry aneurysms (10 to 30 percent) to a normal asymptomatic life period (Figs 13.138 and 13.139).

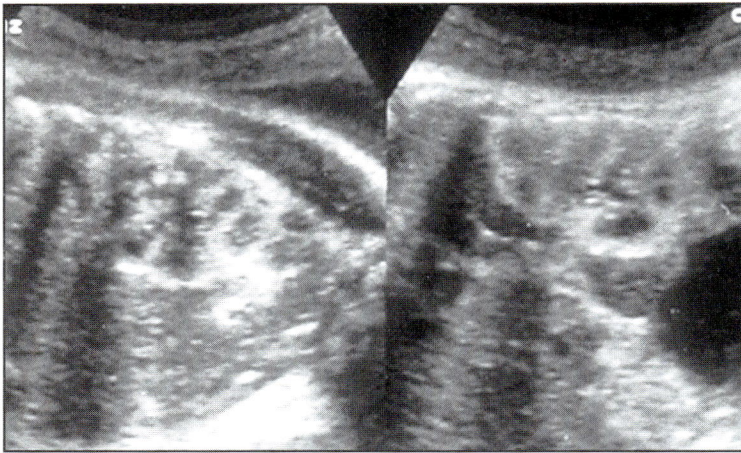

Fig. 13.138

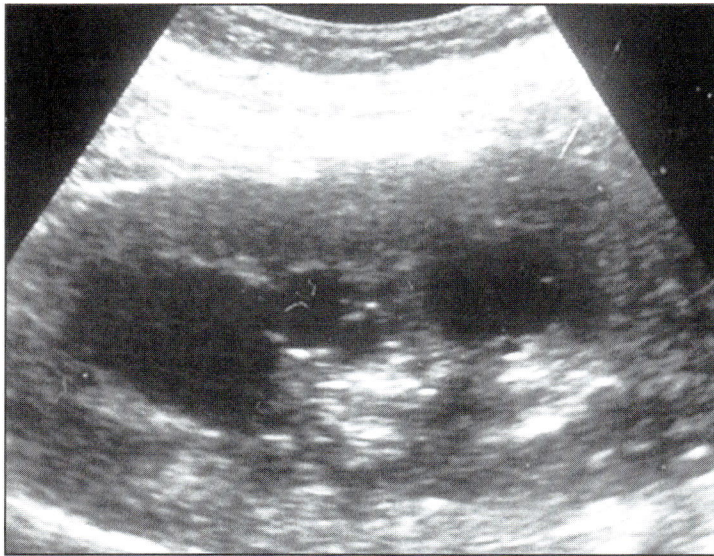

Figs 13.138 and 13.139: Adult polycystic kidney disease. Brightly echogenic kidneys with accentuation of the corticomedullary junction and a small bladder with decreased fluid

Potter Type IV

According to the Potter's classification, type IV results from a urethral obstruction[67] developing later in fetal life, compared with type II which is a consequence of early obstruction. Urinary tract obstruction can increase pressure during nephrogenesis and can lead to renal dysplasia and irreversible renal damage, with reduced renal function. The kidneys are often slightly enlarged and, depending on the extent of the involvement, megacysts, hydroureter and cortical renal cyst can be seen. Hydronephrosis may be the consequence of the obstruction on several levels: Urethra, vesicoureteric orifice, ureteropelvic junction or vesicoureteric reflux. The dilatation depends on the degree of obstruction, and may vary from a mild to a severe form.

The characteristic sonographic sign is a sonolucent cystic dilatation of the caliceal system with reniform shape. It can be seen even in early pregnancy at the end of the first trimester. In this condition, oligohydramnios is usually present later in pregnancy. Color Doppler ultrasound with pulsatility index (PI)

measurements of renal artery blood flow fail to show a significant difference between mild and severe pathology,[72] in spite of the obvious change in renal blood flow (Figs 13.140 and 13.141).

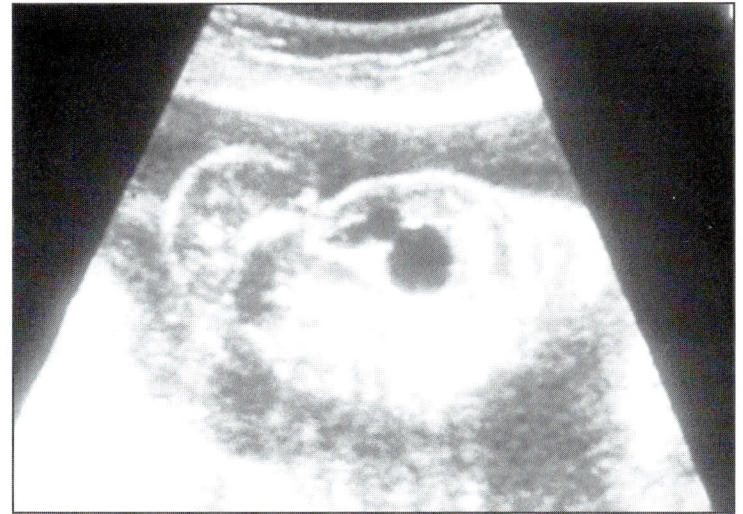

Fig. 13.140

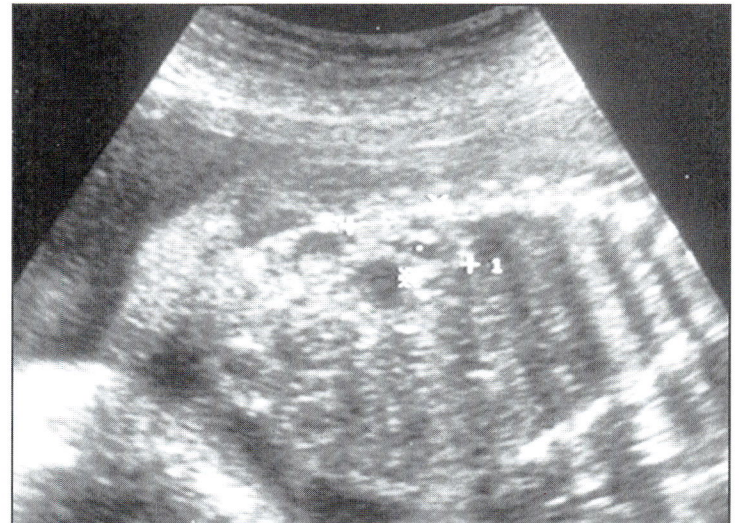

Figs 13.140 and 13.141: Obstructive cystic dysplasia. Peripheral cortical cysts and echogenic parenchyma

Abnormally Dilated Fetal Bladder

A dilated fetal bladder may be the consequence of a posterior urethral valve (PUV), urethral agenesis or stricture, persistence of cloaca and megacystitis-microcolon-hypoperistalsis syndrome.

Posterior Urethral Valve

Posterior uretheral valve (PUV) occurs only in males and is the single most common cause of fetal bladder obstruction (1:5000 males).[73] The role of hereditary factors in PUV is unclear. The PUV has been classified into three types. The most frequent is type I, which is caused by hypertrophied mucosal folds which arise from the posterior urethra near the entrance of the ejaculatory ducts. Type II has finger-like membranous projections proximal to the neck of the bladder and does not cause obstruction. Type III is a result of abnormal canalization of the urogenital membrane, and has a membrane with a small perforation. Valves may arise at any time during fetal life, causing partial or total obstruction of urinary drainage. Only 25 percent of affected babies are diagnosed during pregnancy, and 50 percent during the first year of life.[73]

In the most severe form of PUV, the fetal bladder becomes dilated, filling the entire abdomen and elevating the diaphragm. Oligohydramnios often characterizes this severe form, and, together with an elevated diaphragm, prevents appropriate pulmonary development, leading to pulmonary hypoplasia.

Sonographic signs include: Oligohydramnios, proximal urethral dilatation, a large bladder with thick walls, and a typical keyhole-shaped appearance. Hydronephrosis is present in 64 to 93 percent of the fetuses.[74] In 13 percent of cases, one kidney is nonfunctional, and 15 to 30 percent of affected males need dialysis or transplantation.[75]

Active antenatal management can preserve kidney function to the end of pregnancy.[76,77] Affected fetuses may benefit from open fetal surgery, i.e. marsupialization of the bladder. The alternative treatment includes use of double pigtailed catheters which allow drainage of the urine into the amniotic fluid. This operation has been frequently complicated by catheter displacement and blockage.

Indications for therapy should fulfill certain criteria: early diagnosis (up to the 24th week), preserved renal function (sodium < 100 mg/dl, chloride < 90 mg/dl, osmolality < 210 mOsm/dl), and progressive oligohydramnios. Early treatment prevents pulmonary hypoplasia, but 30 to 50 percent of children require renal transplantation because of dysplastic kidneys.[78]

Affected fetuses with the most severe form of the posterior urethral valve develop prune belly syndrome, characterized by dilated urinary bladder, lax abdominal wall and undescended testicles. On the transaxial scan through the fetus, the distended abdomen appears as a huge sonolucent area filled with the enlarged bladder and ureters. It is believed that some of the features of prune belly syndrome occur secondary to a primary mesodermal defect of the abdominal wall and urinary tract.

Other anomalies associated with PUV are: Hypospadia, cryptorchidism, patent ductus arteriosus, cardiac defects, tracheal hypoplasia and chromosomal abnormalities (Figs 13.142 to 13.146).

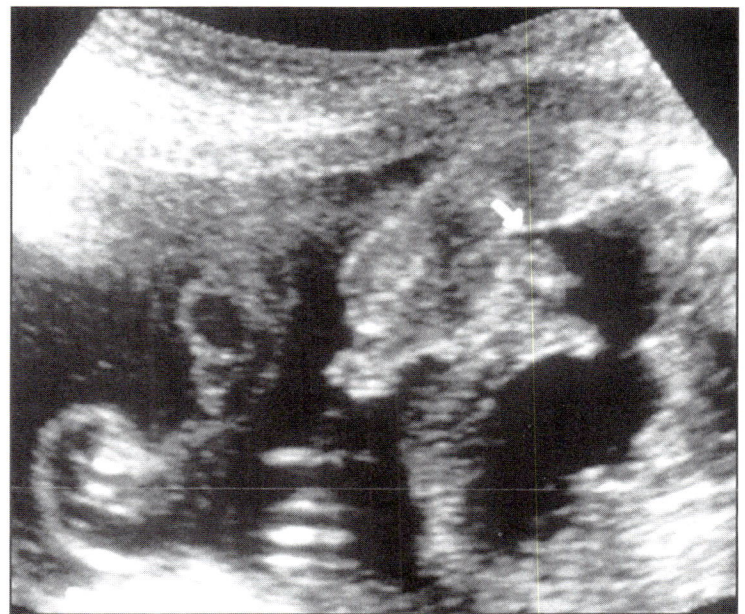

Fig. 13.142: Distal obstruction: The kidney had moderate dilatation

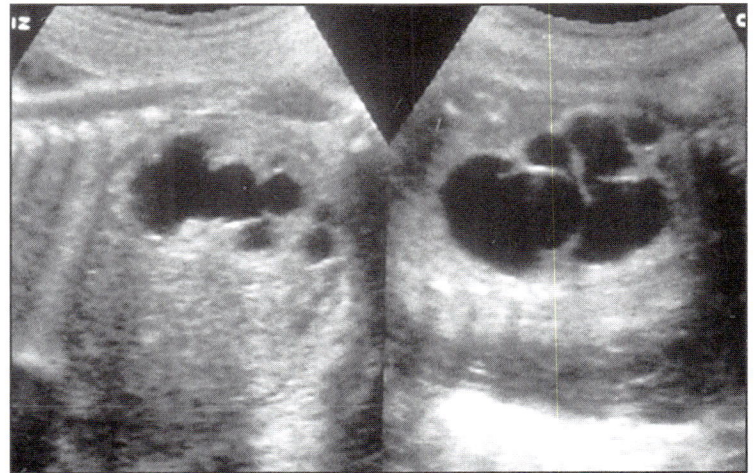

Fig. 13.143: Distal obstruction: Dilated bladder and key hole deformity the posterior urethra

Urethral Stenosis

Urethral stenosis, stemming from incomplete fusion of the urogenital sinus and penile urethra, is the second cause of bladder outlet obstruction. It occurs more commonly in male fetuses and has increased risk for associated nonrenal anomalies. Sonographic findings and consequences to the upper urinary tract are similar to those in PUV.

Agenesis of the Urethra

Agenesis of the urethra is a very rare anomaly. The affected fetus is stillborn or dies immediately after delivery because of pulmonary hypoplasia. The ultrasound picture is characterized by severe early oligohydramnios, an abnormally dilated bladder with urinary ascites, dilatation of the upper urinary tract, kidney dysplasia and pulmonary hypoplasia.

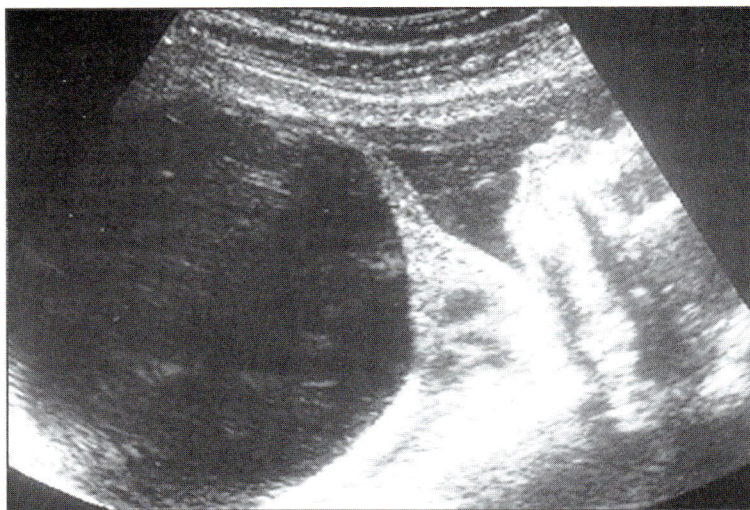

Fig. 13.144

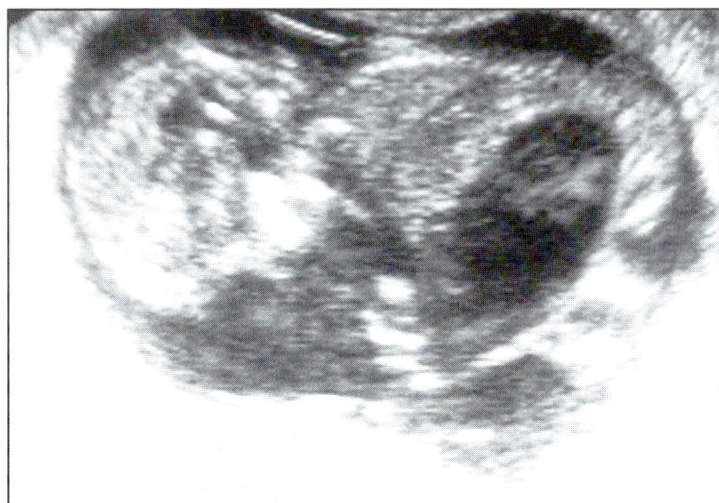

Fig. 13.145

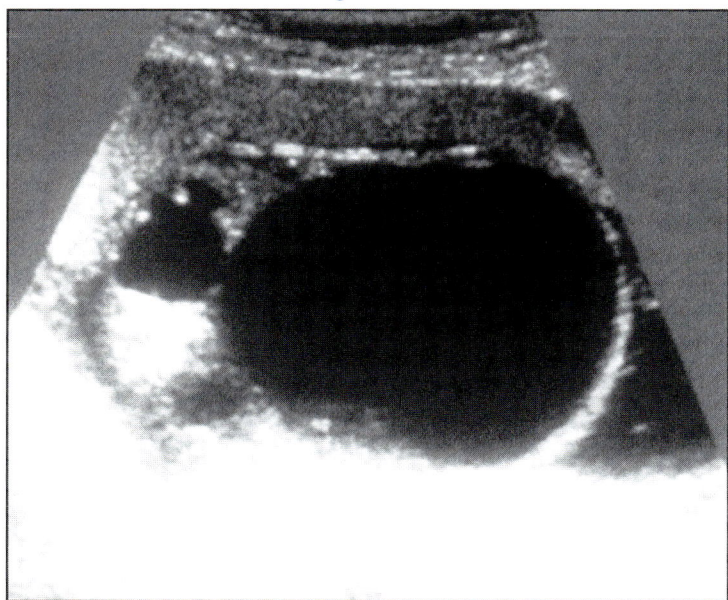

Figs 13.144 to 12.146: Axial plane through the fetal abdomen demonstrating fetal megacystitis. The kidney had moderate dilatation

Cloacal Persistence

Cloacal persistence is a result of non-separation of the bladder, vagina and rectum during the 5th week after conception. This space is a blind cystic pouch into which the gastrointestinal and upper urinary tracts drain, and which will progressively dilate with consequent dilatation of the ureters and renal calices. It is associated with imperforate anus, genital ambiguity, and urethral abnormalities, and secondary renal dysplasia and pulmonary hypoplasia.

Megacystitis-microcolon-intestinal Hypoperistalsis Syndrome

Megacystitis-microcolon-intestinal hypoperistalsis syndrome is characterized by a large bladder with thick walls, and distention of the small bowel, including the duodenum. The amniotic fluid volume is normal or increased, which may help differentiate this condition from PUV. The kidneys appear hydronephrotic, sometimes multicystic. It is believed that the cause of this condition is a defect of the receptor on the smooth muscle of the urinary and gastrointestinal tracts.[79]

Bladder Extrophy

Bladder extrophy is a rare anomaly which occurs in 1 : 25 000 births. A ventral defect in the abdominal wall is located inferior to the insertion of the umbilical cord, involving the bladder wall. The urinary bladder cannot be visualized because of a constant lack of urine and its drainage into the amniotic fluid.

This condition causes progressive dilatation with bilateral hydronephrosis, cystic dysplasia and possible rupture, with a worse prognosis.

Ureteropelvic Junction Obstruction

The ureteropelvic junction is a frequent site of urinary tract obstruction. The causes include fibrous adhesions, kinks, bands, ureteral valves, aberrant vessels, abnormal ureteral insertion and an unusual shape of the pyeloureteral outlet[80] or dysfunction due to a deficiency of the longitudinal muscle fibers.[81]

This condition is bilateral in 30 percent of cases with an asymmetrical involvement of the kidneys. A unilateral condition more commonly affects the left side, and in 27 percent it is associated with other urinary (vesicoureteric reflux, a contralateral non-functioning kidney or agenesis, bilateral obstructed megaureter, hypospadias),[82-84] and extraurinary (Hirschprung's disease, cardiovascular anomalies, neural tube defects, etc.) anomalies in 19 percent.[85] In the extreme cases of ureteropelvic junction, a urinoma or urinary ascites may be present, with a poor prognosis.

In unilateral cases, prognosis is good. There is no need for premature labor or for intervention, even immediately after birth.

The management of bilateral ureteropelvic junction obstruction is based on gestational age, amniotic fluid volume and the condition of the kidneys, as well as on their function after exclusion of associated anatomical and chromosomal abnormalities. If the kidney function is in danger, intervention is justified.

Pyelectasis

Pyelectasis or dilatation of the renal pelvis may occur secondarily to any mild anomaly of the urinary tract below the level of the pyelon. Its severity is gauged by the size of the renal pelvis in the anteroposterior (AP) diameter.

Mild pyelectasis, AP diameter to 5 mm, may be associated with a normal outcome and is a common finding among normal fetuses, but has a higher incidence among fetuses with Down syndrome.[86] Corteville and co-workers[87] reported that the incidence of pyelectasis among fetuses with Down syndrome was 17 percent, compared with 2 percent in normal controls; therefore, they suggest that an AP diameter of 4 to 7 mm warrants postnatal follow-up.[88] An AP diameter of 10 mm or more is consistent with an obstruction etiology, and is likely to lead to hydronephrosis.[89] Since the sonography is especially accurate for fluid-filled lesions, on ultrasound screen, the pyelectasis appears as a sonolucent keyhole structure with diameter variants.

According to Benacerraf, approximately 3.3 percent of fetuses with pyelectasis with an AP diameter of 4 mm and more may have chromosomal abnormalities, including trisomy 21, and 25 percent of fetuses with Down syndrome have pyelectasis of 4 mm and more.[86] In a scoring system for detection of second trimester fetuses with Down syndrome, pyelectasis is given one point, similar to short bones or bright bowel.[90] This association has to be discussed with parents because of the need for additional tests and possibly fetal karyotyping (Figs 13.147 to 13.154).

Megaureter

Megaureter, a dilated ureter with or without dilatation of the renal pelvis, is more common in males and is involved in 92 percent of in utero urinary tract obstructions. It is a sporadic disease and may be caused by obstruction to the flow of urine, by vesicoureteric reflux, and by some other conditions as an indirect consequence of the primary disease (diabetes insipidus, infection). Incompetence at the ureterovesicle junction results in reflux and, in turn, dilatation of the proximal renal system.

Megaureter may be associated with unilateral renal agenesis, a complete or incomplete duplex system, or an ectopic kidney.

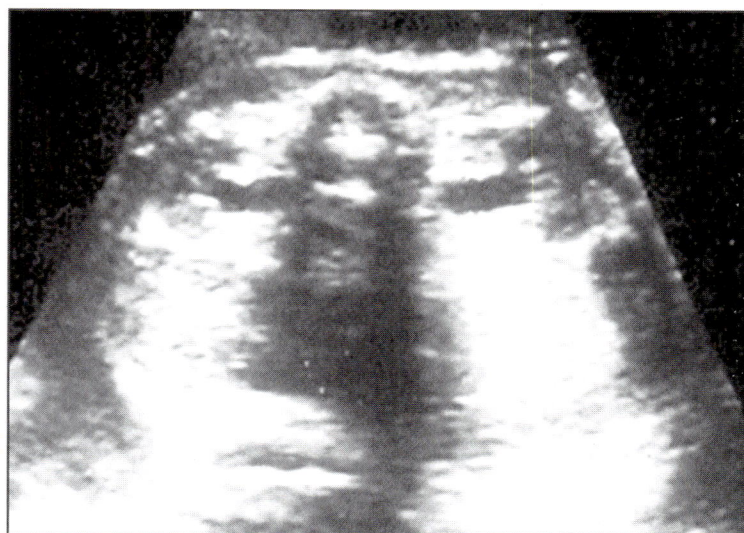
Fig. 13.147

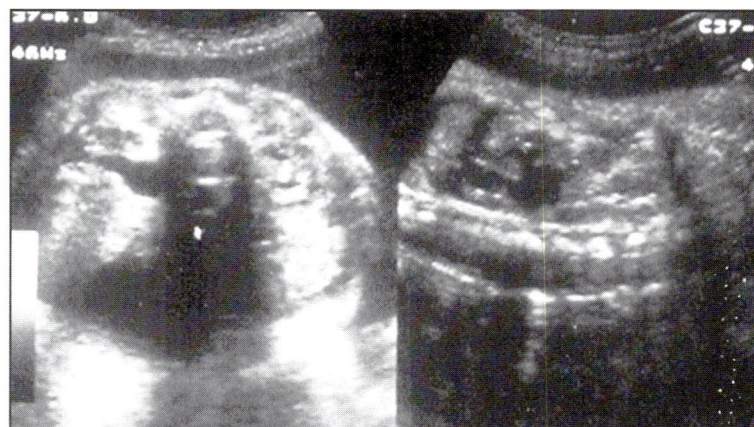
Figs 13.147 and 12.148: Ureteropelvic junction obstruction: Mild dilatation of the renal pelvis

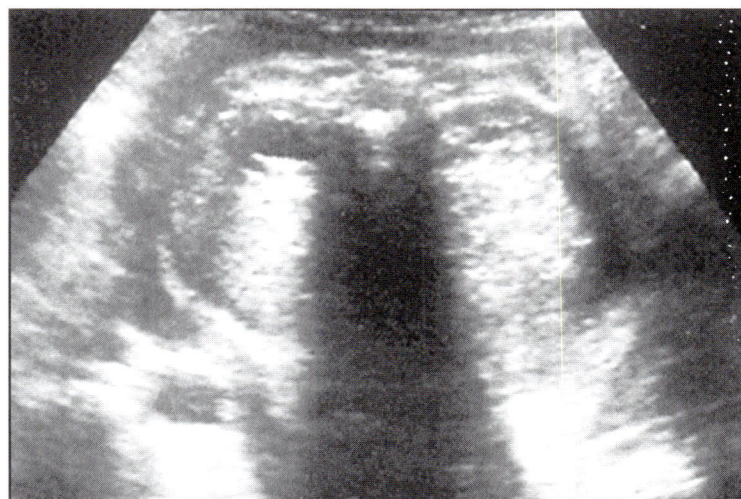
Fig. 13.149

In the normal condition ureters are rarely visible. Megaureters are seen as hypoechogenic intra-abdominal structures that can be traced back to the renal pelvis.

Unilateral changes neither require aggressive treatment, nor does bilateral involvement with normal amniotic fluid volume. If there is bilateral hydronephrosis with oligohydramnios, the prognosis is poor. If there is normal amniotic fluid volume,

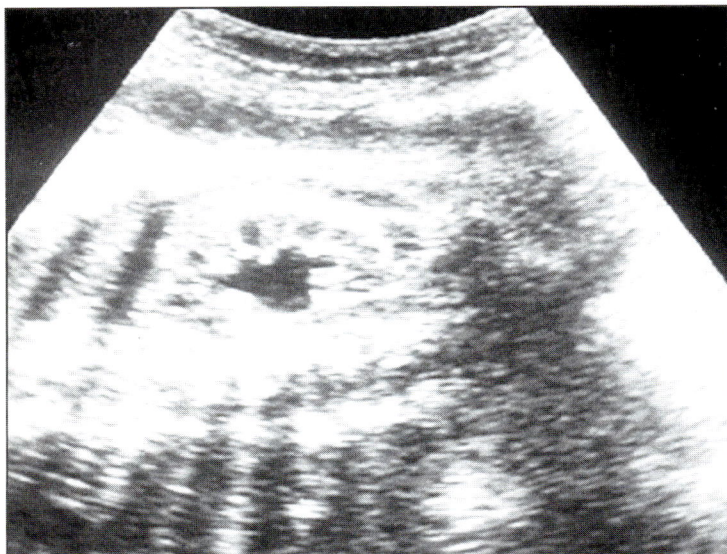

Figs 13.149 and 12.150: Ureteropelvic junction obstruction: Moderate dilatation of the renal pelvis

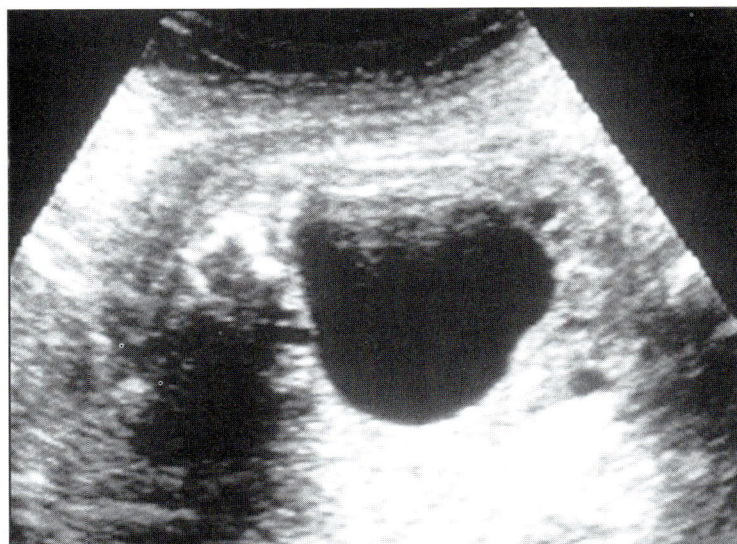

Fig. 13.153: Ureteropelvic junction obstruction: Hydronephrosis. Severe dilatation of the renal pelvis and calices. Enlarged kidney

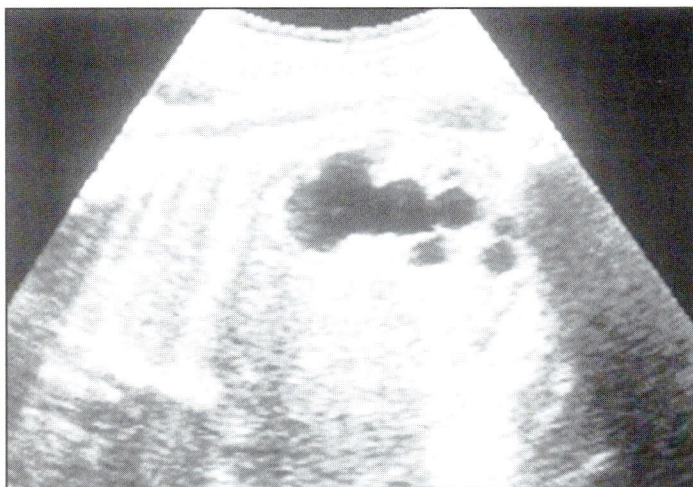

Fig. 13.151

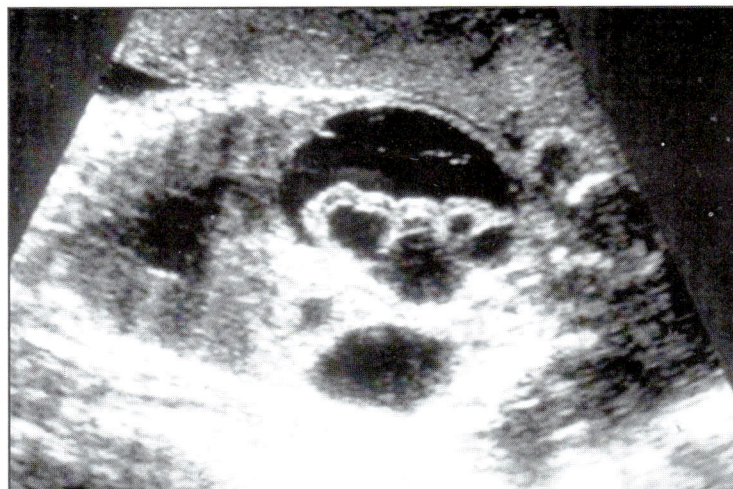

Fig. 12.154: Ureteropelvic junction obstruction: Urinoma. Notice the thinning of the cortex

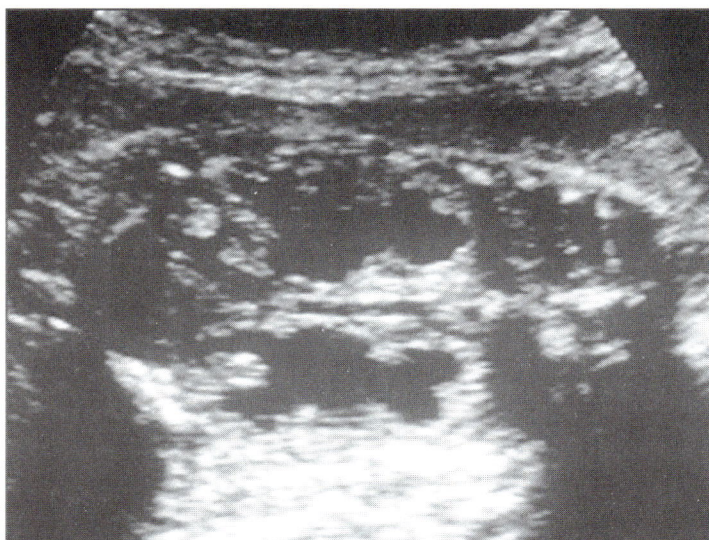

Figs 13.151 and 12.152: Ureteropelvic junction destruction: Moderate dilation of the collecting system and the renal pelvis

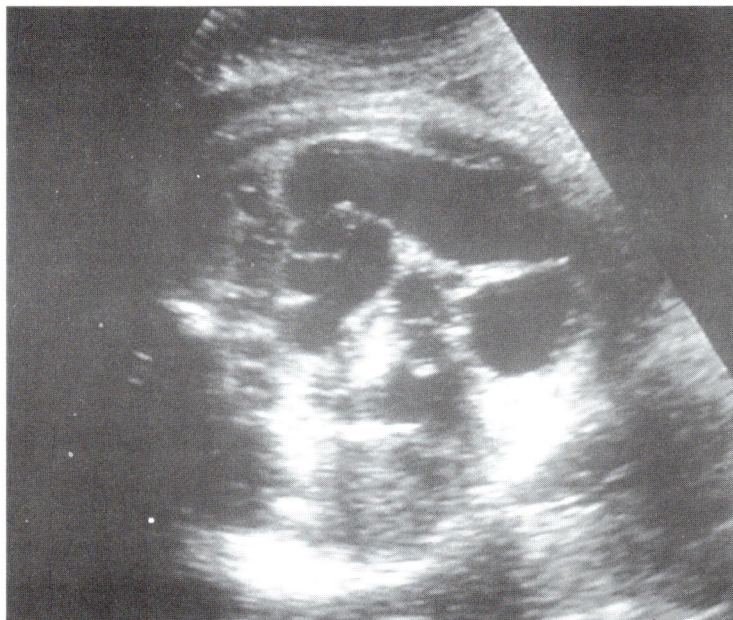

Fig. 13.155

prenatal invasive treatment usually is not justified, but postnatal assessment should be performed (Figs 13.155 to 13.157).

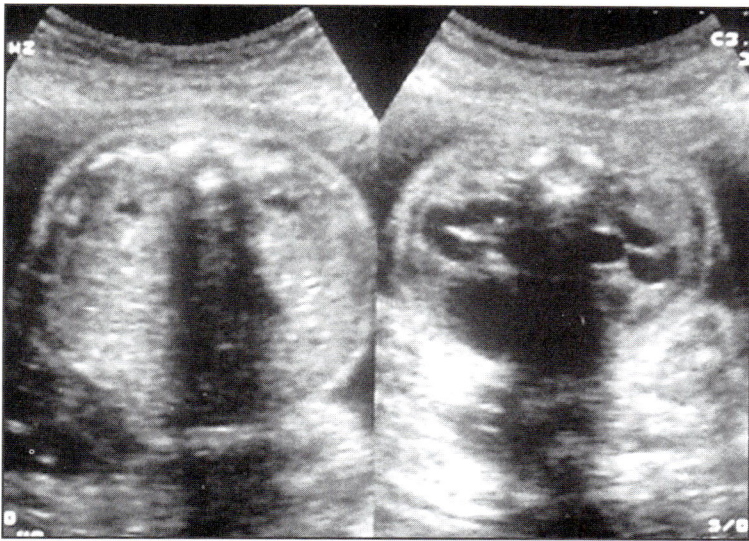

Fig. 13.156

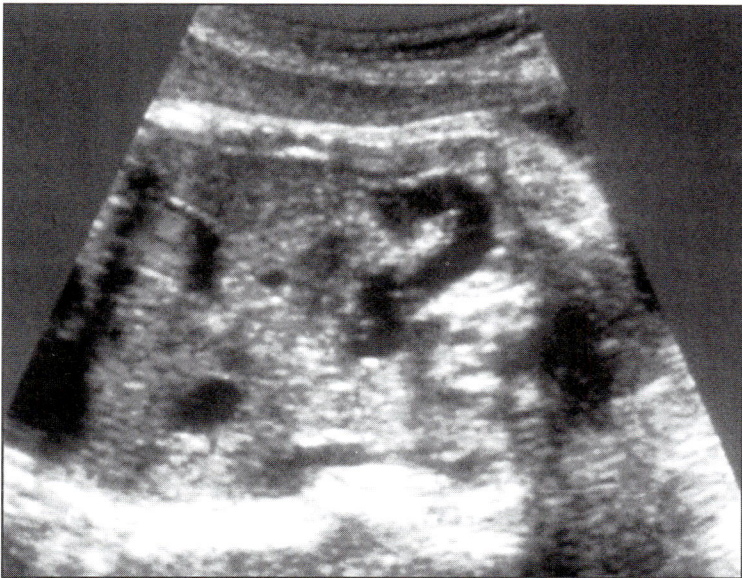

Figs 13.155 to 13.157: Ureteropelvic junction obstruction: Dilatation of the ureters

Vesicoureteral Reflux

The incidence of vesicoureteral reflux in the newborn is approximately 1 percent.[91,92] It may be primary or secondary, as a consequence of an obstructive process, and is sometimes mixed. It is important to recognize whether it is a primary or secondary condition, because of the different outcomes. Antenatal diagnosis can be of significant value because timely and appropriate treatment can save kidney function.

In the past the diagnosis of vesicoureteral reflux was made by X-ray and contrast medium; now it is possible to make a sonographic diagnosis by percutaneous vesicoinfusion.[93] Using this technique, it is possible to make a proper diagnosis on each side separately, and to obtain a better estimate of renal function in the unilateral condition. Quintero and coworkers[93] included vesicoinfusion as part of the work-up of fetuses with a suspicion of lower obstructive uropathy.

Horseshoe Kidney and Empty Renal Fossa

Fusion of the poles of the left and right kidneys results in a horseshoe kidney, which is associated with a higher incidence of urinary infections and stone formation in postnatal life. At autopsy the incidence is 1:500 to 1:1000.[94] Antenatal diagnosis is difficult in the case of lower fusion, which can be diagnosed with serial transverse scans.

Unilateral renal agenesis, ectopic kidney and cross-fused ectopic kidney give the picture of an empty renal fossa (Figs 13.158 to 13.162).[95]

Renal Duplication Anomalies

Duplex kidneys are one of the most common major congenital abnormalities of the urinary tract (approximately 1 percent of live births). The sensitivity of antenatal diagnosis is low because the sonographers are not familiar with this condition. The typical signs of renal duplex anomalies as follows:[96]

1. Longer diameter of the kidney in the sagittal view including the upper pole.
2. Cyst-like structure surrounded by a rim of renal parenchyma in the upper pole of the kidney.
3. Kidney with two separate renal pelves that do not communicate.
4. Dilated ureter, usually draining the upper pole.
5. Echogenic cystic structure in the bladder.

If the sonographer is looking for these typical signs, the sensitivity of antenatal diagnosis will be significantly higher (Figs 13.163 to 13.170).

Tumors of the Kidney

Tumors of the kidney are rare. In fetal life, the congenital mesoblastic nephroma and the Wilms' tumor can be detected. The ultrasound image is very similar: a unilateral or commonly bilateral solid mass which arises from the renal fossa and compresses kidney tissue. The congenital mesoblastic nephroma may show necrosis and hemorrhage. Differentiation between these two tumors and teratoma is not possible. Color Doppler may help in making the diagnosis, but its usefulness in the antenatal period is not yet known.

Adrenal Gland Tumor

The adrenal gland consists of the medulla and cortex, which is more pronounced during fetal life and decreases in size after birth. Adrenal glands can be seen in the 10th week of pregnancy as hypoechoic rings with central hyperechoic echoes. The

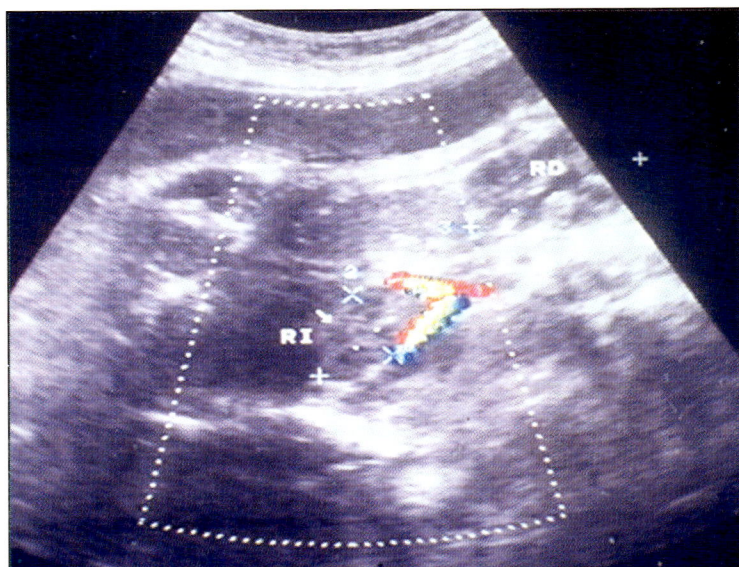

Fig. 13.158

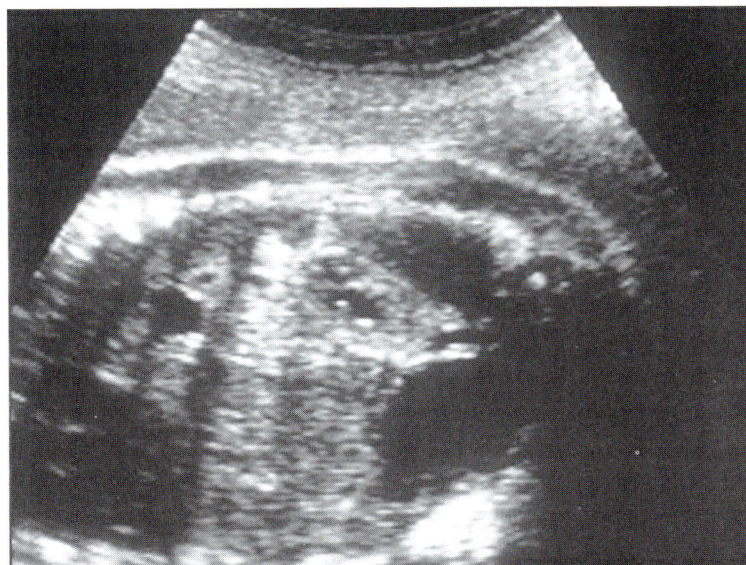

Fig. 13.160

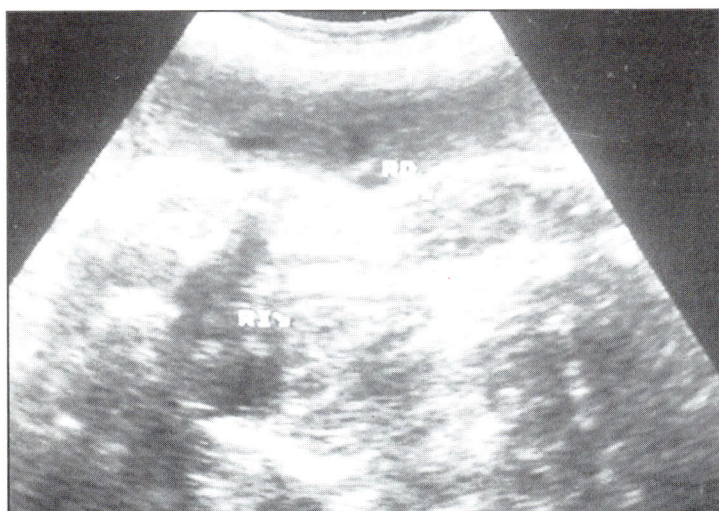

Fig. 13.161

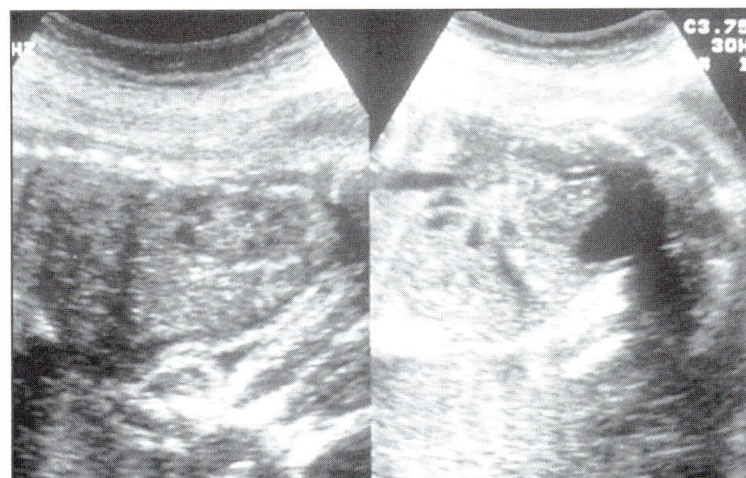

Figs 13.158 and 13.159: Ectopic kidney: Ectopic pelvic kidney between iliac arteries

anterior part of the left adrenal gland is adjacent to the aorta. The inferior vena cava lies in front of the right adrenal gland. The size from 20 weeks to term ranges from 2 to 9 mm in mean thickness and from 7 to 24 mm in mean width.[97]

Congenital Adrenal Neuroblastoma

Congenital adrenal neuroblastoma is the most common abdominal tumor found in newborns (13.3% of all perinatal neoplasms).[98] The discrepancy between the incidence of neuroblastoma in stillbirths and in infants in the first 3 months of life, and that of clinically manifested disease, suggests that either the neuroblastoma is not a true tumor, or that it has a spontaneous regression.

The tumor appears as a mixed cystic and solid mass in the upper part of the kidney, sometimes with calcifications, and can be mixed with Wilms' tumor, renal mesoblastic nephroma, multicystic kidney or retroperitoneal teratoma.

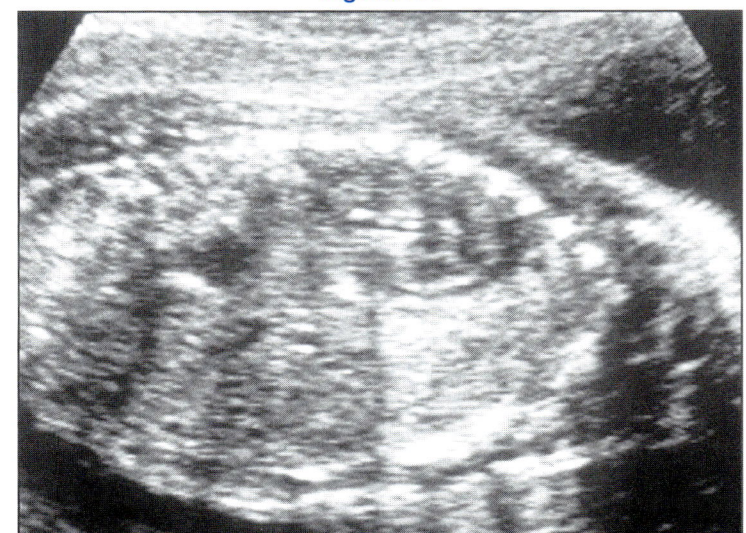

Figs 13.160 to 13.162: Ectopic kidney: Ectopic pelvic kidney (Figs 13.160 and 13.161). Ectopic kidney in the thorax (Fig. 13.162)

Obstetric management depends on the clinical course. Usually the treatment is conservative, with the possibility of cesarean section because of a large tumor and dystocia. In rare circumstances premature delivery is necessary because of rapid tumor growth (Figs 13.171 and 13.172).

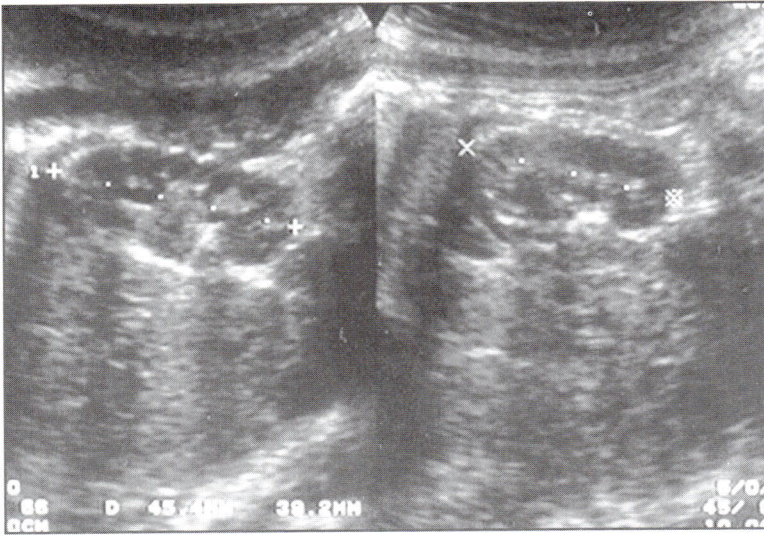

Fig. 13.163

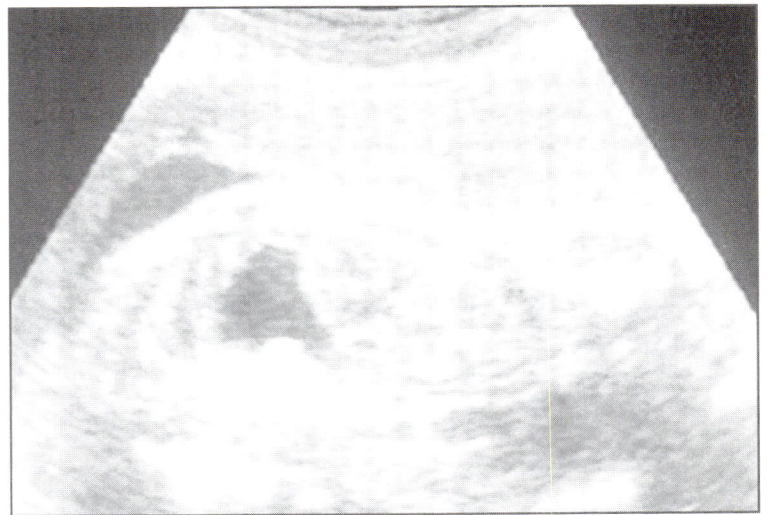

Fig. 13.164

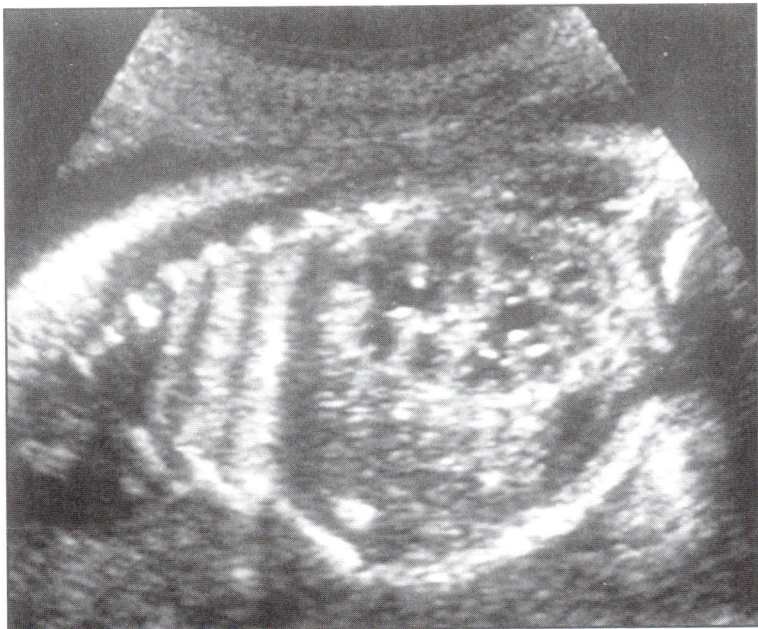

Fig. 13.165

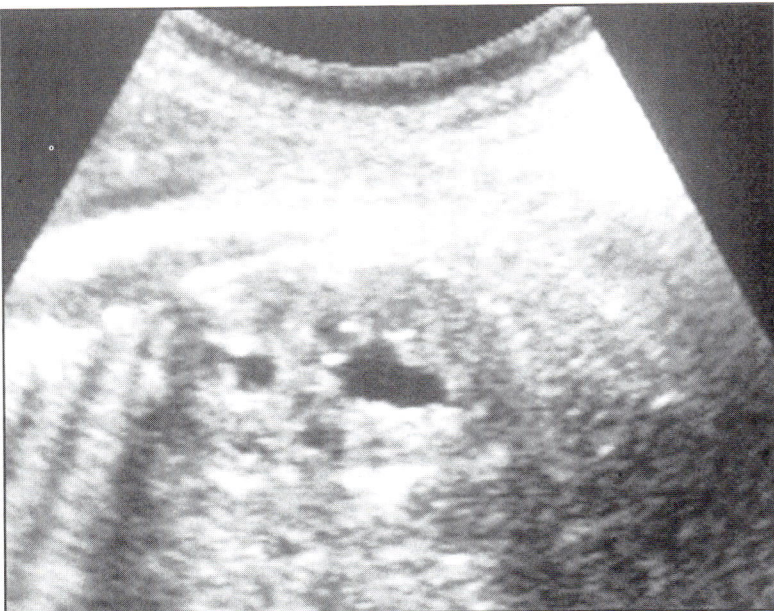

Fig. 13.166

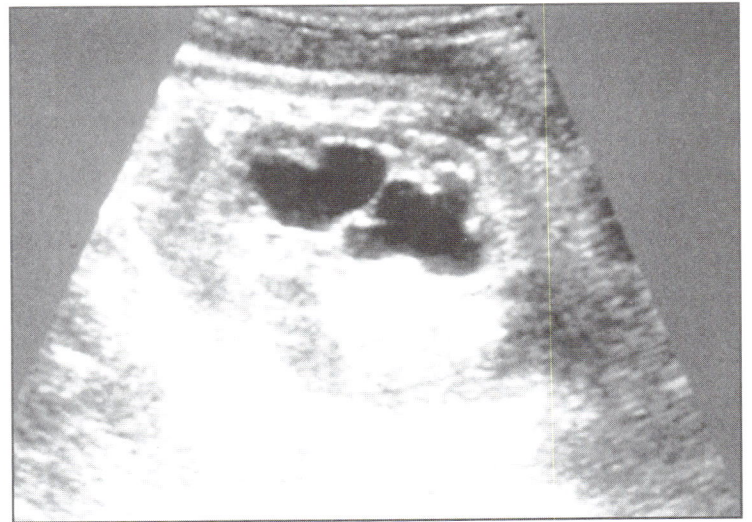

Figs 13.163 to 12.167: Duplex kidney. A sagittal scan through a duplex kidney shows two collecting systems

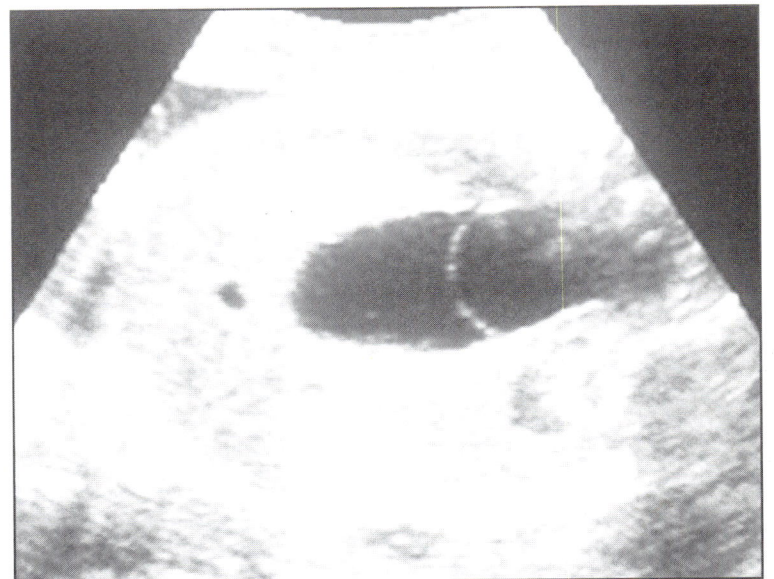

Fig. 13.168

GENITAL ANOMALIES

The genital anomalies include from the fetal ovarian cysts, the hydrocolpos and hydrometrocolpos, in the case of female genitals,

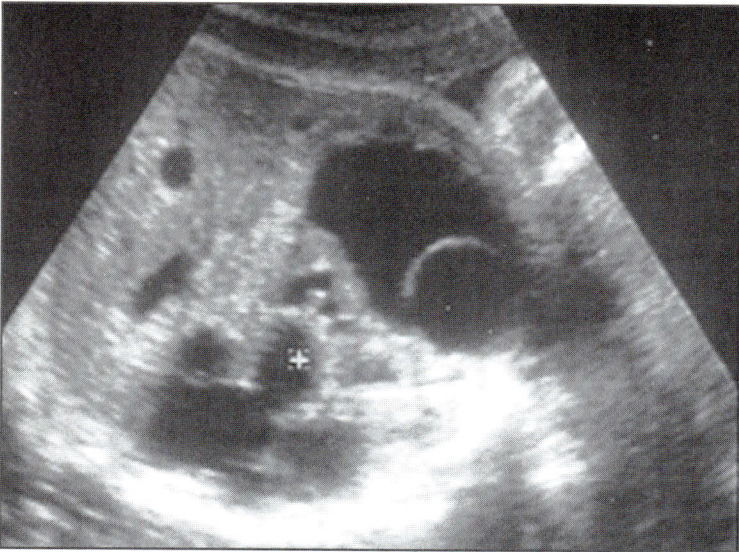
Fig. 13.169

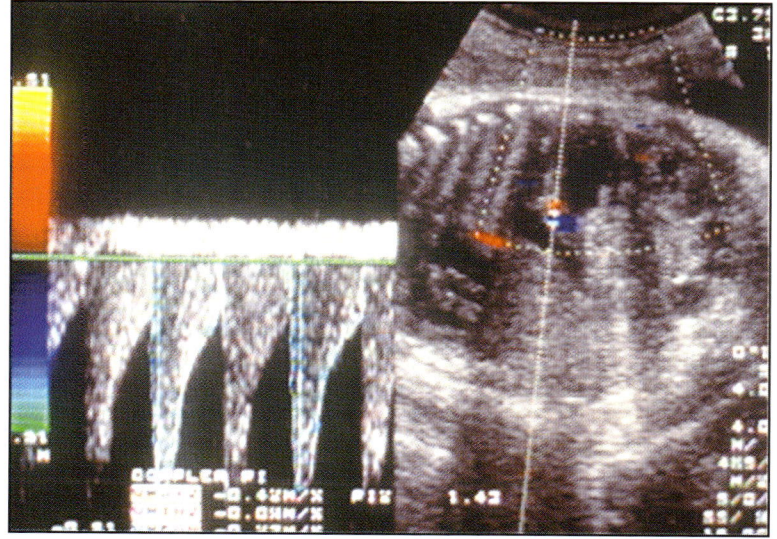
Figs 13.171 and 13.172: Neuroblastoma: Tumor solid and heterogenous. Color Doppler shows artery blood flow

been benefitted extraordinarily by the introduction of the color Doppler (Figs 13.173 to 13.189).

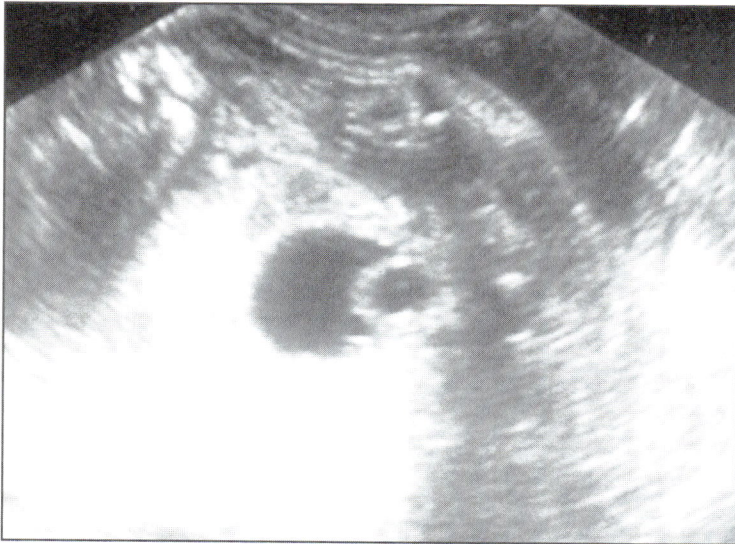
Figs 13.168 to 13.170: Ectopic ureterocele in the bladder

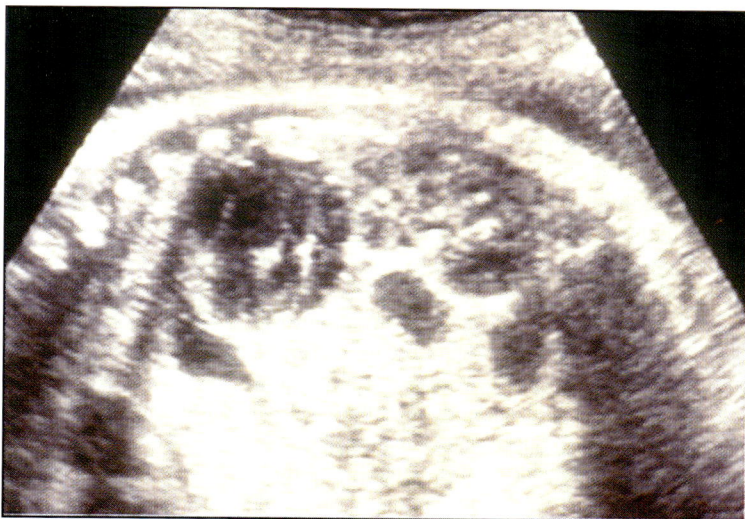
Fig. 13.173: Genital anomaly: Male fetus

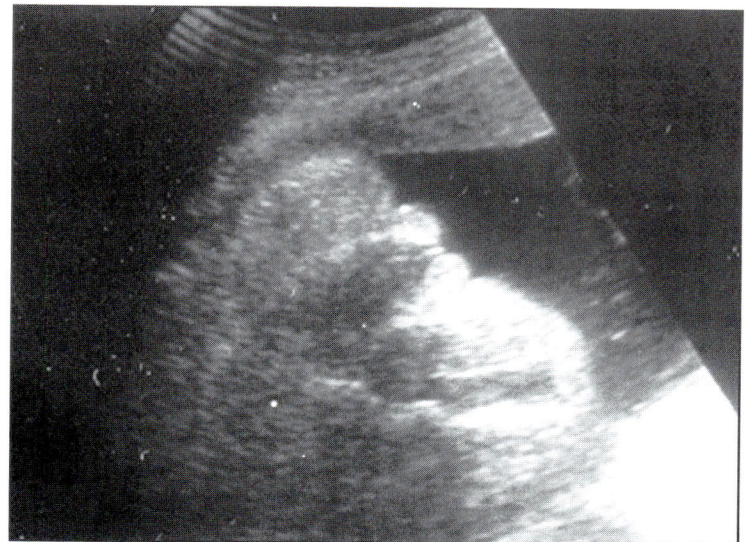
Fig. 13.171

to the fetal hydrocele, the ambiguous genitalia or the hypospadias in the case of male genitals. In some of these suppositions, like the case of the hypospadias, its diagnosis has

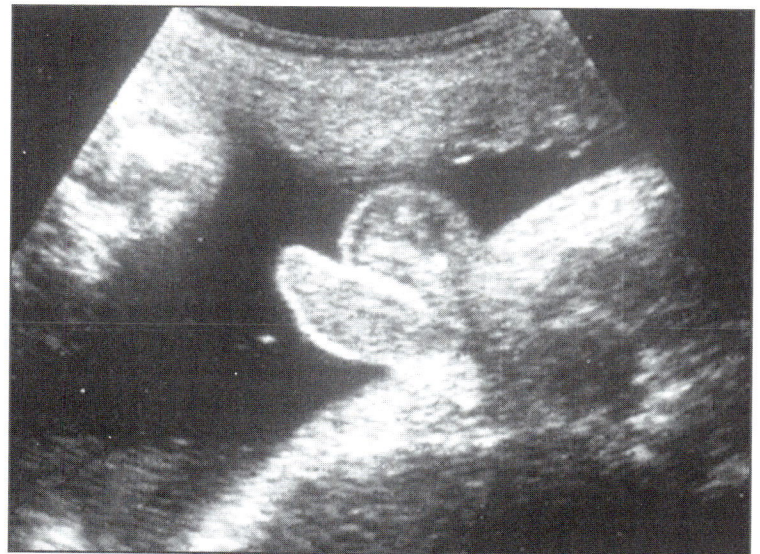
Fig. 13.174: Genital anomaly: Female fetus

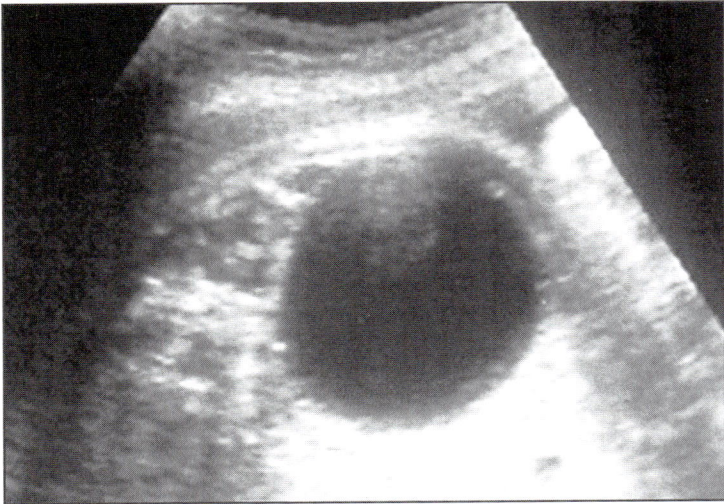

Fig. 13.175

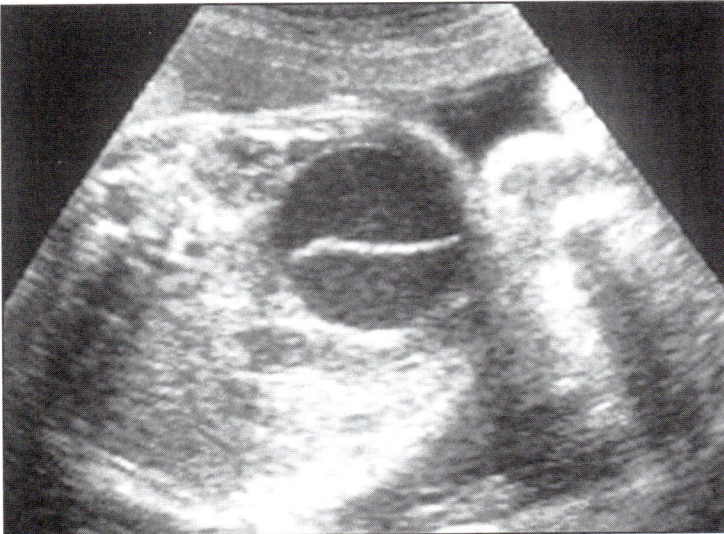

Fig. 13.176

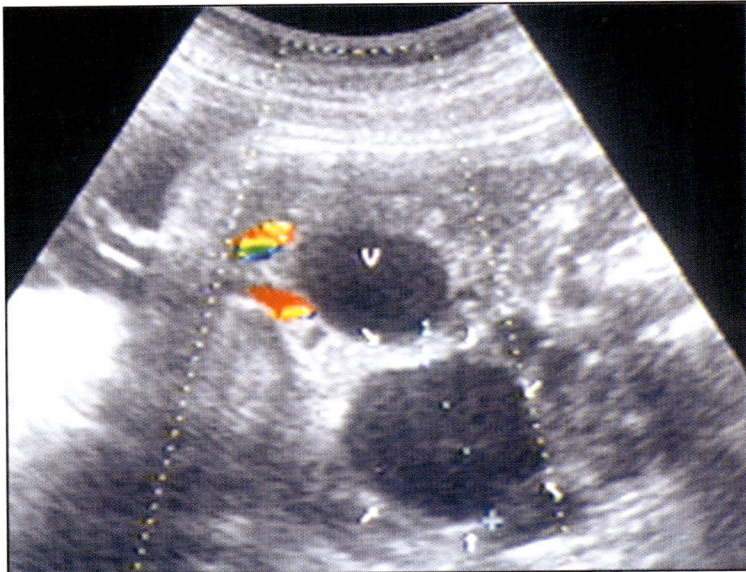

Fig. 13.177

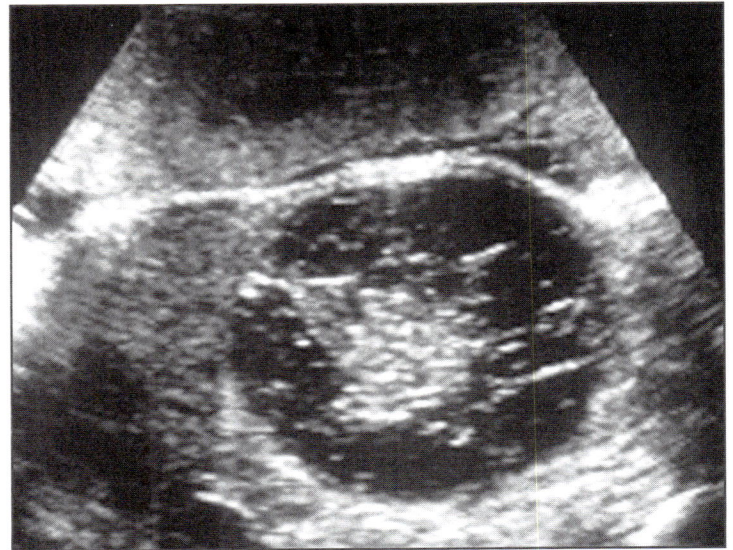

Figs 13.175 to 13.178: Ovarian cyst. The ultrasound exam showed a cystic lesion in the fetal abdomen. The cystic mass lying between the liver and bladder (Figs 13.175 and 13.176). Ovarian cyst, hemorrhagic (Figs 13.177 and 13.178)

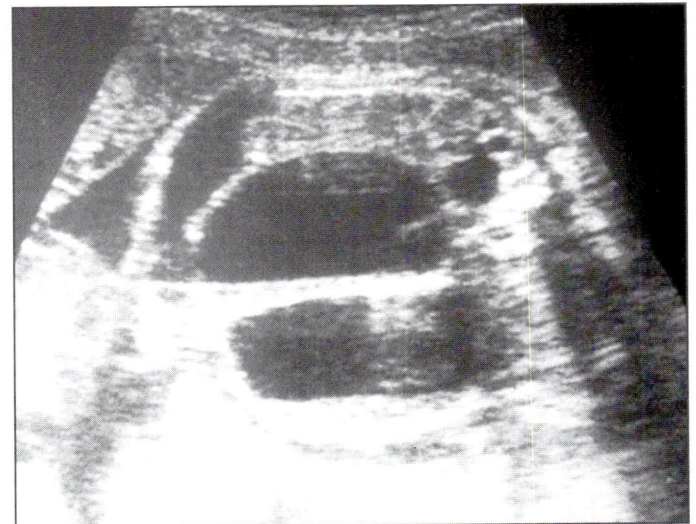

Fig. 13.179

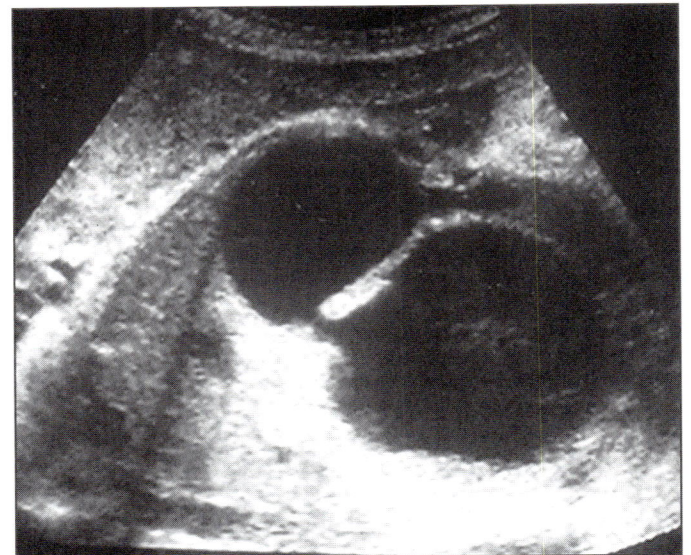

CONCLUSIONS

Prenatal diagnosis of urinary tract abnormalities allows difficult decisions to be made early. In lethal conditions such as bilateral renal agenesis, termination of the pregnancy is offered. In the obstructive uropathies, early intervention with shunts or open

Figs 13.179 and 12.180: Hydrometrocolpos. Distention of the vagina and also the uterine cavity caused by accumulation of watery-mucoid fluid due to the obstruction of the genital orifice (Fig.13.179). Bilobulated cystic tumor in the lower abdomen of the fetus (Fig. 13.180).

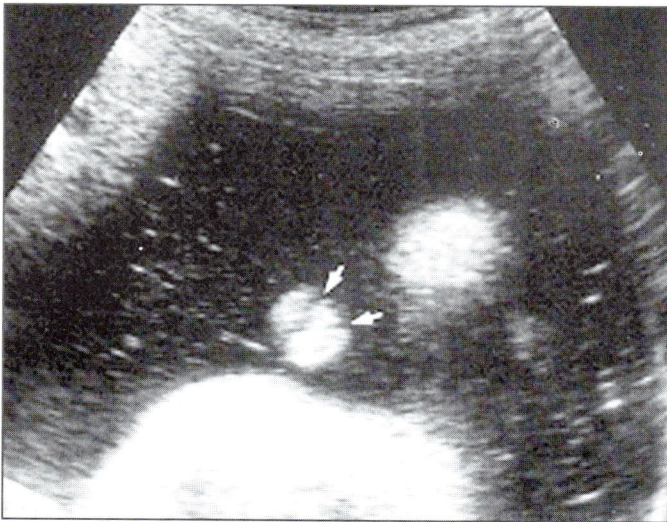

Fig. 13.181

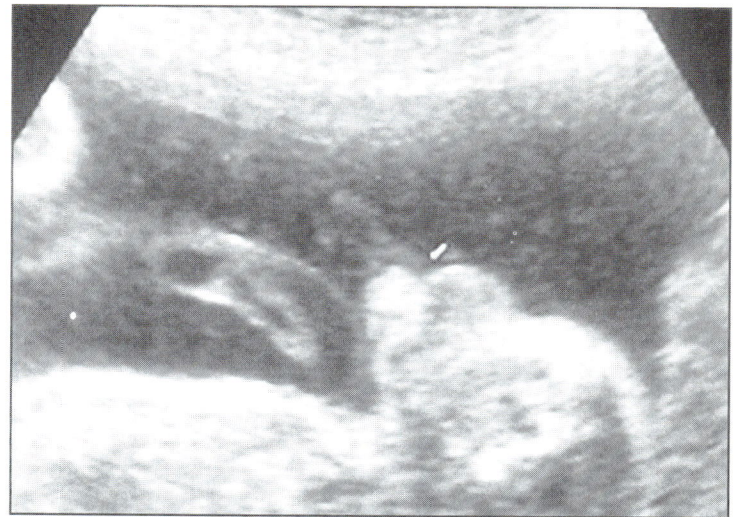

Figs 13.181 to 13.184: Hypospadias: The short curved penis due to the chordae. The first image also shows the tulip sign

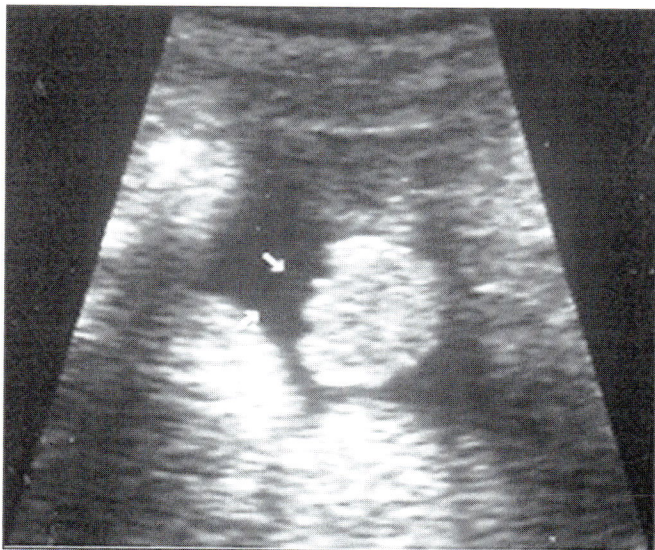

Fig. 13.182

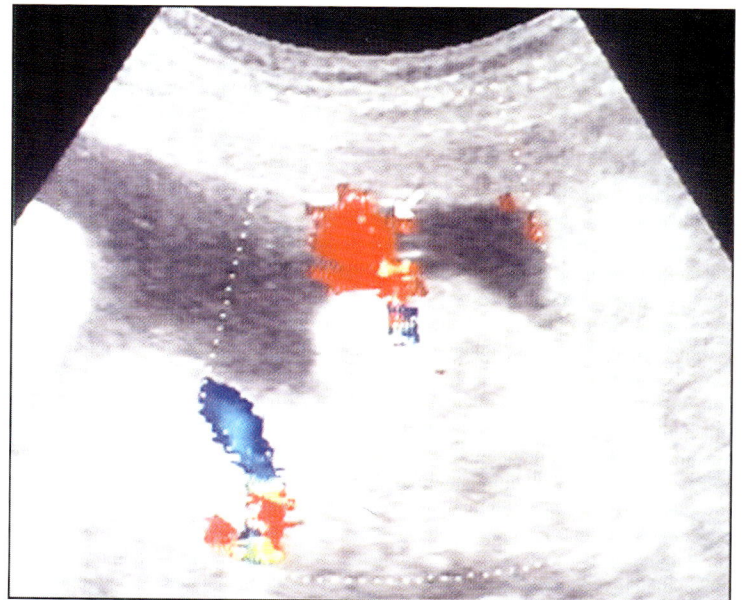

Fig. 13.185

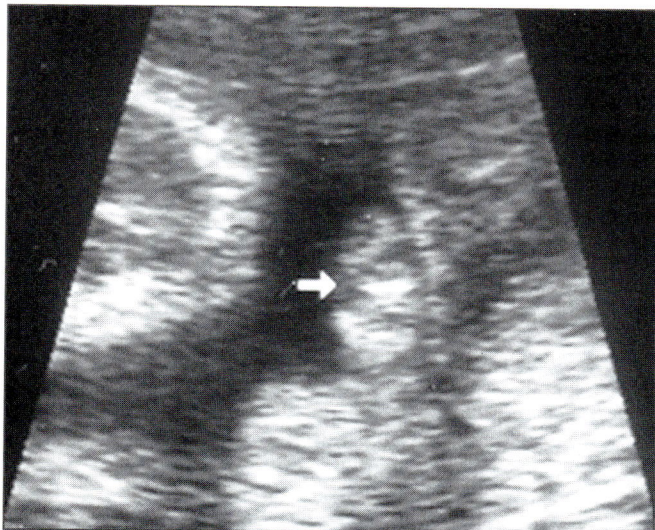

Fig. 13.183

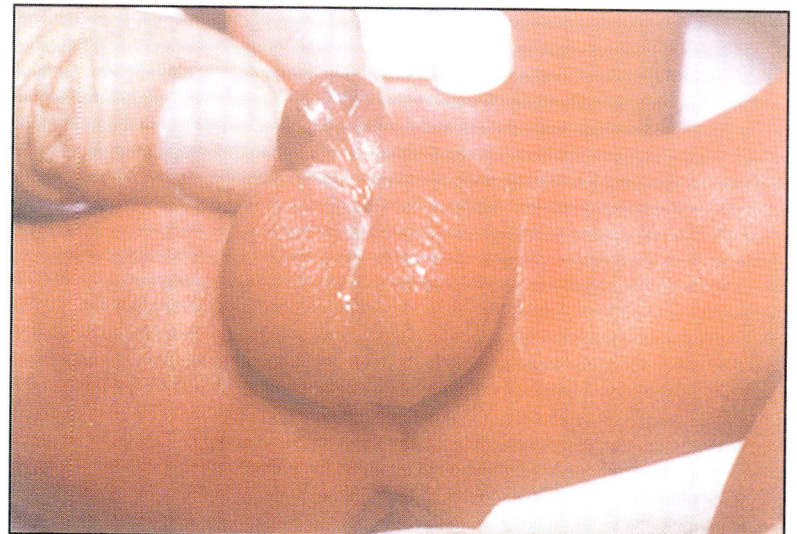

Figs 13.185 and 13.186: Hypospadias: Images showing the mictional fluid through ventral urethral opening

surgery can prevent the development of the Potter sequences including kidney dysfunction and pulmonary hypoplasia with limb and face deformities. Some prospective studies[88,91,92] have shown that, despite normal renal function at birth, the disease is progressive and children very often need dialysis and transplantation. Also, associated anomalies including trisomies should be excluded.

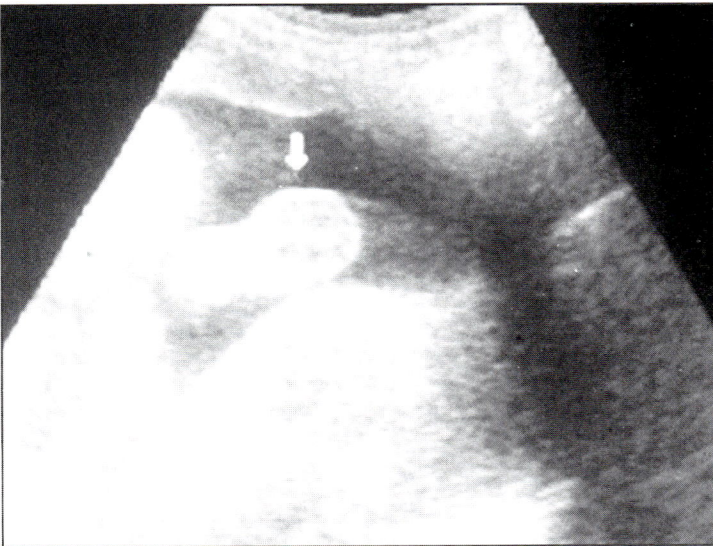

Fig. 13.187: Cryptorchidism: An undescended testicle in the inguinal canal

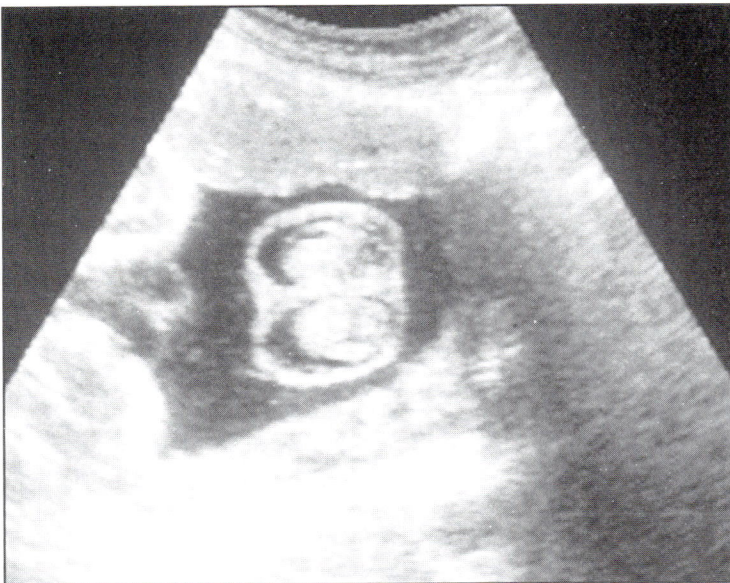

Fig. 13.188

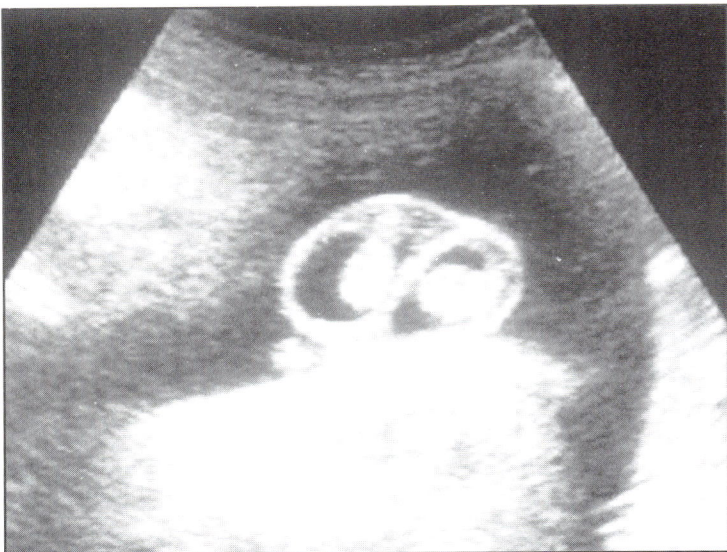

Figs 13.188 and 13.189: Hydrocele: A collection of serous fluid in a sacculated cavity. In practice the term is mostly used to describe a fluid collection in the tunica vaginalis testis (Fig. 13.188). Enlarged scrotal sac with a "half moon" of fluid surrounding the testis (Fig. 13.189).

Pulmonary hypoplasia caused by prolonged oligohydramnios poses a serious problem. Antenatal differentiation between lethal and non-lethal pulmonary hypoplasia is still doubtful, especially using lung biometry techniques.[99] The future will show whether color Doppler can help in this situation.[100] Only with all these data can appropriate treatment for the affected fetus be offered to the parents.

SKELETON MALFORMATIONS

A Muñoz, JM Carrera, E Scazzocchio, M Echevarria

INTRODUCTION

Although sonographic imaging of the fetal skeleton is possible very early, only a small proportion of skeleton abnormalities may be identified in the early second trimester.[101, 102]

It is very important to focus the attention on the following parameters: biometry of long bones, grade of bone density, bowing or fractures, aspect of the spine, appearance and number of digits, and fetal movements.

The long bones are recognizable from the end of the first trimester, and the metacarpals and metatarsals from the 16th week. But the phalanges are identifiable only from 18th to 19th weeks. The scapula, clavicle, humerus, radius and ulna, as well as the femur, tibia and fibula, are easily identified.[103] Especially important, and easy, is the measurement of femur.

The skeletal dysplasias, limb abnormalities and ossification disturbances are very numerous but in this section we will describe only the more frequent abnormalities: hypoplasia/aplasia of long bones, positional anomalies (Figs 13.190 to 13.192), hand anomalies, thanatophoric displasia, achondroplasia, osteogenesis imperfecta and arthrogryposis.

LIMB DEFICIENCY

A careful biometry is necessary for detecting anomalies such as *limb shortening* and establishing a variety of dysplasias according to the segment involved: predominantly rhizomelic, mesomelic, acromelic, etc.[104]

On the other hand, the examination of each bone is fundamental to exclude *absence or hypoplasia of individual bones*: fibula, tibia, radius, scapula, clavicle, etc (Figs 13.193 and 13.194).

Frequently the only identifiable anomaly is the absence of an extremity or a segment of an extremity. Approximately 50 of these limb reduction defects are simple transverse reduction deficiencies of one forearm or hand without associated

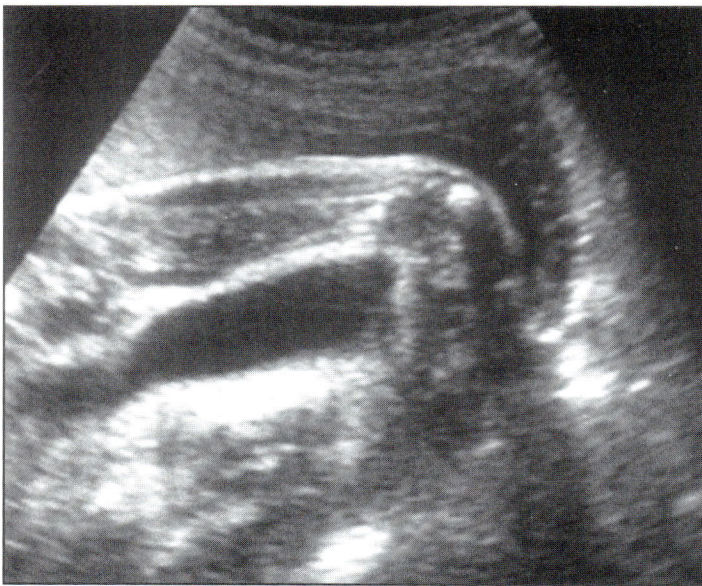

A

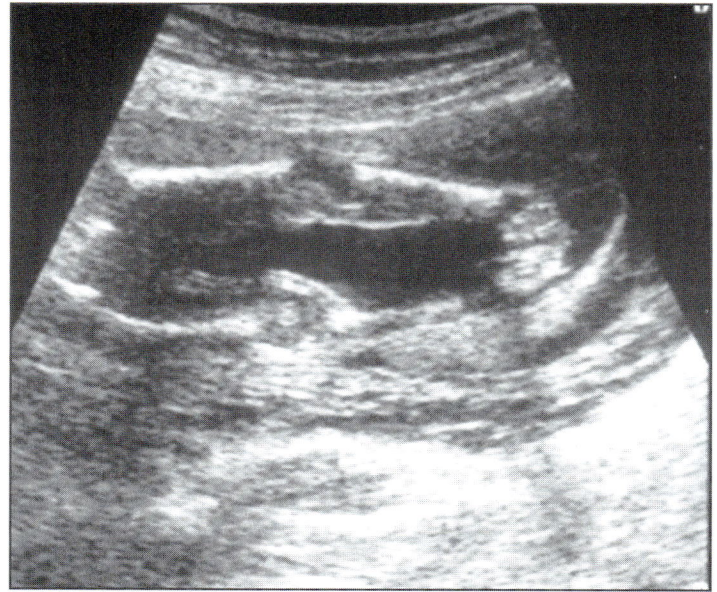

B

Figs 13.190A and B: Foot anomalies: A. Unilateral talipes equinovarus. There are various angulations of the heel, ankle equinus, and forefoot abduction and supination. B. The leg and unilateral talipes. Abnormal foot posture occurs in bone dysplasias; in deformations most commonly due to oligohydramnios; as part of many primary malformation syndromes; and in secondary malformations due to neuromuscular disease[105]

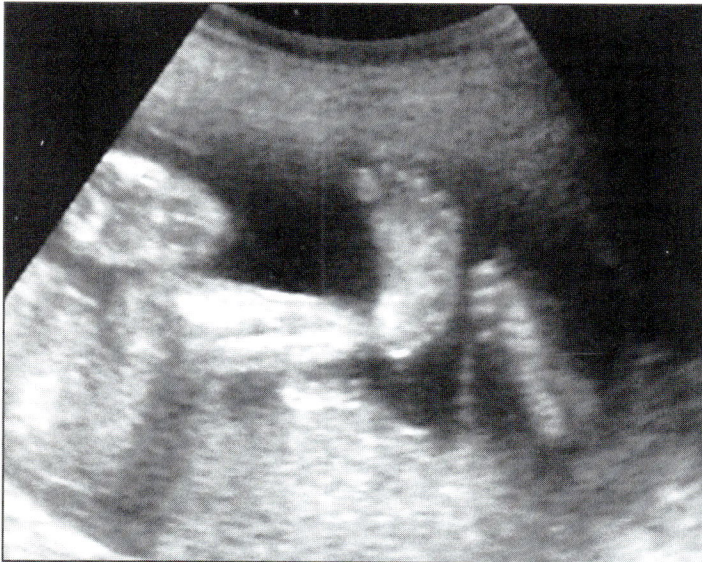

Fig. 13.191: Foot anomalies: Sagittal view of the foot, see a club foot

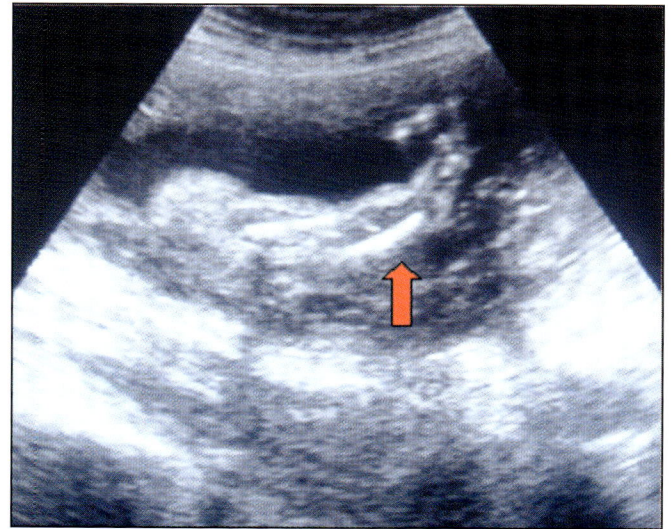

A

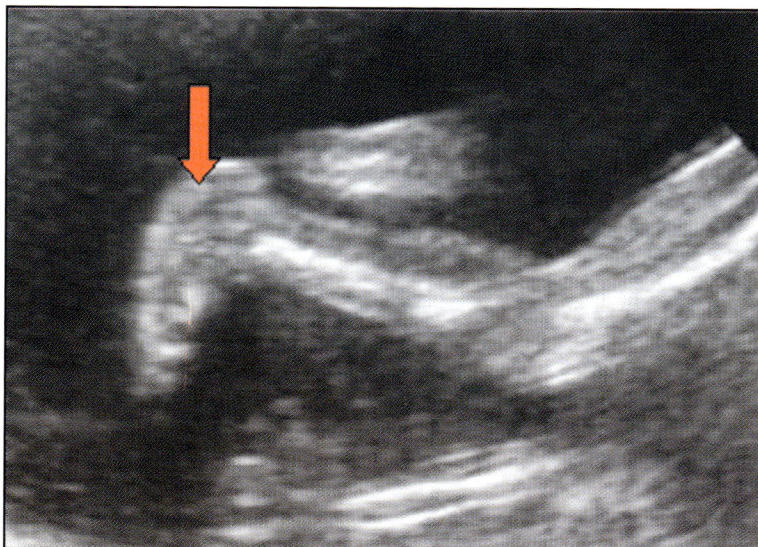

Fig. 13.192: Foot anomalies: Rocker-bottom foot is a foot with prominent heel and convex sole. Occurs in kariyotype anomalies

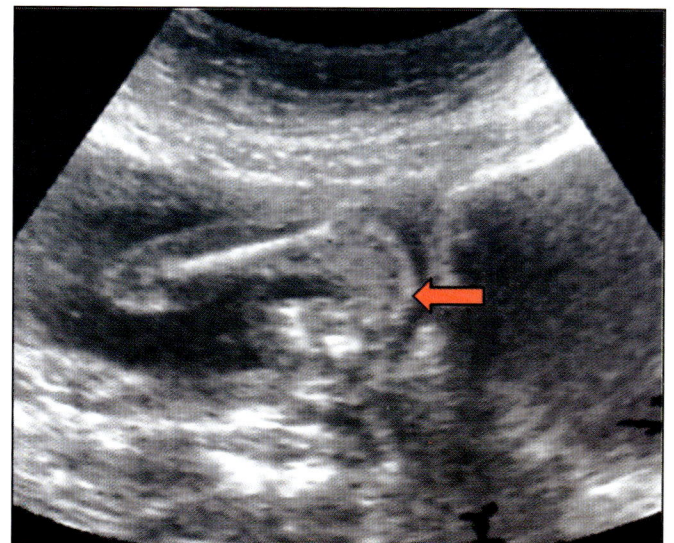

B

Figs 13.193A and B: Redial ray aplasia: A. Shortened forearm with only one bone. B. Acute medial deviation of the wrist and hand is also demonstrated

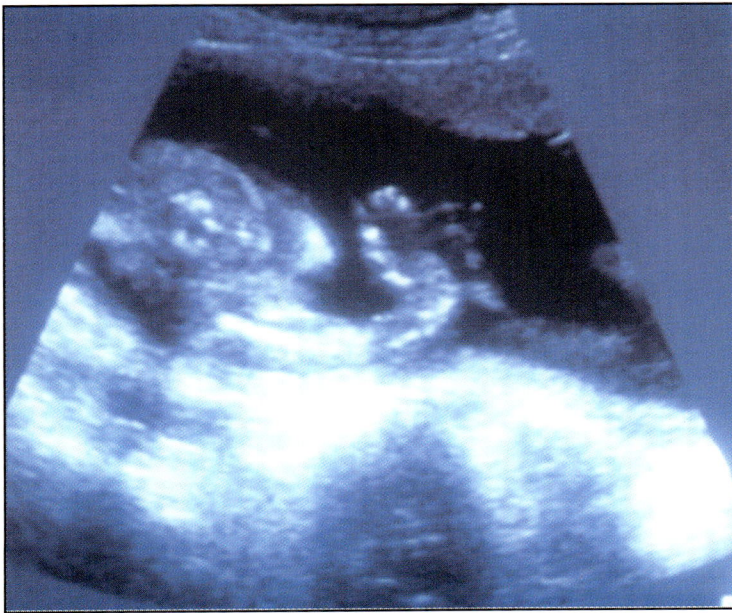

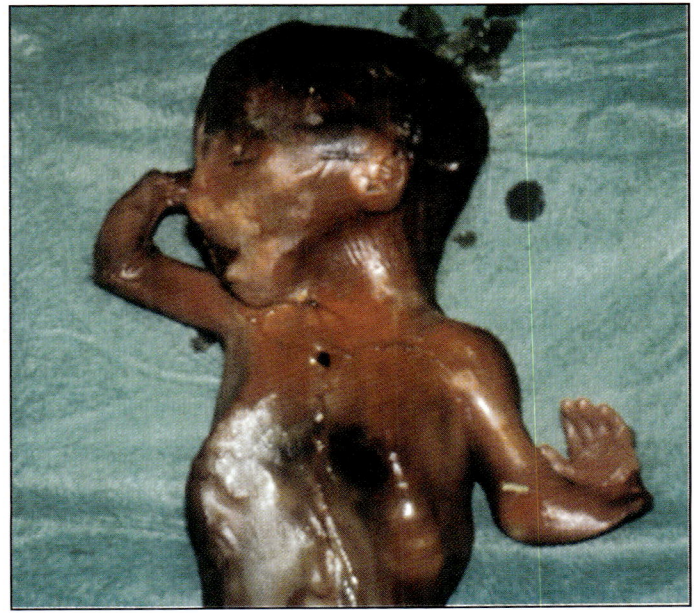

Figs 13.194A and B: Radial ray aplasia: A. Radial ray abnormalities (radial hypoplasia or aplasia) may be seen in: Holt-Oram syndrome. B. The fetus with medial deviation of the wrist and hand. Holt-Oram syndrome

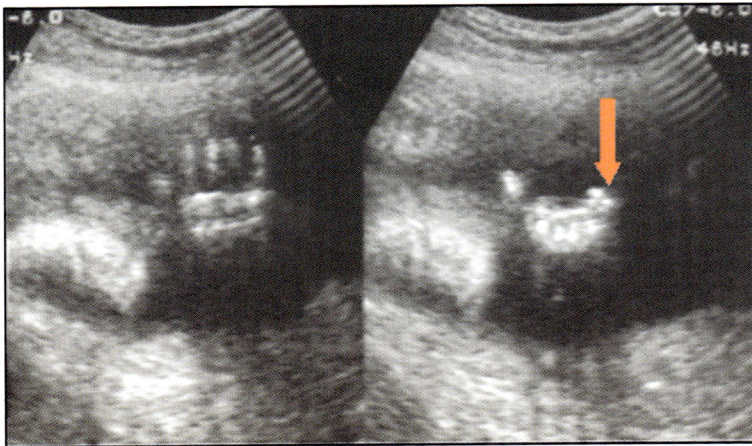

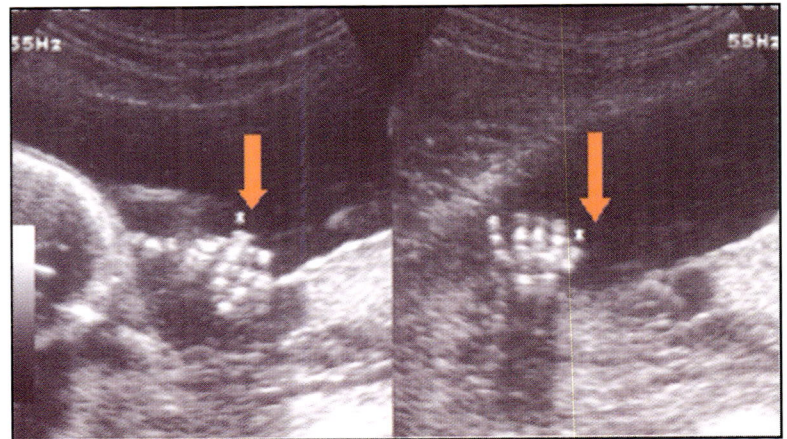

Figs 13.195A and B: Hand anomalies: A. Unilateral postaxial polydactyly. B. Postaxial polydactyly with two phalanges

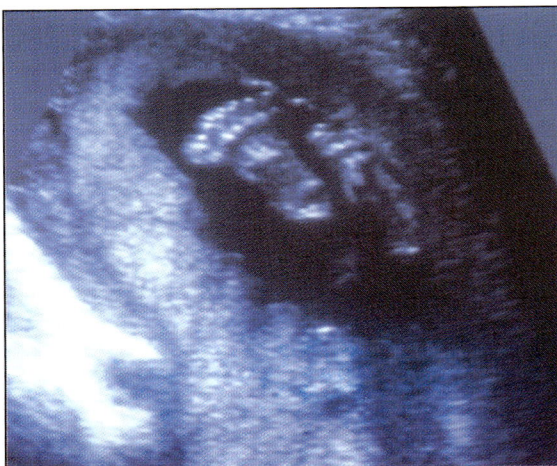

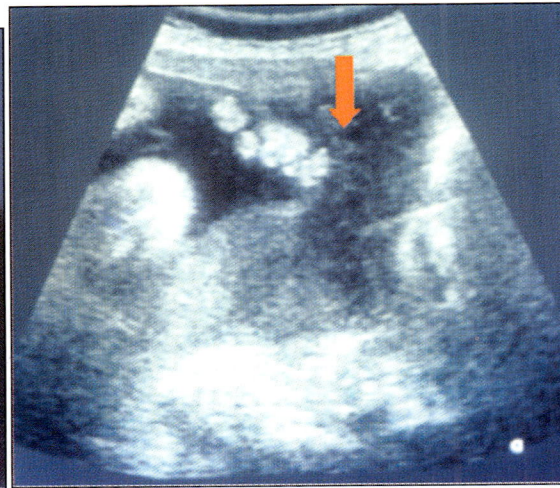

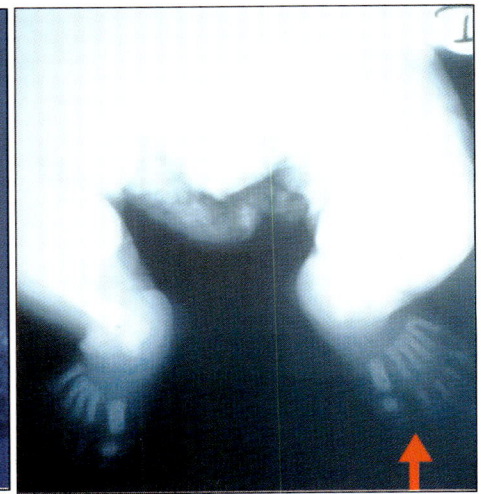

Figs 13.196A to C: Foot anomalies. A. Polydactyly postaxial foot. B. Frontal view: 6 fingers on the foot. C. X-ray: Postaxial extradigit on the right foot

anomalies. The rest of cases consist of multiple reductions deficiencies with 23 percent of them associated with additional anomalies in several organs.[105]

Isolated *amputation of an extremity* can be due to several etiologies: amniotic band syndrome, vascular accident or exposure to a teratogen. In this case the anomaly is sporadic and the risk of recurrence is negligible.

But limb deficiencies may present as a part of a specific syndrome, for example: Hanhart's syndrome (aglossia-adactylia syndrome), Möbius sequence (paralysis of cranial nerves, micrognathia, postural abnormalities and limb reductions), Robert's syndrome, etc. One of more known entity syndromes is *TAR syndrome* (thrombocytopenia, and absent radius).

Congenital short femur can be classified into five groups: type I (simple hypoplasia of the femur), type II (short femur with angulated shaft), type III (short femur with coxa vara), type IV (absent or defective proximal femur), and type V (absent or rudimentary femur).[104]

ALTERATIONS OF THE HANDS AND FEET

By means of sonography it is possible to diagnose several alterations of the hands and feet, that form part of multiple skeletal dysplasias. For example: polydactyly, syndactyly and clinodactyly, and malpositions (Figs 13.195 to 13.198).

Polydactyly refers to the presence of an excess of five digits. On the contrary, *syndactyly* refers to soft tissue or bony fusion of adjacent digits. *Clinodactyly* consists of deviation of digits. The sonographic diagnosis is possible.

There are several malpositions of the foot. Some of most frequent are: Clubfoot, Rocker-Bottom feet, etc.

The ultrasonographic criteria for the diagnosis of *clubfoot* are based on the imaging of the fetal feet and toes in a plane which is parallel to the lower leg.[106]

The Rocker-Bottom feet consist in a deformation of talus and calcaneum. The sonographic appearance is a prominent heel with a convexity of the foot.

ACHONDROPLASIA

This condition is characteristic for: rhizomelic dwarfism, limb bowing, enlarged head and lordotic spine. The bones of the hands and feet are short with trident-shaped hands.

The prenatal diagnosis is possible from 25 weeks (Fig. 13.199). Before that, it is difficult due to the fact that shortness of the long bones does not occur until after 24 weeks.[107] Achondroplasia is the most common nonlethal skeletal dysplasia.

THANATOPHORIC DYSPLASIA

Thanatophoric dysplasia is the most common lethal skeletal dysplasia. The main pathological findings are: extreme rhizomelia, narrow thorax and a large head with prominent forehead (Figs 13.200 to 13.202). Usually are described two types: type I, with typical bowed "telephone receiver" femur without cloverleaf skull, and type II with cloverleaf skull and short, straight long bones.[108]

The ultrasonographic appearance depends on the specific variety but in all the cases the association of cloverleaf skull and micromelia is specific for thanatophoric dysplasia.

OSTEOGENESIS IMPERFECTA

The main sonographic findings are: absence of reduced mineralization of the skull, multiple fractures and angulations of the long bones.[101, 109] There are four types: type I (or van der Hoeve syndrome) is characterized by the classic triad of blue sclera, bone fragility and hearing loss, but the fractures appear after the birth; type II, with multiples fractures in utero and severe dwarf; type III is characterized by blue sclera and multiple fractures at birth, and finally, type IV is the mildest form. Long bones are of normal length. Types I and IV are autosomal dominant and the prognosis is much better than in type II and III that are autosomal recessive.

Nowadays all the types can be diagnosed by ultrasonography (Figs 13.203 and 13.204).

ARTHROGRYPOSIS

Arthrogryposis multiple congenita (ACM) refers to multiple joint contractures in the fetus and neonate (Figs 13.205 and 13.206). In fetuses with this abnormality, clubhand and clubfoot are observed.[101, 110] The absence of movement referred to as fetal akinesia/hypokinesia, is noted in different joins. This anomaly results in contractures. The most frequent etiology is a neurogenic disorder followed by myopathic disorder.[111]

ECHOCARDIOGRAPHY IN EARLY PREGNANCY

*Carmina Comas, Josep M Martínez,
Alberto Galindo, Carlos Millán*

ABSTRACT

Within the last decade, two significant events have contributed to the increasing interest in early fetal echocardiography. First, the introduction of high-frequency vaginal ultrasound probes allows detailed visualization of cardiac structures at early stage of gestation, making early detection of fetal malformations possible.

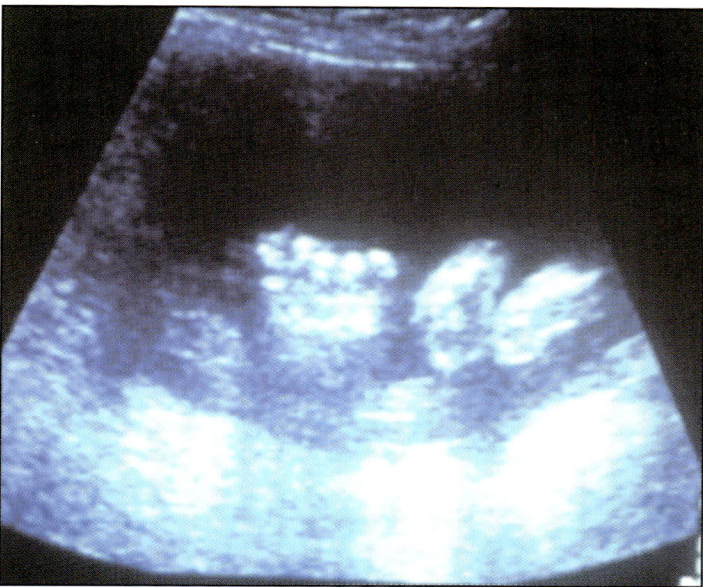

Fig. 13.197: Hand anomalies: Clenched hand: Pathologic correlation with overlapping digits

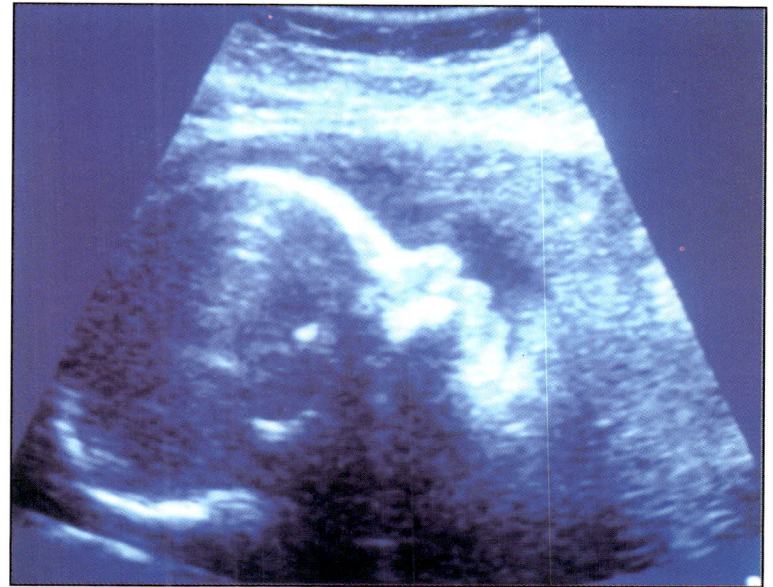

A

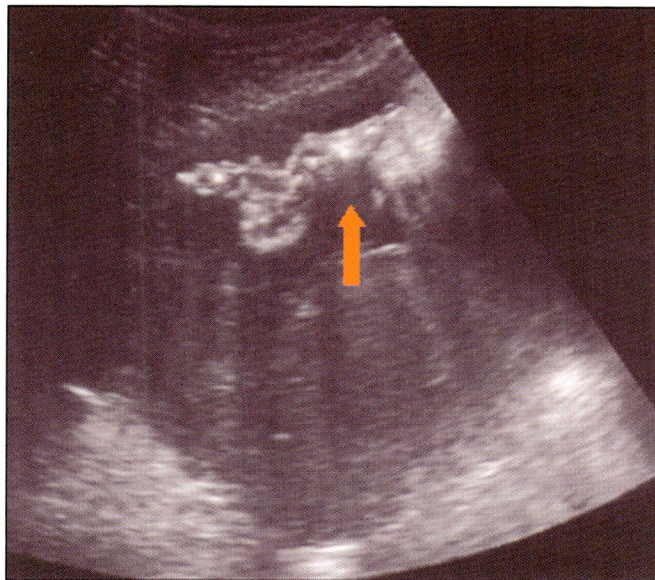

B

Figs 13.198A and B: Hand anomalies: A. Ectrodactyly: defect in midhand. The common name of this is "lobster-claw" deformity. B. Ectrodactyly: At both hands, images demonstrate a paucity of fingers with fused fingers

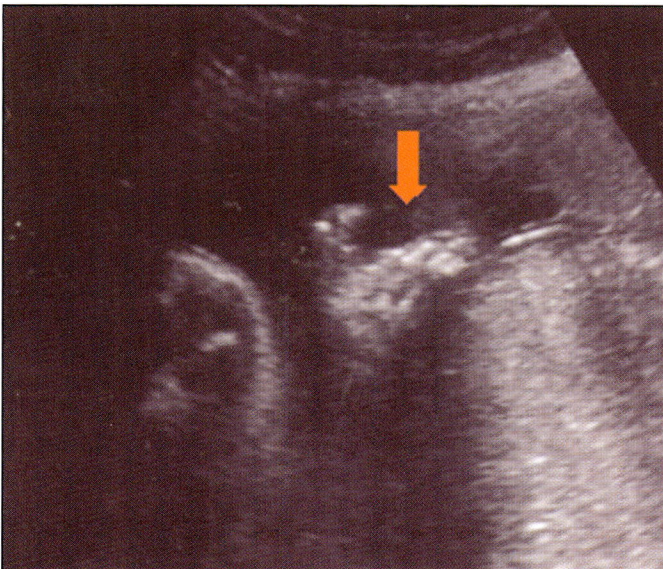

Fig. 13.199: Achondroplasia: Frontal bossing and low nasal bridge

Second, the close relationship observed between some first trimester sonographic and Doppler markers and congenital heart defects allows an early identification of a high-risk group at 11th to 14th weeks of gestation. In this context, from the early 1990s, many authors have examined the potential role of the transvaginal approach to obtain earlier diagnosis of fetal cardiac malformations. Further studies have appeared in the literature showing that early transvaginal echocardiography in experienced hands is a fairly sensitive investigative tool. Although some malformations are detected as early as 11th week of gestation, the optimal gestational age to perform the early scan is at least 13th week of gestation. Transvaginal ultrasound is the preferred approach, although most of the authors agree that results can be improved if transabdominal ultrasound is also incorporated. The further application of color Doppler enhances visualization. The sensitivity and specificity of early fetal echocardiography for the detection of heart anomalies is acceptable compared to the ones obtained by mid-gestational echocardiography, showing a slight reduction in detection rates and an increase in false-positive and negative rates. The cardiac anomalies detected at this early stage of pregnancy are mainly defects involving the four-chamber view, indicating that defects solely affecting the outflow tracts are difficult to diagnose in the first trimester of pregnancy. Heart defects diagnosed early in pregnancy tend to be more complex than those detected later, with a higher incidence of associated structural malformations, chromosomal abnormalities and spontaneous abortions. The neonate follow-up or postmortem examination in case of termination of pregnancy are essential to assess the actual role of early fetal echocardiography. At present, early fetal echocardiography is a promising technique, which can be of considerable value for patients at high-risk. This technique is, however, currently limited to a few specialized centers.

The aim of this review is to explore the possibilities of examining the fetal heart at this early stage of pregnancy. This article also present our experience in the first multicenter trial in early fetal echocardiography performed in Spain. In accordance with other studies, this experience stresses the usefulness of early echocardiography when performed by expert operators on fetus specifically at risk for cardiac defects. Our review of these additional 48 cases contributes to the expanding literature on the ability of transvaginal ultrasonography to detect fetal heart defects in early pregnancy.

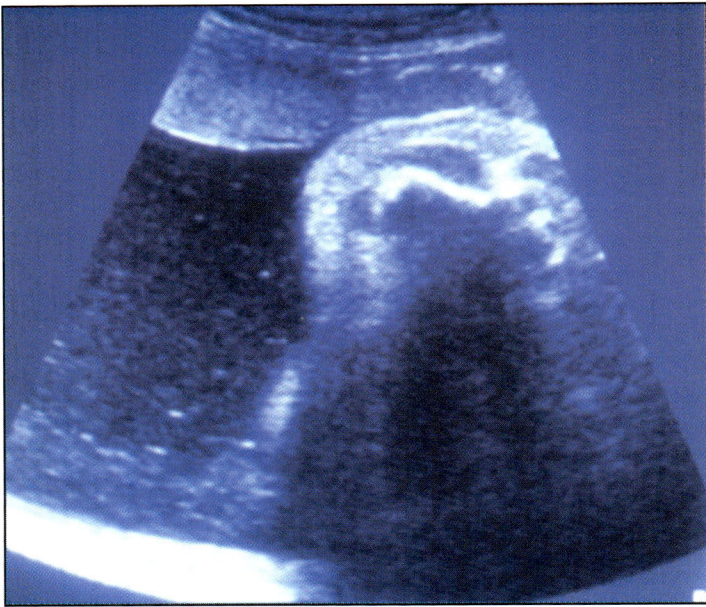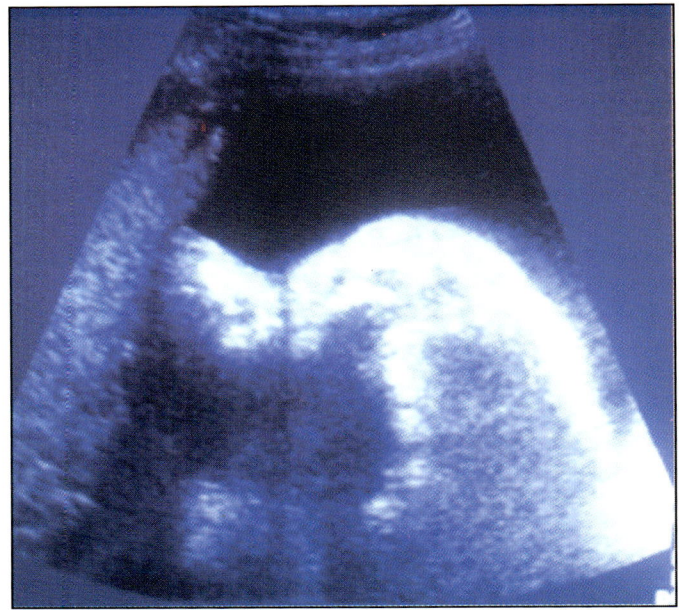

A B

Figs 13.200A and B: Thanatophoric dysplasia: A. Short and bowed femur. B. The severe micromelia of limbs

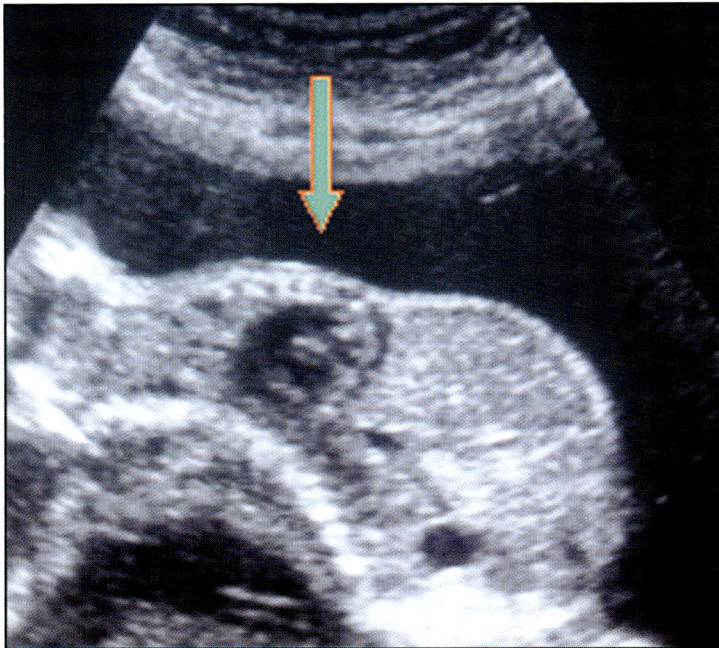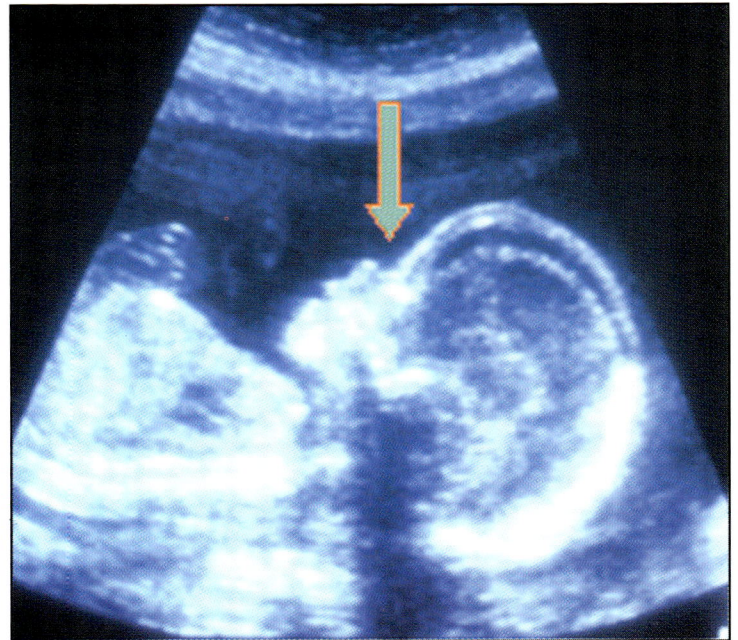

A B

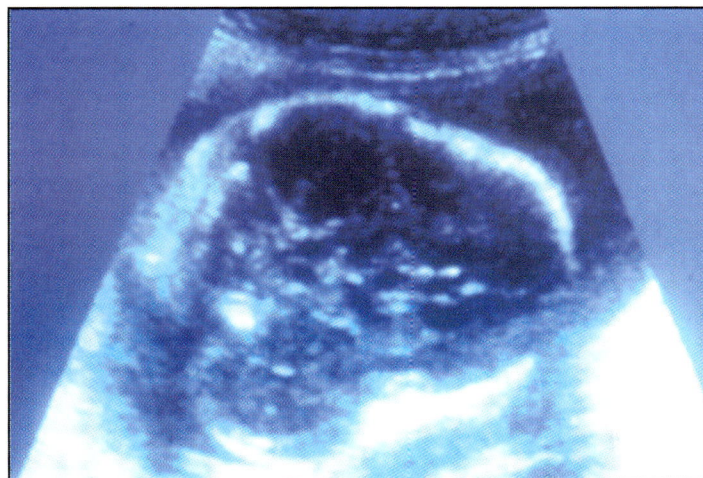

C

Figs 13.201A to C: Thanatophoric dysplasia: A. Comparison of size of the chest and abdomen. B. Frontal bossing. Depressed nasal bridge. C. Cloverleaf skull

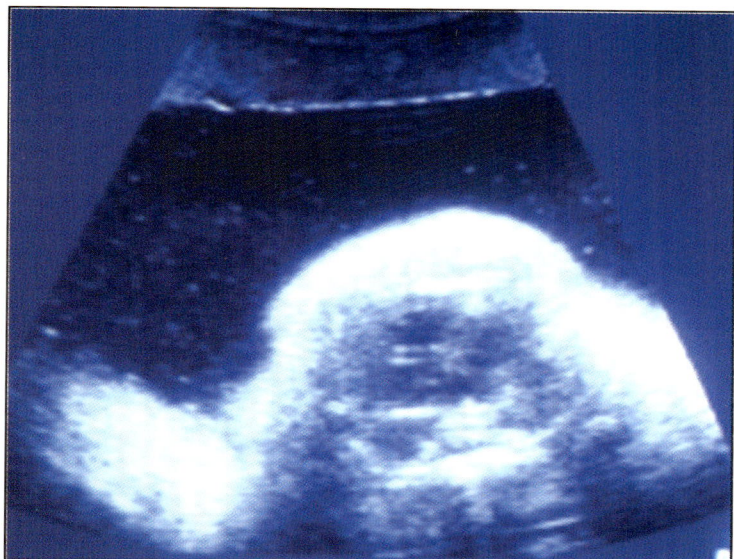

A

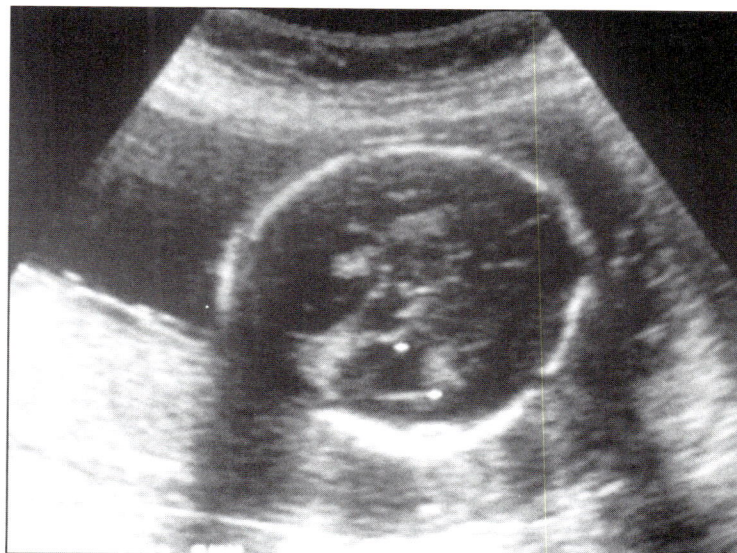

B

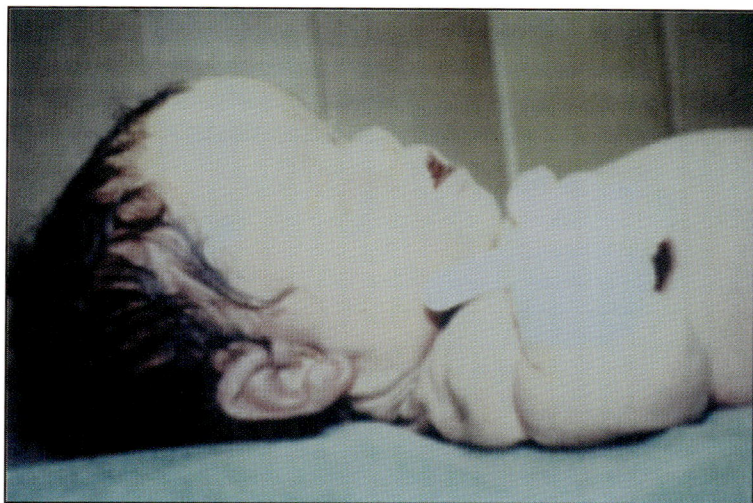

C

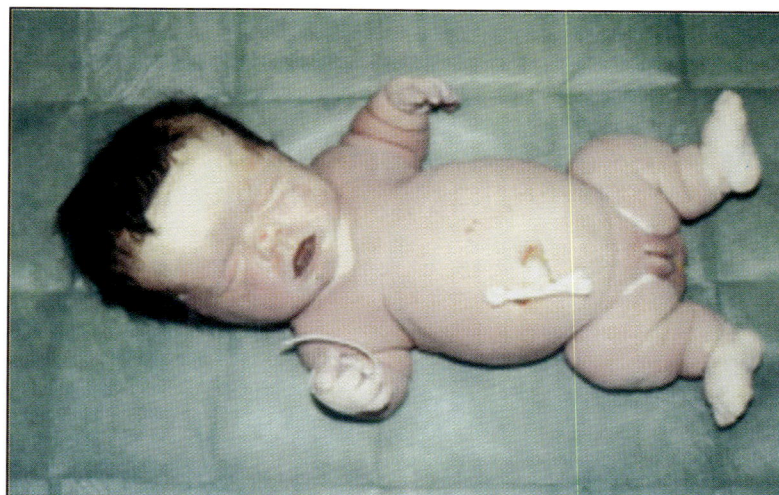

D

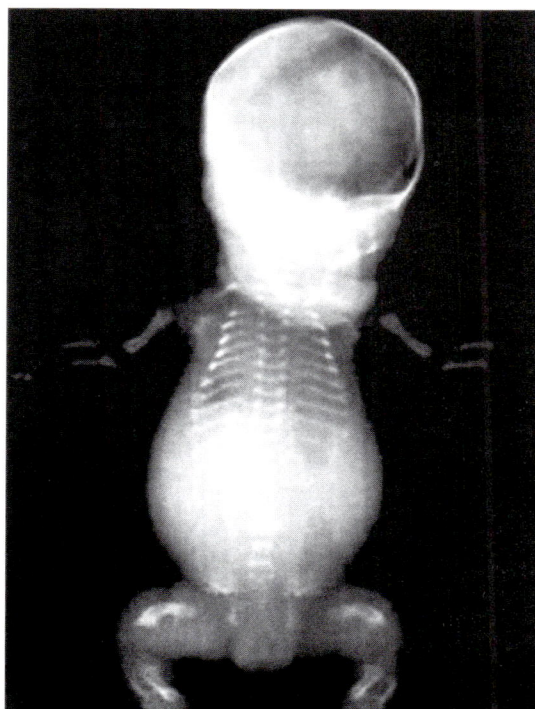

E

Figs 13.202A to E: Thanatophoric dysplasia: A. Sagittal scan narrow chest. B. Ventriculomegaly. C. The newborn: Frontal bossing. D. The newborn. Note the short limbs. E. X-ray after birth. Note the short and bowed femur and narrow chest.

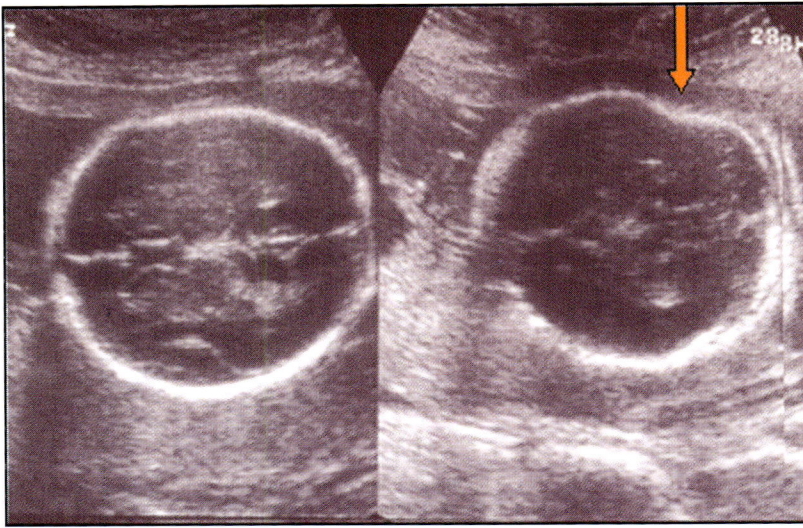

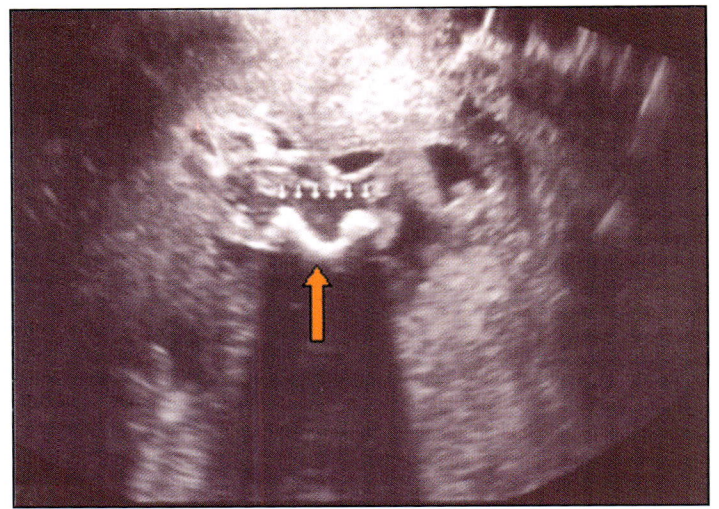

A

B

Figs 13.203A and B: Osteogenesis imperfecta: A. The skull is readily compressible even with moderate transducer pressure. Increased visualization of the intracranial structures. B. Bone with a wrinkled appearance caused by callus formation

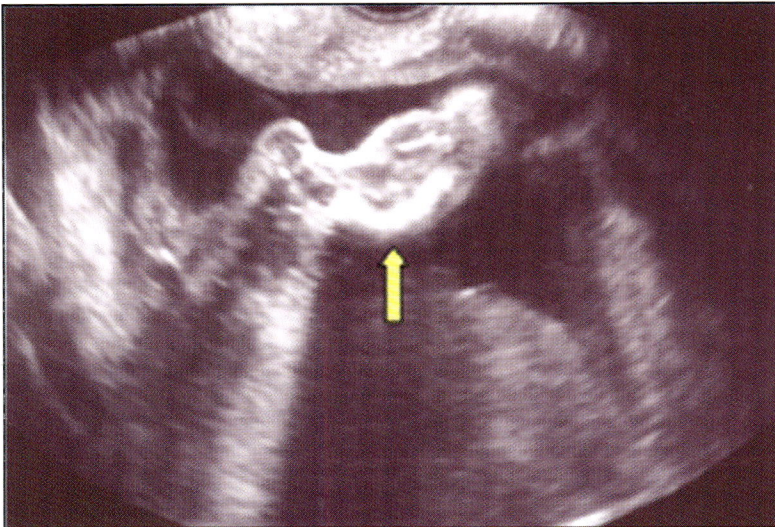

A

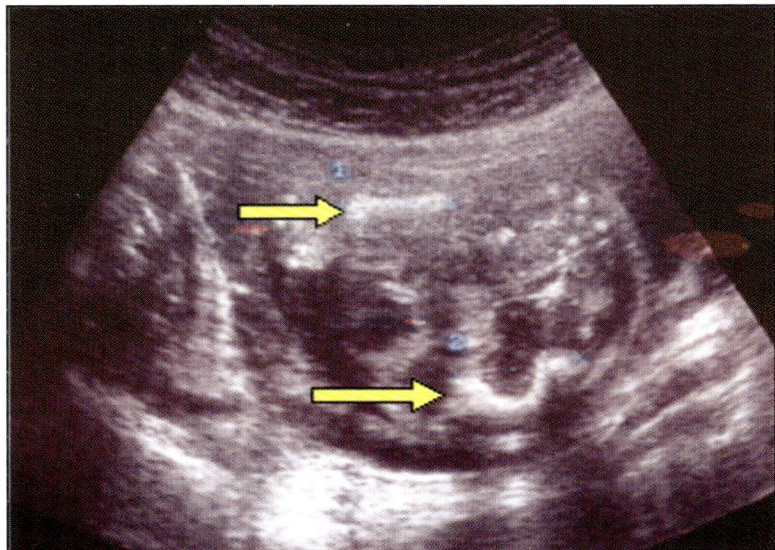

B

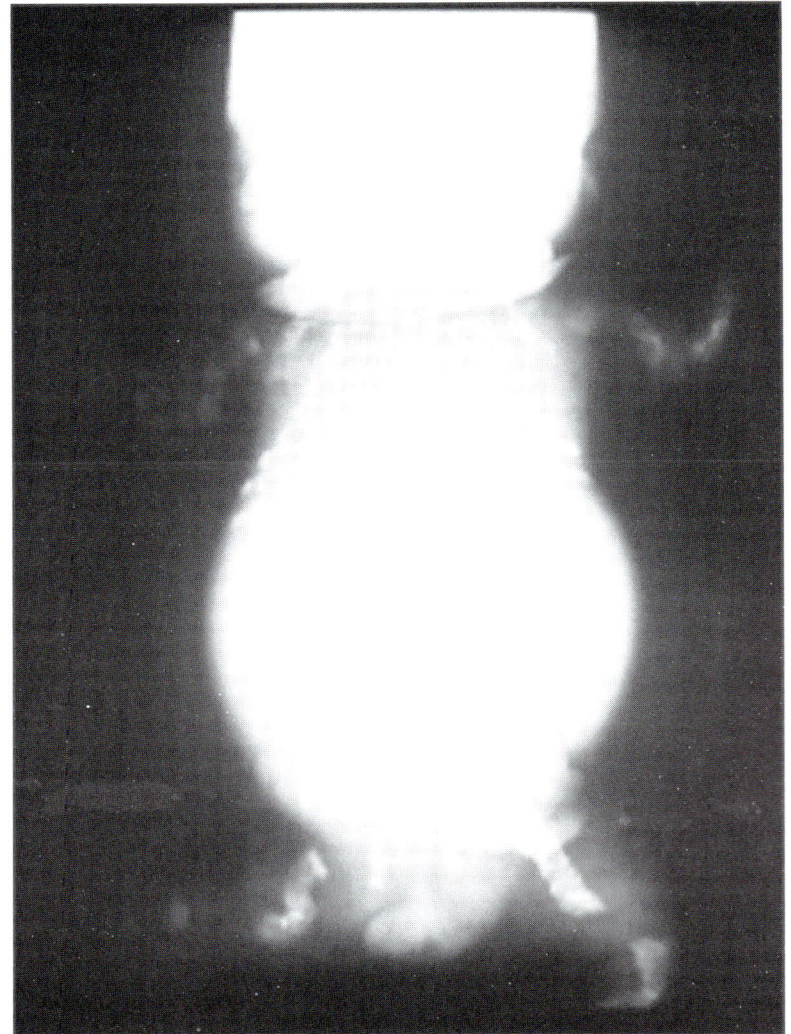

C

Figs 13.204A to C: Osteogenesis imperfecta: A. Bone shortening and angulation, due to multiple fracture. B. Fractured long bones with wrinkled appearance caused by callus formation. C. X-ray of the fetus. Note the poor mineralization and the numerous fractures

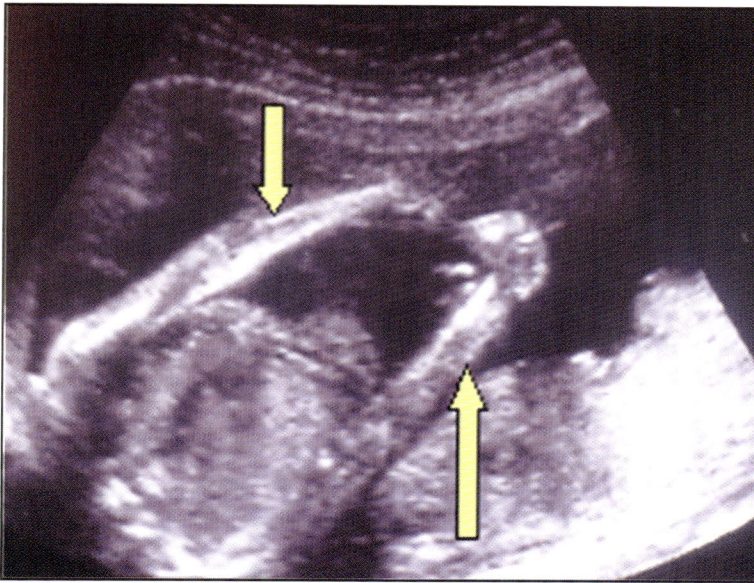

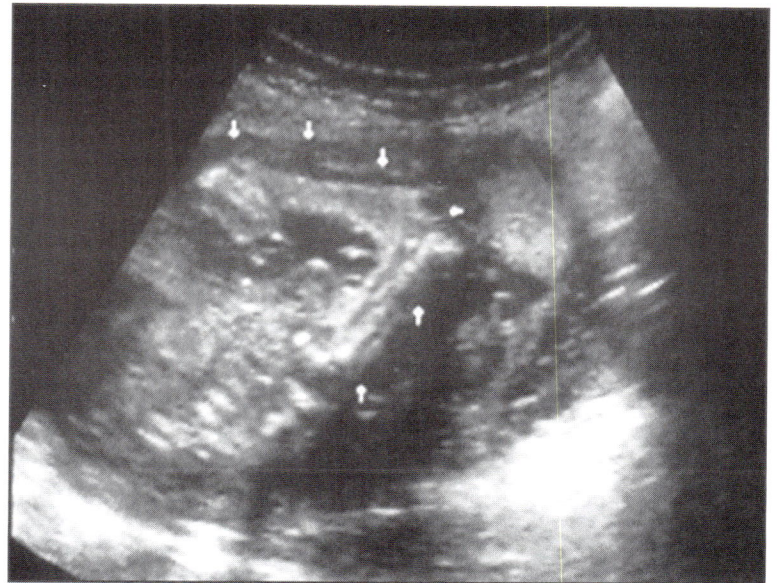

Figs 13.205A and B: Arthrogryposis: A. Joint contractures and rigidity the arms, clenched hand.
B. Noted were fixed limb, clubbed feet and clenched hands

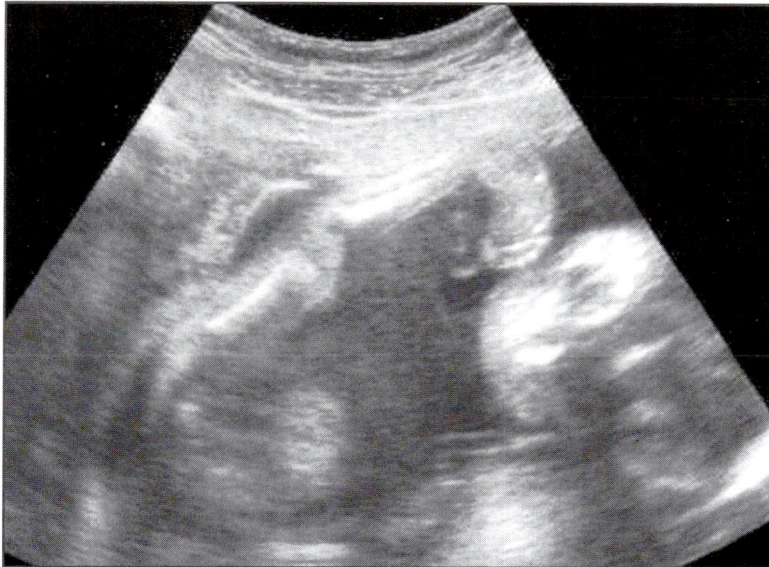

Fig. 13.206: Arthrogryposis: Abnormal foot posture and fixed limbs

INTRODUCTION

Prenatal detection of fetal congenital heart defects (CHDs) remains the most problematic issue of prenatal diagnosis.[112] Major CHDs are the most common severe congenital malformations, with an incidence of about 5 in a thousand live births, whenever complete ascertainment is done and minor lesions are excluded.[112, 113] Congenital heart anomalies have a significant effect on affected children's life with up to 25 to 35 percent mortality rate during pregnancy and the postnatal period, and it is during the first year of life, when the 60 percent of this mortality occurs. Moreover, major CHDs are responsible for nearly 50 percent of all neonatal and infant deaths due to congenital anomalies, and it is likely to be significantly higher if spontaneous abortions are considered. Although CHDs use to appear isolated, they are frequently associated with other defects, chromosomal anomalies and genetic syndromes. Their incidence is 6 times greater than chromosomal abnormalities and 4 times greater than neural tube defects.[112-114]

Most major CHDs scan be diagnosed prenatally by detailed transabdominal second trimester echocardiography at 20th to 22nd weeks of gestation.[112, 114-117] The identification of pregnancies at high-risk for CHDs needing referral to specialist centres is of paramount importance in order to reduce the rate of overlooked defects.[117,118] However, the main problem in prenatal diagnosis of CHDs is that the majority of cases take place in pregnancies with no identifiable risk factors. Therefore, there is wide agreement that cardiac ultrasound screening should be introduced as an integral part of the routine scan at 20th to 22nd weeks. When applied to low-risk population, scrutiny of the four chamber view allows only the detection of 40 percent of the anomalies while additional visualization of the outflow tracts and the great arteries increase the rate up to 60 to 70 percent.[114-116]

Recently, the finding of an increased nuchal translucency[119,120] or an altered ductus venosus blood flow[121,122] at 10th to 14th weeks of gestation have been associated with a high-risk for CHDs and their prevalence increase exponentially with the thickness of nuchal translucency[119] regardless the fetal karyotype. Since earlier diagnosis of congenital malformations is increasingly demanded, the option of an early fetal echocardiography must be taken into account.[123-125] The use of high-frequency vaginal ultrasound probes along with substantial improvements in magnification and processing of the imaging, together with the introduction of color Doppler, have extensively contributed to the development of the technique, allowing better visualization of cardiac structures earlier in pregnancy.[123, 126,127]

Although most of the groups perform early fetal echocardiography between 13th and 16th weeks of gestation, we can name it as so when performed before the 18th week of gestation. Despite several studies that stated that fetal heart examination could be incorporated in first or early second trimester examinations, its use is currently still limited to a few specialized centers.

TECHNICAL ISSUES

Regarding early fetal echocardiography, some institutions use predominantly the transvaginal (TV) approach[125, 128-133] while others prefer the transabdominal one.[134-137] Most of the authors reporting early fetal echocardiography prefer the TV approach due to its increased resolution associated with higher frequency transducers and also because given that equivalent tranducers frequencies, the TV probes provide better quality images.[138] However, most importantly, authors with background training as pediatric cardiologists are more likely to use the transabdominal approach in contrast with most of obstetricians, who are well used to the TV route. The superiority of transvaginal sonography is usually well accepted before the 14th week. Between the 15th and 18th weeks both transabdominal and transvaginal routes seem to offer similar advantages and disadvantages, and beyond the 18th week the transabdominal echocardiography seems to achieve better results.[112, 116, 127, 138, 139]

The combination of two-dimensional echocardiography with color Doppler flow imaging proved generally helpful, in particular by visualization of blood flow on both great arteries and of two divided ventricular inflows. The addition of color Doppler flow studies provides substantial improvement in the diagnostic accuracy of early echocardiography, as was also shown by DeVore for transabdominal sonography in the second half of pregnancy.[140]

When performing early fetal echocardiography, we firstly recommend to scan by the TV route, following the examination by the transabdominal probe when a complete study is not possible. The highest frequency must always be used, whatever the route is chosen. Obviously, a high-resolution realtime ultrasound has to be used. For color Doppler evaluation, the energy output levels have to be lower than 50 mW/cm^2 spatial peak-temporal average. Since color Doppler is dissipated over a wide area of interest, thermal effects resulting from Doppler insonation should not be a matter of concern, unlike pulsed Doppler in which the whole energy of the beam is focused at a specific location. Besides, the embryonic developmental of the heart has been completed by the time the scan is performed.

ULTRASOUND ANATOMY OF THE NORMAL HEART

Embryonic heartbeat can be detected as early as the 5th week of gestation, and normal development of its function shows an increasing heart rate from 80 to 90 beats per minute at 5th week of gestation to 170 to 180 beats per minute at the end of the 9th and 10th weeks. As pregnancy progresses, the control of the heart rate matures with increasing vagal dominance, and the baseline rate declines to 145 to 155 beats per minute with the appearance of beat to beat variation, most likely resulting from the functional adaptation to the development of the heart and autonomic nervous system maturation, and remains more or less constant during the rest of intrauterine life.[141,142]

The structural development of the heart begins on day 16 and it is finished by the 10th week. Early fetal echocardiography has the same goals that the standard one, and we advocate to perform it in a segmental approach. The first objective of the examination is to assess the normality of the four-chamber view through a transverse section of the fetal chest: normal situs solitus; normal size and axis of the heart in relation to the chest; both atria equal in size, with the foramen ovale flapping within the left atrium; both ventricles equal in size and contractility; atrial and ventricular septa are of normal appearance; tricuspid and mitral valves are normally inserted, opening and closing together. Color and pulsed Doppler are particulary useful to confirm normal inflow to the ventricles and to detect turbulent flow or jets suggesting valve regurgitation. It is useful to assess the four chambers in different views: apical, basal and long axis with the interventricular septum perpendicular to the ultrasound beam in order to visualize better the integrity of the septum. Then, the origin and double crossing of the great arteries must be correctly identified: the left ventricle outflow tract, with the continuity between the interventricular septum and the anterior wall of the ascending aorta; the right ventricle outflow tract, more superior, anterior, almost perpendicular to the axis of the ascending aorta and connecting to the descending aorta in the three vessels view. Color Doppler is also of help to better visualize the outflow tracts confirm anterograde flow through the semilunar valves and great arteries, and makes easier the examination of both aortic and ductal arches and their confluence. Pulsed Doppler may be used to assess blood flow through the aortic and pulmonic valves in order to confirm normal anterograde flow and to detect very high velocities suggesting valve stenosis. Finally, color and pulsed Doppler are also very useful to identify normal systemic and pulmonary venous return. Figures 13.207 to 13.216 illustrate images obtained at early fetal scan by 2D echocardiography and color Doppler in a structurally normal heart. In our experience, the average duration of the complete fetal cardiac scan is over 15 minutes. It essentialy depends on the gestational age at the examination, and can be even shorter if there is a favorable fetal lie. In our setting, a subsequent transabdominal echocardiography is scheduled for all our patients at 20th to 22nd weeks of gestation.

Most of the authors agree that the best window of time to perform the early echocardiography is between the 13th and 16th weeks of gestation, since a complete cardiac examination is rarely achieved before the 13th week of gestation.[125, 128, 129, 131-133, 137] Articles on early fetal echocardiography demonstrate an increase in visualization rates of the four-chamber view and the outflow tracts in the last decade, with visualization rates greater than 90 percent at 13th week of gestation.[139] To maximize the reduction of uninterpretable examinations, early fetal echocardiography should be preferably performed at 13 completed weeks of gestation. Using current technology, the four-chamber view and the outflow tracts are often demonstrated by two-dimensional echocardiography only, but color Doppler imaging enhances and makes the identification of the structures faster, increasing the succes rate of the examination, and allows even earlier identification of the structures.

DIAGNOSIS OF CONGENITAL HEART DEFECTS

The first diagnosis of a CHD by early echocardiography was reported by Gembruch et al[143] in 1990. A complete atrioventricular canal defect, with complete heart block and atrioventricular valve regurgitation was diagnosed at 11 weeks + 4 days' gestation using a 5-MHz transvaginal probe. The same year, Bronshtein et al[144] reported the diagnosis of a ventricular septal defect with overriding aorta and a further case of an isolated ventricular septal defect with pericardial effusion, both cases at 14th week of gestation. Since then, an increasing number of case reports and series on the early diagnosis of CHD have been reported, both in high-risk and low-risk population. Tables 13.6 and 13.7 summarize some of the largest and most significant studies on the detection of CHD using early fetal echocardiography in high-risk and low-risk pregnancies.[125, 128-133, 135-137, 145-150] Obviously, studies in unselected population report less encouraging results, with lower visualization rates and detection rates. The largest series so far is the one published by Bronshtein et al.[131] They report the diagnosis of 173 cases of CHD over 36,323 fetuses evaluated by transvaginal ultrasound at 11th to 17th weeks of gestation over a 14-year period of time, with 99 percent of scans performed at 14th to 16th weeks of gestation and 86 percent of them in low-risk population. Recently, two institutions went further and reported their experience performing the echocardiography as early as between 10th and 13th weeks of gestation.[133, 137]

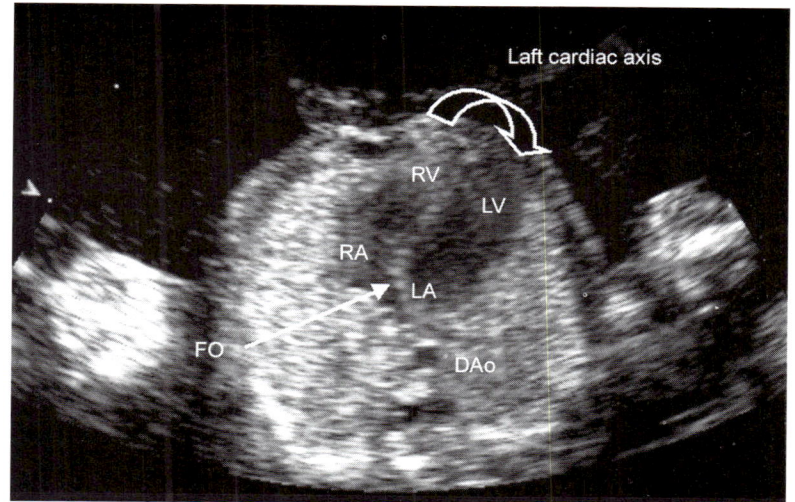

Fig. 13.207: Early fetal echocardiography by 2D in a structurally normal heart. The 4-chamber view: normal situs solitus; normal size and axis of the heart in relation to the chest; both atria equal in size, with the foramen ovale flapping within the left atrium; both ventricles equal in size and contractility; atrial and ventricular septa are of normal appearance; tricuspid and mitral valves are normally inserted. RV right ventricle; LV: left ventricle; RA: right atrium; LA: left atrium; FO: foramen ovale; DAo: descending aorta

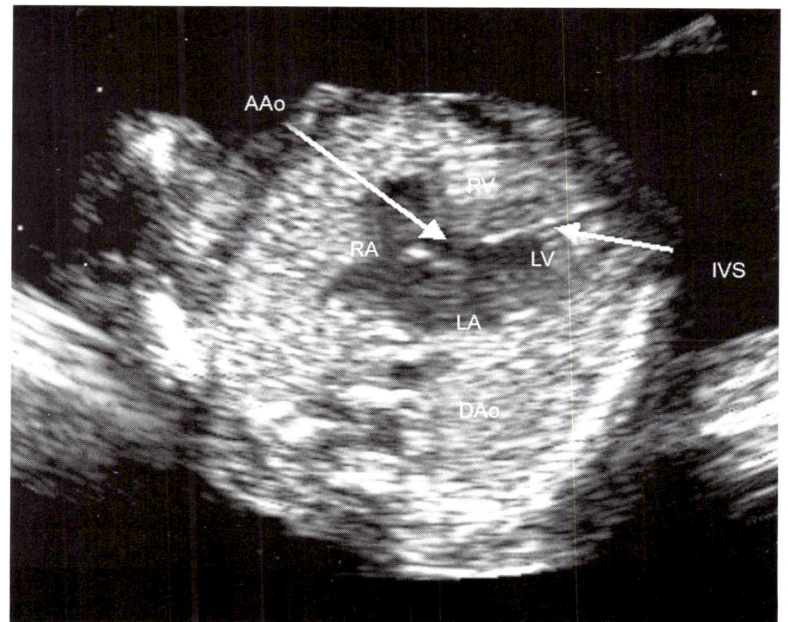

Fig. 13.208: Early fetal echocardiography by 2D in a structurally normal heart. The 5-chamber view: left ventricle outflow tract in the long axis view showing the continuity between the interventricular septum and the anterior wall of the ascending aorta. RV right ventricle; LV: left ventricle; RA: right atrium; LA: left atrium; AAo: ascending aorta; DAo: descending aorta; IVS: interventricular septum

The most frequent fetal heart anomalies diagnosed at early echocardiography are summarized in Table 13.8 (true positive cases).[125, 129-132, 135-137, 145, 146, 148, 150] Note that only the main anomaly for each fetus is presented in the table, even though some fetuses had several cardiac anomalies. It should be noted that defects such a small isolated ventricular septal defect or valvular stenosis are not reported in these studies. Table 13.9 summarize the published cases of cardiac anomaly not detected in early pregnancy (false-negative cases).[125, 130-132, 135-137, 145-148, 150]

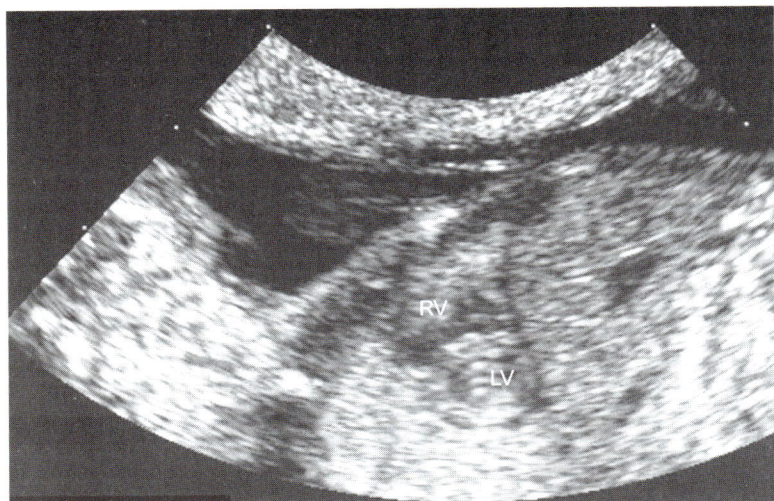

Fig. 13.209: Early fetal echocardiography by 2D in a structurally normal heart. The short axis view, showing an anterior right ventricle and a posterior left ventricle. RV: right ventricle; LV: left ventricle

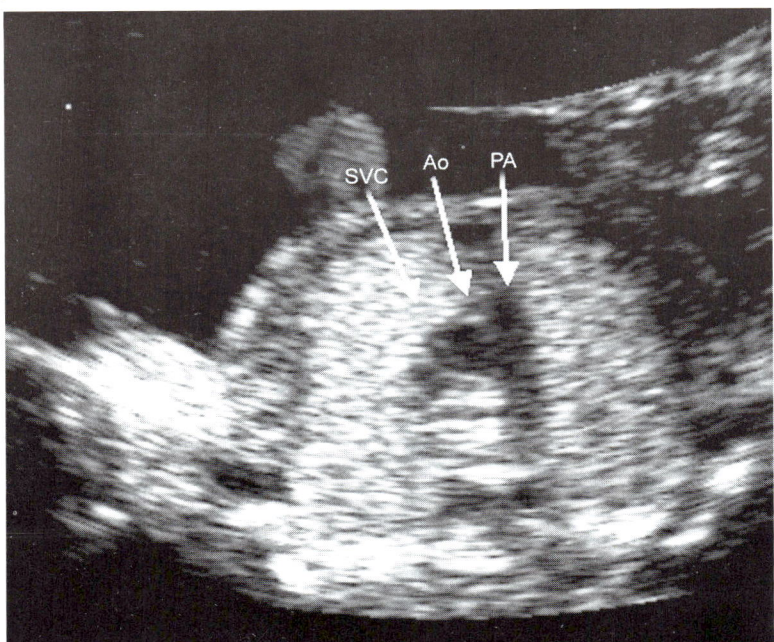

Fig. 13.210: Early fetal echocardiography by 2D in a structurally normal heart. The 3-vessel view: cross-sections of the pulmonary artery, ascending aorta and superior vena cava in a transverse view of upper mediastinum. In normal conditions, the structures in the 3-vessel view are in descending order of size from left to the right. PA: pulmonar artery; Ao: aorta; SVC: superior vena cava

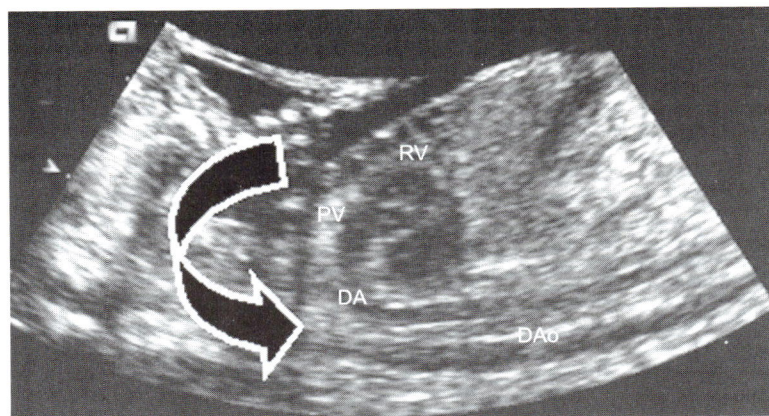

A

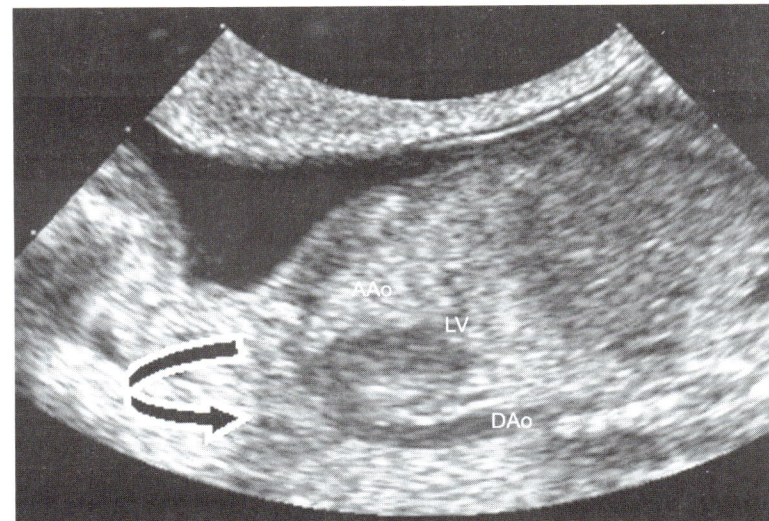

B

Fig. 13.211A and B: Early fetal echocardiography by 2D in a structurally normal heart. The left sagittal view of ductal (A) and aortic arches (B). RV: right ventricle; LV: left ventricle; PA: pulmonar artery; DA: ductus arteriosus; DAo: descending aorta; AAo: ascending aorta

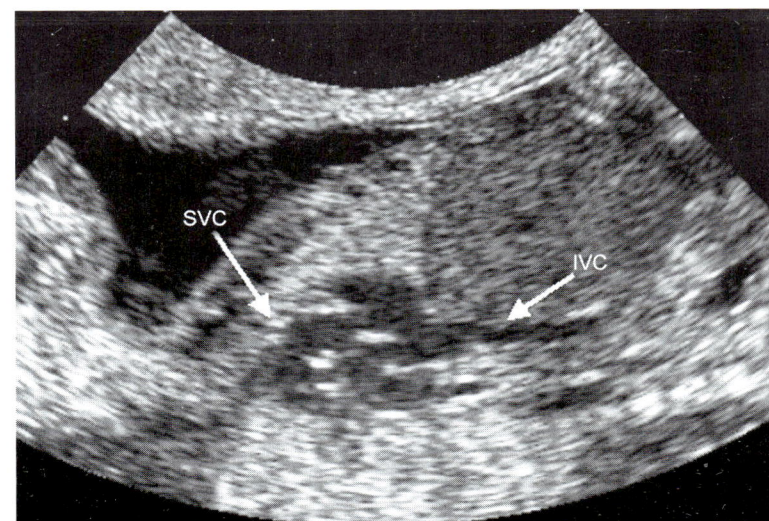

Fig. 13.212: Early fetal echocardiography by 2D in a structurally normal heart. Systemic venous return to the right atrium throws the superior and inferior vena cava. SVC: superior vena cava; IVC: inferior vena cava

The results of these studies support the use of early fetal echocardiography to detect the majority of major CHD in both low-risk and high-risk populations, during the first and early second trimester of pregnancy. The cardiac anomalies detected at this early stage of pregnancy are mainly defects involving the four-chamber view, such as large ventricular septal defects, atrioventricular septal defects and malformations resulting in asymmetry of the ventricles, indicating that defects solely affecting the outflow tracts are difficult to diagnose in the first trimester of pregnancy. Heart defects diagnosed early in pregnancy tend to be more complex than those detected later, with a higher incidence of associated structural malformations, chromosomal

abnormalities and spontaneous abortions. It is widely accepted that the spectrum of CHD diagnosed during prenatal life is different from that observed in postnatal series, with a higher incidence of associated extracardiac lesions and a significant relationship with chromosomal abnormalities in comparison

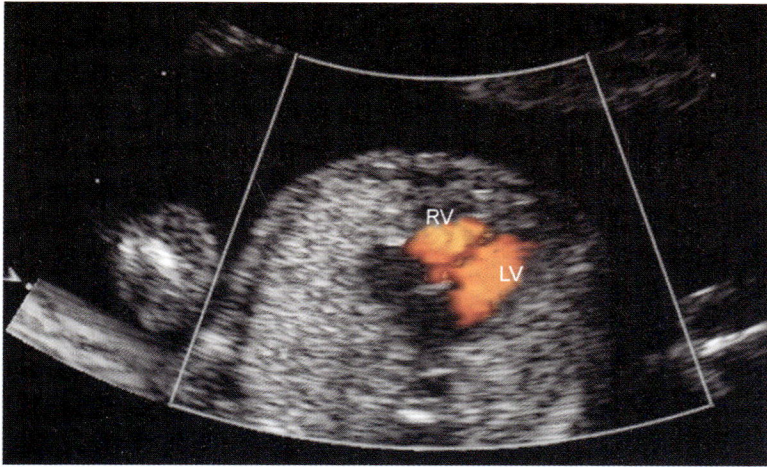

Fig. 13.213: Early fetal echocardiography by 2D and color Doppler in a structurally normal heart. Color Doppler in the 4-chamber view is particulary useful to confirm normal inflow to the ventricles and to detect turbulent flow or jets suggesting valve regurgitation. RV: right ventricle; LV: left ventricle

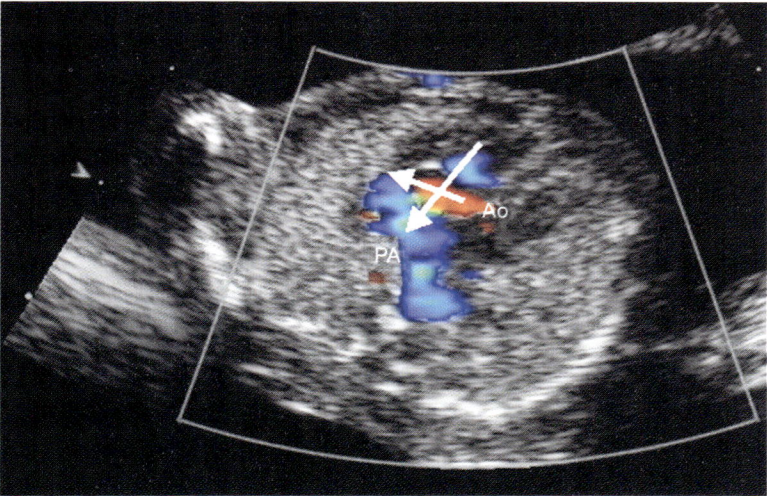

Fig. 13.214: Early fetal echocardiography by 2D and color Doppler in a structurally normal heart. Color Doppler is particulary useful to demonstrate the crossing of the great arteries. Ao: aorta; PA: pulmonar artery

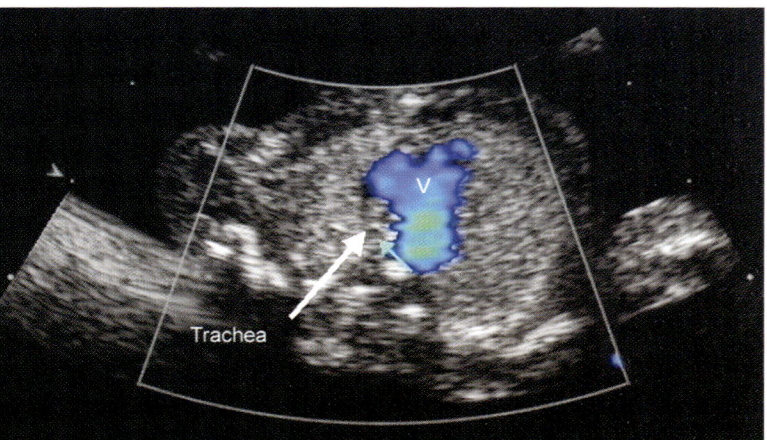

Fig. 13.215: Early fetal echocardiography by 2D and color Doppler in a structurally normal heart. Color Doppler is particulary useful to demonstrate the normal V confluence of the ductal and aortic arches (V sign). Note that normally the trachea is located behind the aortic arch

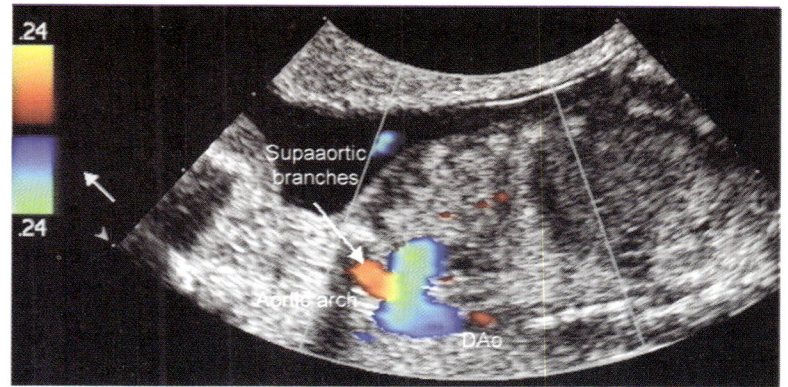

Fig. 13.216: Early fetal echocardiography by 2D and color Doppler in a structurally normal heart. Color Doppler is particulary useful to demonstrate the aortic arch. DAo: descending aorta

with postnatal life.[114-116, 128] Furthermore, when the cardiac defects are detected during the early pregnancy, they use to be even more complex, probably corresponding to the most severe spectrum of the disease[132, 136, 137] and use to cause more severe

hemodynamic compromise in the developing fetus. A common finding is the presence of an hygroma or hydrops associated with CHD, whereas this is not so when the diagnosis is done later in pregnancy.[112, 116, 132] As a result, many of these fetuses are not going to survive long into the second trimester, but this does not argue against early diagnosis. Indeed, when the intrauterine demise of the fetus occurs days or weeks before the delivery, the pathological examination is certainly more difficult to perform. All these considerations should be taken into account when counseling the parents complex CHD.

We have previously published our experience in the first multicenter trial in early fetal echocardiography performed in Spain (Figs 13.217 to 13.221).[132] In accordance with other studies, this experience stresses the usefulness of early echocardiography when performed by expert operators on fetus specifically at risk for cardiac defects. Our review of these additional 48 cases contributes to the expanding literature on the ability of TV ultrasonography to detect fetal heart defects in early pregnancy.

ADVANTAGES AND LIMITATIONS

The first benefit of performing early fetal echocardiography would be an early reassurance of normality in order to relieve anxiety and reduce emotional trauma to the parents at high-risk for CHD. Early prenatal diagnosis of CHD will allow us to optimize the genetic counseling to the parents by permitting further testing such as fetal karyotyping and in those cases with severe defects it may provide the parents with the option of an earlier and safer termination of pregnancy.[124, 125, 128] In selected cases, there is the possibility of pharmacologic therapy. Furthermore, the correct timing and place for delivery may be planned and arranged well in advance.

However, there are certain disadvantages of the early scanning which reduce its diagnostic accuracy compared with the conventional examination at 20th to 22nd weeks of

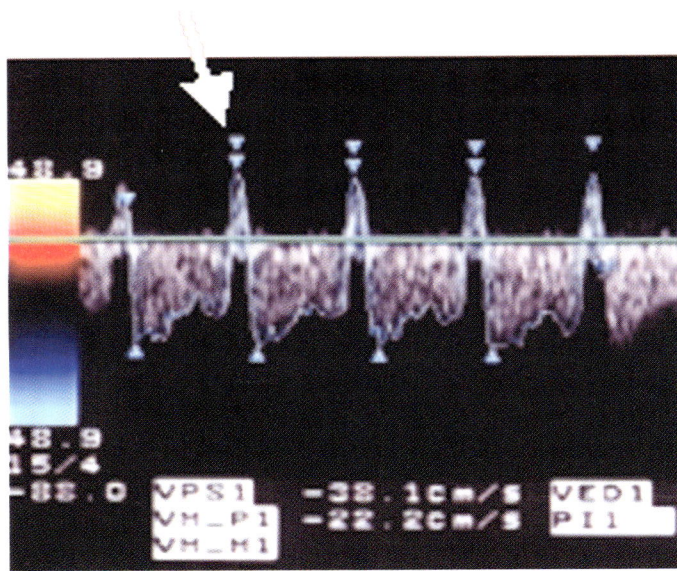

A

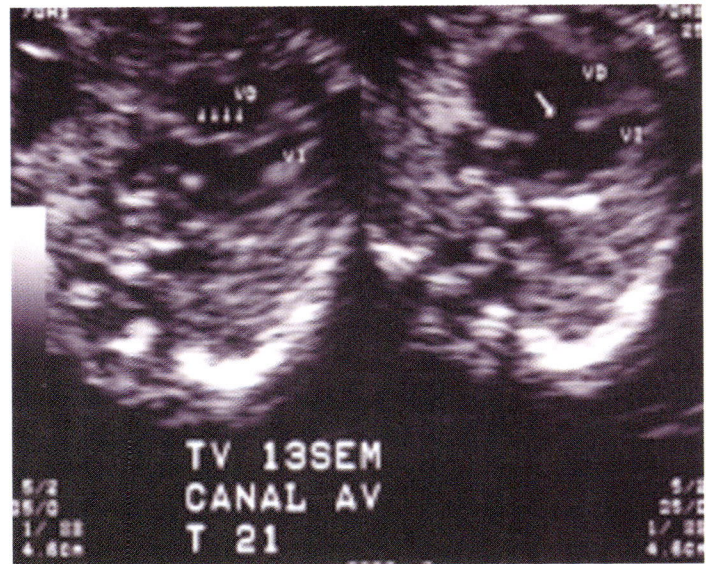

B

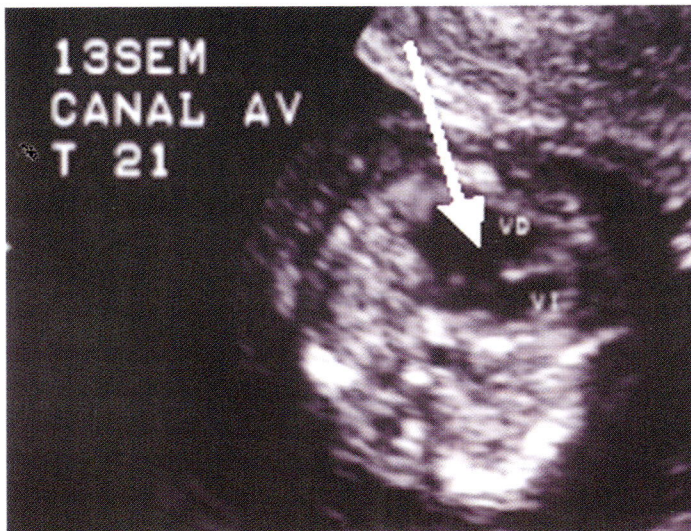

C

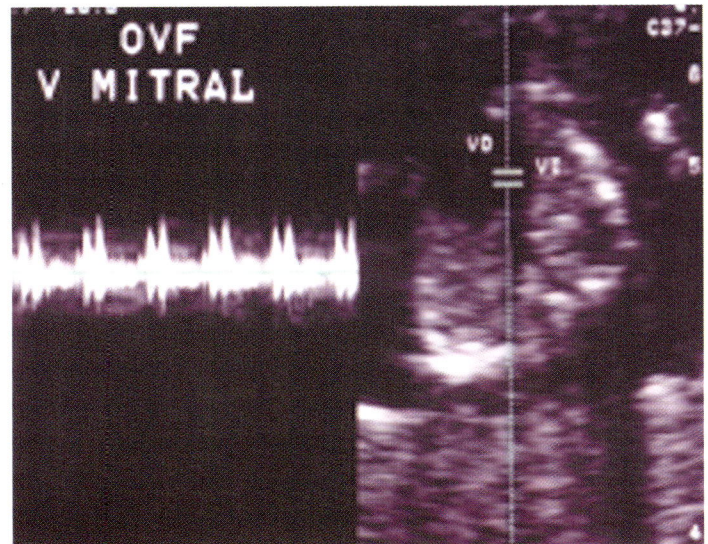

D

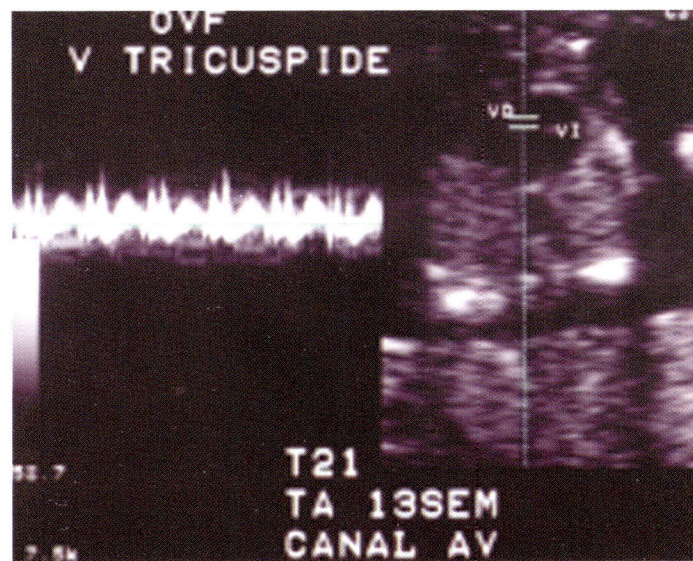

E

Figs 13.217A to E: Atrioventricular septal defect detected at 13th week of gestation in a fetus affected by cystic hygroma and trisomy 21. Note the abnormal reveresed A wave in the ductus venosus (A). Note the ventricular septal defect (B and C). D and E illustrate the mitral and tricuspid diastolic flow, respectively

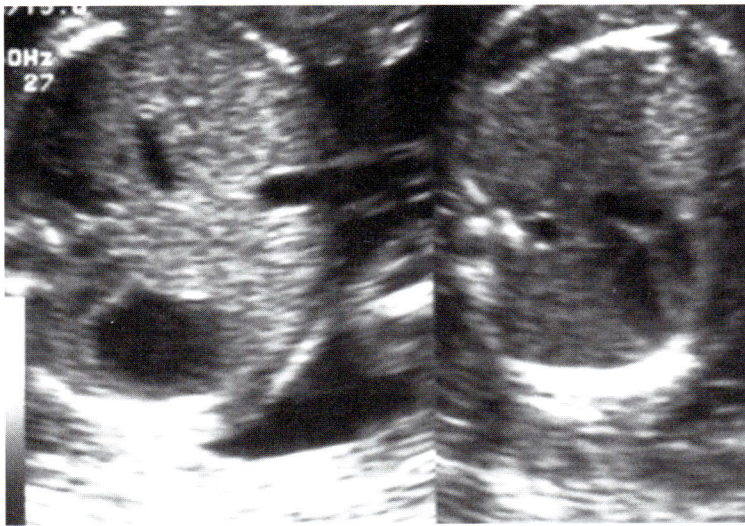

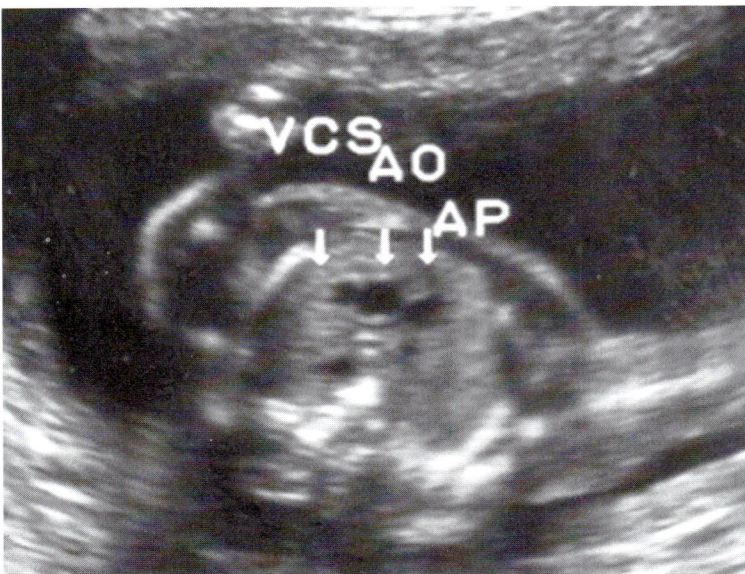

Figs 13.218A and B: Tetralogy of Fallot detected at 16th week of gestation in a fetus affected by cystic hygroma and normal karyotype. Note the left cardiac deviation (A) and the dominance of the aorta compared with the small pulmonary artery at the 3 vessel view in the upper mediastinum (B).

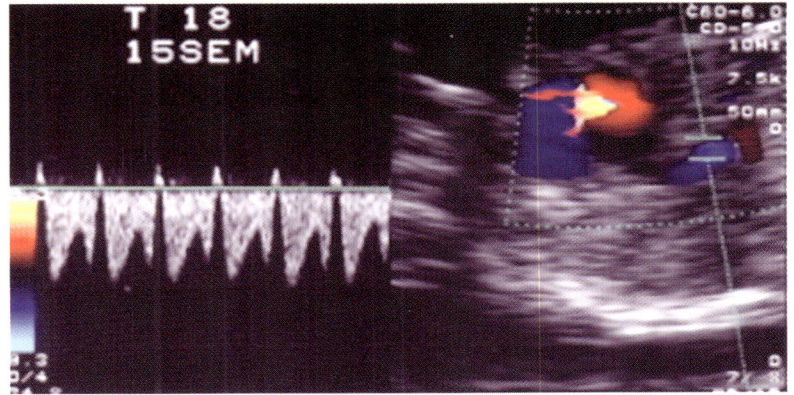

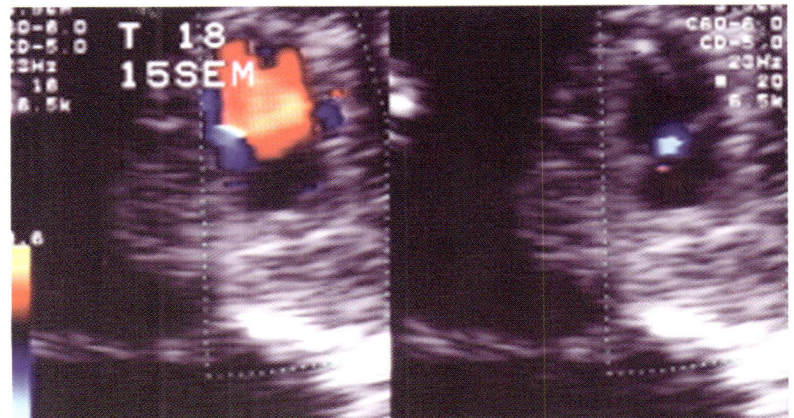

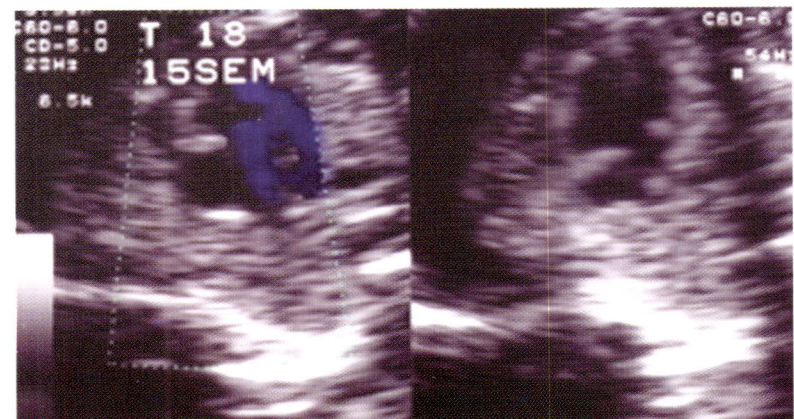

Figs 13.219A to C: Atrioventricular septal defect with unbalanced right ventricle dominance and double outlet right ventricle at 15th week of gestation. Note the abnormal reveresed A wave in the ductus venosus (A), the color Doppler flow through the atrioventricular septal defect with AV regurgitation (B) and the double outlet right ventricle with unbalanced right ventricle dominance (C)

gestation.[112, 116, 124, 125, 128] The transvaginal technique requires a substantial amount of operator experience, yet it cannot be learned from the second trimester examination as the early transabdominal scan. Unfavorable fetal position or limited angles of insonation due to the less mobile capacity of the transvaginal probe may not be overcome. Also, spatial orientation can be challenging by the transvaginal scan. In such cases, we recommend a transabdominal scan that will help us quickly assess the situs and obtain a good spatial orientation. The small size of the fetal heart is an important limiting factor to obtain an optimal sonographic visualization, and also to obtain a successful pathological examination, particularly before the 13th week of gestation. At 13th to 14th weeks of gestation the transverse diameter of the heart at the four-chamber view ranges between 5 and 8 mm, and the great artery diameter at the level of the semilunar valves ranges between

0.8 and 1.8 mm.[116] Moreover, this exploration is more time-consuming and requires a high level of training of the examiner. Finally, the biggest disadvantage of first-trimester echocardiography is the later manifestation of structural and functional changes in some CHDs. Some cardiac lesions are progressive in nature, such as mild pulmonary and aortic stenosis or coarctation and even hypoplastic left heart syndrome. Some obstructive lesions, as a result of a reduced blood flow, may increase the severity of the lesions, resulting in a restricted growth in chambers or arteries. This may be the biggest disadvantage of

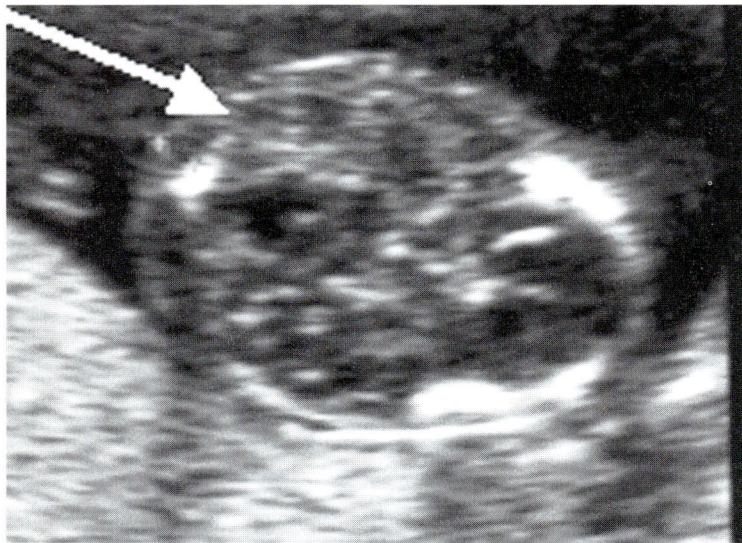

A

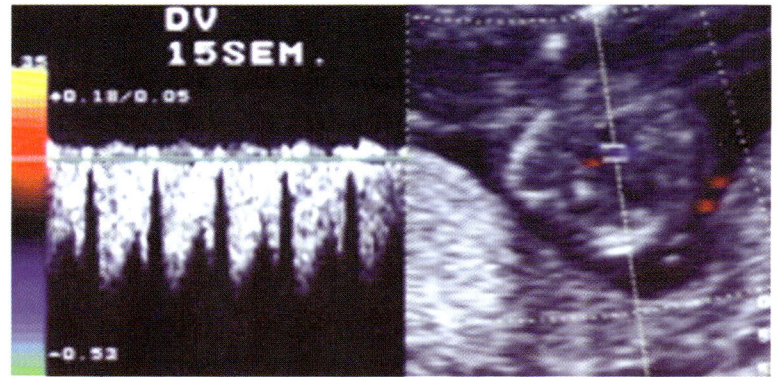

B

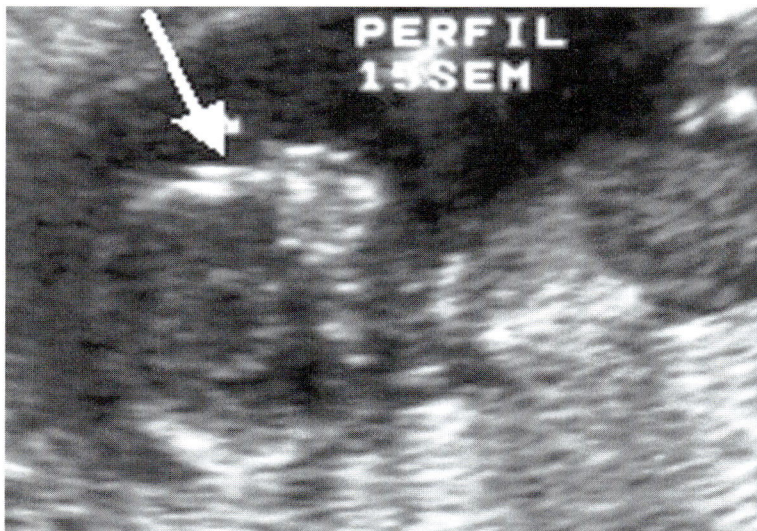

C

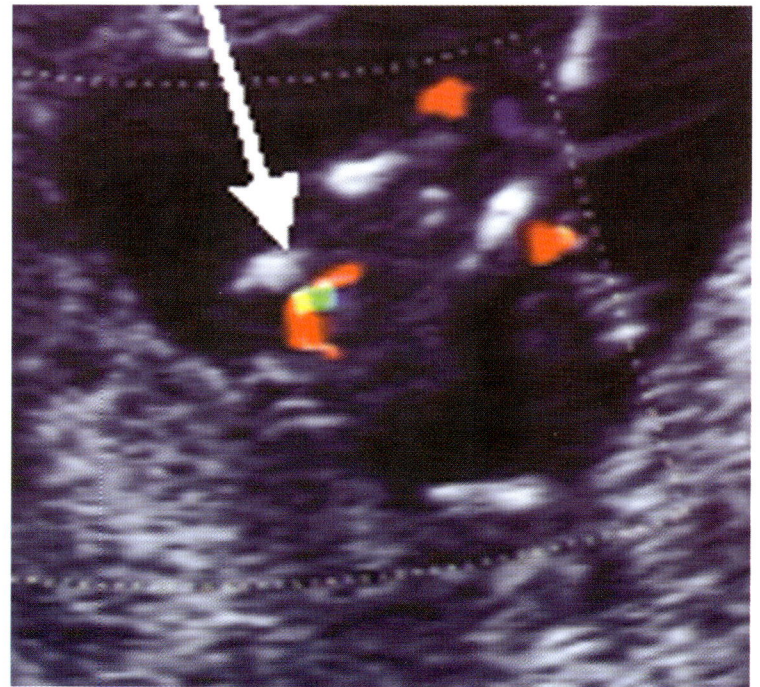

D

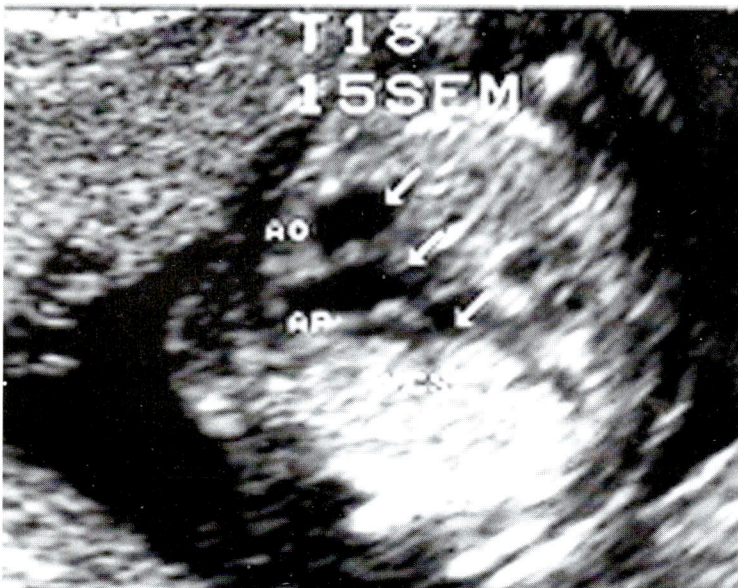

E

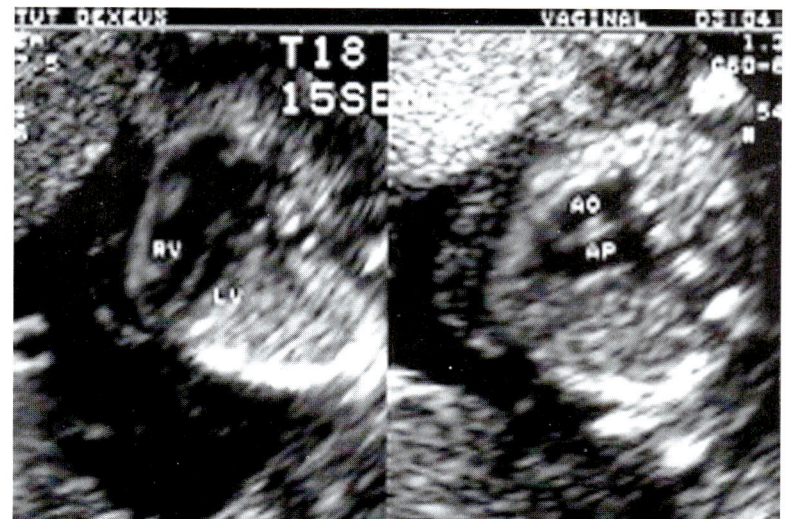

F

Figs 13.220A to F: Hypoplastic left heart and double outlet right ventricle at 15th week of gestation in a trisomy 18. Note the identification of multiples markers of chromosomal abnormality, increased nuchal translucency (A), abnormal ductus venosus flow (B), absent nasal bone (C), single umbilical artery (D). Figure E demonstrates an anterior aorta in the three vessels view. Figure F shows an unbalanced right ventricle dominance with double outlet right ventricle

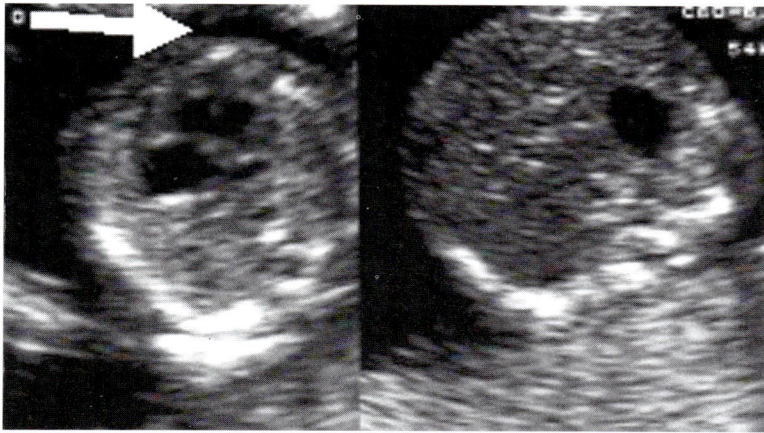

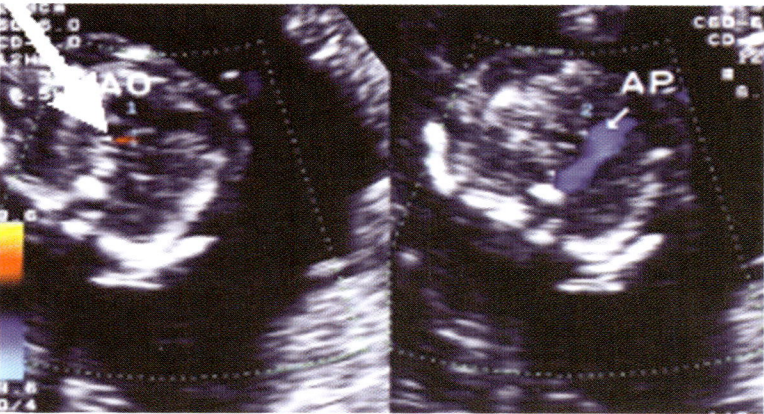

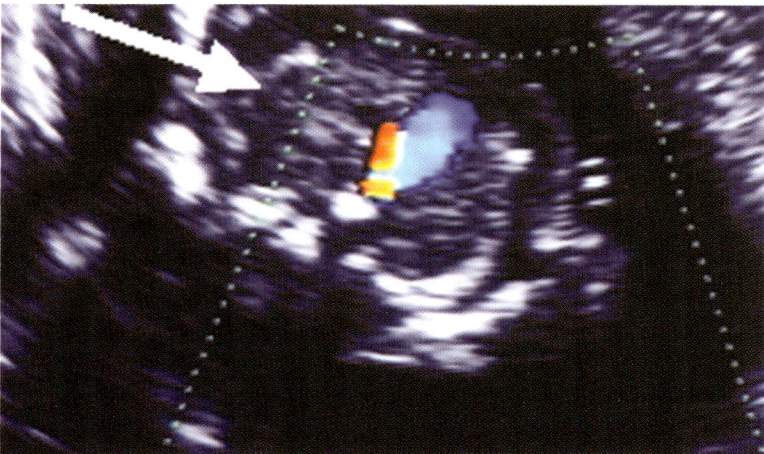

Figs 13.221A to C: Hypoplastic left heart and aortic stenosis at 17th week of gestation in a Turner syndrome. Note the left cardiac axis deviation (A), the severe reduction of the aortic outflow tract compared to the main pulmonary artery (B) and the opposite color flow in the V sign at the upper mediastinum level (C)

performing the early scan. Progression usually is towards a more severe form of lesion that may be sometimes only discernible in the second or even in the third trimester, although in some rare cases a regression to a less severe form may be observed. In this sense, the false-negative cases published in literature are particularly instructive demonstrating these limitations. Another disadvantage of early fetal echocardiography is the possible detection of defects that could resolve spontaneously in later pregnancy, such as muscular venticular septal defects, resulting in unnecessary anxiety in the parents.

Therefore, a normal early examination does not preclude a subsequent abnormal heart development at the second trimester ultrasound, or even in the third trimester or the postnatal period. After a normal early fetal echocardiography, a conventional transabdominal echocardiography at 20th to 22nd weeks of gestation is strongly recommended.

PATHOLOGICAL CONFIRMATION

Pathological confirmation in the case of an early termination of pregnancy or perinatal death is particularly important in those areas where ultrasound diagnosis is most challenging. Only a complete diagnosis will make an individual genetic counseling possible and will validate the accuracy of early fetal echocardiography as a diagnostic technique. Therefore, we advocate that a precise pathological report have to be compulsory for an adequate assessment of the reliability of early fetal echocardiography. This is still a major drawback in most of the studies.[112, 116, 132, 137]

Termination of pregnancy is an option only before 22nd week of gestation in our country. Whenever a termination takes place, it is of vital importance to obtain permission for autopsy in order to confirm the diagnosis and to search for any other associated malformations. Ideally this should be performed by a pathologist who is familiar with the small size of the specimen and with special examination techniques such as dissection microscopy.[116, 132, 133] Current methods of terminating early pregnancies others than using prostaglandins are less recommended because these do not usually allow the retrieval of suitable specimens for appropriate examination to correlate ultrasound and pathological findings. This method allows a more gentle extraction of the embryo or fetus so that a pathological examination for verification of the prenatally diagnosed malformation can be performed. A pathological investigation after TOP following the diagnosis of a CHD should be always recommended, preferably in referral laboratories, being of paramount importance to validate early echocardiography. In particular semilunar valve and aortic arch defects are usually underdiagnosed. We are aware of some cases in which Doppler findings, such turbulent flow and very high velocities, are more reliable to diagnose valve stenosis than pathological examination, even during the second trimester. Indeed, this is a problem and a major challenge not only for ultrasonographers but also for pathologists.

INDICATIONS OF EARLY FETAL ECHOCARDIOGRAPHY

Since most CHDs are detected in low-risk pregnancies, and knowing the high prevalence of heart defects in a nonselected population (incidence of CHD in low risk population 1/238,[131]

Table 13.6: Results of early fetal echocardiograpy to diagnose cardiac defects in high-rish population (only series with at least 10 cardiac defects diagnosed)

Author, year	Route	GA	Success	Risk	N	Cases	11-16 wk	20-22 wk
Gembruch, 93[125]	TV	11-16	90.3 percent	High	114	13	92 percent	100 percent
Zosmer, 99[135]	TA	13-17		High	323	27	89 percent	96.3 percent
Simpson, 00[136]	TA	12-15	98.7 percent	High	229	17	76 percent	94 percent
Huggon, 02[137]	TA	10-14	86.8 percent	High	478	68	94 percent	
Haak, 02[133]	TV	10-13	95.5 percent	High	45	13	54 percent	
Bronshtein, 02[131]	TV	11-17	> 99 percent	High	6175	46	>90 percent	
Comas, 02[132]	TV	12-17	94.6 percent	High	337	48	79 percent	96 percent
Lopes, 03[150]	TV	12-16	94.9 percent	High	275	37	89 percent	

Route: Main approach. TV: transvaginal, TA: transabdominal
GA: Range of gestational age at scan, in weeks
Success: Visualization success rate for the complete early fetal echocardiograpy
N: Total number of pregnancies scanned
Cases: Total number of cardiac defects (pre- and postnatally)
11-16 wk: Percentage of the cardiac defects identified at early echocardiograpy
20-22 wk: Percentage of the cardiac defects identified at mid-trimester echccardiograpy

Table 13.7: Detection rate of cardiac defects at early ultrasound to screen for congenital malformations in low-risk population

Author, year	GA	Success	Risk	Normal	Cases	11-16 wk	20-22 wk
Achiron, 94[129]	13-15	98 percent	Low	660	6	50 percent	50 percent
Hernadi, 97[145]	12		Low	3991	3	33 percent	100 percent
D'Ottavio, 97[146]	13-15		Low	3490	8	25 percent	80 percent
Yagel, 97[128]	13-16	99 percent	Low	6924	66	64 percent	81 percent
Economides, 98[147]	12-13		Low	1632	3	0 percent	33 percent
Whitlow, 99[148]	11-14		Low	6443	10	40 percent	60 percent
Guariglia, 00[149]	10-16		Low	3592	11	18 percent	56 percent
Rustico, 00[130]	13-15	<50 percent	Low	4785	41	10 percent	32 percent
Bronshtein, 02[131]	11-17	99 percent	Low	30148	127	97 percent	99 percent

GA: Range of gestational age at scan, in weeks
Success: Visualization succes rate for the extended cardiac examination (4 chambers + outflow tracts)
Normal: Total number of pregnancies screened
Cases: Total number of cardiac defects (pre- and postnatally)
11-16 wk: Percentage of the cardiac defects identified at early scan
20-22 wk: Percentage of the cardiac defects identified at mid-trimester scan

some authors suggest that an early detailed cardiac examination should be performed in all pregnant women.[128, 131] Indeed, very few cardiac defects have been identified in the pregnancies in which a family history was the main indication for the early fetal echocardiography, which is consistent with the recurrence rate of 2 to 3 percent for siblings. The main value of the early scan in such family-risk cases lies in the reassurance that it gives to the parents. As we have previously stated, in most of the studies the early echocardiography is somewhat less reliable and may result in a higher false-negative and false-positive results in comparison with the 20th to 22nd weeks transabdominal echocardiography. Besides, early echocardiography is most time-consuming and requires a high level of expertise of the examiner. Therefore, it is difficult to offer this scan as a screening test to the general population. In this context, the identification of a high-risk collective is of paramount importance.

Currently, the importance of the aforementioned limitations of early fetal cardiac examination justifies restriction of its use to fetuses at high risk of having cardiac anomalies.[116, 121, 125, 129, 132,133,137] The indications proposed for early fetal echocardiography are as follows:

• Increased nuchal translucency (>95th or 99th centile) is the main indication of referral in all recently reported studies
• Abnormal ductus venosus blood flow, regardless the measurement of the nuchal translucency
• Fetuses affected by other structural malformations: hygroma, hydrops, omphalocele, situs inversus, arrhythmia
• Suspected cardiac anomalies at screening ultrasound
• Pregestational diabetes of the mother
• High-risk family, with a previously affected child, a first-degree relative affected by a congenital heart disease or a genetic disease in which CHD are common
• Women at high risk of chromosomal abnormality declining invasive test for karyotyping
• Pregnancies affected by a chromosomal abnormality.

Currently, as long as the sensitivity, specificity and predictive value of early echocardiography is still unclear, this examination should be generally reserved for patients at high-risk for CHD.

Table 13.8: Fetal heart anomalies diagnosed at early echocardiography
(true-positive cases at early fetal echocardiography)

TRUE +	A	B	C	D	E	F	G	H	I	J	K	L	M	N	O	P	Q	R	OVERALL
Gembruch, 93[125]				6		1	1				2		2						12
Zosmer, 99[135]			3	3	2	1	4	2	3	1			4				1		24
Rustico, 00[130]			2			1	1	1											5
Simpson, 00[136]			3	2				3	2				2	1					13
Huggon, 02[137]			5	29		12	9	1			1			1	1	1			60
Bronshtein,02[131]	4	1	4	13	2	9	25		31*	22	5		18		17	3	2	13	169
Comas, 02[132]			4	8		10	4	1	3		2	2	1			3			38
Achiron, 94[129]				2					2		1				1	1	1		8
Hernadi, 97[145]						1													1
D'Ottavio, 97[146]							2										2		4
Whitlow, 99[148]					1		1									1			3
Rustico, 00[130]	1						2		1										4
Lopes, 03[150]			2	6		11	5	1	1	1	1	3	2						33
OVERALL	4	2	21	71	5	46	54	9	43	24	12	5	29	2	19	9	6	13	374

A Abnormal veno-atrial connections
B Atrial septal defects
C Tricuspid atresia or dysplasia
D Atrioventricular septal defect
E Single ventricle
F Ventricular septal defects
G Aortic atresia, aortic stenosis, hypoplastic left heart
H Pulmonary atresia or stenosis
I Tetralogy of Fallot
J Transposition of great arteries
K Truncus
L Double outlet right ventricle
M Aortic arch anomalies
N Isomerism
O Myocardiopathy
P Ectopia cordis
Q Complex cardiac defect, others
R Vascular ring
* This series include cases with tetralogy of Fallot and double outlet right ventricle

Table 13.9: Fetal heart anomalies not detected at early echocardiography
(false-negative cases at early fetal echocardiography)

FALSE	A	B	C	D	E	F	G	H	I	J	OVERALL
Gembruch, 93[125]					1						1
Hernadi, 97[145]	1			1							2
D'Ottavio 97[146]	1				3	2			1		7
Economides, 98[147]	1					1	1				3
Whitlow, 99[148]	2	1				2	1	1			7
Zosmer, 99[135]					1	1			1		3
Rustico, 00[130]	1				4	1	2		1		9
Simpson, 00[136]	3									1	4
Comas, 02[132]	4	1			3	1	1				10
Huggon, 02[137]	2		2			1			2		7
Bronshtein, 02[131]					1	1		1	1		4
Lopes, 03[150]	3								1		4
OVERALL	18	2	2	1	13	10	5	3	6	1	61

A Ventricular septal defects
B Atrial septal defects
C Abnormal veno-atrial connections
D Tricuspid atresia or dysplasia
E Atrioventricular septal defect
F Aortic atresia, aortic stenosis, hypoplastic left heart
G Tetralogy of Fallot
H Transposition of great arteries
I Aortic arch anomalies
J Myocardiopathy

However, only the accumulation of results from carefully collaborative studies as the present series will clear define the role of early transvaginal echocardiography.

CONCLUSIONS

Fetal echocardiography performed by expert operators is reliable for an early reassurement of normal cardiac anatomy.

1. Transvaginal sonography enables *good visualization of fetal heart earlier in gestation*. The four-chambers view and the extended examination to the great vessels can be imaged in almost 100 percent at 13th and 14th weeks of gestation. Less than 5 percent of patients will need a repeated scan because of inadequate visualization.

2. The *combination of transvaginal and transabdominal routes* and the application of color Doppler enhances visualization.

3. Most CHDs are detected in *low-risk population*. As we cannot perform a targetted fetal echocardiography as a screening test, we need to improve the identification of high-risk group pregnancies. Increased nuchal translucency at 10th to 14th weeks of scan and, may be, ductus venosus blood flow assesment seem to be the newest and most promising risk factors for fetal CHD, and may be particularly useful during the first trimester.

4. Currently, early fetal echocardiography *should be offered to high-risk pregnancies*. Some authors advocate routine early extended cardiac examination in low-risk pregnancies. At present, as long as the sensitivity, specificity and predictive value of early echocardiography is still unclear, this examination should be generally reserved for patients at high-risk for CHD.

5. Whenever a normal heart is diagnosed in the early scan, it has to be supplemented with the *conventional transabdominal examination at 20th to 22nd weeks of gestation*.

Fetal echocardiography performed by expert operators is reliable to diagnose most major structural heart defects in the first and early second trimesters of pregnancy.

1. Cardiac defects diagnosed *early in pregnancy tend to be more complex* than those detected later on and use to cause more severe hemodynamic compromise in the developing fetus.

2. Many CHDs can be detected *at the beginning of the second trimester*.

3. The *incidence of associated structural malformations, chromosomal abnormalities and spontaneous abortions* is significantly *high*.

4. A *complete work-up* including pathological and karyotype evaluation should be warranted in order to provide parents with a proper genetic counseling, which is extremely difficult to obtain if spontaneous loss of the pregnancy occurs.

5. The *small size of specimens* at this time of gestation renders pathological examination difficult and requires high expertise and careful inspection, irrespective of the technique used for termination.

6. Clinical *follow-up in the neonate and postmortem examination* if termination of pregnancy is undertaken are essential to assess the actual role of early fetal ecocardiography.

REFERENCES

Ultrasonographic Prenatal Diagnosis of Malformations

1. Levi S, Hyjazi Y, Schaaps JP, et al. Sensitivity and specificity of routine antenatal screening for congenital anomalies by ultrasound. The Belgian Multicentric study. Ultrasound Obstet Gynecol 1991;1:102-10

Normal Anatomy and Malformations of the Fetal Central Nervous System

2. The nervous system. In Moore KL, Persaud TVN, Shiota K (Eds): Color Atlas of Clinical Embryology. Philadelphia, USA: WB Saunders 1994;209-20.
3. Pooh RK, Maeda K, Pooh KH, Kurjak A. Sonographic assessment of the fetal brain morphology. Prenat Neonat Med 1999;4:18-38.
4. Jeanty P, Dramaix-Wilmet M, Delbeke D, et al.Ultrasonic evaluation of fetal ventricular growth. Neuroradiology 1981;21:127.
5. Johnson MK, Dunne MG, Mack LA, et al. Evaluation of fetal intracranial anatomy by static and realtime ultrasound. J Clin Ultrasound 1980;8:311.
6. Pretorius DH, Drose JA, Marco-Johnson ML. Fetal lateral ventricular ratio determination during the second trimester. J Clin Ultrasound 1986;5:121.
7. Smith PA, Johansson D, Tzannatos C, et al. Prenatal measurement of the fetal cerebellum and cisterna cerebellomedullaris by ultrasound. Prenat Diag 1986;6:133.
8. Pilu G, DePalma L, Romero R, et al. The fetal subarachnoid cisterns: an ultrasound study with report of a case of congenital communicating hydrocephalus. J Ultrasound Med 1986;5:365.
9. Chervenak FA, Isaacson G, Lorber J. Anomalies of the fetal head, neck and spine: ultrasound diagnosis and management. Philadelphia: W.B. Saunders, 1988;pp. 17-36.
10. Campbell S, Johnstone FD, Holt EM, May P. Anencephaly: early ultrasonic diagnosis and active management. Lancet 1972;2:1226-7.
11. Murken JD, Stengel-Rutkowski S, Schwinger E. Prenatal diagnosis of genetic disorders. Stuttgart: Ferdinand Enke, 1979;.pp. 94-192.
12. ChervenakFA, Farley MA, Walter L, et al. When is termination of pregnancy during the third trimester morally justifiable? N Engl J Med 1984;310:501.
13. Chervenak FA, Berkowitz RL, Romero R, et al. The diagnosis of fetal hydrocephalus. Am J Obstet Gynecol 1983;147:703-16.
14. Chervenak FA, Duncan C, Ment LR, et al. The outcome of fetal ventriculomegaly. Lancet 1984;2:179-82.
15. Cardoza JD, Filly RA, Podarsky AE. The dangling choroid plexus: a sonographic observation of value in excluding ventriculomegaly. Am J Radiol 1988;151:767-70.
16. Benacerraf BR, Birnholz JC. The diagnosis of fetal hydrocephalus prior to 22 weeks. J Clin Ultrasound 1987;15:531-6.
17. Benacerraf BR. Fetal hydrocephalus: diagnosis and significance. Radiology 1988;169:858-9.
18. Chervenak FA, Jeanty P, Cantraine F, et al. The diagnosis of fetal microcephaly. Am J Obstet Gynecol 1984;149:512.
19. Chervenak FA, Rosenburg JC, Brightman R, et al. A prospective study of the accuracy of ultrasound in predicting fetal microcephaly. Obstet Gynecol 1984;69:908.
20. Chervenak FA, Isaacson G, Mahoney MJ, et al. The obstetric significance of haloprosencephaly. Obstet Gynecol 1984;63:115.
21. Chervenak FA, Isaacson G, Hobbins JC, et al. The diagnosis and management of fetal holoprosencephaly. Obstet Gynecol 1985;66:322.
22. Chervenak FA, Isaacson G, Mahoney MJ, et al. Diagnosis and management of fetal cephalocele. Obstet Gynecol 1984;64:86.
23. Chervenak FA, Isaacson G, Rosenberg JC, Kardon NB. Antenatal diagnosis of frontal cephalocele in a fetus with ateleosteogenesis. J Ultrasound Med 1986;5:111.
24. Hobbins JC, Grannum PAT, Berkowitz RL, et al. Ultrasound in the diagnosis of congenital anomalies. Am J Obstet Gynecol 1979;134:331.
25. Pearce JM, Little D, Campbell S. The diagnosis of abnormalities of the fetal central nervous system. In Saunders RC, James AE (Eds): The Principles and Practice of Ultrasonography in Obstetrics and Gynecology (3rd edn.). Norwalk: Appleton-Century-Crofts, 1985;pp. 246-8.

26. Nicolaides KM, Campbell S, Gabbe SG, Guidetti R. Ultrasound screening for spina bifida: cranial and cerebellar signs. Lancet 1986;2:72.

27. Crudleigh P, Pearce JM, Campbell S. The prenatal diagnosis of transient cysts of the fetal choroid plexus. Prenat Diagn 1984;4:135.

28. Nicolaides KM, Rodeck CG, Gosden CM. Rapid karyotyping in non-lethal malformations. Lancet 1986;1:283.

29. Comstock CH, Culp D, Gonzalez J, et al. Agenesis of the corpus callosum in the fetus: its evolution and significance. J Ultrasound Med 1985;4:613.

30. Comstock CH. Agenesis of the corpus callosum in the fetus: diagnosis and significance. Female Patient 1991.

31. Chervenak FA, Isaacson G, Lorber J. Anomalies of the fetal head, neck and spine. Ultrasound diagnosis and management, Philadelphia: W.B. Saunders, 1988;pp 152-210

32. Pooh RK, Pooh KH. The assessment of fetal brain morphology and circulation by transvaginal 3D sonography and power Doppler. J Perinat Med 2002;30:48-56.

33. Pooh RK, Pooh KH. Fetal neuroimaging with new technology. Ultrasound Review Obstet Gynecology 2002;2:178-81.

Face and Neck

34. Bronshtein M, Zimmer EZ, Blumenfeld Z. Early sonographic detection of fetal anomalies. In Kurjak A, (Ed.):Textbook of Perinatal Medicine. Parthenon Publishing: London 1998; pp 263-80.

35. Bronshtein M, Blumenfeld I, Kohon J, et al. Detection of cleft lip and palate by early second trimester transvaginal sonography. Obstet Gynecol 1994;84:73-6.

36. Jeanty P, Cautraine F, Cousaert E, et al. The binocular distance: a new way to estimate fetal age. J Ultrasound Med 1984;3:241-3.

37. Romero R, Pilu G, Jeanty P, Ghidini A, Hobbins JC. Ocular abnormalities. In Romero R, Pilu G, Jeanty P, Ghidini A, Hobbins JC, (Eds.): Prenatal Diagnosis of Congenital Anomalies. Norwalk CT: Appleton Lange, 1988.

38. Zimmer EZ, Bronshtein M, Ophir E, et al. Sonographic diagnosis of fetal congenital cataracts. Prenat Diag 1993;13 :503-4.

39. Gaary EA, Rawnsley E, Martin-Pedilla M, et al. In utero detection of fetal cataracts. J Ultrasound Med 1993;12:234-6.

Thorax

40. Buln DI, Soal HM, Allen JF, et al. Cystic hygroma and congenital diaphragmatic hernia: early prenatal sonographic evaluation of Fryn's syndrome. Prenat Diagn 1992;12:867-75.

41. Adzick NS, Harrison MR, Glick PI, et al. Diaphragmatic hernia in the fetus prenatal diagnosis and outcome in 94 cases. J Pediatr Surg 1985;20:357-61.

42. Leberge JM, Flageole H, Pugash D, et al. Outcome of the prenatally diagnosed congenital cystic adenomatoid lung malformation. Fetal Diag Ther 2001;16(3):178-96.

43. Papp Z. Ultrasound examination of the fetal thorax. In Kurjak A, Chervenak FA, (Eds): Textbook of Ultrasound in Obstetrics and Gynecology. Jaypee Brothers: New Delhi, 2004; pp 272-9.

44. Stocker JT, Madewell JE, Drake RM. Congenital cystic adenomatoid malformation of the lung. Classification and morphological spectrum. Hum Path 1977;8:155.

45. Longarek MT, Laberge JM, Dauseran J, et al. Primary fetal hydrothorax : natural history and management. J Pediatr Surg 1989;24:573-6.

Anterior Abdominal Wall Defects

46. Timor-Tritsch IE, Warren WB, Peisner DB, et al. First trimester midgut herniation: a high frequency transvaginal sonographic study. Am J Obstet Gynecol 1989;161:831-3.

47. Bowerman RA. Sonographic of fetal midgut herniation: normal size criteria and correlation with CRL. J Ultrasound Med 1993;5:251-4.

48. Guzman ER. Early prenatal diagnosis of gastroschisis with transvaginal ultrasounography. Am J Obstet Gynecol 1990;162:1253-4.

49. Kushir O, Izguierlo I, Vigil D, et al. Early transvaginal sonographic diagnosis of gastroschisis. J Clin Ultrasound 1990;18:194-7.

50. D'Addario V, Di Cagno L, Tamburo R. Malformations of the gaastrointestinal system. In Kurjak A, Chervenak FA, (Eds): Textbook of Ultrasound in Obstetrics and Gynecology. Jaypee Brothers: New Delhi, 2004, pp 290-7

51. Ginsberg NE, Cadkin A, Strom C. Prenatal diagnosis of body stalk anomaly in the first trimester of pregnancy. Ultrasound Obstet Gynecol 1997;10:419-21.

52. Takeuchi K, Fujita I, Nakajima K, et al. Body stalk anomaly: prenatal diagnosis. Int J Gynaecol Obstet 1995;51:49-52.

Genitourinary Tract Malformations

53. Livera LN, Brookfield DSK, Egginton JA, Hawnaur JN. Antenatal ultrasonography to detect fetal renal abnormalities: a prospective screening programme. Br Med J 1989;298:1421-3.

54. Sabbagha RE. Renal abnormalities. In Sabbagha RE, (Ed.): Diagnostic Ultrasound Applied to Obstetrics and Gynecology. Philadelphia: JB Lippincott Company,1994;pp:523-38.

55. Mahony BS, Filly RA. The genitourinary system in utero. Clin Diagn Ultrasound 1986;18:1-6.

56. Rosati P, Guariglia L. Transvaginal sonographic assessment of the fetal urinary tract in early pregnancy. Ultrasound Obstet Gynecol 1996:7:95-100.

57. Bronshtein M, Kushnir O, Ben-Rafael Y, et al. Transvaginal sonographic measurements of fetal kidney in the first trimester of pregnancy. J Clin Ultrasound 1990;18:299-301.

58. Chitty LS, Altman DG, Henderson A, Campbell S. Appendix 1: Fetal biometry. In Chervenak FA, Isaacson GC, Campbell S, (Eds): Ultrasound in Obstetrics and Gynecology. Boston, Toronto, London: Little Brown and Co., 1993;1784-5.

59. Kurjak A, Kirikinen F, Latin V. Ultrasonic assessment of fetal kidney function in normal and complicated pregnancies. Am J Obstet Gynecol 1981;141:266-70.

60. Wilkins IA, et al. The nonpredictive value of fetal urine electrolytes: preliminary report of outcomes and correlations with pathologic findings. Am J Obstet Gynecol 1987;157:694-8.

61. Sadler TW. In Sadler TW (Ed.): Langman's Medical Embryology: Urogenital System. Baltimore, Hong Kong, London, Sydney: Williams and Wilkins, 1990;pp260-96

62. Doroshow LW, Abeshouse BS. Congenital unilateral solitary kidney; report of 37 cases and a review of the literature. Urol Surv 1961;11:219–26

63. Carter CO. The genetics of urinary tract malformations. J Genet Hum 1984;32:23-9.

64. Harmon CR. Maternal furosemide may not provoke urine production in the compromised fetus. Am J Obstet Gynecol 1984;150:322-3.

65. Osathanondt V, Potter EL. Pathogenesis of polycystic kidneys. Arch Pathol 1964;77:459-65.

66. Zerres K, Volpel MC, Weiss H. Cystic kidneys. Hum Genet 1984;68:104-35.

67. Potter EL. Normal and Abnormal Development of the Kidney. Chicago: Year Book Medical Publishers, 1972;pp154-81.

68. Simpson JI, Sabbagha RE, Elis S, et al. Failure to detect polycystic kidneys in utero by second trimester ultrasonography. Hum Genet 1982;60:295-9.

69. Reeders ST, Breuning MH, Davies KE, et al. A highly polymorphic DNA marker linked to adult polycystic kidney disease on chromosome 16. Nature (London) 1985;317:542-4.

70. Reeders ST, Zerres K, Gal A. Prenatal diagnosis of autosomal dominant polycystic kidney disease with a DNA probe. Lancet 1986;2:6-8.

71. Greene LF, Feinzaig W, Dahlin DC. Multicystic dysplasia of the kidney: with special reference to the contralateral kidney. J Urol 1971;103:482-7.

72. Gudmundsson S, Neerhof M, Weoner S, et al. Fetal hydronephrosis and renal artery blood velocity. Ultrasound Obstet Gynecol 1991;1:413-8.

73. King LR. Posterior urethra. In Kelalis PP, King LR, Belman AB, (Eds): Clinical Pediatric Urology, (2nd edn). Philadelphia: Saunders, 1985:527-46

74. Hayden SA, Russ PD, Pretorius DH, et al. Posterior urethral obstruction: prenatal sonographic findings and clinical outcome in fourteen cases. J Ultrasound Med 1988;7:371.

75. Egami K, Smith, EDA. A study of the sequelae of posterior urethral valve. J Urol 1982;127:84.

76. Golbus MS, Harrison MR, Filly RA. In utero treatment of urinary tract obstruction. Am J Obstet Gynecol 1982;142:383.

77. Kurjak A, Latin V, Mandruzzato GP, et al. Ultrasound diagnosis and perinatal management of fetal genito-urinary abnormalities. J Perinat Med 1984;12:291.

78. Estes JM, Adzick NS, Harrison MR. Antenatal open surgery for the abnormal fetus. In Sabbagha RE, (Ed): Ultrasound Applied to Obstetrics and Gynecology, (3rd edn). JB Lippincott, 1993;557-69.

79. Penman DG, Lilford RI. The megacystis–microcolon–intestinal hypoperistalsis syndrome: a fatal recessive condition. J Med Genet 1989;26:66.

80. Hanna MK, Jeffs RD, Sturgess J, et al. Ureteral structure and ultrastructure. Part II. Congenital ureteropelvic junction obstruction and primary obstructive megaureter. J Urol 1976;116:725.

81. Antonakopoulos GN, Fuggle WI, Newman I, et al. Idiopathic hydronephrosis. Arch Pathol Lab Med 1985;109:1097.

82. Johnston JH, Evans JP, Glassberg KI, et al. Pelvic hydro-nephrosis in children: a review of 219 personal cases. J Urol 1977;117:97.

83. Drake DP, Stevens PS, Eckstein HB. Hydronephrosis secondary to ureteropelvic obstruction in children: a review of 14 years experience. J Urol 1978;119:649.

84. Ahmed S, Savage JP. Surgery of pelviureteric obstruction in the first year of life. Aust NZ J Surg 1985;55:253.

85. Lebowitz RL, Griscom NT. Neonatal hydronephrosis: 146 cases. Radiol Clin North Am 1977;15:49.

86. Benacerraf BR, Mandell J, Estroff JA, et al. Fetal pyelectasis, a possible association with Down syndrome. Obstet Gynecol 1990;76:58-60.

87. Corteville JE, Dicke JM, Crane JP. Fetal pyelectasis and Down syndrome: is genetic amniocentesis warranted? Obstet Gynecol 1992;79:770-2.

88. Corteville JE, Gray DL, Crane JP. Congenital hydronephrosis: correlation of fetal ultrasonographic findings with infant outcome. Am J Obstet Gynecol 1991;165:384-8.

89. Langer B, Imeoni U, Montoya Y, et al. Antenatal diagnosis of upper urinary tract dilatation by ultrasonography. Fetal Diagn Ther 1996;11:191-8.

90. Benacerraf BR. The second trimester fetus with Down syndrome: detection using sonographic features. Ultrasound Obstet Gynecol 1996;7:147-55.

91. Scott J, Lee R, Hunter E, et al. Ultrasound screening of newborn urinary tract. Lancet 1991;338:1571-3.

92. Hiraoka M, Kasuga K, Hori C, Sudo M. Ultrasonic indicators of ureteric reflux in the newborn. Lancet 1994;343:519-20.

93. Quintero RA, Johnson MP, Aria F, et al. In utero sonographic diagnosis of vesicoureteral reflux by percutaneous vesicoinfusion. Ultrasound Obstet Gynecol 1995;6:386-9.

94. Sherter DM, Culen JBH, Thompson HO, et al. Prenatal sonographic findings associated with a fetal horseshoe kidney. J Ultrasound Med 1990;9:477-9.

95. Jeanty P, Romero R, Kepple D, et al. Prenatal diagnosis in unilateral empty renal fossa. J Ultrasound Med 1990;9:651-4.

96. Abuhamad AZ, Horton CE, Horton H, Evans AT. Renal duplication anomalies in the fetus: clues for prenatal diagnosis. Ultrasound Obstet Gynecol 1996;7:174-7.

97. Jeanty P, Chervenak F, Grannum P, et al. Normal ultrasonic size and characteristics of the fetal adrenal glands. Prenat Diagn 1984;4:21-8.

98. Isaacs H Jr. Perinatal (congenital and neonatal) neoplasms: a report of 110 cases. Pediatr Pathol 1985;3:165-216.

99. Vintzileos AM. Prenatal detection of lethal pulmonary hypoplasia (opinion). Ultrasound Obstet Gynecol 1996;7:163-4.

100. Laudy JAM, Gaillard JLJ, van den Anker JN, et al. Doppler ultrasound imaging: a new technique to detect lung hypoplasia before birth? A case report. Ultrasound Obstet Gynecol 1996;7:189-92.

Skeleton Malformations

101. Bronshtein M, Keret D, Deutsch M, et al. Transvaginal sonographic detection of skeletal anomalies in the first early second trimester. Prenat Diagn 1993;13:597-601.

102. Bronshtein M, Zimmer EZ, Blumenfeld Z. Early sonographic detection of fetal anomalies. In Kurjak A (Ed): Textbook of Perinatal Medicine. Parthenon Publishing: London, 1998, pp 263-80.

103. Papp Z. Atlas of Fetal Diagnosis. Elsevier: Amsterdam, 1992; pp 195-97.

104. Sherer DM, Ghezzi F, Cohen J, Romero R. Fetal skeletal anomalies. In R (Eds): Sonography in Obstetrics and Gynecology, (6th ed). Fleisher A, Manning FV, Jeanty Ph, Romero Appleton and Lange: 1996;

105. Bod M, Creizel A, Lenz W. Incidence at birth of different types of limb reduction abnormalities in Hungary 1975-1977. Hum Genet 1983;65:27.

106. Jeanty P, Romero R, d'Alton M, et al. In utero sonographic detection of hand and foot deformities. J Ultrasound Med 1985;4:595-601.

107. Kurtz AB, Filly RA, Wapner RJ, et al. In utero analysis of heterozygous achondroplasia: variable time of onset as detected by femur length measurements. J Ultrasound Med 1986;5:137.

108. Yang SS, Heidelberger KP, Brough AJ, et al. Lethal short-limbed chondrodysplasia in early infancy. In Rosenberg HS, Boland RP(Eds): Perspectives in Pediatric Pathology. Chicago: Year Book. Medical Publishers, 1976; 3-I.

109. D'Ottavio G, Tamaro LT, Mandruzzato G. Early prenatal ultrasonographic diagnosis of osteogenesis imperfecta. Am J Obstet Gynecol 1993;169:384-5.

110. Bui TH, Lindholm H, Demir N, et al. Prenatal diagnosis of distal arthrogyposis type I by ultrasonography. Prenat Diagn 1992;12:1047-53.

111. Thompson GH, Bilenker RM. Comprehensive management of arthrogyposis multiplex congenita. Clin Orthop 1985;194-6.

Echocardiography in Early Pregnancy

112. Campbell S. Isolated major congenital heart disease (Opinion.). Ultrasound Obstet Gynecol 2001;17:370-9.

113. Mitchell SC, Korones SB, Berendes HW. Congenital heart disease in 56,109 births. Incidence and natural history. Circulation 1971;43:323-32.

114. Allan L, Sharland G, Milburn A, Lockhart S, Groves A, Anderson R, Cook A. Prospective diagnosis of 1006 consecutive cases of congenital heart disease in the fetus. J Am Coll Cardiol 1994;23:1452-8.

115. Allan LD. Fetal cardiology. Curr Op Obstet Gynecol 1996;8:142-7.

116. Gembruch U. Prenatal diagnosis of congenital heart disease. Prenat Diagn 1997; 17:1283-98.

117. Todros T. Prenatal diagnosis and management of fetal cardiovascular malformations. Curr Opin Obstet Gynecol 2000;12:105-9.

118. Levi S, Schaaps JP, De Havay P, et al. End result of routine ultrasound screening for congenital anomalies. The Belgian Multicentric study 1984-92. Ultrasound Obstet. Gynecol 1995;5:366-71.

119. Hyett J, Perdu M, Sharland G, Snijders R, Nicolaides KH. Using nuchal translucency to screen for major cardiac defects at 10-14 weeks of gestation: population based cohort study. Br Med J 1999;318:81-5.

120. Devine PC, Simpson LL. Nuchal translucency and its relationship to congenital heart disease. Semin Perinatol 2000;24:343-51.

121. Matias A, Huggon I, Areias JC, Montenegro N, Nicolaides KH. Cardiac defects in chromosomally normal fetuses with abnormal ductus venosus blood flow at 10-14 weeks. Ultrasound Obstet Gynecol 1999;14:307-10.

122. Bilardo CM, Müller MA, Zikulnig L, Schipper M, Hecher K. Ductus venosus studies in fetuses at high risk for chromosomal or heart abnormalities: relationship with nuchal translucency measurement and fetal outcome. Ultrasound Obstet Gynecol 2001;17:288-94.

123. Johnson P, Sharland G, Maxwell D, Allan L. The role of transvaginal sonography in the early detection of congenital heart disease. Ultrasound Obstet Gynecol 1992;2:248-51.

124. Bronshtein M, Zimmer EZ, Gerlis LM, Lorber A, Drugen A. Early ultrasound diagnosis of congenital heart defects in high-risk and low-risk pregnancies. Obstet Gynecol 1993;82:225-9.

125. Gembruch U, Knopfle G, Bald R, Hansmann M. Early diagnosis of fetal congenital heart disease by transvaginal echocardiography. Ultrasound Obstet Gynecol 1993;3:310-7.

126. Achiron R, Tadmor O. Screening for fetal anomalies during the first trimester of pregnancy: transvaginal versus transabdominal sonography. Ultrasound Obstet Gynecol 1991;1:186-91.

127. D'Amelio R, Giorlandino C, Masala L, et al. Fetal echocardiography using transvaginal and transabdominal probes during the first period of pregnancy: a comparative study. Prenat Diagn 1991;11:69-75.

128. Yagel S, Weissman A, Rotstein Z, Manor M, Hegesh J, Anteby E, Lipitz S, Achiron R. Congenital heart defects: natural course and in utero development. Circulation 1997;96:550-5.

129. Achiron R, Rotstein Z, Lipitz S, Mashiach S, Hegesh J. First trimester diagnosis of congenital heart disease by transvaginal ultrasonography. Obstet Gynecol 1994;84:69-72.

130. Rustico MA, Benettoni A, D' Ottavio G et al. Early screening for fetal cardiac anomalies by transvaginal echocardiography in an unselected population: the role of operator experience. Ultrasound Obstet Gynecol 2000;16:614-9.

131. Bronshtein M, Zimmer Z. The sonographic approach to the detection of fetal cardiac anomalies in early pregnancy. Ultrasound Obstet Gynecol 2002;19:360-5.

132. Comas C, Galindo A, Martínez JM, Carrera JM, Gutiérrez-Larraya F, De la Fuente P, Puerto B, Borrell A. Early prenatal diagnosis of major cardiac anomalies in a high-risk population. Prenat Diagn 2002;22:586-93.

133. Haak MC, Twisk JWR, van Vigt JMG. How successful is fetal echocardiographic examination in the first trimester of pregnancy?. Ultrasound Obstet Gynecol 2002;20:9-13.

134. Carvalho JS, Moscoso G, Ville Y. First trimester transabdominal fetal echocardiography. Lancet 1998;351:1023-7.

135. Zosmer N, Souter VL, Chan CS, Huggon JC, Nicolaides KH. Early diagnosis of major cardiac defects in chromosomally normal fetuses with increased nuchal translucency. Br J Obstet Gynecol 1999;106:829-33.

136. Simpson JM, Jones A, Callaghan N, Sharland GK. Accuracy and limitations of transabdominal fetal echocardiography at 12-15 weeks of gestation in a population at high risk for congenital heart disease. Br J Obstet Gynecol 2000;107:1492-7.

137. Huggon IC, Ghi T, Cook AC, Zosmer N, Allan LD, Nicolaides KH. Fetal cardiac abnormalities identified prior to 14 weeks' gestation. Ultrasound Obstet Gynecol 2002;20:22-9.

138. DeVore GR. First trimester fetal echocardiographic: is the future now?. Ultrasound Obstet Gynecol 2002;20:6-8.

139. Haak MC, van Vugt JM. Echocardiography in early pregnancy: a review of the literature. J Ultrasound Med 2003;22:271-80.

140. DeVore GR. Color Doppler examination of the outflow tracts of the fetal heart: a technique for identification of cardiovascular malformations. Ultrasound Obstet Gynecol 1994;4:463-71.

141. Wladimiroff JW, Seelen JC. Doppler tachometry in early pregnancy. Development of fetal vagal function. Eur J Obstet Gynecol Reprod Biol 1972;2:55-63.

142. Schats R, Jansen CAM, Wladimiroff JW. Embryonic heart activity: appearance and development in early human pregnancy. Br J Obstet Gynaecol 1990;97:989-94.

143. Gembruch U, Knopfle G, Chatterjee M, Bald R, Hansmannn M. First-trimester diagnosis of fetal congenital heart disease by transvaginal two-dimensional and Doppler echocardiography. Obstet Gynecol 1990;75:496-8.

144. Bronshtein M, Siegler E, Yoffe N, Zimmer EZ. Prenatal diagnosis of ventricular septal defect and overriding aorta at 14 weeks' gestation using transvaginal sonography. Prenat Diagn 1990;10:697-705.

145. Hernadi L, Torocsik M. Screening for fetal anomalies in the 12th week of pregnancy by transvaginal sonography in an unselected population. Prenat Diagn 1997;17:753-9.

146. D'Ottavio G, Meir YJ, Rustico MA, Pecile V, Fischer-Tamaro L, Conoscenti G, et al. Screening for fetal anomalies by ultrasound at 14 and 21 weeks. Ultrasound Obstet Gynecol 1997;10:375-80.

147. Economides DL, Braithwaite JM. First trimester ultrasonographic diagnosis of fetal structural abnormalities in a low risk population. Br J Obstet Gynaecol 1998;105:53-7.

148. Whitlow BJ, Chatzipapas IK, Lazanakis ML, Kadir RA, Economides DL. The value of sonography in early pregnancy for the detection of fetal abnormalities in an unselected population. Br J Obstet Gynaecol 1999;106:929-36.

149. Guariglia L, Rosati P. Transvaginal sonographic detection of embryonic-fetal abnormalities in early pregnancy. Obstet Gynecol 2000;96:328-32.

150. Lopes LM, Brizot ML, Lopes MAB, Ayello VD, Schultz R, Zugaib M. Structural and functional cardiac abnormalities identified prior to 16 weeks'gestation in fetuses with increased nuchal translucency. Ultrasound Obstet Gynecol 2003;22:470-8.

14

*D Varga, G Azumendi, N Vecek,
C Millan, A Kurjak*

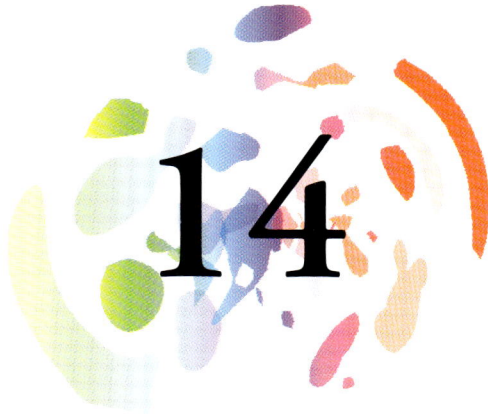

Basic Principles of 3D and 4D Sonography

INTRODUCTION

Three-dimensional (3D) sonography enables 3D imaging of 3D structures. Since human body and organs are 3D structures this type of imaging is the most appropriate for its confidential visualization. Organ structure and spatial relationships are simultaneously visualized, facilitating recognition of spatial anomalies. Using this type of imaging, fetal spatial anomalies such as clubfoot and spine deformations (scoliosis, kiphosis) were for the first time depicted on single image. For the same result with two-dimensional sonography, it was necessary to visualize several sections and reconstruct spatial images in examiner's mind. Stated in other words, delicate functions that examiner had to perform in his own mind are performed by machine. Recognition of spatial anomalies with two-dimensional sonography was the question of examiner mental capacity and art, whereas with three-dimensional sonography is simple routine task.

Moreover, in polymalformed fetuses two anomalies such as omphalocele with foot amelia or omphalocele with kyphosis can be visualized on single image. In those situations, three-dimensional imaging offers plastic reconstruction of fetal external anatomy (surface rendering) that enables to the parents to see and understand fetal condition quickly, totally and easily. This facilitates parental decision on fetal future and necessity for pregnancy termination. On the other hand, in parents who faced with polymalformed fetus in previous pregnancy, confirmation of normal fetal anatomy in subsequent pregnancy with plastic comprehensive image as direct proof results in parents tension relief.

Although 3D images are more informative than two-dimensional, disadvantages limited its application in clinical praxis included long processing period needed for image generation and condition that required the absence of fetal movements during scanning period. Because of that 3D technology was very time-consuming and not suitable for every day routine work.

If one performs two-dimensional sonography, true 3D structures can be represented in the form of single two-dimensional sectional planes. This disadvantage was compensated by fast image generation and analysis of organ of interest from multiple sections. Since, two-dimensional imaging does not require high processing capacity for fast image generation, realtime sonography was possible by low capacity processor.

The efforts were concentered to increase the speed of data processing in order to create three-dimensional imaging in realtime. This goal was nearly achieved after the advent and introduction of very fast microprocessors with high capacity of data processing. Fast generation of 3D images was precondition for introduction of 3D sonography in every day praxis and four-dimensional sonography (4D US).

Four-dimensional ultrasound has recently been introduced in clinical practice, overcoming the limitations of three-dimensional sonography (3D US). The most prominent limitation of three-dimensional technology is related to the static reconstruction of fetal anatomy. Three-dimensional image freezes the object and therefore does not provide information on movements or any information about dynamic changes of the object of interest. Moreover, fetal movements were significant source of image artefacts. There were requirements to produce technique which will enable possibility of performing three-dimensional imaging in a realtime mode. This technique can also be called live three-dimensional ultrasound (3D US) or four-dimensional ultrasound (4D US), as coined by a manufacturer, because time becomes a parameter within the three-dimensional imaging sequence.

Four-dimensional sonography is characterized by spatial visualization in almost realtime. From technical point of view this visualization is based on the continuous data acquisition by volume scanning with generating of surface spatial image. Modern machines are capable of the 20 volume scans in second associated with surface rendering and image display at frame rate of 12 images in second. Such presented images create movie. In contrast to the three-dimensional sonography, four-dimensional sonography is characterized by continuous volume scanning with creation of surface rendered image, whereas 3D US is characterized by single volume scanning.

Implementation of this new technology is still challenging for perinatologist. At present, it has been recognized that benefits of new technology can be achieved in the evaluation of fetal heart, fetal behavior and in invasive procedures.

Understanding of technical aspects of 4D US is important for proper using of 4D and for obtaining its full potential. In this chapter we systematically present the most important technical details needed for performing 4D sonography.

3D AND 4D IMAGING

Rapid development of digital ultrasound systems allows 3D image reconstructions and lately 4D realtime inspection of anatomical regions and pathological changes. Three-dimensional images are static and do not provide information of movements and dynamic changes of the object of interest (Figs 14.1 and 14.2).[1] Moreover, fetal movements are the source of significant artefacts and volume scanning should be performed during fetal inactive phase. Stated in other words, whenever fetus is active, qualitative 3D image is unobtainable. This fact limits usage of classic 3D ultrasound. Four-dimensional overcomes above mentioned disadvantage, making possible to obtain qualitative 3D image regardless of fetal movements. Only limiting factor for 4D sonography is quantity of adjacent amniotic fluid.

The acquisition of volume datasets is performed by 2D scans with special transducers (linear, convex, transvaginal) designed for 2D scans, 3D and realtime 4D volumes.[2] Realtime 4D mode is obtained from simultaneous volume acquisition and computing of 3D images. At this time it is possible to speak of multi-dimensional ultrasound.[3,4] The movement of the ultrasound beam over the region of interest (ROI) is automatically. Such design enables simplified 3D and 4D acquisition. Ultrasound probes include scanning mechanism moved by built in

electromotor. Processing speed allows continuous acquisition and processing of 4D volumes. Special endocavitary and transvaginal probes supports also working in Doppler modes and harmonic imaging. Supported applications are Gynecology, Obstetrics, Fetal Cardiology, and Urology.

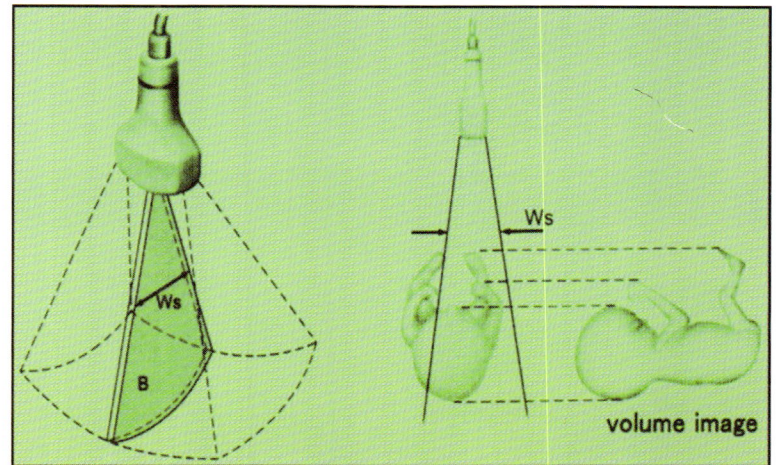

Fig. 14.1: Volume imaging. Slice width (Ws) is widened by a defocusing lens attached to the surface of a conventional probe (Adapted from reference no.4, with permission)

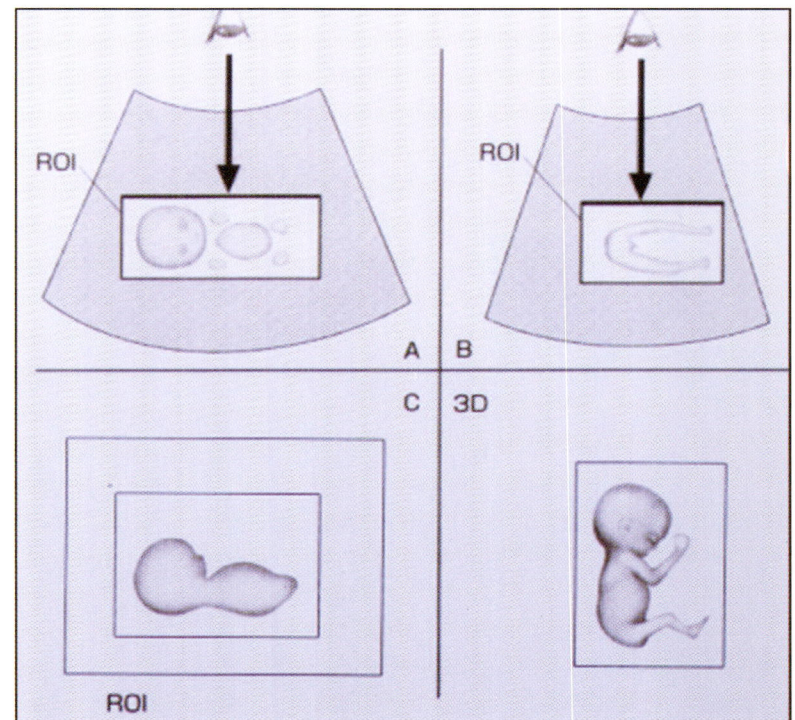

Fig. 14.2: Relation between three orthogonal planes and a 3D image (Adapted from reference no.4, with permission)

STARTING A 3D AND 4D MODE

The volume acquisition begins with a 2D image and superimposed volume box. The start 2D image is the central 2D image of the volume. According to dimensions of the volume box, volume scan sweeps between the margins of the volume box. The volume box is set to frame region of interest (ROI) (Fig. 14.3). During the 3D and 4D acquisition sweep time depends on the volume box size, scan quality and adjusted scan parameters such as depth, number of focuses and other parameters which affect B-mode image frame rate.[4]

1. Orientation in realtime 2D mode.
2. Selection of region of interest (ROI).
3. Starting the volume scan. Volume data are shown in a multiplan display on the monitor (transverse, sagittal and coronal) (Figs 14.4 and 14.5)

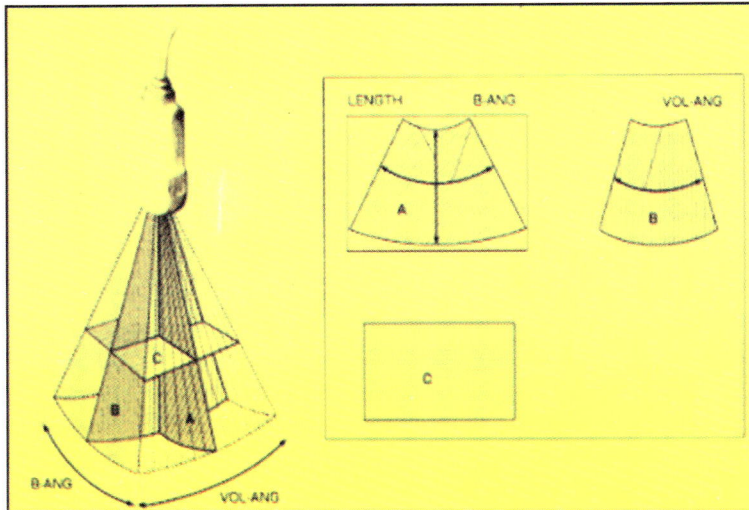

Fig. 14.3: Relation between three orthogonal planes and a 3D image (Adapted from reference no.4, with permission)

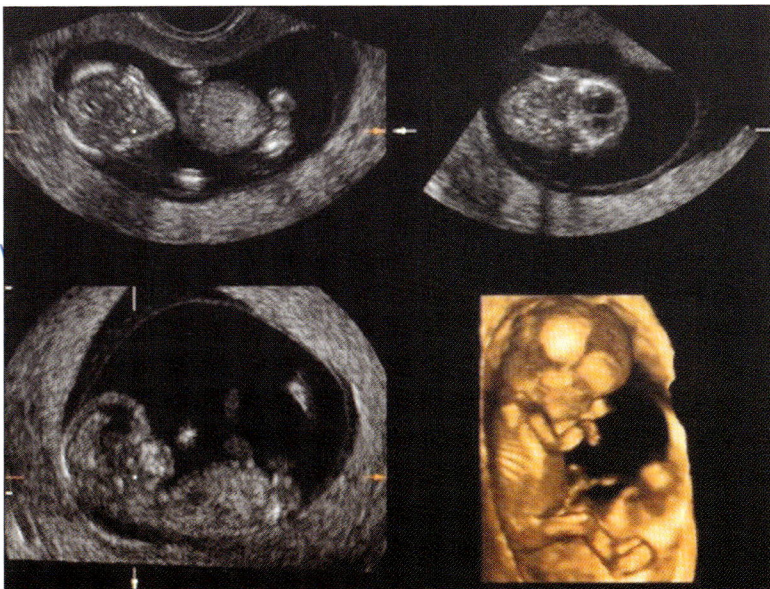

Fig. 14.4: Three orthogonal plane sections of a fetus are displayed simultaneously

3D AND 4D RENDERING

Pixel is the smallest element of 2D images while voxel is the smallest information unit in 3D and 4D imaging. Volume rendering provide visualization of animated voxel-based images on two-dimensional screen. Thanks to instant computer technology development and fast data transmission, volume acquisition and data processing are accelerated to enable 3D

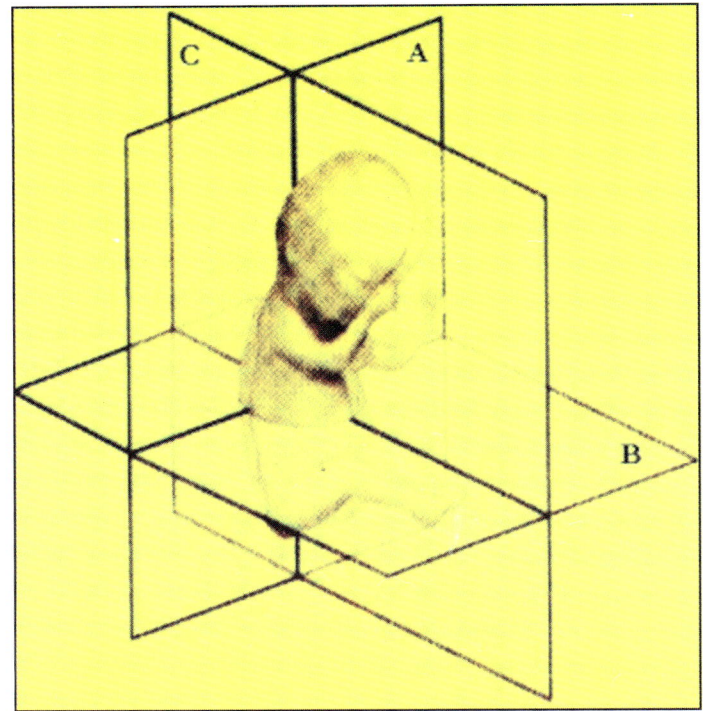

Fig. 14.5: Three orthogonal plane display of fetus (Adapted from reference no.4, with permission)

rendering in realtime (4D) (Fig. 14.6). Fast volume data processing enables calculation of 5 to 30 volumes per second depending on the system hardware and size of the render box. As 4D imaging is not really a realtime, there is always some delay as a result of time needed to reconstruct 3D image from 2D scans. It is always desirable to achieve as many volumes per second (volume rate) as possible. Number of volumes per second is some kind of trade of between image quality and frame rate. 3D and 4D image quality mostly depends on 2D image quality. Prior to volume acquisition it is important to achieve best 2D image quality, adjusting: depth, focus position and number of focuses, frequency and gain. Using CFI and Power Doppler Imaging adjusting velocity (PRF), wall filter, persistence and Doppler gain is important. All 2D image artefacts will be also present on 3D and 4D image reconstruction.

Good 4D image acquisition depends on following important points: region of interest (ROI) size and volume box size, ROI position or direction of view and accessibility to the object. The render box determines the contents that will be rendered. Structures that are not selected by volume box will be cut from 3D reconstruction.

Region of interest can be sized, moved and rotated in all directions arbitrary by operator. Volume data can be acquired from different 2D modes: gray scale imaging, CFI and power Doppler imaging. There are different rendering modes available: Surface, Transparent (maximum, minimum, X-ray) and Light, some of them can be active simultaneously in realtime.

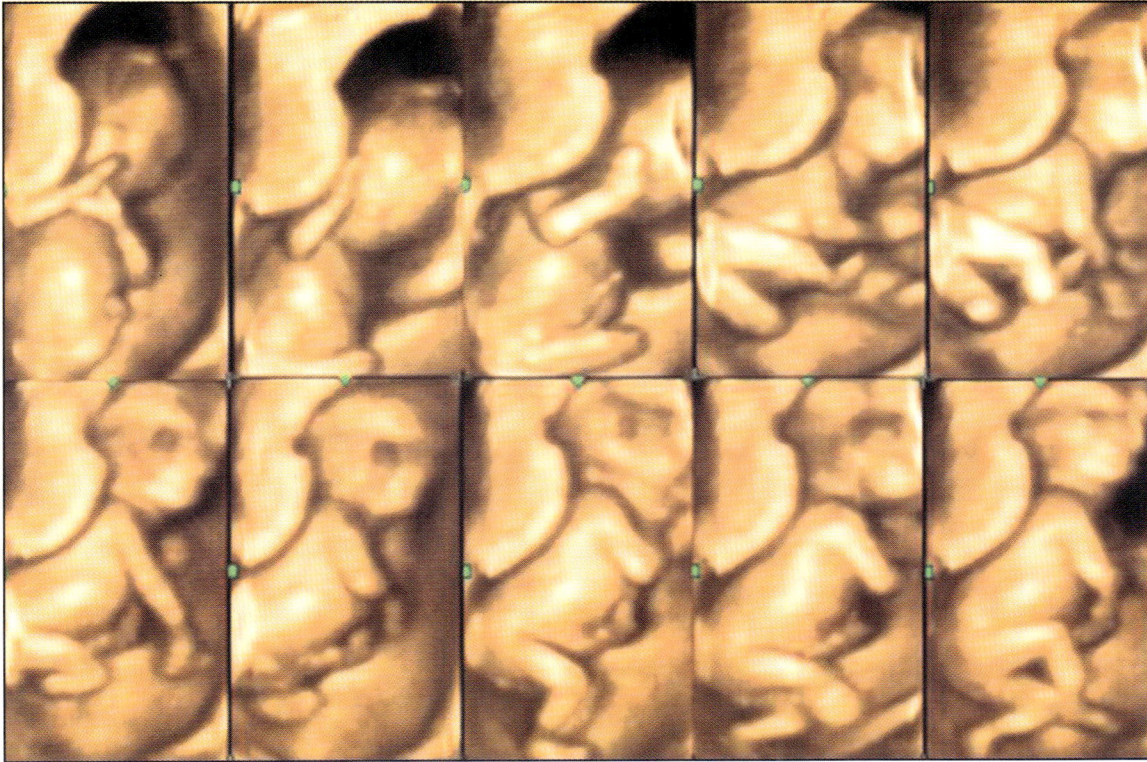

Fig. 14.6: 4D ultrasound sequence of the fetus at 12th week of gestation showing general movements. The complex movements of the limb, trunk and head are clearly visible and cause a shift in fetal position

Volume rendering is a process of visualization 3D structures on animated 2D screen. Render modes determine how 3D image will be presented on screen.

SURFACE RENDERING OR GRAY SCALE RENDERING

In the surface rendering mode, only signals from the surface of region of interest (ROI) are extracted and displayed in the plastic appearance (Fig. 14.7). Surface rendering examination of fetus focuses sonographer's attention exclusively on fetal external anatomy. This mode is capable of clear visualization of fetal normal surface anatomy or surface anomalies such as encephalocele, spina bifida, cleft lip/palate and abdominal wall and limb defects. Furthermore, visualization spatial relationship between surface structures enables accurate diagnosis of subtle malformations and anomalies such as bilateral cleft lips, myelomeningocele, omphalocele, overlapping fingers, arthrogryposis or others malformation (Figs 14.8 to 14.12).

Surface rendering gives best result when ROI structures are surrounded by fluid or hypoechoic tissue. Selecting the threshold level, voxels with gray values below the threshold value selected are not shown on reconstructed image. Selecting threshold parameter influences quality of surface rendered image.

Surface image can be displayed in "textural" mode. The gray values can be colored by different color maps, but most successful map for 3D/4D image is "body heat" map. Texture mode can

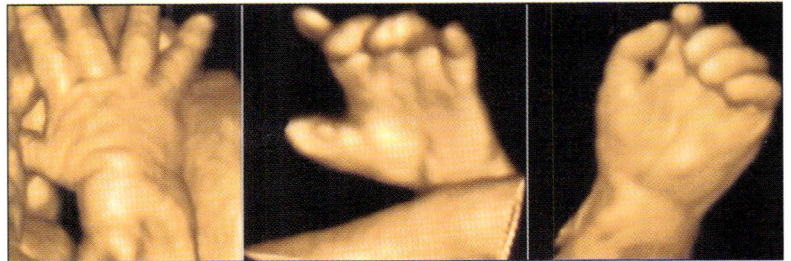

Fig. 14.7: 3D surface rendering of the normal hand movement. Note the alteration of the palm position.

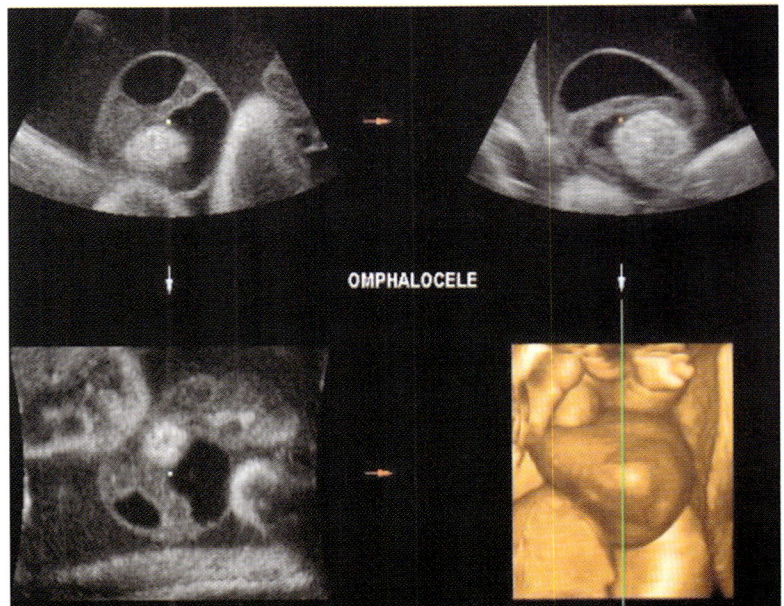

Fig. 14.8: 3D orthogonal sections from fetus with omphalocele are displayed simultaneously

also be "smoothed," showing smooth surfaces on 3D/4D reconstructions.[4-7] Texture and smooth surface display are

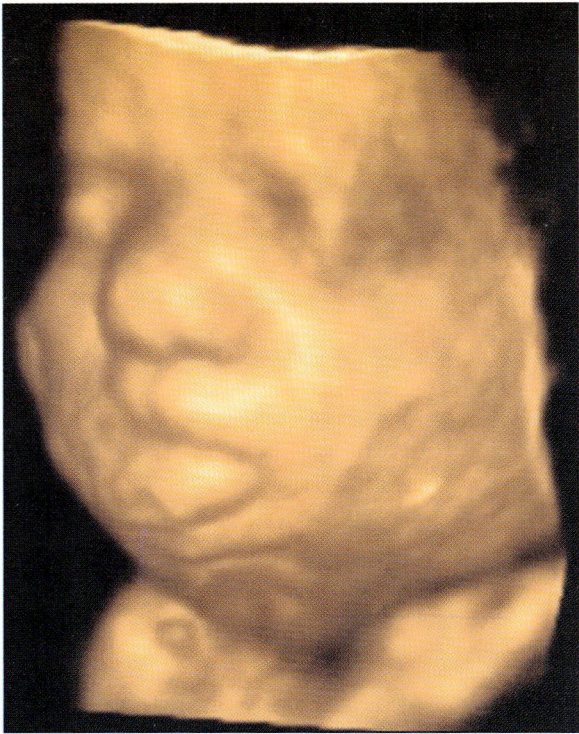

Fig. 14.9: 3D surface rendering of macroglossia

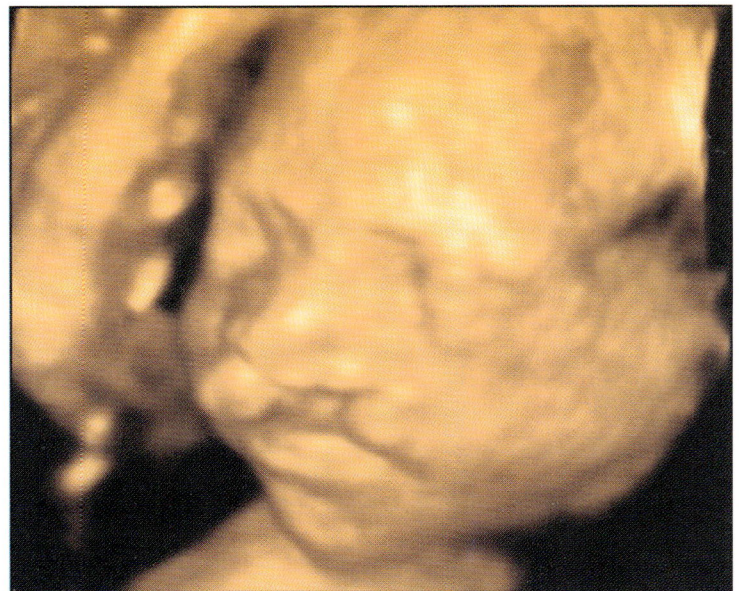

Fig. 14.11: 3D surface rendering of bilateral cleft lips

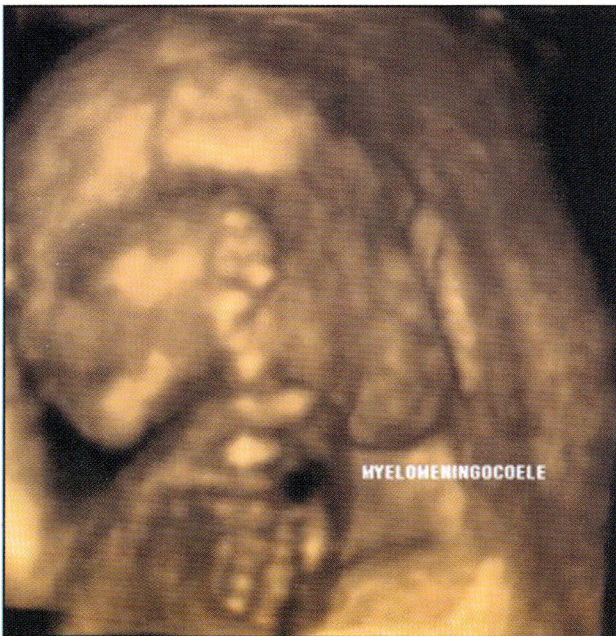

Fig. 14.10: 3D surface rendering of myelomeningocele

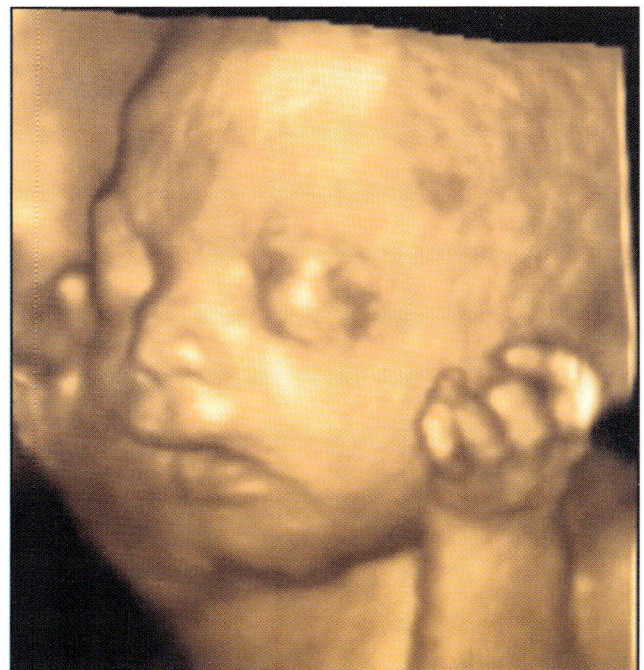

Fig. 14.12: 3D surface rendering of arthrogryposis of the fingers showing rigid and fixed posture

suitable for use in applications like: fetal face, fetal ear, abdominal wall, genitals, umbilical cord or other structure (Figs 14.13 to 14.17). Surface can be displayed in "light" mode. Closer structures are brighter while distant structures are displayed darker. Variation of the light mode is "gradient light mode" showing virtual illumination from spot light source.[8]

TRANSPARENT MODE

In transparent mode, contrary to surface mode, only the signals from the inner layers of ROI are extracted providing spatial reconstruction of internal structure of ROI. According to echogenicity of extracted signals there are two sub-modalities: maximum and minimum mode (Figs 14.18 A to C). In maximum mode only the signals of highest echogenicity, whereas in minimum mode only the signals of lowest echogenicity are extracted from the entire volume. In transparent mode only maximum gray values are displayed. This mode is suitable for visualization of fetal bones, endometrium and breast.[4]

MINIMUM MODE

Minimum gray values are displayed for visualization of vessels, cystic structures and parenchyma of different organs (Figs 14.19).[9]

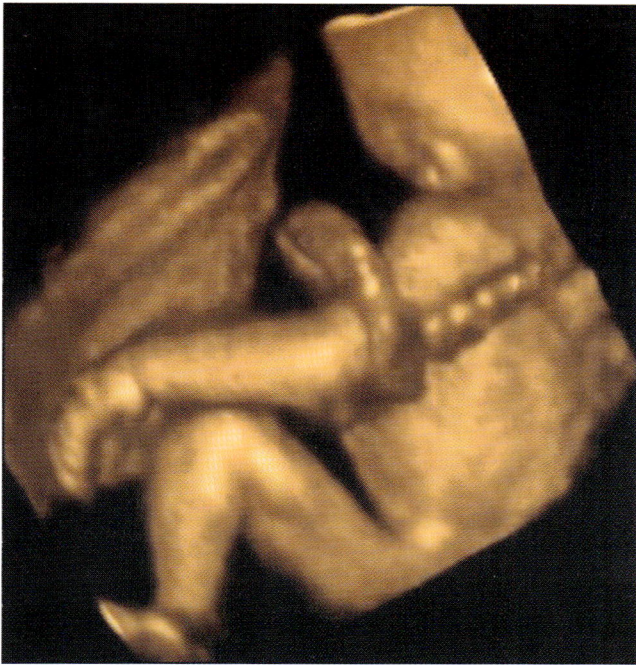

Fig. 14.13: 3D surface rendering of umbilical cord around the arm

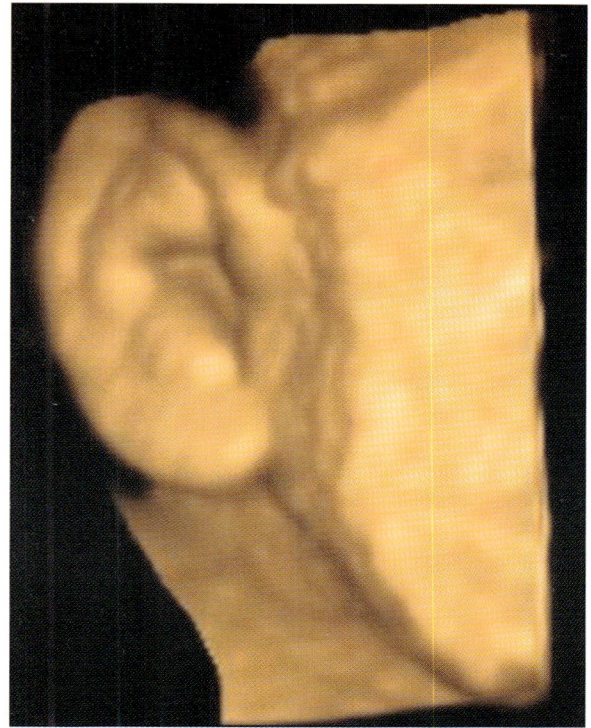

Fig. 14.14

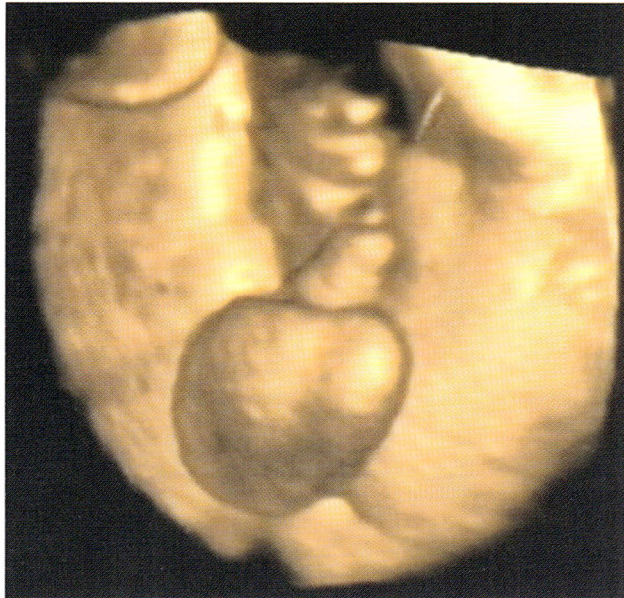

Figs 13.14 and 13 15: 3D surface rendering of fetal genitals

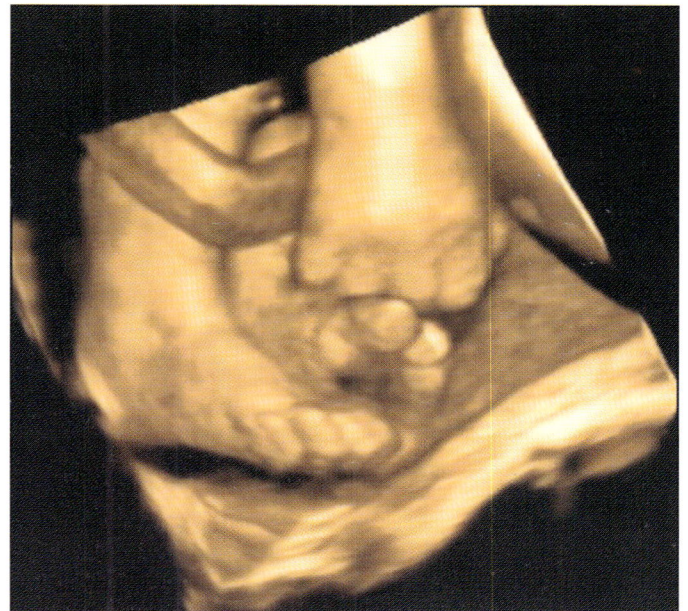

Fig. 14.16: 3D surface rendering showing ear structure

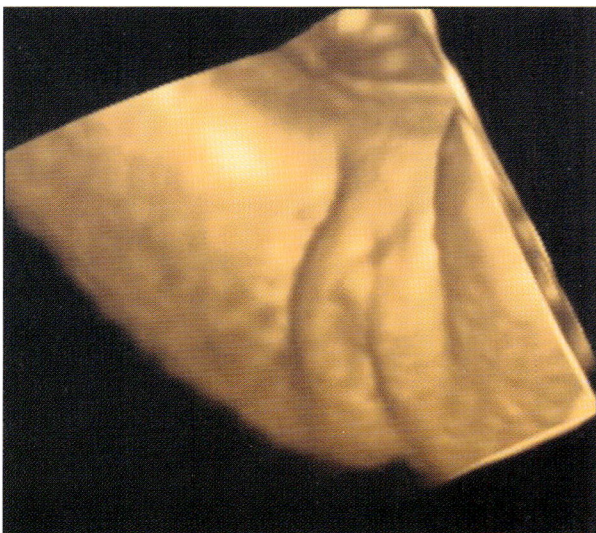

Fig. 14.17: 3D surface rendering showing fetal feet surrounded by umbilical cord and fetal hand

MAXIMUM MODE

Maximum gray values are displayed. Maximum mode is suitable for visualization of fetal bone structures.[10] It is the method of choice for imaging of the spatial relationships between bones. Moreover, this modality offers an option of complete visualization of curved bones such as ribs or clavicle on single image.

Evaluation of complete skeleton, particularly thoracic skeleton in the developing fetuses often is difficult with 2D US because of curvature of the bones. Ribs can be completely observed using the 3D US transparency mode. This modality reduces the echogenicity of soft tissues, leaving behind echogenic structures,

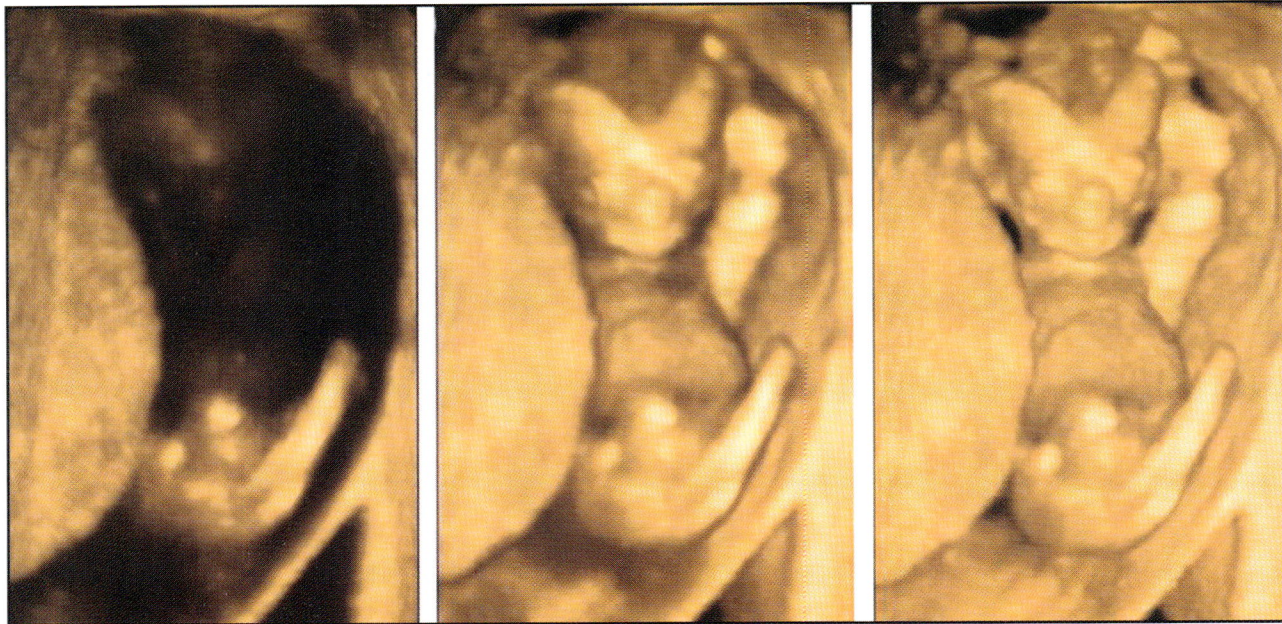

Figs 14.18A to C: Comparison of echogenicity of 3D images of a fetus at 12th week. (A) the fetus cannot be seen in the gestational sac because the threshold is set too low; (B) the fetus, amniotic membrane can be seen when the threshold is set properly; (C) the image is seen with the high threshold

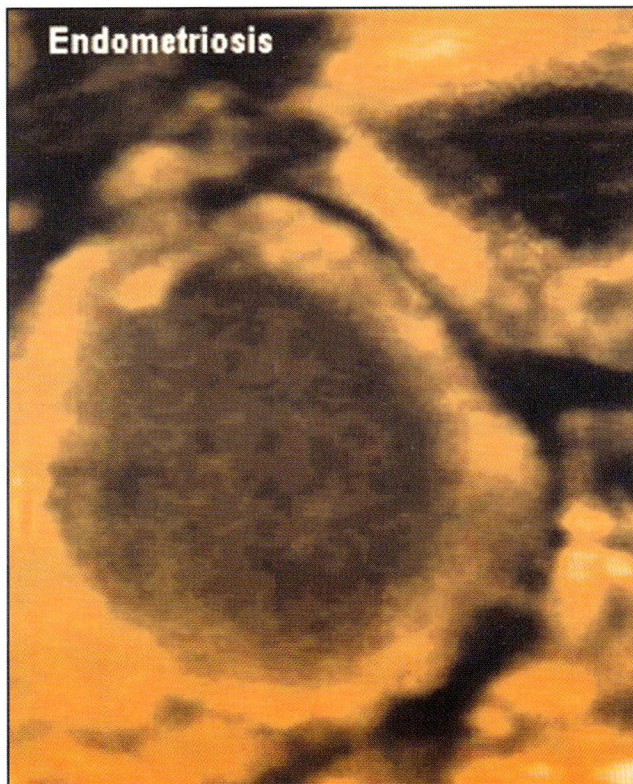

Fig. 14.19: 3D image of endometrial cyst in the ovary sets in minimum mode

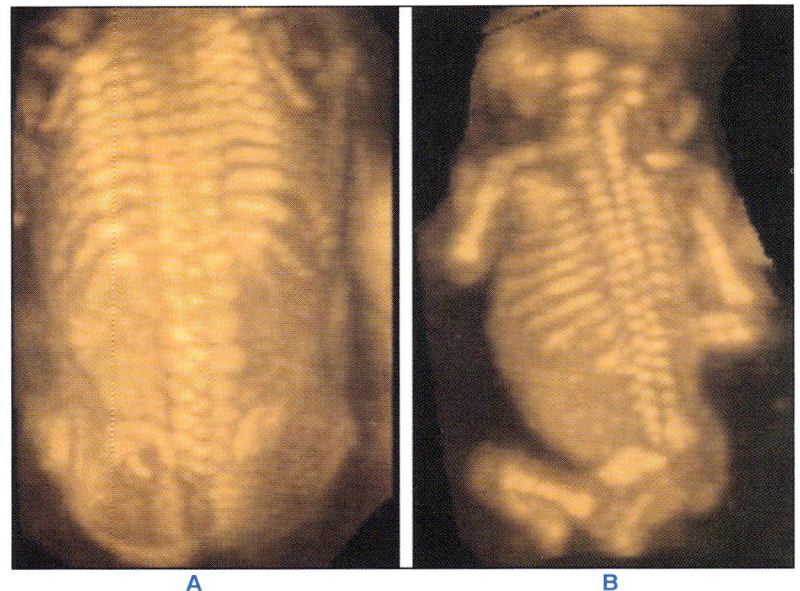

Figs 14.20 A and B: 3D maximum mode showing the vertebral column

namely the bones (Figs 14.20 A and B). The curvature and relationship of the rib ends to the vertebral bodies and the anterior chest wall can be demonstrated as well as the entire length.

The vertebral column is originally curved anteroposteriorly. If it is pathologically curved laterally, it is impossible to display the whole vertebral column in single sectional image by 2D US. The advantage of 3D ultrasound is the ability to visualize both curvatures at the same time. Anomalies such as scoliosis,

kyphosis, lordosis and spina bifida may be overlooked by 2D ultrasound, but are easy to recognize by using three-dimensional maximum mode. Congenital malformations of fetal spine can be identified easier using 3D surface and transparent mode reconstruction together. Specific vertebral body level may be accurately identified by simultaneous evaluating of axial planes of the spine within the volume rendered image. It is difficult to acquire the entire spine in a single volume and thus multiple volumes are often necessary to evaluate the spine completely.

Extremities consist of three parts: proximal, medial and distal. With this mode all three segments and spatial relationships between them could be analyzed in three dimensions. Therefore, the deviation of normal anatomical axis such as pathological angulations of hands and foots can be excluded by 3D US examination.[10]

Three-dimensional analysis of fetal extremities can be performed in two modes. If one interests spatial relationship between segments of fetal extremity then surface rendering mode should be used (see Fig. 14.8A). However, if in the focus of interest is relationship between bone elements of fetal extremity, then transparent mode should be used (see Fig. 14.8B). Combining these two modalities a more detailed analysis of fetal anatomy can be performed. This illustrates that fetal skin, subcutaneous tissue and bone structures can be evaluated. As fingers are clearly visible in the surface mode, this technique is very useful in demonstrating the normal morphology of these structures (see Fig. 14.9).

Spatial relations between medial and distal segment of fetal leg can be assessed on surface rendering mode. Normal anatomical axis and her deviations can be confirmed. The number and position of toes are clearly demonstrated on surface mode (see Fig.14.10). On such image toes can be counted and also pathological angulations can be conformed or excluded with higher confidence.

Using two modalities of the three-dimensional ultrasound step by step we can evaluate fetal foot from external appearance to complex bone inner and intratopographic relations (see Fig. 14.11). Surface of the skin and external spatial relations are shown on surface rendering image (see Fig. 14.12). Complex anatomy of bone elements is confirmed on transparent mode image.

VOLUME CONTRAST IMAGING (VCI)

Using 4D it is possible to make high contrast 2D images. The render algorithm is a combination of surface texture mode and minimum transparency 4D mode. It is possible to display couple of millimeters thin volume slice showing very good contrast between different tissues (Fig. 14.21). User can define thickness of slice that is scanned using 4D image rendering. Reconstructed image is showing improved tissue contrast. The VCI is used for better visualization of nodular or diffuse lesions in parenchyma of organs such as liver and spleen.

SPATIO-TEMPORAL IMAGE CORRELATION (STIC), FETAL CARDIO

Spatio-Temporal Image Correlation (STIC) is a new method for clinical investigation of the fetal heart. The reconstructed volume scan offers a user friendly technique to acquire data from the fetal heart and its visualization in a 4D sequence. The

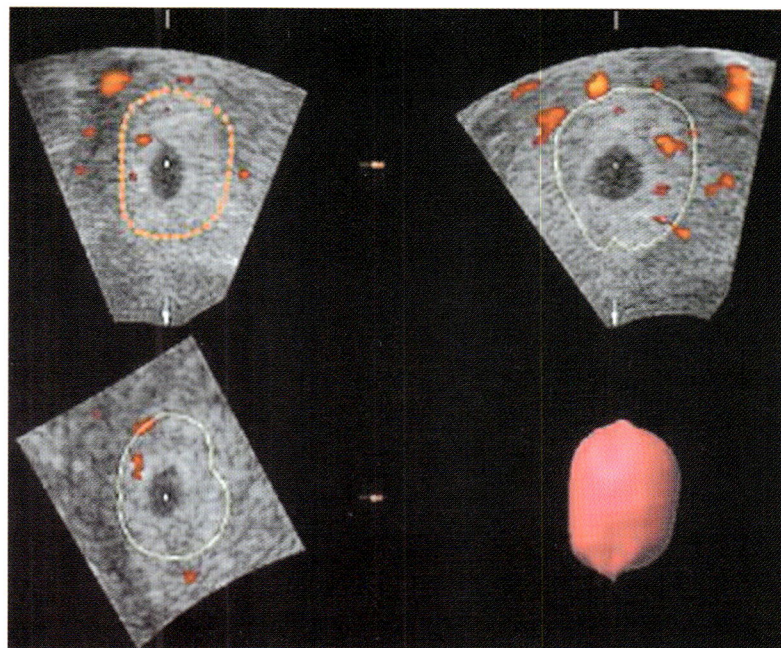

Fig. 14.21: Measurement of the chorionic volume in early pregnancy. The outlines of chorion were traced on some sectional images. A 3D image by surface rendering is displayed (lower right) and its volume is calculated automatically

volume acquisition is functioned in two ways: First, data is performed by a single, automatic volume sweep. In the second step the system examines the data in proportion to their spatial and temporal domain and processes a 4D sequence. This sequence presents the heart beating in realtime in a multiplanar display. After the volume acquisition, the heart can be assessed off-line, without being dependent on patient.[11]

REMOVING OVERLAYING STRUCTURES

This option is called Magic-Cut or The Electronic scalpel. During 3D and 4D scanning in most cases there are structures that are interfering or are superimposed to the reconstructed image. Magic-Cut tool enables successful removal of overlaying structures using 3D imaging. Unwanted structures can be cut off from the image in all three directions along x,y,z axes. Lately, there is also a possibility of using this tool to remove some structures from realtime 4D volumes. The cutting tool enables the operator to have improved visibility to the object from all directions.[13]

ADVANTAGES AND POSSIBILITIES OF 4D AND 3D IMAGING

3D and 4D ultrasound as new methods in ultrasound diagnostic have numerous advantages in comparison to classical gray scale imaging.[13] Reduced study time, faster examination procedure, and increased perspective from volume data provides better qualitative and quantitative information about selected area.

APPLICATIONS AND ADVANTAGES OF 4D ULTRASOUND

1. *Obstetrics*
   - Fetal morphology, malformation, agenesis
   - Bone shape abnormalities: Spina bifida, dwarfism, cleft palate, cleft lip
   - Skeletal dysplasia
   - Fetal heart: better correlation between valves, chambers and vessels; volume calculation of heart cavities; atrial and ventricular communication; assessment of valvular function
   - Variety of fetal volume evaluation: Urinary bladder, stomach, cyst
   - Fetal biopsy: umbilical blood sampling punctures with precision, amniocentesis, kidney dilatation, uropathy
   - Fetal movement and mimic: Normal and abnormal fetal gestures; evaluation of fetal sleep and awakening, hand and feet motion, eyelid, limbs and mouth motion
   - Fetal neuromyopathy genetic diseases: fetal reactivity/tonicity
   - Cord insertion using power-Doppler and 3D
   - Frontal bones.

2. *STIC and fetal cardio*
   - Fast, efficient assessment
   - Information acquired can be stored allowing processing of reproducible views
   - Simultaneous visualization of 2 to 3 planes: Easier for obstetrician to learn spatial orientation of fetal heart
   - Better correlation between valves, chambers and vessels
   - Volume calculation of heart cavities
   - Better access to heart pathology: Left ventricular and right ventricular outflow tracts; opening and closing of the foramen ovale
   - Atrial and ventricular communication: Ventricular wall can be seen in relation to the chambers or cutaway the top of the atria and look into the ventricles using Magicut tool or analyze septum alone
   - VSD and relation to pulmonary artery
   - Diagnose fetal heart defects in utero and prepare conditions for later treatment.

3. *Gynecology*
   - Exact volume measurement of endometrial hyperplasia (3/4D)
   - Virtual hysteroscopy (3D/4D), using slicing technique
   - Exact volume measurement of cysts (post-menopausal), polyps, myoma or fibroma
   - Exact localization and measurement of ovarian and endometrial tumors
   - Gynecological tumor monitoring after treatment (chemotherapy)
   - Contrast media use to check tumor vascularization and blood supply
   - Gynecological contrast media for tumor follow-up (4D)
   - Placental abnormalities (placenta previa).

4. *Breast and small parts*
   - 4D biopsy in all 3 planes, exact placement of the needle
   - Breast tumor volume evaluation
   - Breast tumor treatment monitoring (chemotherapy)
   - Skin tumor infiltration evaluation
   - Contrast media use on breast tumors (4D)
   - Sectional planes to define margins of different tumors.

5. *Urology*
   - 4D biopsy
   - Needle visualization in all 3 planes
   - Evaluation of the prostate parenchyma due to addition of coronal plane
   - Prostate and urinary bladder volume measurement and prostatic or bladder
   - Tumors
   - Correct positioning of urinary catheter
   - Exact assessment of the post-micturitional residue.

6. *Internal medicine*
   - Precise evaluation of acute abdominal syndrome
   - 4D biopsy (liver, kidney)
   - Excellent evaluation of parenchyma/tumor volumes
   - Lithiasis localization in the urethra during renal colic (3D, C-plane)
   - Contrast media use in abdominal tumor (kidney, liver)
   - Evaluation of cholecystitis
   - Abdominal tumor volume follow-up and monitoring in 3D
   - Tumor location and vascularization during chemotherapy
   - Obstruction determination in icterus mechanism.

7. *Pediatrics*
   - Neonatal brain, 3-plane view of chamber symmetry; volume measurements
   - Color or power-angio vessel correlation
   - Hip measurement.

8. *Data review and networking*: Volume data sequences can be stored on hard disk of ultrasound unit or at different media (CD-R, MO) in various formats: 2D image, 2D cine (selected sequence of 2D images), 3D volume (sequence of 3D rotating images) and 4D volume. Since the complete volume data set

is saved, it is possible to review saved examinations without any loss of image quality. Stored data can be interactively processed with additional 3D reconstruction possibility.

3D and 4D provides additional aspects to conventional 2D sonography. The main advantage of ultrasound in general is dynamic imaging of human body. 4D imaging is following this tradition pointing dynamic changes inside body and organs. Using 4D ultrasound in Obstetrics it is possible to monitor quality and quantity of fetal movements on 3D realtime reconstructed images.

CONCLUSIONS

Understanding technical aspects of 4D US is important either for proper using of 4D or for obtaining its full potential. Furthermore, image post-processing should be considered as a part of examination. Sometimes, an additional information about ROI can be provided with post-processing.

Undoubtedly, 4D US is the technology of future whose potential still needs to be discovered and evaluated. For proper evaluation of benefits of four-dimensional sonography full range of its options should be used. The knowledge of basics and principles of 3D US is precondition for its successful application of 4D US, because 4D US is based on three-dimensional imaging. In contrast to the classic two-dimensional imaging,

after 3D image is obtained it can be processed in order to improve image quality and to obtain additional information. Postprocessing includes rotation of surface rendered image and magic cut.

REFERENCES

1. Kurjak A, Azumendi G, Vecek N, et al. Fetal hand movements and facial expression in normal pregnancy studied by four-dimensional sonography. J Perinat Med 2003; 31(6): 496-508.
2. Hu W, Wu MT, Liu CP, et al. Left ventricular 4D echocardiogram motion and shape analysis. Ultrasonics 2002; 40(1-8): 949-54.
3. Kossoff G. Basic physics and imaging characteristics of ultrasound. World J Surg 2000; 24(2): 134-42.
4. Baba K. Development of 3D Ultrasound. In Kurjak A, Chervenak F (Ed): Textbook of Ultrasound in Obstetrics & Gynecology. New Delhi: Jaypee Publishing, 2004: pp 27-42.
5. Timor-Tritsch IE, Platt LD. Three-dimensional ultrasound experience in obstetrics.Curr Opin Obstet Gynecol 2002; 14(6): 569-75.
6. Lee W. 3D fetal ultrasonography. Clin Obstet Gynecol 2003; 46(4): 850-67.
7. Arzt W, Tulzer G, Aigner M. Real time 3D sonography of the normal fetal heart-clinical evaluation. Ultraschall Med 2002; 23(6): 388-91.
8. Yanagihara T, Hata T. Three-dimensional sonographic visualization of fetal skeleton in the second trimester of pregnancy. Gynecol Obstet Invest 2000; 49(1): 12-6.
9. Mangione R, Lacombe D, Carles D, et al. Craniofacial dysmorphology and three-dimensional ultrasound: a prospective study on practicability for prenatal diagnosis.. Prenat Diagn 2003; 23(10): 810-8.
10. Kurjak A, Hafner T, Kos M, et al. Three-dimensional sonography in prenatal diagnosis: a luxury or a necessity? J Pernatal Med 2000; 28(1): 194-209.
11. De Vore GR, Falkensammer P, Sklansky MS, et al. Spatio-temporal image correlation (STIC): new technology for evaluation of the fetal heart. Ultrasound Obstet Gynecol 2003; 22(4): 380-7.
12. Vinals F, Poblete P, Giuliano A. Spatio-temporal image correlation (STIC): a new tool for the prenatal screening of congenital heart defects. Ultrasound Obstet Gynecol 2003; 22(4): 388-94.
13. Kurjak A, Vecek N, Hafner T, et al. Prenatal diagnosis: what does four-dimensional ultrasound add? J Perinat Med 2002; 30(1): 57-62.

15

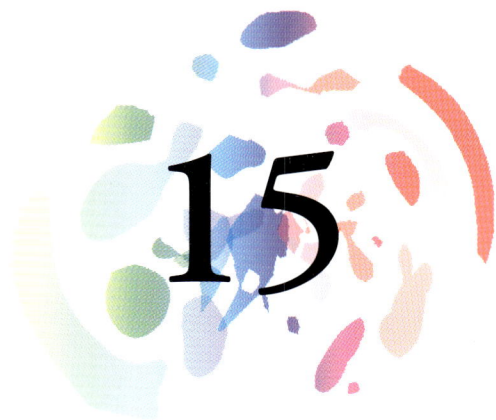

G Azumendi, A Kurjak, JM Carrera, W Andonotopo, E Scazzocchio

3D and 4D Sonography in the Evaluation of Normal and Abnormal Fetal Facial Expression

INTRODUCTION

The face is the anatomical structure that clearly demonstrates the utility and advantages of three-dimensional (3D) and four-dimensional (4D) ultrasound. It is difficult to find a book about ultrasound published during the last few years that does not include a 3D picture about the fetal face on its cover. Even in a text dedicated to gynecological ultrasound, it is usual to find a 3D picture of a fetal face helping illustrate the potential of such a new technology.

Practically all the pioneering studies on 3D ultrasound provide an example of three-dimensional fetal face reconstruction.[1-29] We have all taken our first steps in 3D ultrasound by exploring the fetal face and our main aim has always been to obtain good pictures of this anatomic structure. It is, therefore, a good opportunity to elaborate on the role of 3D and 4D ultrasound of the fetal face (Figs 15.1 to 15.118).

ADVANTAGES AND LIMITATIONS OF 3D ULTRASOUND

The study of the fetal face is of great importance in prenatal medicine because some facial and encephalic structures share the same embryologic origin. This is why every malformation detected at the facial level must necessitate the corresponding study at encephalic level.[30,31] We all recognize the thought of De Meyer and colleagues, who said, 'The face predicts the brain'.[32] In the ever-increasing body of knowledge on this topic, there are papers that demonstrate some advantages of 3D ultrasound compared with the use of 2D ultrasound in perinatal medicine, mainly in the study of the fetal face.[18,19,32,33] Three-dimensional ultrasound shows perspectives that cannot be obtained with 2D ultrasound and depicts the anatomy in the most appropriate and comprehensive position.[34] This standardized display of images helps us obtain a better understanding of the fetal anatomy for both the parents and less-experienced doctors. Because of its curvature and small anatomical details, the fetal face can be visualized and analyzed only to a limited extent with 2D sonography.[35,36] The entire face cannot be seen on a single image. Three-dimensional ultrasound provides a spatial reconstruction of the fetal face and simultaneous visualization of all facial structures such as the fetal nose, eyebrows, mouth, jaws, dental germs and eyelids (Figs 15.11 and 15.12).[28,33-37]

Advantages

Improved Maternal-fetal Bonding

Steiner and colleagues have stated that, for many parents, the image taken by 2D ultrasound is abstract, whilst with 3D ultrasound the features of the baby are instantly recognized, regardless of whether they are normal or not, which allows parental bonding with the baby.[38] This is one of the unquestionable benefits of 3D ultrasound over 2D.[18,22,39,40] In a few papers in which no other real benefits are found with the use of 3D, the reinforcement of the affective bonding is unchallengeable.[40] Three-dimensional images give the mother more security and a deeper vision of the psychological aspects of ongoing pregnancy.[41] It has also been noted that these positive and close affective bonds between the mother and the fetus can help her stop smoking or end any other potentially harmful habits.[42]

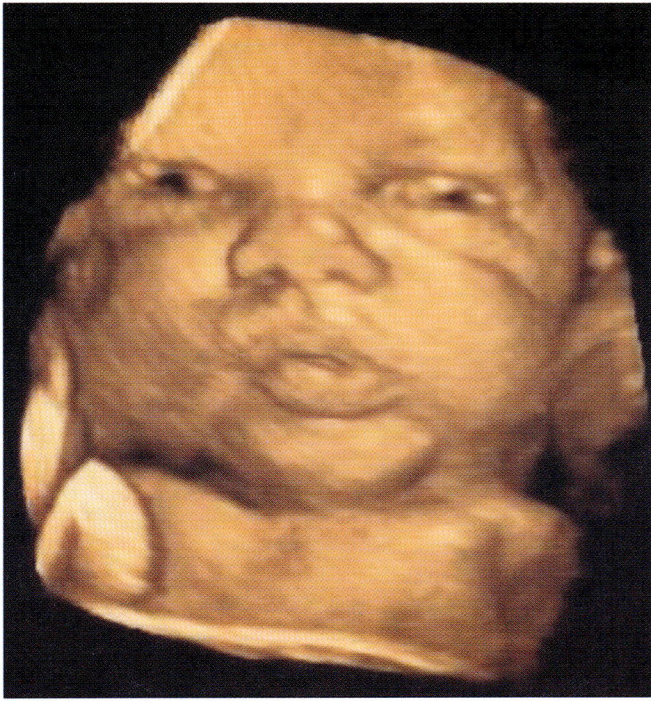

Fig. 15.1: 3D scan of a fetus showing complete face profile at 33rd week of gestation. Eyelids are opened and surface of facial features are discernible

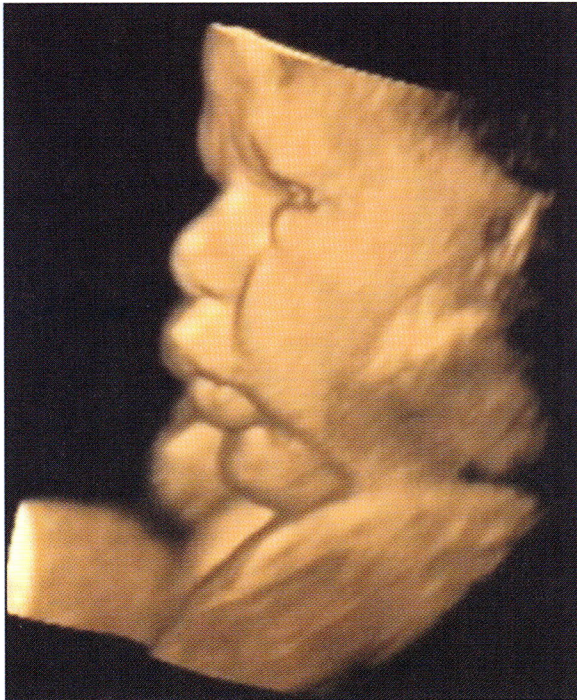

Fig. 15.3: 3D scan of a fetus with semi-profile position showing contours of both eyelids and surrounding soft tissue structures such as nose and cheeks

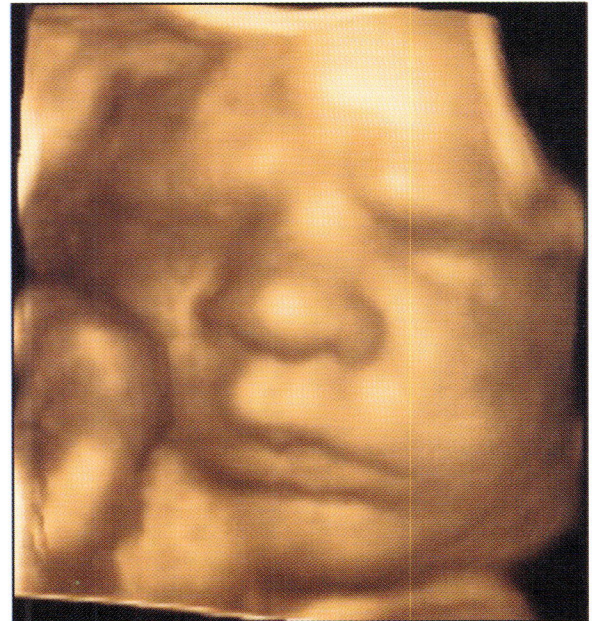

Fig. 15.2: 3D scan of a fetal profile showing facial contours of the facial muscle

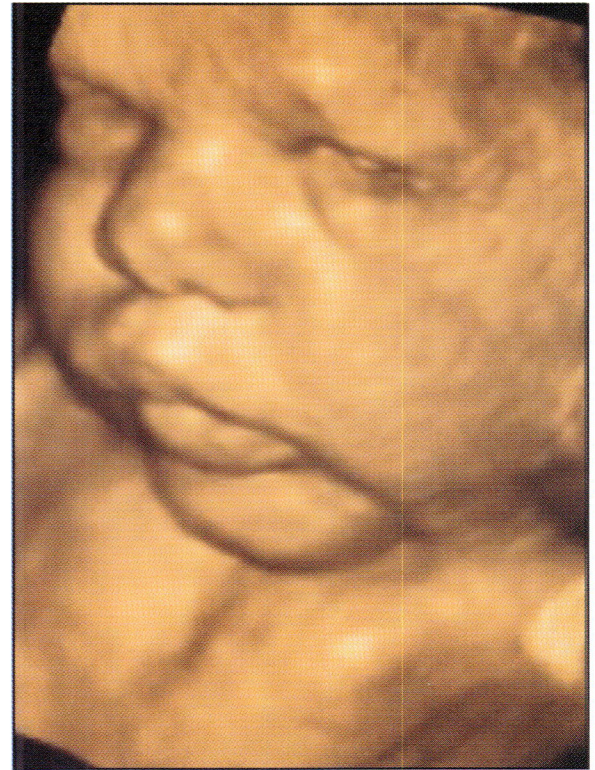

Fig. 15.4: 3D image shows alteration of the facial expression of the fetus. The fetus seems to be glumness

Improvement in Identifying Anomalies

The improvement in the identification of anomalies by the performance of images in perspectives and planes that cannot be obtained with 2D ultrasound has proved vital. It is precisely stated that most fetal face deformations have been diagnosed with 3D ultrasound whilst they had gone unnoticed with 2D ultrasound. Ultrasound cases of micrognathia, cleft lip (Figs 15.88 to 15.93), mid-facial hypoplasia, orbitary hypoplasia, facial dysmorphea, defects in the cranium ossification and auricular dysplasia have been picked up.[18,22,31,32] Some of these abnormalities have been diagnosed in the 3D presentations and some others in the planes not available with conventional 2D ultrasound. By allowing evaluation of the volume millimeter by millimeter and in three perspectives, it is possible to study the upper lip in coronal and axial images and the palate in the axial plane. Three-dimensional ultrasound assists by visualizing the

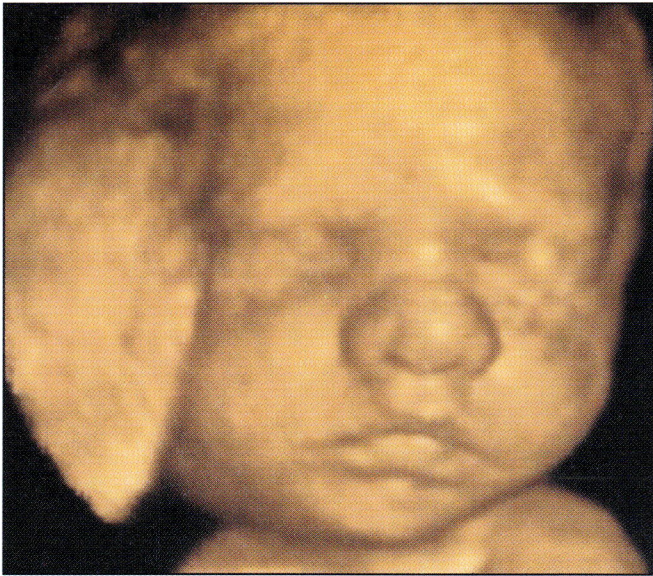

Fig. 15.5: This image shows alteration of the facial expression. The movements of the facial musculature caused the fetus seems to be sleeping

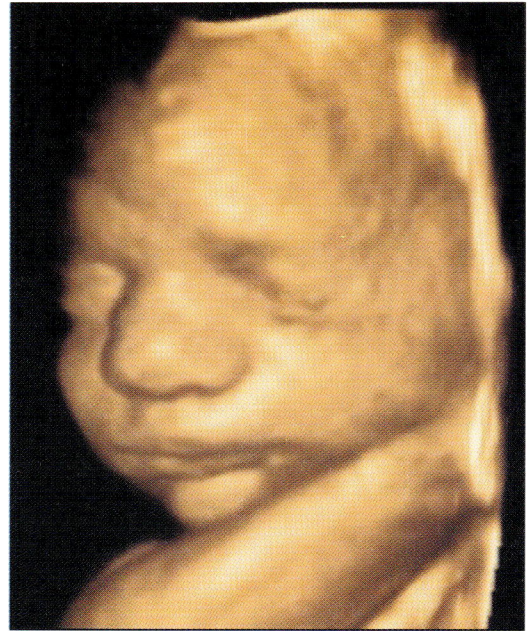

Fig. 15.6: Sleeping expression of the fetus is clearly visible

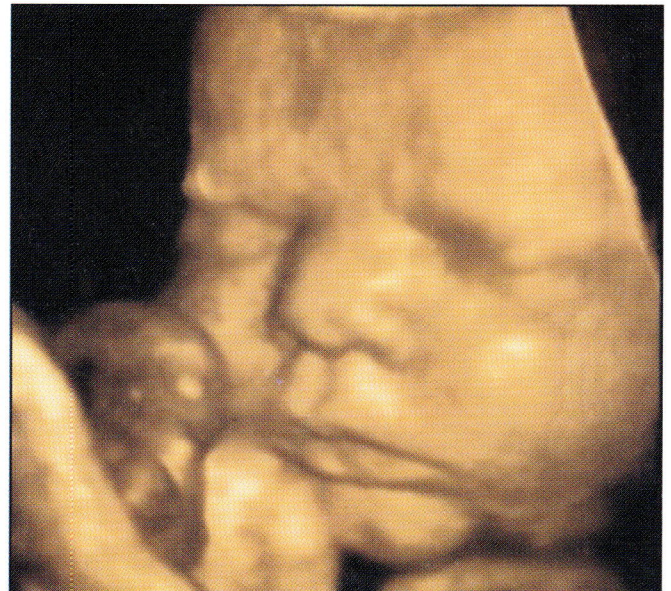

Fig. 15.7: Other facial expression of the fetus showing mouth opening

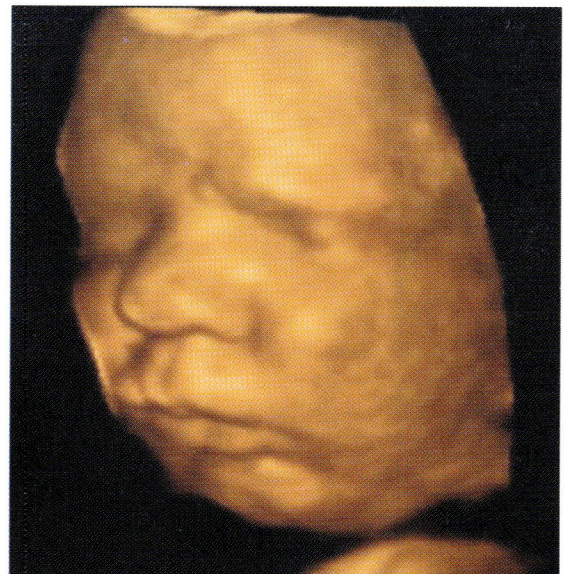

Fig. 15.8: Surface rendering by 3D demonstrates the facial contours of the lips and nose. The fetus seems to be sleeping

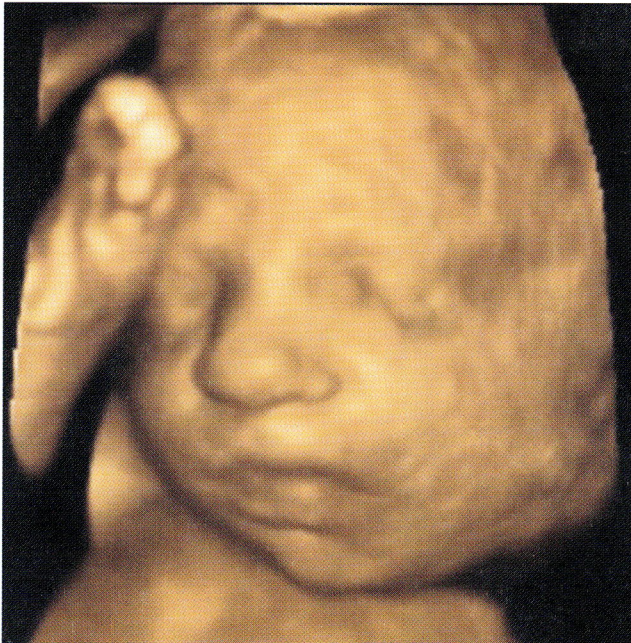

Fig. 15.9: Facial expression showing distortion of the facial muscles. The fetus seems to be angry

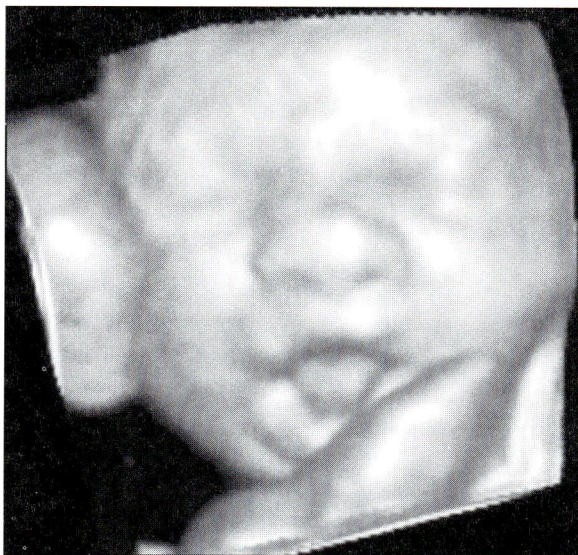

Fig. 15.10: Semi-profile expression of the facial contour

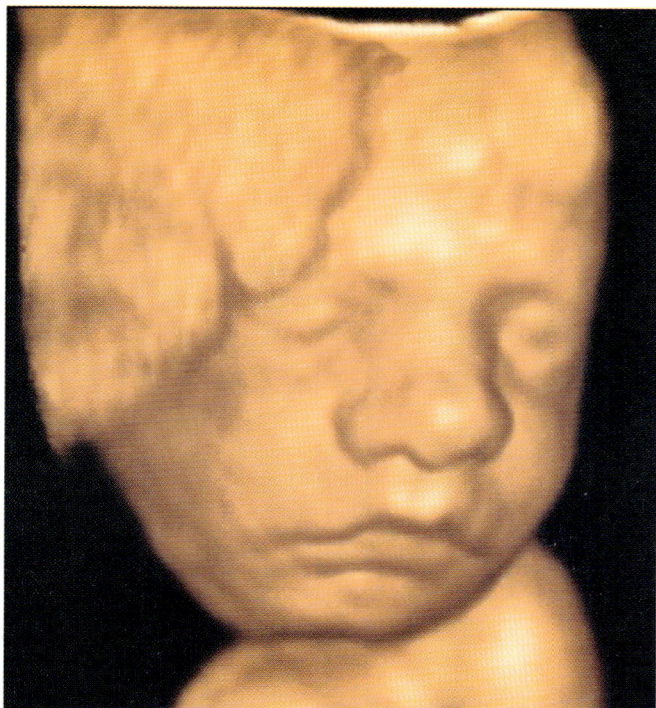

Fig. 15.11: Semi-profile surface rendering showing the contours of the fetal face, eyelids and nose

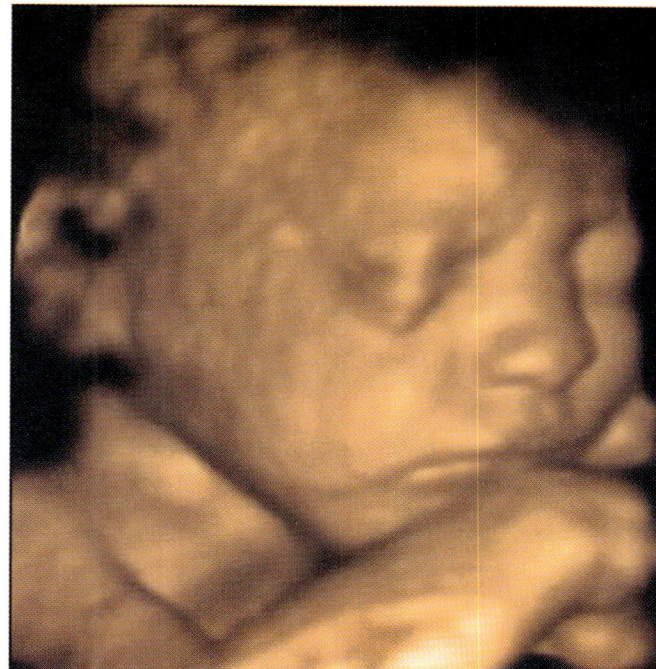

Fig. 15.13: The entire face is discernible, with clear visualization of nostrils, right ear and eyelids. The fetal hand is positioned in front of the mouth

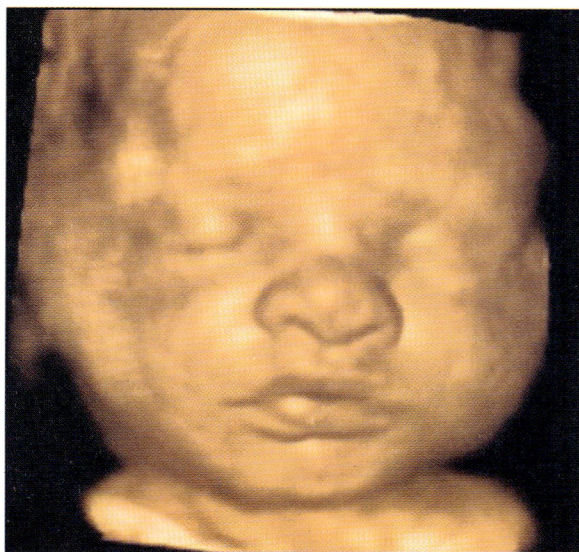

Fig. 15.12: Complete profile of surface rendering showing movements of the bilateral part of eyebrows is clearly visible

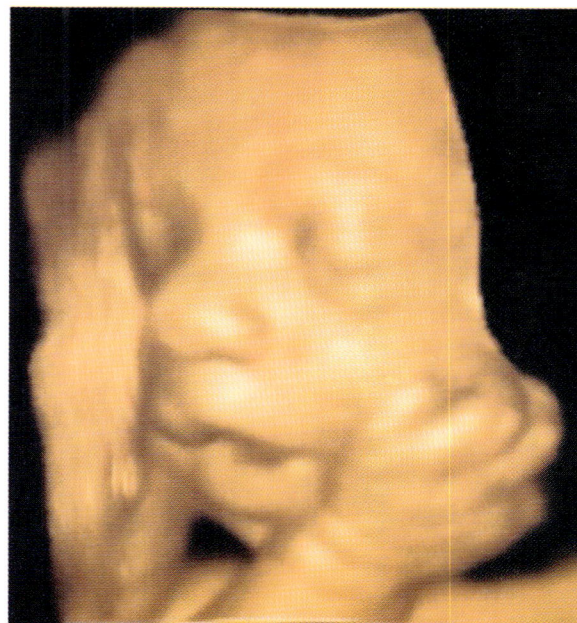

Fig. 15.14: 3D surface rendering showing opening of the mouth and movements of eyebrows

facial profile in the correct axis, which is not always obtainable on a 2D image.[43] Merz and colleagues analyzed the effect of 3D facial profile reconstruction on 125 fetuses.[22] They found that 30.4 percent of the profiles were turned 3 to 20 degrees from the real one. Therefore, in only 69.6 percent of the cases was the true profile obtained with 2D ultrasound. The magnitude of this discovery cannot be disputed, since previously those anomalies could not be detected or were overdiagnosed. Several papers state the clear superiority of 3D ultrasound for the study of the fetal face in both normal and abnormal conditions[1-7,9-15,17-20,22-29,44,45], although some authors do not find these differences so significant.[40]

Improved Assessment of Extent and Location of Fetal Anomalies

Assessment of the extent and location of fetal anomalies can be improved by using 3D ultrasound[18,28,32,46] (Figs 15.81 to 15.97). A cleft lip and/or a cleft palate are often difficult to diagnose with 2D ultrasound, or at least it has been difficult to precisely evaluate their extent, especially if the operator has little experience or lacks anatomic references with the appropriate image plane. In the RADIUS study, 7,685 low-risk fetuses were studied and only three of nine cleft lips were prenatally identified.[47] Using 3D ultrasound, the operator can evaluate the front alveolar ledge or the primary palate in the appropriate axial plane, using the

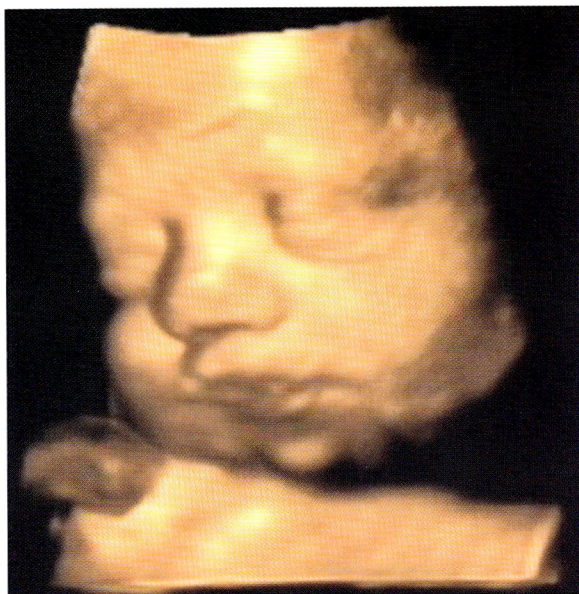

Fig. 15.15: Surface rendering of the facial contour showing expression of the sleeping fetus

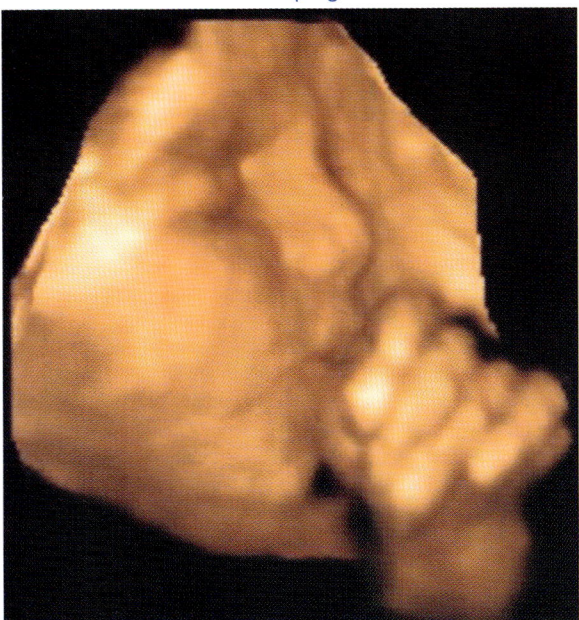

Fig. 15.17: Semi-profile position showing facial contour of the fetal lips which cause the change in facial expression

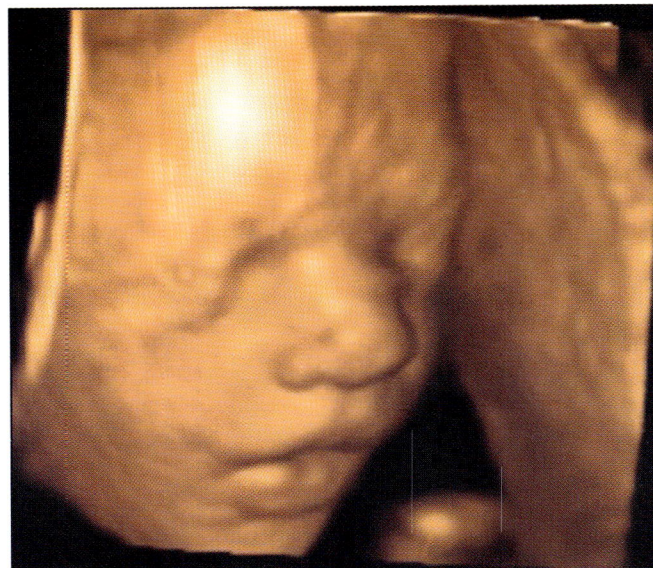

Fig. 15.16: Semi-profile position of the fetus showing eyelids opening and all facial features

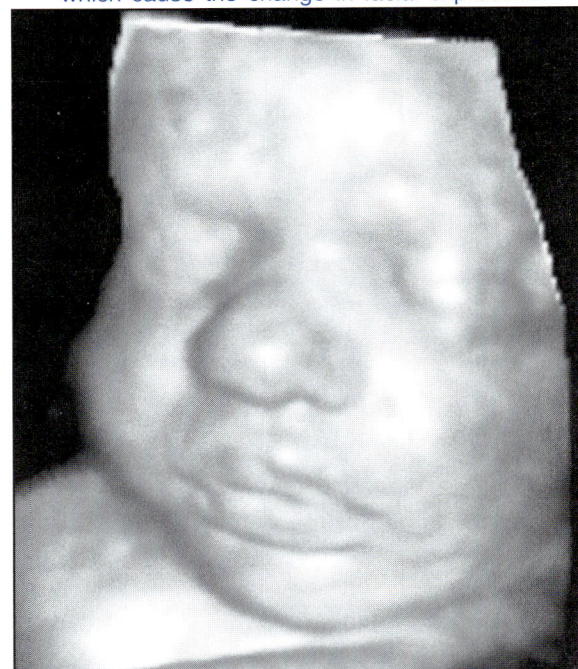

Fig. 15.18: Surface rendering demonstrates clear visualization of facial anatomical structures

correct reconstruction or the sagittal planar image as a reference, and can then move on to the parallel axial images. This possibility for studying axial or frontal parallel planes of the fetal face is not obtained with 2D ultrasound. It is extremely useful to show the anomaly to both relatives and trainee doctors in order to assist their decision regarding future diagnostic and therapeutic options.[14,18,22,23,28,33,48]

Four-dimensional Ultrasound

Four-dimensional ultrasound has some additional advantages such as the ability to study fetal activity in the surface-rendered mode, and is particularly superior for fast fetal movements.[49] With 2D ultrasound, fetal movements such as yawning, swallowing and eyelid movements cannot be displayed

simultaneously, whilst, with 4D sonography, the simultaneous facial movements can be clearly depicted.[50] There are several types of jaw movement patterns, such as isolated jaw movement, sucking and swallowing, which can be observed by 2D ultrasound.[51] The variable amplitudes of jaw opening and speed characterize isolated jaw movements (Fig. 15.3). Yawning can be observed as a movement pattern identical to that seen in infants, children and adults: slow opening, prolonged wide opening of the jaws followed by quick closure, with simultaneous retroflexion of the head. With 4D ultrasound, it is now feasible to study a full range of facial expressions including smiling, crying, scowling and eyelid movement.[50,52]

The observation of the facial expression may be of scientific and diagnostic value and this scientific approach opens an

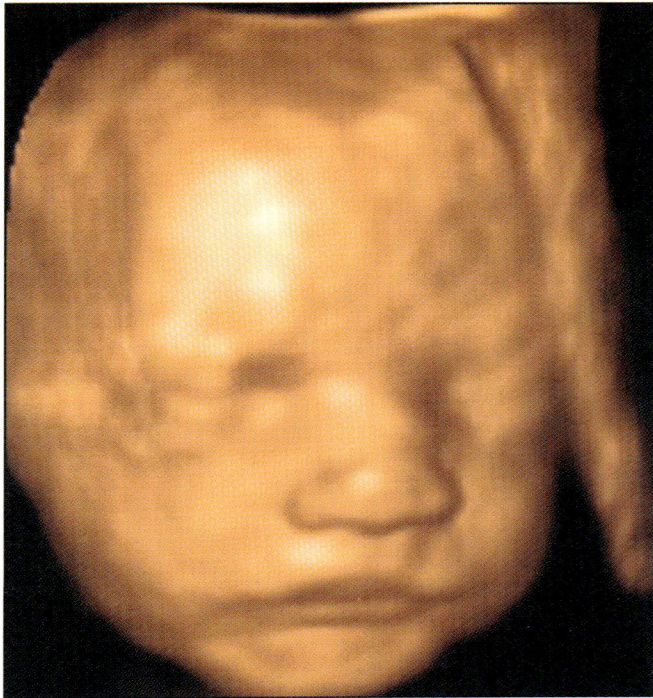

Fig. 15.19: 3D surface rendering of complete profile showing discernible contour of facial musculatures

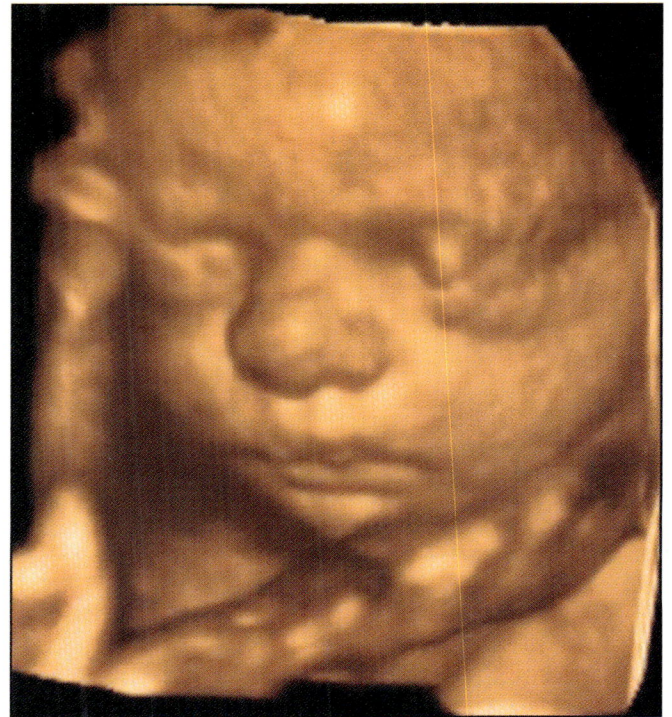

Fig. 15.21: Complete profile of the fetus showing the facial contour. Even the umbilical cord is observable surrounded the fetal neck

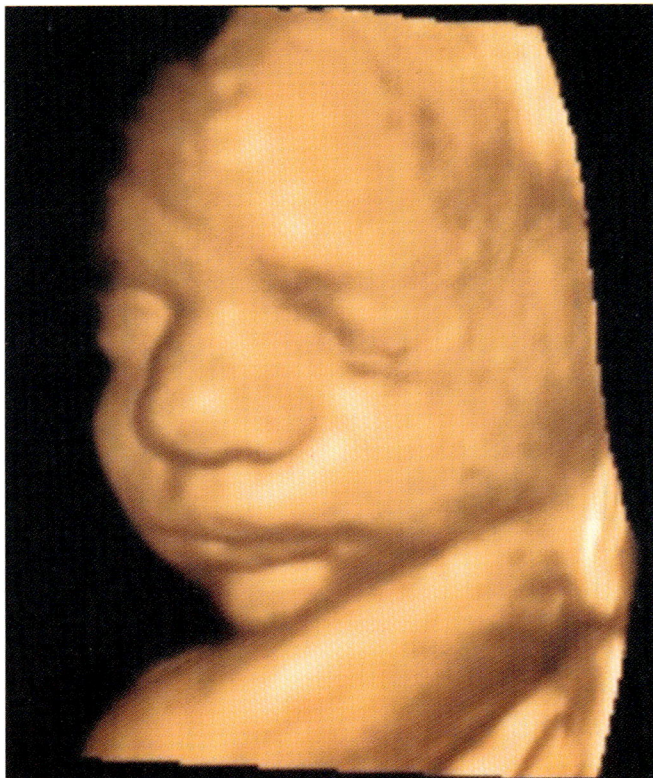

Fig. 15.20: Semi-profile surface rendering showing sleeping expression of the fetus

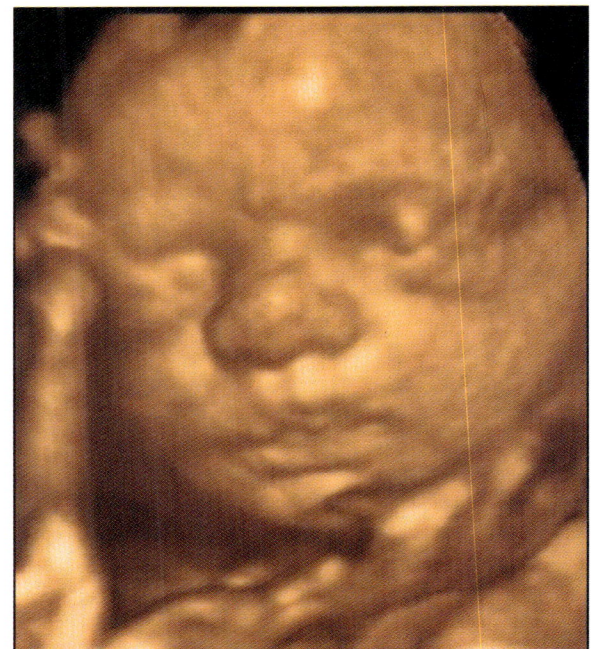

Fig. 15.22: 3D surface rendering shows sleeping expression of the fetus. Note the nuchal cord around the neck is cleary visible

entirely new field. There are many unanswered questions. When do facial expressions start ? Which expression dominates and at what gestational age do they occur ? An important diagnostic aim of the observation of facial expression is prenatal diagnosis of facial paresis. The criterion for the diagnosis is asymmetrical facial movement and detection of the movements limited to only one side of the face. Unfortunately during the relaxed phase, it is not possible to evaluate the status of the facial nerve.

Therefore, during the active phase, the fetus should be scanned by 4D ultrasound. Since the origin of the facial expression can be external, the sonographer should be aware of this pitfall. For example, force of the fetal hand can alter the facial expression on one side of the face, causing asymmetry (Fig. 15.80). This kind of asymmetry, however, should be differentiated from pathological features such as unilateral facial paresis (Fig. 15.6). We believe that the largest challenges for 4D ultrasound are in the unexplored areas of parental and fetal behavior.[53-55] Two-dimensional realtime ultrasound and 4D

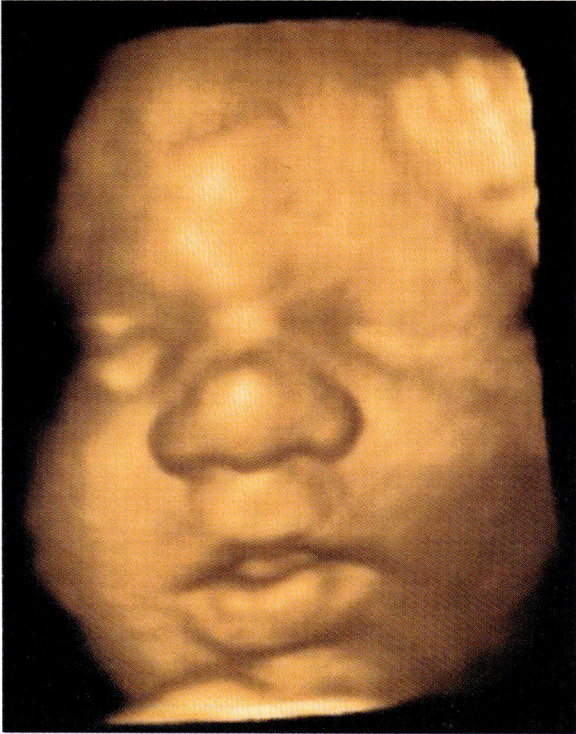

Fig. 15.23: Asymmetry of the facial expression caused by changing in lateral parts of the cheek

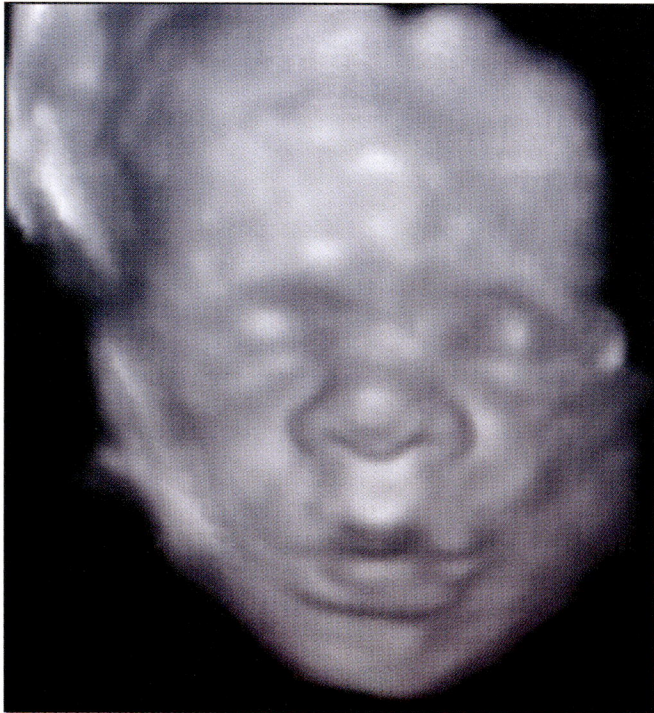

Fig. 15.25: Fetal profile by f3D surface rendering showing the facial texture

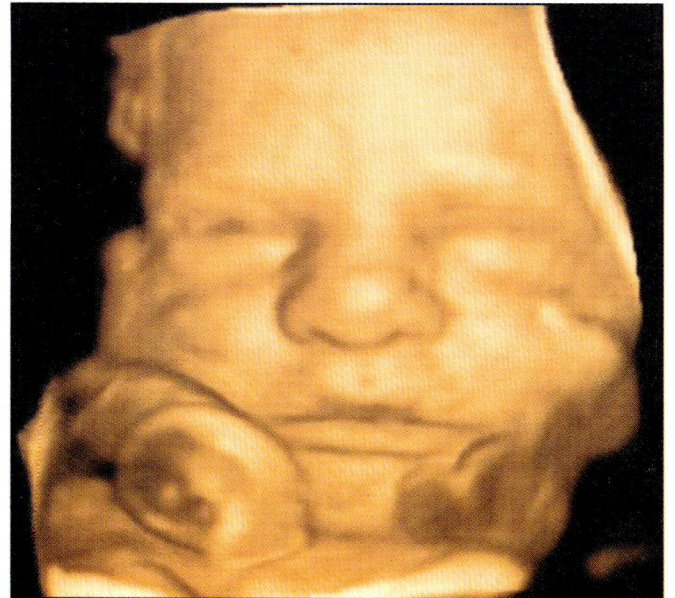

Fig. 15.24: Changing of the facial expression due to the movements of the bilateral parts of eyebrows

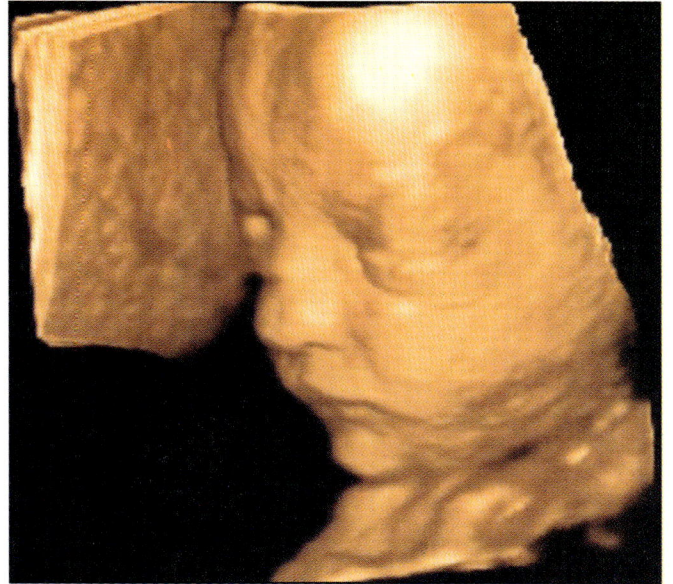

Fig. 15.26: Surface rendering demonstrates the beginning of opening of the right fetal eyelids

patterns in the third trimester between 30th and 33rd weeks of gestation in 10 gravidas.[56] The continuity between fetal and neonatal behavior have been published recently from Zagreb, Barcelona and Malaga groups.[57]

Limitations

As with any new technique, there are some limitations. Failure rates are reported in obtaining high-quality images in surface mode under certain circumstances such as oligohydramnios or the shadowing by hands, feet, umbilical cord or placenta (Fig. 15.34). Under these circumstances, it is advisable to re-examine the reconstructions together with the planar data of the same volume, in order to evaluate the direction of the ultrasound beam that is more visible on planar images than on those

sonography are complementary methods used for evaluation of fetal movements. It is clear that the quality of each fetal movement can be visualized and evaluated more reliably by 4D ultrasound. It appears that there are still not enough prospective studies that may clarify or prove real benefits of 3D ultrasound in daily practice and there is an urgent need for randomized control studies.[40] Our group have been evaluating fetal behavioral

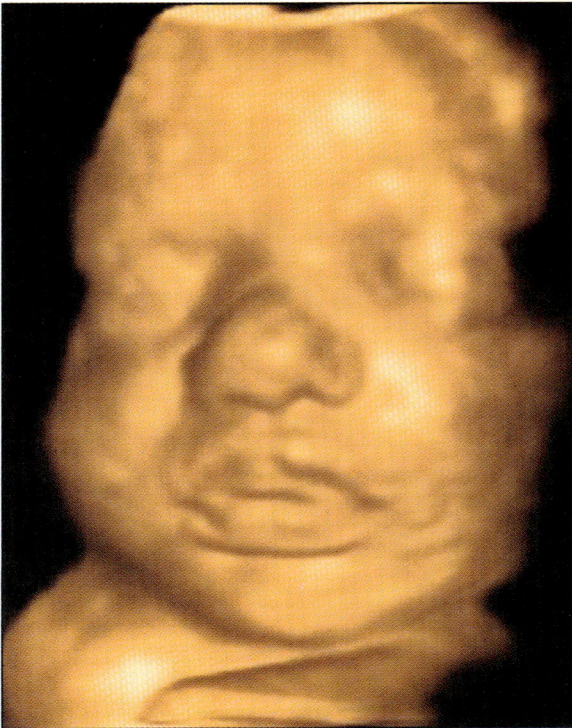

Fig. 15.27: Surface rendering of complete profile of the facial contour

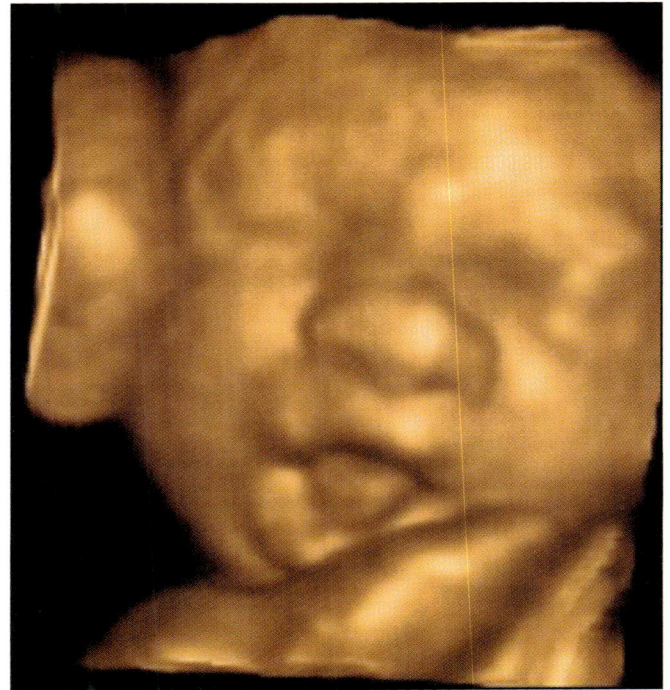

Fig. 15.29: 3D scan of the fetus in complete profile showing opening of the mouth. Note clear demonstration of the fetal lips

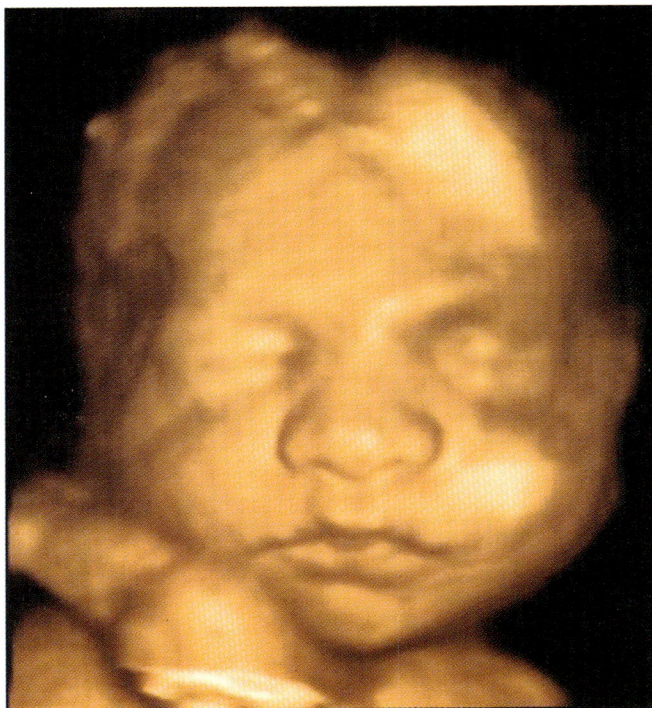

Fig. 15.28: Sleeping expression is clearly visible on this image

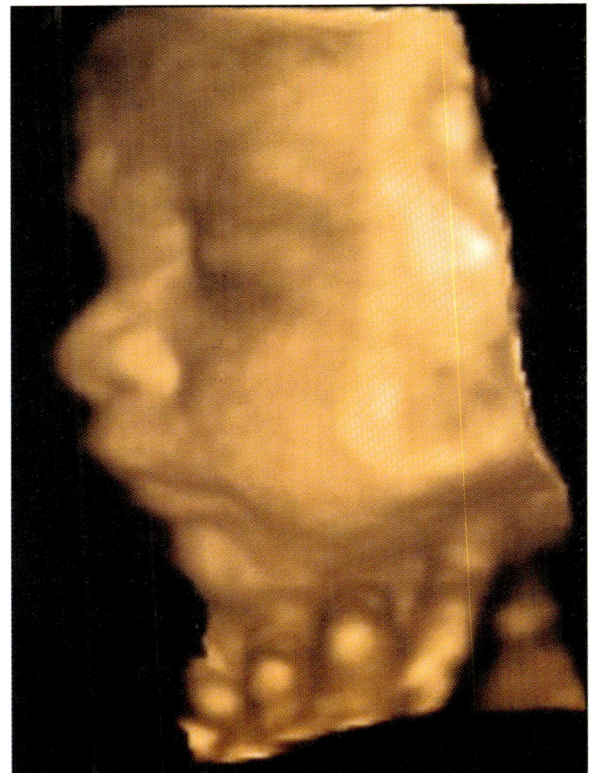

Fig. 15.30: Profile of the fetus by 3D surface rendering, with clear visualization of small anatomical features from the fingers

reconstructed. One report described how a totally normal fetal face appeared to have a cleft lip due to the shadow of the umbilical cord adjacent to the upper lip on the multiplanar images.[46] Sometimes, we have difficulties in identifying other surface features such as fingers and toes because they are frequently opposed to the wall of the uterus. An additional limitation of 4D ultrasound, at least for the moment, is the inability to display fetal movements that are too quick (within 1 to 2 sec) and subtle fetal movements such as those of breathing. However, many of these limitations may disappear in the near future as more powerful equipment is developed and appears on the market.

ASSESSMENT OF FETAL FACIAL EXPRESSION

We had classified several facial expressions at least to 8 different activities.

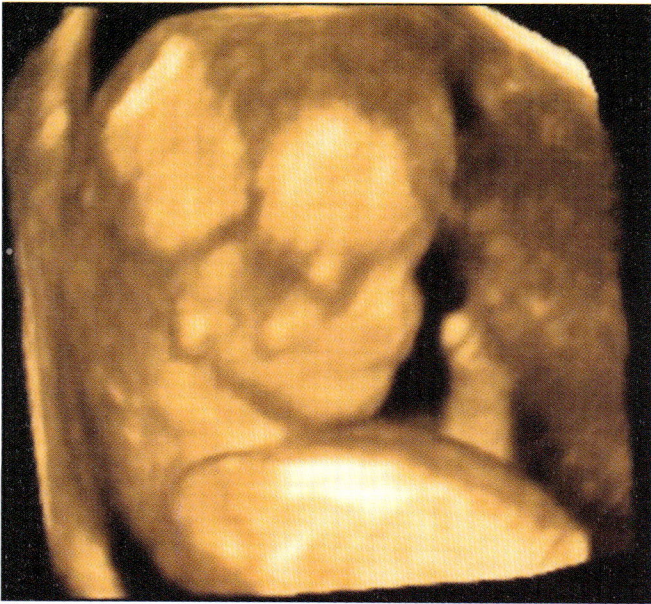

Fig. 15.31: 3D surface rendering of the facial contour in early pregnancy. Facial structures have reached an adequate degree of development in order to start studying them for diagnostic purposes

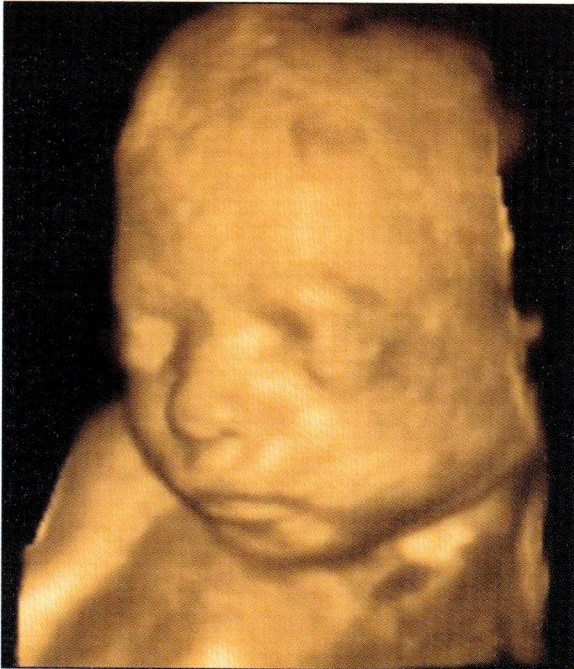

Fig. 15.32: High quality of fetal facial image could be obtained in the surface rendering mode when other structures is not shadowing the fetal face

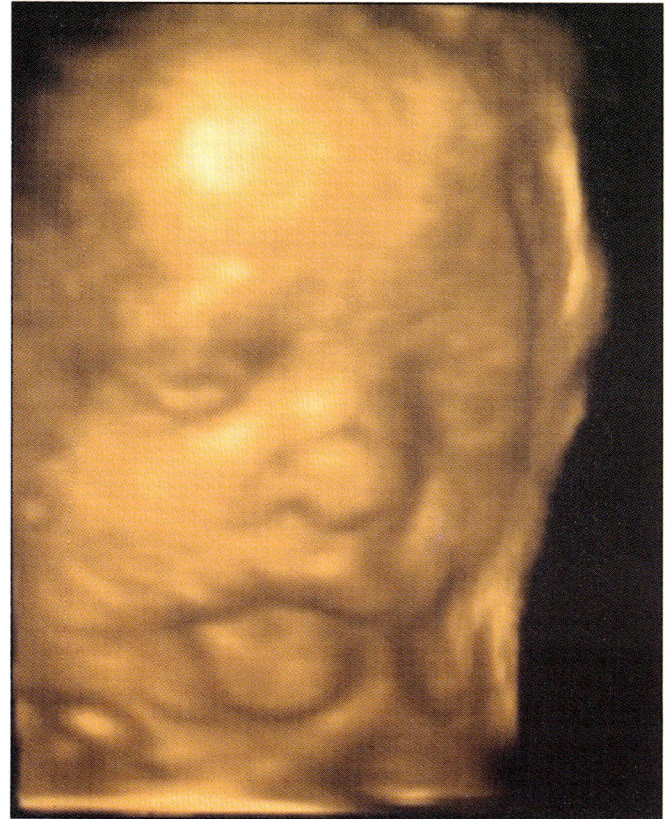

Fig. 15.33: 3D scan of the fetus in semi-profile position showing expulsion of the tongue

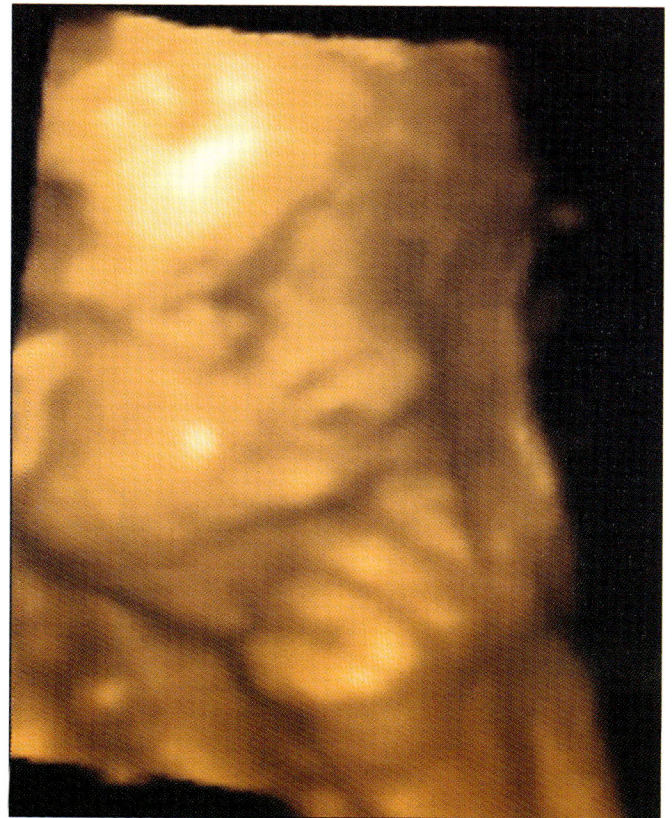

Fig. 15.34: 3D scan of the fetus in semi-profile position, the eyelids are opened and the surfaces of all visible facial features are discernible. The fetus seems to be observing the surrounding environment

Classification of Facial Patterns

1. *Yawning*: This movement is similar to the yawn observed after birth: An involuntary wide opening of the mouth, with maximal widening of the jaws followed by quick closure often with retroflexion of the head and sometimes elevation of the arms. This movement pattern is non-repetitive (Figs 15.54 and 15.55).

2. *Swallowing*: Indicating that the fetus is drinking amniotic fluid. Swallowing consists of displacements of tongue and/or larynx. Swallowing activity develops earlier than sucking in the course of fetal development (Fig. 15.115).

3. *Sucking*: Rhythmical bursts of regular jaw opening, and closing at a rate of about one per second. Placing the finger or thumb on the roof of the mouth behind the teeth and

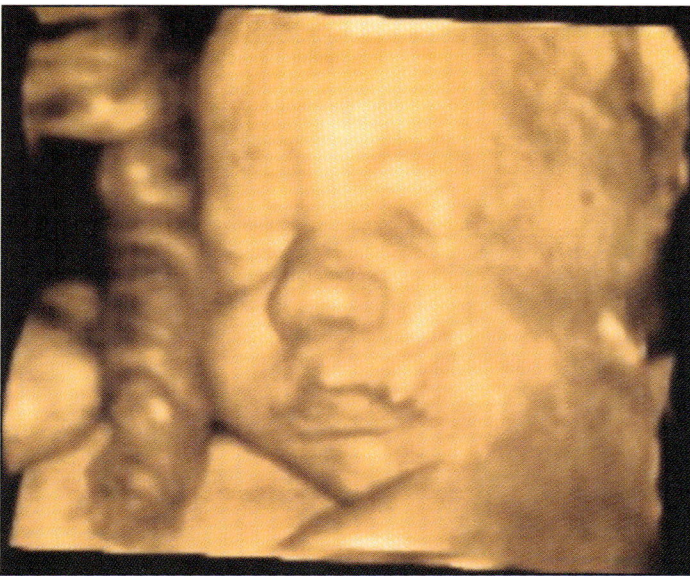

Fig. 15.35: 3D ultrasound of the fetus in the third trimester of gestation. Note clear demonstration of surrounding structure such us umbilical cord

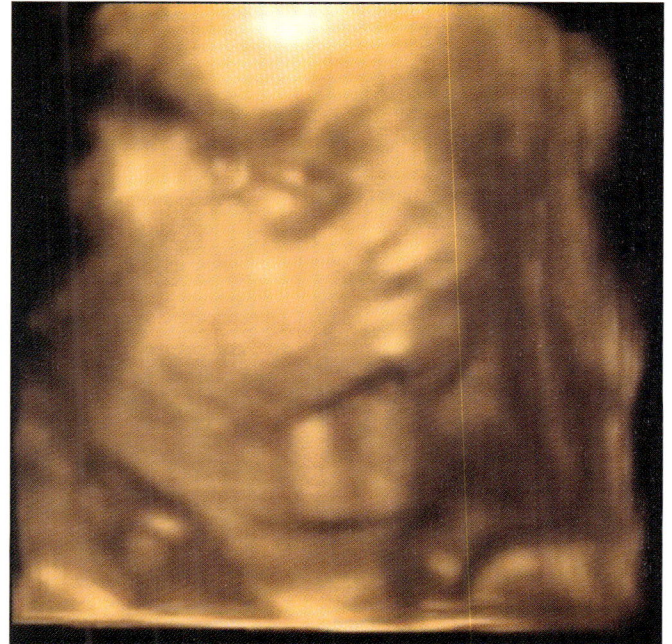

Fig. 15.37: 3D surface rendering shows the expulsion of the tongue and change of the facial expression due to eyelids opening

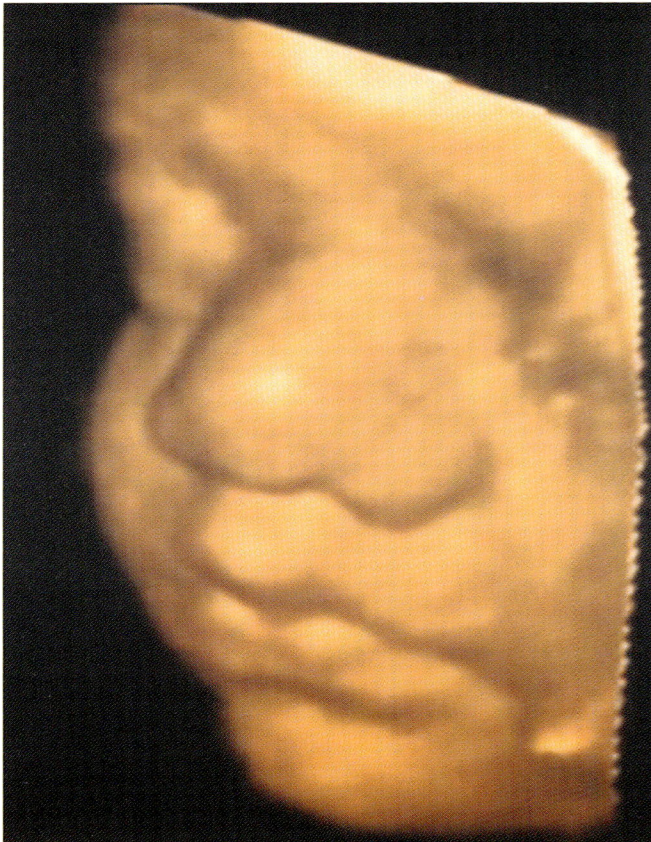

Fig. 15.36: 3D scan of the fetus in semi-profile position demonstrates clearly facial anatomy such as nose, mouth and eyelids

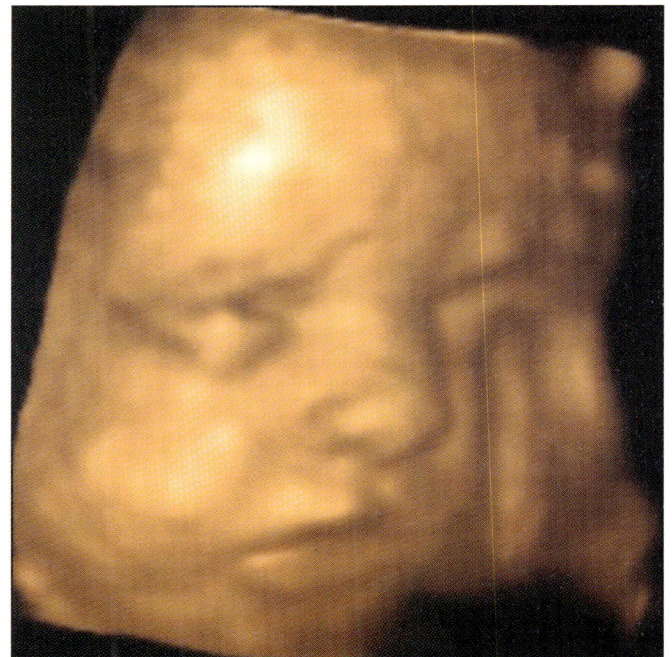

Fig. 15.38: Eyelids opening and clearly observable anatomy of the eyes such as the eyeballs

sucking with lips closed. Thumb sucking is a very frequent fetal behavioral pattern (Fig. 15.52).

4. *Smiling*: A facial expression characterized by turning up the corners of the mouth (Fig. 15.50).

5. *Tongue expulsion*: A facial expression characterized by expulsion of the tongue (Fig. 15.33).

6. *Grimacing*: The wrinkling of the brows or face in frowing to express of displeasure (Figs 15.103 and 15.104).

7. *Mouthing*: A facial expression characterized by mouth manipulation to investigate an object. Mouthing is most common in fetus and it may develop into a persistent, stereotyped behavior pattern (Fig. 15.113).

8. *Isolated eye blinking*: A reflex that closes and opens the eyes rapidly. Brief closing of the eyelids by involuntary normal periodic closing, as a protective measure, or by voluntary action (Figs 15.16 and 15.110).

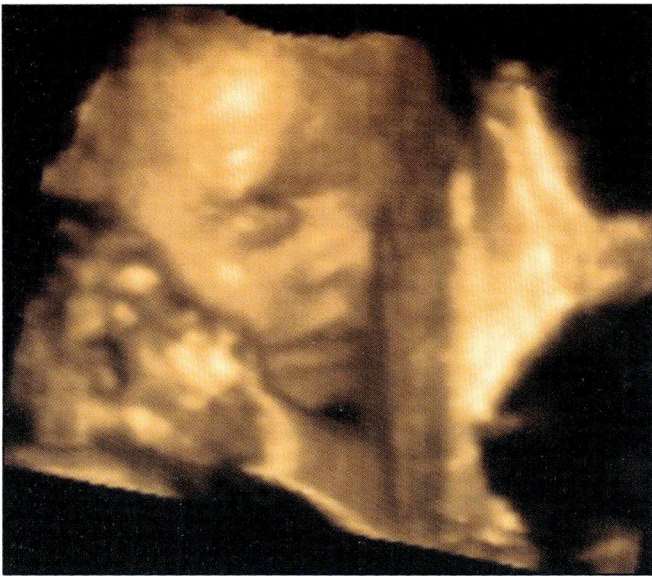

Fig. 15.39: The fetal hand is positioned on the right side of the fetal cheek and the entire face is discernible, with clear visualization of the eyeballs

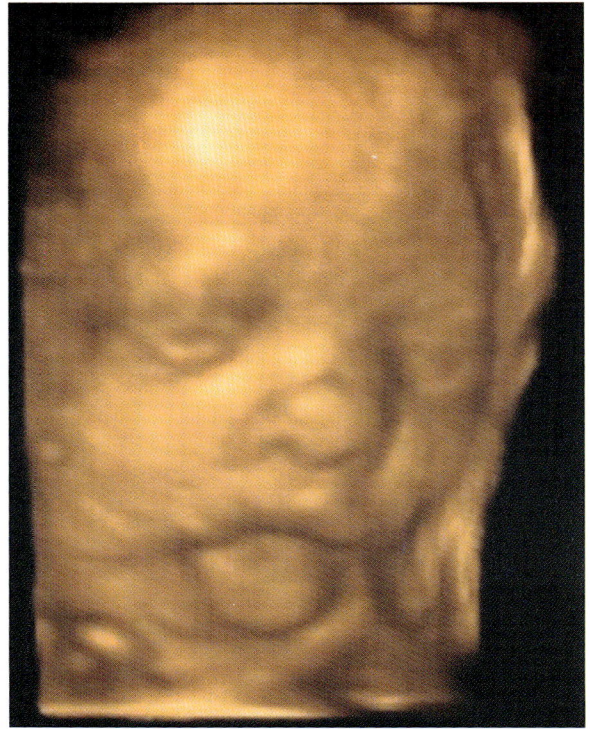

Fig. 15.40: Nuchal cord image around the fetal neck is obtained by 3D surface rendering

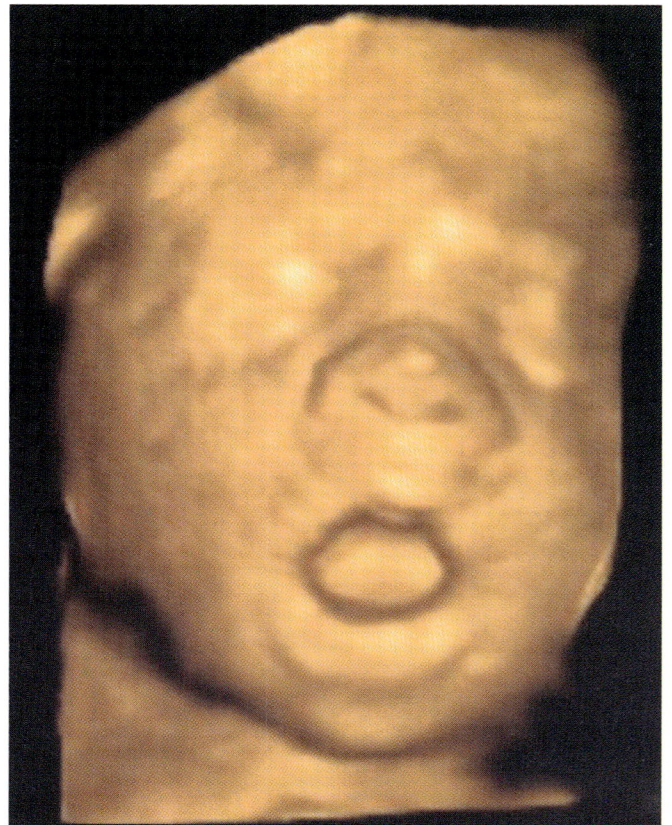

Fig. 15.41: Change in fetal expressions demonstrating opening of the mouth

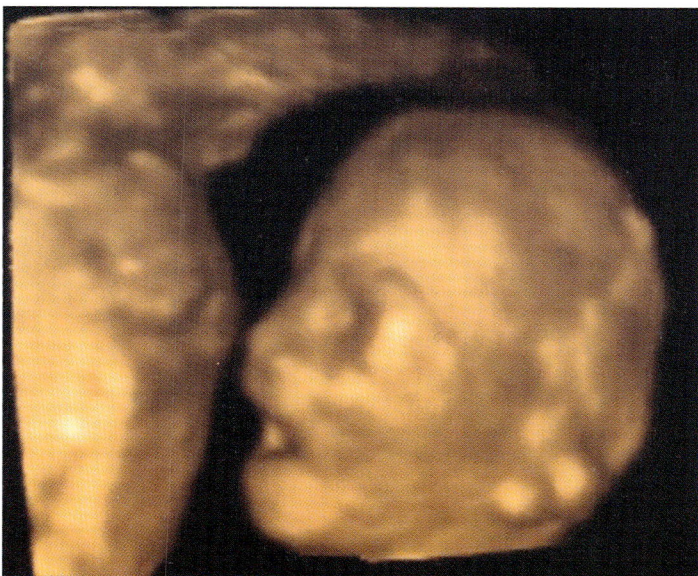

Fig. 15.42: Change in fetal expression due to expulsion of the tongue

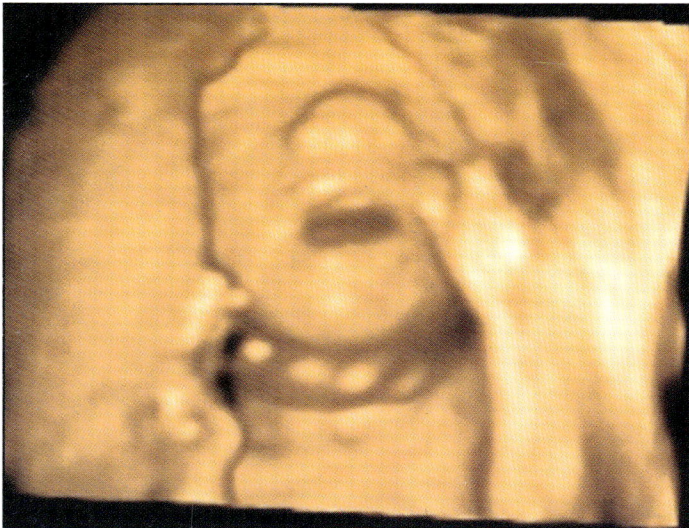

Fig. 15.43: Opening of the mouth is cleary visible

OPTIMUM CONDITIONS FOR 3D SCANNING OF THE FETAL FACE

For 3D visualization of the fetal face, the surface mode is generally used. This normally needs a shorter training period with acceptable results in a relatively limited period of time. It must be said, however, that the achievement of appropriate images

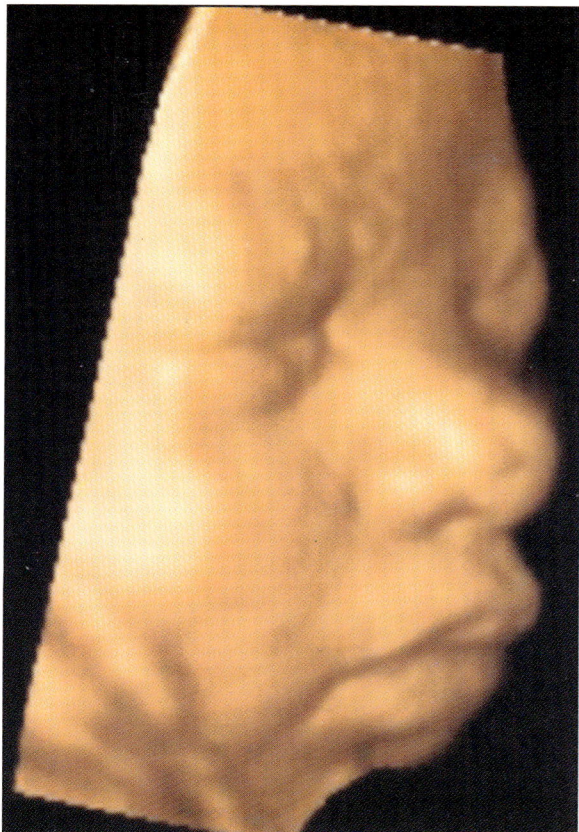

Fig. 15.44: High quality of semi-profile facial contour demonstrate the lips, nostrils and forehead

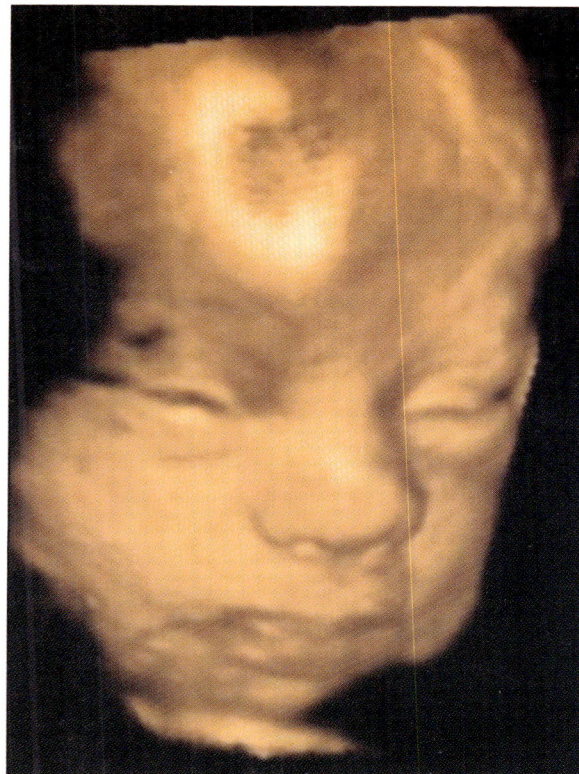

Fig. 15.46: 3D image shows the beginning of opening of the eyelids

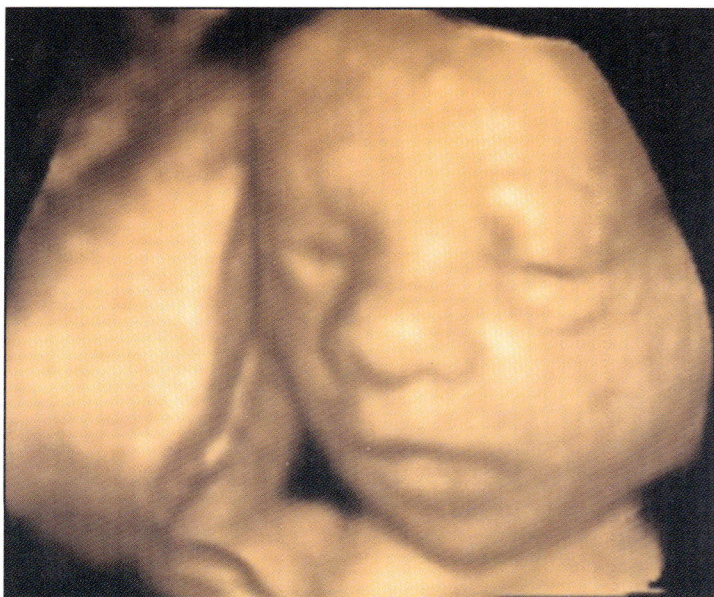

Fig. 15.45: Surface rendering demonstrates the beginning of opening of the eyelids. Note the fetus seems to be observing something in the left side

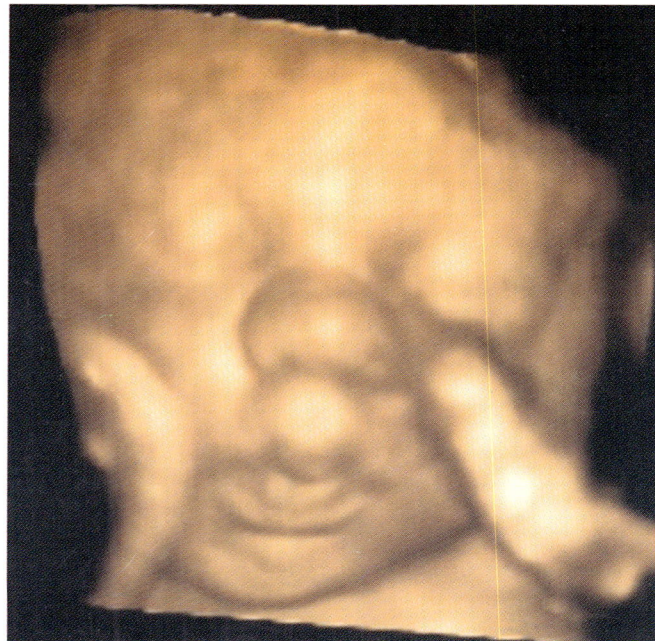

Fig. 15.47: Alteration of the facial expression is clearly visible on this image which illustrates the surrounding influence, altering the facial expression on one side

requires a set of previous conditions without which our results would probably be discouraging. It is clear that one of the great, advantages of 3D ultrasound is that the information remains captured as a volume and it is possible to reconstruct the recorded image and modify all the adjustments as if the patient was still present. This enables us to manipulate the image, re-rotate it three-dimensionally and achieve another 3D reconstruction from the data already taken. There are also electronic scalpels, which

assist by cutting off and eliminating all parts that can hide or distort the area we wish to study. With these facilities, we can improve the 3D reconstruction made from an image that is less than favorable.

Appropriate Gestational Age to Visualize the Fetal Face

The appropriate gestational age is neither too early (as the facial structures are not sufficiently developed) nor too late (the relative

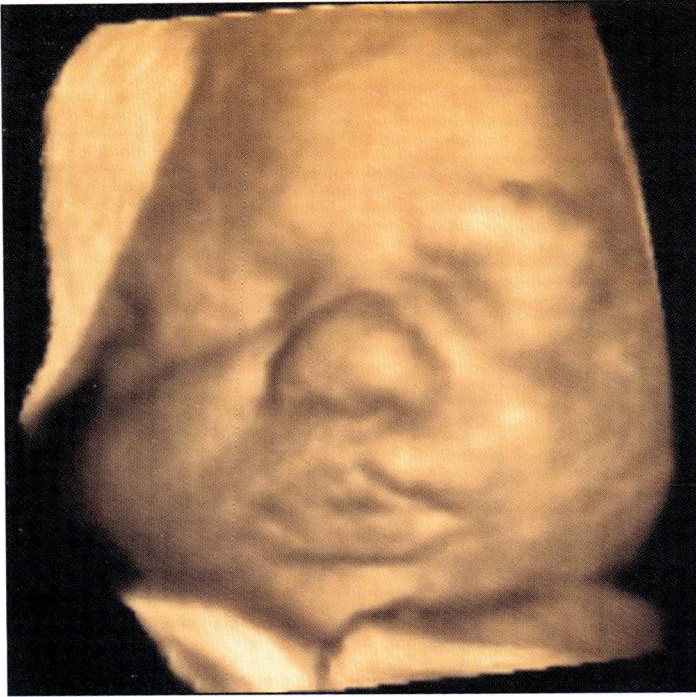

Fig. 15.48: 3D surface rendering of the fetal face shows alteration of the facial expression. Movement of the lateral side of facial musculature causes transient and slight asymmetry. However, it shoud be differentiated from pathlogical features such as unilateral paresis

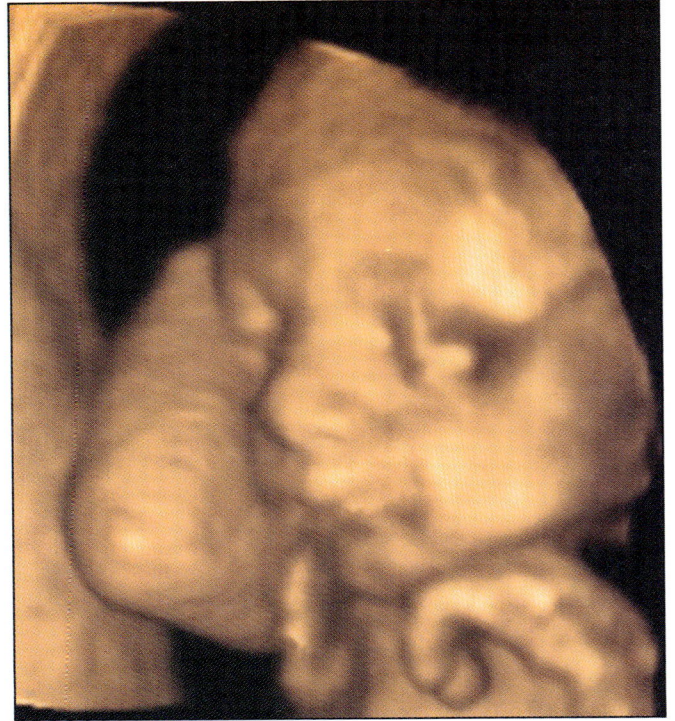

Fig. 15.50: The change of the facial expression due to turning up the corners of the mouth. The fetus appears to be smiling

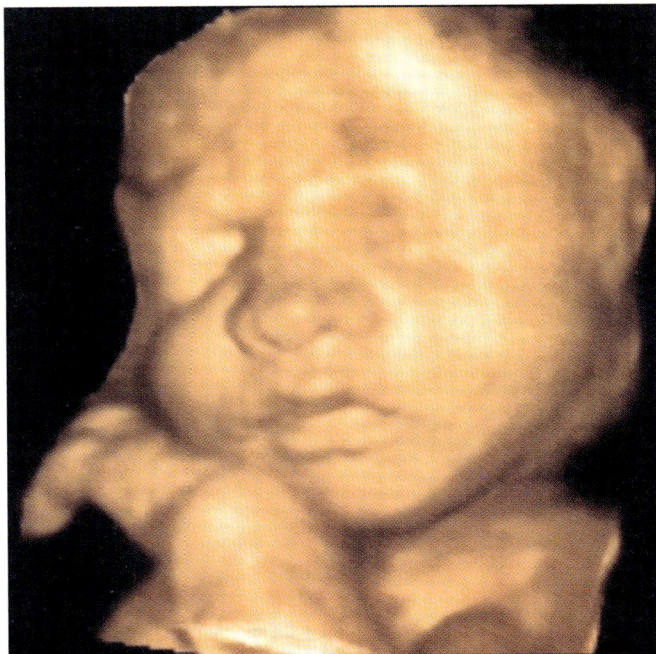

Fig. 15.49: The subtle alteration of the facial expression is clearly visible on this image which illustrates influence of the fetal hand

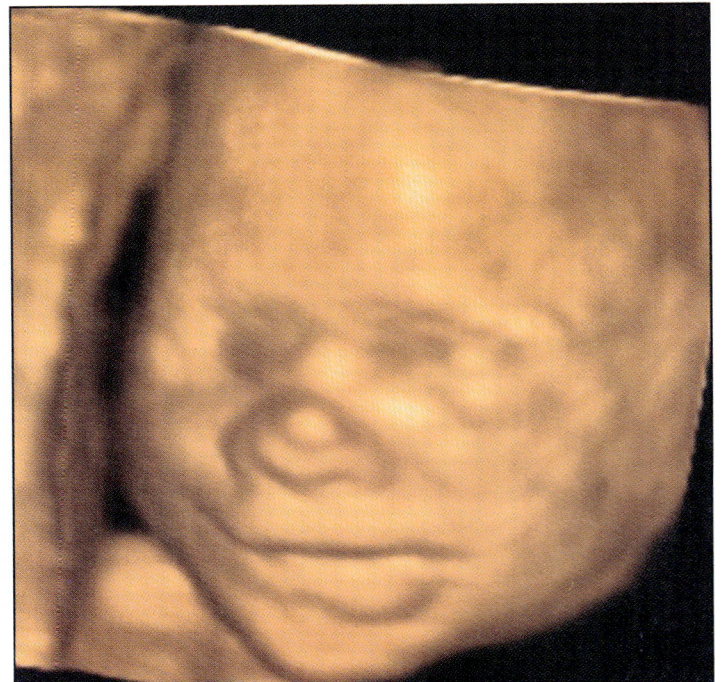

Fig. 15.51: A facial expression characterized by turning up the corners of the mouth. The fetus seems to be smiling

lack of space available during the last gestational weeks might hinder an appropriate visualization of the fetal face, due to its immediate closeness to the uterine wall, the placenta or the fetal extremities). From weeks 13 to 14, facial structures have reached an adequate degree of development in order to start studying them for diagnostic purposes. This may still be too early to show the mother any images if we support, at this stage, the contribution of the scan to reinforce the affective bonds between the fetus and the future parents. Our experience shows that it is

counterproductive to show the 3D image of the fetal face to the parents during the first trimester. For most parents, the image appears to be strange and it can create a distorted image of their child, which will not reinforce the affective bonds. It could indeed create anxiety. From weeks 18 to 19, we can obtain 3D reconstruction of the fetal face which is starting to show clear facial features[58] and these can be shown to the parents. From this moment and until week 35 or 36, we can obtain 3D reconstructions of the facial surface in a high percentage of

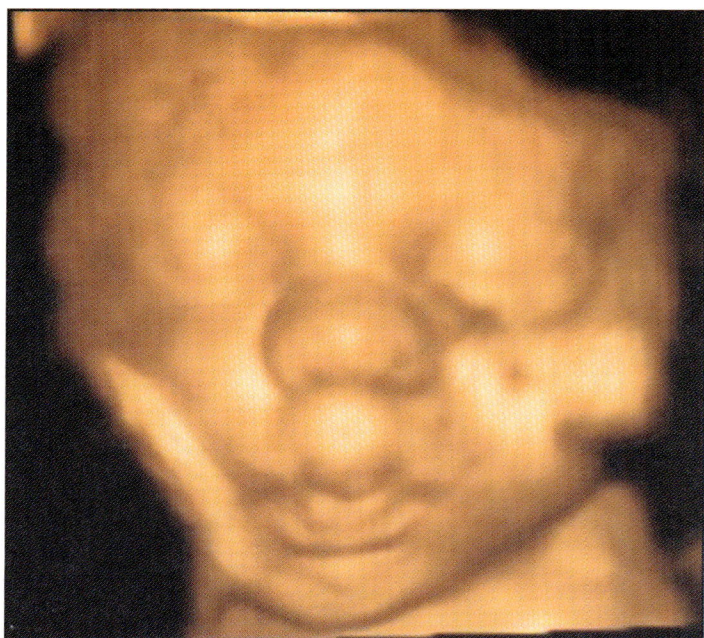

Fig. 15.52: A facial expression characterized by mouthing expression. This is most common in fetus and it may develop into a persistent, stereotyped behavior pattern

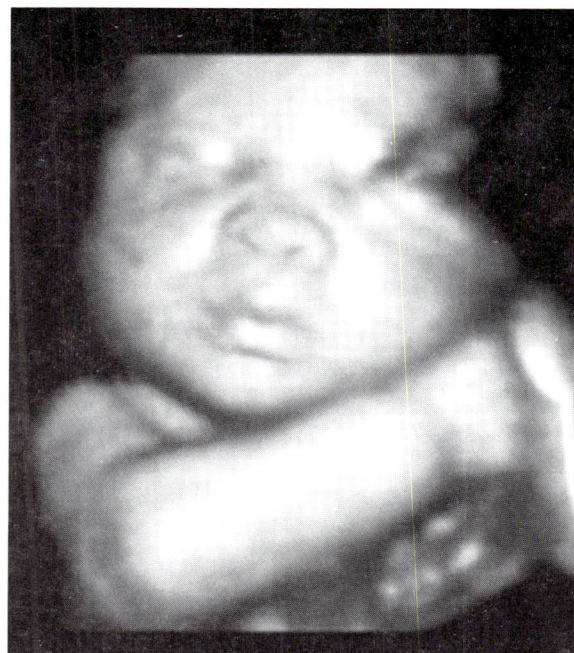

Fig. 15.54: The entire face is discernible, with clear visualization of the right arm positioned on the left shoulder

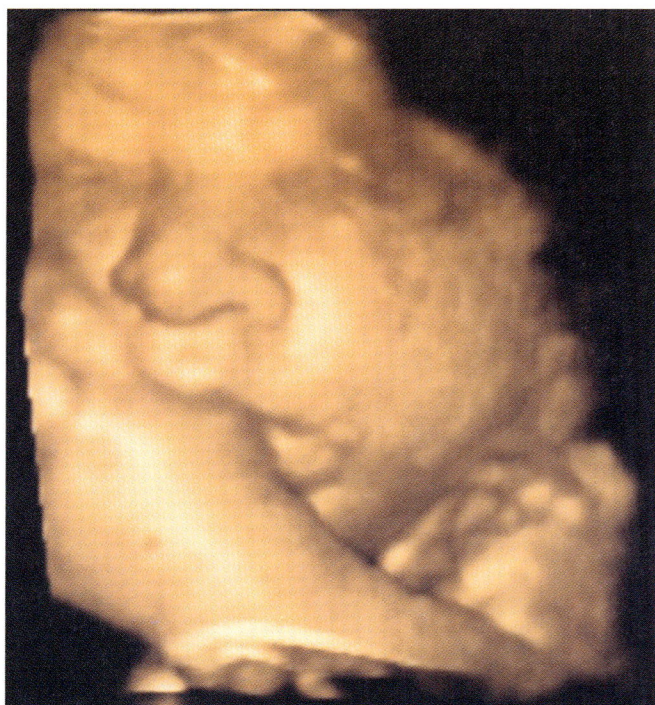

Fig. 15.53: The fetus is placing the finger or thumb on the roof of the mouth behind the teeth and sucking with lips closed. Thumb sucking is a very frequent fetal behavioral pattern

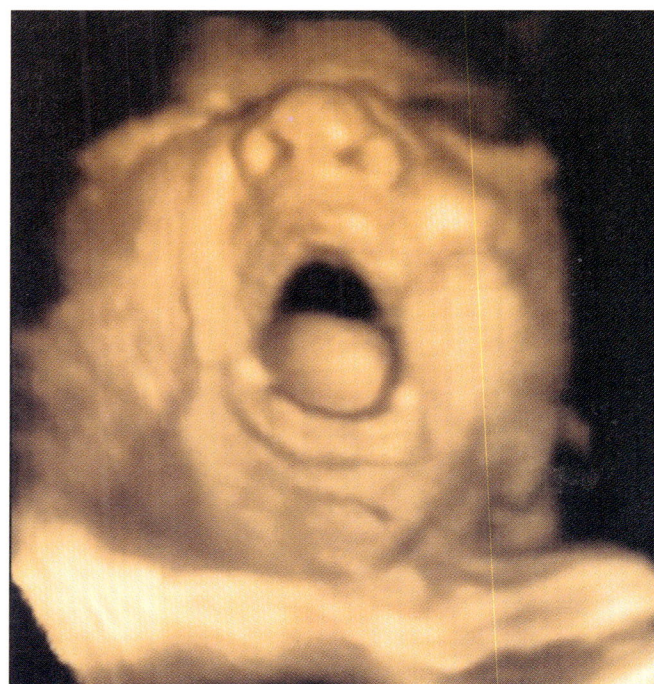

Fig. 15.55: Yawn expression is defined as an involuntary wide opening of the mouth, with maximal widening of the jaws followed by quick closure

Favorable Fetal Position

mothers. Experience and much patience are needed to wait for the fetus to adopt an appropriate position for this type of scanning.[59] We think that the most favorable age for 3D scanning of the fetal face is from weeks 23 until 30. During this period of gestation, we have succeeded in visualizing the face three-dimensionally in a high percentage of the cases (higher than 70 %) without extending the length of the prenatal 2D ultrasound scan.

To obtain the best images, the probe has to be moved so that the face of the fetus is facing the probe surface. In addition, it is very important for the fetal face not to be in contact with other structures such as the uterine wall, the placenta or fetal extremities. Sometimes, it will be of much assistance to stimulate the fetus using the free hand over the abdominal wall. The fetus may then change position and move away from the structures that prevent correct visualization. Once the correct position is

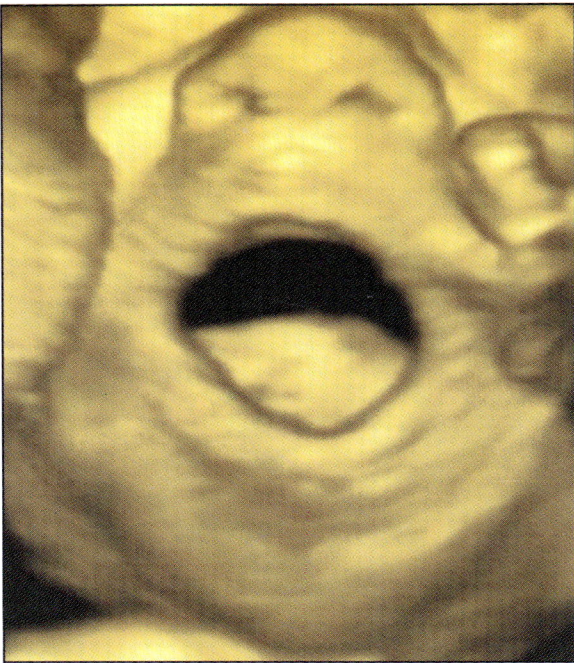

Fig. 15.56: 3D surface rendering of fetal yawning. This movement is often followed by retroflexion of the head and sometimes elevation of the arms

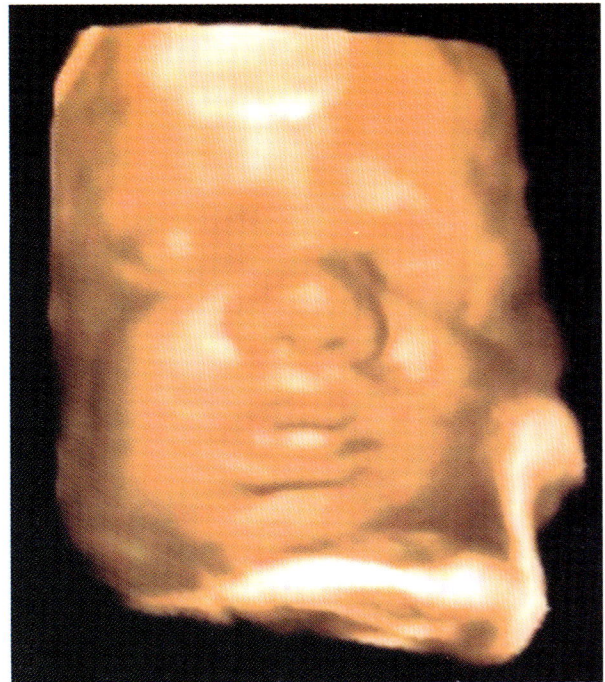

Fig. 15.58: Full profile of the fetal face showing distinct contour of facial musculature

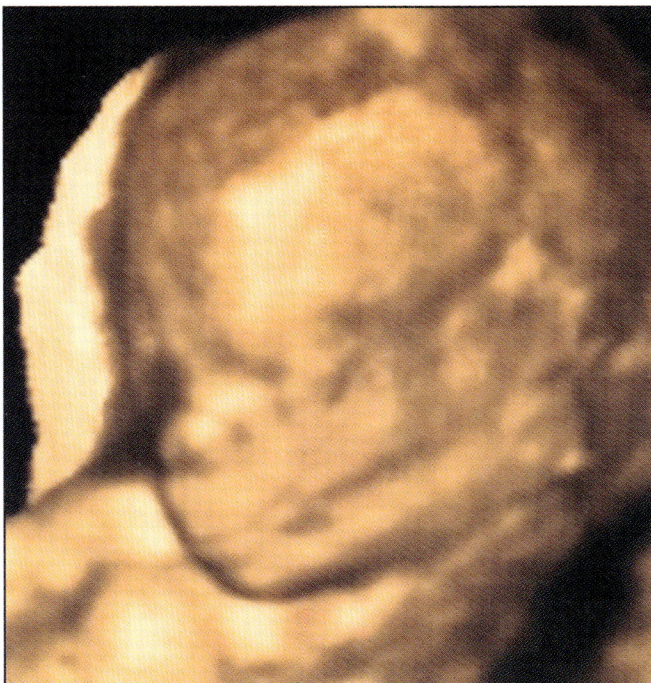

Fig. 15.57: 3D scan of facial expression in the second trimester of gestation is adequate enough for diagnostic purpose

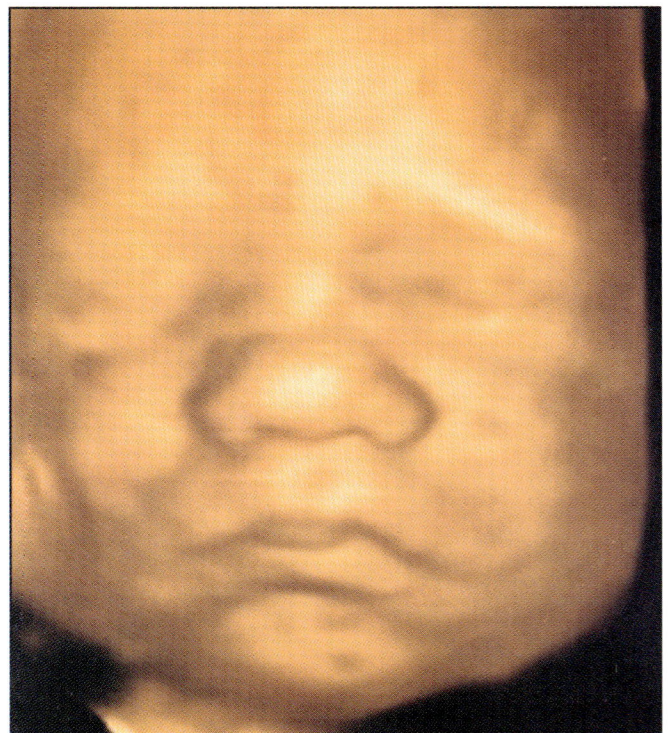

Fig. 15.59: Both of the eyes and the mouth are closed and the fetus appears calm

obtained, the capture box is placed over the reference line in the closest possible way to the fetal face. We will have to wait for the baby to keep still, if we seek a static 3D reconstruction, or to make facial movements (yawning, suctioning, lids opening) if we seek a 4D scanning.

Post-processing of the Image

In addition to these previous requirements, one should not forget that, after capturing the image, there are many adjustment possibilities. Amongst all the tools we have at the moment, the

most useful one is the electronic scalpel, which allows us to eliminate all areas that are of no interest, and also those which disturb the demonstration of the structure that we wish to visualize. This tool can be used in both multiplanar and 3D images. The control of all these adjustments, possibilities and tools does take time, but, the final achievement of images shown will surely compensate for all our efforts.

Once we have acquired this experience, we can verify that, while all the procedures stated here are very complicated and

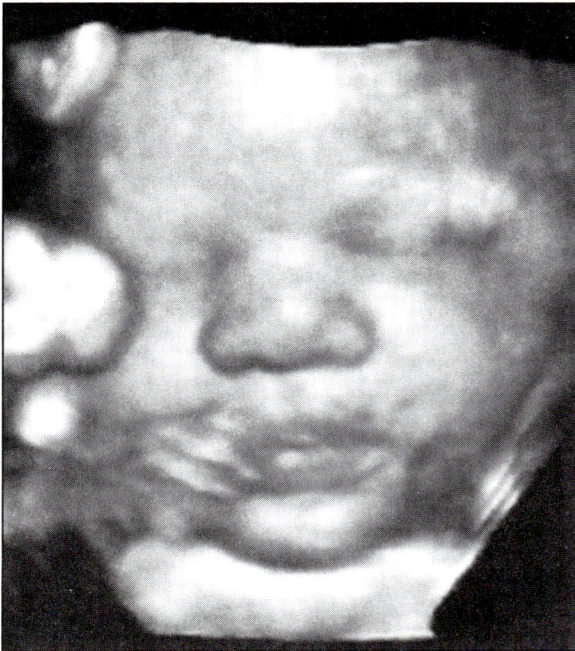

Fig. 15.60: Calm and tranquil expression of the fetus obtained by 3D technique

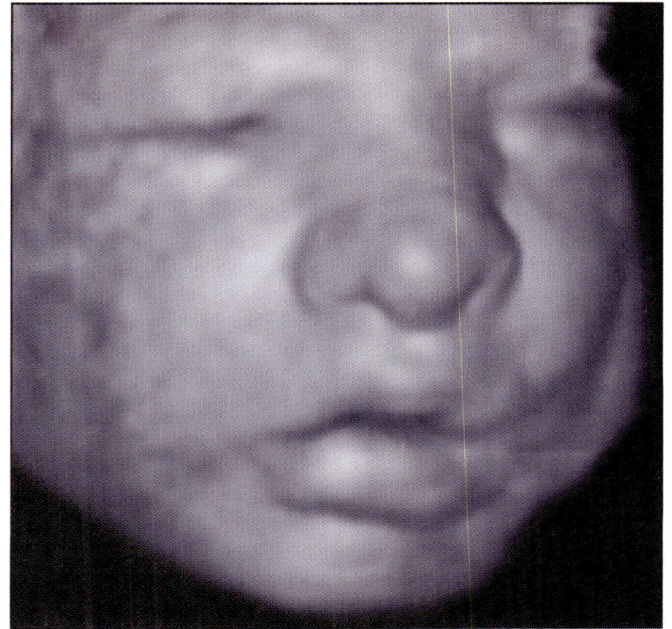

Fig. 15.62: Surface rendering shows the beginning of eyelids opening. Note clear demonstration of the facial contour of the fetal lips

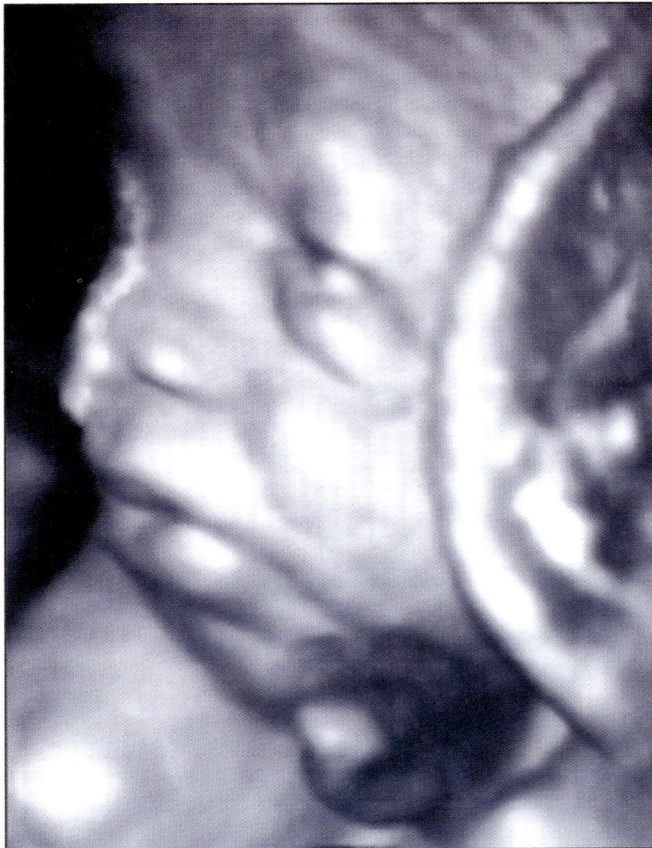

Fig. 15.61: 3D scan of the fetus in semi-profile image. The eyelids are opened and the surfaces of all visible facial features are distinctly clear

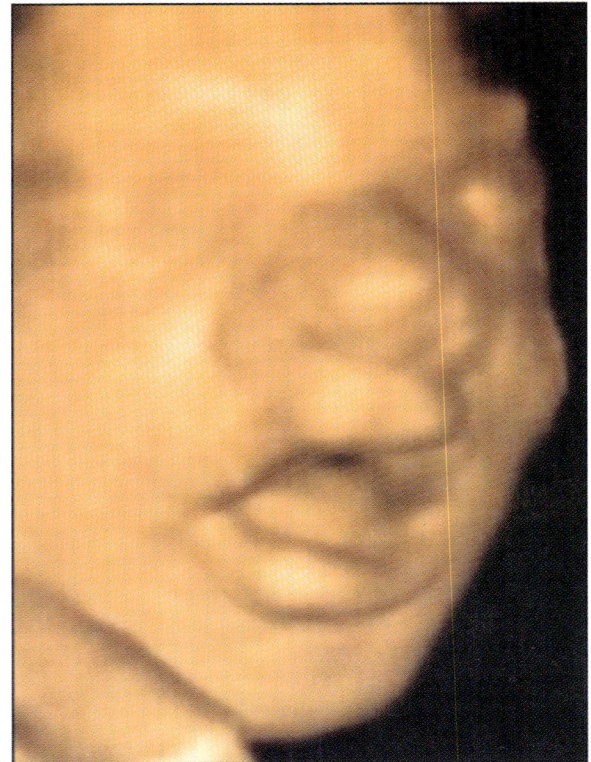

Fig. 15.63: The beginning of opening of the fetal mouth

complex, with time they become relatively easy and, in fact, require only a few seconds to adjust the equipment and just a few minutes to re-touch the 3D reconstruction. Usually, we start the conventional scanning and, when we acquire a favorable position of the fetal face, we interrupt the 2D exploration and capture the image for 3D reconstruction, following which 2D ultrasound study is then continued. With this procedure, we can achieve 3D visualization of the fetal face without adding more than 3 or 4 min to the complete length of the usual ultrasound scanning.

CONCLUSIONS

Three-dimensional ultrasound offers the possibility of studying the fetal face in a more global way than conventional two-dimensional ultrasound. In normal cases, the images obtained

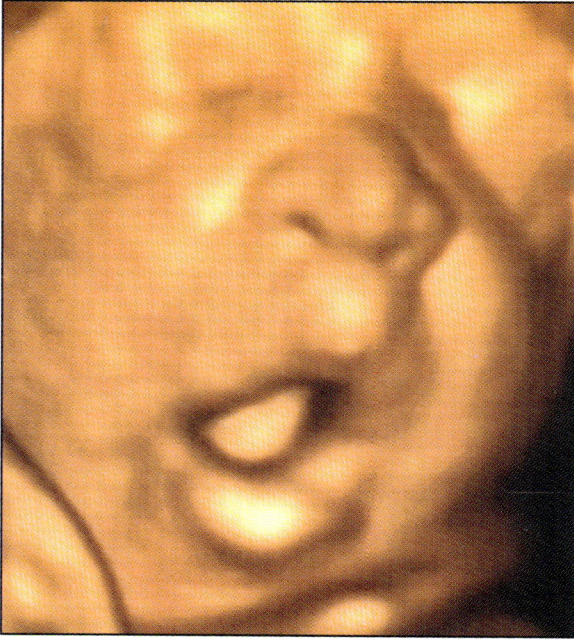

Fig. 15.64: The ending of maximal opening of the mouth

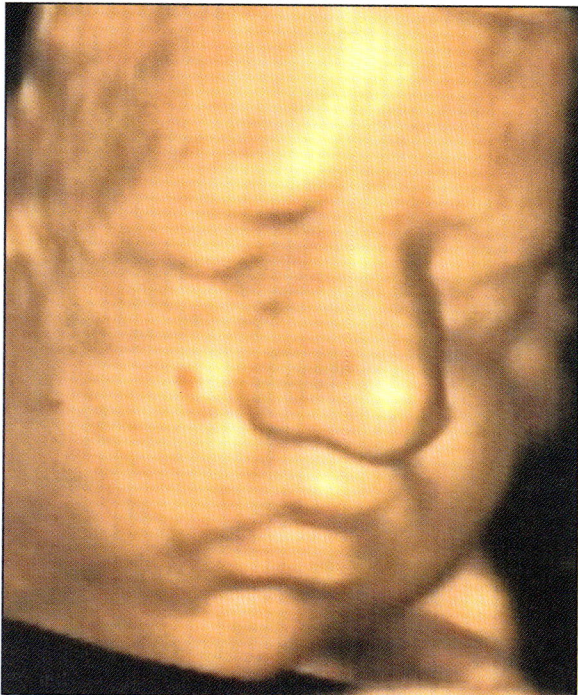

Fig. 15.66: Calm expression of the fetus is obtained by 3D surface rendering

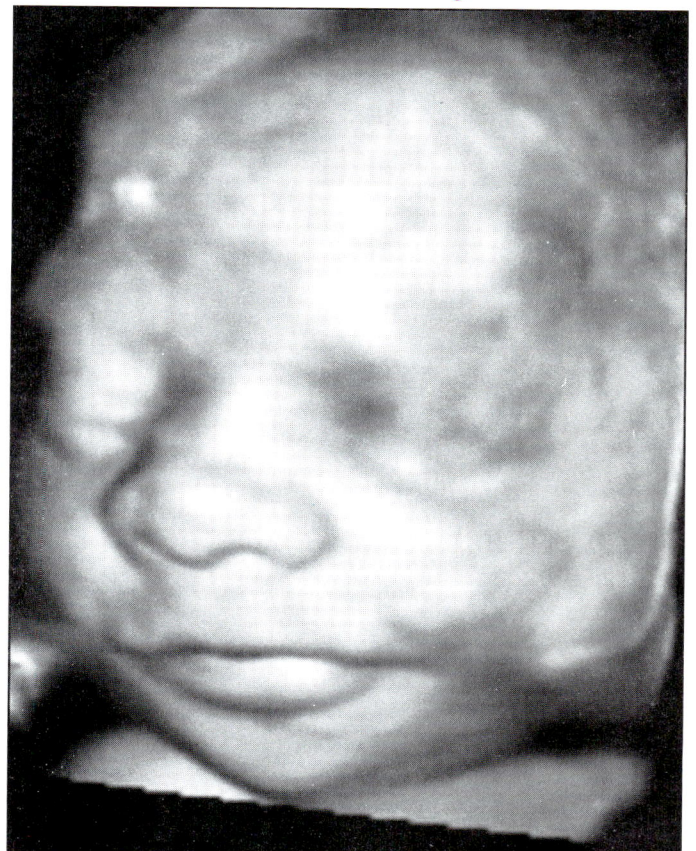

Fig. 15.65: The change of the facial expression due to movements of the lateral parts of the eyebrows and the facial musculature between them is clearly visible

help transmit a feeling of calmness to the parents and reinforce the affective bonds with their child. In pathological cases, three-dimensional ultrasound can help parents and other doctors involved to take a more realistic view of the problem. It is expected that the use of this novel technology will provide parents with the knowledge to have a better judgement whilst taking decisions. Four-dimensional ultrasound has enormous potential in perinatal research. This technique is still in its infancy but there is much scope for investigation of fetal anatomy as well as fetal behavior. This technique should assist us in the better understanding of

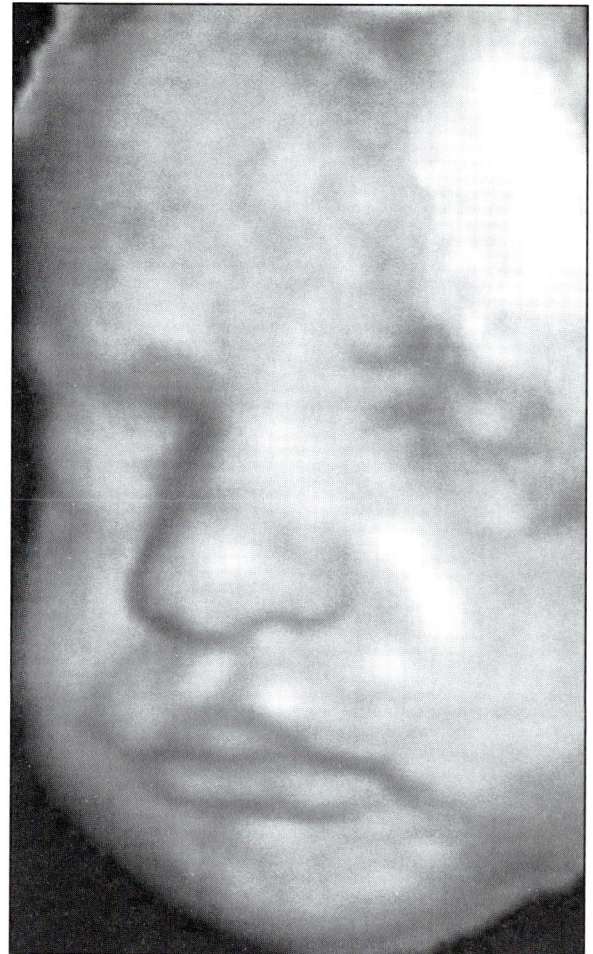

Fig. 15.67: Smiling expression of the fetus. Both of the lateral side of the mouth is turning up

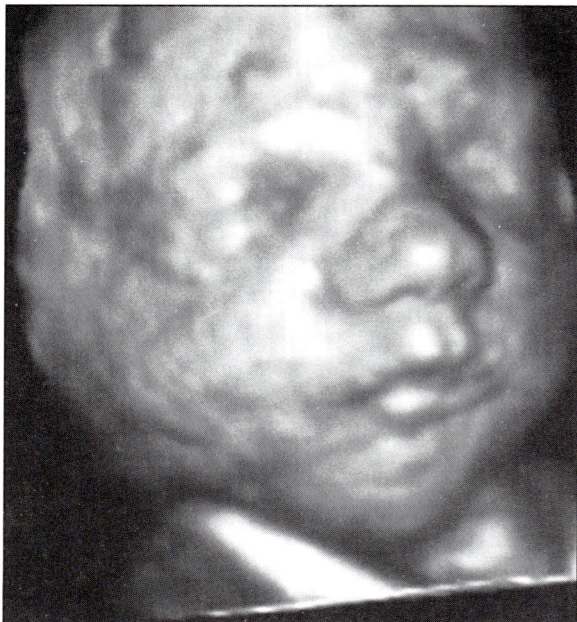

Fig. 15.68: The fetus appears to be calm in this 3D image

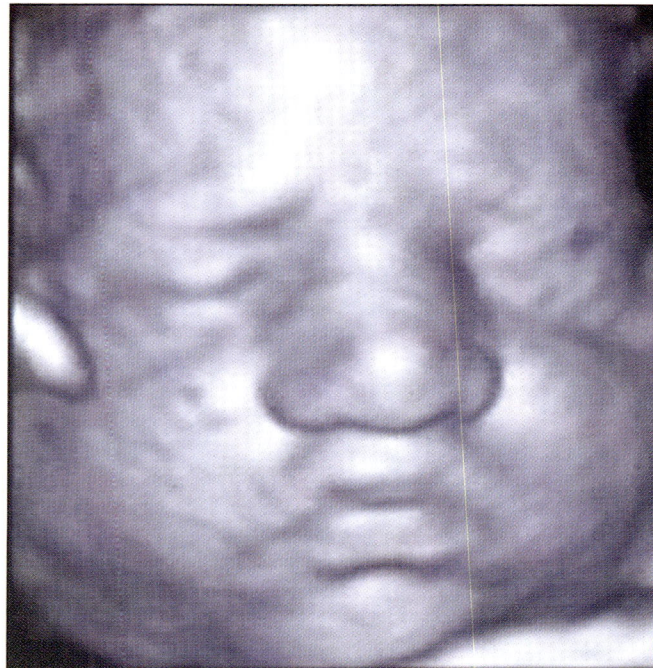

Fig. 15.70: The frontalis muscle also can be responsible for the appearance of grimacing. However, the main agent responsible for the appearance of scowling is the corrugator muscle. The fetus seems to be sad.

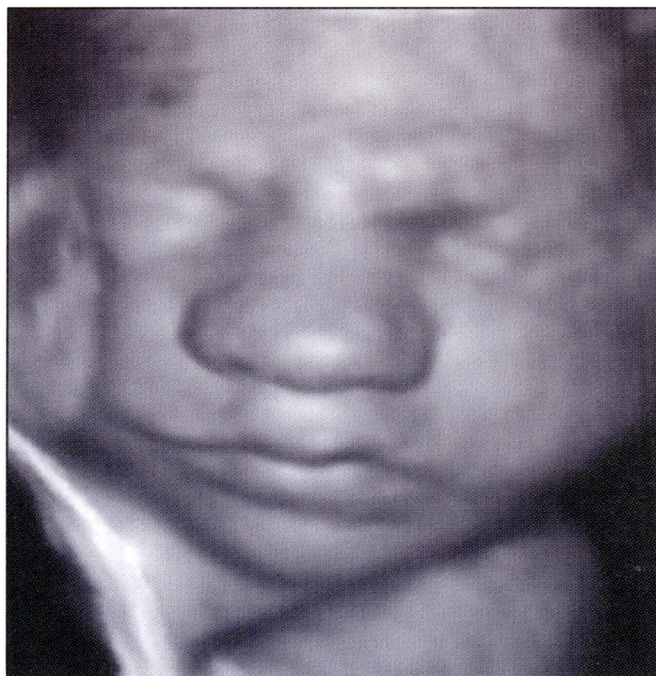

Fig. 15.69: Grimacing expression demonstrated by 3D surface rendering

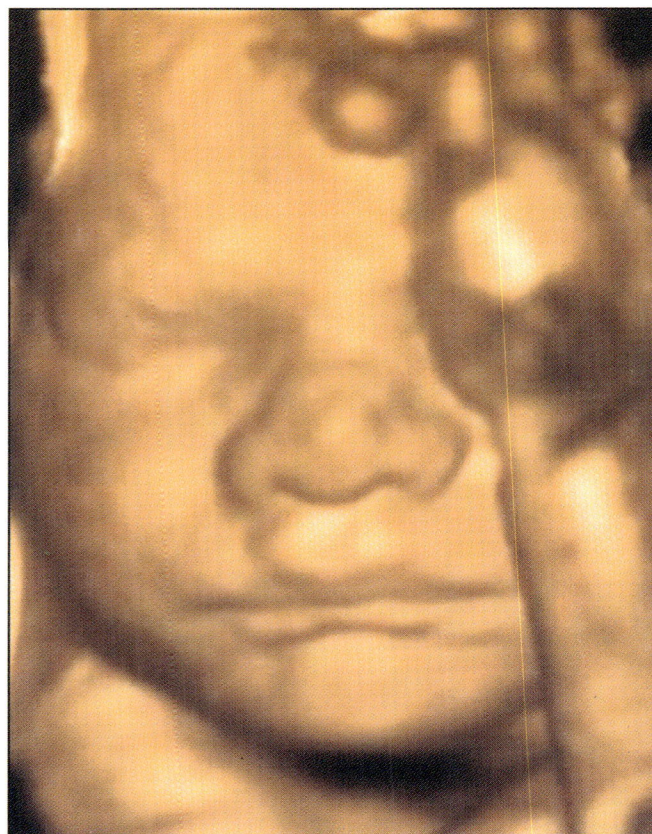

Fig. 15.71: Both of the mouth and eyes are closed and fetus appears tranquil

both the somatic and functional development of the early embryo and the fetus.

REFERENCES

1. Baba K, Okai T, Kozuma S. Real-time processable three-dimensional fetal ultrasound. Lancet 1996; 348:1307.

2. Baba K, Satoh K, Sakamoto S, Okai T, Ishi IS. Development of an ultrasonic system for three-dimensional reconstruction of the foetus. J Perinat Med 1989; 17:24.

3. Baba K, Okai T, Kozuma S, Taketani Y, Mochizuki T, Akahane M. Real-time processable three-dimensional US in obstetrics. Radiology 1997;203:571-4.

4. Bonilla-Musoles F, Raga F, Osborne N, Blanes J. Ecografia tridimensional en Obstetncia y Ginecologia. Obstet Ginecol Espan 1994;3:233-50.

5. Bonilla-Musoles F, Raga F, Blanes J, Osborne N, Siles CH. Three-dimensional ultrasound in reproductive medicine: preliminary report. Hum Reprod Update 1995,1:4 item 21 CDRom.

6. Bonilla-Musoles F, Machado L. Ultrasonidos y Reproduccion. Cuadernos de Medicina Reproductiva, No 2. Madrid: Panamericana Ed., 1999;6.

7. Devonald KJ, Ellwood D, Cnffiths K, et al. Volume imaging: three-dimensional appreciation of the fetal head and faceJ J Ultrasound Med 1995,14:919-26.

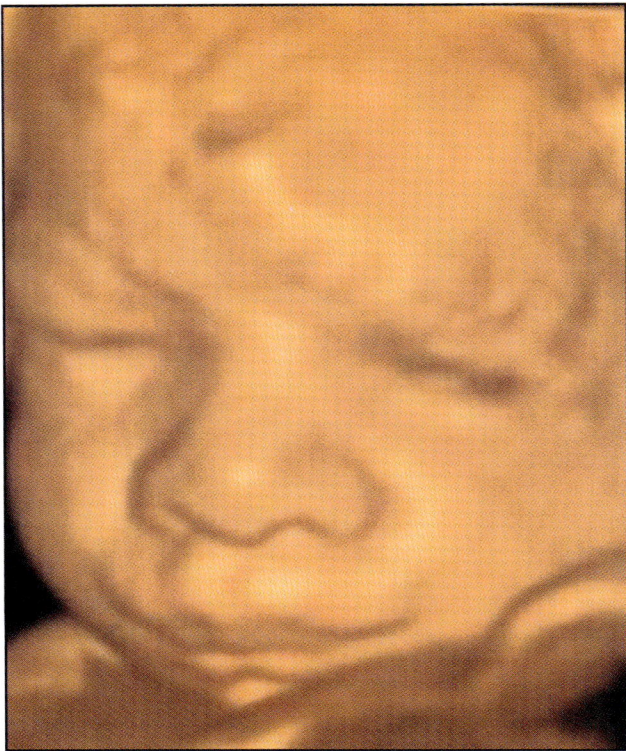

Fig. 15.72: The fetus seems trying to manipulate something with mouth in this 3D image

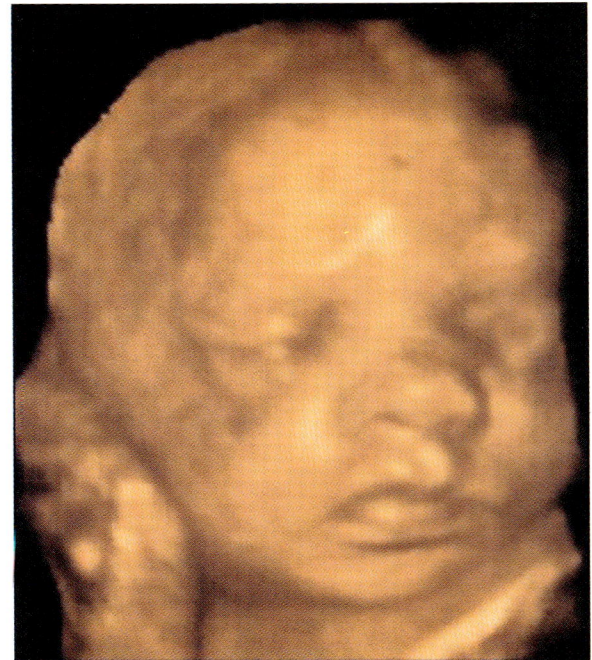

Fig. 15.74: High quality of full profile of the fetal expression shows sleeping expression

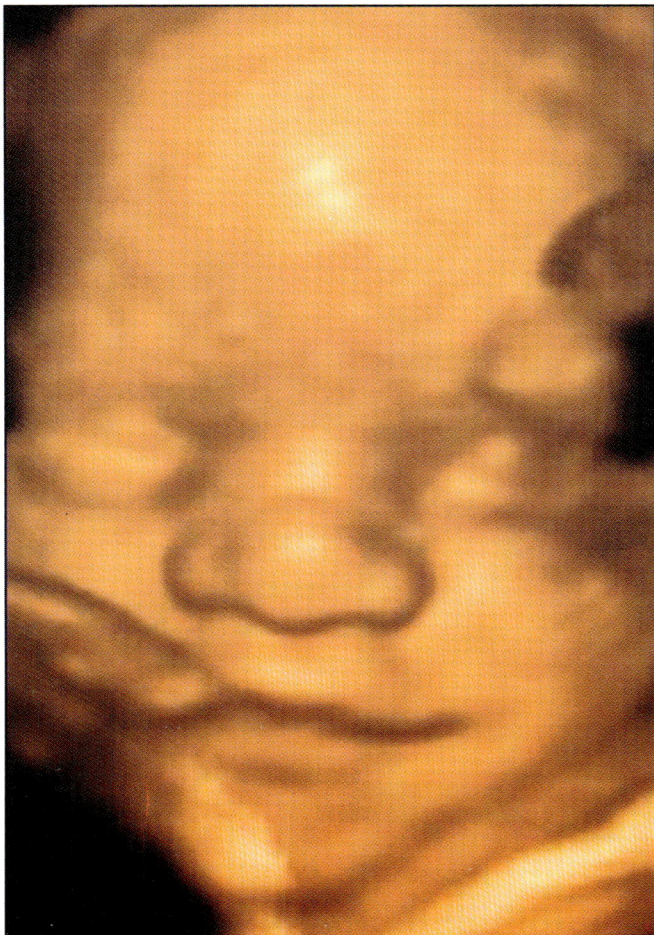

Fig. 15.73: Smiling expression is obtained by 3D surface technique

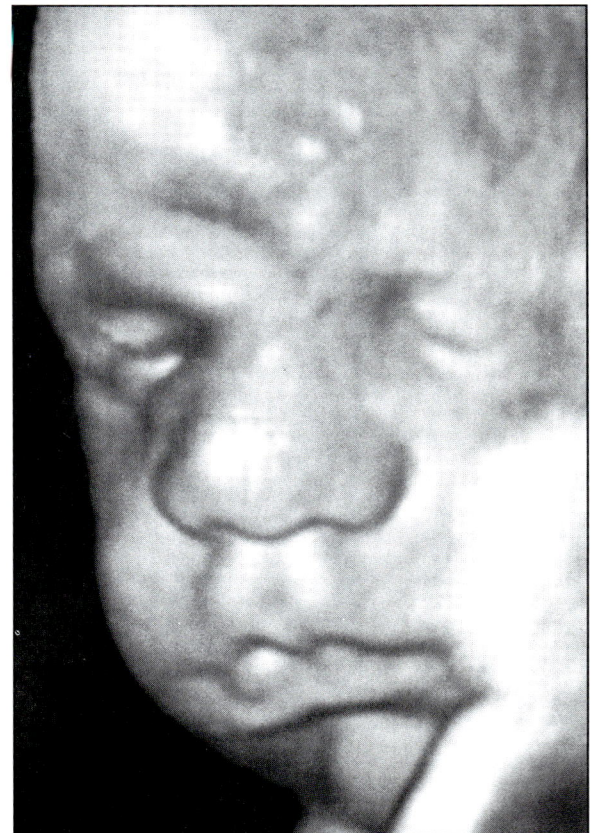

Fig. 15.75: Asymmetry of the facial expression due to movement of lateral side of the fetal facial musculature

8. Hull AD, Pretorius DH. Fetal face: what we can see using two-dimensional and three-dimensional ultrasound. Semin Roentgenol 1998;33:369-74.

9. Hata T, Yonehara T, Aoki S, Manabe A, Hata K, Miyazaki K. Three-dimensional sonographic visualization, of the fetal face. Am J Roentgenol 1998; 170:481-3.

10. Kelly IMC, Cardener JE, Lees WR. Three-dimensional fetal ultrasound. Lancet 1991;339:1062-4.

11. Kelly IMC, Cardener JE, Brett AD, Richards RR, Lees WR. Three-dimensional US of the fetus. Work in progress. Radiology 1994; 192:253-9.

12. Kratochwil A. Versuch der 3-dimensionalen Darstellung in der Ceburtshilfe. Ultraschall Med 1992; 13:183-6.

13. Kuo HC, Chang FM, Wu CH, Yao BL, Liu CH. The primary application of three-dimensional ultrasonography in obstetrics. Am J Obstet Gynecol 1992; 166:880-6.

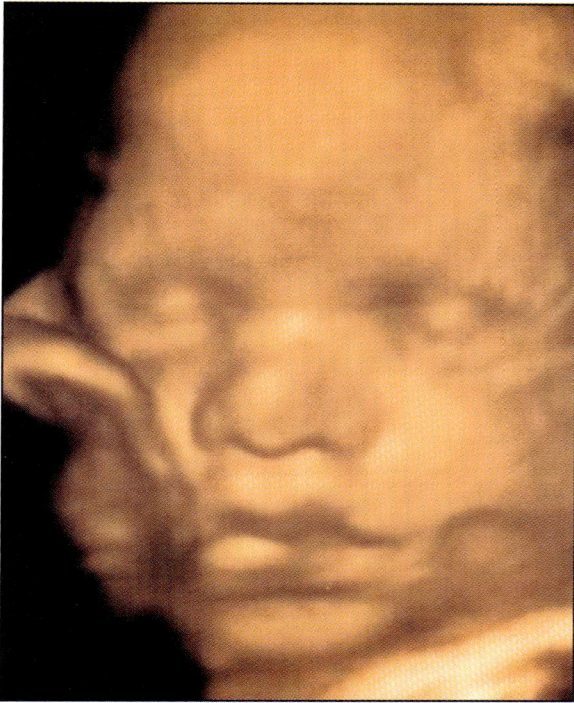

Fig. 15.76: Sleeping expression is cleary depicted

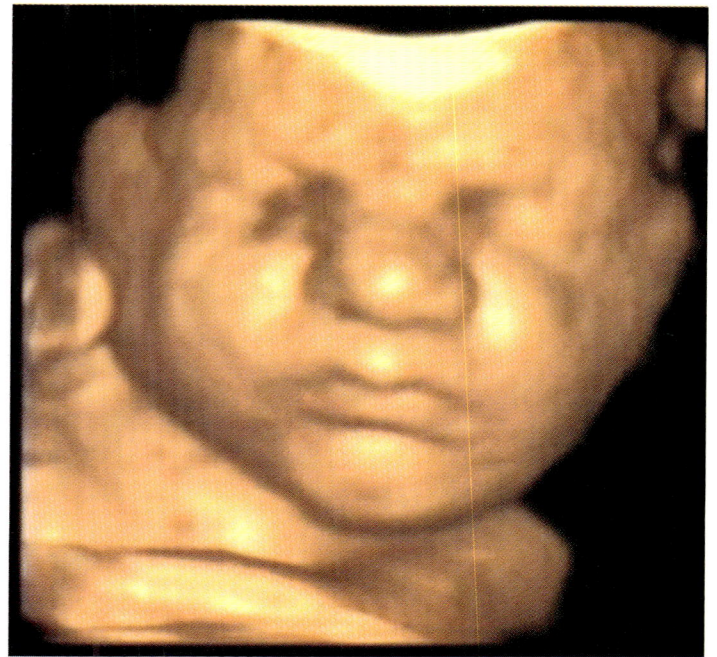

Fig. 15.78: The fetus in this 3D image seems to be displeasure

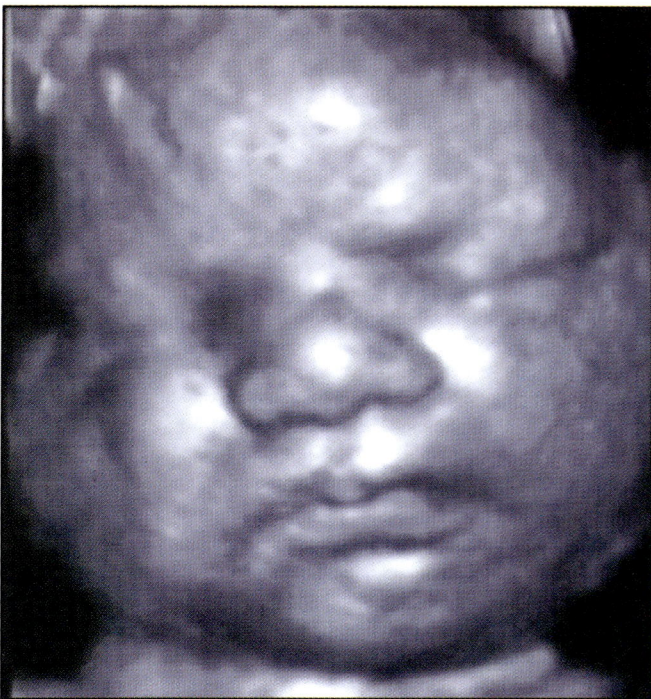

Fig. 15.77: Grimacing expression is obtained by surface rendering technique

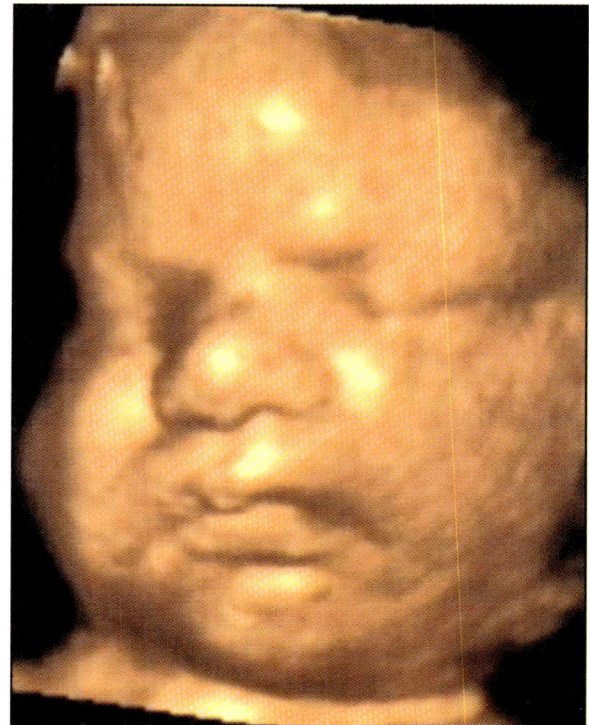

Fig. 15.79: 3D surface rendering demonstrates grimacing expression

14. Lee A, Deutinger J, Bernaschek C. Three-dimensional ultrasound: abnormalities of the fetal face in surface and volume rendering mode. Br J Obstet Gynaecol 1995;102:302-6.

15. Levaillant JM, Benoit B, Bady J, Rotten D. Echographie tridimensionelle apport technique et clinique en echographie obstetricale. Reprod Humaine Hormone 1995;3:341-7.

16. Ludomirski A, Khandelwal M, Uerpairojkit B, Reece EA, Chan L. Three-dimensional ultrasound' evaluation of fetal facial and spinal anatomy. Am J Obstets Gynecol 1996;174(Suppl):318.

17. Manabe A, Hata T, Aoki S, et al. Three-dimensional sonographic visualization of fetal facial anomaly. Acta Obstet Gynecol Scand 1999;78:917-8.

18. Merz E, Bahlmann F, Weber C. Volume scanning in the evaluation of fetal malformations: a new dimension in prenatal diagnosis. Ultrasound Obstet Gynecol 1995;5:222-7.

19. Merz E, Bahlmann F, Weber C, Macchiella D. Three-dimensional ultrasonography in prenatal diagnosis. J Perinat Med 1995;23:213-22.

20. Merz E. Einsatz der 3D-Ultraschalltechnik in der pranatalen Diagnostik. Ultraschall Med 1995; 16: 154-61.

21. Merz E. Three-dimensional ultrasound in the evaluation of fetal anatomy and fetal malformations. In Chervenak FA, Kurjak A, (Eds): Current Perspectives on the Fetus as a Patient. London: Parthenon-Publishmg 1996; pp 75-87.

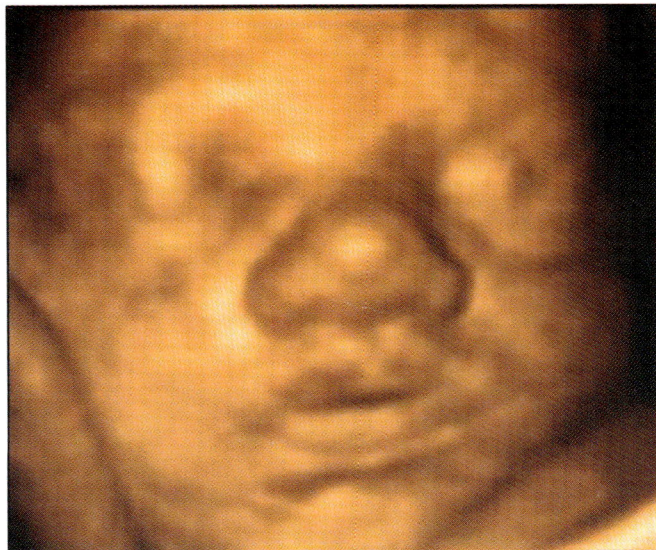

Fig. 15.80: 3D surface rendering shows the clearly contour of fetal face

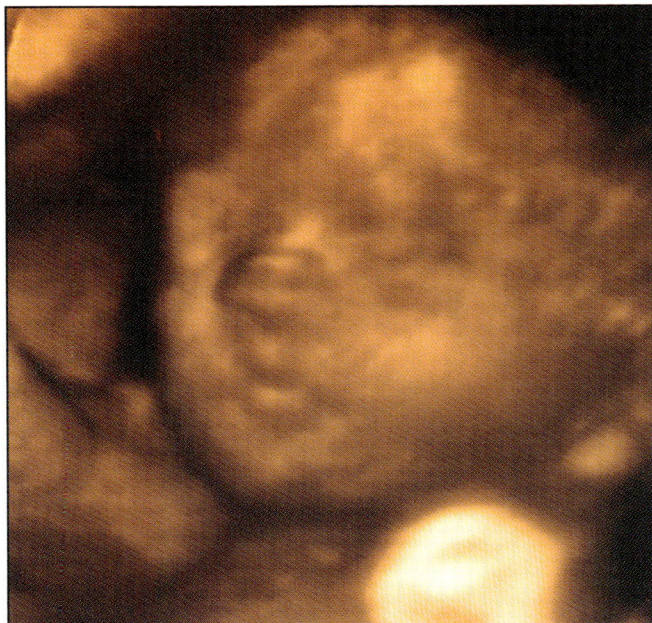

Fig. 15.81: 3D ultrasound of the fetus shows alteration of the facial expression. This kind of asymmetry, however, should be differentiated from pathological features such as unilateral facial paresis

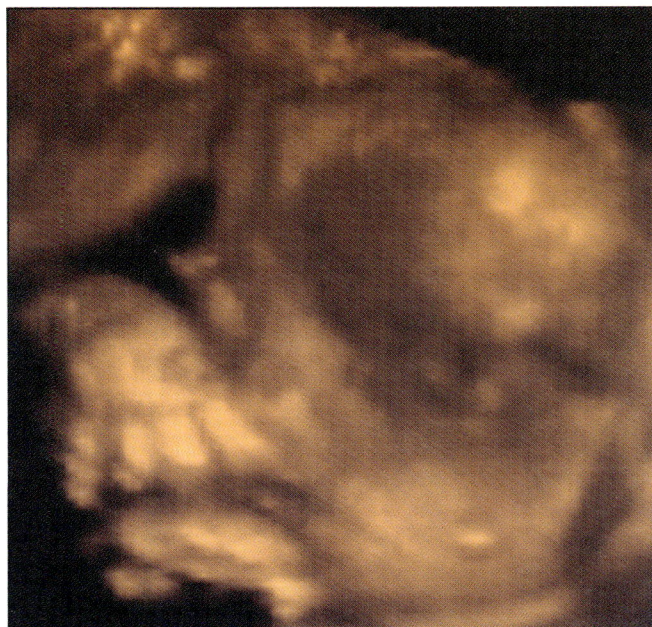

Fig. 15.82: 3D surface rendering of the fetus with trisomy 18 shows the round face

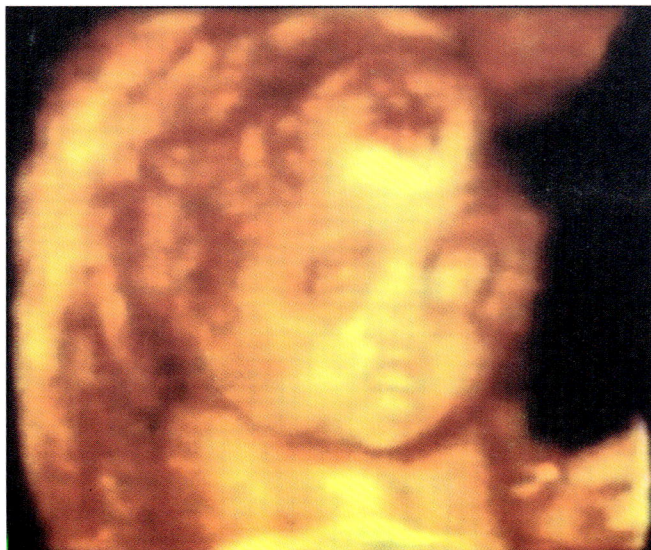

Fig. 15.83: 3D surface rendering of the fetus with trisomy 18

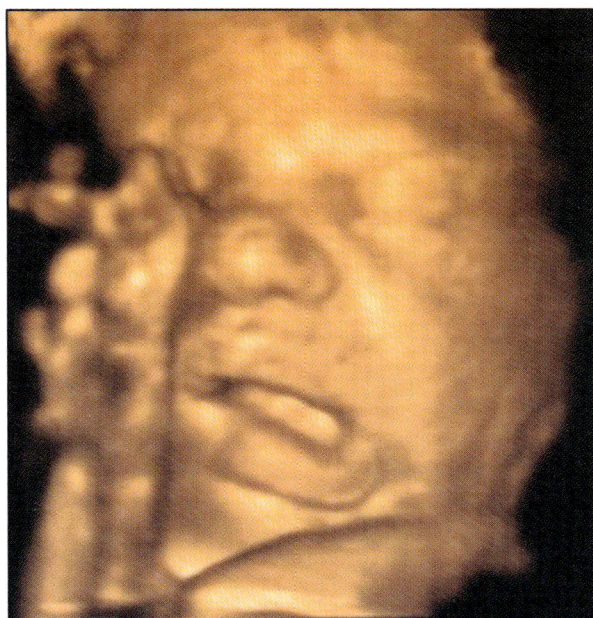

Fig. 15.84: Facial expression and hand movement of the fetus with trisomy 18

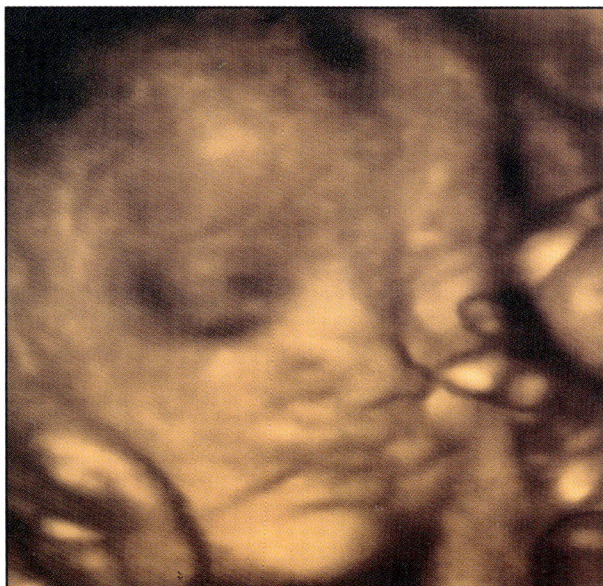

Fig. 15.85: 3D surface rendering of the fetus with thanatophoric dysplasia

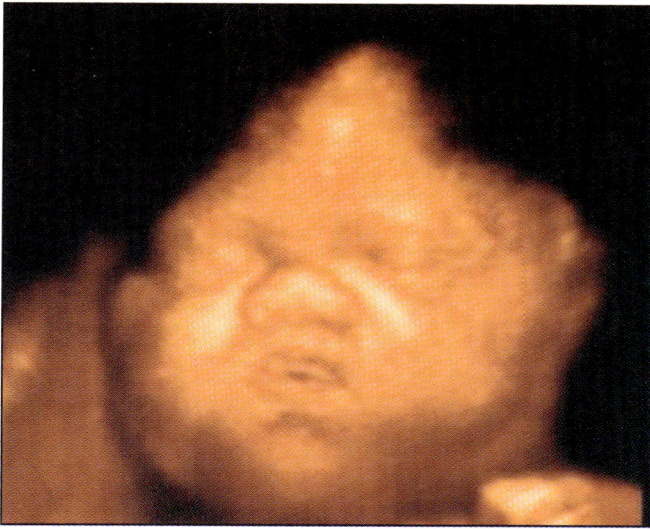

Fig. 15.86: 3D image of the fetus with thanatophoric dysplasia

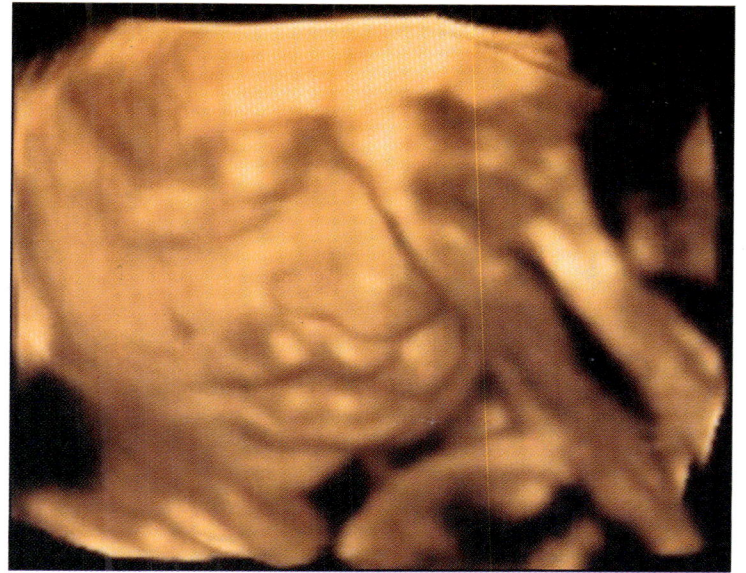

Fig. 15.89: 3D ultrasound image of a fetal face in the fetus with bilateral cleft lip

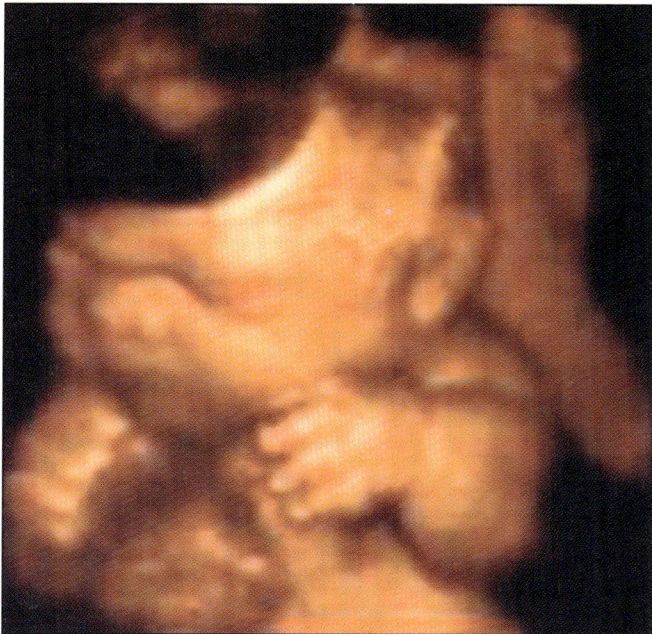

Fig. 15.87: 3D surface rendering of the fetus with osteochondrosis dysplasia

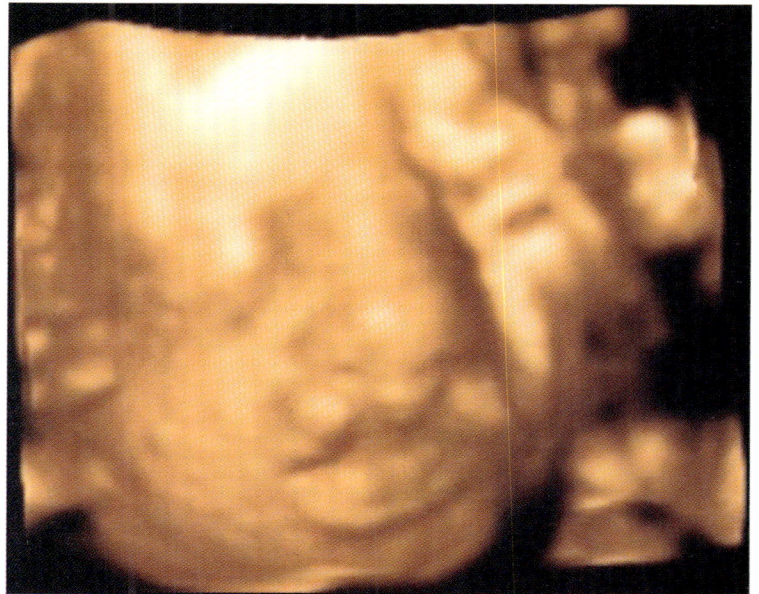

Fig. 15.90: 3D ultrasound of a fetus with bilateral cleft lip

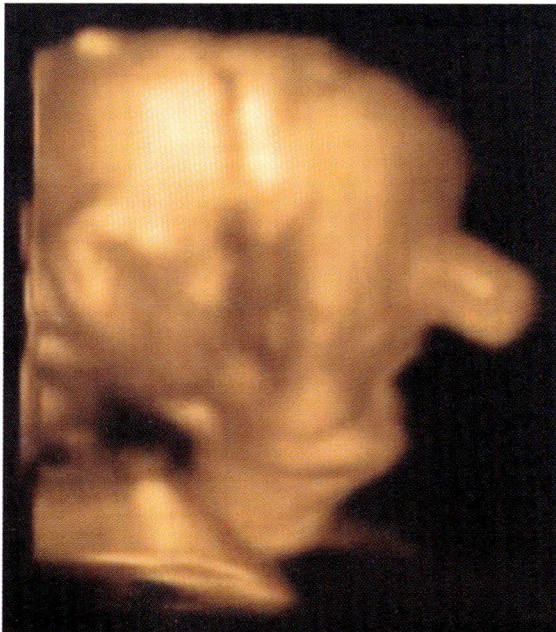

Fig. 15.88: 3D surface rendering of the fetus with proboscis

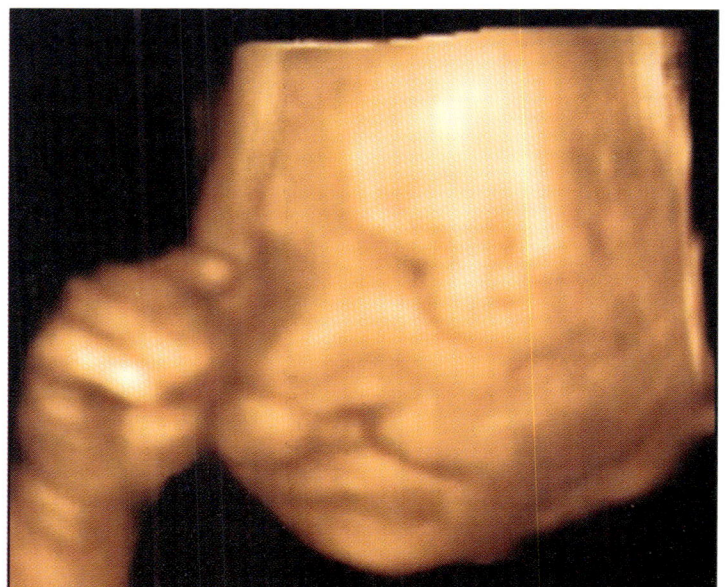

Fig. 15.91: Cleft lip is clearly visible by 3D surface rendering. The exact location and surrounding affected structure are visible

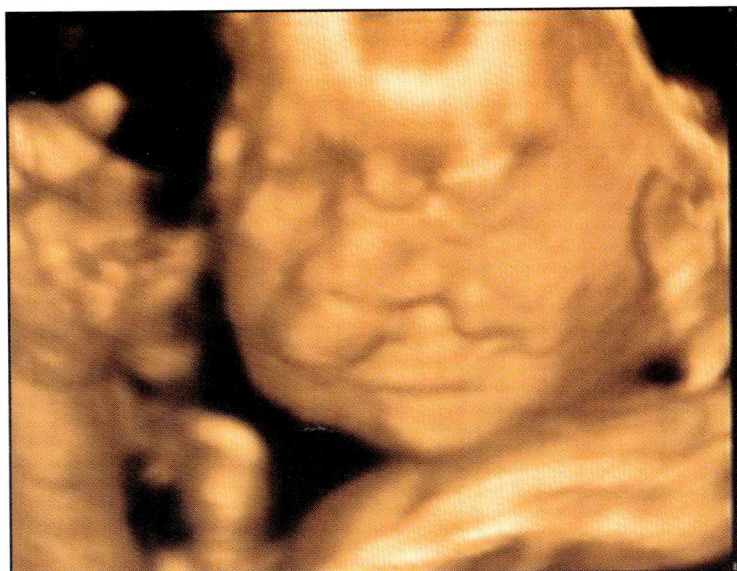

Fig. 15.92: 3D surface rendering of a fetus with unilateral cleft lip

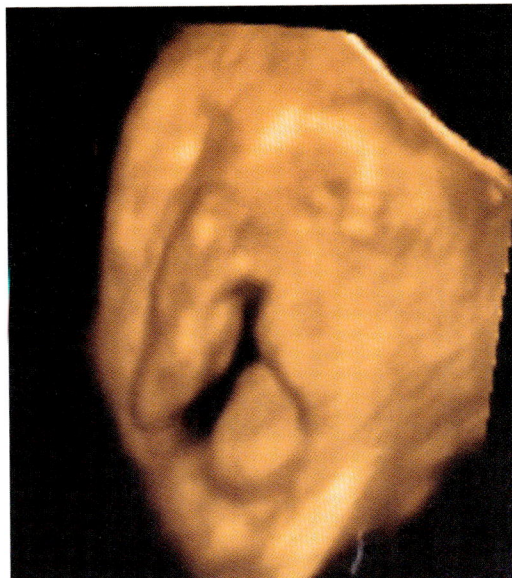

Fig. 15.95: 3D surface rendering demonstrates fetus with labiopalatoschisis

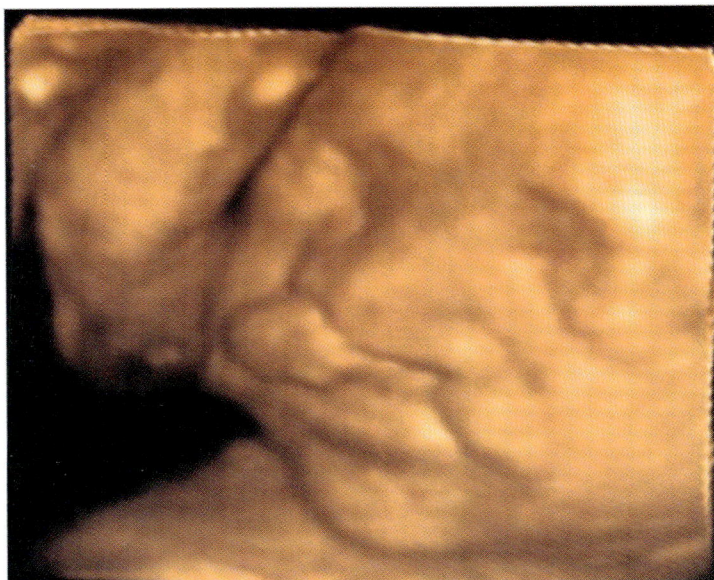

Fig. 15.93: 3D scan of a fetus with a unilateral cleft lip

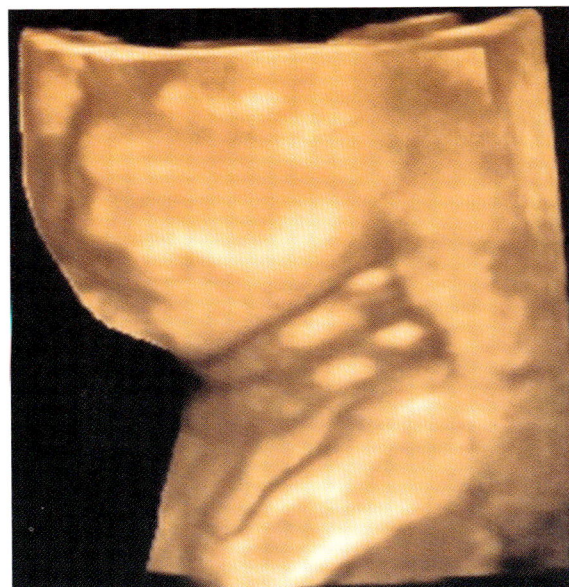

Fig. 15.96: 3D surface rendering of the nuchal cord

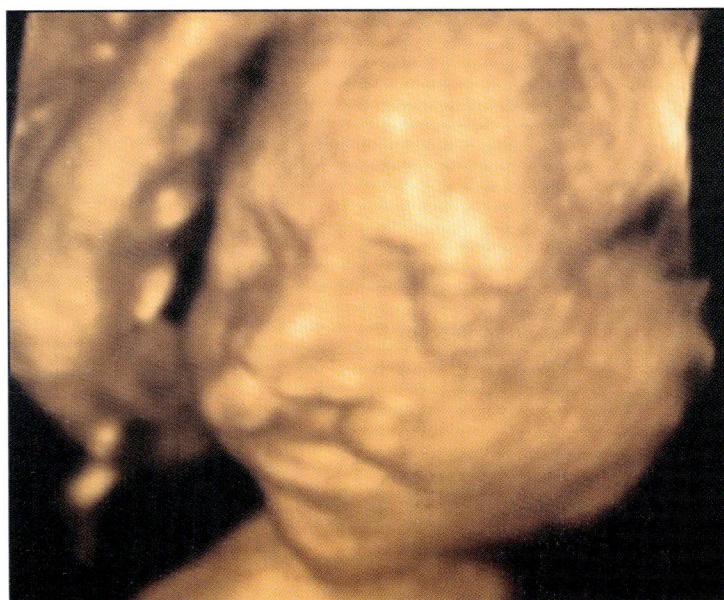

Fig. 15.94: 3D surface rendering of facial expression of the fetus with unilateral cleft lip

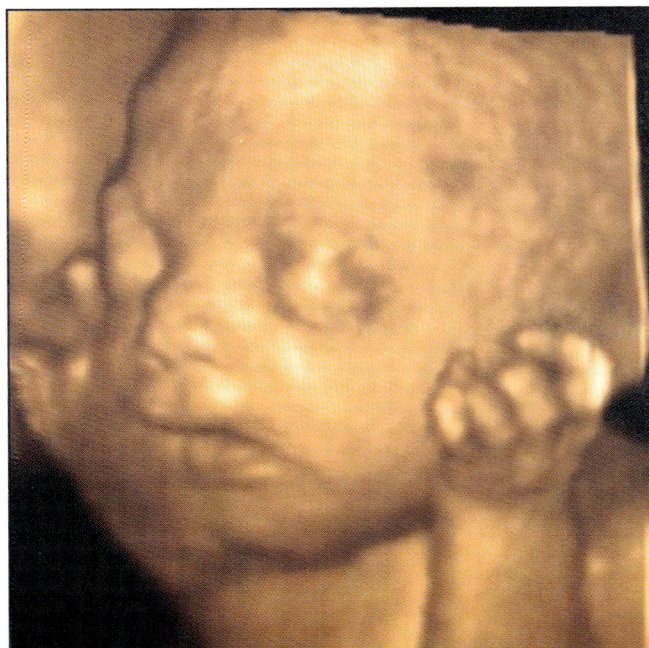

Fig. 15.97: 3D surface rendering shows the facial expression of the fetus with arthrogryposis

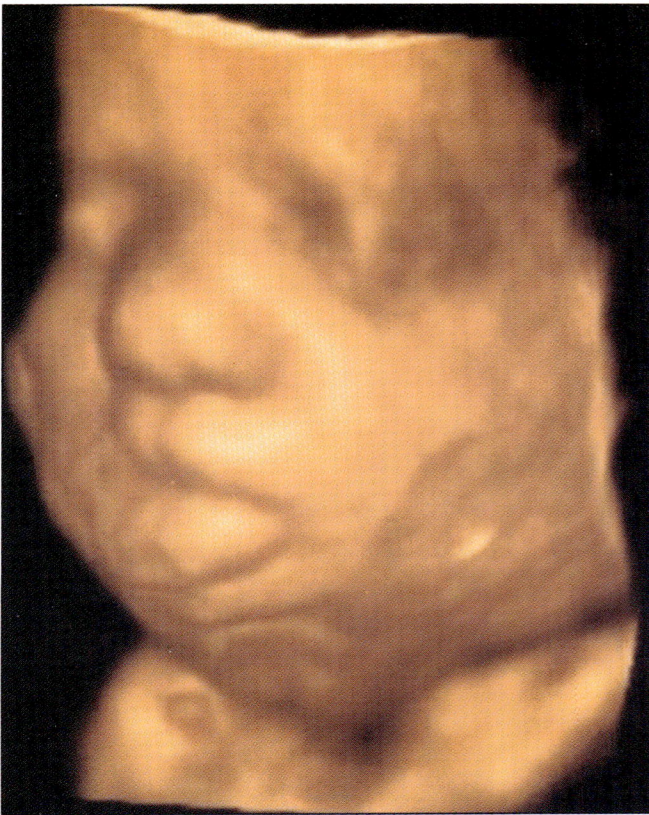

Fig. 15.98: 3D surface rendering of the fetus with macroglossia

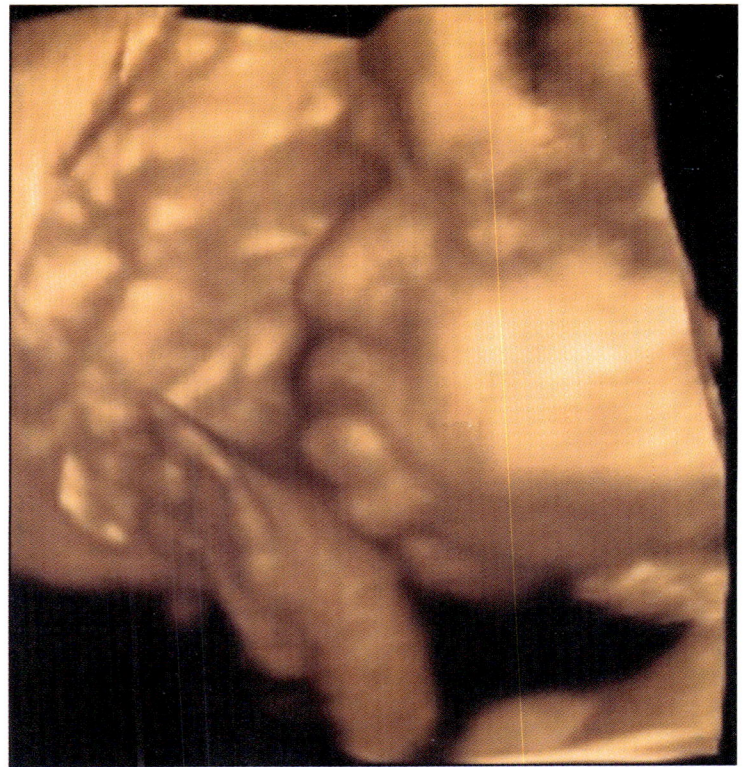

Fig. 15.99: 3D surface imaging showing fetus with macroglossia

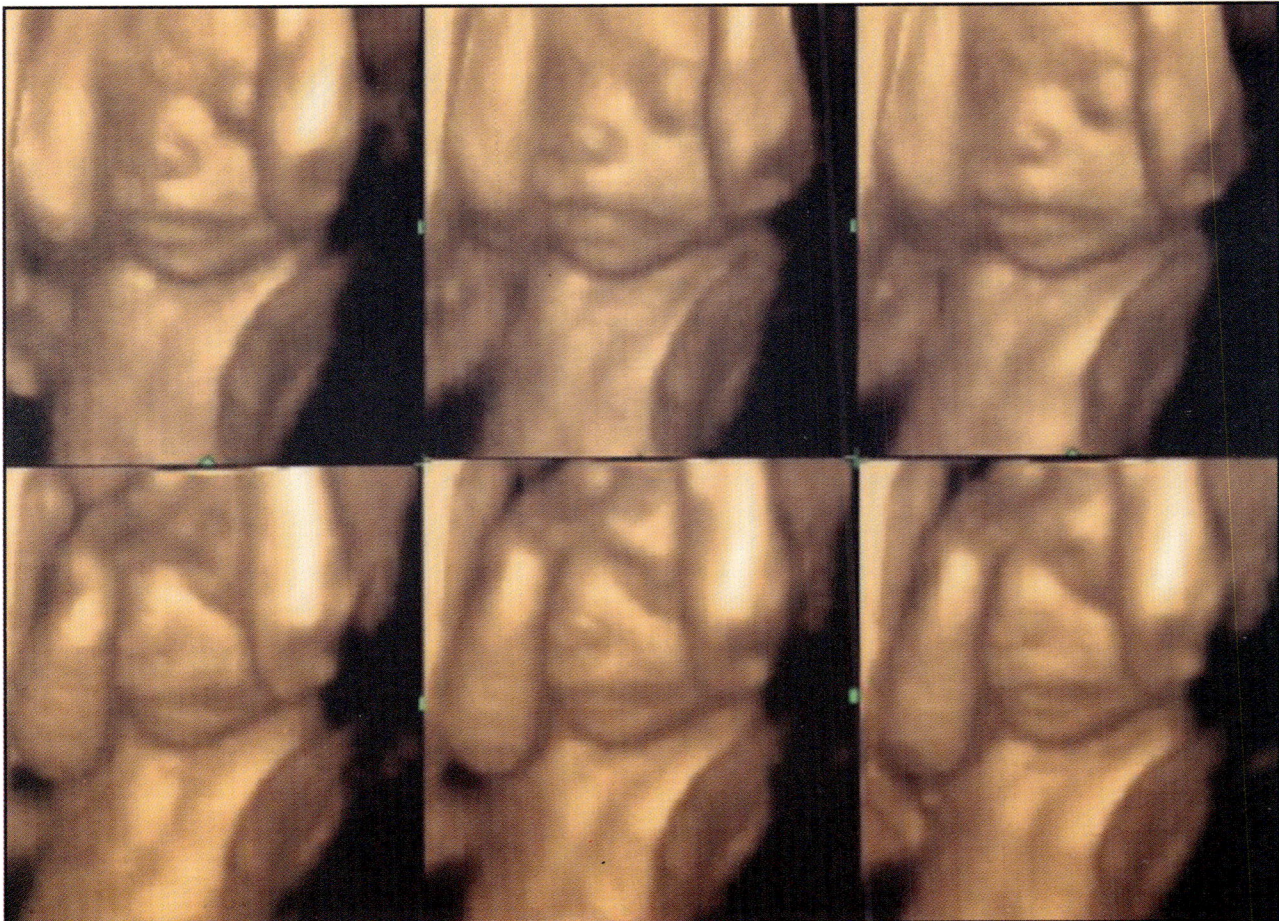

Fig. 15.100: 4D sequence demonstrates alteration in facial expression and movement of the hands beside the head

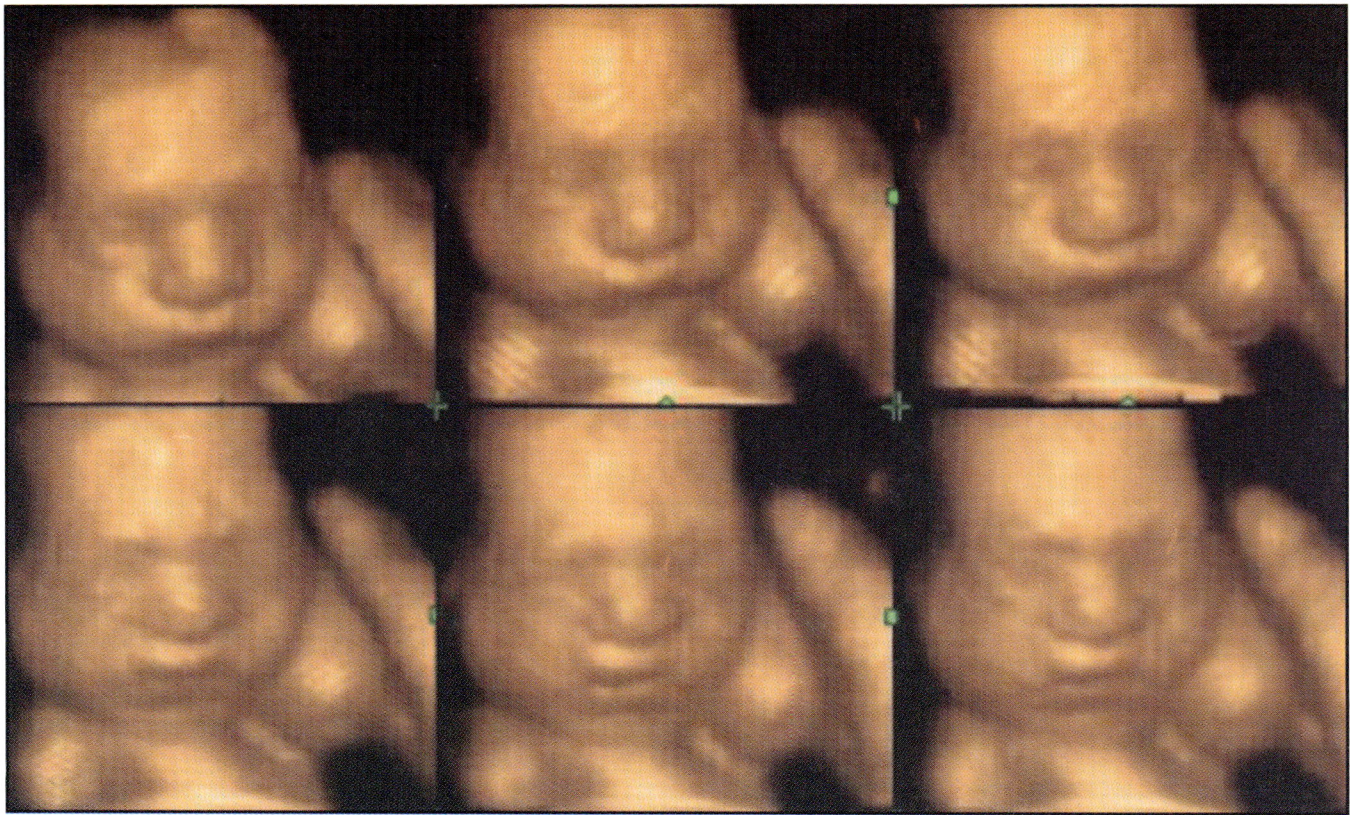

Fig. 15.101: 4D sequence demonstrates grimacing expression of the fetus

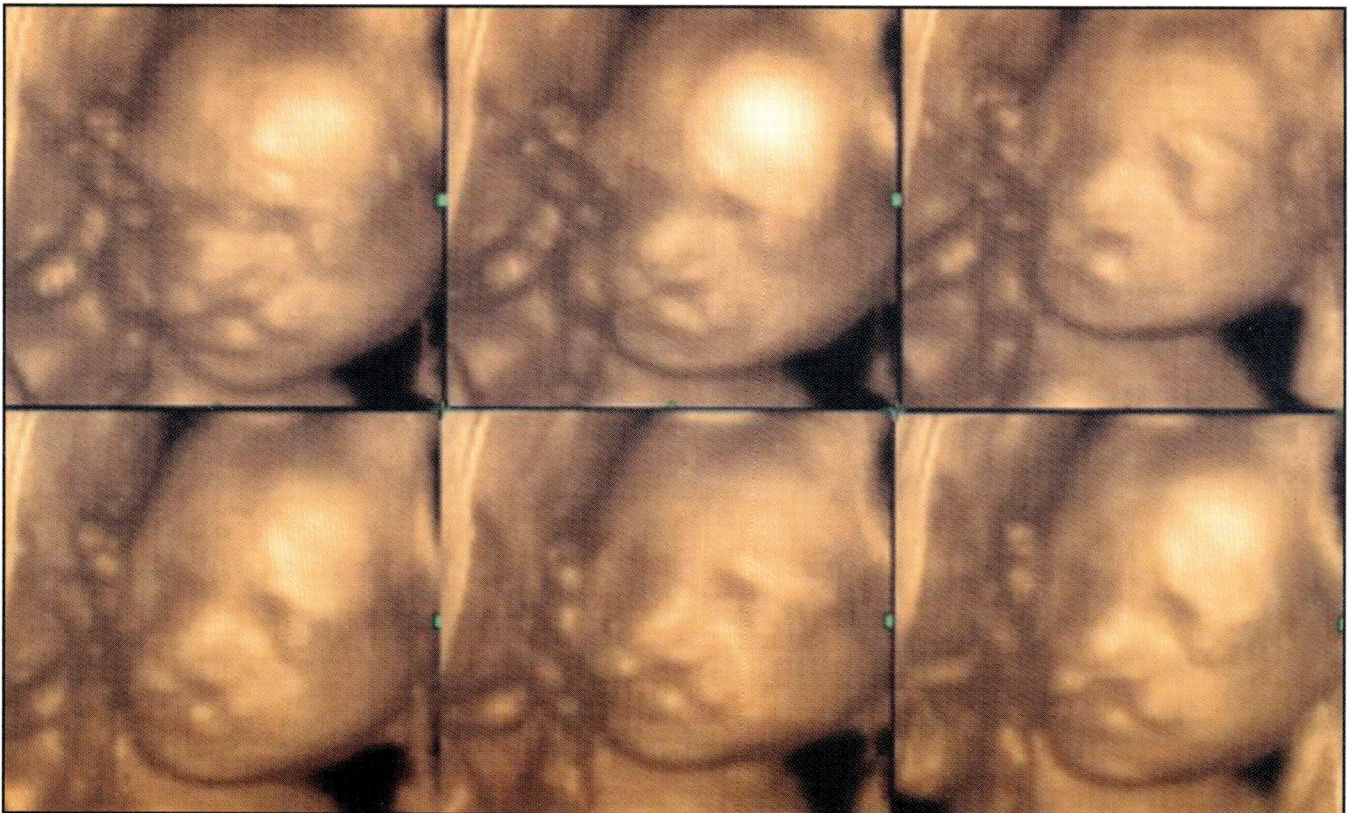

Fig. 15.102: 4D sequence shows changing in the facial expression in the fetus with unilateral cleft lip

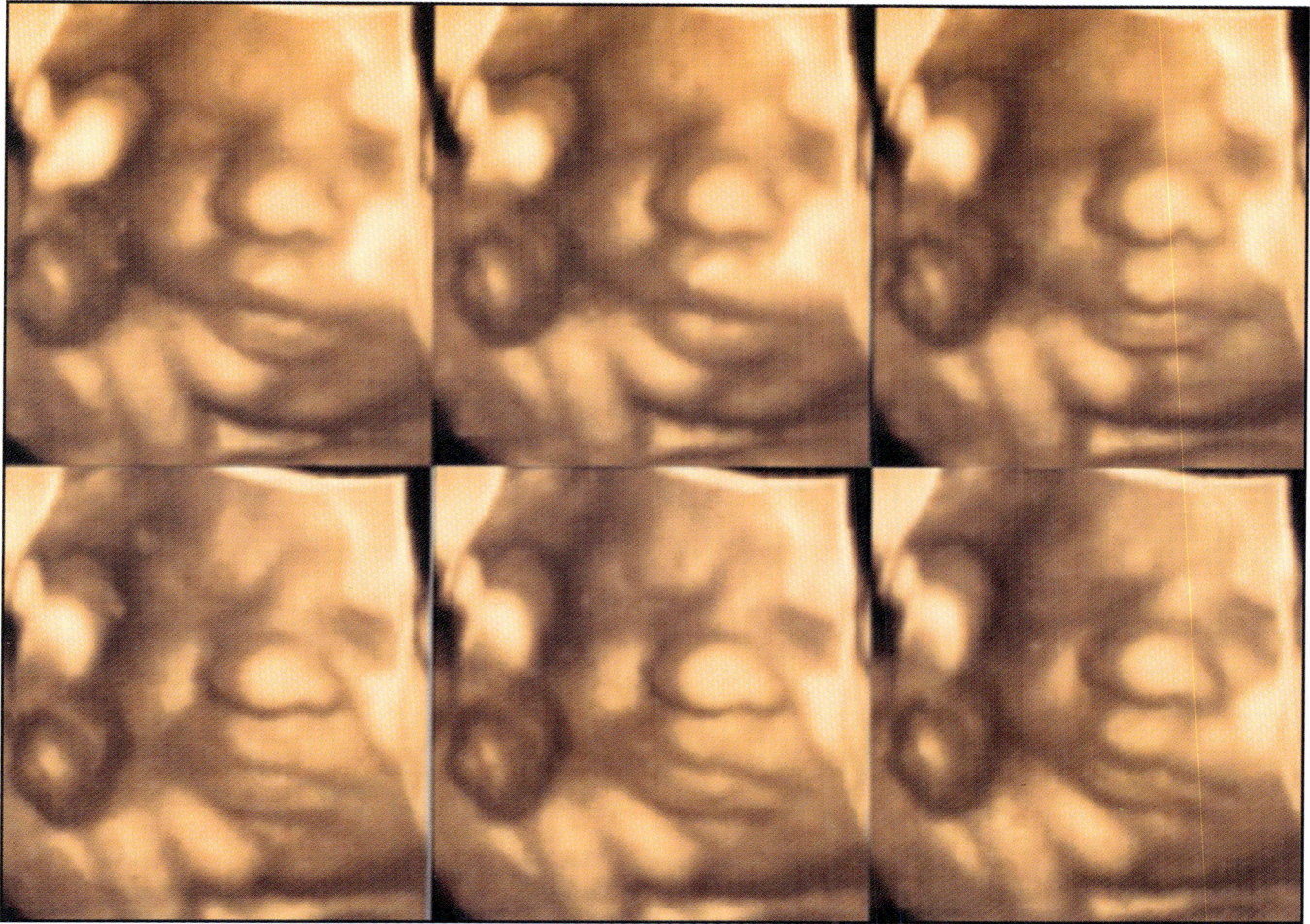

Fig. 15.103: Grimacing expression of the fetus shows the wrinkling of the brows or face

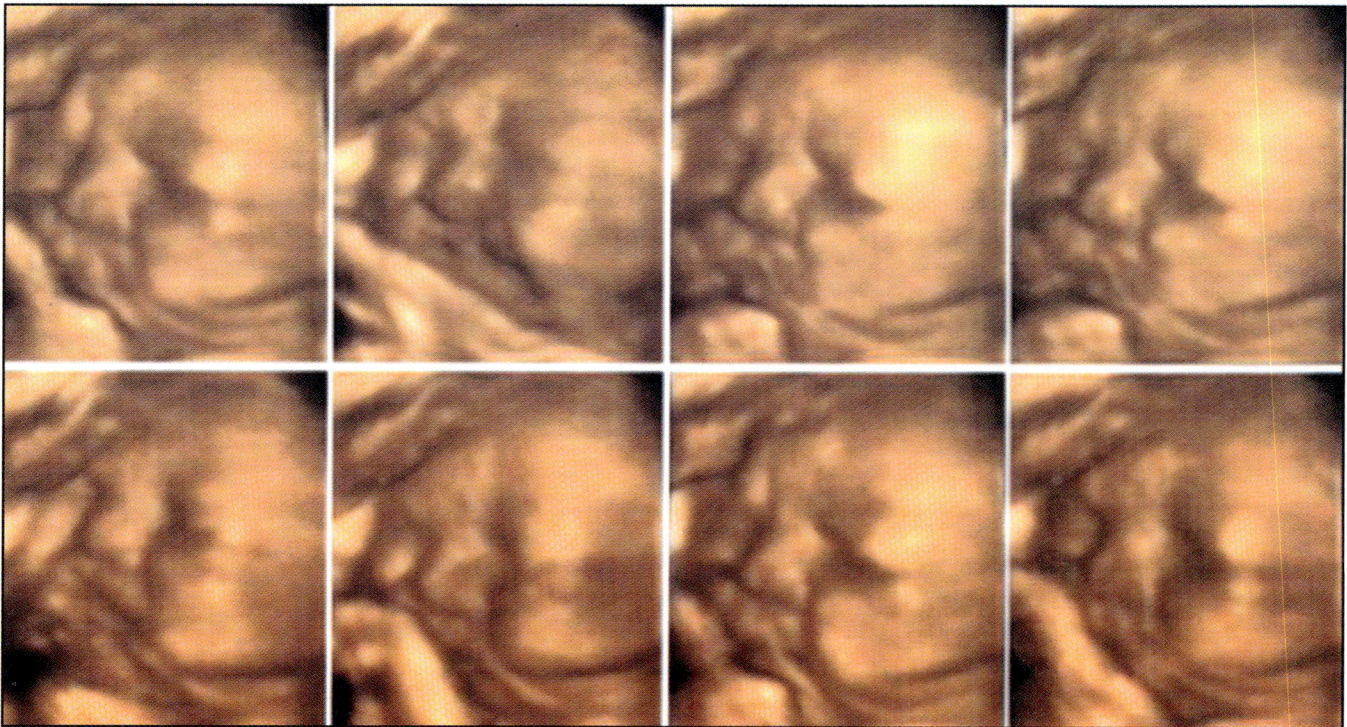

Fig. 15.104: The fetus seems to express displeasure in this 4D sequence

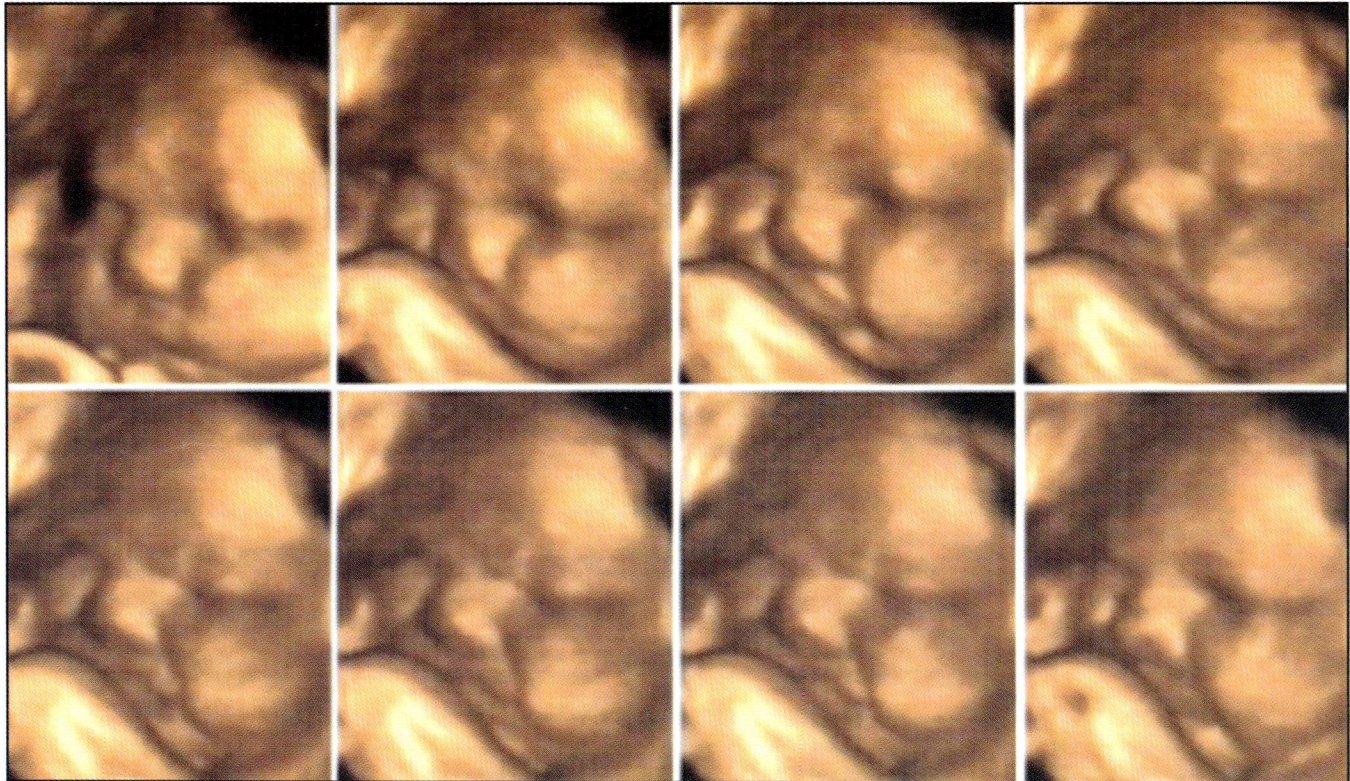

Fig. 15.105: 4D sequence shows wrinkling of the brows or face

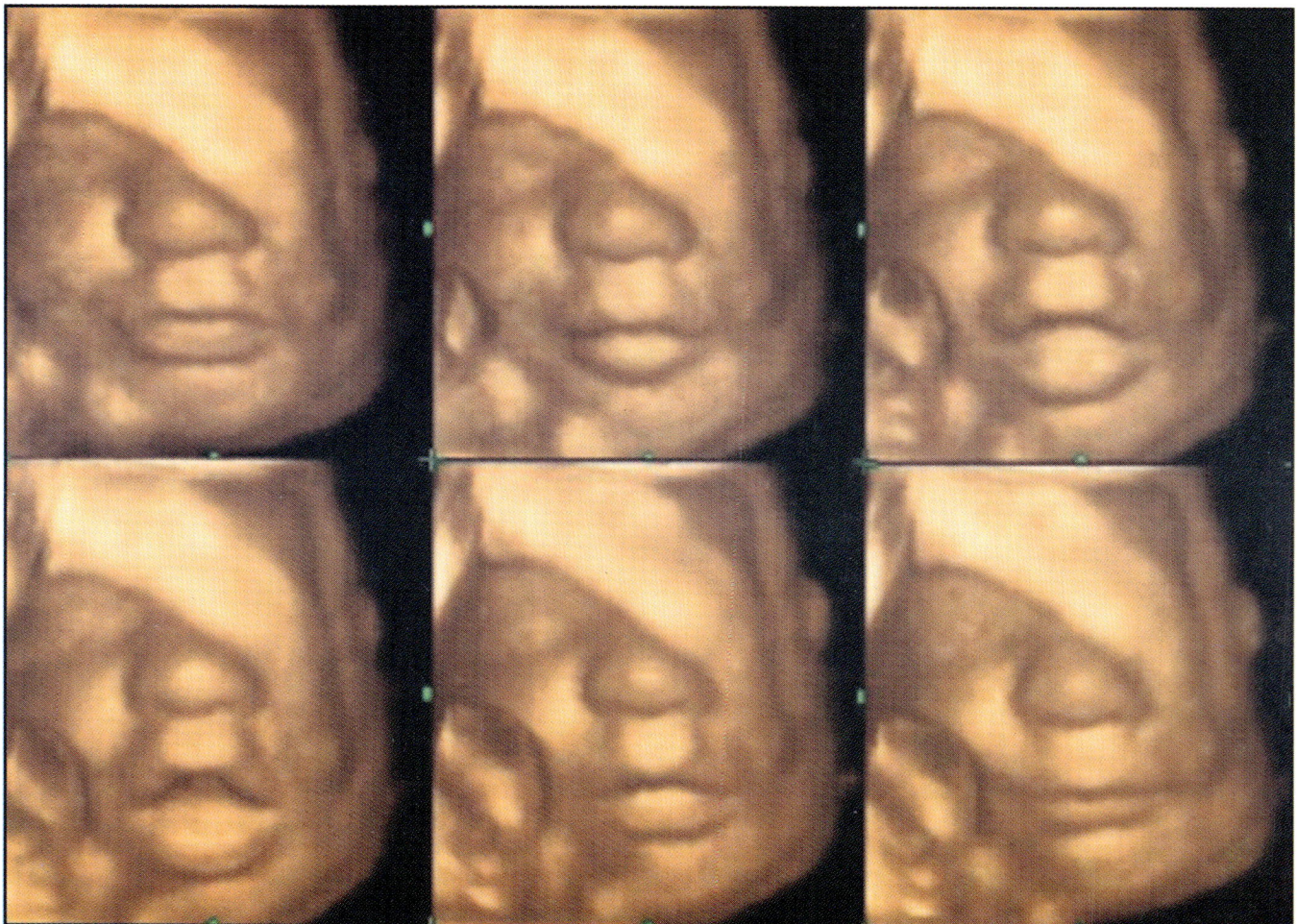

Fig. 15.106: Mouthing expression is obtained by 4D technique

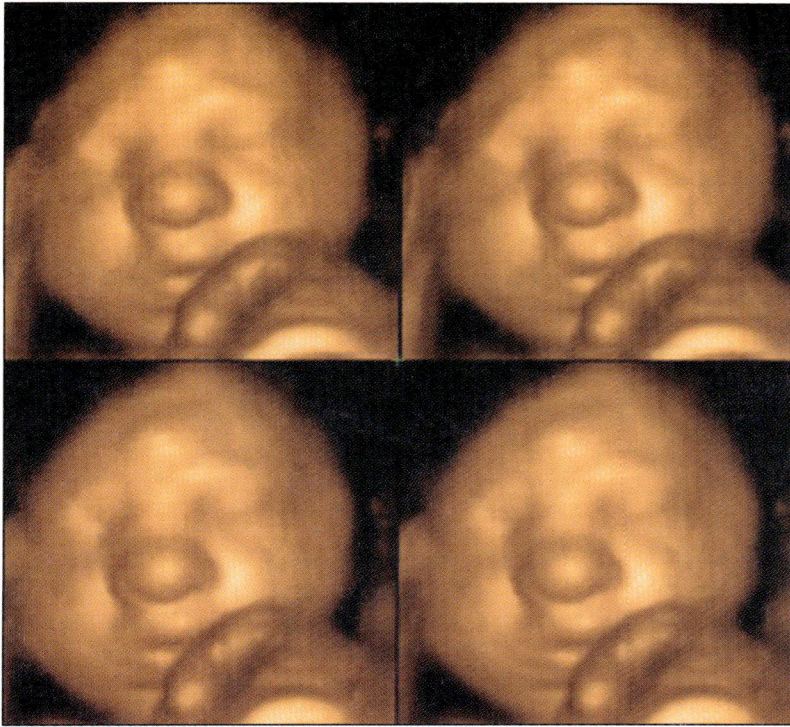

Fig. 15.107: 4D sequence shows mouthing expression

22. Merz E, Weber C, Bahlmann F, Miric-Tesanic D. Application of transvaginal and abdominal three-dimensional ultrasound for the detection or exclusion of malformations of the fetal face. Ultrasound Obstet Gynecol 1997;9:237-43.

23. Mueller CM, Weiner CE Yankowitz J. Three-dimensional ultrasound in the evaluation of fetal head and spine anomalies. Obstet Gynecol 1996; 88: 372-8.

24. Nelson TR, Pretonus DH. Three-dimensional ultrasound of fetal surface features. Ultrasound Obstet Gynecol 1992;2:166-74.

25. Pretorius DH, Nelson TR, Jaffe JS. Three-dimensional US of the fetus. Radiology 1990;177:194.

26. Pretorius DH, Nelson TR. Three-dimensional ultrasound imaging in patient diagnosis and management: the future. Ultrasound Obstet Gynecol 1991;!:381-3.

27. Pretorius DH, Nelson TR. Prenatal visualization of cranial sutures and fontanelles with three-dimensional ultrasonography. J Ultrasound Med 1994;13:871-6.

28. Pretonus DH, Johnson DD, Budonck NE, Jones MC, Lou KV, Nelson TR. Three-dimensional ultrasound of the fetal lip and palate. Radiology 1997; 205(P) (Suppl):245.

29. Steiner H, Merz E, Staudach A. Three-dimensional fetal facing. Hum Reprod Update 1995;l:item 6

30. Hegge FN, Prescott CH, Watson PT. Fetal tadal abnormalities identified during sonography. J Ultrasound Med 1986;5:679-88.

31. De Meyer V, Zeman W, Palmer CC. The face predicts the brain: diagnostic significance ot medial tacial anomalies for holoprosencephaly (archinencephaly). Pediatrics 1964; 34:256-8.

32. Hamper UM, Trapanotto V, Sheth S, DeJong MR, Caskey CI. Three-dimensional US: preliminary clinical expenence. Radiology 1994;191:397.

33. Pretorius DH, House M, Nelson TR, Hollenbach KA. Evaluation of normal and abnormal lips in fetuses: comparison between three and two dimensional sonography. Am J Roentgenol 1995;165:1233-7.

34. Nelson TR, Downey DB, Pretorius DH, Fenster A. Ecografia 3D en Obstetrida en Ecografia 3D. Madrid: Marban, 2000.

35. Hepper PC, Shannon FA, Dornan JC. Sex differences in fetal mouth movements. Lancet 1997;350:1820.

36. Kozuma S, Okai T, Ryo F, et al. Ditterential developmental process of respective behavioral states in human fetuses. Am J Perinatol 1998;15:203-8.

37. Ulm MR, Kratochwil A, Ulm B, Solar P, Aro C, Bernaschek G. Three-dimensional ultrasound evaluation of fetal tooth germs. Ultrasound Obstet Gynecol 1998;12:240-3.

38. Steiner H, Staudach A, Spitzer D, Schaffer H. Three-dimensional ultrasound in obstetrics and gynaecology: technique, possibilities and limitations. Hum Reprod 1994;9:1773-8.

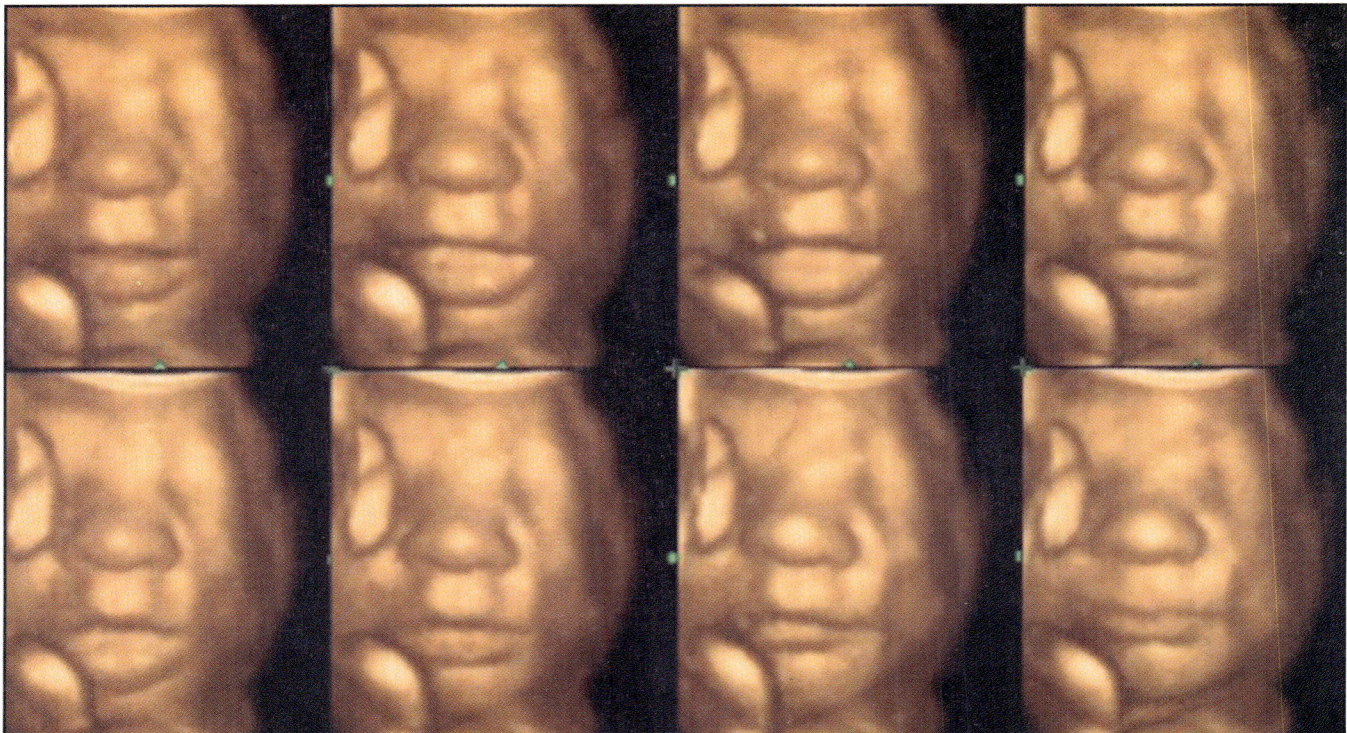

Fig. 15.108: A facial expression characterized by mouthing expression

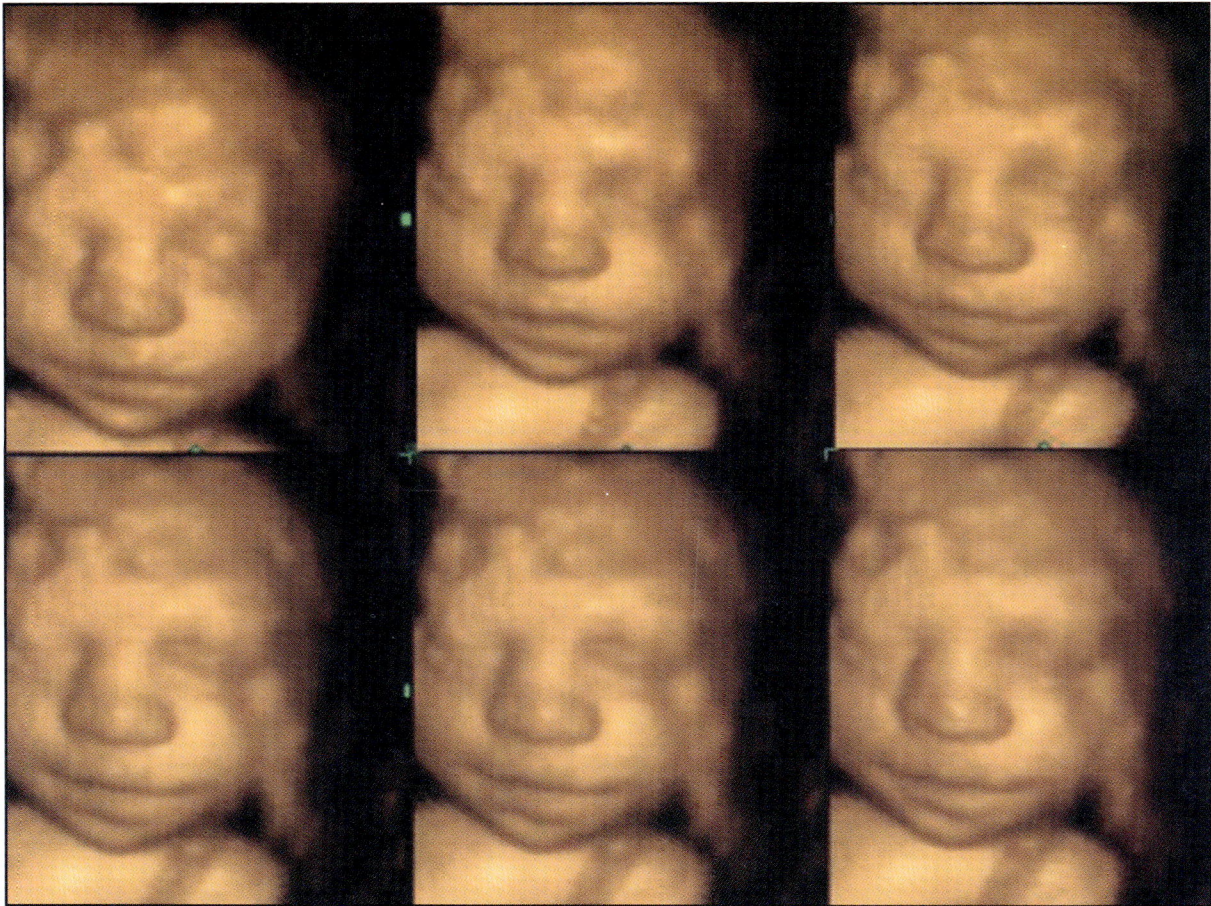

Fig.15.109: This image is showing change in the lateral side of the mouth which results in smiling expression

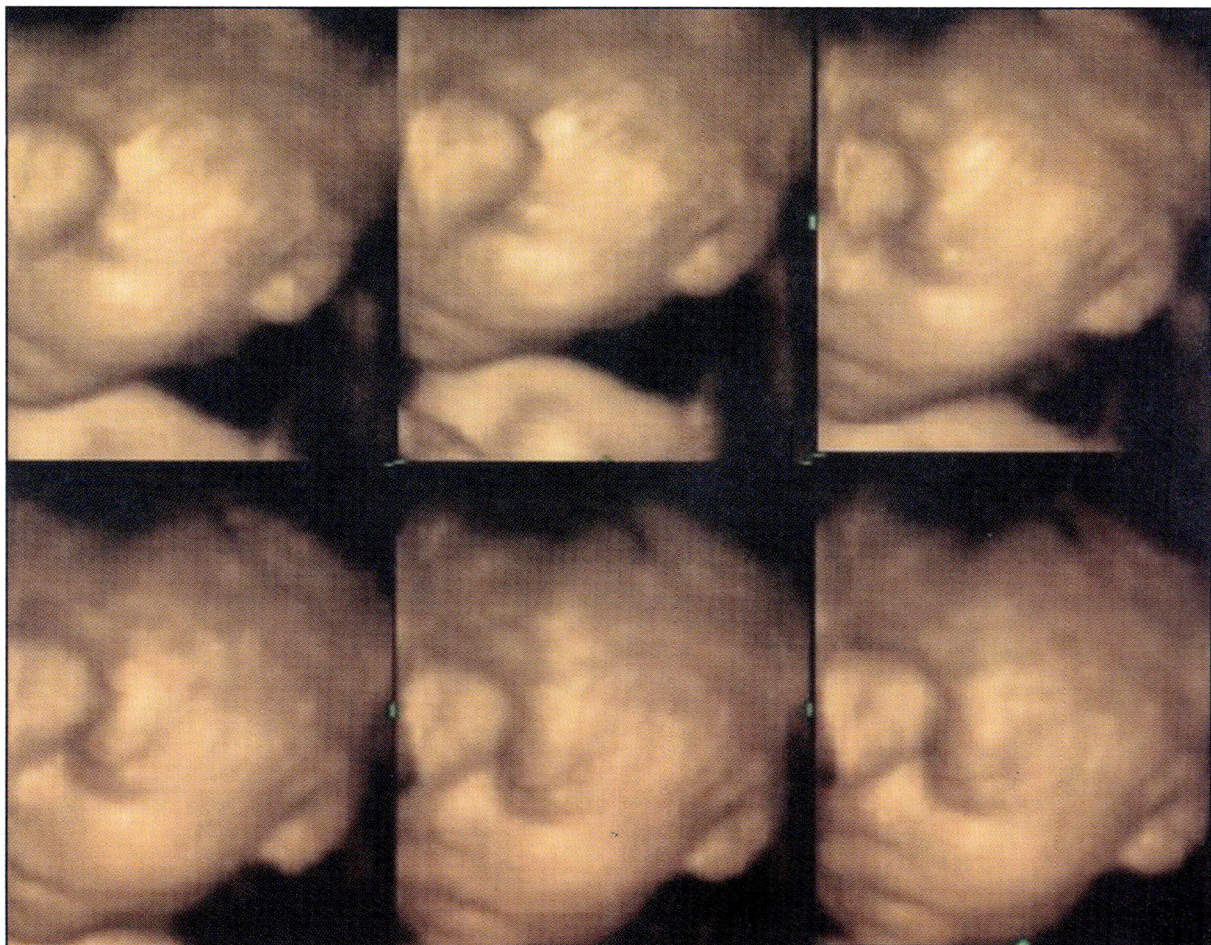

Fig. 15.110: 4D images show a brief closing of the eyelids by involuntary normal periodic closing

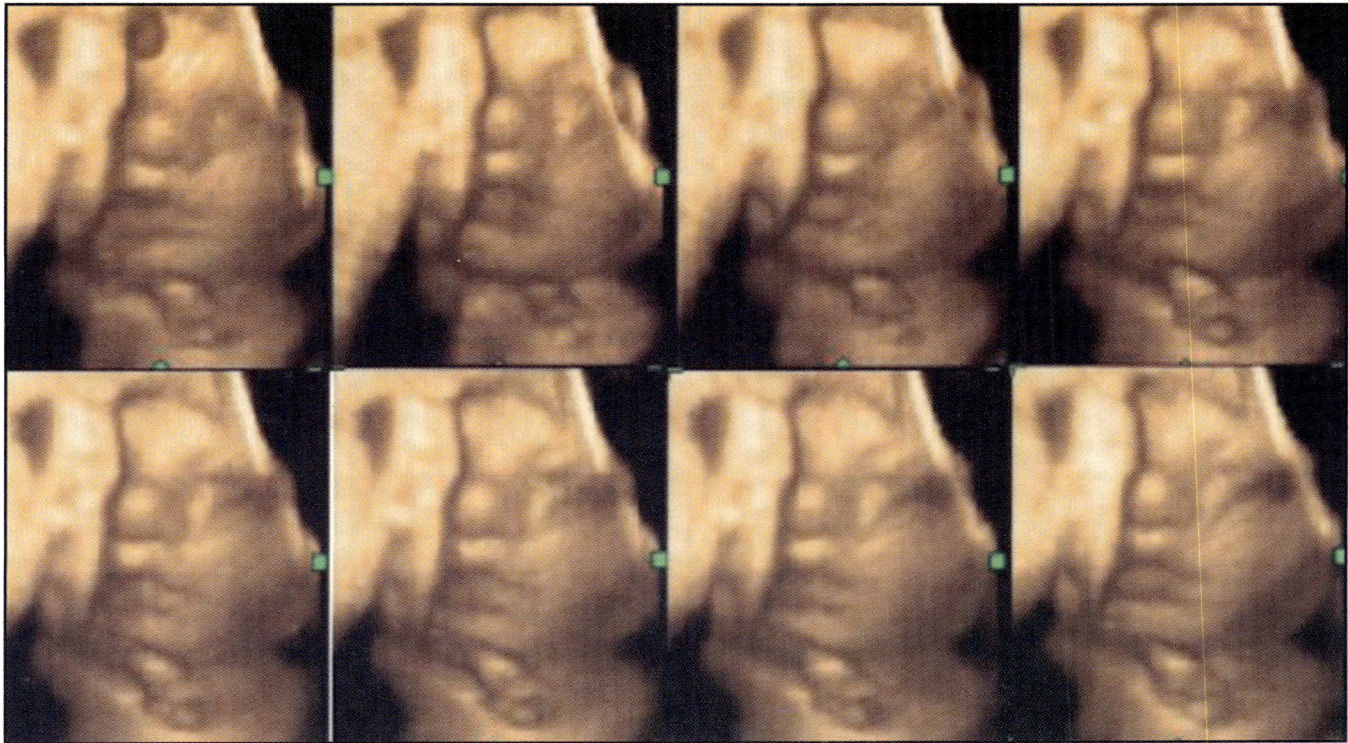

Fig. 15.111: 4D sequence showing a reflex that closes and opens the eyes rapidly

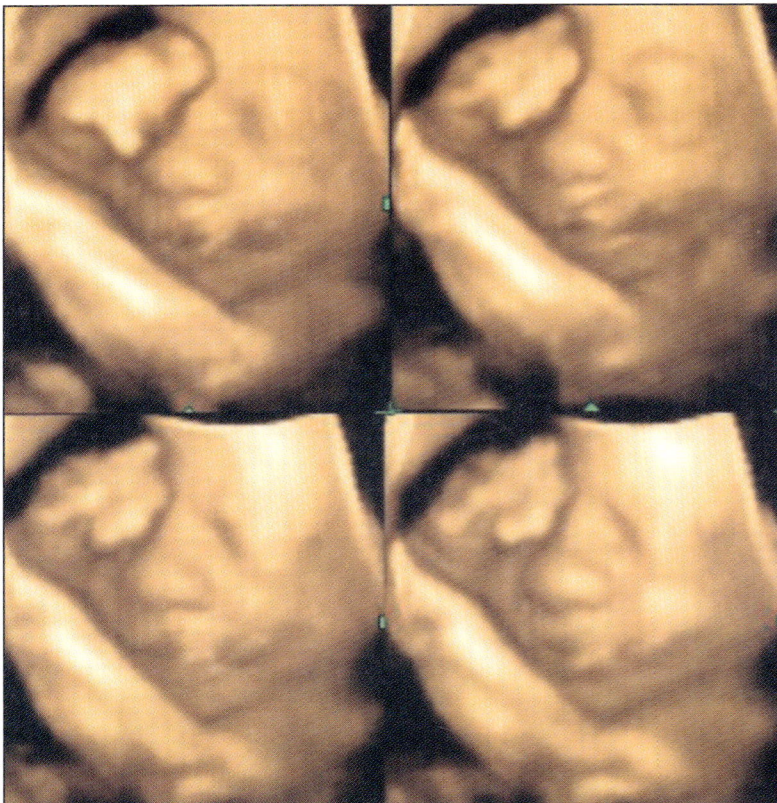

Fig. 15.112: 4D sequence characterized by mouthing expression

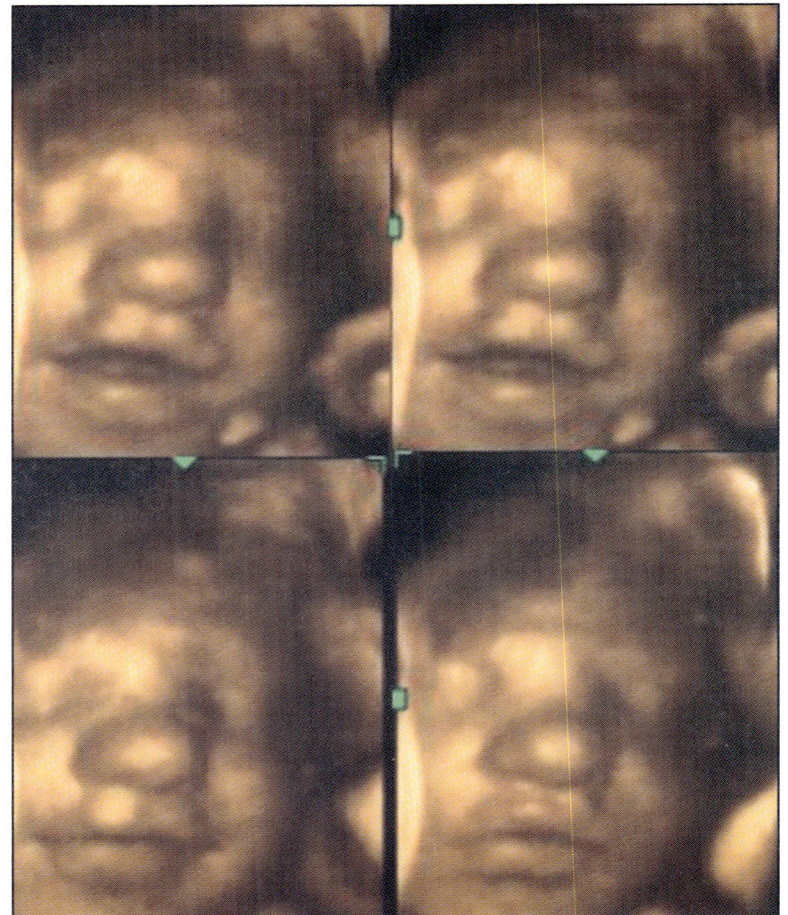

Fig. 15.113: 4D imaging characterized by turning up the corners of the mouth. The fetus seems to be smiling

39. Merz E, Weber G, Bahlmann AF, Macchiella D. Transvaginale 3D-Sonographie in der Gynaekologie. Gynaekologe 1995;28:270-5.

40. Schart A, Chazwiny MF, Steinbom A, Baier P, Sohn C. Evaluation of two-dimensional versus three-dimensional ultrasound in obstetric diagnostics: a prospective study. (Fetal) Diagn Ther 2001;16:333-41.

41. Maier B, Steiner II, Wienerroither H, Staudach A. The psychological impact of three-dimensional fetal imaging on the fetomaternal relationship. In Baba K, Jurkovic D, (Eds). Three-dimensional Utlrasound in Obstetrics and Cynecology. Lancaster: Parthenon Publishing, 1997:pp67-74.

42. Pretonus DH. Maternal smoking habit modification via fetal visualization. University of California Tobacco Related Disease Research Program. Annual Report to the California State Legislature, 1996:76.

43. Merz E. 3-D Ultrasound in Obstetrics and Gynecology. Philadelphia: Lippincott Williams and Wilkins, 1998.

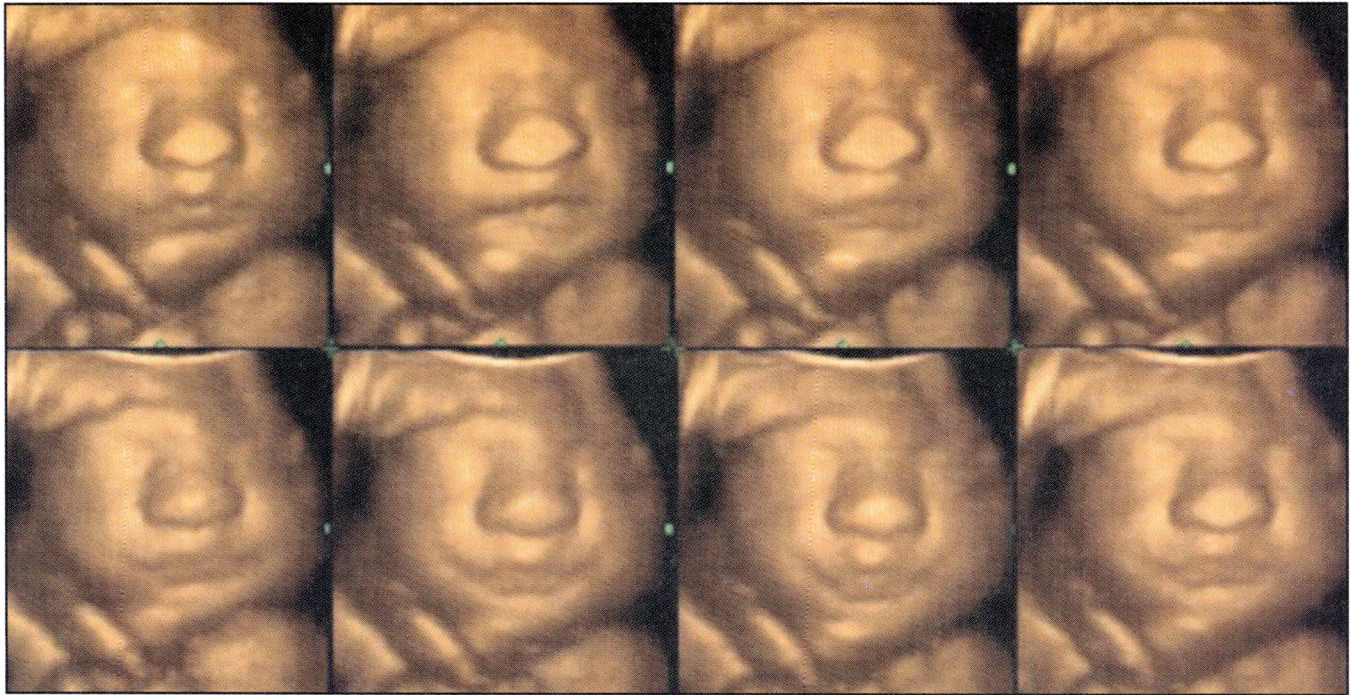

Fig. 15.114: 4D sequence characterized by mouth manipulation to investigate an object. Mouthing is most common in fetus and it may develop into a persistent, stereotyped behavior pattern

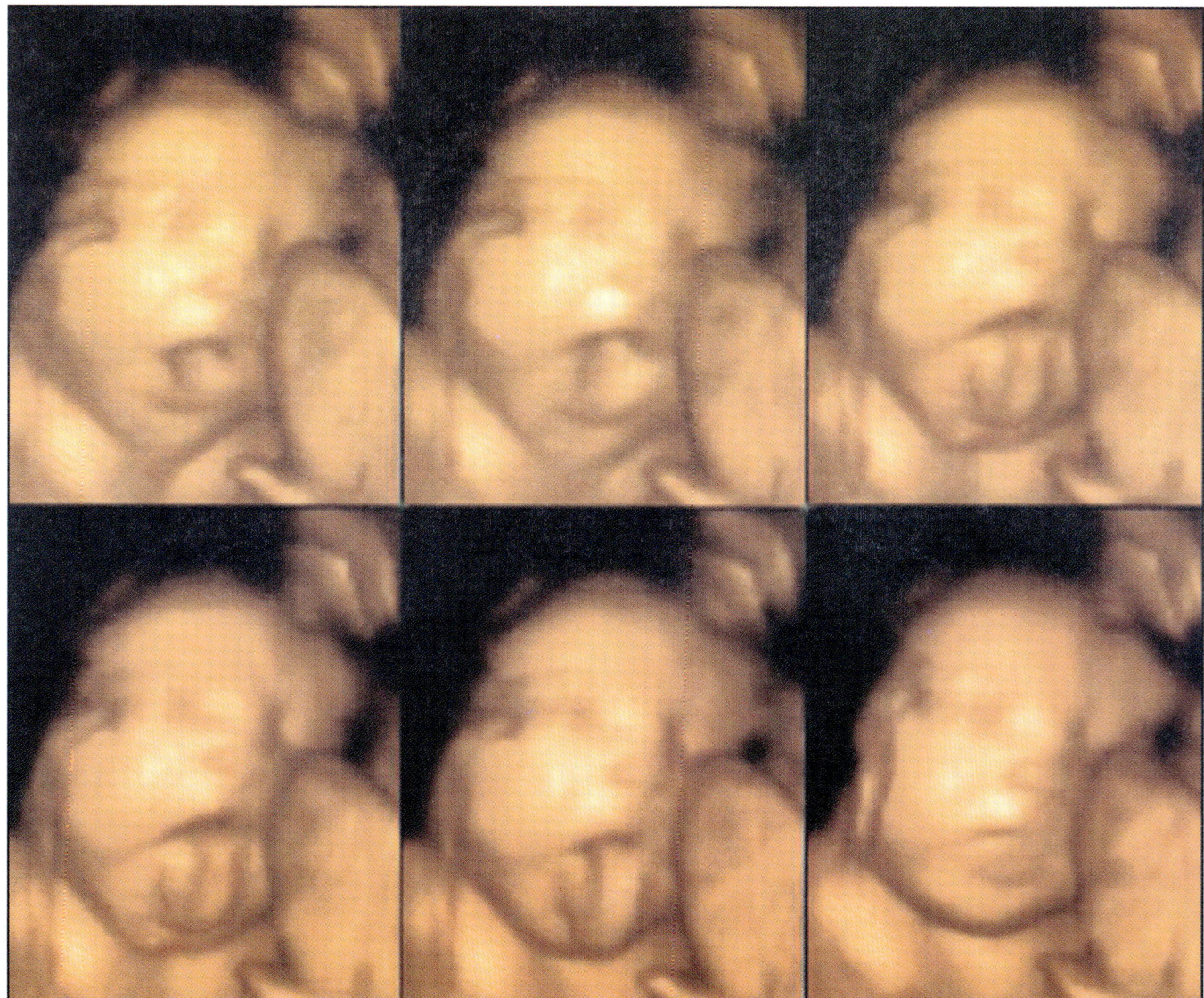

Fig. 15.115: 4D sequence demonstrates the beginning and the ending of tongue expulsion

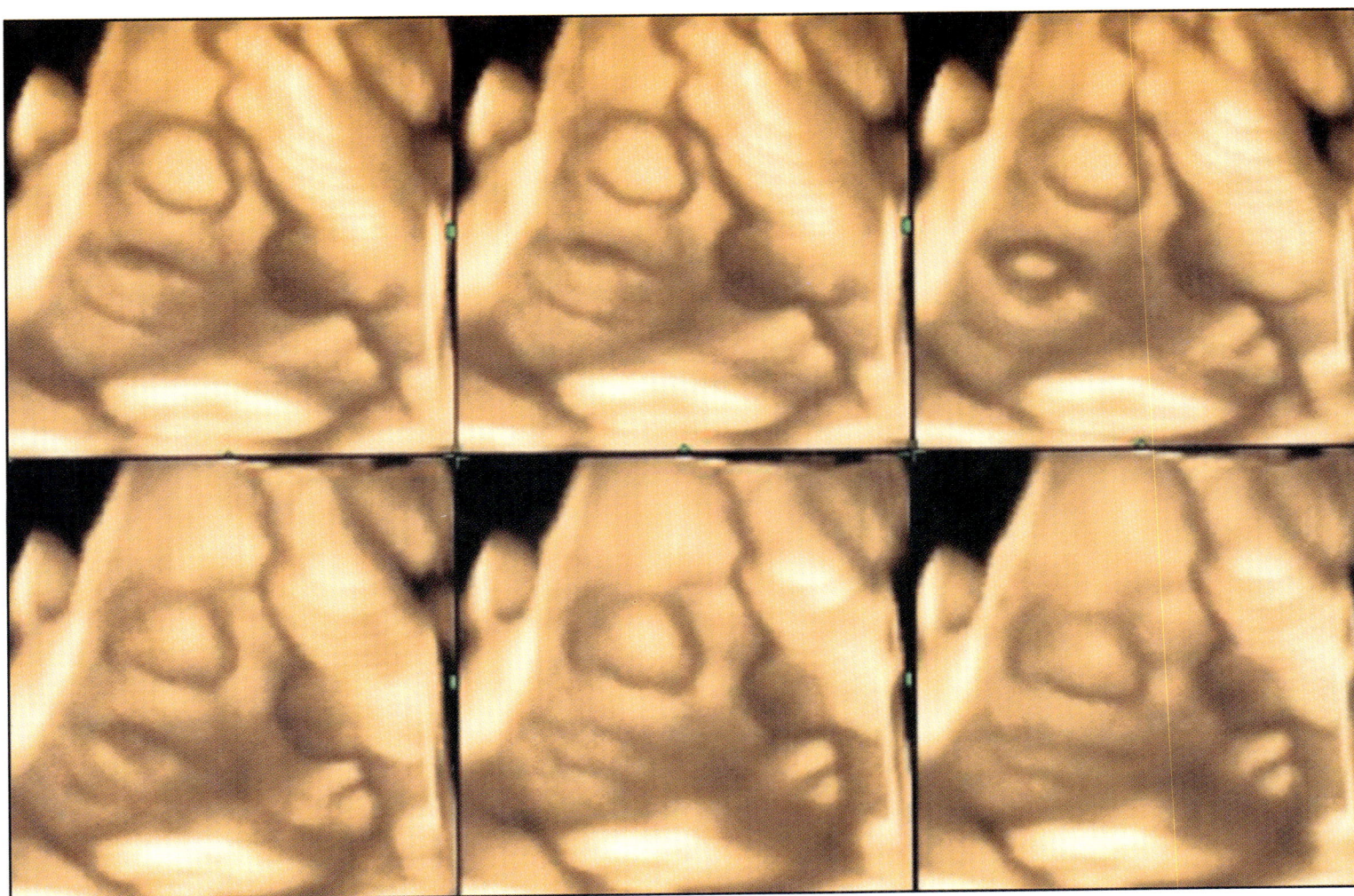

Fig. 15.116: 4D sequence shows mouth opening. The fetus demonstrates drinking and swallowing of the amniotic fluid

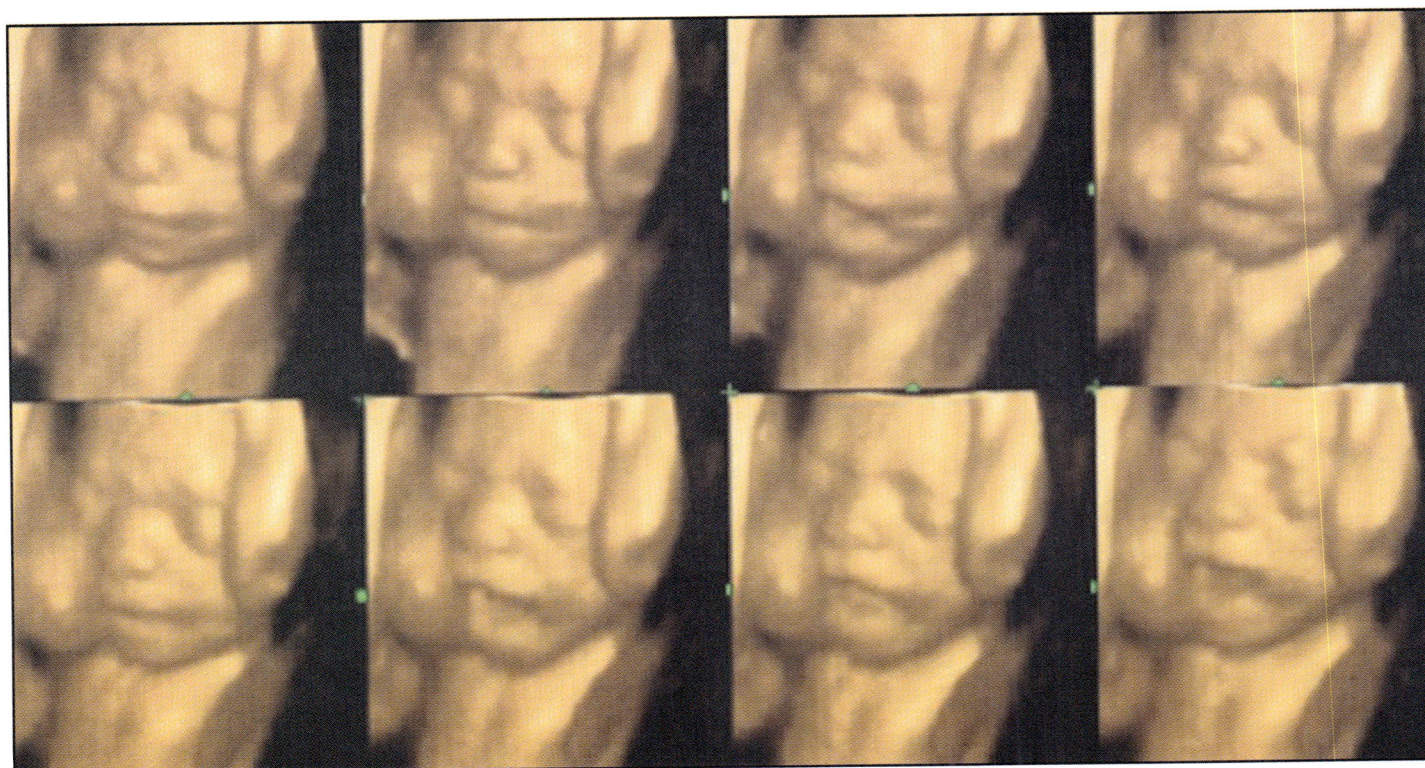

Fig. 15.117: 4D sequence demonstrates mouth opening and hand movement of both of the hands beside the head

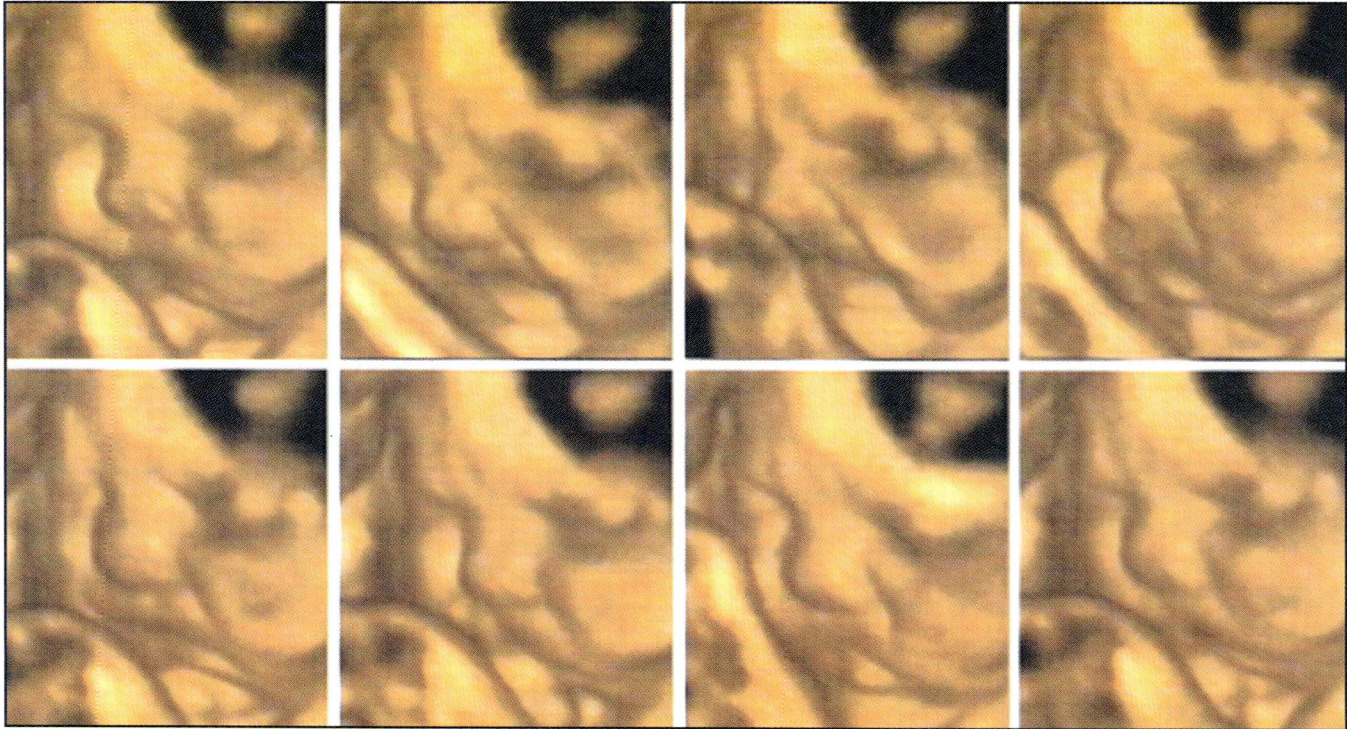

Fig. 15.118: 4D sonography sequence demonstrates changing in the facial expression. The fetus seems to be angry

44. Lees WR, Gardener JE, Gilliams A. Three-dimensional US of the fetus. Radiology 1991;181:131-2.

45. Ludomirski A, Ucrpairojkit B, Whiteman VE, Reece EA, Chu GP, Chan L. New technology in three-dimensional obstetrical ultrasonography: technique, advantages and limitations. Am J Obstet Gynecol 1996;174(Suppl):328.

46. Pretonus DH, Richards RD, Budorick NE, et al. Three-dimensional ultrasound in the evaluation of tetal anomalies. Radiology 1997;205(P)(Suppl):245.

47. Crane JP LeFevre ML, Winbom RC, et al. A randomized trial of prenatal ultrasonographic screening: impact on the detection, management, and outcome of anomalous fetuses. Am J Obstet Gynecol 1994;171: 392-9.

48. Pretorius DH, Nelson TR. Fetal face visualization using three-dimensional ultrasonography. J Ultrasound Med 1995;14:349-56.

49. Lee A. Four-dimensional ultrasound in prenatal diagnosis; leading edge in imaging technology. Ultrasound Rev Obstet Gynecol 2001;1:194-8.

50. Kozuma S, Baba K, Okai T, Taketani. Y. Dynamic observation ot the fetal face by three-dimensional ultrasound. Ultrasound Obstet Gynecol 1999;13:283-4.

51. Roodenburg PJ, Vladimiroff IW, van Es A, Prechtl HFR. Classification and quantitative aspect of tetal movements during the second half of normal pregnancy. Early Hum Dev 1991;25:19-35.

52. Campbell S. 4D or not 4D: that is the question. Ultrasound Obstet Gynecol 2002;19:1-4.

53. Kurjak A, Vecek N, Kupesic S, Azumendi C, Solak M. Four-dimensional sonography: how much does it improve perinatal practicei. In Carrera JM, Kurjak A, Chervenak FA, (Eds): Controversies in Perinatal Medicine. London: Parthenon Publishing, 2003.

54. Kurjak A, Vecek N, Hatner T, Bozek T, Funduk Kurjak B, Ujevic B. Prenatal diagnosis: what does tour-dimensional ultrasound add. J Perinat Med 2002; 30:57-62.

55. Kuno A, Akiyama M, Vamashiro C, Tanaka H, Yamagihara T, Hata T. Three-dimensional sonographic assessment ot fetal behavior in the early second trimester of pregnancy. J Ultrasound Med 2001; 20:1271-5.

56. Kurjak A, Azumendi G, Vecek N, et al. Fetal hand movements and facial expression in normal pregnancy studied by four-dimensional sonography. J Perinat Med 2003;31:496-508.

57. Kurjak A, Stanojevic M, Andonotopo W, et al. Behavioral pattern continuity from prenatal to postnatal life—a study by four-dimensional (4D) ultrasonography. J Perinat Med 2004;32: 346-53.

58. Hohlteld J. Le diagnostic prenatal des feintes labio-palatines. Med Foct Echographie Gynecol 1995; 22:4-15.

59. Bonilla-Musoles F, Machado LE, Osborne NC. Ecograha tridimensional en Obstetricia en el nuevo milemo. Madrid: Marco Crafico, 2000.

**A Kurjak, W Andonotopo,
G Azumendi, N Vecek, B Funduk**

16

Normal and Abnormal Fetal Hand Movements Studied by 4D Sonography

INTRODUCTION

As described earlier, four-dimensional sonography (4D US) provides a new tool for observation of the different movements. The developmental pattern of hand movement concerning the first phase seen by 4D US was described elsewhere.[1-4] However, the differentiation of hand movement concerning the second phase was not reported. Therefore, this topic was in the focus of interest in the current study.

In the early second trimester 4D US provides simultaneous visualization of all four extremities and enables confidential recognition of isolated arm movement and its direction. Because of limitations of 2D US only five types of isolated hand movements are described. They include: hand to head, hand to trunk, hand to foot, hand to fluid and hand to the uterine wall.[5] If one perfoms 4D US hand to head movement can be divided into seven subgroups: hand to head, hand to mouth, hand near mouth, hand to face, hand near face, hand to eye and hand to ear. We have determined the incidence of each subtype of isolated hand to head movement between 13th and 16th weeks of gestation (Figs 16.1 to 16.101).

NORMAL FETAL HAND AND FINGER POSITIONING IN EARLY PREGNANCY

Pooh and Ogura had examined 65 normal fetuses by 3D and 4D US to investigate the natural course of fetal hand and finger positioning.[6] Each appearance of fingers, thumb and wrist was confirmed by viewing on three orthogonal planes. They stated that at 9th week and the beginning of 10th week, fetal hands were located in front of the chest and no movements of wrists

and fingers were visualized (Figs 16.4 to 16.6). Fetal digits including thumbs are located on the same layer at this stage. From the middle of 10th week of gestation, active arm movements were observed associated with active body and lower limb movement (Figs 16.10 and 16.11). Despite active movements of glenohumeral and elbow joints at this stage, wrist and finger movements were not visualized in most cases. At 11th week, a change of finger positioning was seen. At this stage, all fetuses still opened their palms, but five digits were no longer on the same layer. Mild adduction of the thumb and atonic fingers were observed and the palm appearance was clearly different from that at 9th and 10th weeks (Figs 16.4 to 16.6). At 12th week of gestation, fetuses started to clench and unclench their fists (Figs 16.12 and 16.13), but the fist at 12th week seemed to be mild compared with that observed at 13th to 15th weeks. After 13th week, the number of clenching and unclenching fists increased and this movement was often observed. Independent movement of each finger was seen after 13th week of gestation and it appeared to increase in activity and strength.[6]

FETAL HAND AND FINGER POSITIONING IN CASES WITH CENTRAL NERVOUS SYSTEM DISEASES

Fetal hand movements and finger positioning may be influenced by abnormal central nervous system (CNS) development as well as musculoskeletal and peripheral nervous system development. Recently Pooh and Ogura had used 3D and 4D US examination focusing on fetal hand or finger positioning and movements in six cases of CNS diseases, including alobar holoprosencephaly,

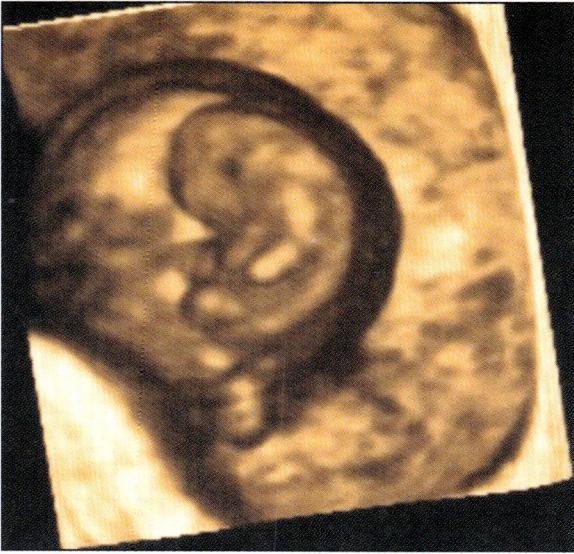

Fig. 16.1: Embryo at 7th week of gestation. The fetal hands are located beside the abdomen and no movements of hands are visualized

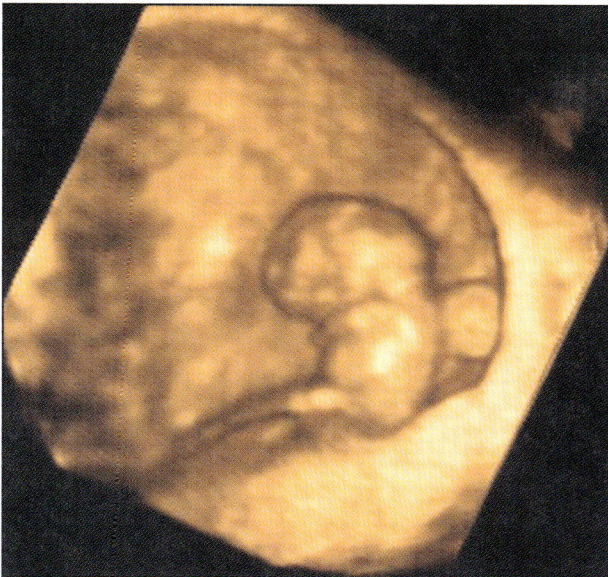

Fig. 16.2: Embryo at 7th week of gestation demonstrated no movements of hands

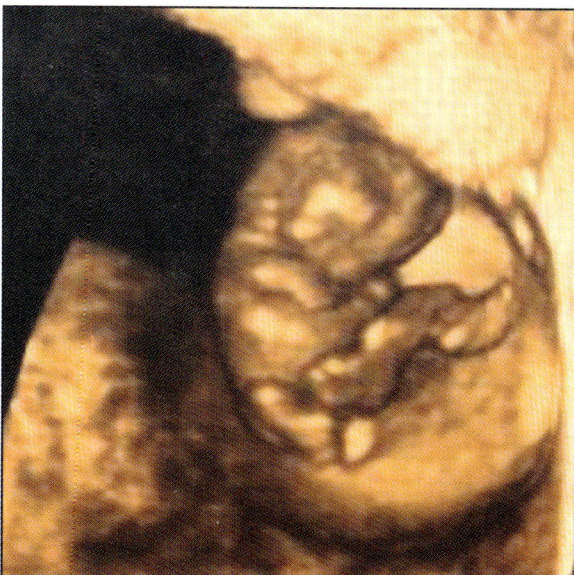

Fig. 16.3: Fetus at 8th week of gestation. The fetal hands are located in front of chest and no movements of wrist and fingers are visualized

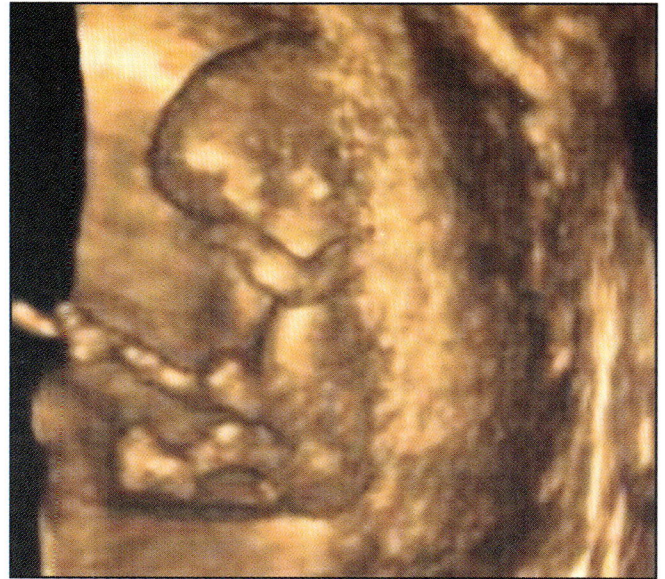

Fig. 16.4: Fetus at 9th week of gestation. The fetal hands are located in front of chest. No movements of the hands are visualized

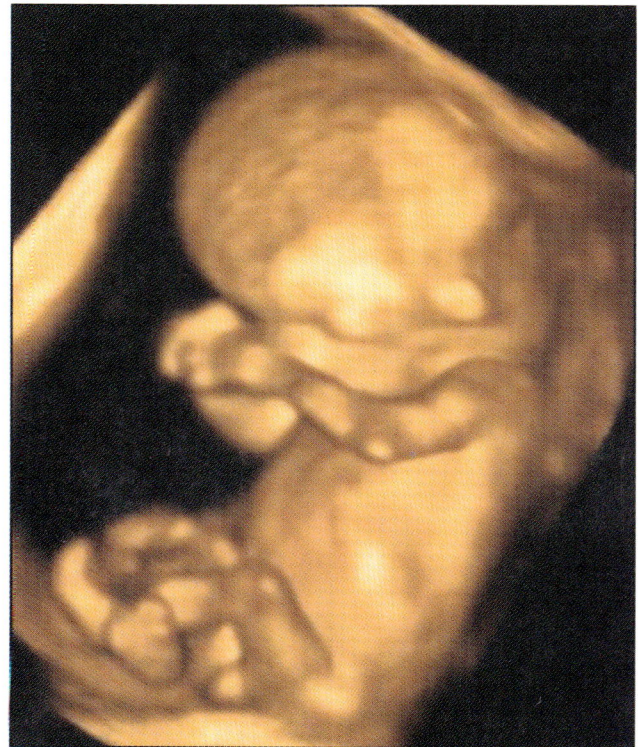

Fig. 16.5: Fetus at 9th week of gestation. No movements of the hands are visualized. Note the wrist and fingers are on the same level

hydrocephaly due to aqueduct obstruction, secondary hydrocephalus with Chiari type II malformation and lumbosacral myeloschisis, exencephaly with incomplete cranial defect, complete anencephaly and Dandy–Walker malformation in the first half of pregnancy.[6] In those cases with CNS abnormalities, fetal hand/finger positioning and movements were demonstrated normally. However, it would be prudent to assume that there is a relationship between a CNS abnormality and fetal behavior including hand/finger positioning and movement. Further multicentric studies are needed before final conclusion.

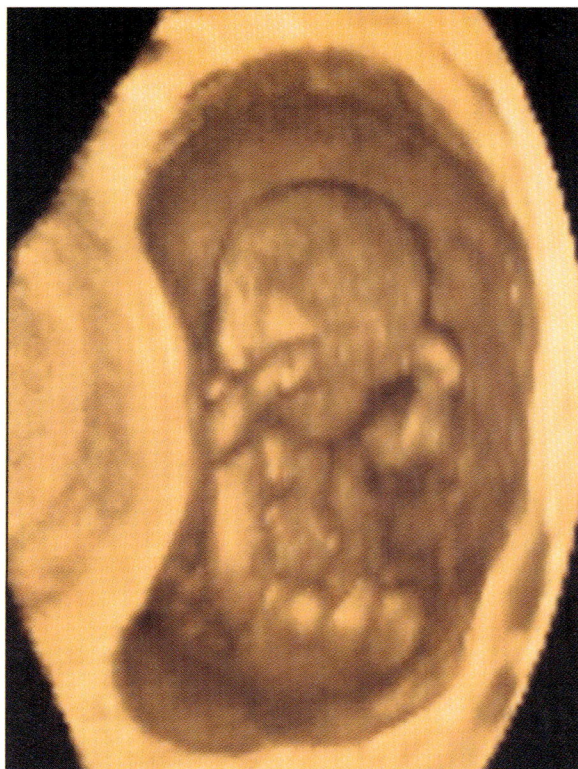

Fig. 16.6: Fetus at 9th week of gestation showing no movements of the hands

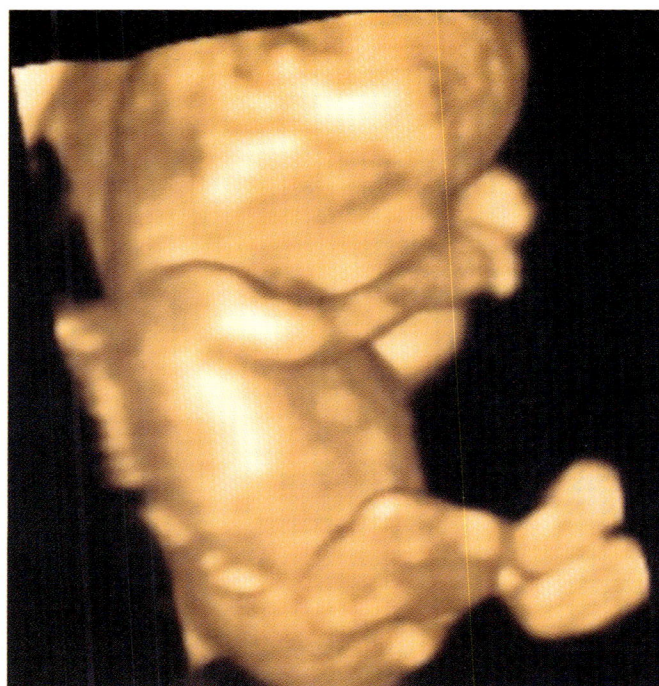

Fig. 16.8: Fetus at 10th week of gestation. The fetal hands are moving directly to the face. Note the movements of wrist and fingers are depicted

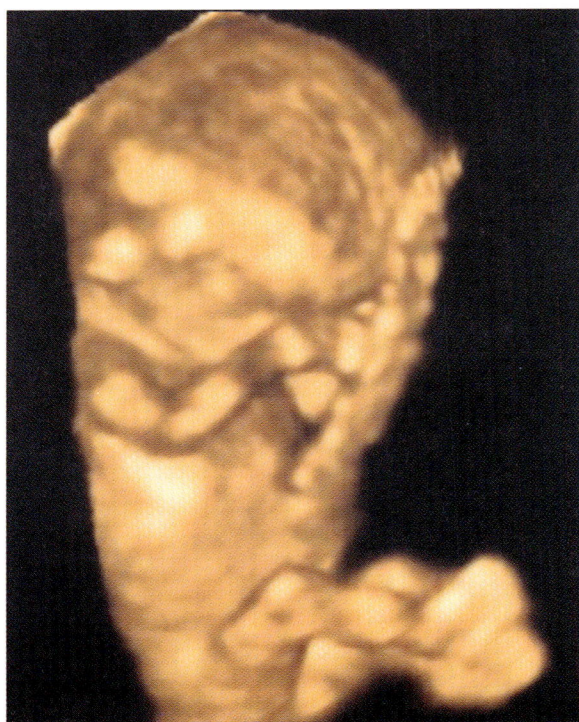

Fig. 16.7: Fetus at 10th week of gestation. The fetal hands are located in front of chest. The wrist and fingers are clearly visualized without movements

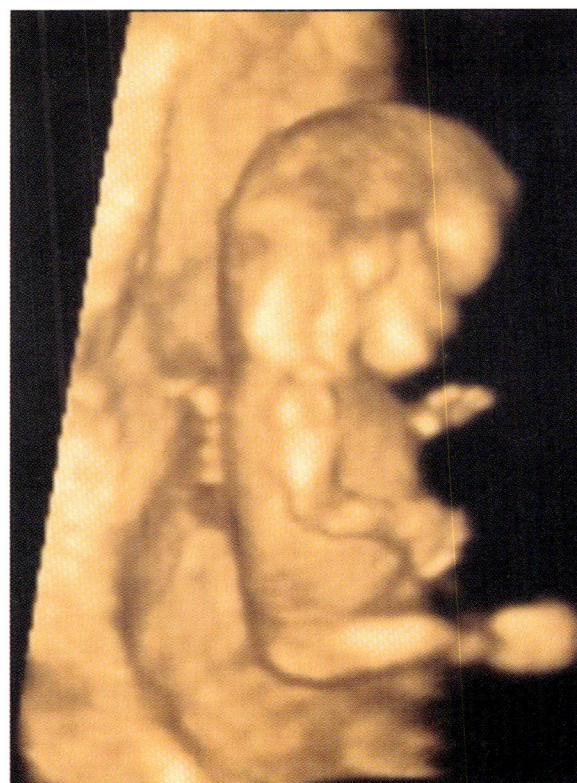

Fig. 16.9: Fetus at 11th week shows opening of the palms, five digits are no longer on the same level

ABNORMAL POSITIONING AND CONTRACTURE OF FETAL HAND/ FINGERS

It has been shown that limb deformity and abnormal hand/finger positioning are known to be associated with chromosomal aberration and/or syndromic diseases.[6] Paluda and colleagues evaluated the relationship of the fetal hand to the forearm in the second and third trimesters by two-dimensional ultrasound, and reported that an abnormal fetal wrist position was associated with a high incidence of karyotype and movement abnormalities.[7] Kos and coworkers reported three-dimensional detection of limb deformity.[8] An overlapping finger is a well known hand deformity often observed in cases of trisomy 18. The overlapping finger is formed from muscle variations along

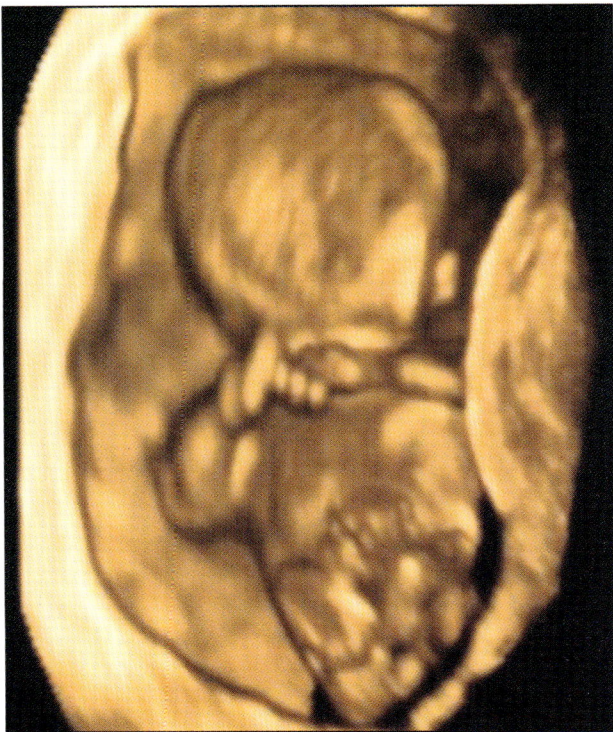

Fig. 16.10: Fetus at 11th week still opens the palms. Note the five digits are not on the same level. Mild adduction of the thumb was observed and the appearance was clearly different from that at 9th and 10th weeks

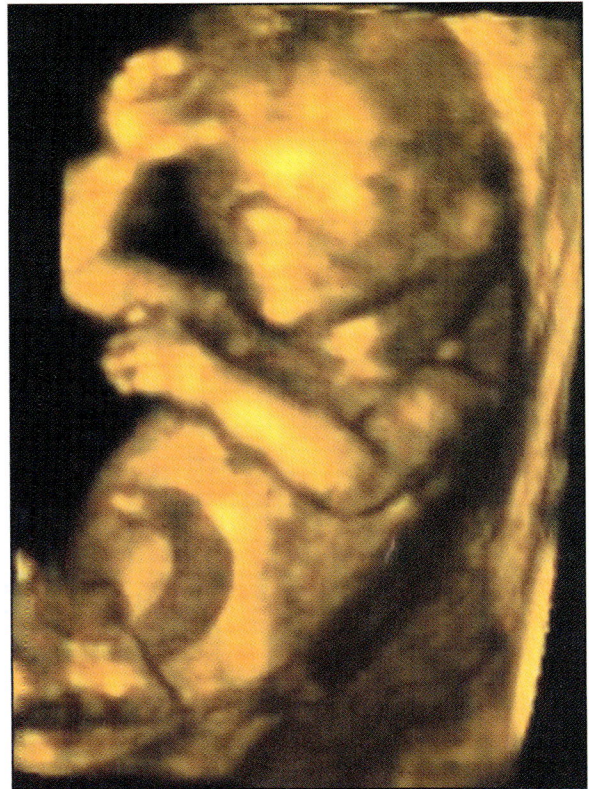

Fig. 16.12: The fetus at 12th week. Active arm movements are associated with active body and lower limb movements

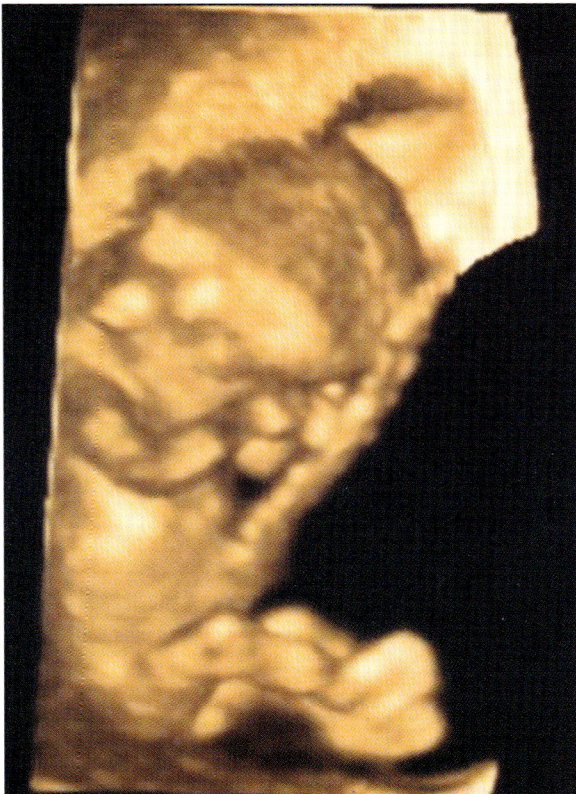

Fig. 16.11: The fetus at 11th week. Hand movement in direction to the face is demonstrated

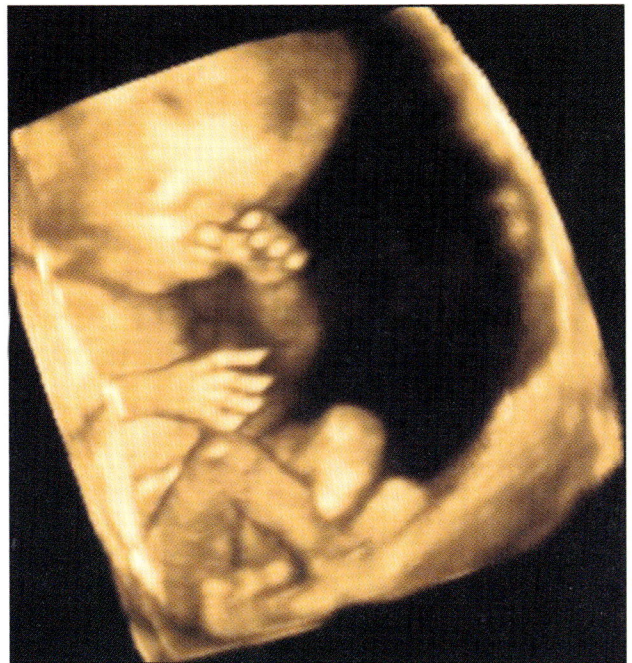

Fig. 16.13: The fetus at 12th week. Note the unclenching visualization of wrist and fingers is clearly depicted. The appearance of the opening palms was different from that at 9th and 10th weeks

the radial margin of the forearm and hand, absence of the thenar muscles, anomalous tendons and attachments and fusions among the arm/forearm flexor group. These variations result in radial or ulnar displacement of the tendons of the extensor digitorum and digiti minimi, with overlapping of the fourth and fifth fingers radially and the index finger in an ulnar direction. However, it has not been clarified when and how the fetal fingers are flexed, overlapped and contracted. Quintero and associates performed transabdominal thin gauge fetoscopy at 12th and 14th gestational weeks in a case of trisomy 18.[9] They observed that finger malposition was not apparent at 12th week, but evident at 14th week, and concluded that malpositioning of the fingers

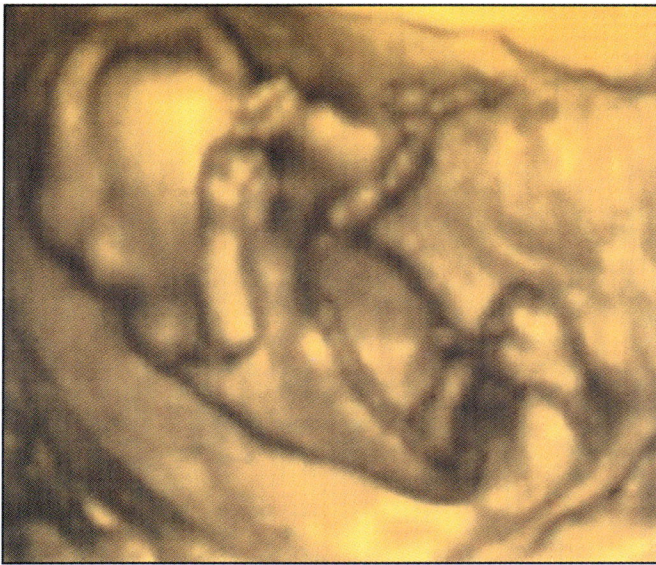

Fig. 16.14: The fetus at 13th week. Note clenching the fist movement at 13th week. The number of clenching and unclenching fist increased from this gestational age

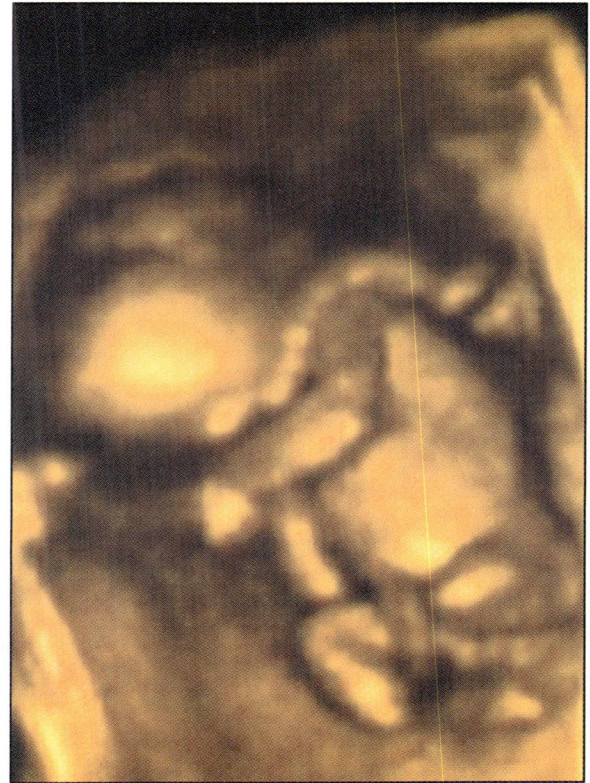

Fig. 16.16: The same fetus from the previous Figure 16.15 shows the hand movement on the umbilical cord

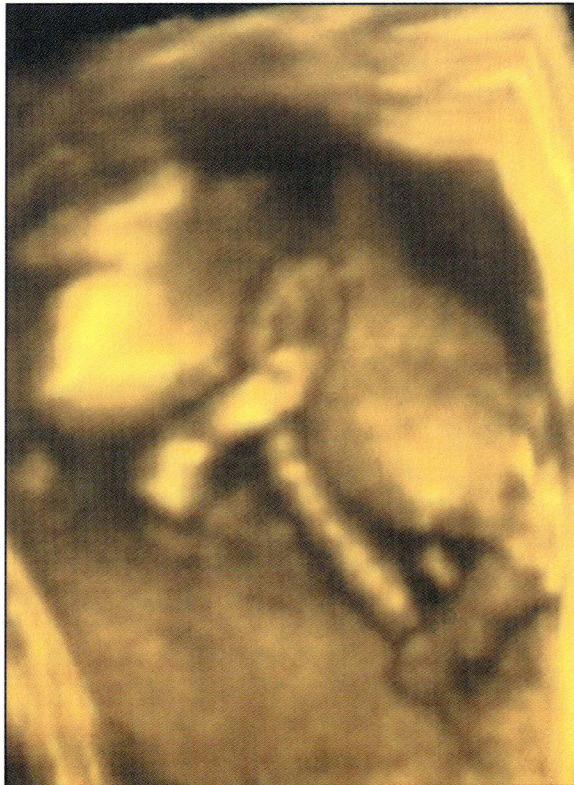

Fig. 16.15: The fetus at 13th week of gestation. Note the umbilical cord is between the left arm and the fetal shoulder

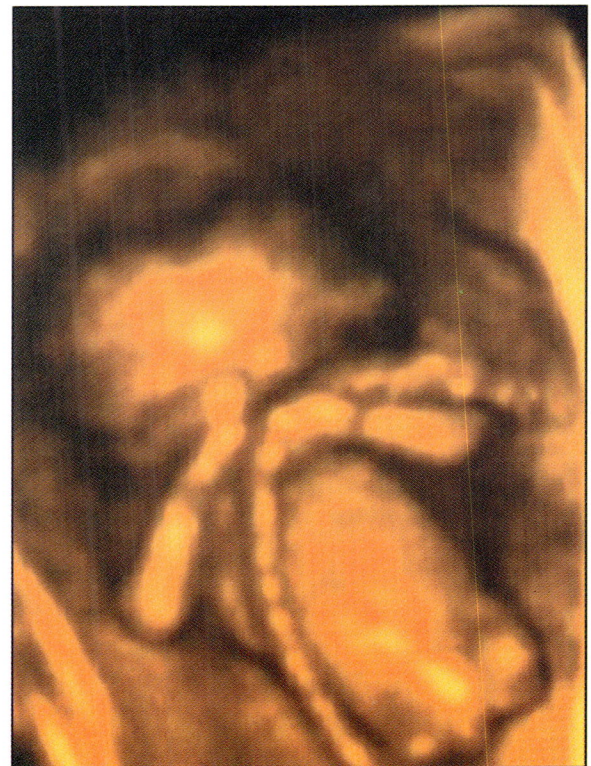

Fig. 16.17: The fetus at 13th week of gestation. The fetus seems trying to grasp the umbilical cord

in trisomy 18 occurs some time between 12th and 14th weeks of gestation. Normal extended fingers were demonstrated at 11th week. A clenched fist without overlapping fingers was depicted at 12th week and overlapping fingers were clearly detected at 17th week of gestation. From both the case of Quintero and colleagues and our case, it is suggested that overlapping of fingers may not occur before 13th week of gestation. However, we had another interesting case of trisomy 18 with left wrist malposition. In this case, on referral because of nuchal translucency at 11th

week, abnormal left hand appearance was demonstrated and wrist malposition already formed was strongly suspected. Serial three/four-dimensional ultrasound examination confirmed wrist malposition before amniocentesis at 16th week (Figs 16.91 and 16.95). This case had an abnormal palmar flexion instead of

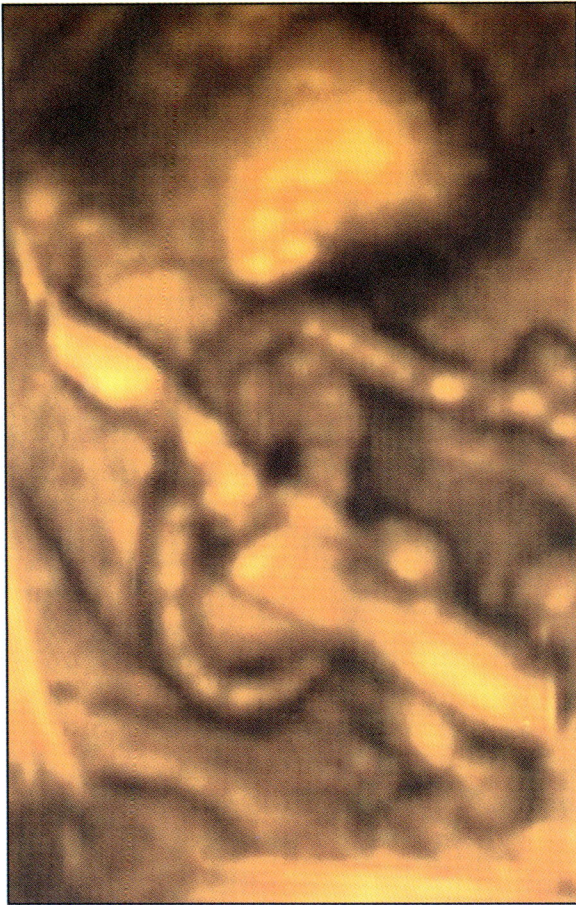

Fig. 16.18: The fetus at 13th week. Note the hand movements are visualized and the fetus seems trying to flee from the umbilical cord

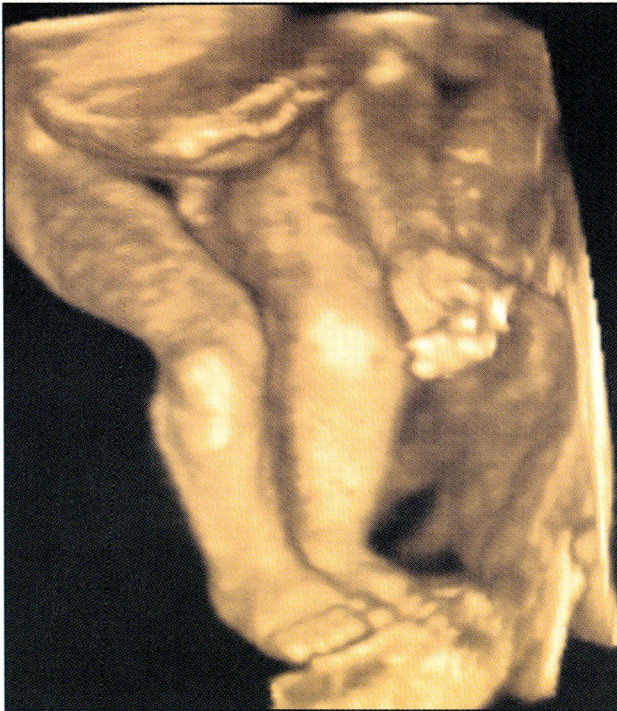

Fig. 16.20: Fetus at 18th week demonstrated the hand movement direction to the left knee. Note the umbilcal cord is surrounding the upper left arm

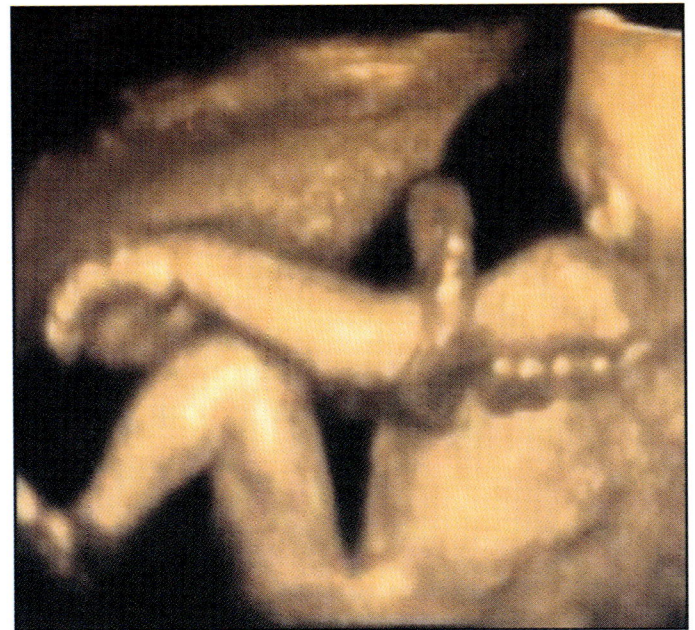

Fig. 16.19: Fetus at 16th week of gestation shows the hand movement direction to the left knee

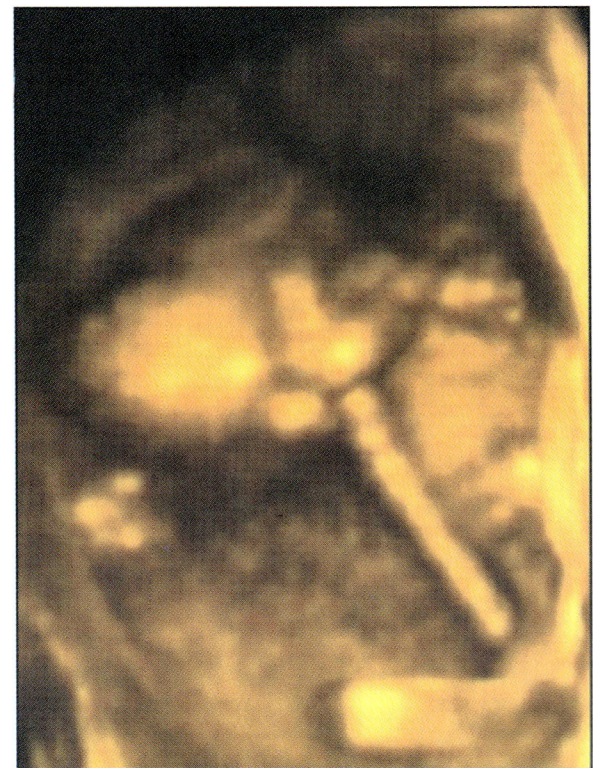

Fig. 16.21: Fetus at 13th week. Note the hand movement in grasping the umbilical cord

overlapping fingers. From this case, it is indicated that there may be a different mechanism associated with other muscular and tendon variations to cause abnormal palmar/ wrist flexion at an earlier stage than that of abnormal digital flexion such as overlapping fingers.

ZAGREB EXPERIENCE

Zagreb group has analyzed a total of 15 fetuses in uncomplicated pregnancies at 13th to 16th weeks by 4D US.[1] For visualization of the fetal hand movements, transducer was positioned so that

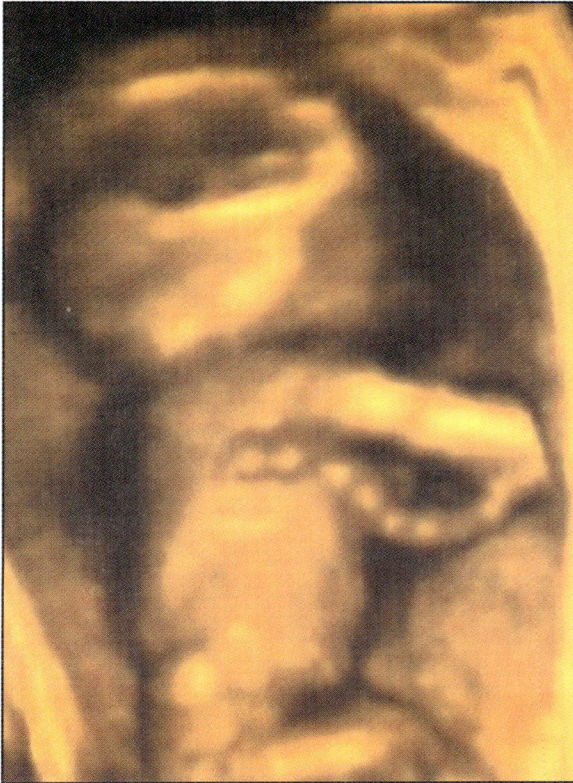

Fig. 16.22: Fetus at 13th week. Note the left hand of the fetus dragged along the umbilical cord

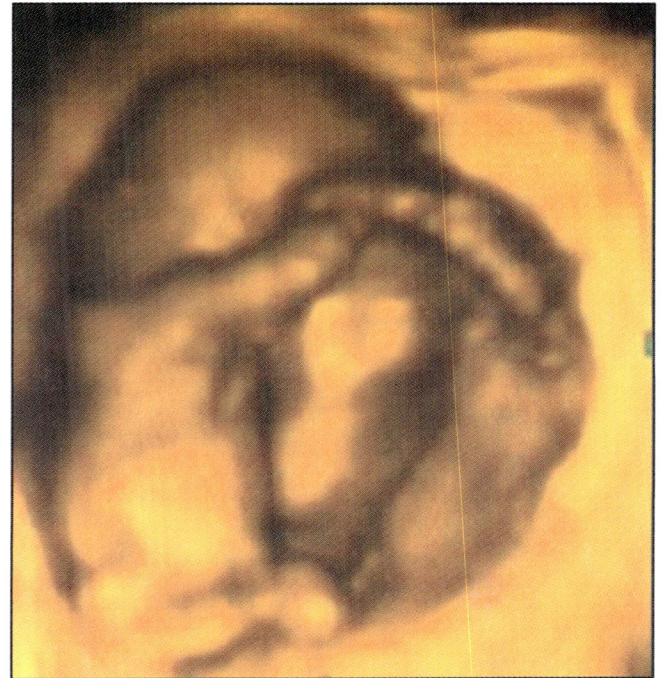

Fig. 16.24: Fetus at 13th week demonstrated hand movement on the umbilical cord

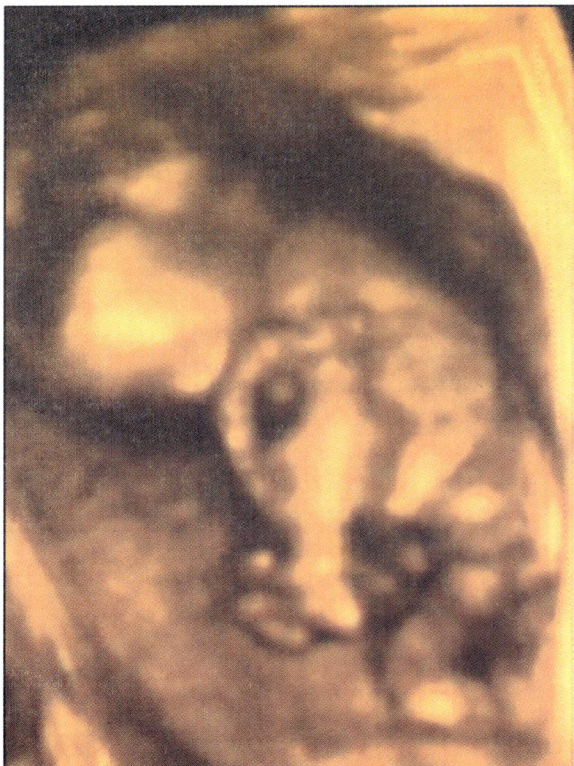

Fig. 16.23: Fetus at 13th week shows extension from both of the hands in the longitudinal axis

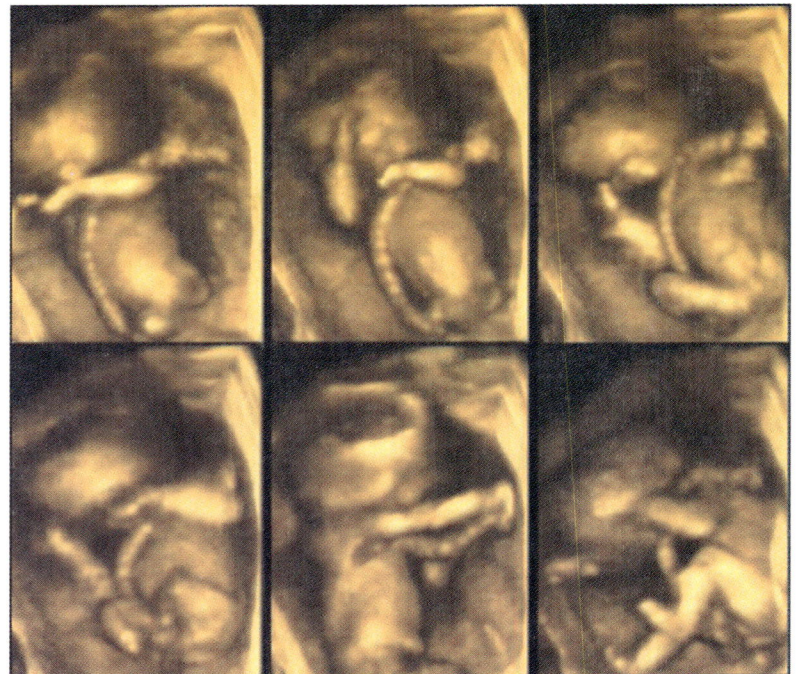

Fig. 16.25: 4D sequence demonstrated active hand movement and movement of the elbow joints at the 13th week of gestation

a sagittal section of fetal trunk including head, thorax and abdomen was obtained. Each fetus was documented for 15 minutes by 4D US. Gestational age was estimated from the first day of the last menstrual period and confirmed by first trimester sonographic examination. In the first part of study gestational age was determined using BPD measurement. Fetuses were divided into following groups: the first consisted of fetuses between 12th and 13th weeks, the second of fetuses between 14th and 15th weeks and the third group of fetuses between 16th and 17th weeks.[1]

Our group had characterized seven types of hand movement. They include:

1. Hand to head — when hand movement ends as contact of fingers with parieto-occpitalo-temporal region of the head (Fig. 16.73).

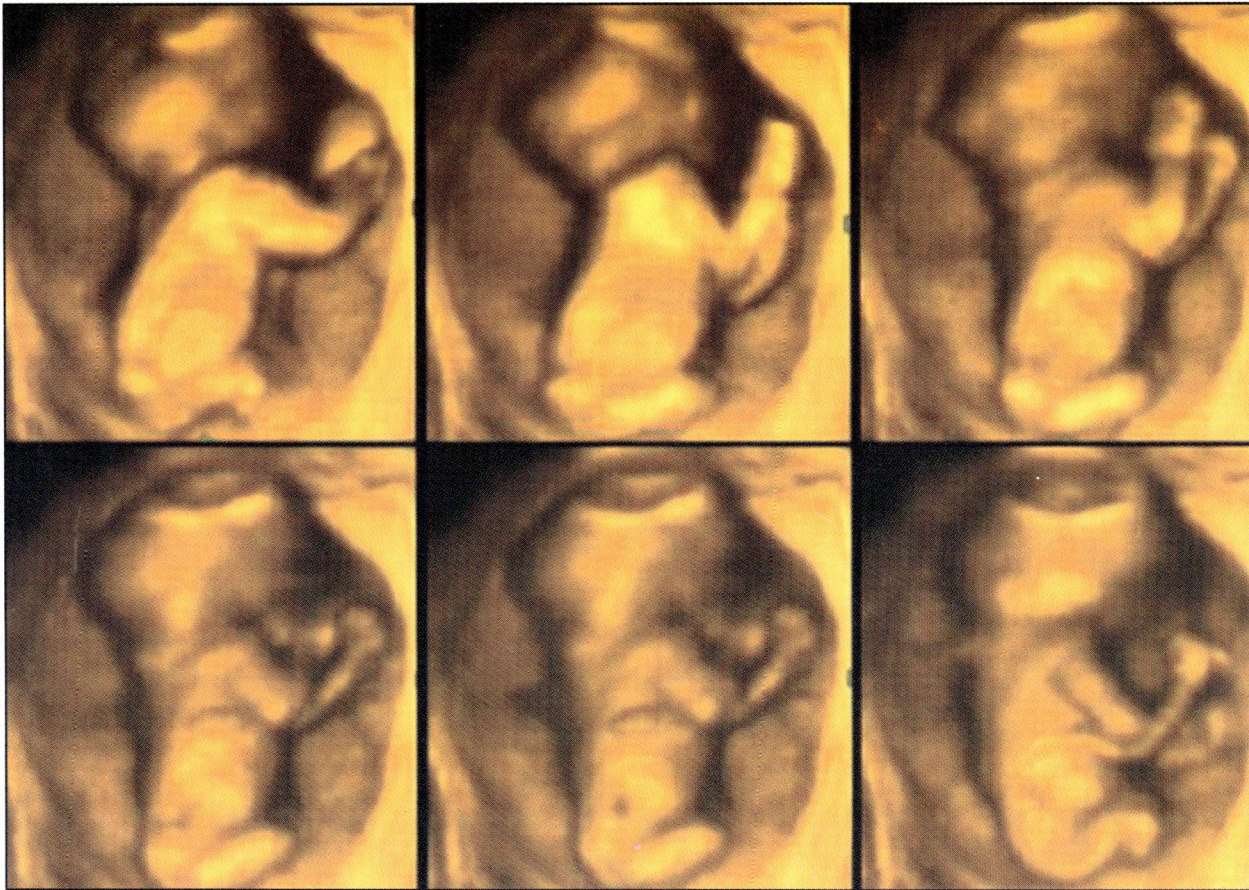

Fig. 16.26: 4D sequence depicted the hand movement in the direction to the uterus wall

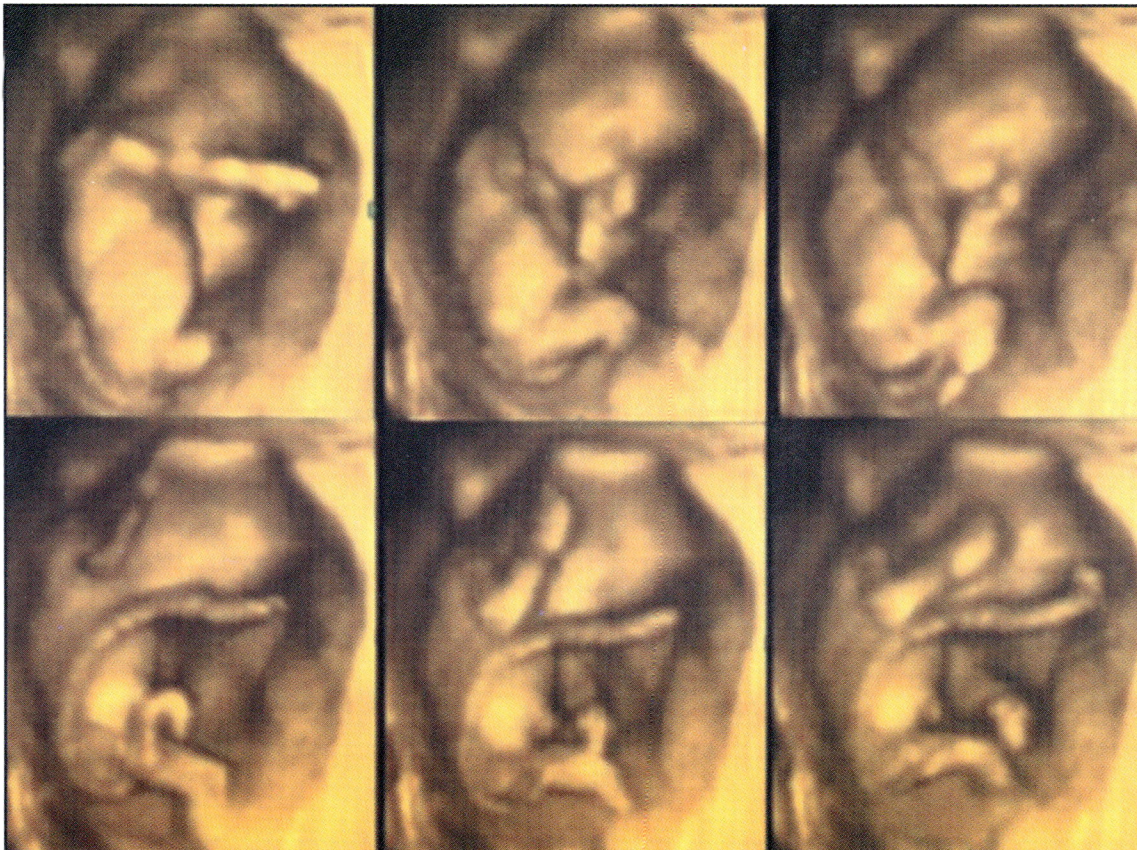

Fig. 16.27: 4D sequence demonstrated extension and flexion of the hand from the fetus at the 13th week

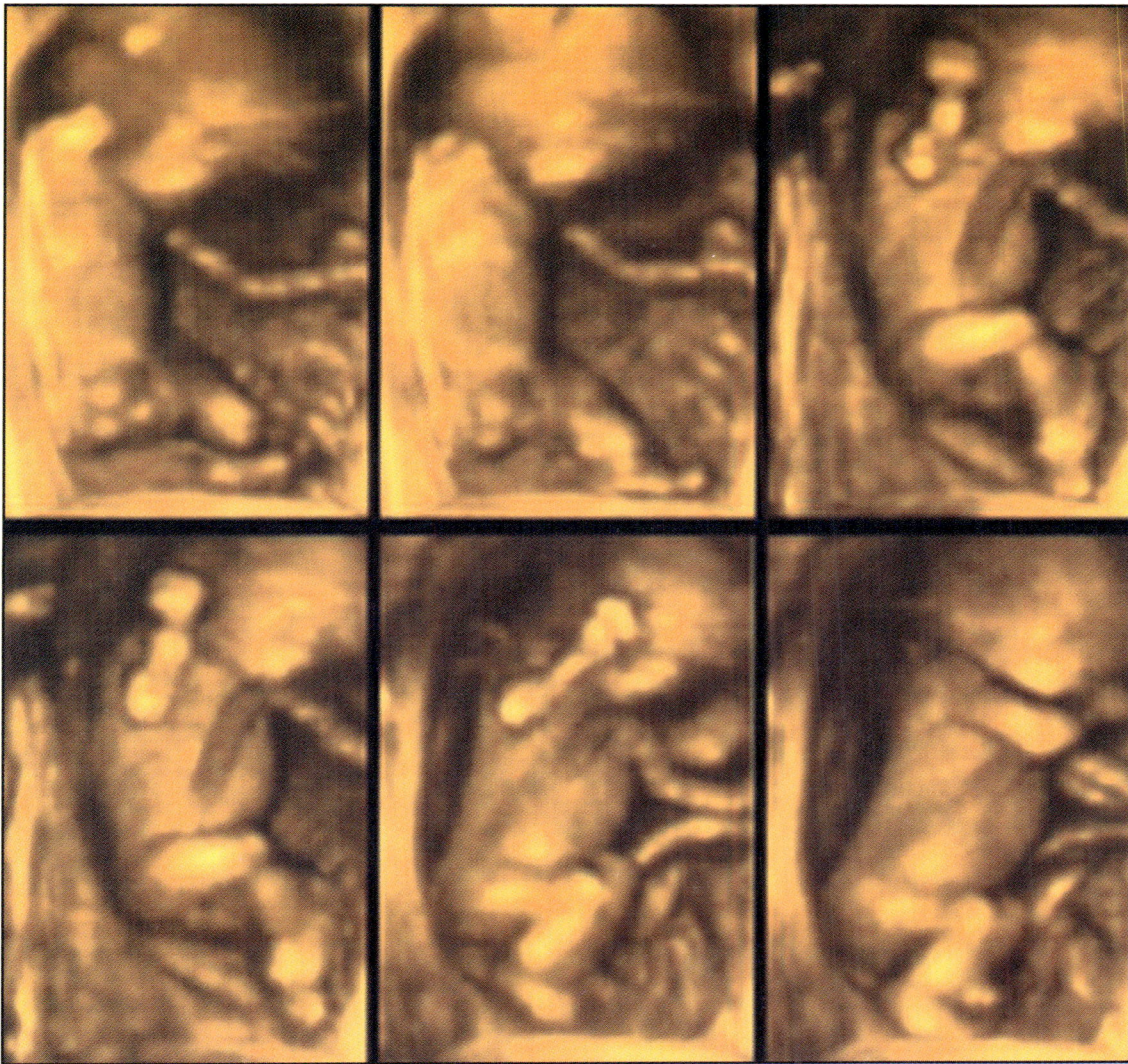

Fig. 16.28: 4D sonography imaging shows hand movements in the direction to the head of the fetus at 13th week

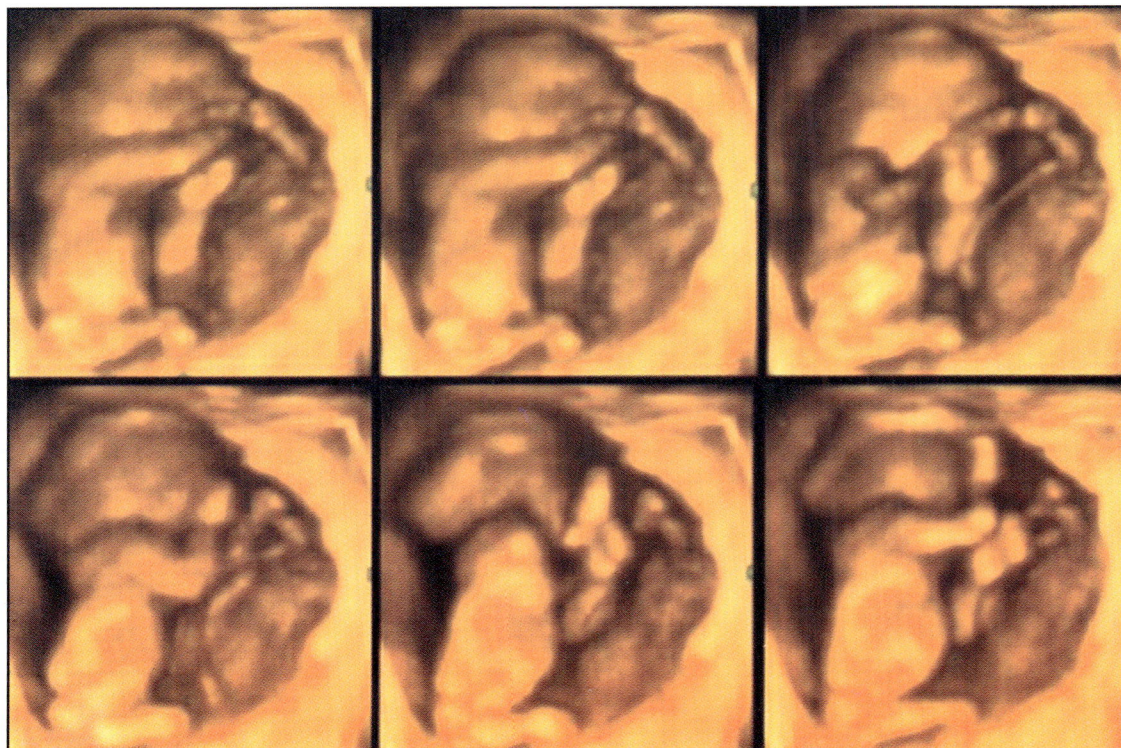

Fig. 16.29: 4D sonography imaging shows hand movements from the fetus in attempting to release from the umbilical tie

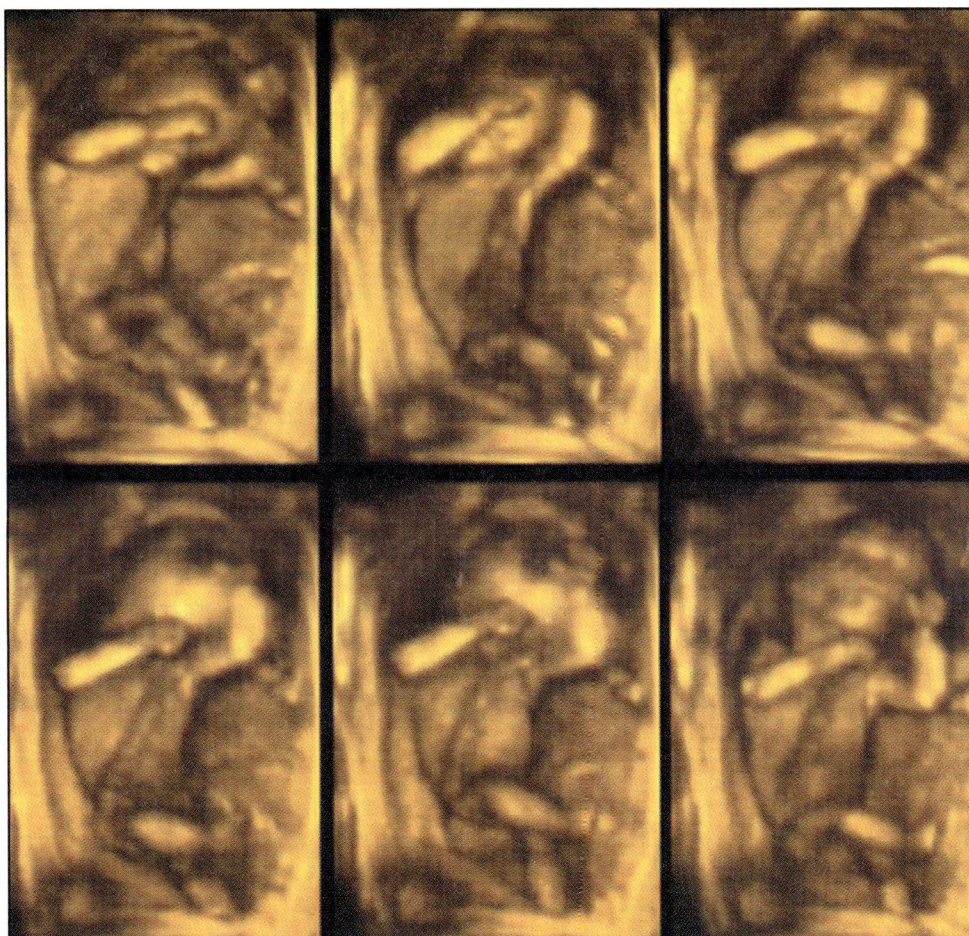

Fig. 16.30: 4D sonography imaging demonstrated hand movements direction to the head

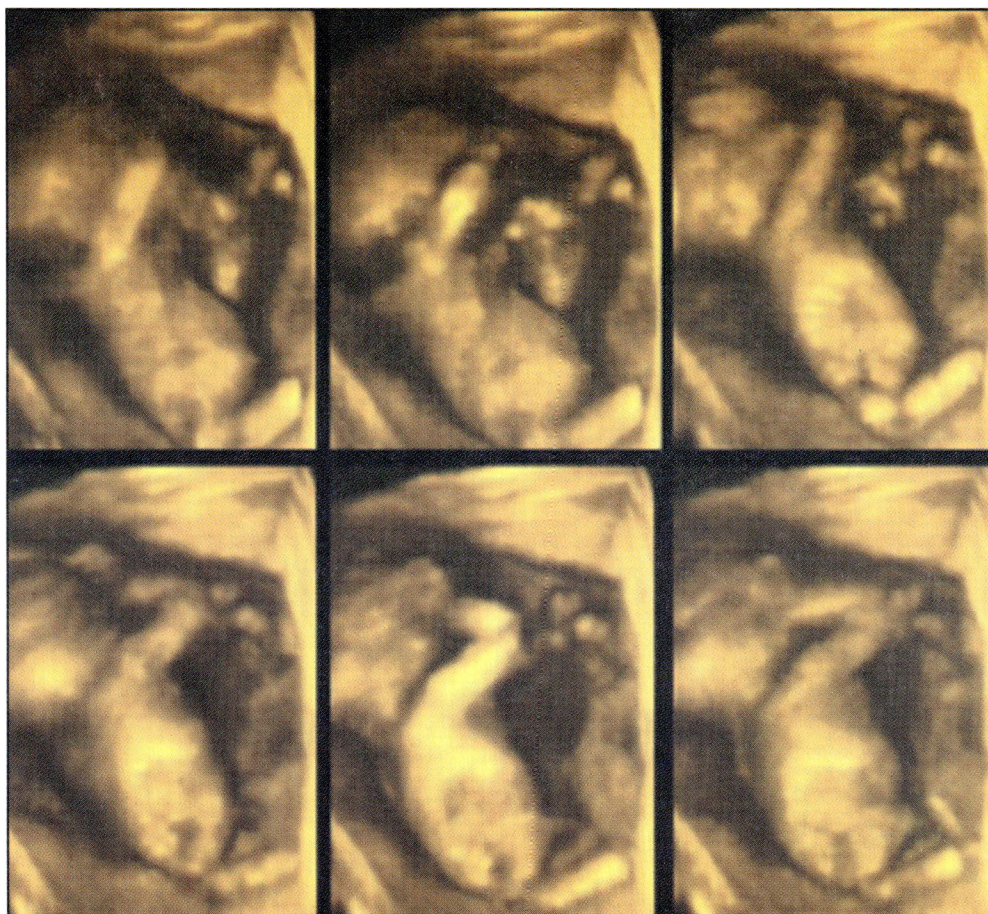

Fig. 16.31: 4D sequence shows the hand direction and elbow joints movement to the uterine wall

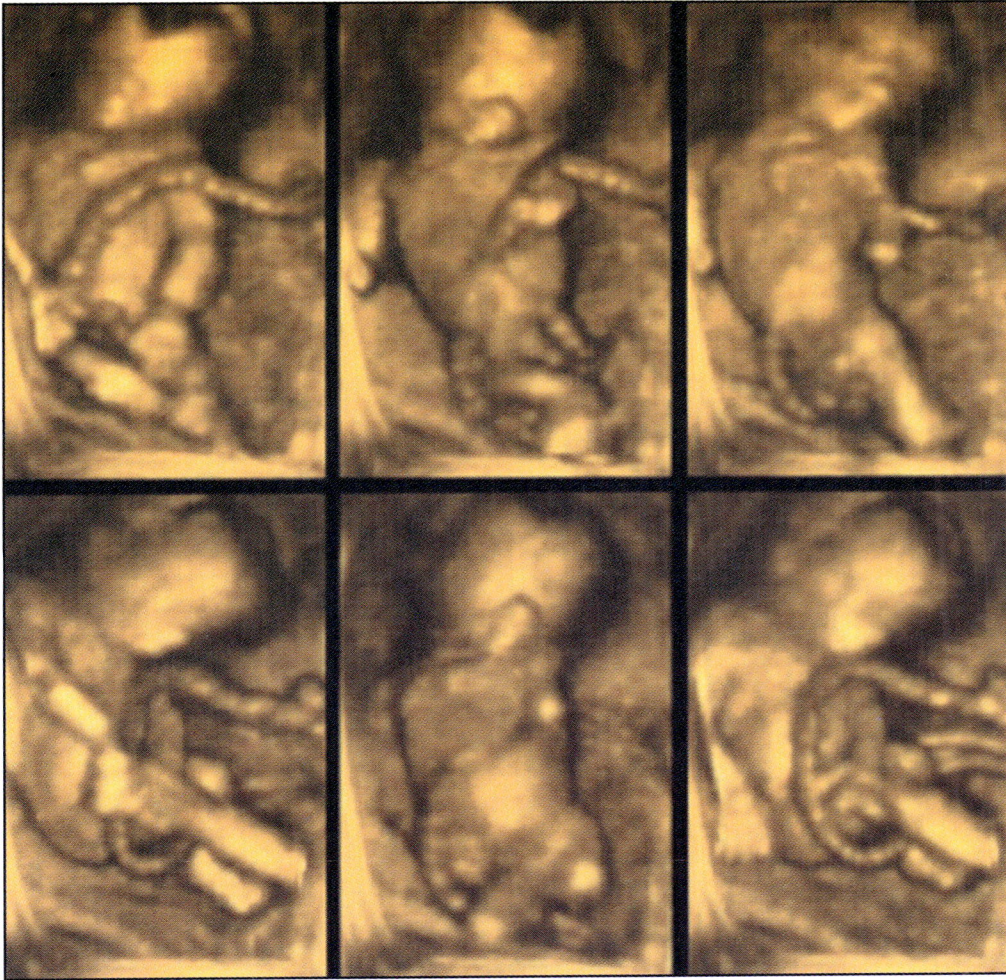

Fig. 16.32: 4D sequence demonstrated the fetus at 13th week still plays with the umbilical cord

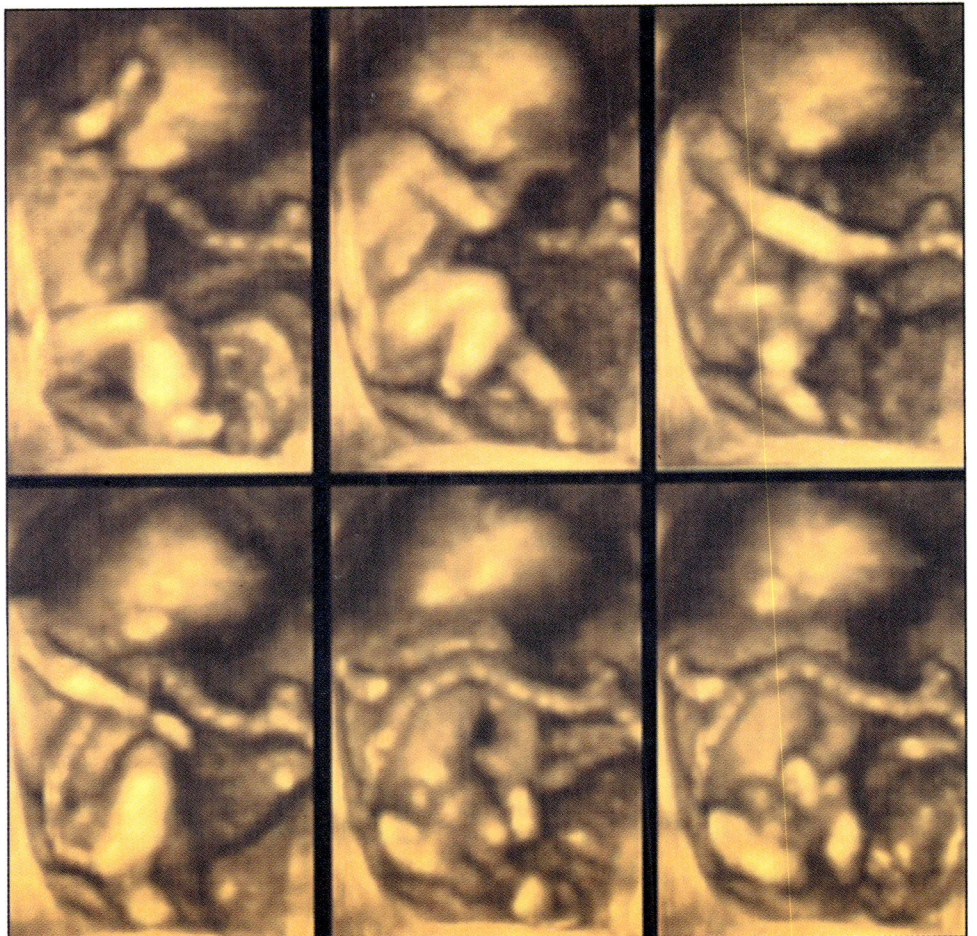

Fig. 16.33: 4D sequence shows the fetus at 13th week is tried to manipulate the umbilical cord

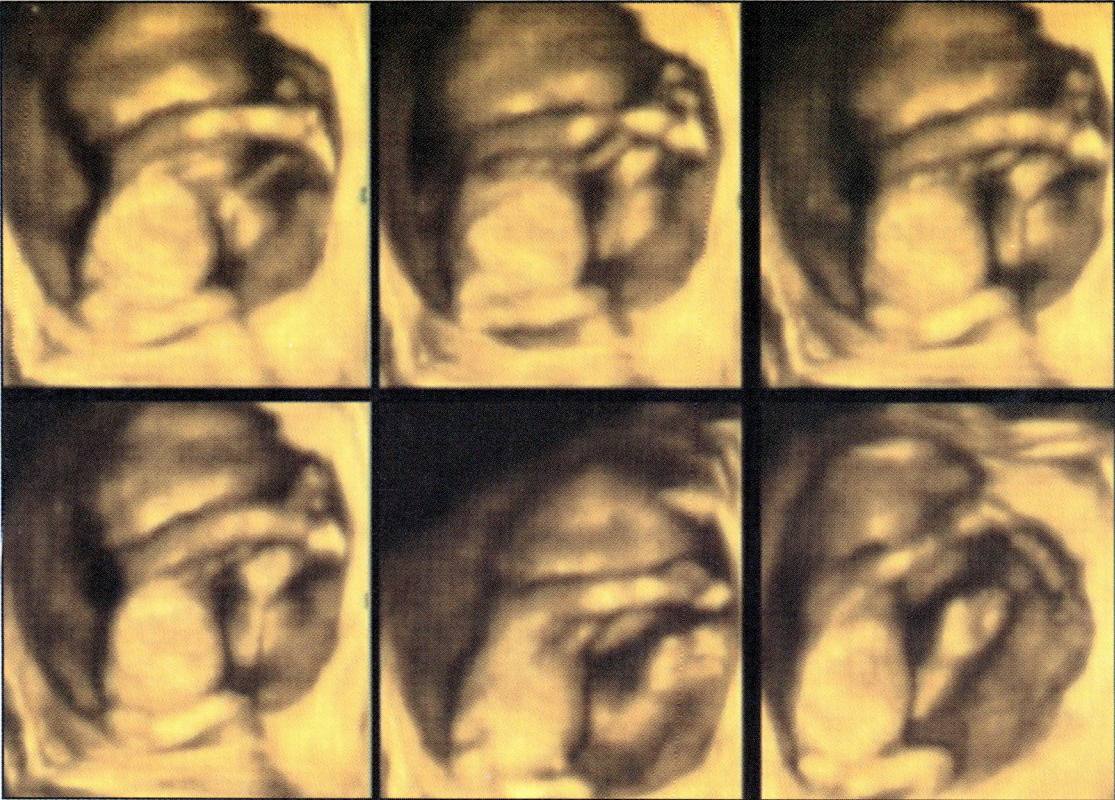

Fig. 16.34: 4D imaging demonstrated hand movements directly extended to the uterine wall

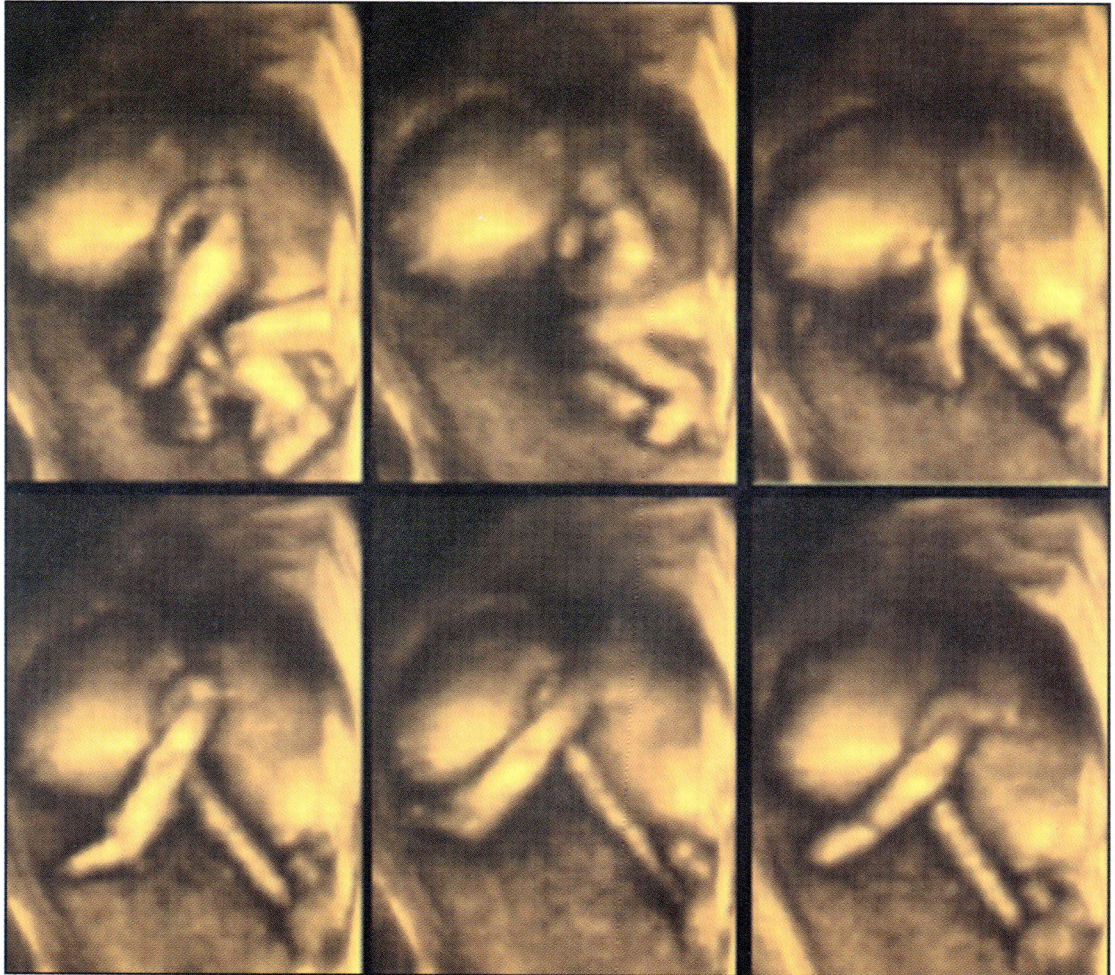

Fig. 16.35: 4D imaging shows the left arm of the fetus turned up. The fetus seem to be raising the umbilical cord

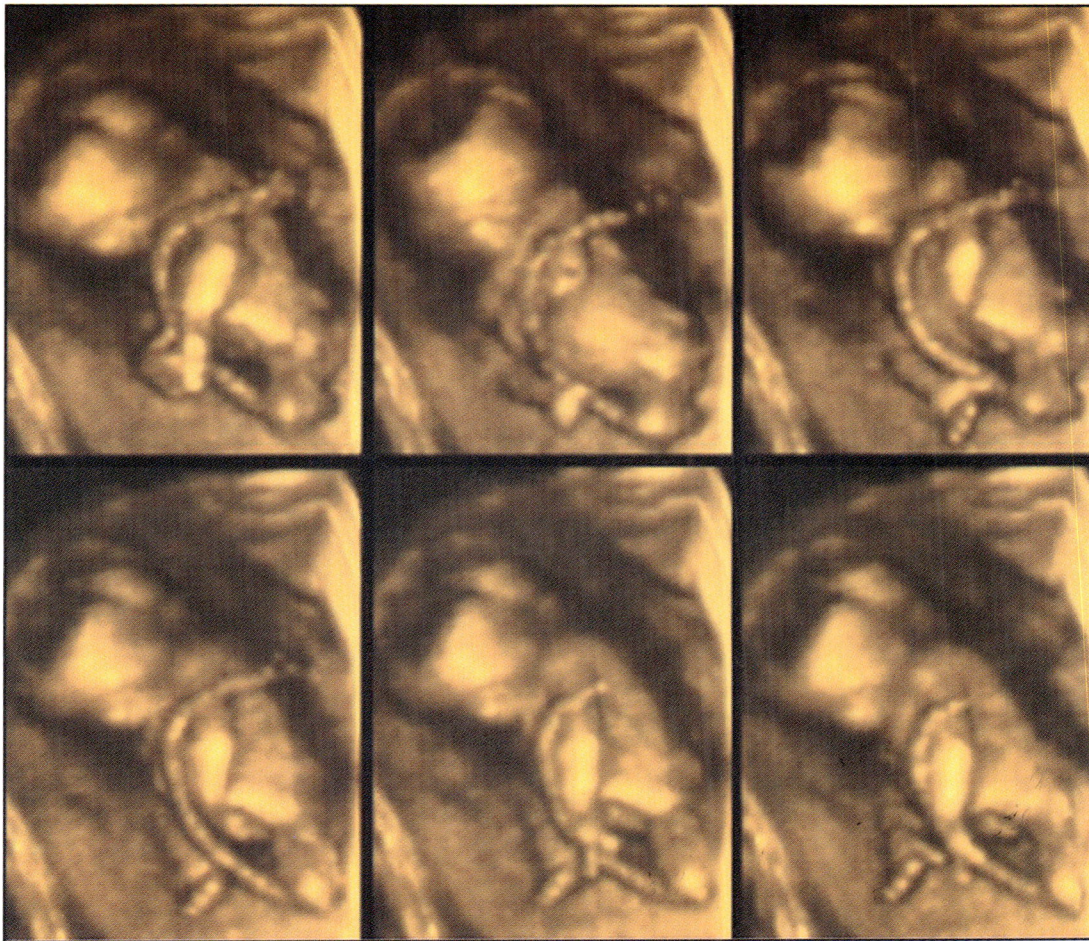

Fig. 16.36: 4D imaging of the fetus shows active arm movement when trying to release from the umbilical tie

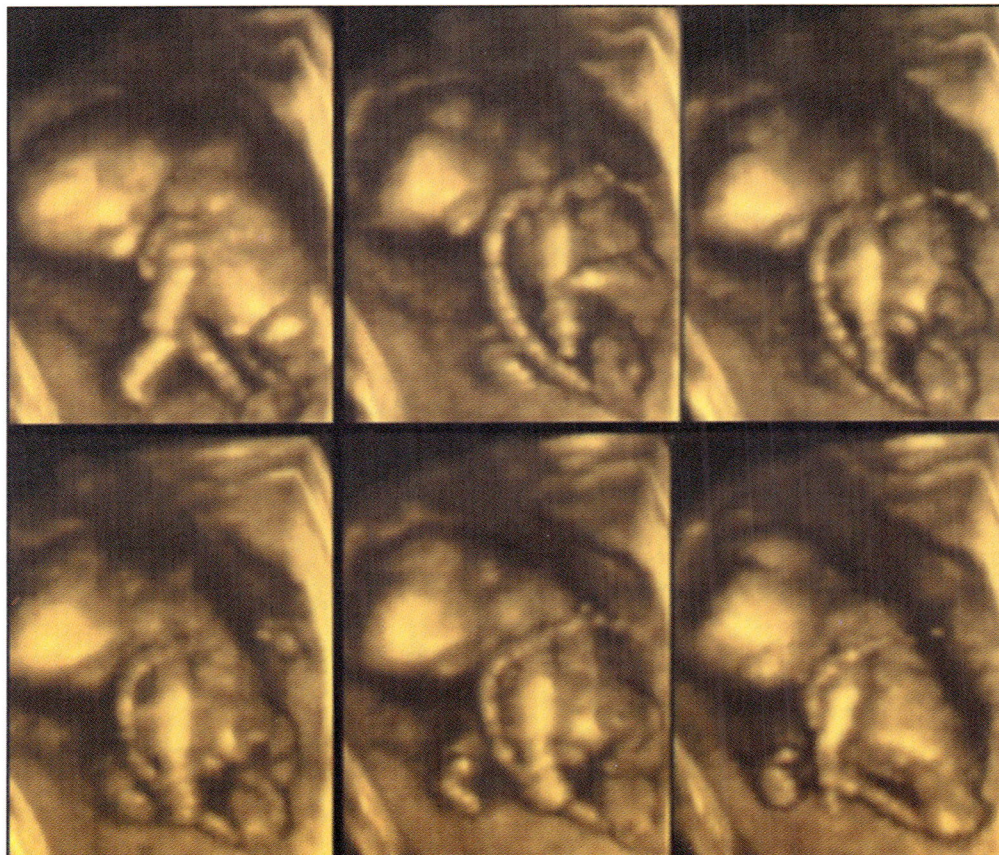

Fig. 16.37: 4D imaging of the fetus shows extension of the arms side by side from the umbilical cord

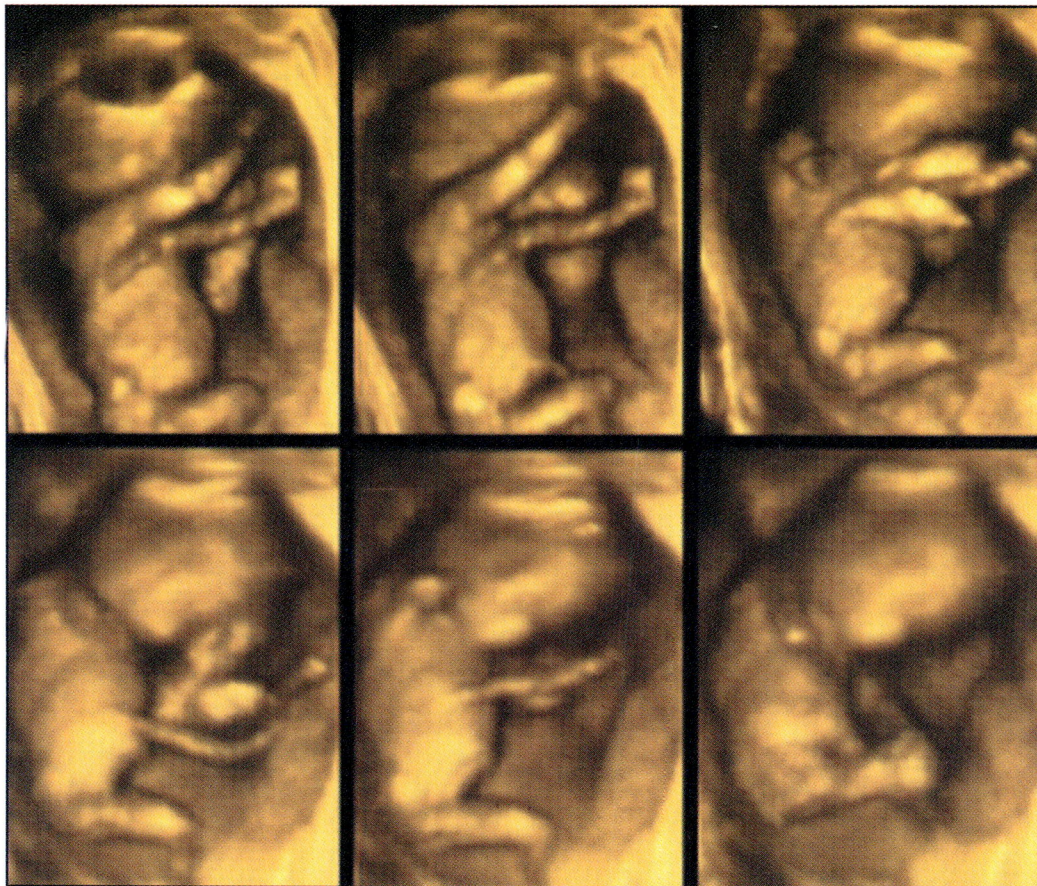

Fig. 16.38: 4D imaging of the fetus demonstrated hand movements in the direction to the uterine wall

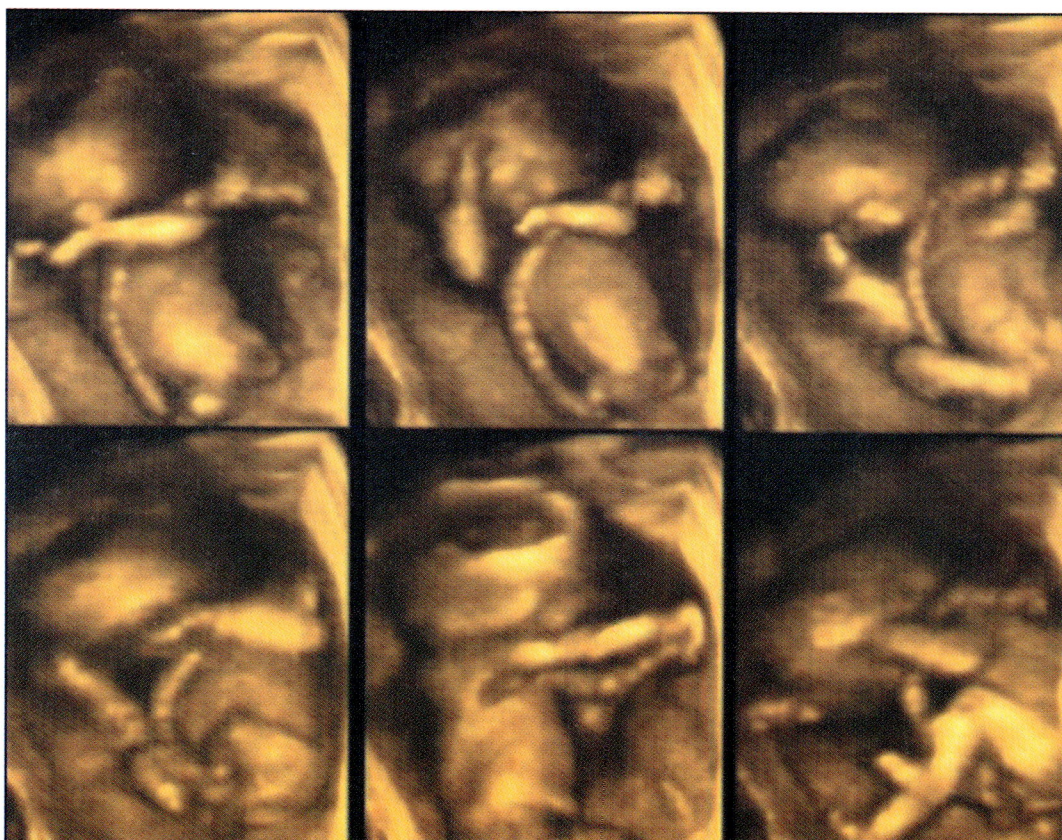

Fig. 16.39: 4D imaging of the fetus at 13th week in manipulating the surrounding environment such as umbilical cord and uterine wall

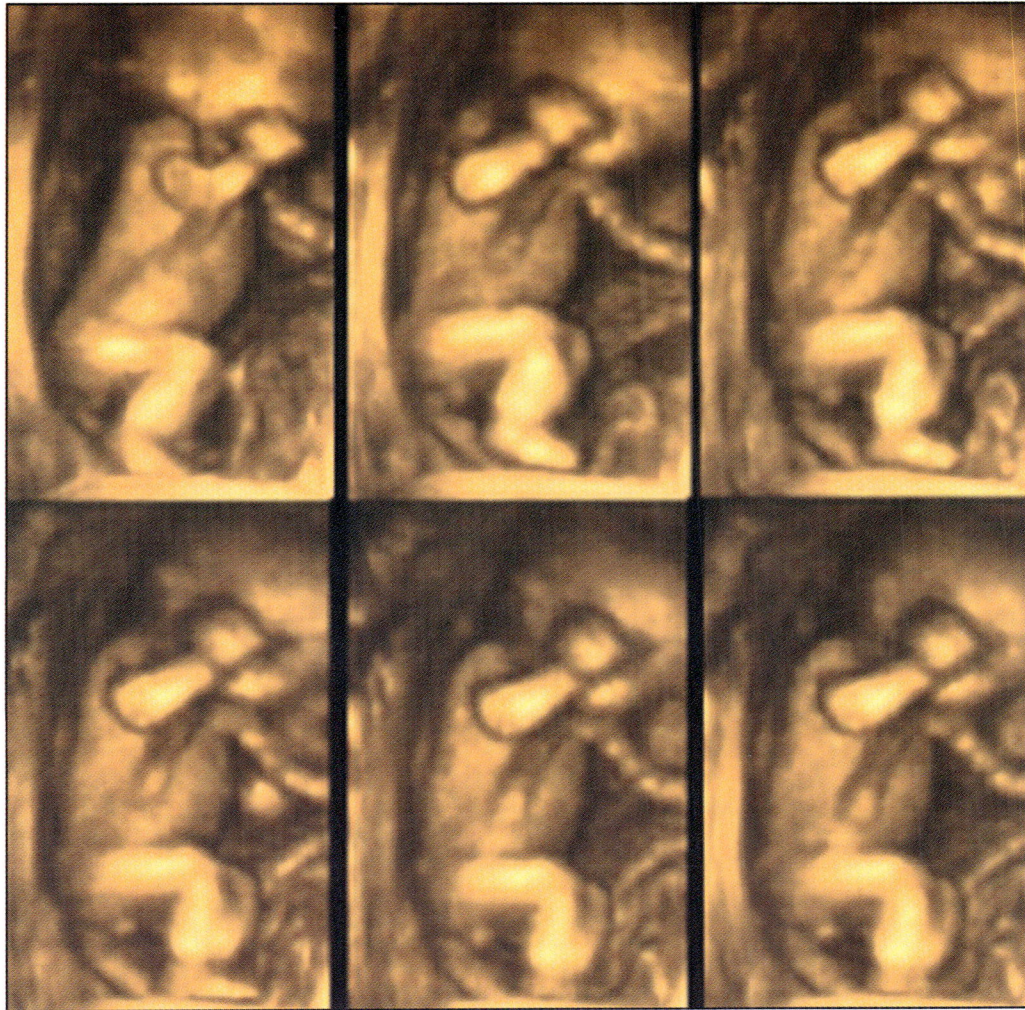

Fig. 16.40: Hand movement directed to the fetal face is clearly visualized

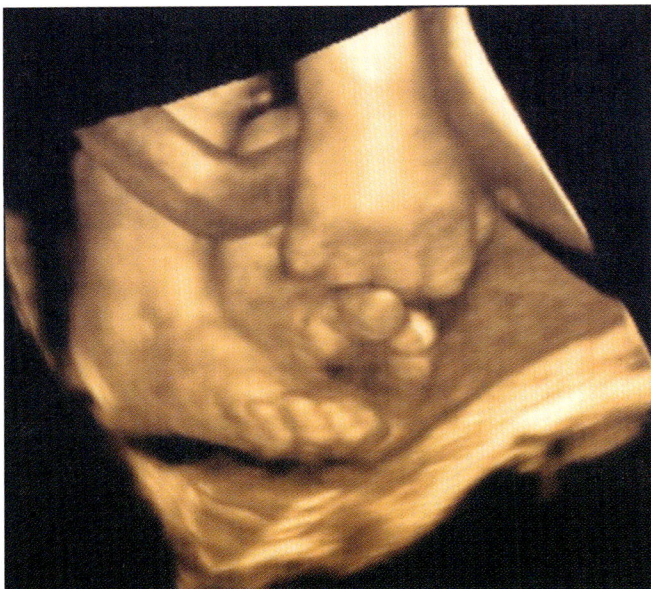

Fig. 16.41: Hand movement directed to the feet is clearly depicted by 3D surface rendering

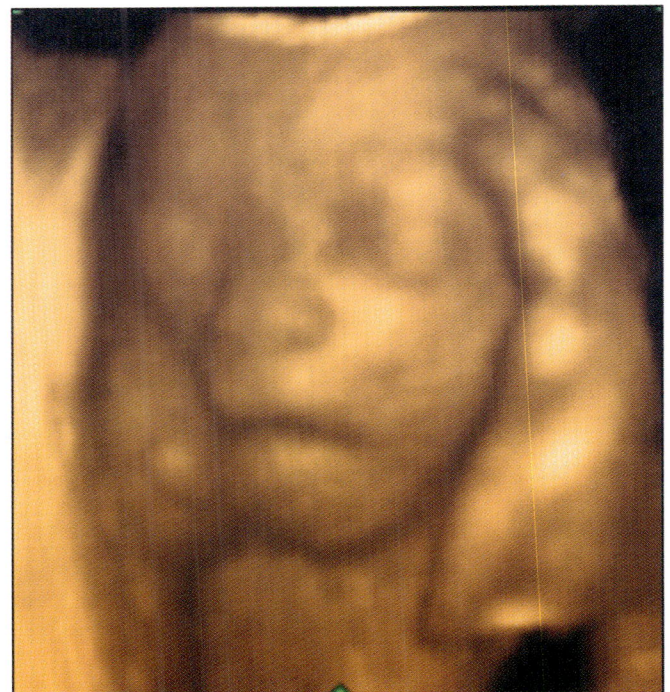

Fig. 16.42: Hand movement directed to the head is clearly visualized in the fetus at 19th week of gestation

2. Hand to mouth — when hand movement ends as contact of thumb or finger and the mouth, touch of the lips or or touch of the immediate oral region (Fig. 16.70).

3. Hand near mouth — when movement ends with fingers in fluid between nose and sholders/nipples or between both shoulders. Hands must be below eyes within ears, less a hand away from mouth (Fig. 16.44).

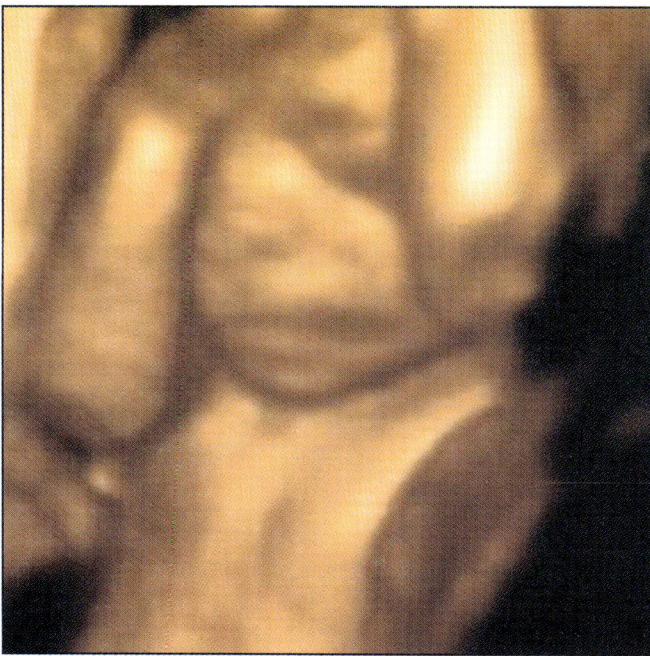

Fig. 16.43: Hand movements directed to the head is obtained by 3D scan

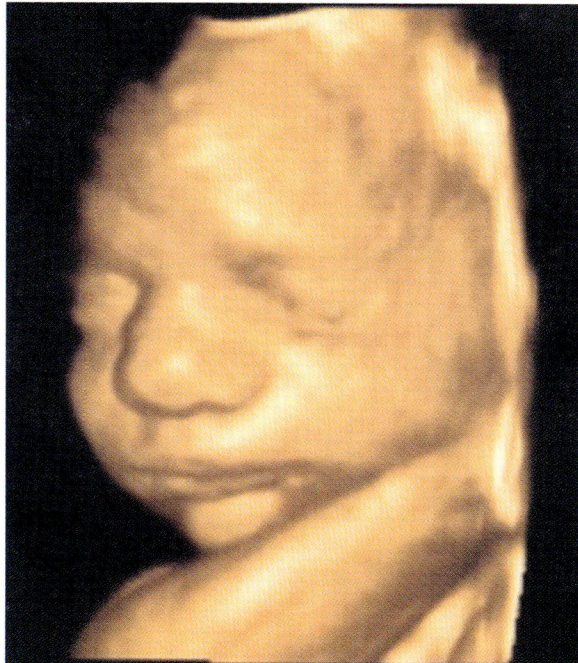

Fig. 16.44: 3D surface rendering shows hand movement directed to the left shoulder

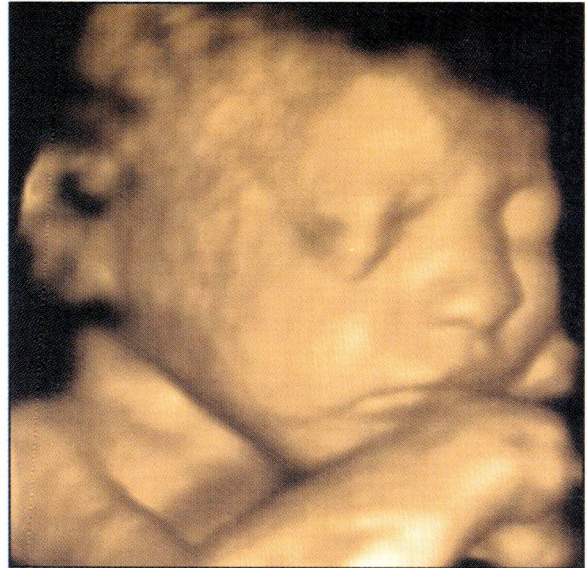

Fig. 16.45: 3D surface rendering shows hand to mouth direction

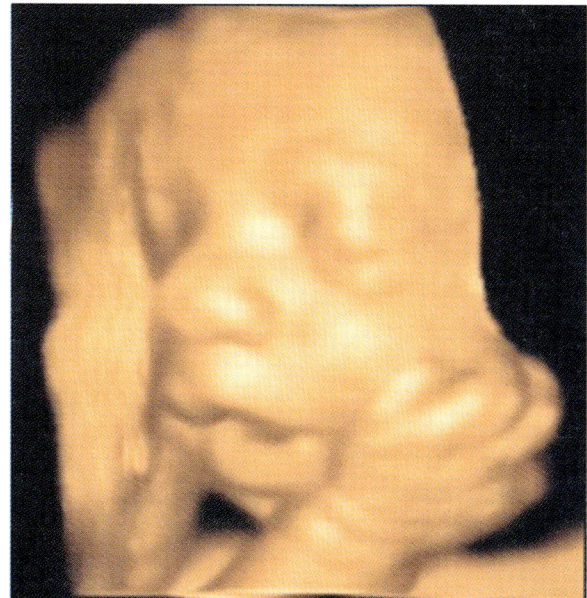

Fig. 16.46: 3D surface rendering shows hand to face direction

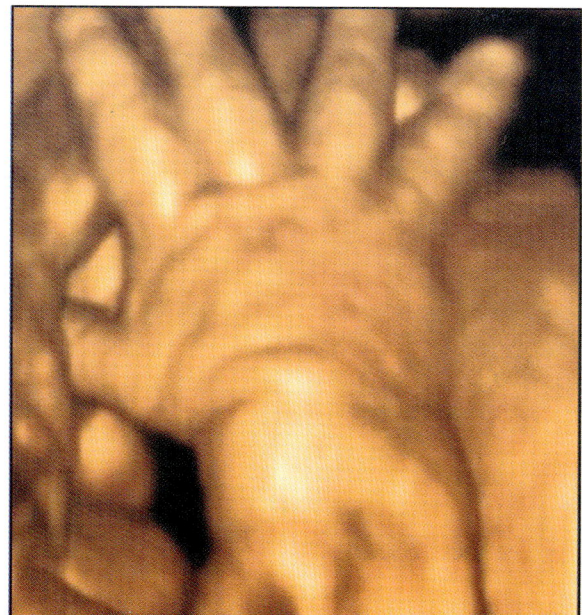

Fig. 16.47: 3D surface rendering shows the opening palms. Note the surface anatomical structure of the fingers are distinctly visualized

4. Hand to face — when movement ends with hand in contact with the face (cheeks, chin, forehead) (Fig. 16.60).
5. Hand near face — when movement ends with finger in fluid in front of the face but not in mouth region (Fig. 16.55).
6. Hand to eye — when movement ends as hand or palm or fingers in eye region (Fig. 16.75).
7. Hand to ear — when movement ends as hand contact with the ear (Fig. 16.72).

Our recent study has shown that during the second and third trimesters it is possible to study total fetal behavioral activities. This may stimulate multicentric studies of the fetal behavior and

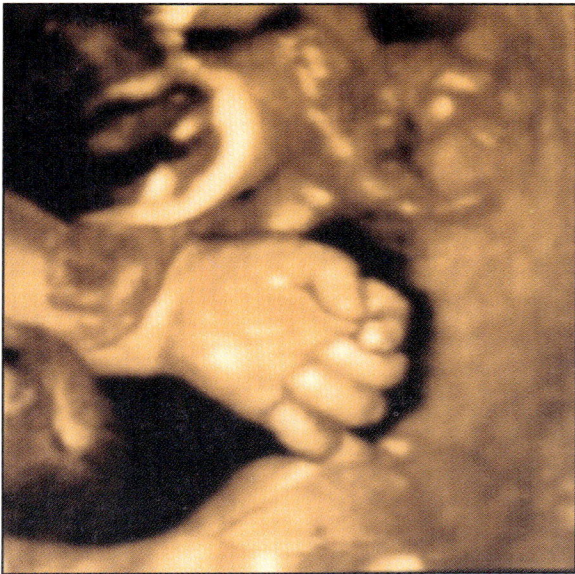

Fig. 16.48: 3D surface rendering shows the fetal palms

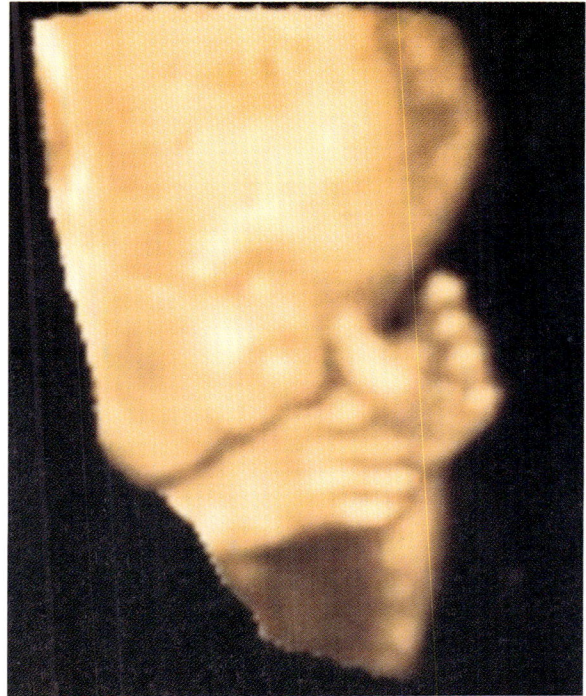

Fig. 16.50: 3D scan shows both of the hand in front of the face

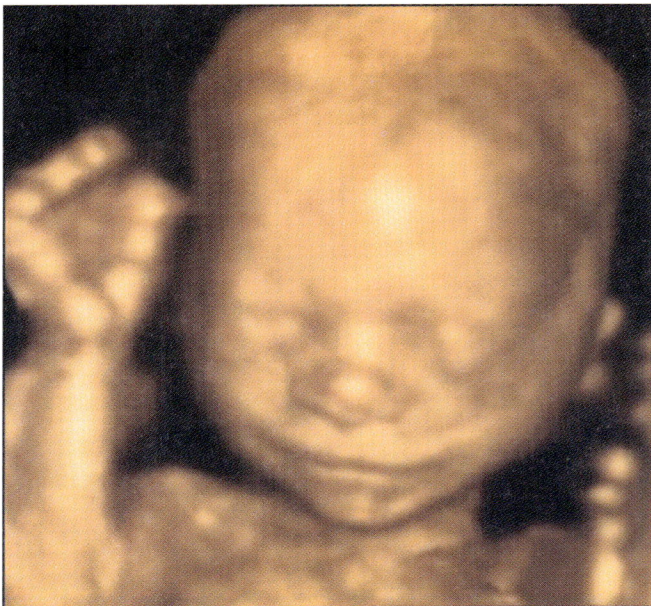

Fig. 16.49: 3D scan shows the fetus raised the right arm in front of the face

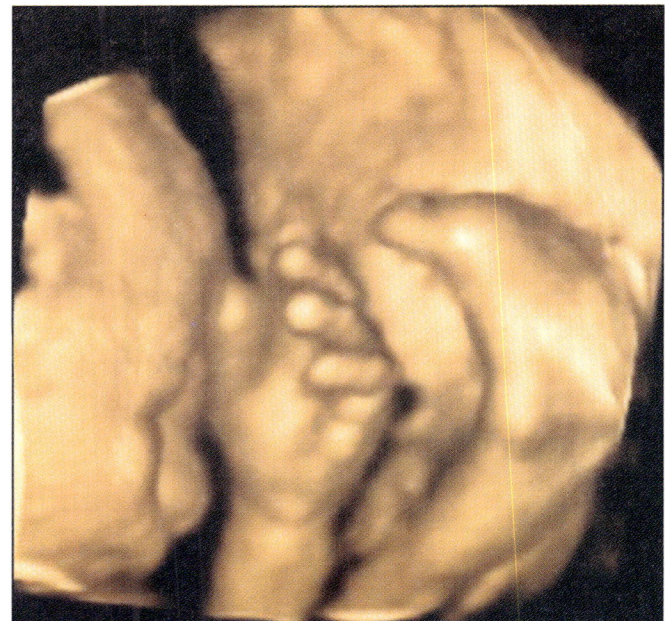

Fig. 16.51: Hand to head movement is visualized by 3D technique

responsiveness as a sign of neurological maturation. In the long-term fetal behavioral studies may become a mean of assessing fetal wellbeing.[1,4] Such a collaborative study is under way in Zagreb, Barcelona and Malaga.

It has been established that the amount of isolated arm movements decreased gradually from 13th through 16th weeks (Fig 16.102A). All recordings have been made during 15 minutes interval. The incidence varied between 50 and 120 with a median value of 60 at 13th week, 17 and 27 with a median value of 23 at 14th week, 0 and 6 with a median value of 2 at 15th week, 18 and 28 with a median value of 25 at 16th week. The highest range was registered at 13th week of gestation. Data from Figure 16.102B demonstrate the incidence of hand to head movement pattern. Note a decrease in their incidence, followed by a plateau

at 14th week of gestation. The incidence varied from 4 to 29 at 13th week and from 0 to 7 at 16th week of gestation. Figure 16.102C shows the incidence of hand at mouth movement between 13th and 16th weeks of gestation. The incidence varied between 0 and 4 with a median value of 2 at 13th week, and between 0 and 2 with a median value of 2 at 16th week. The highest range was found at 15th week of gestation. At 13th week a plateau was observed and stayed present until 16th week. Although this plateau was evident, mild fluctuations occurred. In contrast to most other movement patterns, hand near mouth movements decreased gradually from 13th week onwards with a single fluctuation in 14th week (it varied between 0 and 3 with

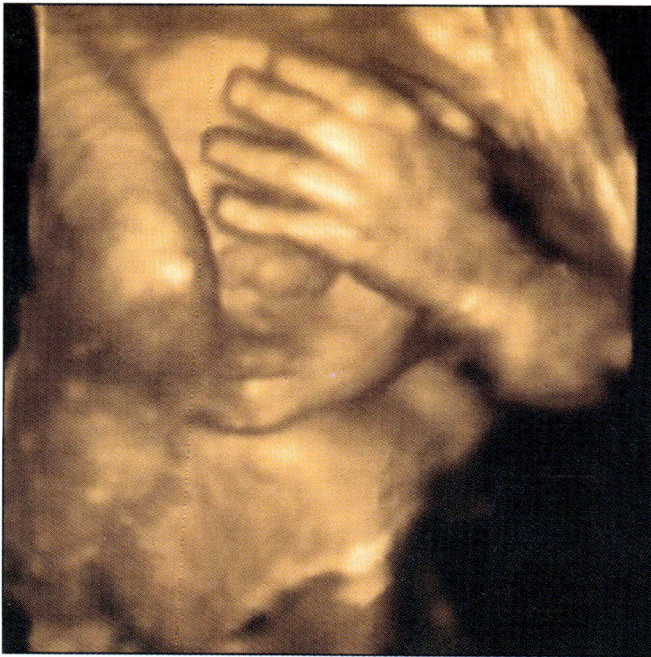

Fig. 16.52: Hand to head movement is clearly demonstrated

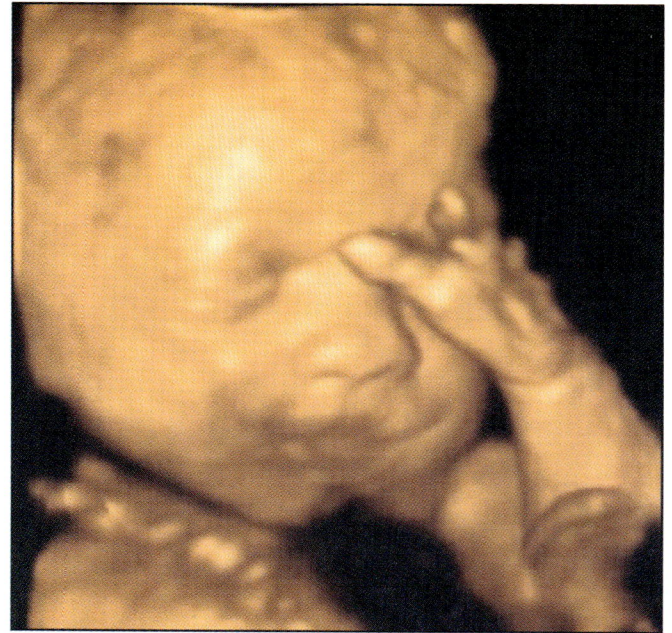

Fig. 16.54: Hand to eye movement is demonstrated by 3D surface rendering

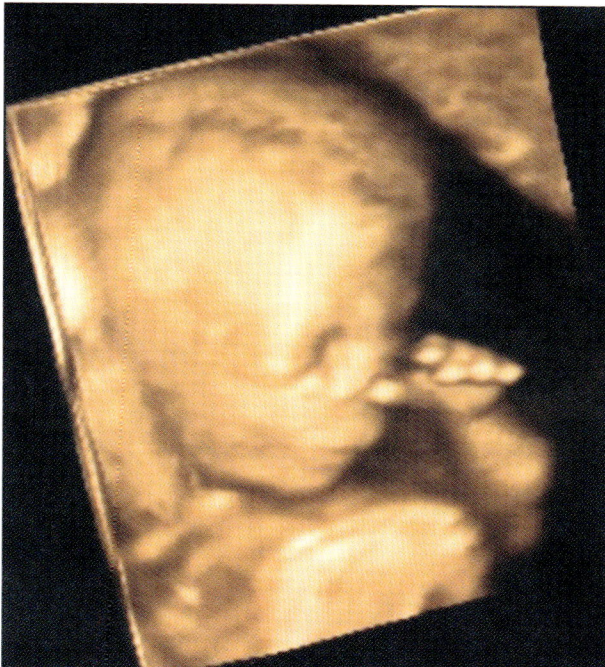

Fig. 16.53: Hand movement in front of the nose is clearly visualized

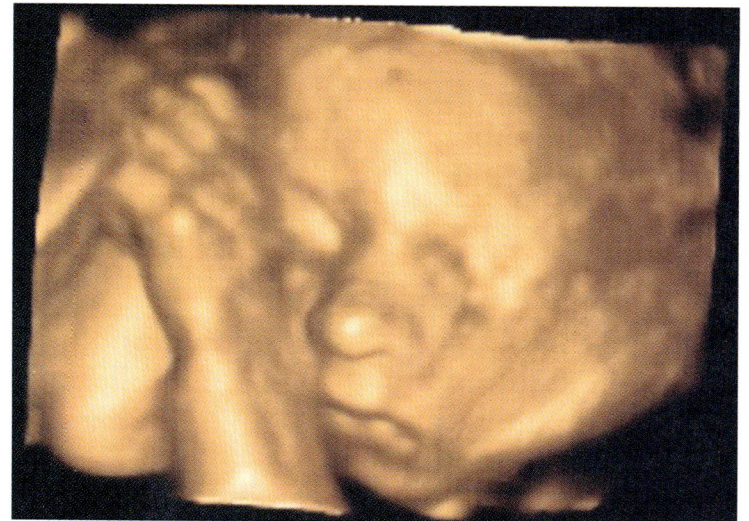

Fig. 16.55: 3D surface rendering shows both of the hands side by side from the right of the face

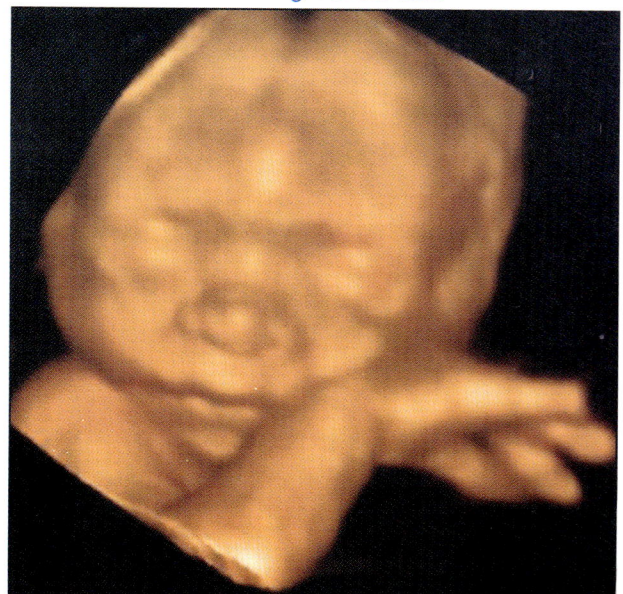

Fig. 16.56: 3D surface rendering shows the hand movement to the fetal face

a median value of 1). Figure 16.102D lists the incidence of these hand movement patterns. The incidence of hand to face movement is characterized by decrease at 14th week followed by a plateau (Fig 16.102E). From 13th week hand near face movement pattern was visible in all 15 fetuses with an incidence of 2 to 9 and a median value of 8. At 16th week the range was from 1 to 7 with a median value of 3. Although plateau was observed, mild fluctuation was evident, especially at 15th week. From Figure 16.102F, we can recognize that the incidence of hand near face movement is stable between 13th and 16th weeks of gestation with slight increase at 14th and 15th weeks. At 13th week the range was the widest from 0 to 12, with the median

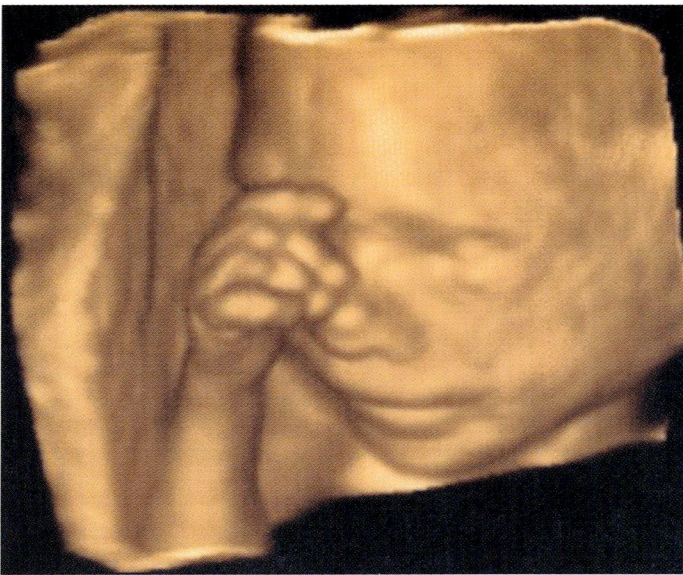

Fig. 16.57: 3D surface rendering shows the hand movement to the nose

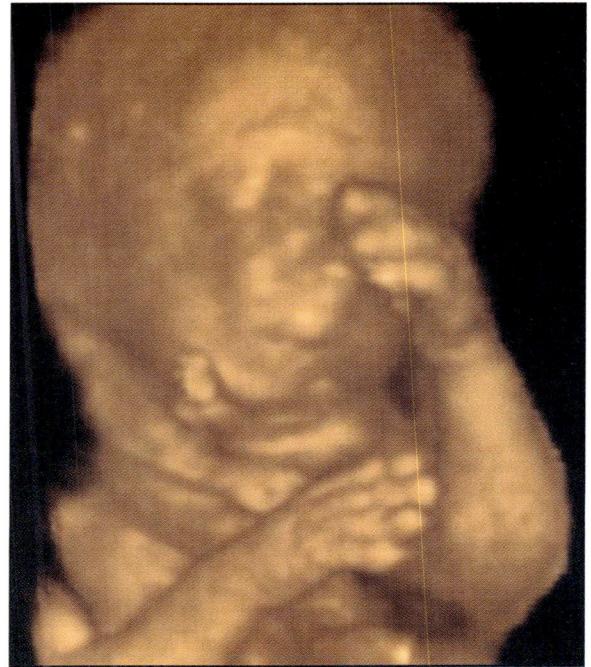

Fig. 16.58: 3D surface rendering demonstrated right hand movement beside the head

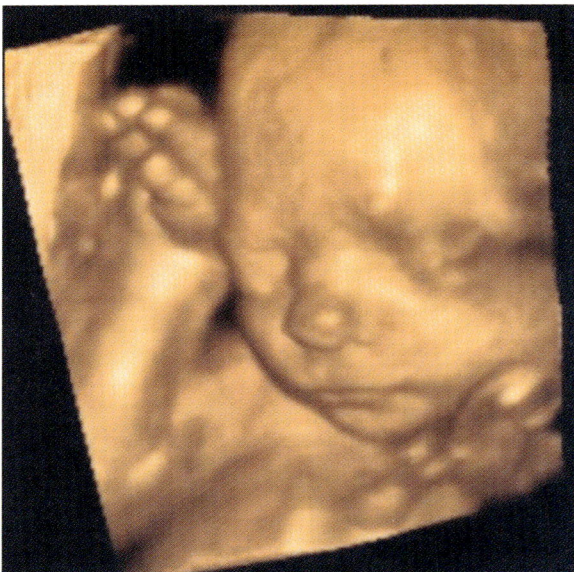

Fig. 16.59: 3D surface rendering of the opening palms in the direction to the fetal face

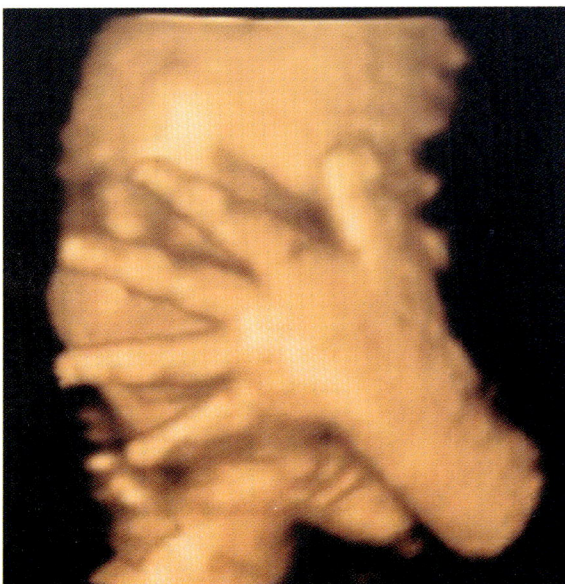

Fig. 16.60: 3D surface rendering shows hand to face movement

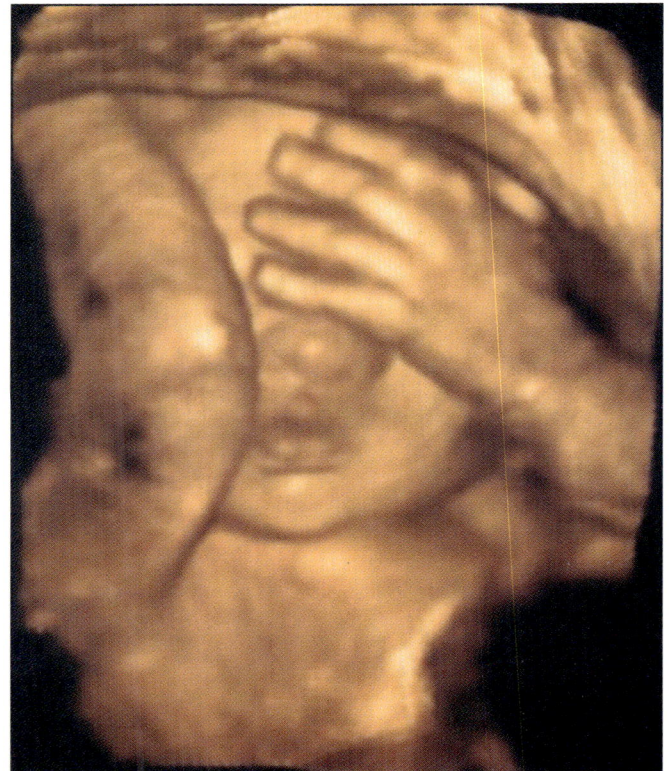

Fig. 16.61: Fetal hand movement to the fetal face is clearly demonstrated

value of 3. The incidence of hand to ear showed rapid trend of decrease between 13th and 16th weeks (Fig 16.102G). The incidence varied between 4 and 12 with a median value of 8 at 13th week, and 0 and 3 with a median value of 0 at 16th week. The incidence of hand to eye movement pattern showed same developmental trend such as hand to head and hand to face movement patterns. In Figure 16.102H, decrease of incidence followed by plateau is shown. At 13th week the incidence was between 4 and 12 occurrences per 15 minutes observation time

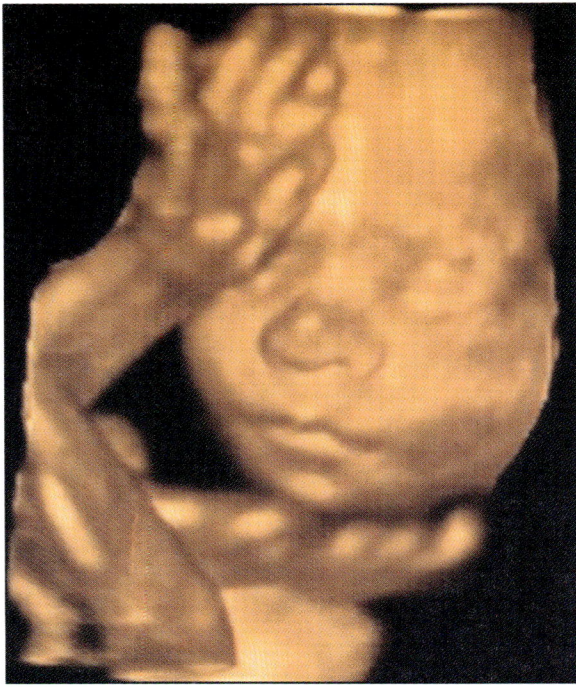

Fig. 16.62: Fetal hand movement to the face

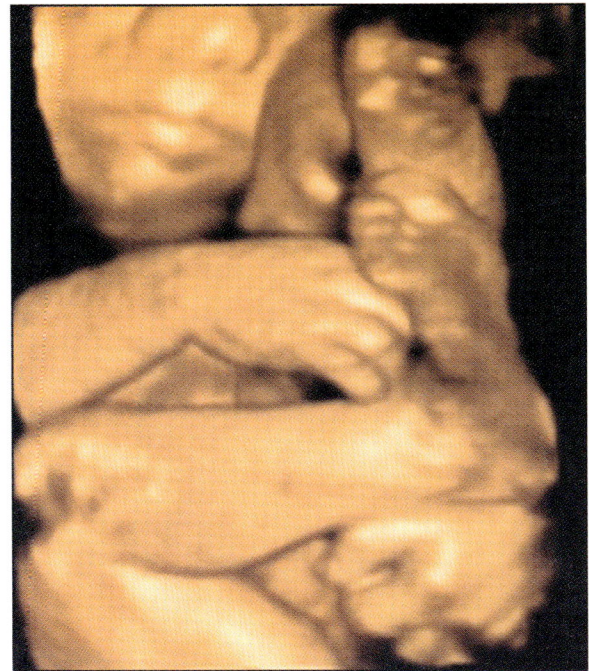

Fig. 16.63: 3D surface rendering shows both of the hands are directed in front of the face

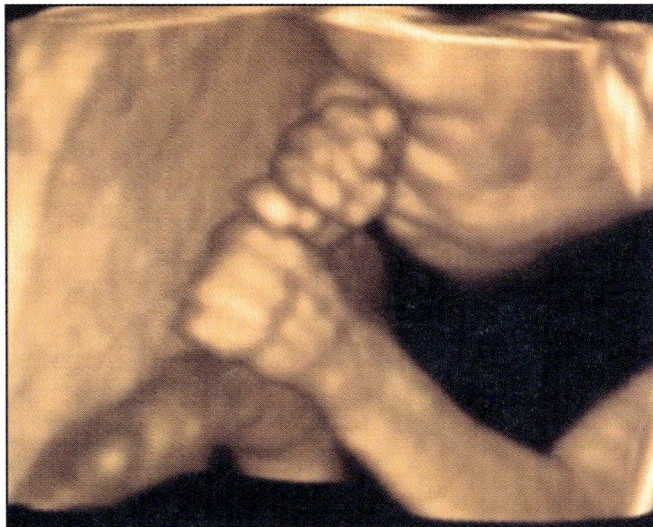

Fig. 16.64: 3D surface rendering demonstrated hand to face movement

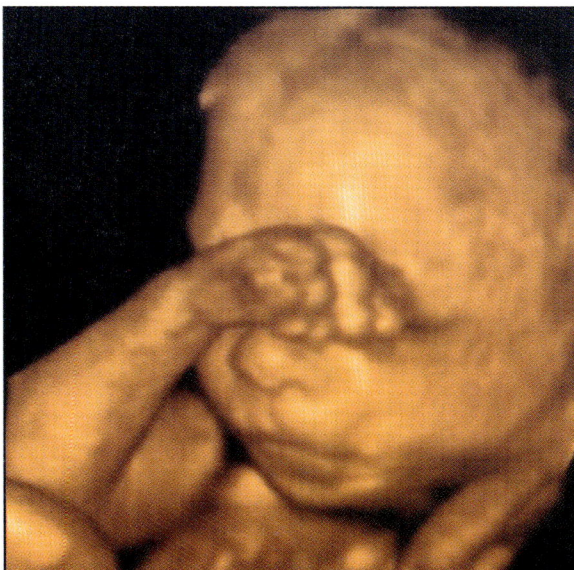

Fig. 16.65: Both of the hands are positioned in front of the chest

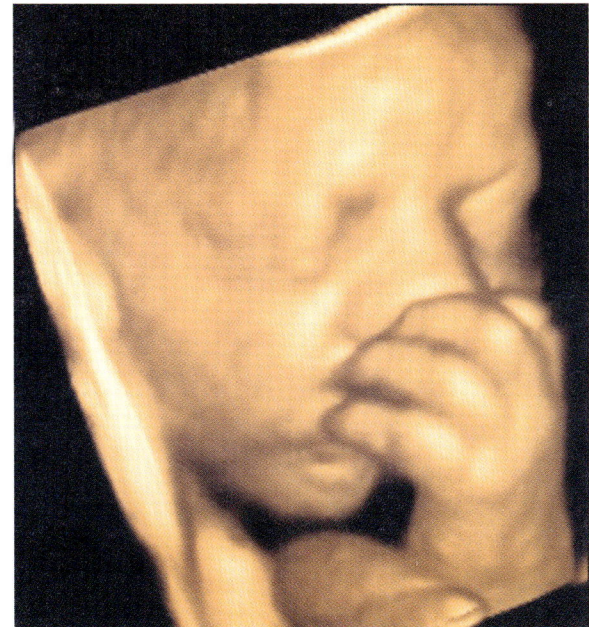

Fig. 16.66: 3D scan shows the left hand is directed to the nose

with a median value of 8. At 16th week the range was from 0 to 3 with a median value of 1.[1]

Hand movements appeared to be directed to a body part or the uterine wall.[5] One of the movements toward the body part is hand to face contact. It is impossible to measure the exact number and to determine the exact direction of hand in this pattern with realtime 2D US due to the limitation that the scanning plane only allows viewing of a section of facial area.[10]

It is well known that a clear view of important area may only be obtainable for a few moments. For these reasons, the advent of 4D scanning is a significant advance which for the present time should be realistically considered. Clinical research about possible applications is still missing. Our study clearly shows

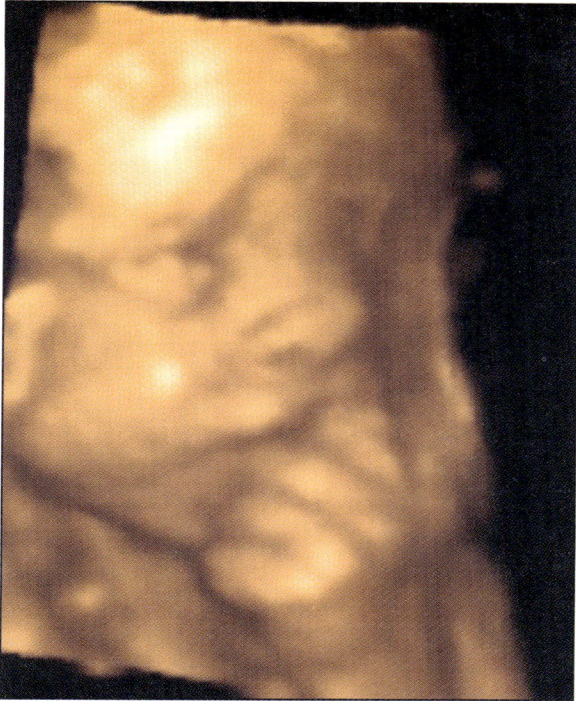

Fig. 16.67: 3D scan shows the hand directed to the mouth

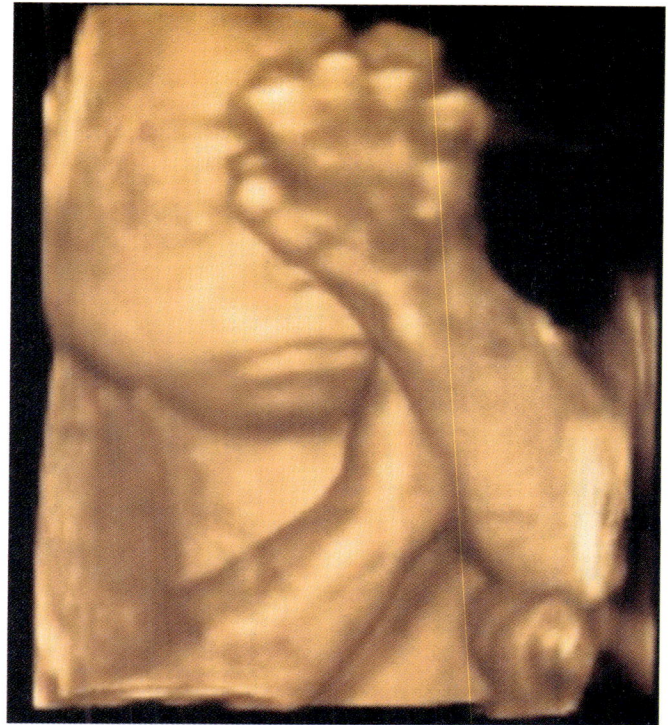

Fig. 16.69: 3D surface rendering shows the right hand is positioned on the left shoulder while the left hand is raised with opening palms

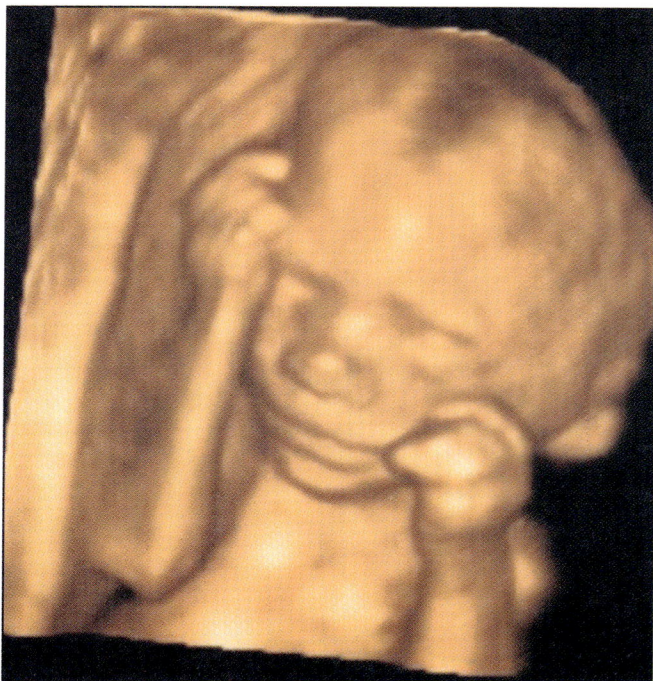

Fig. 16.68: 3D scan showing both of hands directed to the face

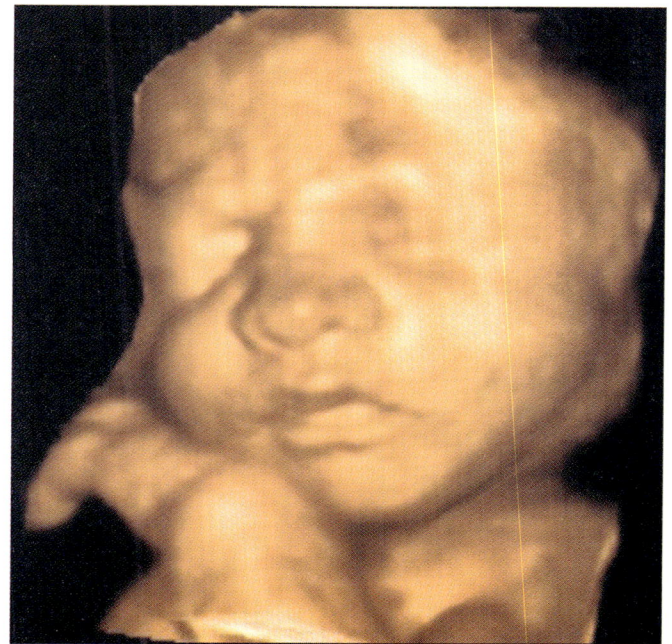

Fig. 16.70: 3D surface rendering shows the left hand is directed to the right cheek

incomparable clear observations of the simultaneous movements of the head, body and all four limbs and extremities.[2]

The advantage of 4D over realtime 2D US is that isolated hand movement can be confidentially determined. Two-dimensional sonography easily recognizes hand movements associated with body movements, whereas there are problems in recognition and differentiation of the isolated hand movements and hand movements associated with leg movements. In this situation 4D US is the method of choice for reliable recognition of the isolated hand movements.[2]

Another advantage of 4D US is precise assessment of the direction of the hand movement and target of the fingers. Realtime 2D US provides tomographic image of fetal head and visualization of hand movement in two dimensions. Four-dimensional sonography provides surface rendered image of the fetal head and visualization of hand movements in three dimensions that allows further differentaiation of hand to head movements.[2]

The incidence of isolated arm movement increases gradually from 8th through 19th weeks.[2] Such a discordance of the results

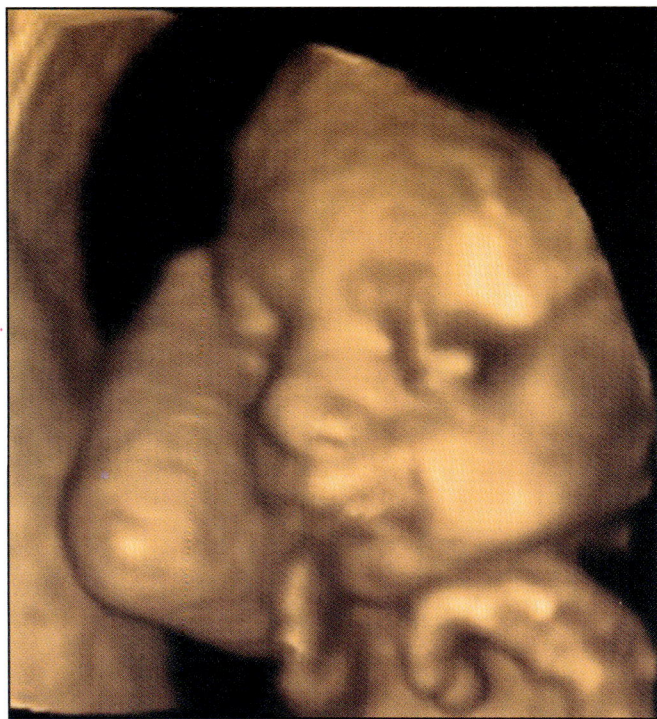

Fig. 16.71: 3D surface rendering demonstrated the right hand movement to the right side of the head

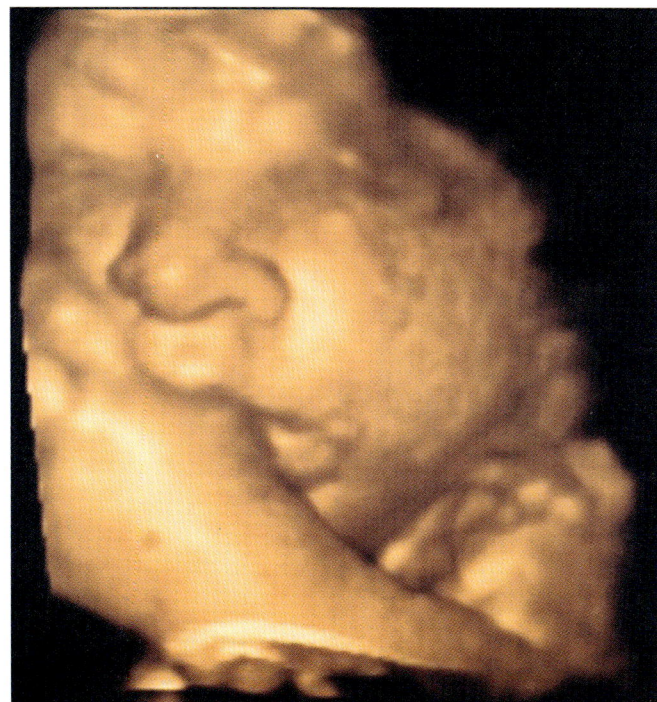

Fig. 16.72: 3D surface rendering demonstrated hand movement to the mouth. The fetus was sucking the thumb

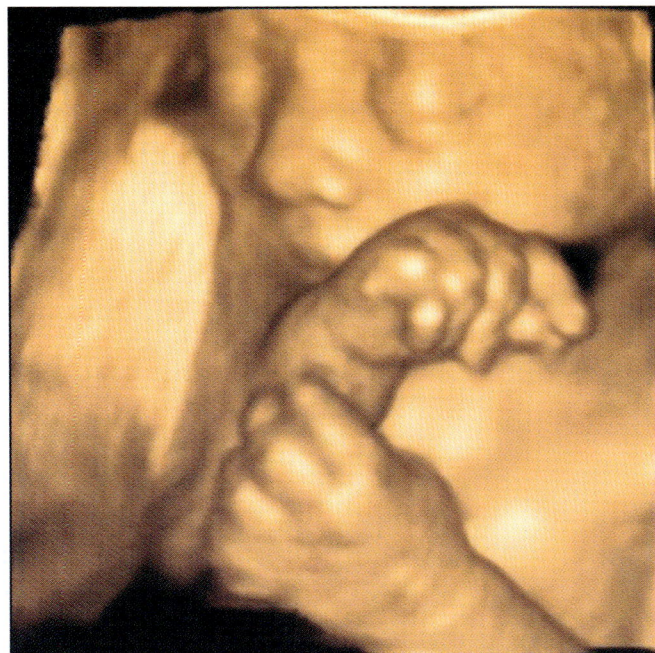

Fig. 16.73: Both of the hands showed in front of the chest by 3D surface rendering

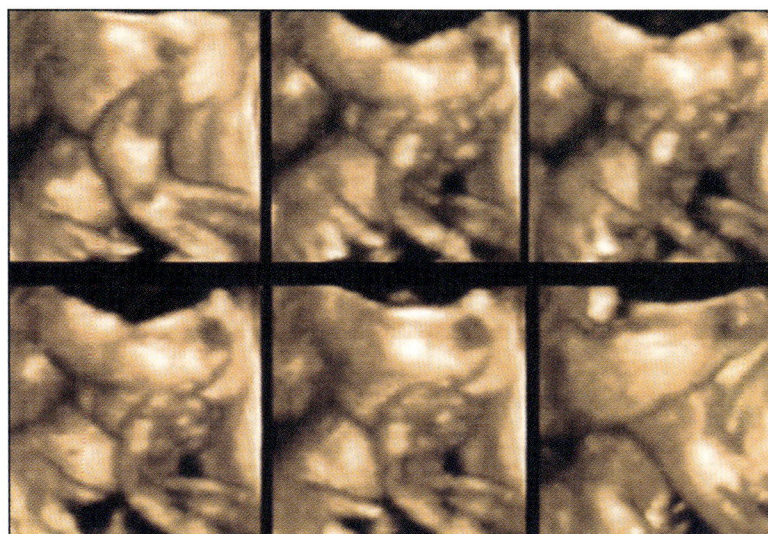

Fig. 16.74: This 4D image demonstrated hand movement to the ear

with those reported by de Vries and coworkers what can be explained with limitations of 4D US. Since 4D US provides only near realtime reconstruction of the intrauterine movements, fast and slow hand movements are not registered. Furthermore, we observed fetuses in a period of 15 minutes, whereas most of the studies with realtime ultrasound were done during a 60-minute time period.

Recently in our unpublished data, we had evaluated fetal behavior especially from the hand movement direction in fetuses with thanatophoric dysplasia, anencephaly, osteochondrosis dysplasia and trisomy 18 by four-dimensional ultrasound (Figs. 16.94,16.96,16.98 and 16.99). From our data, fetal hand movements in anencephalic fetus were visibled only in one direction (hand to head) and it appeared abnormal and monotonous. Isolated arm movement was also observed in anencephalic fetus.[12] The characteristic of movements in the fetuses with CNS malformation showed forceful quality, jerky, and appeared incidentally. While in the normal fetus, all of the movement parameters were qualitatively and quantitatively normal. Decreased variability can be observed in anencephalic fetus. Indeed, the movement of fetuses with abnormal CNS has been observed as lacking in variability.[12] Our result suggests that there was a prominent underlying structure. Movement patterns in anencephalic fetus had a tendency to appear suddenly

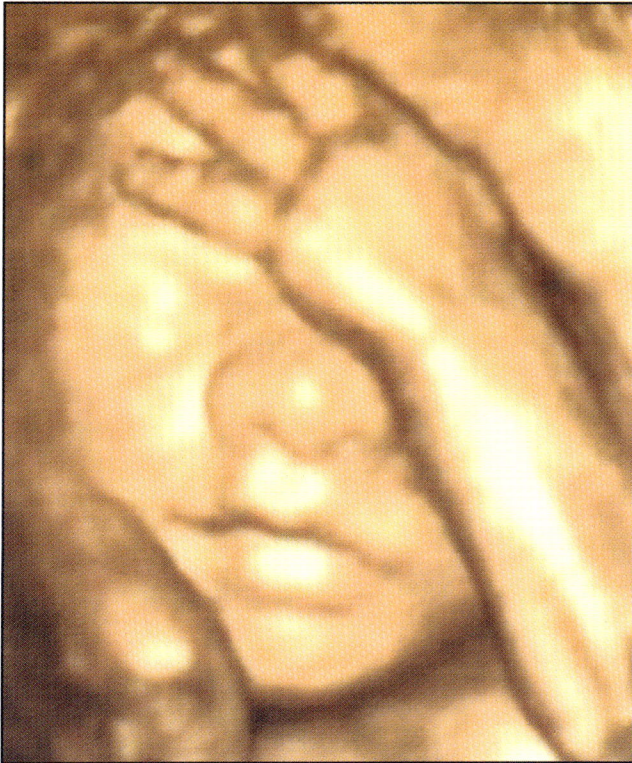

Fig. 16.75

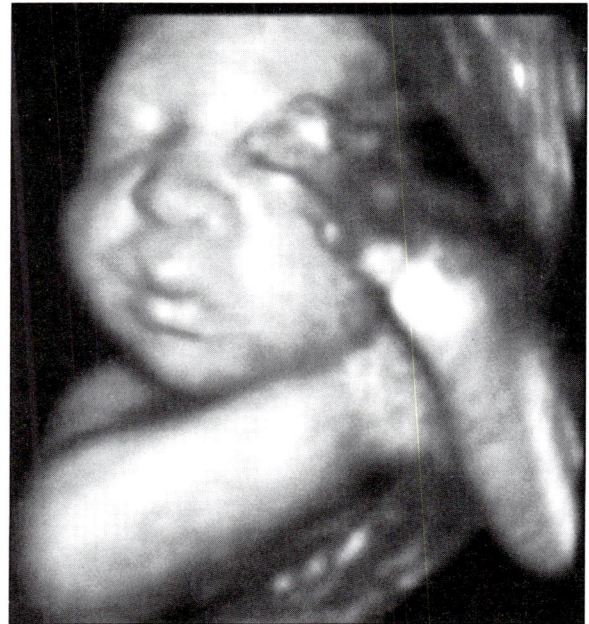

Fig. 16.77: 3D image shows the right hand is directed to the left shoulder while the left hand moved to the eye region

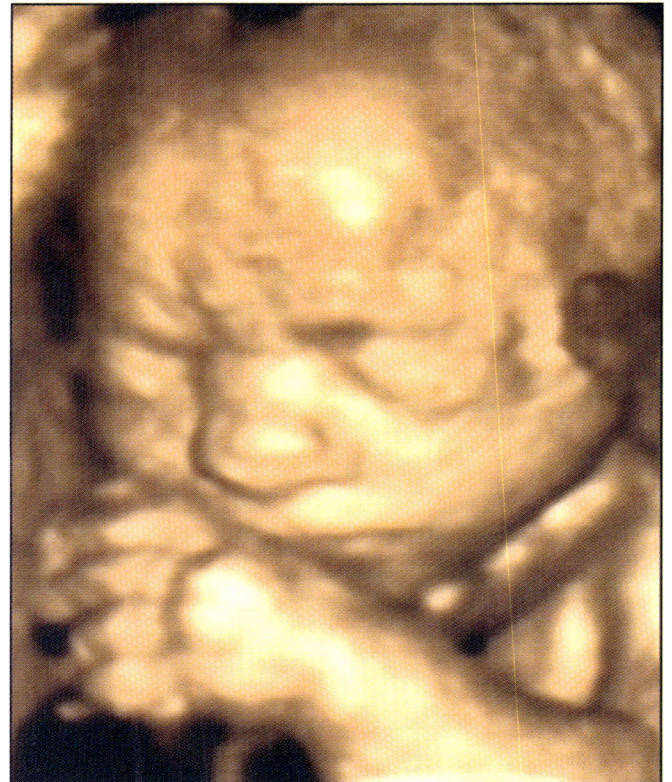

Figs 16.75 and 16.76: 3D surface rendering shows hand movement to the head

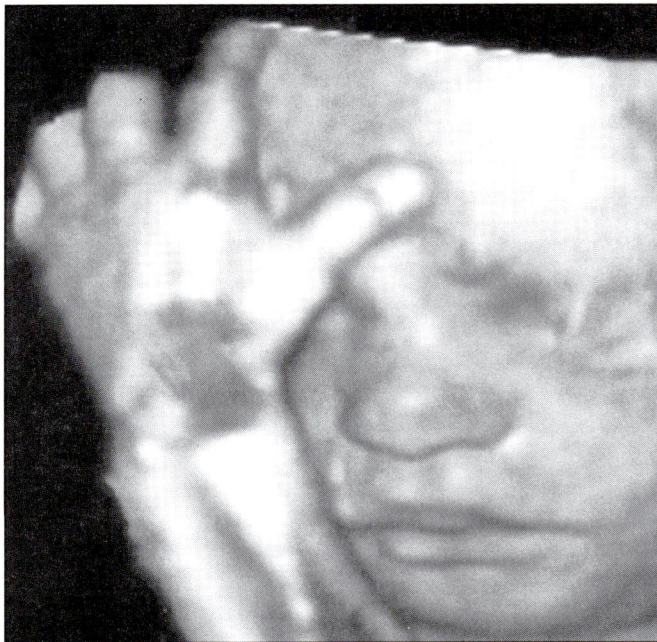

Fig. 16.78: 3D surface rendering showing fetal hand movement in front of the mouth. Note the umbilical cord is surrounding the fetal neck

compared to being sporadically and continuously in normal fetus. It is coming to an end that with malformation of fetal CNS, movement patterns are abnormal and can exist in spite of serious reducing in the quantitiy and change in the fetal CNS (Figs 16.98 and 16.99).[12,13]

We believe that observation not only quantity but the quality of the movements also will bring us to the moment when we might be able to predict the neurologically disabled fetus. However, to achieve this goal there is still long way to go.

CONCLUSIONS

All seven types of hand to head movement can be seen from 13th week of gestation, with mild fluctuation in the incidence. Therefore, the second phase of the increase in the number of axodendritic and axosomatic synapses influences only on the incidence of hand movement. 4D US provides an option of the exact determination of the direction of fetal hand, but determination of the exact number of each type of hand

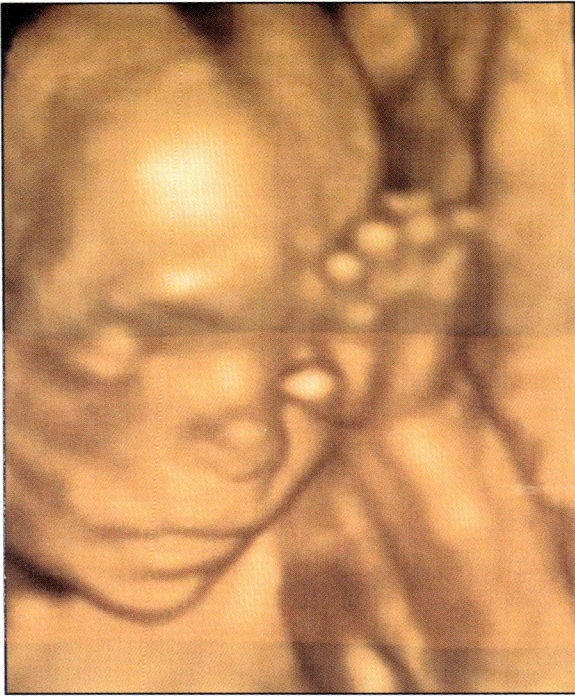

Fig. 16.79: 3D image shows the fetus raised the hand to the eye region

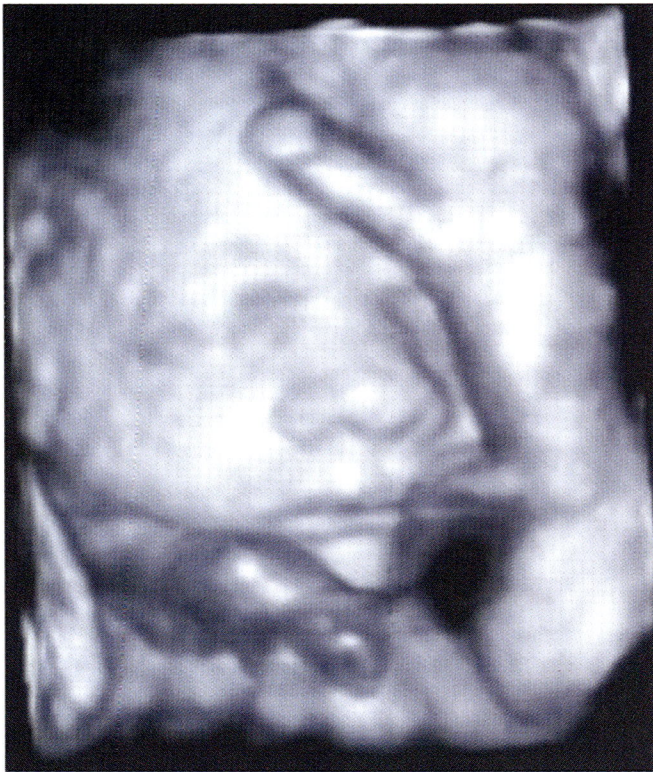

Fig. 16.81: 3D surface rendering shows the right fetal digits pointed the scrotum and penis

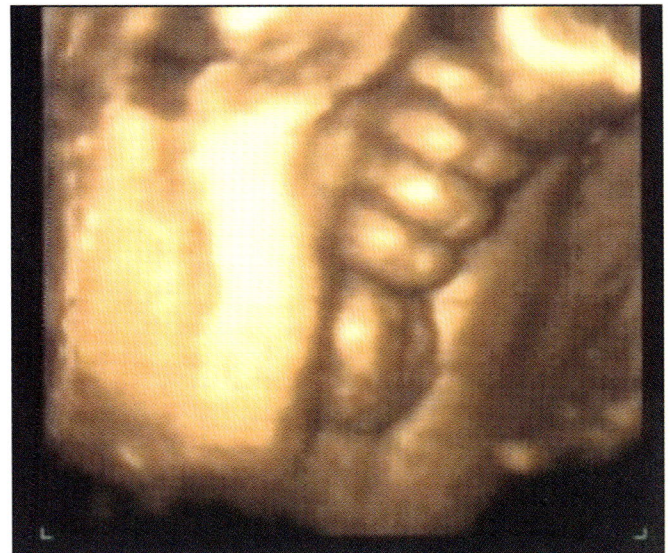

Fig. 16.80: 3D image shows hand to head direction

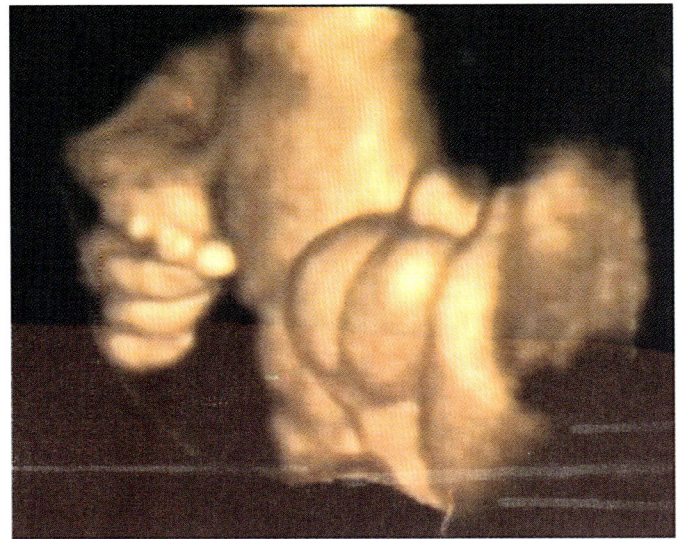

Fig. 16.82: 3D surface rendering demonstrated the fetal penis is grasped by the fetal hand

movements is still unachievable. Further improvements might help us identify the level of neurological maturation of the fetus by careful study of many behavioral activities.

REFERENCES

1. Kurjak A, Azumendi G, Vecek N, et al. Fetal hand movements and facial expression in normal pregnancy studied by four-dimensional sonography. J Perinat Med 2003;31:496-508.
2. Kurjak A, Vecek N, Hafner T, Bozek T, Funduk-Kurjak B, Ujevic B. Prenatal diagnosis: what does four-dimensional ultrasound add? J Perinat Med 2002; 30:57.
3. Kurjak A, Vecek N, Kupesic S, Azumendi G, Solak M. Four dimensional ultrasound: how much does it improve perinatal practice? In Carrera JM, FA Chervenak, Kurjak A (Eds): Controversies in Perinatal Medicine, Studies on the Fetus as a Patient. A CRC Press company : Parthenon Publishing, New York 2003: pp 222-34.
4. Andonotopo W, Stanojevic M, Kurjak A, et al. Assessment of fetal behavior and general movements by four-dimensional sonography. Ultrasound Review of Obstetrics & Gynecology (London) (In Press).
5. Sparling JW, Von Tolt J, Chescheir NC. Fetal and neonatal hand movement. Phys Ther 1999; 79:24.
6. Pooh RK, Ogura T. Normal and abnormal fetal hand positioning and movement in early pregnancy detected by three-and four dimensional ultrasound. Ultr Rev Obst Gyn 20004;4:46-51.
7. Paluda SM, Comstock CH, Kirk JS, et al. The significance of ultrasonographically diagnosed fetal wrist position anomalies. Am J Obstet Gynecol 1996;174:1834-7; discussion 1837-9.
8. Kos M, Hafner T, Funduk-Kurjak B, et al. Limb deformities and three-dimensional ultrasound. J Perinat Med 2002;30:40-7.
9. Quintero RA, Johnson MP, Mendoza G, et al. Ontogeny of clenched-hand development in trisomy 18 fetuses: a serial transabdominal fetoscopicobservation. Fetal Diagn Ther 1999;14:68-70.

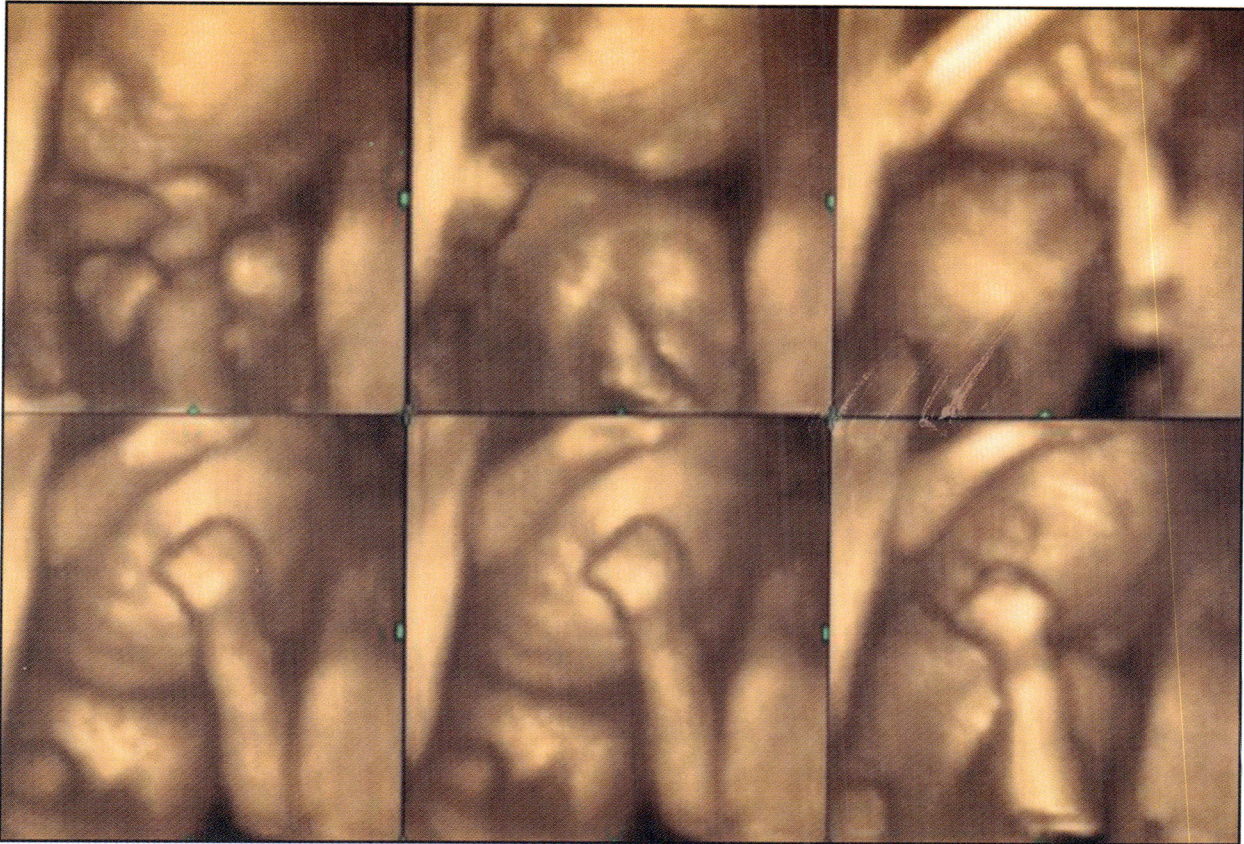

Fig. 16.83: 4D surface rendering shows active arm movements associated with active body movement.

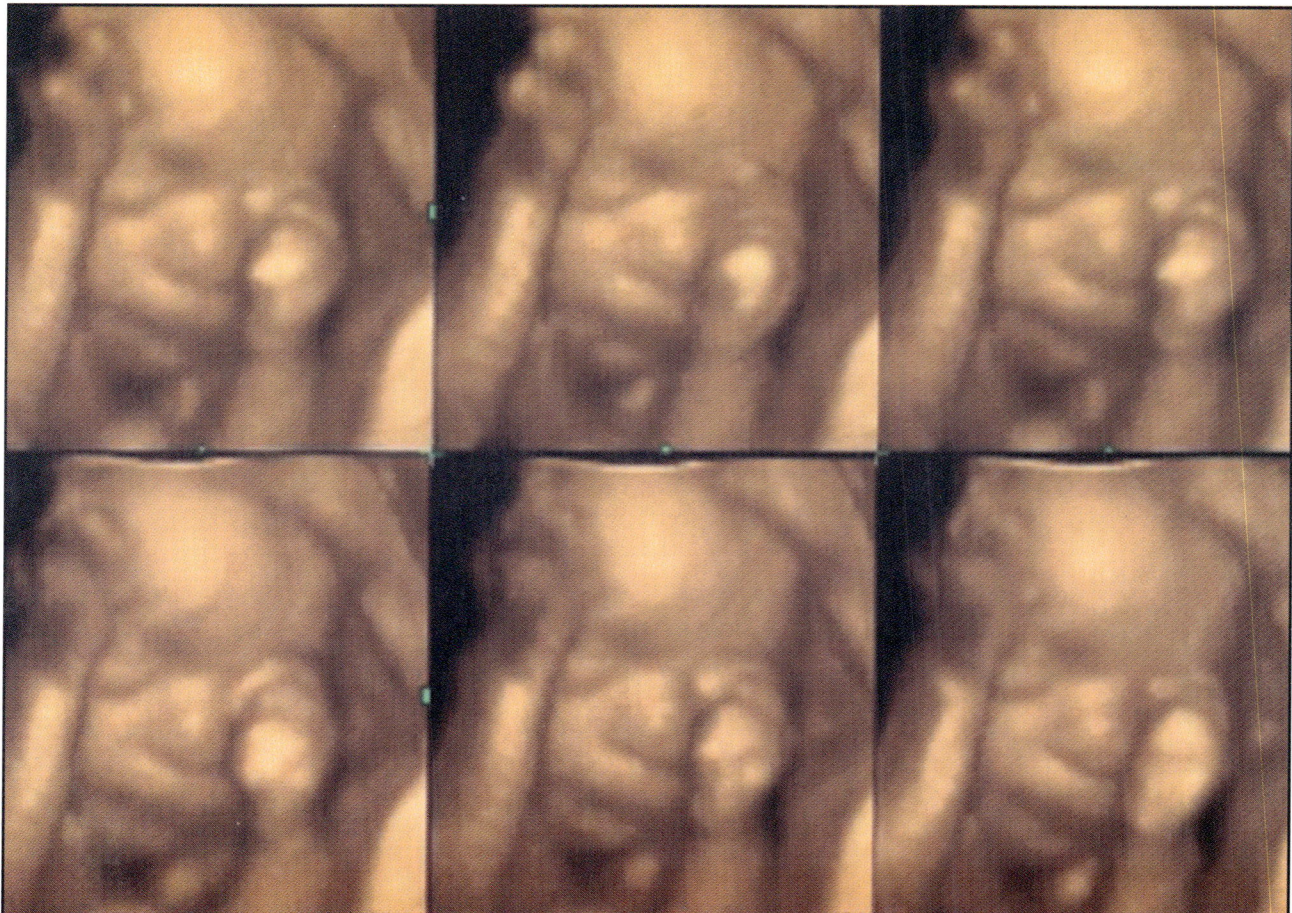

Fig. 16.84: 4D surface rendering demonstrated both of the hands moved in front of the face

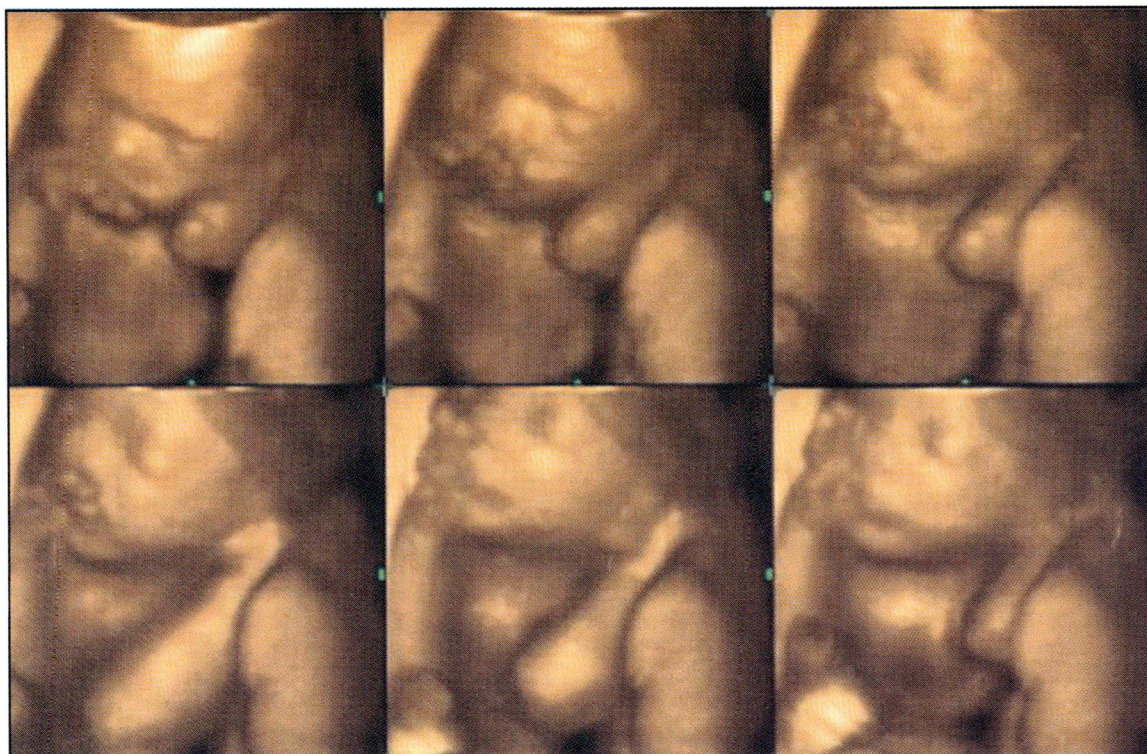

Fig. 16.85: This image shows active movements of the fetal hand and arm movements

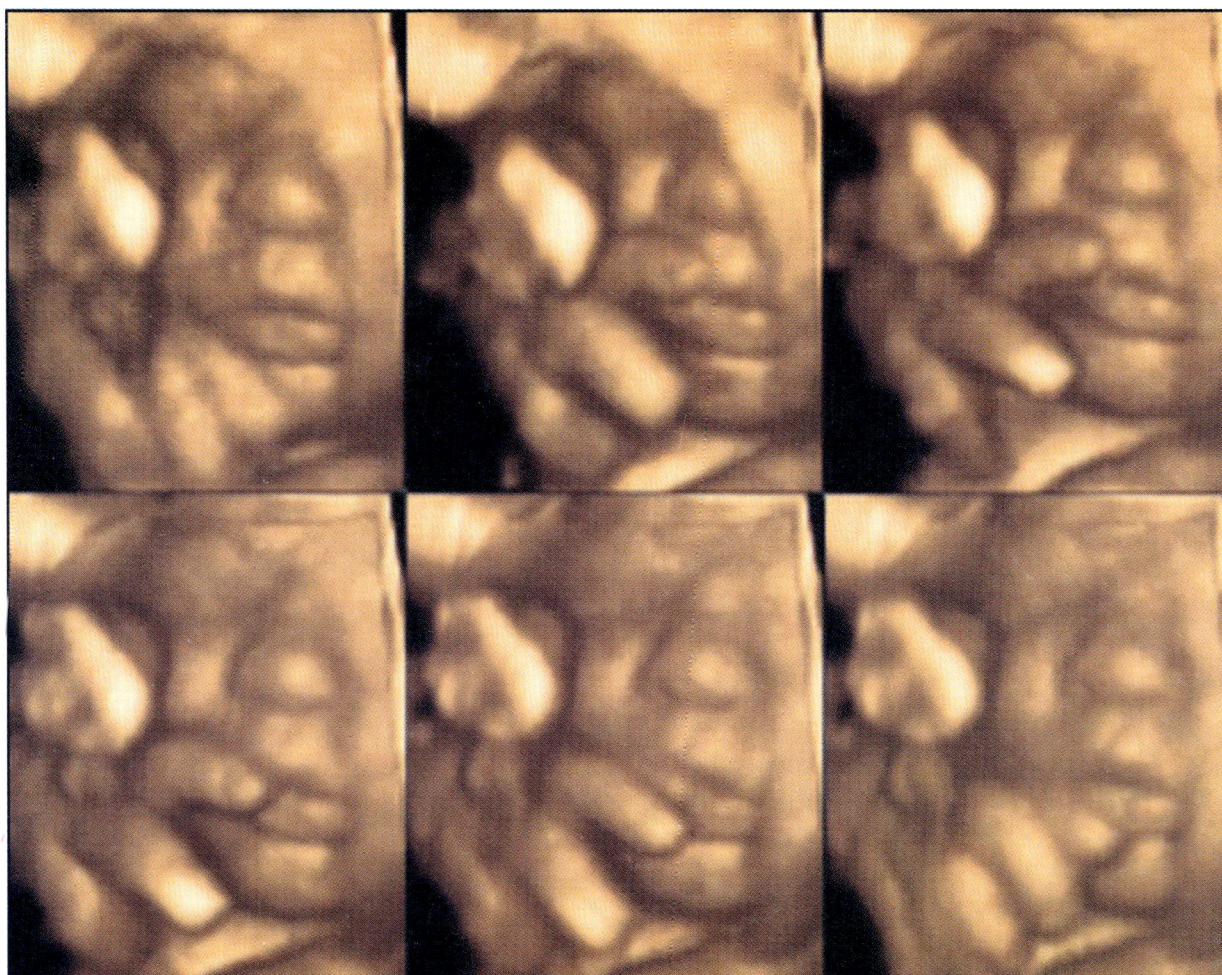

Fig. 16.86: This image demonstrated 4D surface rendering of hand to mouth direction

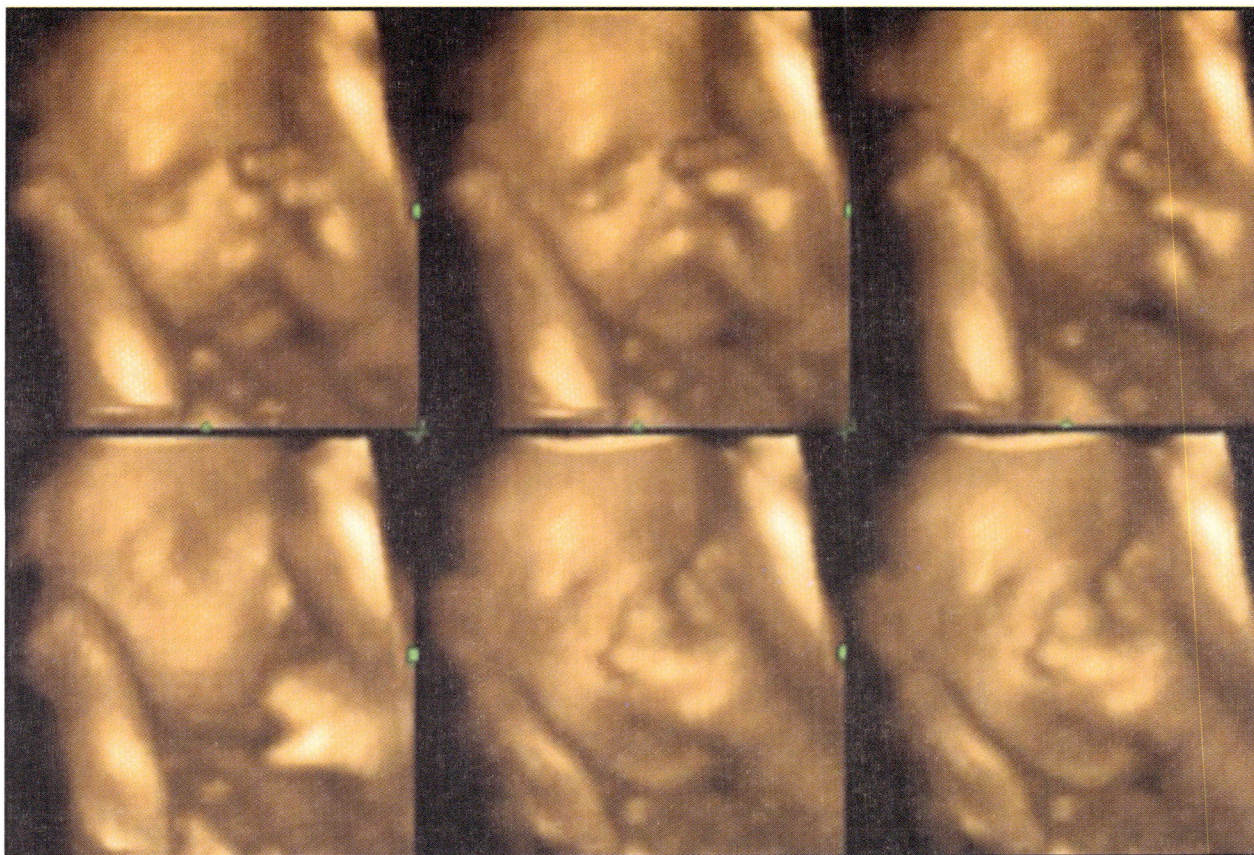

Fig. 16.87: 4D image demonstrated hand movement to the fetal face region. The fetus seems to grasp the nose

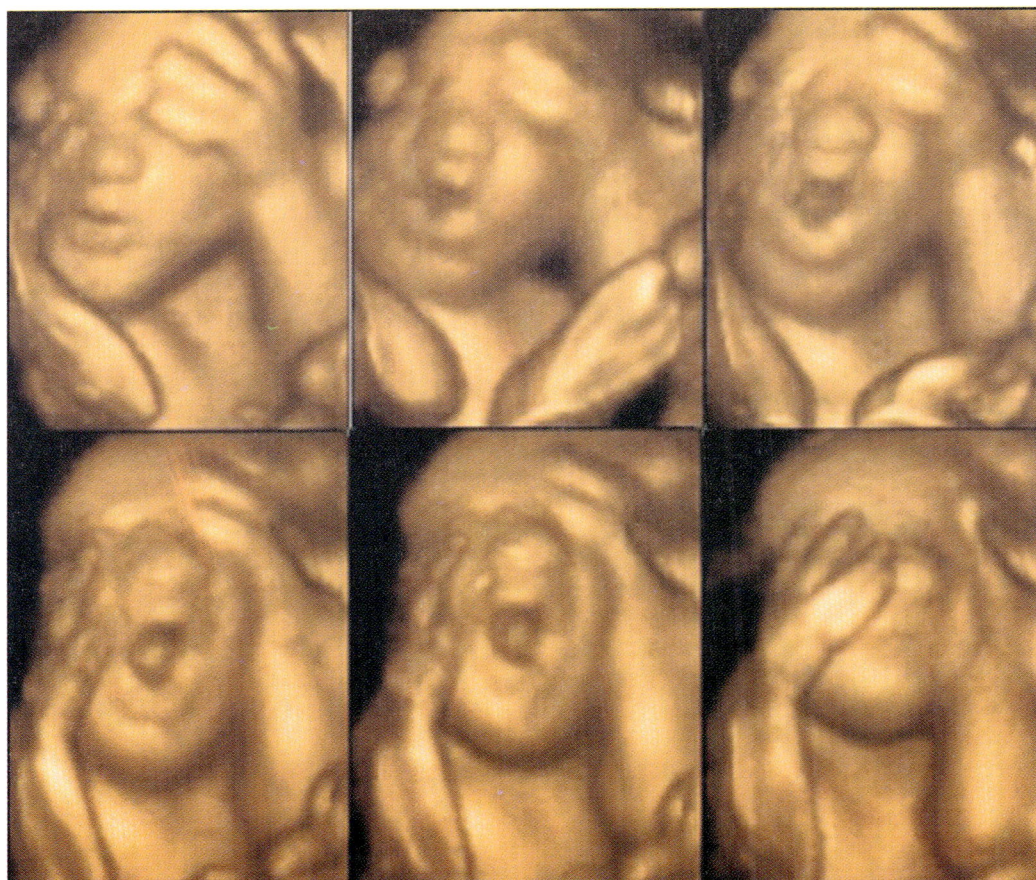

Fig. 16.88: 4D image demonstrated hand movements to the eyes region

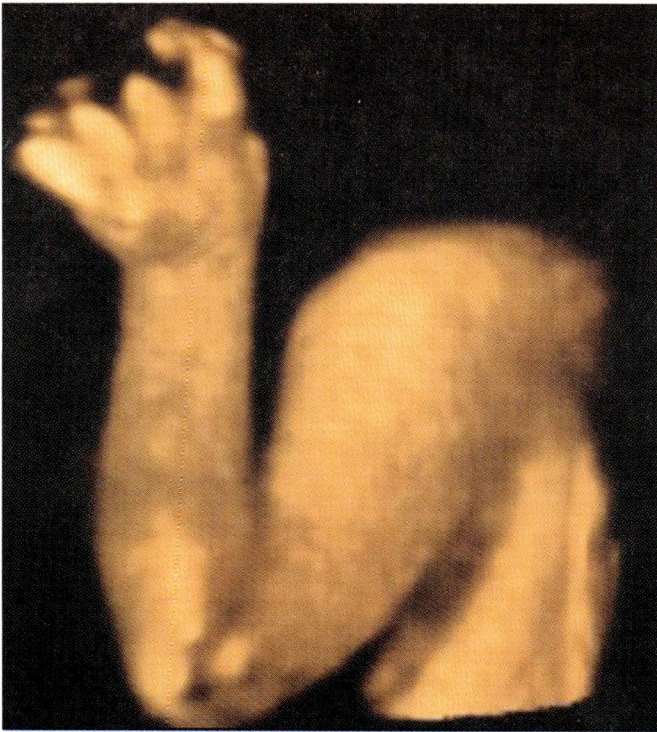

Fig. 16.89: 3D surface rendering shows clench fist of the fetus with arthrogryposis

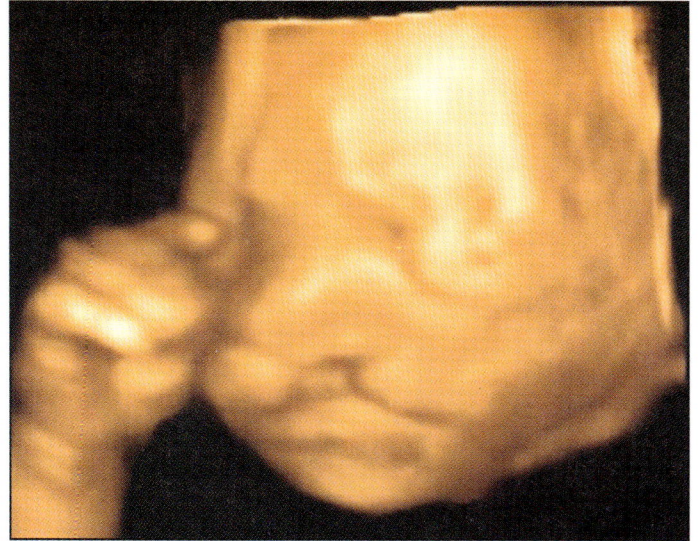

Fig. 16.91: 3D scan shows hand movement to the facial region. Note the unilateral cleft clip

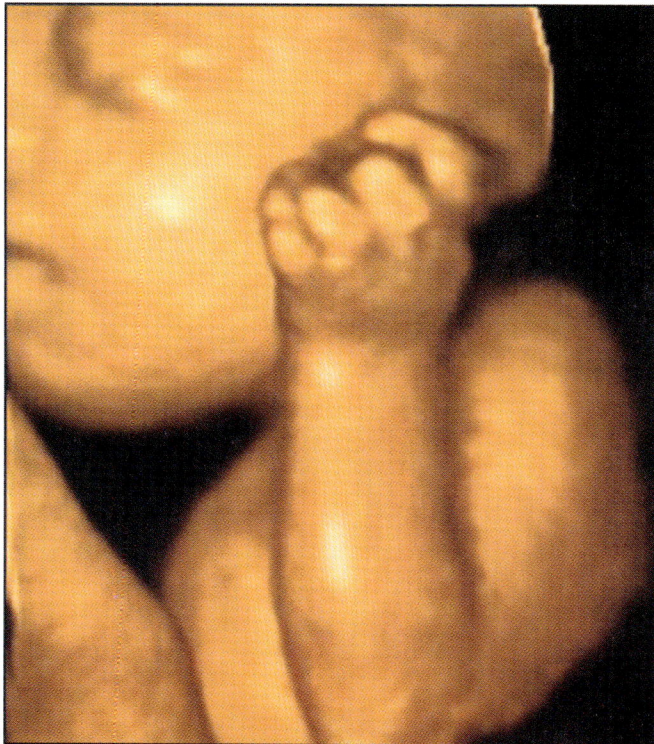

Fig. 16.92: Clenching the fist of the fetus with arthrogryposis is clearly visualized

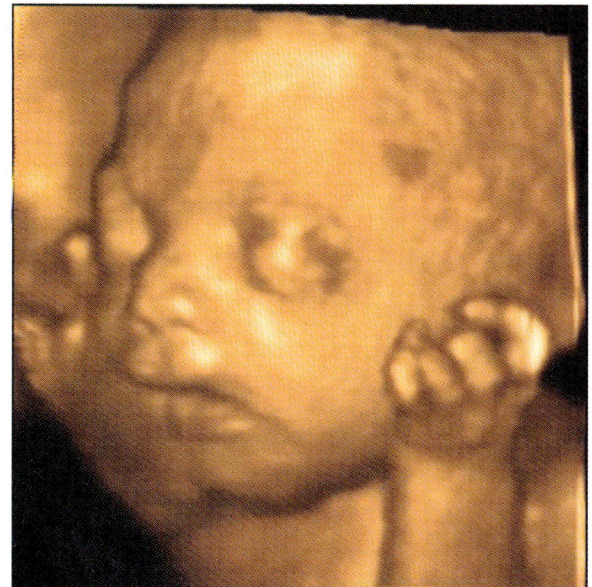

Fig. 16.90: 3D surface rendering demonstrated clench fist of the fetus with arthrogryposis. Note the hand movement directed to the ear

10. Roodenburg PJ, JW Wladimiroff , van Es A, Prechtl HFR. Classification and quantitative aspects of fetal movements during the second half of normal pregnancy. Early Hum Dev 1991; 25:19.

11. de Vries JIP, Visser GH, Prechtl HFR. The emergence of fetal II: quantitative aspects. Early Hum Dev 1985; 12:173.

12. Andonotopo W, Kurjak A, Ivanèiæ-Košuta M. Behavioral of anencephalic fetus studied by 4D sonography. Journal Maternal-Fetal and Neonatal Medicine (London) (In Press).

13. Visser GH, Laurini RN, de Vries JIP, et al. Abnormal motor behaviour in anencephalic fetuses. Early Hum Dev 1985;12:173-82.

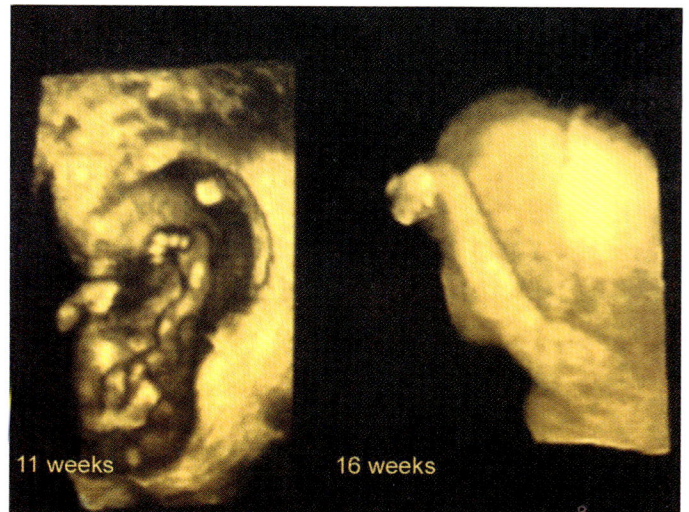

11 weeks   16 weeks

Fig. 16.93: Wrist malpositioning from 11 weeks fetus with trisomy 18 (left). Abnormal left hand appearance is demonstrated. The right panel shows the left wrist malpositioned at 16th week in the case of trisomy 18 (adapted from Reference 6)

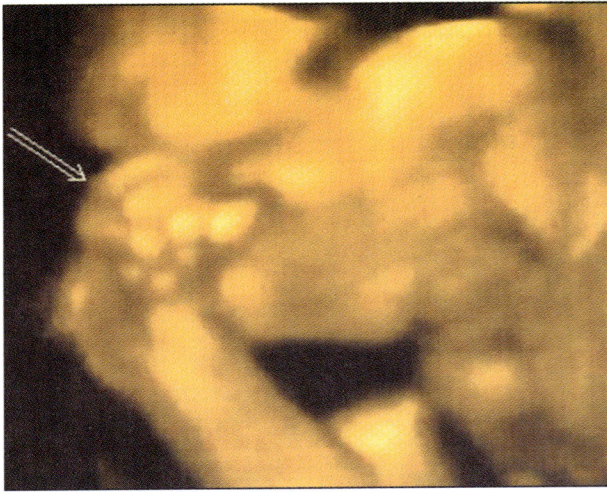

Fig. 16.94: Wrist malpositioning from 22 weeks fetus with trisomy 18 depicted by 3D surface rendering. Note the clenching fist

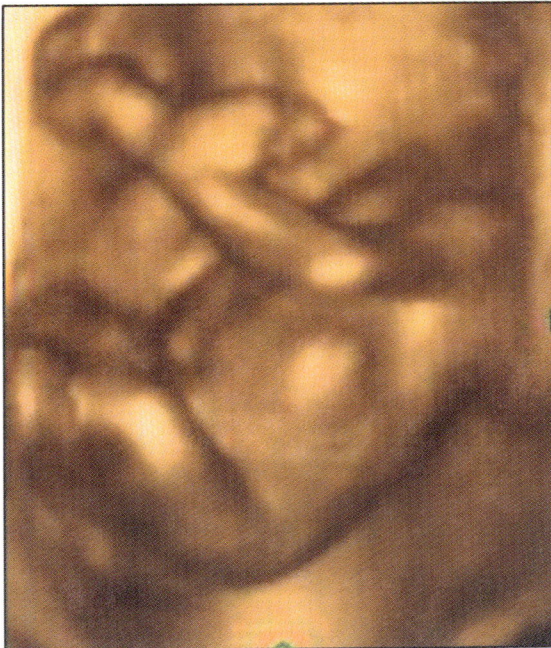

Fig. 16.95: 3D surface rendering of the fetus with trisomy 18 shows movement of hands to the region of face

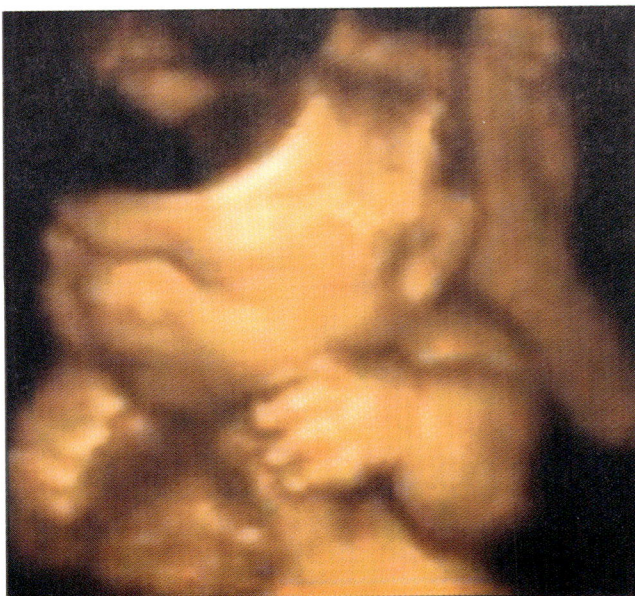

Fig. 16.96: 3D surface rendering of the fetus with osteochondrosis dysplasia showing the short upper extremities moved in front of the chest

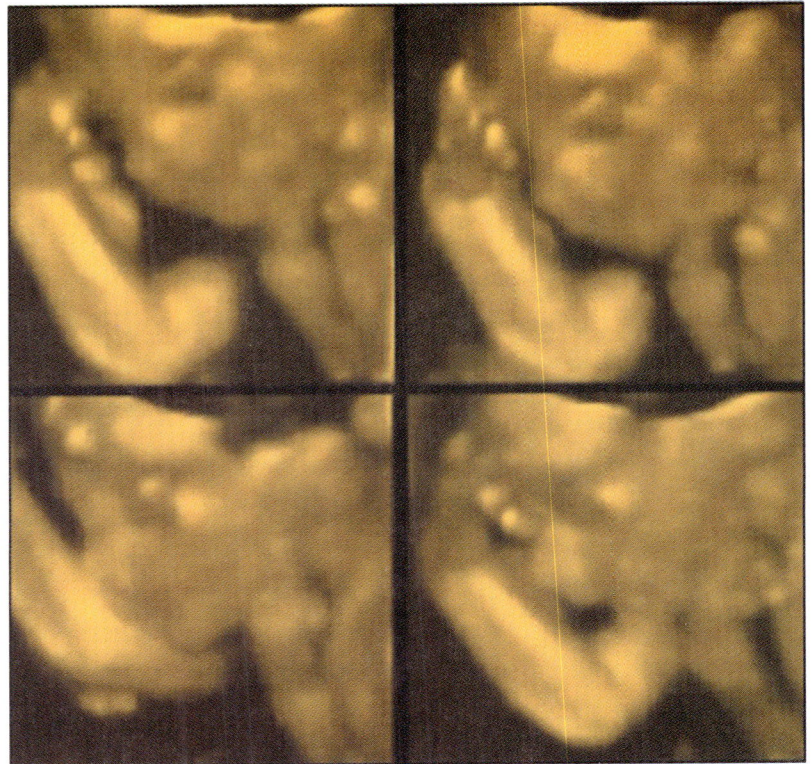

Fig. 16.97: 4D sequence demonstrated wrist malpositioning of the fetus with trisomy 18. Abnormal right hand appearance is demonstrated and wrist malposition already formed was strongly suspected

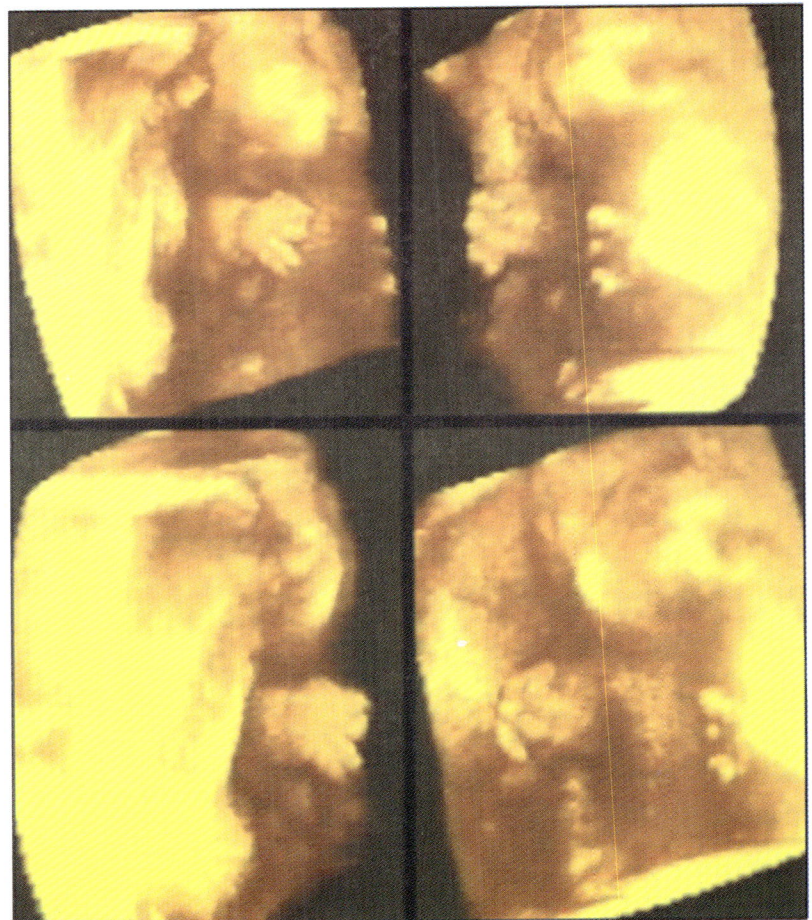

Fig. 16.98: 3D imaging of the hand movements direction in the front of the abdomen from the fetus with thanatophoric dysplasia

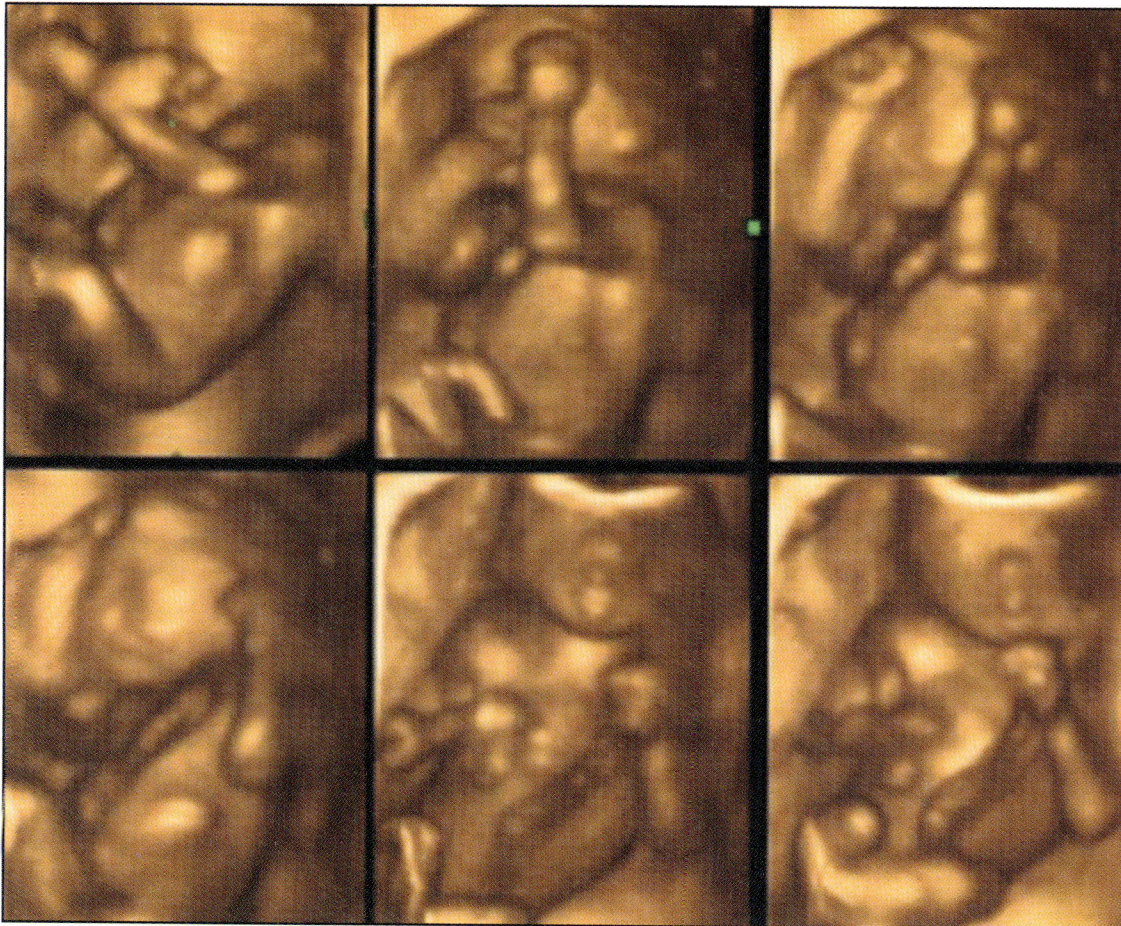

Fig. 16.99: 4D sequence of the fetus with trysomy 18 demonstrated independent hand movements at 20th week of gestation

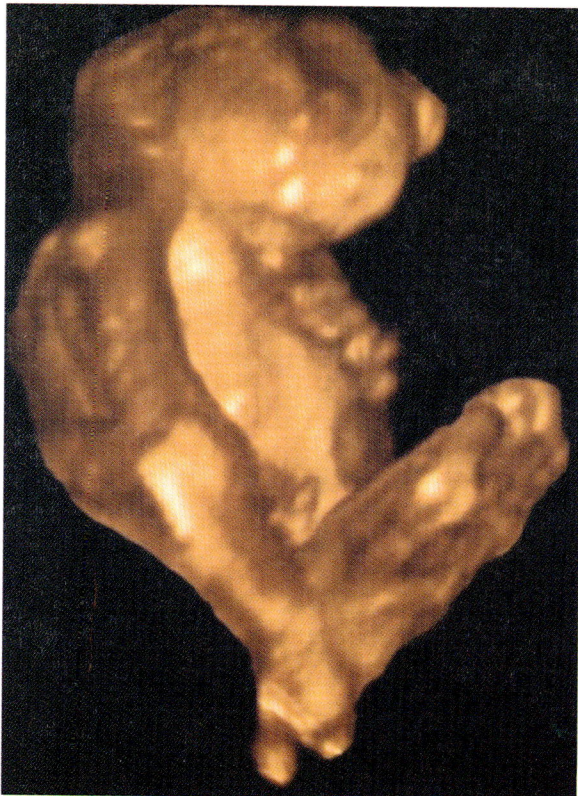

Fig. 16.100: 3D image shows right hand movement extended in the longitudinal axis from the fetus with anencephaly

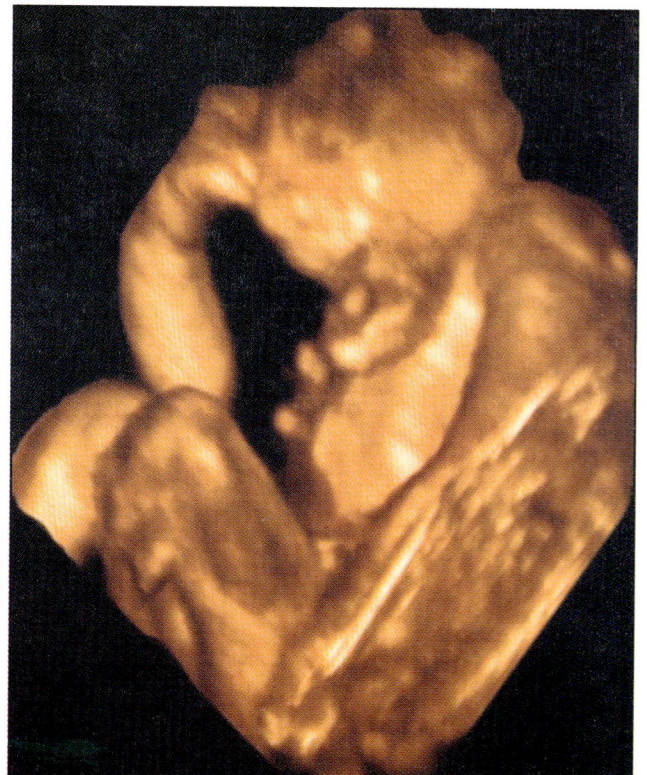

Fig. 16.101: Hand movement directed to the head is clearly visualized in the fetus with anencephaly

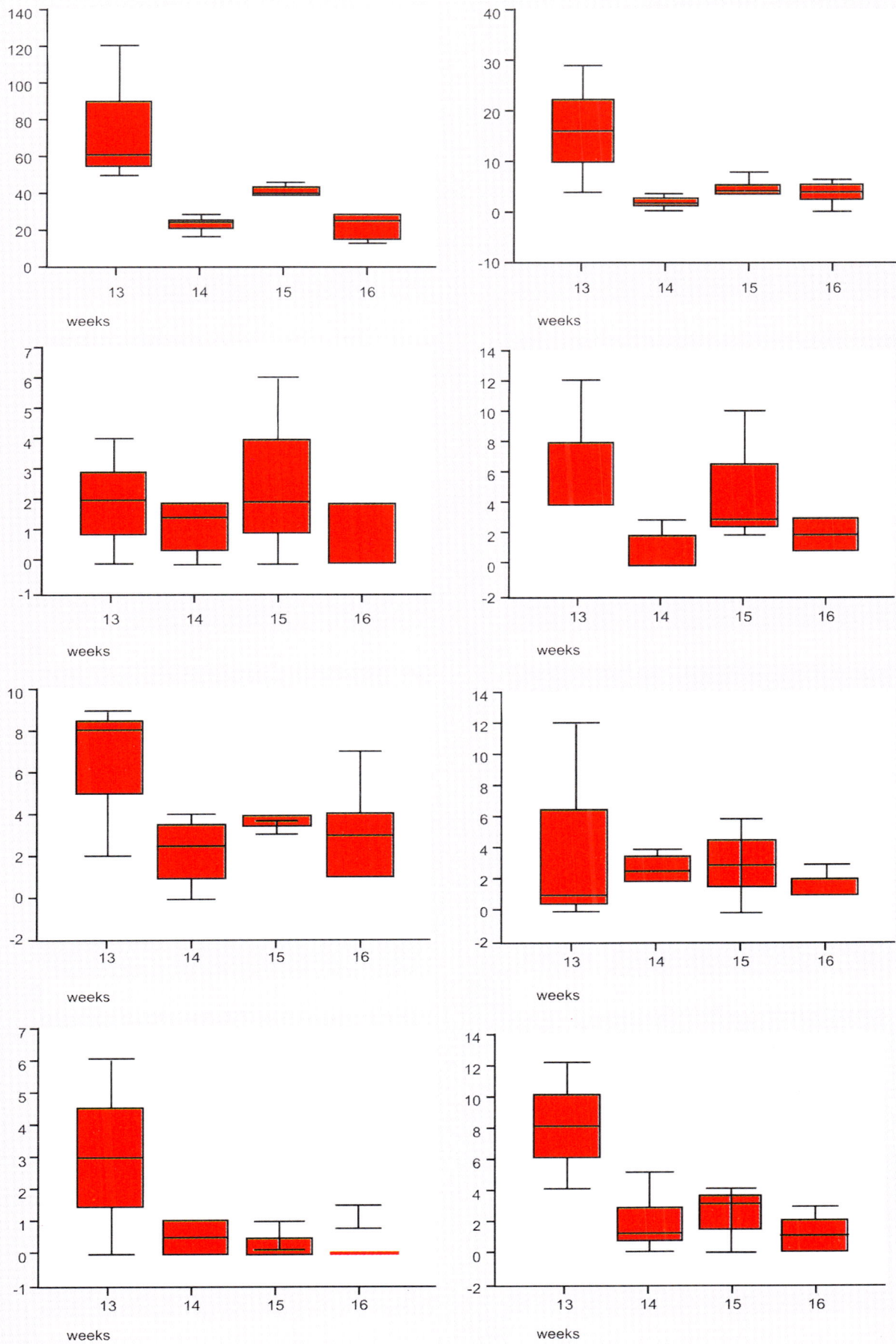

Figs 16.102 A to H: The incidence of several characteristics of hand movements from 13th to 16th gestational weeks showed by 4D sonography. (A) Isolated hand movement, (B) Hand to head movements, (C) Hand to mouth movements, (D) Hand near mouth movements, (E) Hand to face movements, (F) Hand near face movements, (G) Hand to ear movements, (H) Hand to eye movements. Adapted from Reference 1

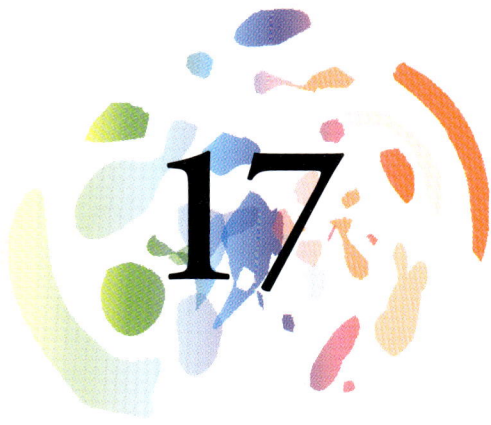

**Milan Stanojevic, Lara Sanchez,
Asim Kurjak, Jose Maria Carrera**

17 Three-dimensional Ultrasound in the Assessment of Neonatal Brain

INTRODUCTION

In the late seventies and early eighties ultrasound has significantly improved diagnosis of many diseases and conditions in newborn infants, enabling better diagnostics, treatment and prognosis of sick newborns.[1-9] It is very important to keep the continuity of the assessment of the brain from fetal to neonatal period.[9,10-12] Two-dimensional (2D) realtime ultrasonography of newborn brain enabling its realtime assessment was an exciting event and a great diagnostic achievement in the late seventies.[1-6] In comparison with radiological X-ray imaging techniques or magnetic resonance it was more convenient, because of unlimited examination frequency of critically sick newborns in the isolates, and less costly, without need for sedation and transportation of infants.[2] Introduction of Doppler studies was a new advancement in the assessment of neonatal brain circulation in the late eighties.[13-15] This technique enabled follow up of brain circulation and its dynamics.[15,16] In the nineties, a new exciting technique of 3D and 4D ultrasonography was developed, depicting neonatal brain in the third dimension.[7-9,15,17-21] When performing 2D ultrasound imaging, sonographers were making three-dimensional reconstruction in their imagination, while development of computer technology enabled more precise and accurate 3D reconstruction from ultrasonic tomograms, and their projection on a 2D plane.[22,23] Surface mode is used for the depiction of the brain surface (gyri and sulci), minimum mode is used for the depiction of the cystic formations, while maximum mode is better for the depiction of calcifications.[22] During the examination there is a possibility of color and power Doppler studies of brain circulation.[16,24] Volumetric measurements of brain structures are sometimes important for follow up of cysts, hydrocephalus, and ventriculomegaly, and could be a promising marker for predicting disturbances of cognitive outcome in preterm infants.[20,25-27]

Brain ultrasound has become the most widely used technique for evaluation of brain morphology and cerebral lesions in neonates.[20,21,28] It can identify not only the presence of lesions but also their type and extent.[29]

PRINCIPLES OF 3D NEUROSONOGRAPHY

3D high-resolution (5 to 8 MHz) sector probe swings mechanically in a fan-like manner during volume acquisition, recording sets of tomograms at fixed angular increments, which are digitalized and saved to the computer memory.[18,20,22,23] Using specialized software, the sonologist can generate orthogonal sets of images in any desired plane through the 3D volume.[18,20,22,23] In addition to the standard sagittal and coronal planes which are traditionally obtained through the anterior fontanel when 2D neurosonography is performed, during 3D neurosonography brain can be viewed in axial plane, which cannot be obtained by conventional 2D imaging through the anterior fontanel.[2,17,20] The obtained images are displayed in three orthogonal planes for multi-planar view analysis with the possibility of data manipulation.[2,17,18,20,22,23,28] For better orientation during multiplanar analysis, dot marker is always positioned in the same structure of the brain in all three orthogonal planes. After multiplanar analysis of neonatal brain, volume rendering of the region of interest (ROI) can be performed, with direct projection of 3D data on a 2D plane.[18,20,22,23] Different modes of volume reconstruction can be used depending on the location of the object of interest. 3D ultrasound consists of: 3D data acquisition, construction of 3D data sets and projection and displaying 3D data on a 2D plane.[18,20,22,23]

INDICATIONS FOR 3D NEUROSONOGRAPHY IN NEWBORN INFANTS

Although 3D brain ultrasonography is safe and low-risk procedure, due to a very limited availability of equipment for 3D neurosonography, which is often connected with the necessity of newborn transportation, benefits and risks of 3D imaging should be taken under consideration. In the institutions where equipment is available and can be transported to the patient, it is method of choice for the depiction of neonatal brain.[8] Indications for 3D neurosonography in the newborn period are the same as for 2D, so whenever 2D is unreliable or doubtful, then 3D is indicated.[2,7-9] The main indications for 3D neurosonography in the newborn period are:

• Intracranial hemorrhage
• Hypoxic-ischemic brain damage
• Inflammatory disorders of the brain and its complications
• Ventriculomegaly and hydrocephaly with volumetric studies
• Congenital brain defects
• Assessment of gestational age.

COMMENTS ON INDICATIONS FOR NEUROSONOGRAPHY IN NEWBORNS

Regular assessment of neurologic maturation in the neonate along with a basic assessment of neurologic optimality at 40th week of gestation is of substantial significance for the future developmental outcome.[30] Many known and unknown perinatal and social risk factors can influence the development of neonatal brain especially in premature infants, although abnormal neurological findings in apparently well neonates can prompt neonatologists to search for ultrasound abnormalities.[13,19,26,27,31,34] A good correlation was found between ultrasound findings and signs of neurological impairment in the neonatal period[1] and later in childhood.[3,29] Cranial ultrasound can be a good predictor of disabling and not disabling cerebral palsy at the age of two years in low birth weight infants[35,36] and it can be in relation with impaired motor function in five-year-old children.[3] Improving survival of very low birth weight infants contributed to the increased incidence of cerebral palsy despite introduction of sophisticated treatment methods of intensive care.[36-38] Brain lesions of the white matter diagnosed by ultrasound were found to be a powerful predictor of disabling cerebral palsy.[36]

The classical description of intraventricular hemorrhage with its grading was given by Papile et al.[39] The prevalence of intracranial hemorrhage in very low birth weight (VLBW) premature infants has had decreasing tendency in the last twenty years from as high as 60 percent at the beginning of eighties, to 25 percent in nineties.[40] In apparently normal full-term newborns intracranial hemorrhage can be detected in 3.5 percent.[31,41] Some new concepts in the pathogenesis of germinal matrix intraparenchymal hemorrhages in premature infants enabled better understanding of pathological events and their prevention.[13,19,26,27,34,42] Multiplanar view and 3D reconstruction of subependymal hemorrhage and hemorrhage grades II, III and IV (according to Papile) are shown in Figures 17.1A and B to 17.4.

Prevalence of periventricular leukomalacia in VLBW infants is 9.2 to 14.9 percent,[43] while the incidence of cystic periventricular leukomalacia is 4.3 to 15.7 percent in preterm infants between 27th and 32th weeks of gestation.[33] The most important pathophysiological factor of the brain white matter damage is inflammation.[32,44,45] Released as a part of the inflammatory cascade, cytokines and other compounds (nitric oxide) cause pronounced vasoactive effects with the consecutive impairment of cerebrovascular regulation and thereby increased risk for ischemic white matter injury.[33] The ultrasonic finding of transient hyperechogenicities of white matter or so called "flares" is transient, resolving spontaneously without any consecutive developmental problems, while cystic periventricular leukomalacia is often associated with an up to 50 percent risk of cerebral palsy.[36,43] Figure 17.5 showing 3D reconstruction and multiplanar view of periventricular flares. Figure 17.6 depicting multiplanar view and 3D reconstruction of cystic periventricular leukomalacia. Comparison of 3D surface rendering and magnetic resonance imaging (MRI) of cystic periventricular leukomalacia with subdural effusion is shown in Figure 17.7.

Despite improved hygienic practices, vaccines and introduction of new anti-inflammatory agents, congenital infections remain an important cause of neurologic morbidity in newborns.[46,47] Among neuroimaging diagnostic procedures ultrasound has an important role in the detection and follow up of neonatal TORCH infections and meningitis.[46,47] Regardless of its etiology, meningitis in VLBW infants is often caused by intrahospital agents.[46,47] The role of postnatal inflammation in the pathogenesis of the brain damage in VLBW infants still remains to be proved, while the role of prenatal inflammation is undoubted in the pathogenesis of cystic PVL.[32,33,36,43] Figure 17.8 depicting multiplanar view and 3D reconstruction of subdural effusion in the course of bacterial meningitis.

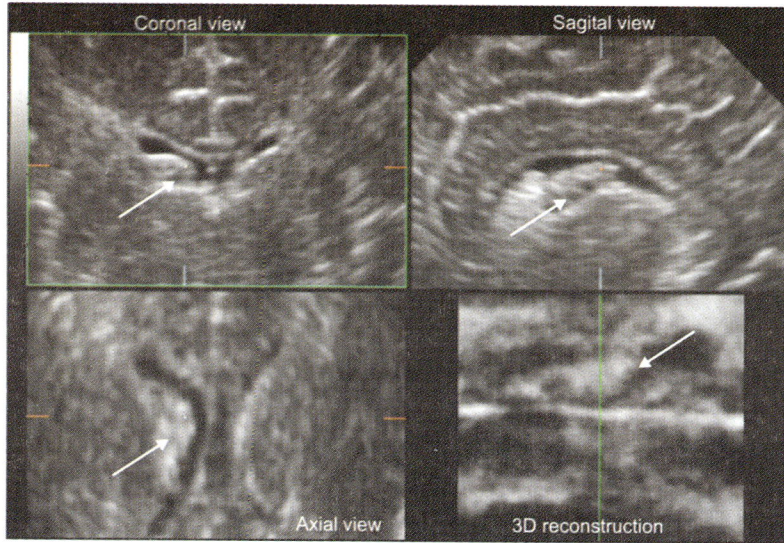

Fig. 17.1A: Multiplanar view and 3D reconstruction of unilateral subependymal hemorrhage (dot on the hemorrhage, unbroken arrow showing hemorrhage)

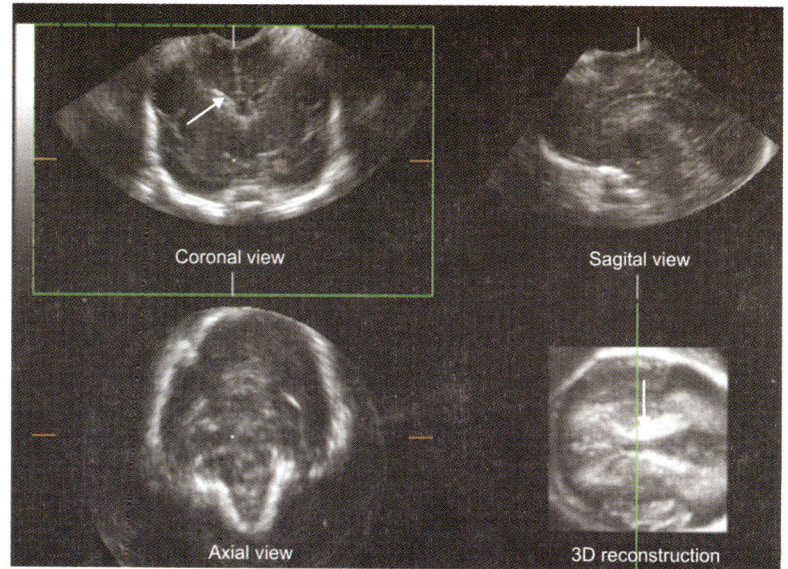

Fig. 17.2: Multiplanar view and 3D reconstruction of intracranial intraventricular hemorrhage grade II (Papile)

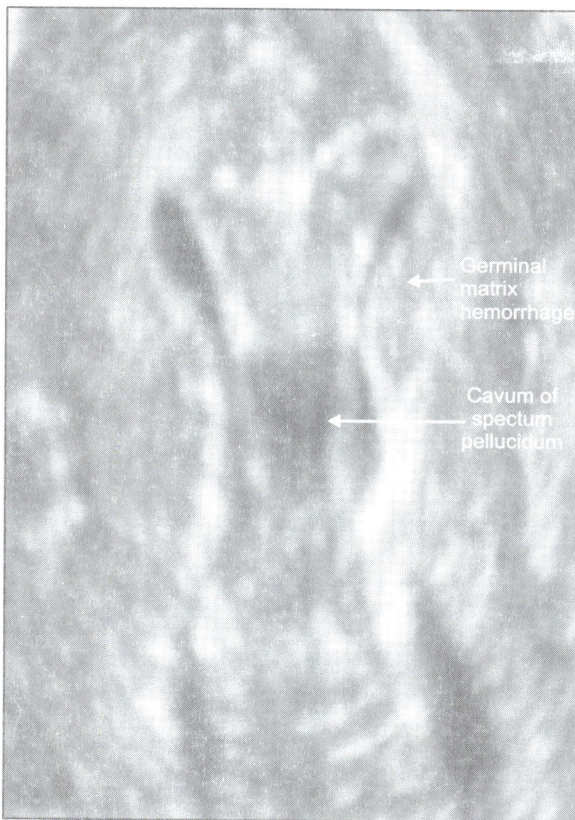

Fig.17.1B: 3D reconstruction of subependymal hemorrhage

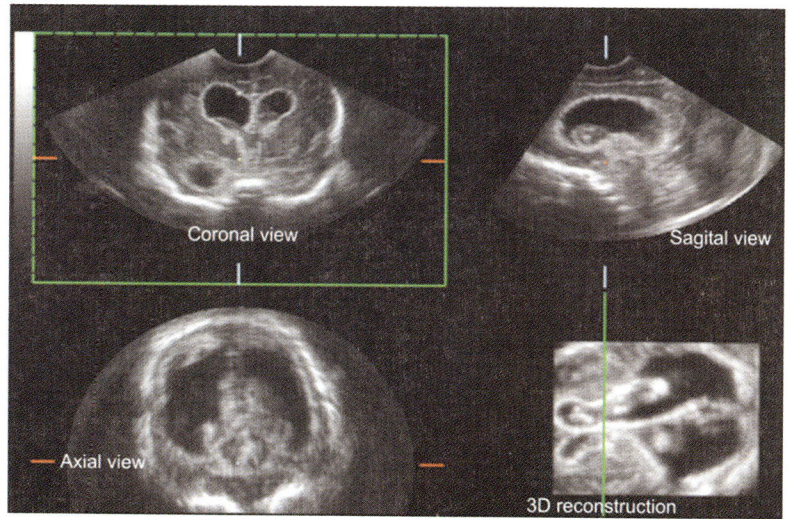

Fig. 17.3: Multiplanar view and 3D reconstruction of intracranial intraventricular hemorrhage grade III (Papile)

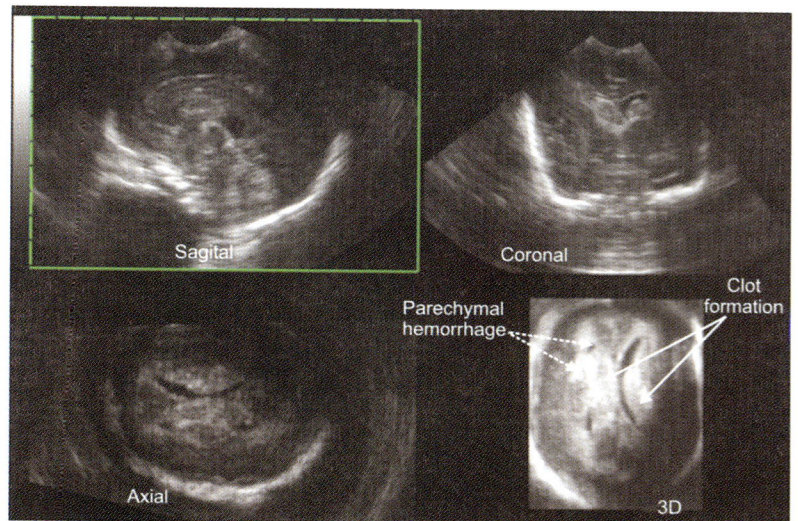

Fig.17.4: 3D reconstruction of parenchymal hemorrhage (Papile grade IV broken arrows)

Although application of different neuroimaging modalities, among which ultrasound is the most important, has enabled prenatal and postnatal detection of hydrocephalus, its management remains a difficult challenge.[48] One major reason for the difficulty is the multifactorial nature of the conditions affecting postnatal outcome in congenital hydrocephalus.[48] New clinicoembryological classification of congenital hydrocephalus reflects both clinical and embryological developmental aspects of the neuronal maturation process in the hydrocephalic infant.[48] Congenital hydrocephalus is one of the most common CNS malformations with an incidence of 0.3 to 0.8 per 1000 births.[38] Ventriculomegaly, defined as an enlargement of the ventricular

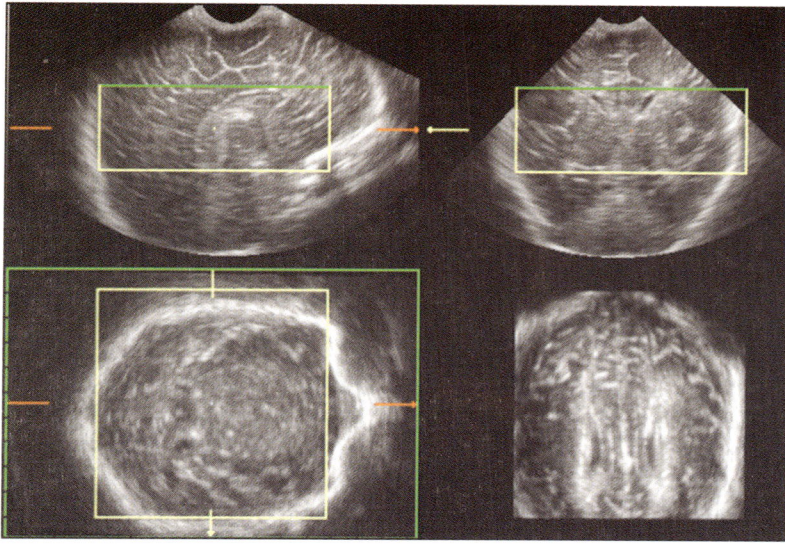

Fig. 17.5: Multiplanar view and 3D reconstruction of periventricular "flares"

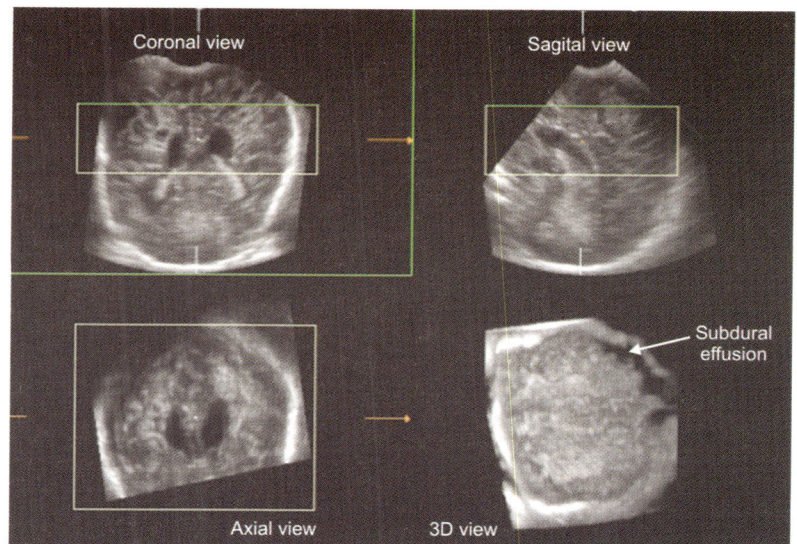

Fig. 17.6: Multiplanar view and 3D reconstruction of cystic periventricular leukomalacia grade III

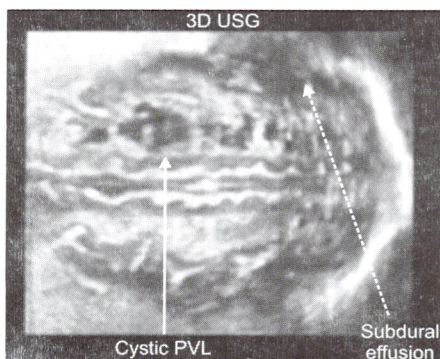

Fig. 17.7: 3D surface rendering and MRI of cystic periventricular leukomalacia with subdural effusion

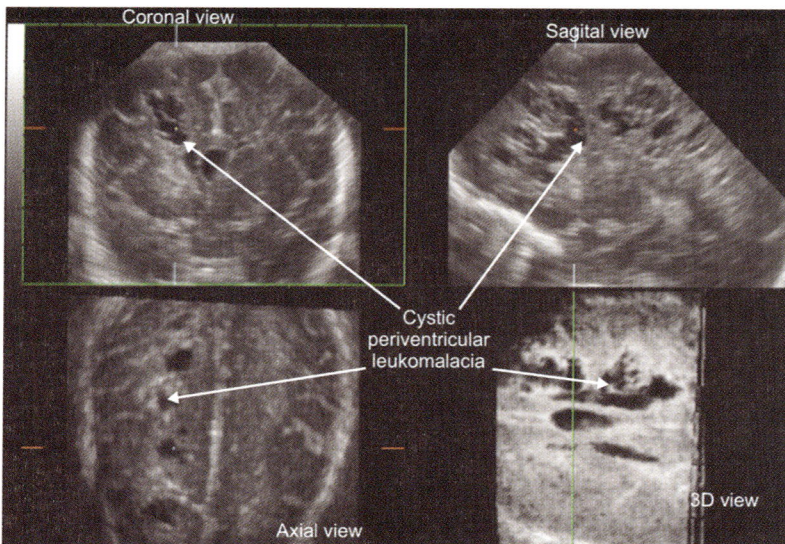

Fig. 17.8: Multiplanar view and 3D reconstruction of subdural effusion in the course of bacterial meningitis

atrium with a width of greater than 1 cm, is often associated with numerous etiologies ranged from the underdevelopment or atrophy of intracranial structures affecting the normal flow of cerebrospinal fluid through the ventricular system to disorders of mendelian inheritance.[38] In one-third ventriculomegaly is connected with additional intracranial lesions, while two-thirds have extracranial anomalies.[38,49] Severe hypertensive hydrocephalus – multiplanar 3D view and MRI depicted in Figure 17.9.

The 3D ultrasound studies of fetal CNS development improved prenatal diagnosis of malformations and other conditions with the sensitivity of up to 80 percent.[10,11,18,21] Nevertheless, postnatal ultrasound still remains important for the detection of prenatally unrecognized conditions and for the postnatal follow-up. Incidence of central nervous system anomalies is estimated to be 0.2 percent.[10] Despite a possibility of a genetic diagnosis of some CNS malformations, detection of mutated genes will not be available in the nearest future as a screening method in clinical practice,[38] and therefore diagnostic ultrasound will remain of great importance. The incidence of some common CNS anomalies like agenesis of corpus callosum is 2 to 3 percent of developmentally disabled individuals.[38] In 57 percent agenesis of corpus callosum is connected with coexisting anomalies, while in 10 percent of cases it is complicated by chromosomal aberrations.[38] Choroid plexus cysts have incidence of 1 to 2 percent in general population.[38] Cysts above 5 mm in diameter have a higher rate of aneuploidy in comparison with cysts between 2 and 5 mm.[38] Figure 17.10 depicts 3D color Doppler of normal pericallosal vasculature excluding agenesis of corpus callosum. Figure 17.11 depicting 3D multiplanar view of choroid plexus cysts (small cyst white-unbroken arrow, large cyst – white dashed arrow).

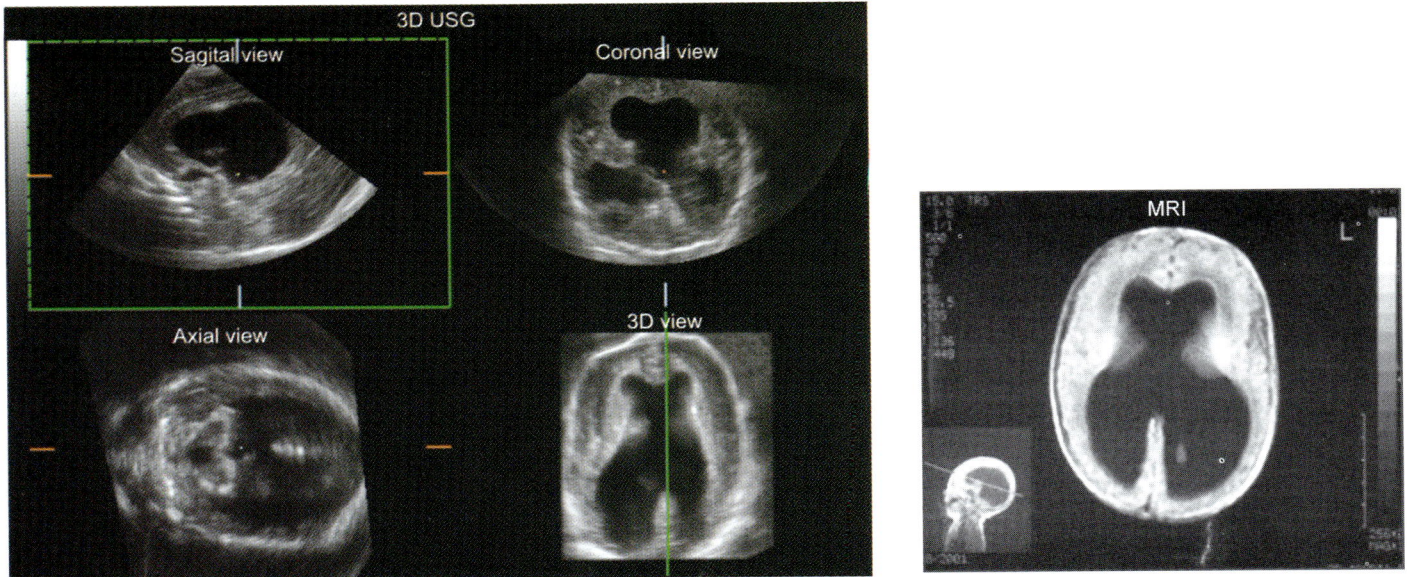

Fig. 17.9: Severe hypertensive hydrocephalus—multiplanar view 3D ultrasonography reconstruction and MRI

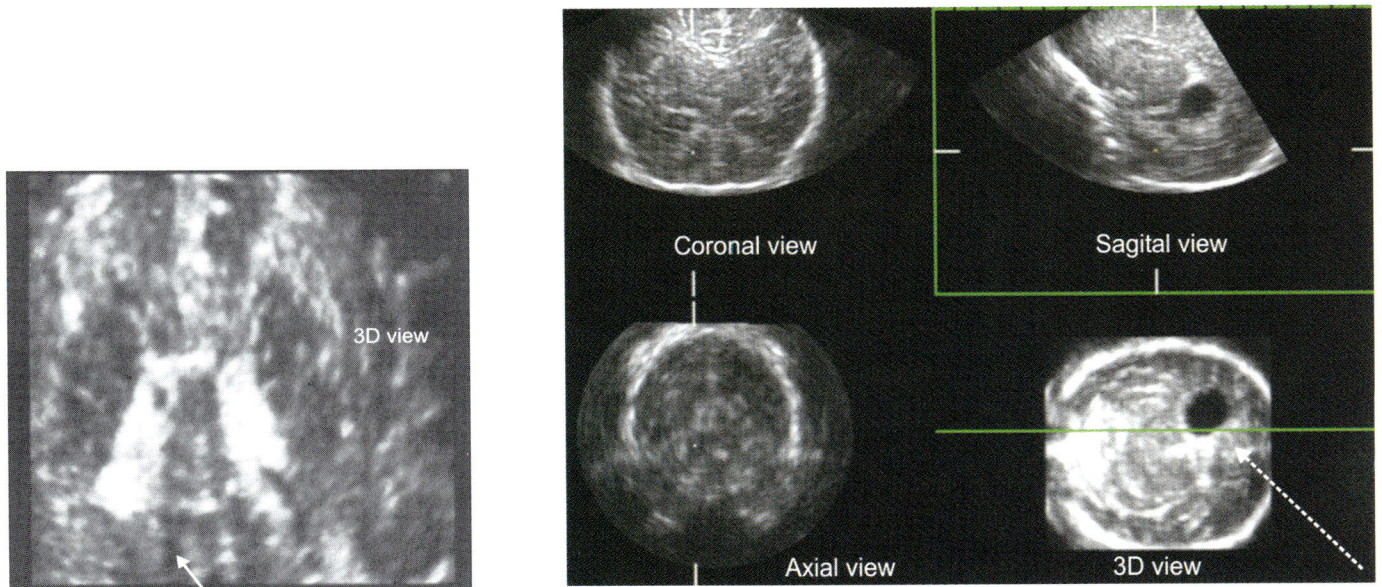

Fig. 17.10: 3D multiplanar view of choroid plexus cysts (small cyst—white unbroken arrow, large cyst—white dashed arrow)

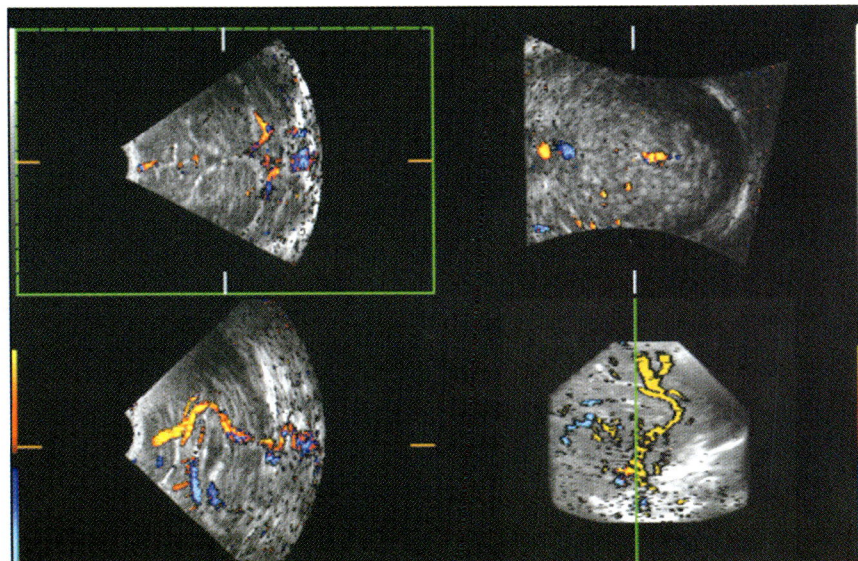

Fig. 17.11: 3D color Doppler of normal pericallosal vasculature

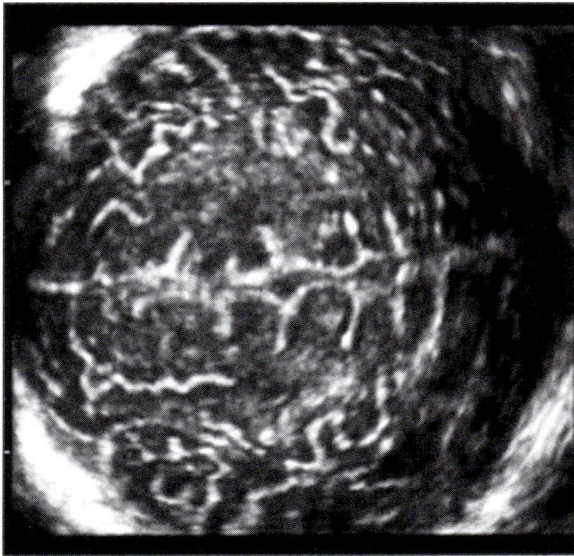

Fig. 17.12: Surface 3D rendering of gyri and sulci of normal brain

There is a need for an easy and accurate clinical method to assess the gestational age in newborns. From the 24th to the 34th weeks of gestation there are important identifiable changes in the cerebral surface, and principal sulci develop and alter in complexity each week.[14,50] After 34th week, as the gyri increase in complexity, distinctive changes are less easy to identify.[14] Ultrasound is a noninvasive method of studying the important changes in the development of neonatal brain with scoring system enabling determination of gestational age.[14,50] Figure 17.12 showing surface 3D rendering of gyri and sulci of normal brain.

CONCLUSIONS

3D neurosonography of neonatal brain has been considered a significant improvement compared to the conventional 2D sonography. Some of the improvements are: shorter time of data acquisition in three orthogonal planes with unlimited number of planes, possibility of comprehensive and thorough analysis of obtained data set, volume rendering, volumetric, color and power Doppler studies. Possibility of sending 3D images, without the necessity of referring the patient is a great achievement of modern technology.[18,20,22] Although 3D neurosonography is still not available as the standard method for the assessment of neonatal brain due to high costs of the equipment, it should become widely available in the nearest future.

REFERENCES

1. Dubowitz LMS, Levene MI, Morante A, Palmer P, Dubowitz V. Neurologic signs in neonatal intraventricular hemorrhage: a correlation with real-time ultrasound. J Pediatr 1981; 99:127.
2. Fischer AQ, Anderson JC, Shuman RM, Stinson W. Pediatric neurosonography. Clinical, tomographic and neuropathologic correlates. A Wiley Medical Publication: New York,Chicester, Brisbane, Toronto, Singapore, 1985.
3. Levene M, Dowling S, Graham M, Fogelman K, Galton M, Philips M. Impaired motor function (clumsiness) in 5-year-old children: correlation with neonatal ultrasound scans. Arch Dis Child 1992; 67:687.
4. Levene MI, Wigglesworth JS, Dubowitz V. Cerebral structure and intraventricular hemorrhage in the neonate: a real-time ultrasound study. Arch Dis Child 1981; 56:416.
5. McNay MB, Fleming JEE. Forty years of obstetric ultrasound 1957-1997:from a-scope to three dimensions.Ultrasound in Med and Biol 1999; 25:30.
6. Nelson TR, Pretorius D. Interactive acquisition, analysis and visualization of sonographic volume data. International Journal of Imaging System and Technology 1997; 8:260.
7. Stanojevic M. Three-dimensional ultrasound in the neonatal period. http://www.sickkids.on.ca/FrontiersinFetalHealth/FFHSeptember2001.asp.
8. Stanojevic M, Hafner T, Kurjak A. Three-dimensional ultrasound – a useful imaging technique in the assessment of neonatal brain. J Perinat Med 2002; 30:74.
9. Stanojevic M, Pooh RK, Kurjak A, Kos M. Thre-dimensional ultrasound assessment of the fetal and neonatal brain. Ultrasound Rev Obstet Gynecol 2003; 3:117.
10. Pilu G, Perolo A, Falco P, Visentin A, Gabrielli S, Bovicelli L. Ultrasound of the fetal central nervous system.Curr Opin Obstet Gynecol 2000; 12:93.
11. Terrone DA, Kenneth GP Jr. Ultrasound in evaluation of the fetal central nervous system. Obst Gynecol Clin North Am 1998; 25:479.
12. Timor-Tritsch IE, Monteagudo A, Mayberry P. Three-dimensional ultrsound evaluation of fetal brain: the three-horn view.Ultrasound Obstet Gynecol 2000; 16:302.
13. Levene MI, de Vries LS. Neonatal intracranial hemorrhage. In Levene MI, Chervenak FA, White M (Eds): Fetal and Neonatal Neurology and Neurosurgery (3rd ed)Churchill Livingstone, 2001; pp339-71.
14. Murphy NP, Rennie J, Cooke RW. Cranial ultrasound assessment of gestational age in lowbirthweight infants. Arch Dis Child 1989; 64:569.
15. Nelson TR, Pretorius DH. 3-dimensional ultrasound volume measurement. Medical Physiscs 1993; 20:227.
16. Kurjak A, Kupesic S, Banovic I, Hafner T, Kos M. The study of morphology and circulation of early embryo by three-dimensional ultrasound and power Doppler. J Perinat Med 1997;27:145.
17. Kampmann W, Walka MM, Vogel M, Obladen M. 3-D sonographic volume measurement of cerebral ventricular system:in vitro validation. Ultrasound Med Biol 1998; 24:1169.
18. Kurjak A, Hafner T, Kos M, Kupesic S, Stanojevic M. Three-dimensional sonography in prenatal diagnosis: a luxury or necessity. J Perinat Med 2000; 28:194.
19. Linder N, Haskin O, Levit O, et al. Risk factors for intraventricular hemorrhage in very low birth weight premature infants: a retrospective case control study. Pediatrics 2003; 111:590.
20. Merz E. Aktuelle technische Möglichkeiten der 3D-Sonographie in der Ginäkologie und Geburtshilfe Ultrashal in Med 1997; 18:190.
21. Monteagudo A, Timor-Tritsch IE, Mayberry P. Three-dimensional transvaginal neurosonography of the fetal brain: 'navigation' in the volume scan. Ultrasound Obstet Gynecol 2000; 16:307.
22. Baba K, Okai T. Basis and principles of three-dimensional ultrasound. In Kurjak A (Ed): Progress in Obstetric and Gynecological Sonography Series. Baba K, Jurkovic D (Series Eds): Three-dimensional ultrasound in obstetrics and gynecology. The Parthenon Publishing Group: New York, London, 1997.
23. Baba K, Satoh K, Sakamato S, Okai T, Ishii S. Development of an ultrasonic system for three-dimensional reconstruction of the fetus. J Perinat Med 1989; 17:19.
24. Peng SS, Lin JH, Lee WT, et al. 3-D power Doppler cerebral angiography in neonates and young infants:comparison with 2-D Doppler angiography. Ultrasound Med Biol 1999; 25:947.
25. Chang CH, Chang FM, YU CH, Ko HC, Chen HY. Assessment of fetal cerebellar volume using three-dimensional ultrasound. Ultrasound in Med 2000; 26:981.
26. Murphy BP, Inder TE, Rooks V, et al. Posthaemorrhagic ventricular dilatation in the premature infant: natural history and predictors of outcome. Arch Dis Child Fetal Neonatal Ed 2002; 87:F37.
27. Osborn DA, Evans N, Kluckow M. Hemodynamic and antecedent risk factors of early and late periventricular/intraventricular hemorrhage in premature infants. Pediatrics 2003; 112:33.
28. Newman PG, Rozycki GS. The history of ultrasound. Surgical Clinics of North America 1998; 78:179.
29. Mercuri E, Dubowitz L, Paterson Brown S, Cowan F. Incidence of cranial ultrasound abnormalities in apparently well neonates on postnatal ward: correlation with antenatal and perinatal factors and neurological status.Arch Dis Child Fetal Neonatal Ed 1998; 79:F185.
30. Amiel-Tison C. Clinical assessment of the infant nervous system. In Leven MI, Chervenak FA, Whittle MJ (Eds): Fetal and Neonatal Neurology and Neurosurgery, (3rd ed). Churchill Livingstone: London, Edinburgh, New York, Philadelphia, St Louis, Sydney, Toronto, 2001.

31. Heibel M, Heber R, Bechinger D, Kornhuber HH. Early diagnosis of perinatal cerebral lesions in apparently normal full-term newborns by ultrasond of the brain. Neuroradiology 1993; 35:85.
32. Leviton A, Dammann O Coagulation, imflammation, and the risk of neonatal white matter damage. Pediatr Res 2004; 55:541.
33. Volpe JJ. Neurobiology of periventricular leukomalacia in the premature infant. Pediatr Res 2001; 50:553.
34. Whitelaw A. Intraventricular haemorrhage and posthaemorrhagic hydrocephalus: pathogenesis, prevention and future interventions. Semin Neonatol 2001; 6:135.
35. Peterson BS, Anderson AW, Ehrenkranz R, Staib LH, Tageldin M, Colson E, et al. Regional brain volumes and their later neurodevelopmental correlates in term and preterm infants. Pediatrics 2003; 111:939.
36. Pinto-Martin J, Riolo S, Cnaan A, Holzman C, Susser MV, Paneth N. Cranial ultrasound prediction of disabling and nondisabling cerebral palsy at age two in low birth weight population. Pediatrics 1995; 95:249.
37. Perlman JM, Risser MB, Broyles RS. Bilateral cystic perivantricular leukomalacia in the premature infant: associated risk factors. Pediatrics 1996; 97:822.
38. Tanak T, Gleeson GJ. Genetics of brain development and malformation. Curr Opin Pediatr 2000; 12:523.
39. Papile LA, Burstein J, Burstein R. Incidence and evolution of subependymal and intraventricular hemorrhage: a study of infants with birth weights less than 1,500 gm. J Pediatr 1978; 92:529.
40. Vohr B, Ment LR. Intraventricular hemorrhage in the preterm infant. Early Human Developmen 1996; 44:1.
41. Larcos G, Gruenwald SM, Lui K. Neonatal subependymal cysts detected by sonography: prevalence, sonographic findings, and clinical significance. Am J Radiol 1994; 162:953.
42. Ghazi-Birry HS, Brown WR, Moody DM, Challa VR, Block SM, Reboussin DM. Human germinal matrix:venous origin of hemorrhage and vascular characteristics. Am J Neuroradiol 1997; 18:219.
43. Dammann O, Leviton A. Duration of transient hyperechoic images of white matter in very-low-birthweight infants: a proposed classification. Developmental Medicine and Child Neurology 1997; 39:2.
44. Wu YW, Colford JM. Chorioamnionitis as a risk factor for cerebral palsy. JAMA 2000; 284:1417.
45. Zupan V, Gonzales P, Lacaze-Masmonteil T, Boithias C, d'Alest AM, Dehan M, Gabilan JC. Periventricular leukomalacia:risk factors revisited. Developmental Medicine and Child Neurology 1996; 38:1061.
46. Bale FB, Murph JR. Congenital infections and nervous system. Pediatr Clin North Am 1992; 39:669.
47. Frank JL. Sonography of intracranial infection in infants and children. Neuroradiology 1986; 28:440.
48. Ot S, Honda Y, Hidaka M, Sato O, Matsumoto S. Intrauterine high-resolution magnetic resonance imaging in fetal hydrocephalus and prenatal estimation of postnatal outcomes with perspective classification. J Neurosurg 1998; 88:685.
49. Nagdyman N, Walka MM, Kampmann W, Stowver B, Obladen M. 3-D ultrasound quantification of neonatal cerebral ventricles in different head positions. Ultrasound Med Biol 1999; 25:895.
50. Huang CC, Yeh TF. Assessment of gestational age in newborns by neurosonography. Early Human Development 1991; 25:209.

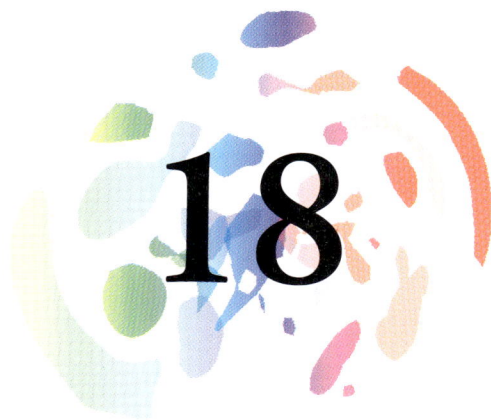

**Luis T Mercé, María J Barco,
Santiago Bau, Sanja Kupesic,
Asim Kurjak**

18

3D Power Doppler Ultrasound in Obstetrics and Gynecology

INTRODUCTION

Three-dimensional power Doppler angiography is an emerging technology in the field of ultrasound and Doppler diagnostics in Obstetrics and Gynecology. Since 1996 there are around 400 publications on 3D ultrasound although no more than a hundred deal specifically with the diagnostic problems getting along with this technique.

From this point of departure our aim is to review in an orderly way all the possible applications of this technology according to the previous reports and our own experience on the subject. We tried to gather the most interesting initial results and the most thought-provoking diagnostic possibilities. We have sought too those images more representative on the subject as required to a real atlas. With a practical purpose the different applications have been classified in Reproductive Medicine, Obstetrics and Gynecology.

As it usually happens with other technologies, the most important thing is the technique itself. Its application offers new and unexpected advantages in the ultrasonic diagnosis in our specialty as the telediagnosis. We will be capable only to obtain an optimal diagnostic result from this technology if we adapt our mentality to these new requirements.

ESSENTIALS OF THREE-DIMENSIONAL POWER DOPPLER

In 1996, Ritchie et al reported the appearance of a new technology to produce three-dimensional angiograms from slices obtained by bidimensional power Doppler. These authors suggest that this new technique will be useful to the assessment of vascular anatomy and blood flow perfusion of the different organs as the kidneys and placenta.[1]

The development of three-dimensional power Doppler ultrasonography or power Doppler angiography is closely linked to the diagnostic abilities of power Doppler and the design of the software capable of representing and properly evaluate the vascularization of the different organs.

3D power Doppler image is essentially characterized by its high sensitivity to depict any vessel, as much the great vessels as the microvascularization.[2] Otherwise conventional color Doppler, this is possible because images are obtained from ultrasound amplitude instead of Doppler frequency. The color map acquired is not affected by the insonation angle and does not show dark zones or aliasing.[3]

VOCAL (Virtual Organ Computer-aided Analysis) is a software developed from a rotational method for the automatic or manual assessment of three-dimensional volumes.[4] This program allows basically: (i) surface definition and characterization by the "surface" or "skin" mode (Fig. 18.1A); (ii) automatic or manual calculation of the volumes of the different structures (Fig. 18.1B); (iii) production of a virtual "shell" of different thickness (Fig. 18.1C) and (iv) automatic calculation of 3D Doppler indices to the assessment of organ vascularization (Fig. 18.1D).[5]

By means of a histogram, the VOCAL program does the automatic calculation of the gray scale and color values from the volume acquired. The three-dimensional volume is made up of units named "voxels" which store all the information about the gray scale and color expressed in an intensity scale from 0 to 100. This way a gray index and three color indices are obtained for the quantitative assessment of the vascularization.[4,5]

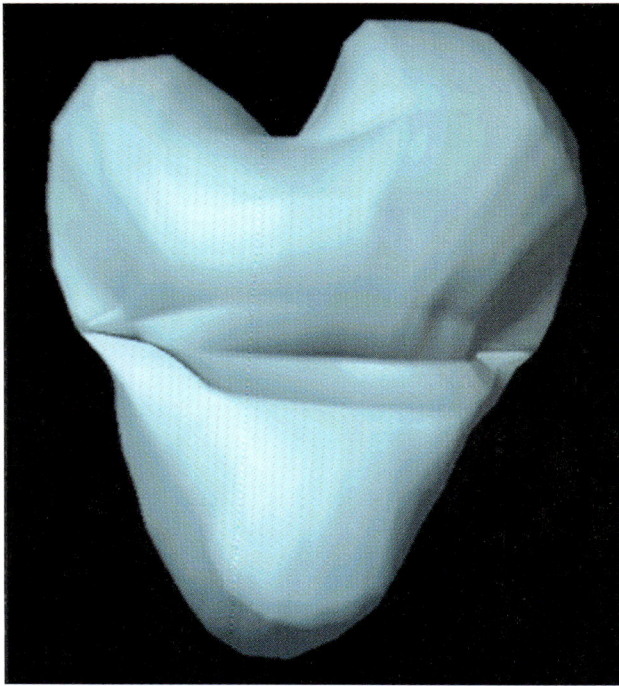

A

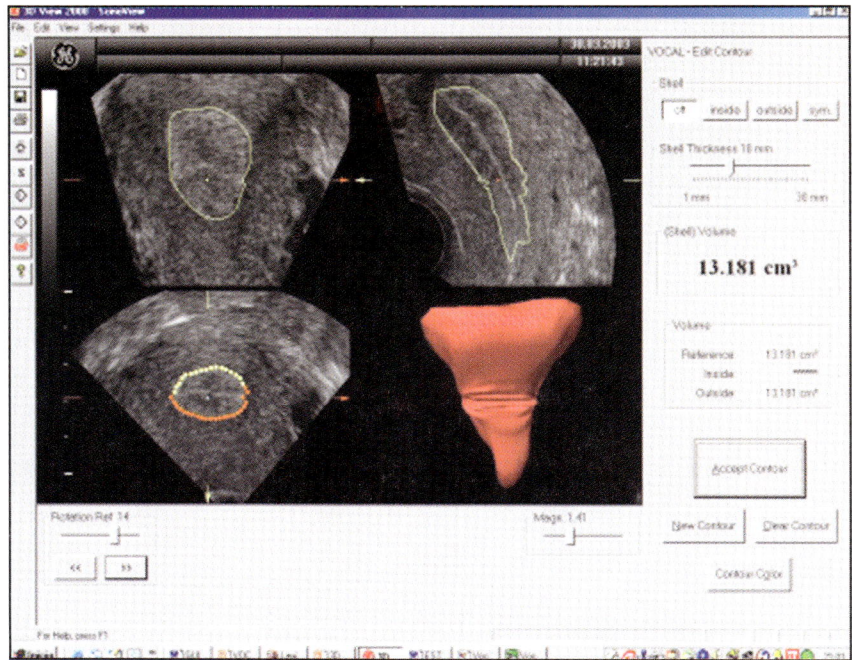

B

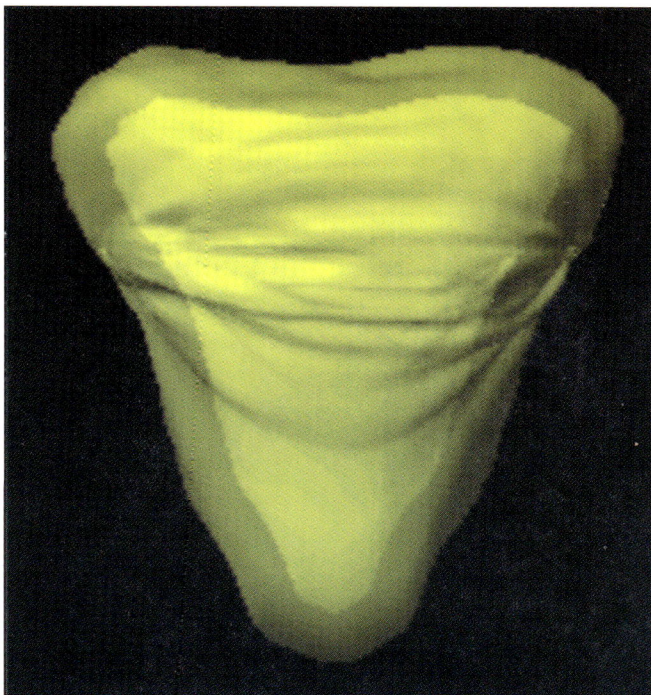

C

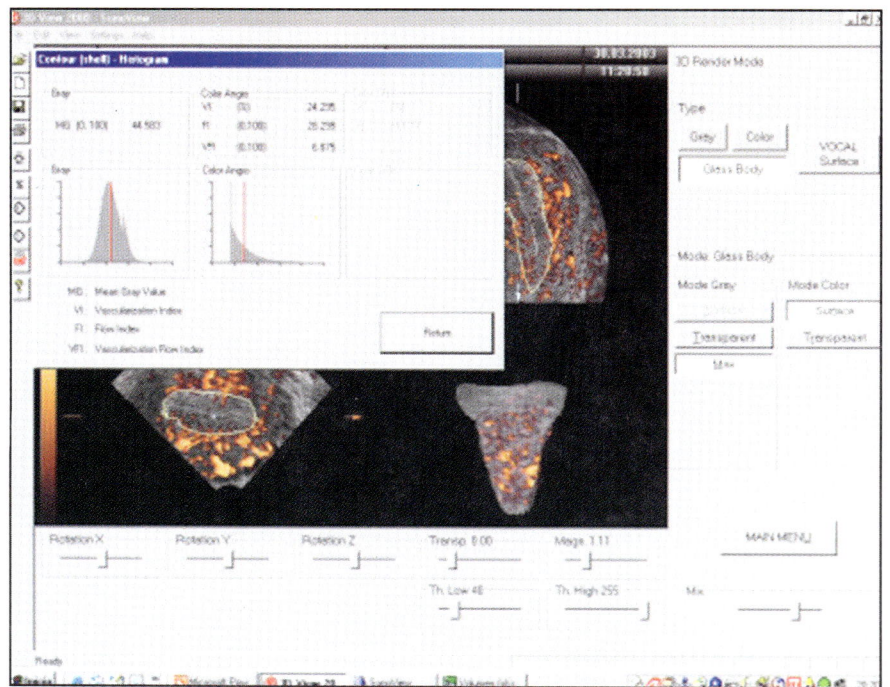

D

Figs 18.1A to D: The three-dimensional treatment program VOCAL allows the definition of the surface of the organs by the "surface" or "skin" mode: (A); the manual or automatic measurement of the volumes from different structures (B) the construction of a virtual "shell" with different thickness (C) and the calculation of 3D Doppler indices to the study of the vascularity (D)

The mean gray (MG) represents the mean gray value among all the gray voxels from the volume acquired. The Vascularization Index (VI) estimates the number of color voxels inside the volume, thus expressing the number of blood vessels as a percentage. The Flow Index (FI) is the average color value from all the color voxels, depicting the mean intensity of the blood flow. The Vascularization Flow Index (VFI) is the average color value out of all the color and gray voxels, meaning the vascularization as

well as the blood flow, in other words, the perfusion inside the region of interest (Figs 18.2A and B).[4,5]

All the above mentioned accounts for VOCAL as an essential program to the right quantitative evaluation of the 3D power Doppler angiography, not forgetting the 3D power Doppler map depicts in a highly precise way the whole tree network. The study of the morphology and architecture of the vascular networks suggests its normality and nature which contributes to the diagnosis of vascular anomalies and tumor vascularization.

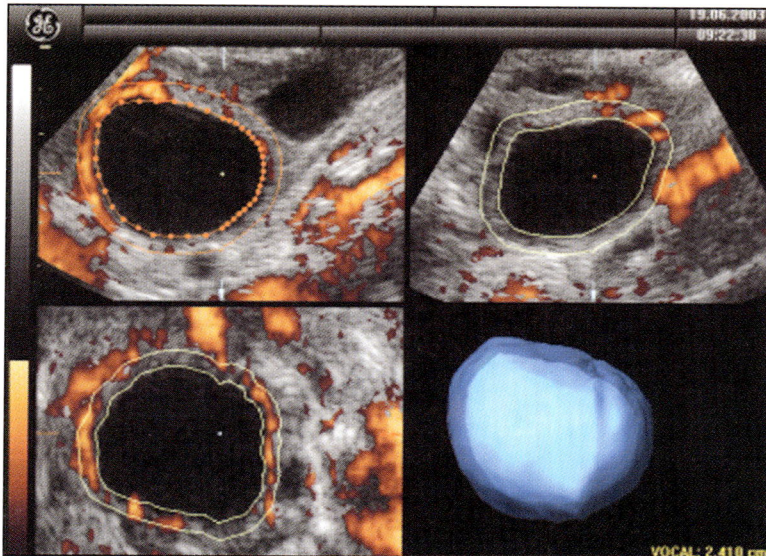

A

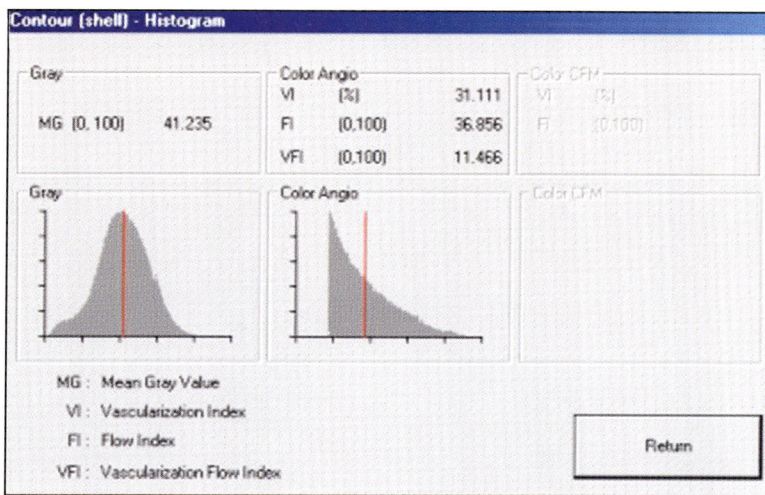

B

Figs 18.2A and B: Study of the perifollicular vascularization with a 2 mm shell in a preovulatory follicle. (A) Multiplanar presentation and volumetric rendering; (B) 3D Doppler indices Histogram: VI: Vascularization Index; FI: Flow Index and VFI: Vascularization Flow Index. The mean gray (MG) histogram is also shown

APPLICATIONS IN REPRODUCTIVE MEDICINE

One of the first clinical applications of 3D power Doppler was in the field of assisted reproductive technologies. It has been basically applied on the study and quantitative evaluation of the ovarian, follicular and endometrial microvascularization as possible markers of ovarian response, oocyte developmental competence and embryonic implantation respectively.

Ovarian Response Markers

Doppler studies have demonstrated that the ovarian blood flow is implied in the recruitment of the follicular cohort during the early follicular phase of the normal ovarian cycle.[6] We have confirmed the intraovarian vascular resistance is correlated to the number of recruited follicles until the dominant follicle is selected (Figs 18.3). It has also been observed that the stromal

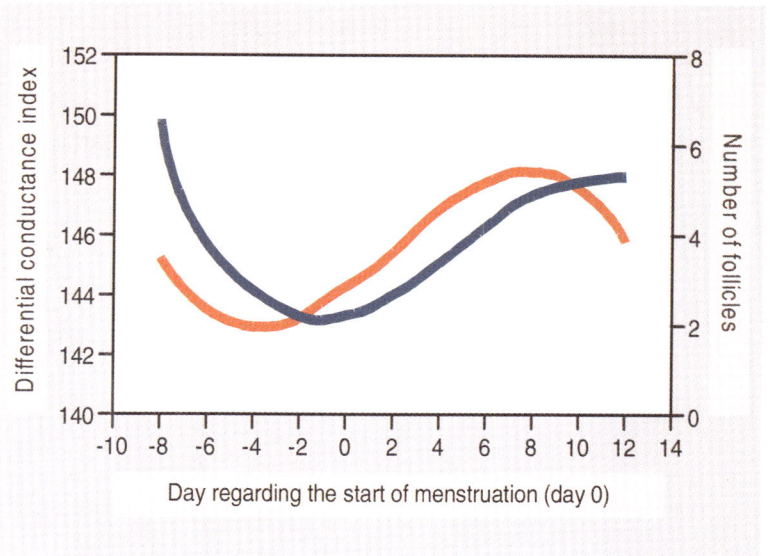

Fig. 18.3: Relationship between the recruited follicles number (red line) and the stromal blood flow assessed by its differential conductance index (blue line) during the luteo-follicular transitional period in 22 normal ovulatory cycles

peak systolic velocity during the early follicular phase is related to the number of oocytes retrieved.[7] When it is higher than 10 cm/s, a greater number of oocytes and a better pregnancy rate are achieved.[8] All these data support the importance of ovarian blood flow as a marker of the ovarian response to the gonadotropin stimulation therapy.

The 3D power Doppler has proven the progressive decrease of the stromal ovarian blood flow from premenopause to postmenopause as the follicular reserve runs out.[9] It has also been demonstrated that 3D Doppler indices are diminished after gonadotropin ovarian stimulation on surgically treated ovaries of endometriosis without differences in the whole ovarian volume but with a number of oocytes retrieved significantly smaller.[10] On the contrary, polycystic ovaries show increased 3D Doppler indices with regard to normal ovaries at the beginning of the menstrual cycle[11] although these differences are not found after the GnRH agonists treatment[12] (Figs 18.4A to D).

The ovaries under controlled hyperestimulation with gonadotropins show significantly higher 3D Power Doppler vascular indices in hyper-responder women[13] and lower in those from the hyporesponders.[14] However, Jarvela et al[15] observed that 3D vascular indices from ovaries after pituitary suppression do not correlate with the number of retrieved oocytes. Our results from the first IVF cycle on 60 infertile patients are similar to the previously exposed. As it is shown on Table 18.1 there is a significant correlation among ovarian volume, number of follicles > 2 mm and all power Doppler indices after pituitary suppression with the number of follicles ≥10 mm on the day of hCG injection and the number of oocytes retrieved. Nevertheless, when a multiple regression analysis is done to predict the number of

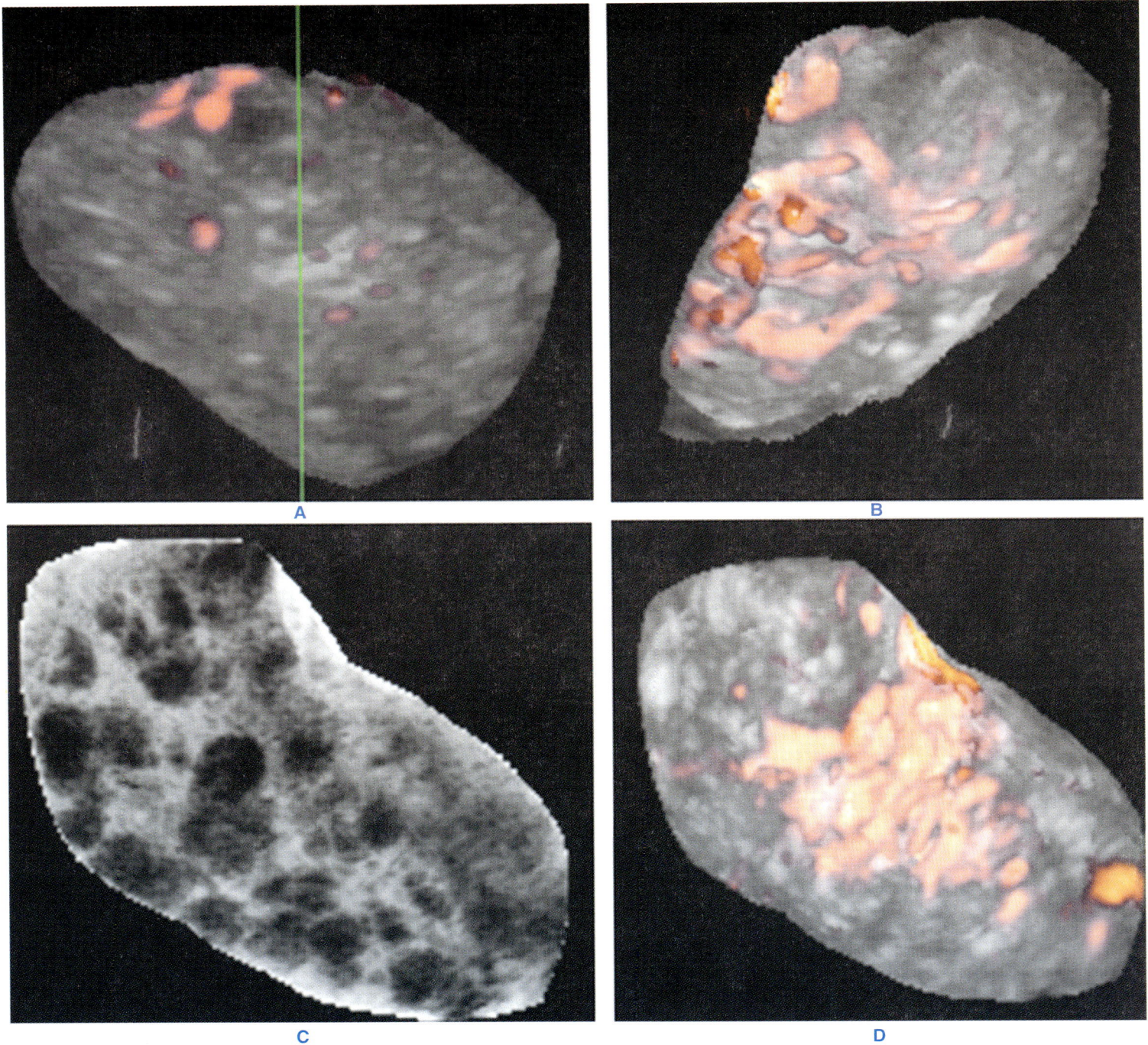

Figs 18.4A to D: Ovarian vascularity after GnRH analogs pituitary suppression with different stromal flow (A and B). Compare with a polycystic ovary showing a vascular network strongly developed

Table 18.1: Correlation coefficients of the sonographic parameters and power Doppler indices after pituitary suppression with the number of recruited follicles and the number of retrieved oocytes in 60 IVF cycles

	No. of follicles ≥10 mm on hCG the day	No. of retrieved oocytes
Ovarian volume	0.46	0.41
Number of follicles > 2 mm	0.52	0.53
Vascularization index	0.36	0.31
Flow index	0.30	0.27
Vascularization flow index	0.34	0.30

All correlation coefficients are significant (P < 0.01)
Only the number of follicles and the ovarian volume reach a statistical significance by multiple regression.

follicles recruited and the number of oocytes retrieved, only the ovarian volume and follicular amount after suppression reach statistical significance. Therefore, the 3D power Doppler study contributes nothing new to predict the ovarian response to the gonadotropin stimulation.

Finally, we have to specify that the ovarian power Doppler indices have a high intra- and interobserver reliability showing intraclass correlation coefficients (ICC) greater than 0.90.[16,17] However, we have found a smaller intraobserver ICC in the ovary under controlled gonadotropin hyperestimulation than the basal ovary after pituitary suppression (Table 18.2).

Table 18.2: Intraobserver differences (mean and SD) and intraclass correlation coefficients for the ovarian volume, number of follicles and 3D Doppler indices by VOCAL calculated in A Plane with 15º rotation step on the day of pituitary suppression confirmation (A) and on the day of hCG administration (B) in IVF cycles (n= 60)

PDA indices		Mean difference	SD	ICC	95% confidence interval CCI
VI	A	−0.55	2.33	0.92	0.96-0.84
	B	−0.17	2.31	0.88	0.94-0.75
FI	A	−0.23	2.00	0.94	0.97-0.88
	B	0.12	2.23	0.84	0.92-0.68
FVI	A	−0.21	1.03	0.91	0.96-0.81
	B	0.004	0.89	0.88	0.94-0.76

VI: Vascularization index; FI: Flow index, FVI: Flow vascularization index; A: After suppression; B: hCG day

Table 18.3: Correlation coefficients of the number of follicles and 3D power Doppler indices on the day of hCG administration with biological laboratory parameters in 87 IVF cycles

	NO	NOM	NOF	NE	NEI	NEM	SCE
NF	0.87[a]	0.70[a]	0.62[a]	0.62[a]	0.26[a]	0.29[a]	0.46[a]
VI	0.31[a]	0.27[a]	0.20	0.21[a]	0.07	0.18[b]	0.08
FI	0.25[a]	0.21[a]	0.08	0.11	0.09	0.12	0.05
VFI	0.32[a]	0.28[a]	0.21[a]	0.21[a]	0.08	0.18[b]	0.09
FV/VI	0.04	0.00	0.09	0.06	0.08	-0.15	0.06
FV/FI	0.73[a]	0.65[a]	0.62[a]	0.59[a]	0.27[a]	0.20[b]	0.40[a]
FV/VFI	0.00	-0.02	0.06	0.03	0.06	-0.15	0.04

NF: Number of follicles > 10 mm on the day of hCG administration; VI: Vascularization index; FI: Flow index; VFI: Vascularization flow index; FV: Follicular volume; NO: Number of retrieved oocytes; NOM: Number of metaphase II oocytes; NOF: Number of fertilized oocytes; NE: Number of developed embryos; NEI: Number of Type I embryos; NEM: Number of multinucleated embryos; SCE: Score of embryos. [a] means $P < 0.01$; [b] means $P < 0.05$

Oocyte Competence Markers

The development of the optimal perifollicular vascular network determines the intrafollicular oxygen concentration, whose deficit has been related to oocyte cytoplasmatic defects, embryos with multinucleated blastomere and abnormal chromosomal arrangement.[18]

Although it is possible to assess the follicular flow as expressed by the peak systolic velocity and perifollicular color map,[19] it is the 3D power Doppler which proves the most precise information about the vascularization and follicular blood flow.[20]

Studies with three-dimensional power Doppler have proven that the perifollicular vascularization of the dominant follicle is greater than the average vascularization of the whole ovary.[21] The 3D vascular indices from the corpus luteum are higher than those from the preovulatory follicle and luteinized unruptured follicle[20] (Figs 18.5A to C). The follicular fluid concentrations of leptine, a follicular angiogenesis related factor, are inversely related to the stromal blood flow index.[10] It has been suggested also that the follicles containing oocytes capable to produce a pregnancy have a perifollicular vascular network more uniform and distinctive.[22]

We have studied the 3D Doppler indices on 87 IVF cycles the day of hCG administration (Figs 18.6A to F). The number of follicles and the ratio between follicular volume and flow index are related to the number of retrieved oocytes, its maturity degree and the capability to fertilize and develop embryos. The relationship between these variables and the biological quality of the embryos has no significance (Table 18.3).

After pituitary suppression, Kupesic and Kurjak[23] observed that when the average stromal blood flow from both ovaries was greater than 11 they achieved a 89 percent fertilization rate and a 50 percent pregnancy rate. When this index was between 11 and 13, the fertilization and pregnancy rates were 75.2 and 47.2 percent respectively. Nevertheless, if the average index from both ovaries was lower than 11, the fertilization rate decreased to 64.3 percent and no pregnancy was achieved. According to our results, the ratio follicular volume/blood flow index on the day of hCG injection is more increased in the women that get pregnant. When this ratio is between 0.40 and 0.60 the pregnancy rate is 39 percent. If it is superior to 0.60 the rate achieved is 52 percent. When it is inferior to 0.40 the rate descends to 21 percent. The pregnancy rate in this group of patients was 39 percent.

Implantation Marker

The endometrial blood flow reflects more properly the uterine receptivity because the endometrium is the place where the embryonic implantation is going to take place.[19] The absence of color map at the endometrial and subendometrial levels leads to a significant decrease of the implantation rate[24,25] whereas the pregnancy rate increases when vessels reach the subendometrial halo and the endometrium.[24,26]

Ultrasonography and 3D power Doppler have the advantage to assess simultaneously the endometrial volume and sub-endometrial and endometrial blood flow. For all the 3D vascular indices from the endometrium and sub-endometrium an excellent intra- and interobserver reproducibility has been observed with intraclass correlation coefficients greater than 0.90[16,17] (Figs 18.7A to D).

3D Doppler indices vary significantly with the menstrual cycle and are characterized by a preovulatory peak and a postovulatory nadir during the embryonic implantation window.[27] The subendometrial flow index on the day of embryo transfer is greater among the group of patients getting pregnant[28] and the subendometrial vascularization-flow index on the day of hCG administration is better than the endometrial volume to predict a pregnancy in IVF cycles.[29] It has also been proven that those

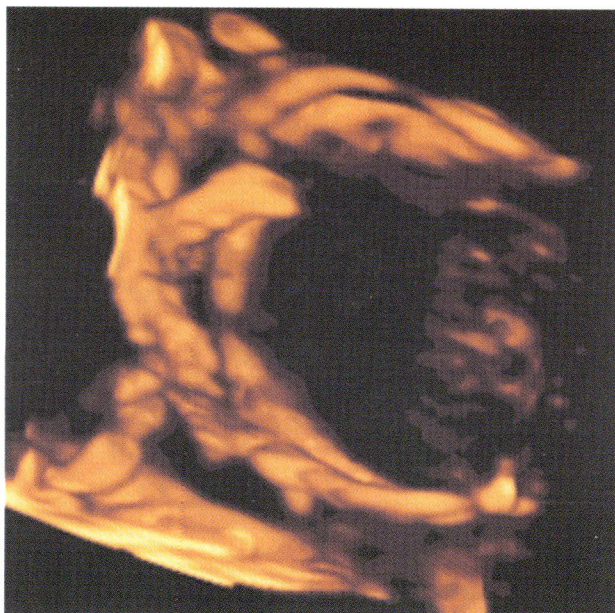

A

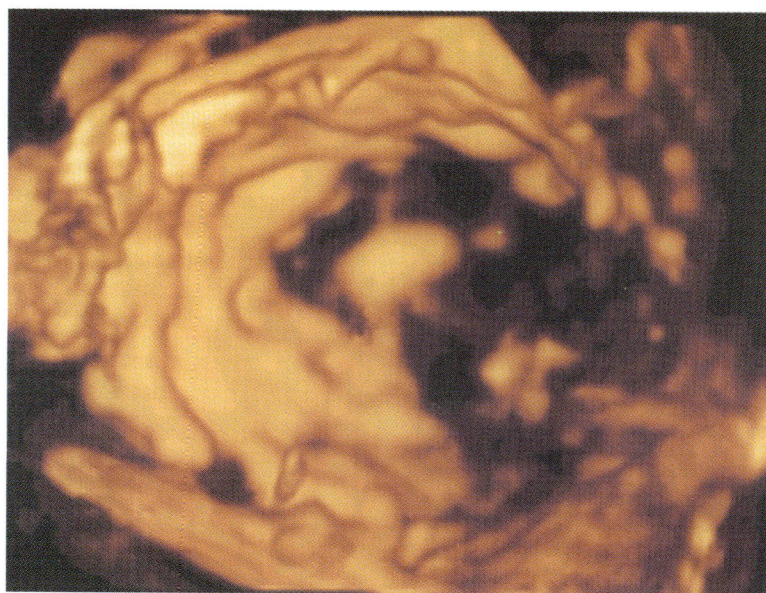

B

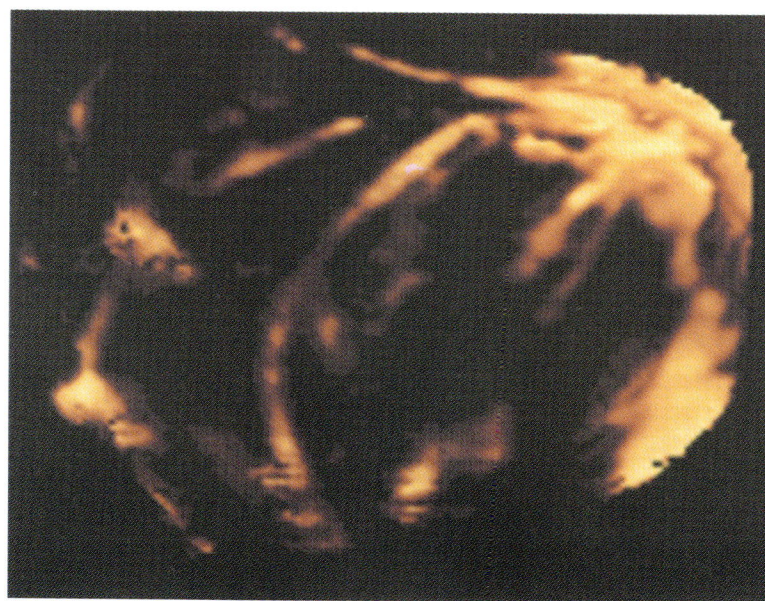

C

Figs 18.5A to C: 3D power Doppler rendering of the vascular network of a preovulatory follicle (A), corpus luteum (B) and luteinized unruptured follicle (LUF). Observe the poor vascularization in LUF as compared with the corpus luteum

patients with a high response to the gonadotropin treatment show lower endometrial and subendometrial 3D vascular indices[30] (Figs 18.8A and B).

According to our results,[20] intermediate 3D Doppler indices on the hCG administration day in IVF cycles are associated to a high pregnancy rate. On the contrary, when the vascularization index is inferior to 10th woman gets no pregnancy. When the blood flow is highly increased, the pregnancy rate decreases without significant difference (Table 18.4).

APPLICATIONS IN OBSTETRICS

Three-dimensional power Doppler can be used in Obstetrics for the study and assessment of the early pregnancy as well as in late gestation.

Table 18.4: Pregnancy rate according to subendometrial 3D power Doppler indices on the day of hCG administration in 40 IVF cycles

3D Power Doppler indices		No cases n (%)	Pregnancy rate n (%)
Vascularization index	<10	5 (12.5%)	0 (0%)
	10-35	18 (45%)	11 (61.1%)
	>35	17 (42.5%)	5 (29.4%)
Flow index	< 28	12 (30%)	1 (8.3%)
	28-34	20 (50%)	12 (60%)
	> 34	8 (20%)	3 (37.5%)
Vascularization flow index	< 6	10 (25%)	1 (10%)
	6-12	17 (42.5%)	10 (58.8%)
	> 12	13 (32.5%)	5 (38.5%)

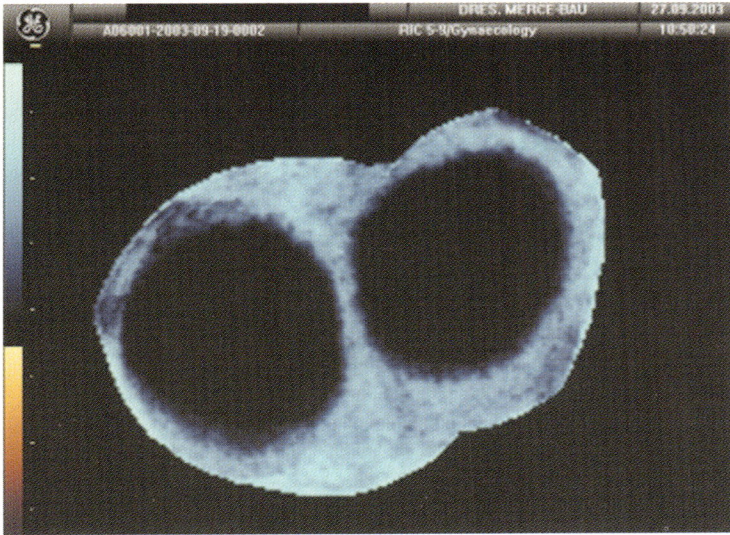

A

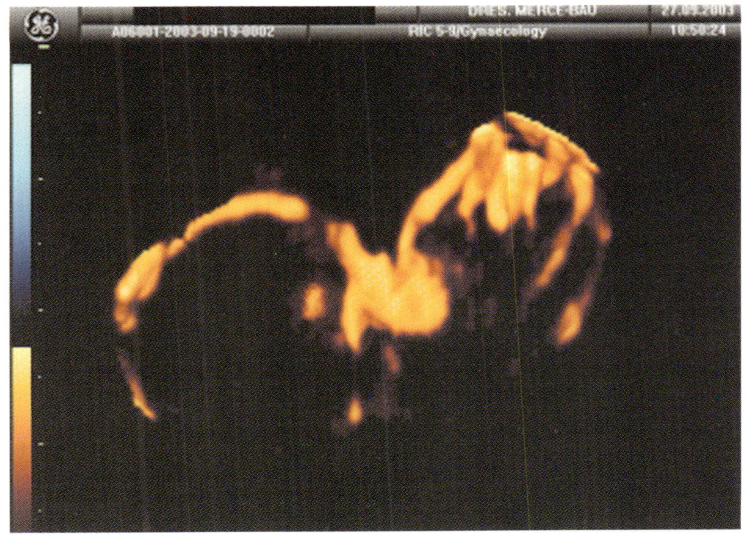

B

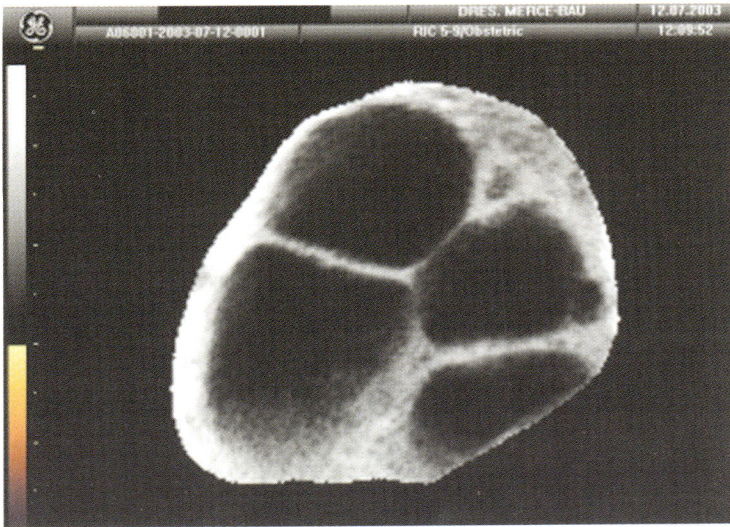

C

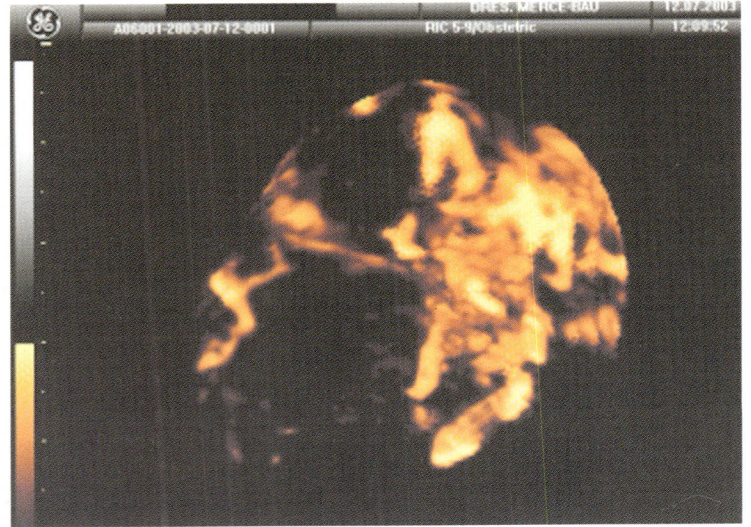

D

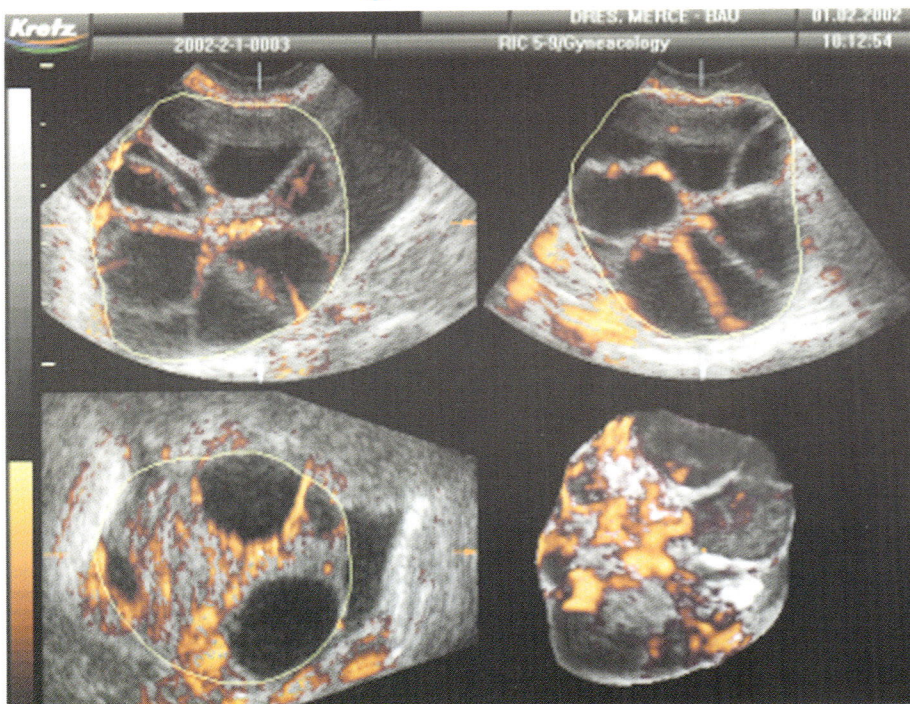

E

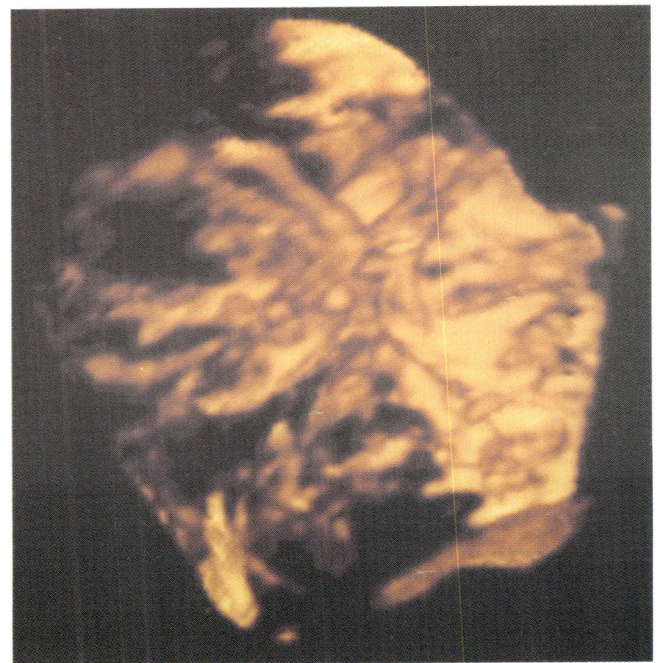

F

Figs 18.6A to F: Vascular network in different follicular growth after ovarian stimulation: (A and B) Bifollicular; (C and D) Polyfollicular; (E and F) Multifollicular

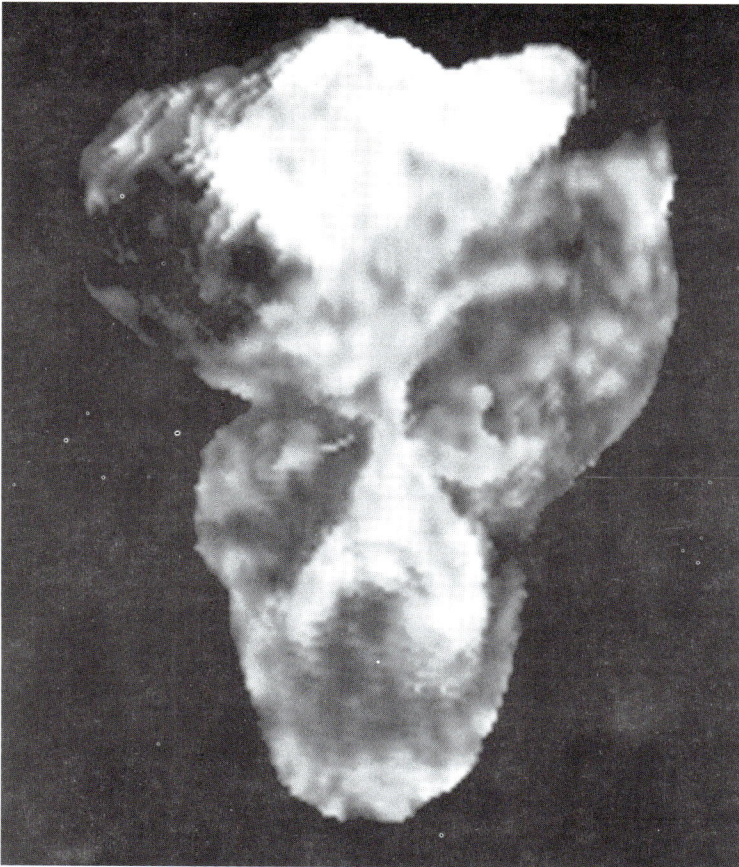

A

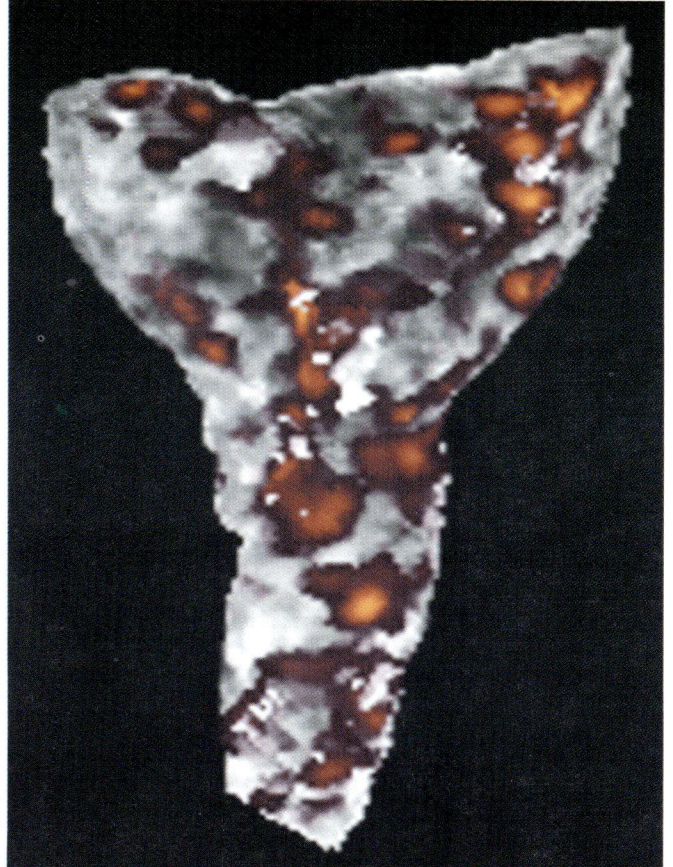

B

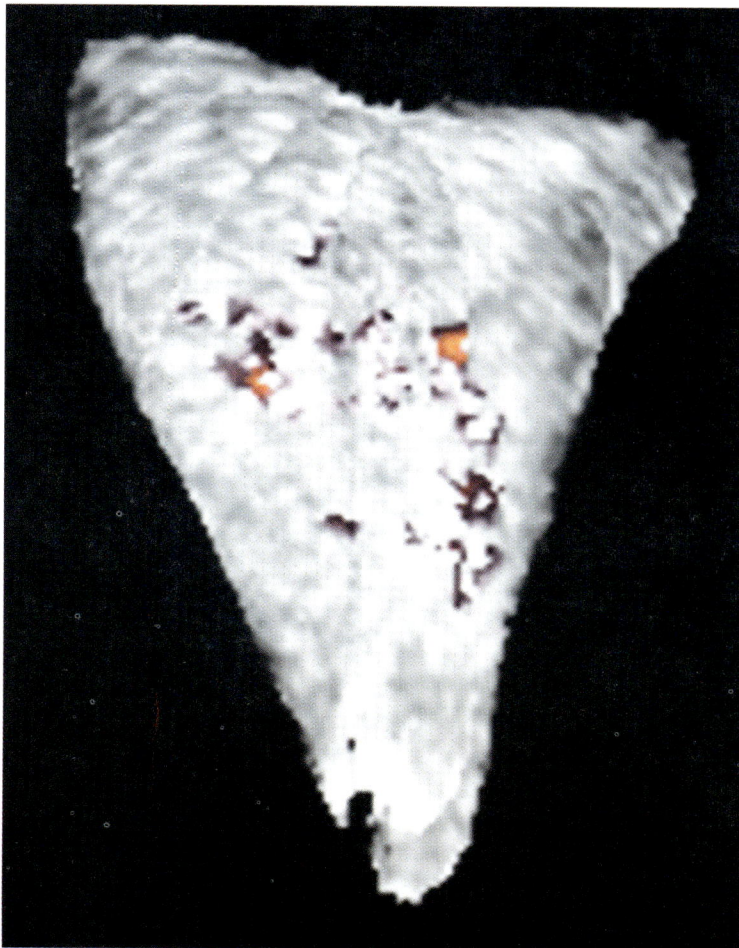

C

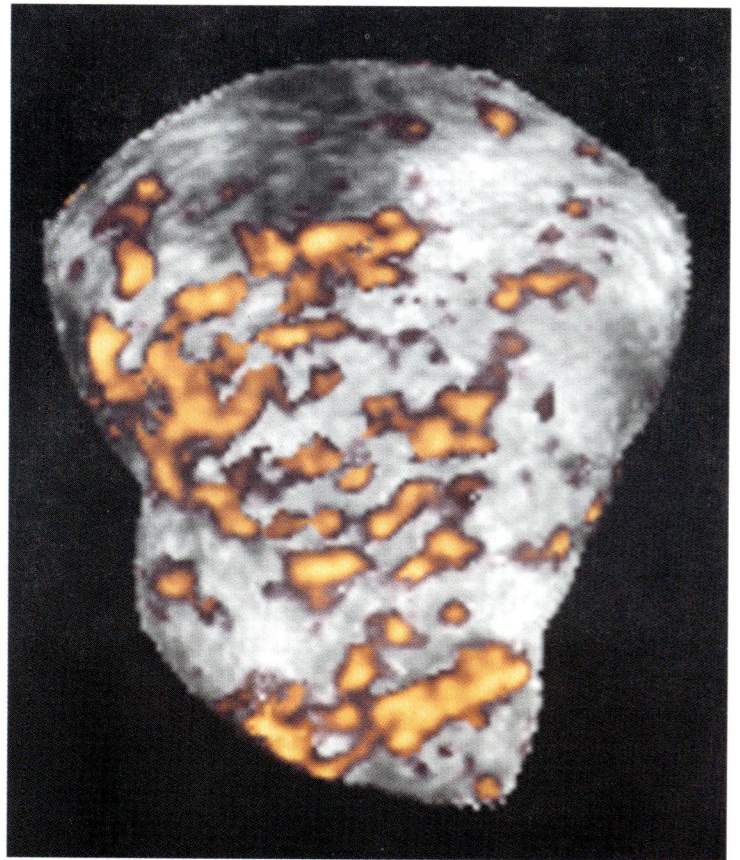

D

Figs 18.7A to D: Endometrial vascularity at different stages of an IVF cycle: A. After pituitary suppression; B. hCG administration day after gonadotropin ovarian stimulation; C. Seven days after oocyte retrieval; D. Fourteen days post-embryo transfer with positive pregnancy test

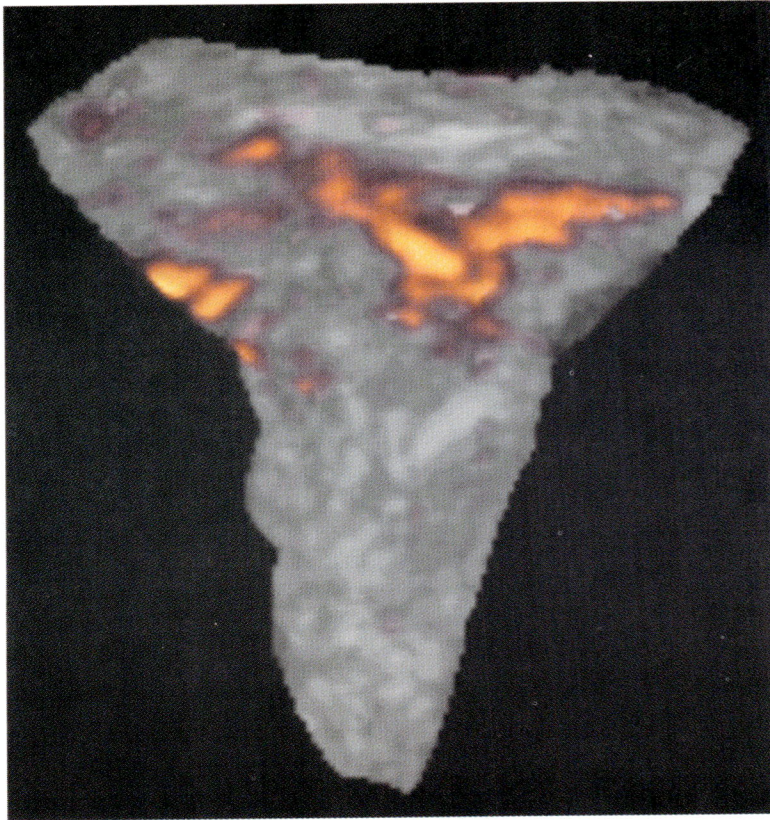

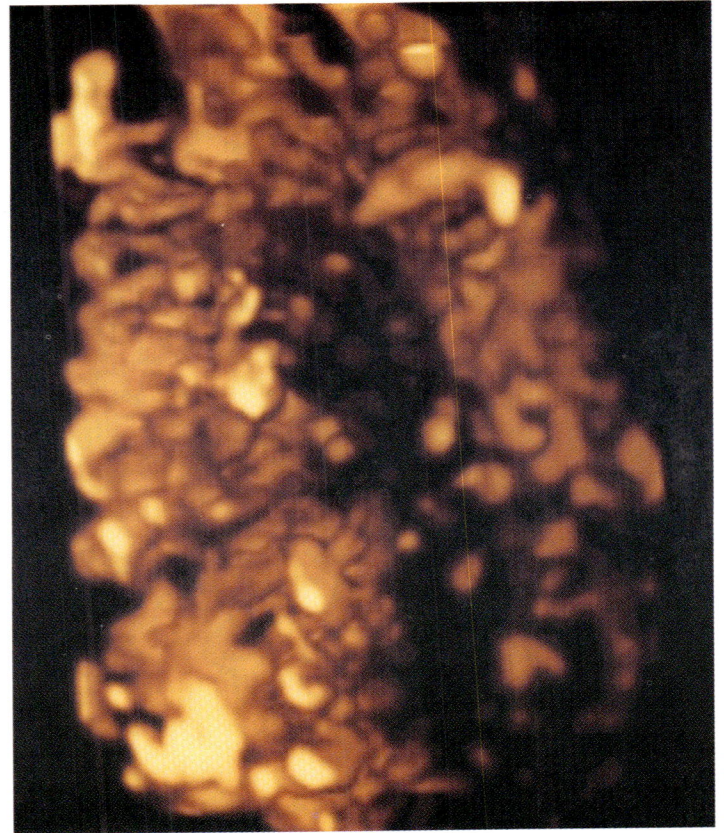

A
B

Figs 18.8A and B: Endometrial (A) and sub-endometrial (B) vascular network rendered by 3D power Doppler

Early Pregnancy

During early pregnancy, transvaginal 3D power Doppler angiography allows the assessment of placental and fetal circulations. The ovarian and uterine circulations can be depicted likewise. Theoretical risks of biological adverse effects of the Doppler ultrasonography during the early gestation must be minimal by applying this technology. 3D power Doppler angiography has a very short time of capture, observing the ALARA principles (As Low As Reasonably Available). Nevertheless, new technical reports are required to allow a more liberal use of 3D Doppler technology during the human first trimester of pregnancy.

Placental Circulation

Power Doppler angiography allows the representation of the whole uterine circulation with its several branches along gestation, although more precisely during the early pregnancy (Figs 18.9A and B).

Around the 4th to 5th weeks in normal gestations it is possible to observe how the spiral arteries approach the gestational sac drawing the picture of a comet— "comet sign" (Figs 18.10A and B). The invasion of radial and spiral arteries by cytotrophoblast is the mechanism to secure a progressive increase of the uteroplacental perfusion. These arteries lose its self-regulation ability and grow in diameter becoming the uteroplacental arteries.[31]

During the first gestational trimester the size of the placenta allows it to be fully included inside the examination field of the 3D transvaginal probe. From the 6th week onwards we can differentiate the uterochorionic circulation, essentially constituted by spiral and radial arteries, from the intrachorionic circulation or, in other words, the intervillous blood flow (Figs 18.11A and B).

Although the VOCAL software is able to assess independently the utero-chorionic and intervillous circulations, we have initially studied the intervillous circulation alone by excluding the retrochorionic one (Figs 18.12A to D). 3D Doppler indices increase gradual and significantly between the 6th and the 12th weeks in normal gestations. These findings confirm the previous results obtained by transvaginal color Doppler[32-34] demonstrating the appearance of intervillous blood flow from the 6th gestational week and no later, at the end of the first trimester as supported by other authors.[35,36] The progressive disappearance of the trophoblastic plugs from the spiral arteries during the first trimester produce an increase in the color Doppler signal from the chorion frondosum (vascularization index) and in its intensity (flow index) what it means an increase in the intervillous blood flow (Figs 18.13A to D).

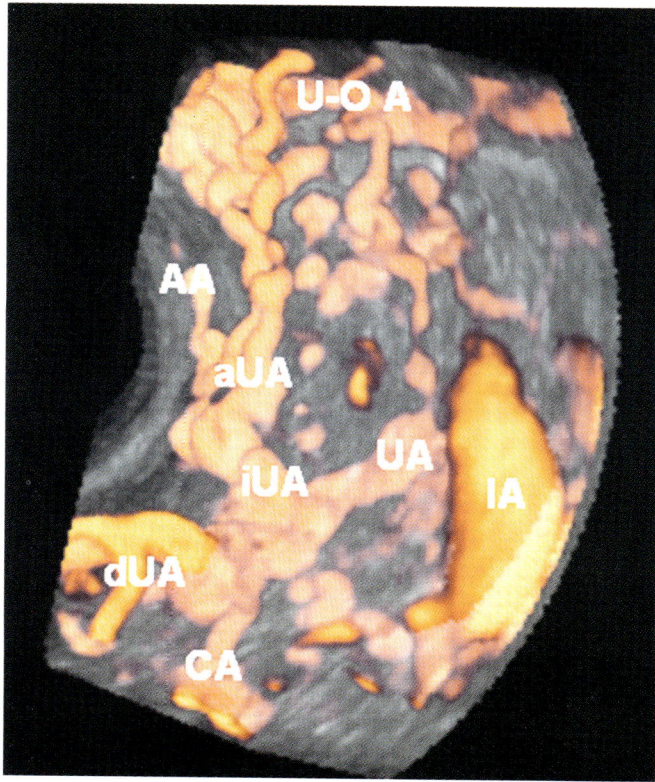

A

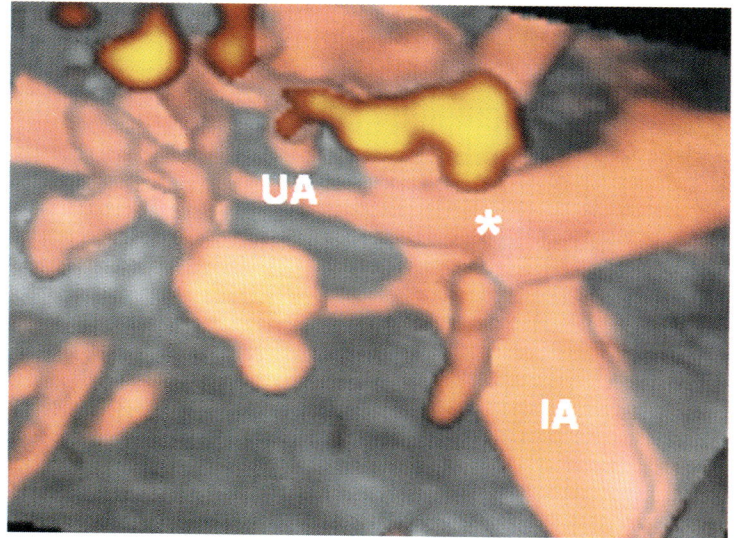

B

Figs 18.9A and B: Uterine circulation at 11 (A) and 20 (B) weeks of amenorrhea. 3D power Doppler angiography depicts the uterine artery and its main branches trajectory. IA: iliac artery; UA: uterine artery; aUA: ascendent branch of the uterine artery; iUA: isthmic part of the uterine artery; dUA: descendent branch of the uterine artery; CA: cervical artery; U-O A: utero-ovarian artery; * uterine and iliac junction at 20th week

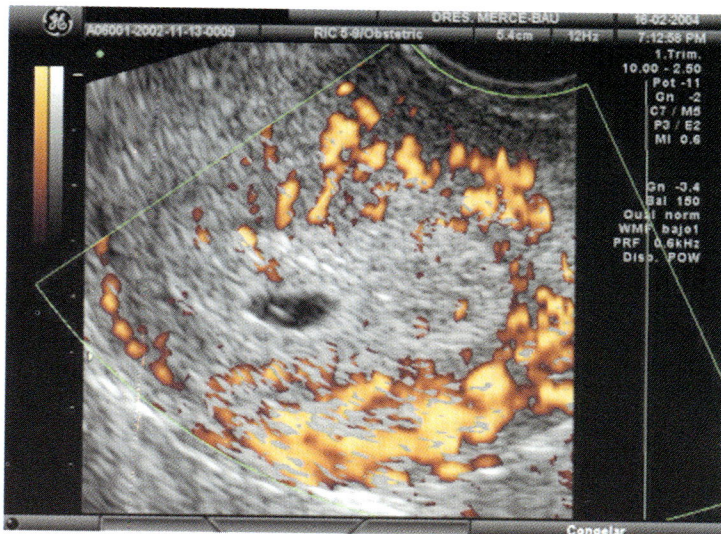

A

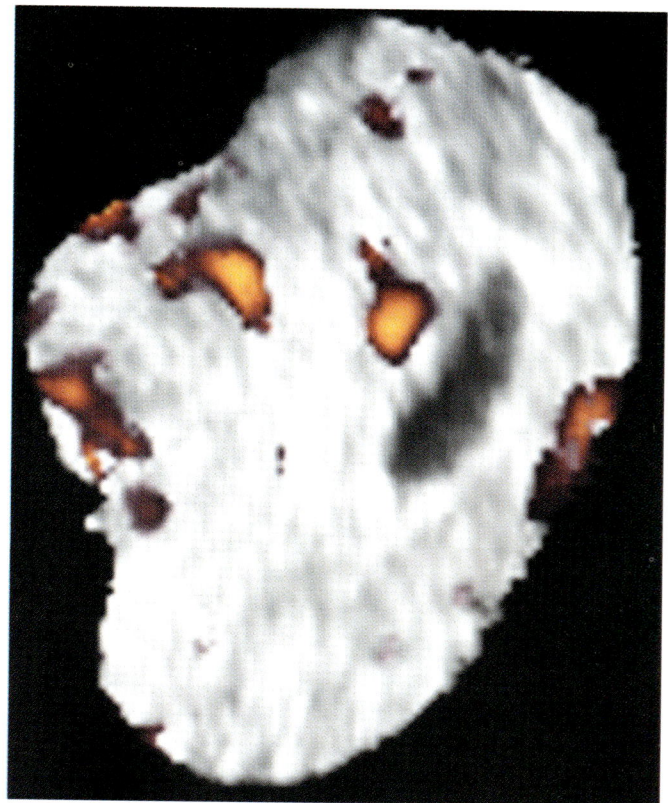

B

Figs 18.10A and B: "Comet" sign produced by early placentation with the transformation of the spiral arteries closer to the gestational sac into uteroplacental arteries. Conventional power Doppler (A) and power Doppler angiography (B) in a 4w + 4d pregnancy

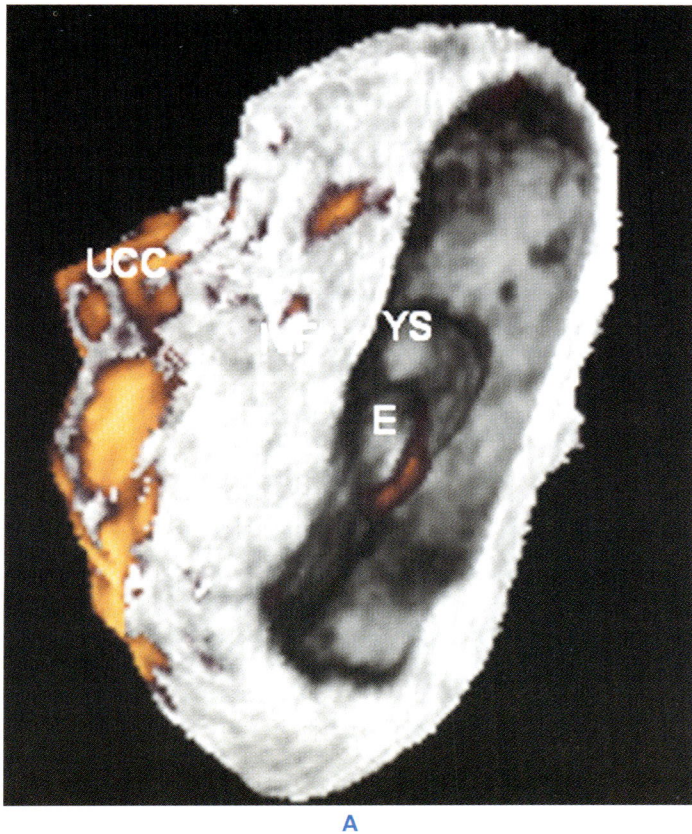

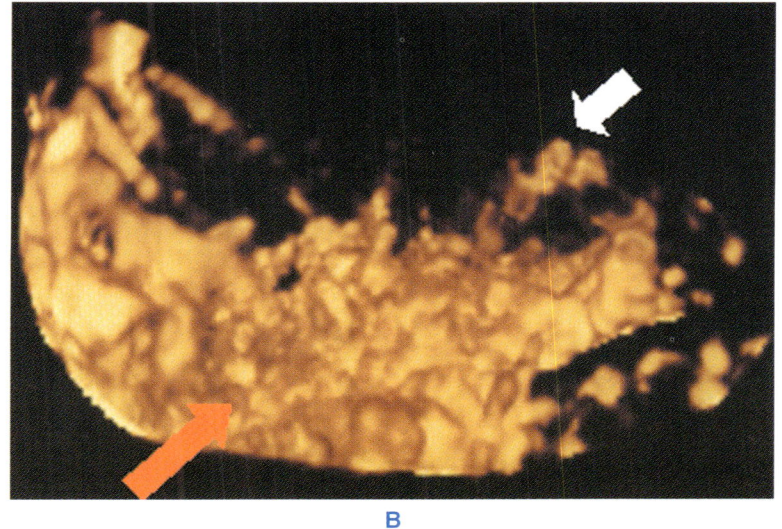

Figs 18.11A and B: A. Volumetric mode and power Doppler angiography of a normal 7 weeks pregnancy. E: living embryo; YS: yolk sac; IVF: intervillous flow; UCC: utero-chorionic circulation. B. Placental circulation at 12th week. Distinct uterochorionic (red arrow) and intervillous (white arrow) circulations can be appreciated

In cases of miscarriage an increase as well as a decrease in the uterochorionic circulation has been reported depending on the natural evolution of the process[37] (Figs 18.14A and B). The intervillous flow is usually increased pointing also to a failure in early placentation.[38] Recently, we have observed that the flow index is greater in those early pregnancies ending in miscarriage than in normal ongoing pregnancies[39] (Fig. 18.15). This fact supports our previous findings demonstrating an increased intervillous velocity in the spontaneous abortion.[37]

Embryonic and Fetal Circulations

Power Doppler angiography is able to depict the circulations in the embryo and the fetus.[40]

At the 6th and 7th weeks we can only see the cardiac signal (see Fig. 18.11A) but progressively the fetoplacental and fetal circulations are rendered by 3D power Doppler. Figure 18.16 shows all the existing circulations in a normal pregnancy at the 8th week. In that moment, it is possible the differentiation between the vessels in the uteroplacental circulation from the uterine nonplacental vessels. The intervillous blood flow, the fetoplacental circulation and the heart can also be observed.

At 10 weeks the development of the embryo/fetal circulation is completed. By means of power Doppler angiography the cerebral vessels and the ductus venosus can be detected (Fig.

18.17). At the end of the first trimester the majority of fetal vessels are visualized, as shown in Figure 18.18.

Luteal Circulation

3D power Doppler allows the assessment of the ovarian circulation during the first gestational trimester too. Conventional color Doppler studies report contradictory results about the luteal blood flow changes during the abnormal early pregnancy.[39] Once more, power Doppler angiography provides a new opportunity to study the luteal circulation in miscarriage and evaluate its diagnostic potential (Figs 18.19A to C).

According to our experience, 3D power Doppler can help to the diagnosis of ectopic pregnancies. Using color and pulsed Doppler sometimes we mix up the luteal and chorionic circulations from an ectopic pregnancy. Three-dimensional representation of the vascular networks of the ectopic gestational sac and the corpus luteum allow the differentiation of both circulations and a more precise diagnosis in these cases (Fig. 18.20).

Late Gestation

During the second and third gestational trimesters all the placental and fetal vessels can beneficiate from 3D power Doppler angiography examination.

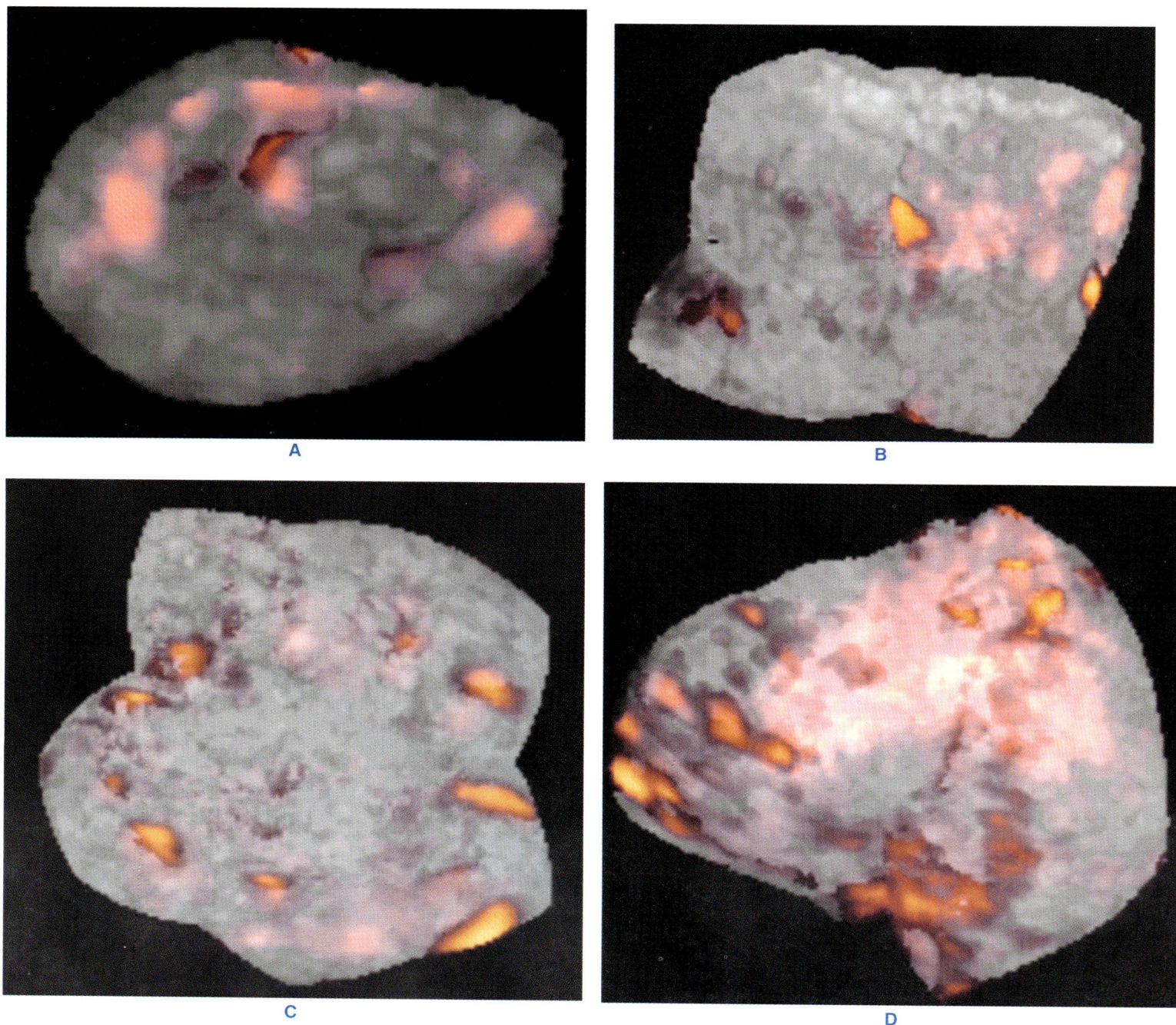

Figs 18.12A to D: Chorion frondosum and intervillous circulation by power Doppler angiography in transparent mode. A. 7 weeks; B. 9 weeks; C. 10 weeks; D. 11 weeks. The progressive increase of intervillous blood flow is clearly depicted

Placental Circulation

In 1998 3D power Doppler image was proposed as a means to individualize placental vessels from the fetal circulation as well as from maternal circulation[41] (Fig. 18.21). Some years later, this method was proven to be superior to bidimensional power Doppler to detect the terminal vascular branches of the fetal circulation in the placental tree.[42] Recently it has been demonstrated that 3D power Doppler angiography can evaluate the normal placental development, investigate the placental anomalies in realtime and has become a new diagnostic method of surveillance and care during gestation.[43]

From the first trimester onward the scanning field of the three-dimensional probe is not able to include the whole placental volume. To overcome this problem we developed the "placental biopsy" method.[44,45] In summary, the aim is the acquisition of a representative sample from the placental vascular tree by application of the VOCAL program and the calculation of the vascular power Doppler indices. The placental sample is usually taken from its central part where the villous vascularization shows the greatest density. Maternal and fetal movements should be avoided during the procedure. Through the multiplanar system, the placental zone with the best color map from the region of interest stored is selected off-line. Finally, in the plane A as working image we set the limits of a virtual reference axis between the basal and chorionic plates (both of them excluded) and the volume of a sphere is automatically obtained by rotation

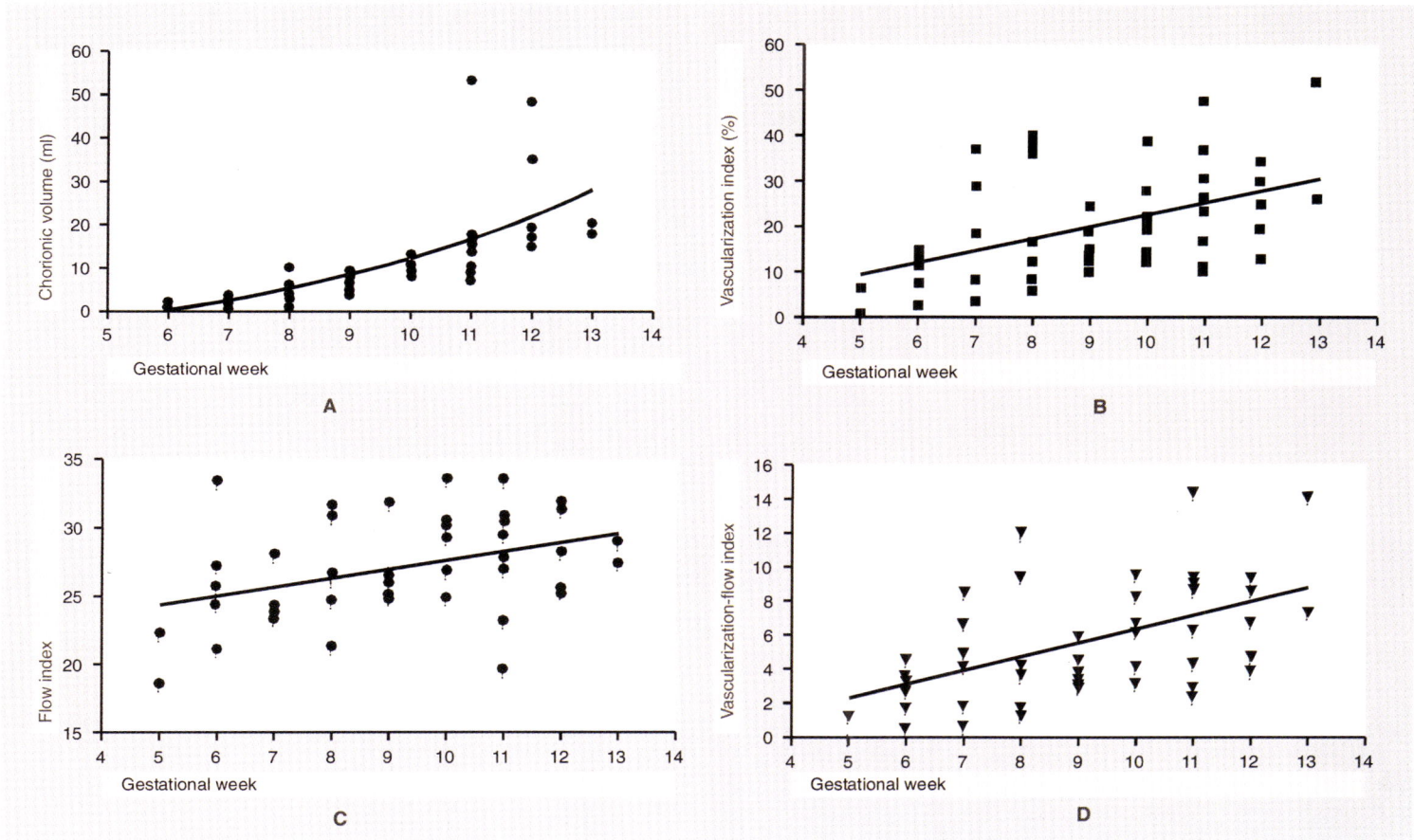

Figs 18.13A to D: Chorionic volume and intervillous blood flow throughout the early normal pregnancy from 46 normal pregnancies: A. Chorionic volume; B. Vascularization index; C. Flow index and D. Vascularization flow index

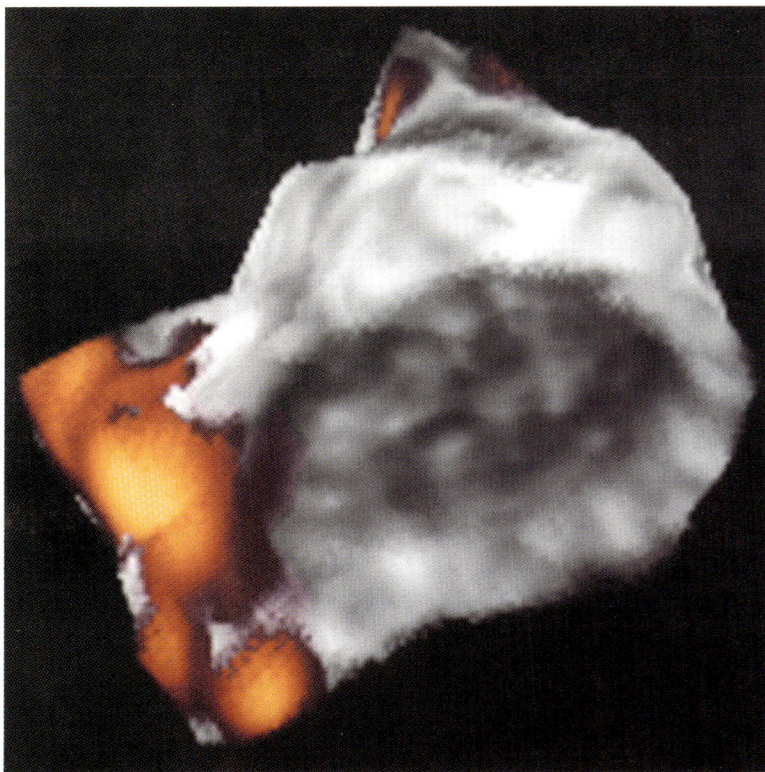

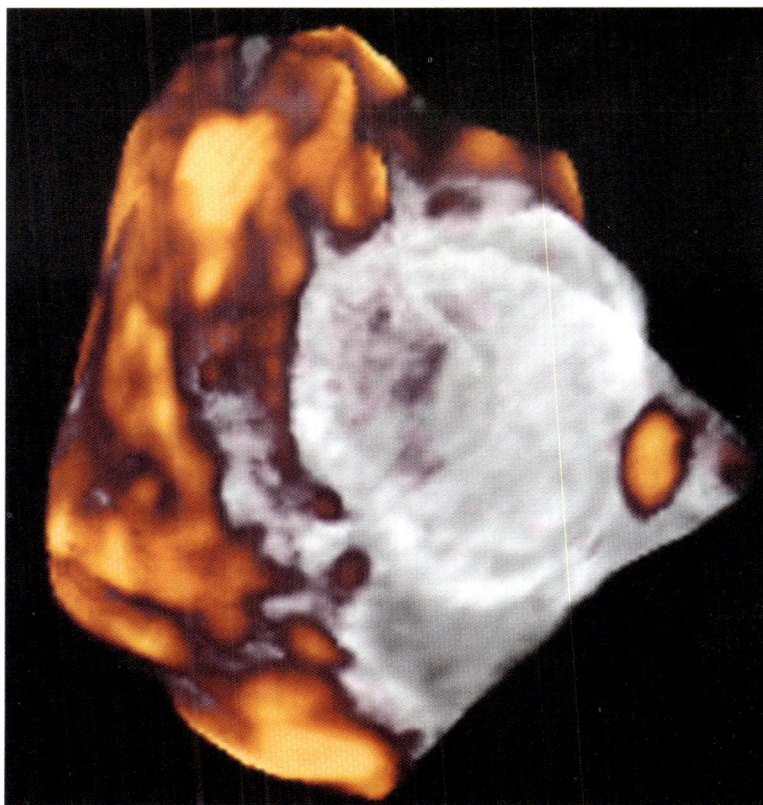

Figs 18.14A and B: Uterochorionic circulation in two 7 weeks miscarriages. Observe the decrease (A) or increase of the utero-chorionic flow as compared with a normal pregnancy of the same gestational age in Figure 18.11A

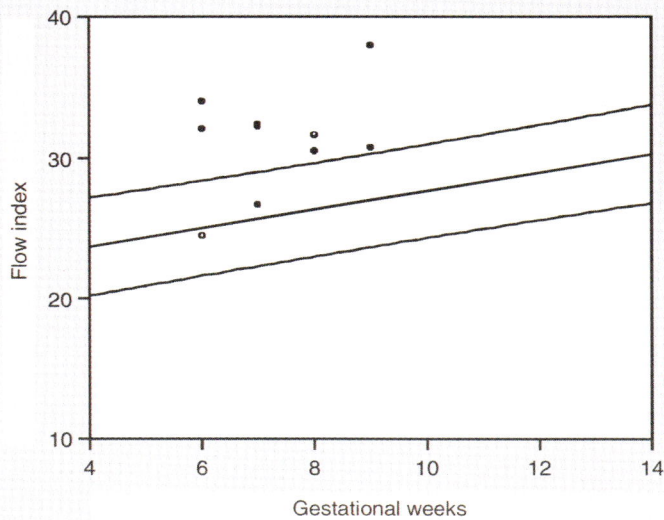

Fig. 18.15: Flow index from the intervillous flow in miscarriage. It is increased comparatively with the reference values in normal gestations

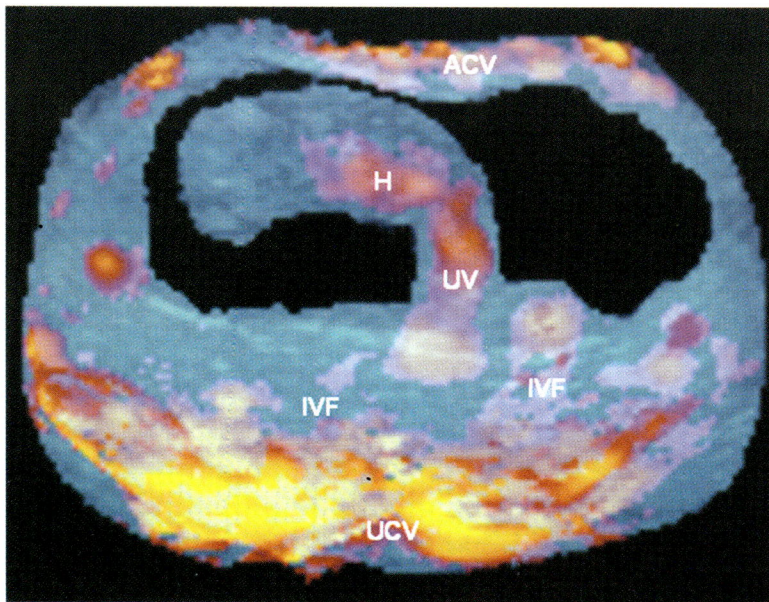

Fig. 18.16: Placental and fetal circulations in a normal 8 weeks pregnancy. UCV: uterochorionic vessels; IVF: intervillous flow; ACV: anti-chorionic vessels; UV: umbilical vessels; H: heart

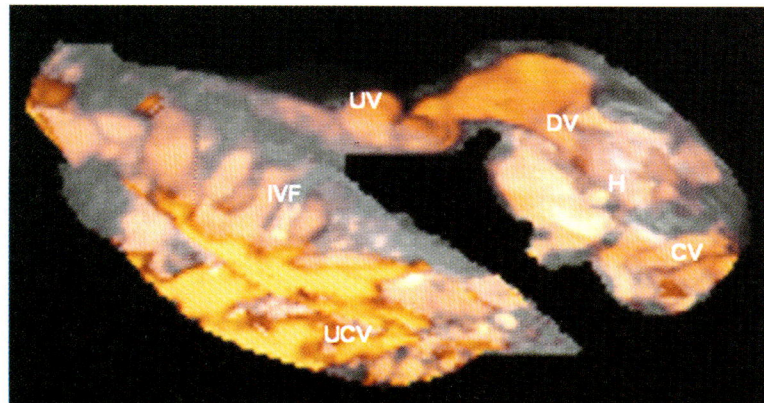

Fig. 18.17: Placental and fetal circulations in a normal 10 weeks pregnancy. UCV: utero-chorionic vessels; IVF: intervillous flow; UV: umbilical vessels; DV: ductus venosus; H: heart; CV: cerebral vessels

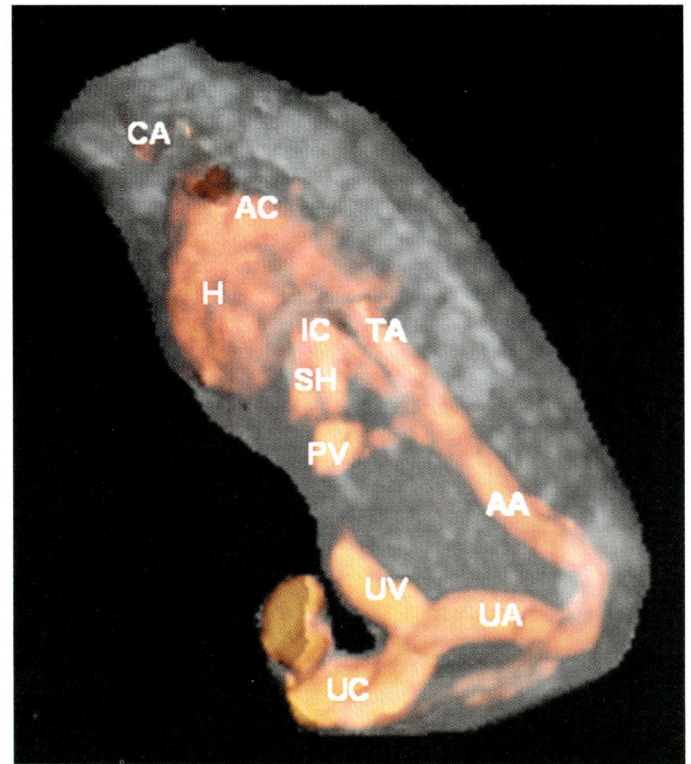

Fig. 18.18: Fetal circulation at 15th week of amenorrhea. UC: umbilical cord; UV: umbilical vein; UA: umbilical artery; PV: portal vein; SH: suprahepatic veins; IC: inferior vena cava; AA: abdominal aorta; TA: thoracic aorta; H: heart; AC: aortic arch; CA: carotid artery

to make the calculations of volume and Doppler indices (Fig. 18.22).

The "placental biopsy" method has a good reproducibility and intraobserver agreement for the 3D Doppler indices. The intraclass correlation coefficient is greater than 0.85 for all the indices studied[44,45] (Table 18.5).

The placental vascular tree shows a progressive growth during normal gestations. Up to weeks 20 the vessels from the chorionic and basal plates are usually depicted being exceptional the visualization of the vascular branches of the fetal villous tree (Figs 18.23A and B). From 20 up to 30th to 32nd week takes place the first and second order vascular villous branches development (Figs 18.23C and D). During the third trimester the vascular villous tree is fully developed and the 3rd order villous vessels can be rendered with a growing thickness and density of their branches[43,44] (Figs 18.23E and F). This pattern of vascular development is very similar to that described in the classical histological studies and even by electronic microscopy.[46]

The placental blood flow assessed by the "placental biopsy" method through the 3D Doppler indices is significantly related to gestational age (Fig. 18.24A). The Flow Index shows a linear and significant increase from 14 to 40 weeks ($r= 0.58$, $p<0.01$) (Fig. 18.24C). On the contrary, the vascularization ($r= 0.29$, $p<0.05$) and vascularization flow Indices ($r= 0.32$, $p<0.01$) show a curve flattening from 30 weeks and a decrease at term

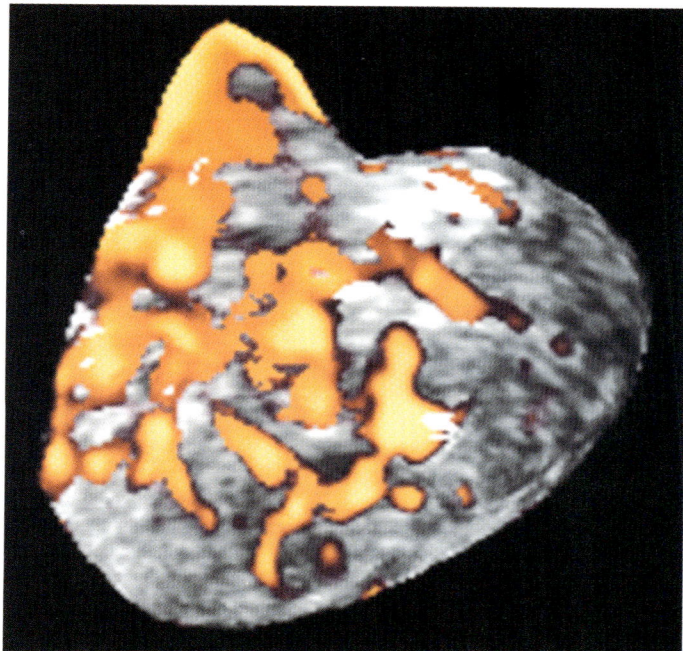

A

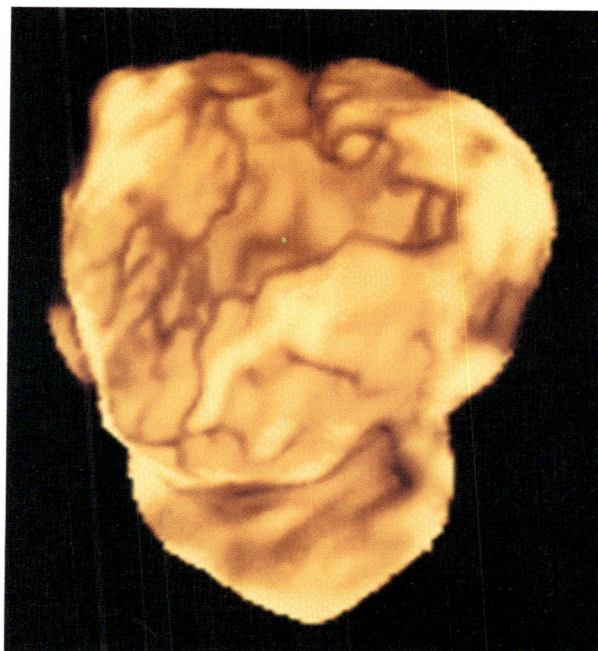

B

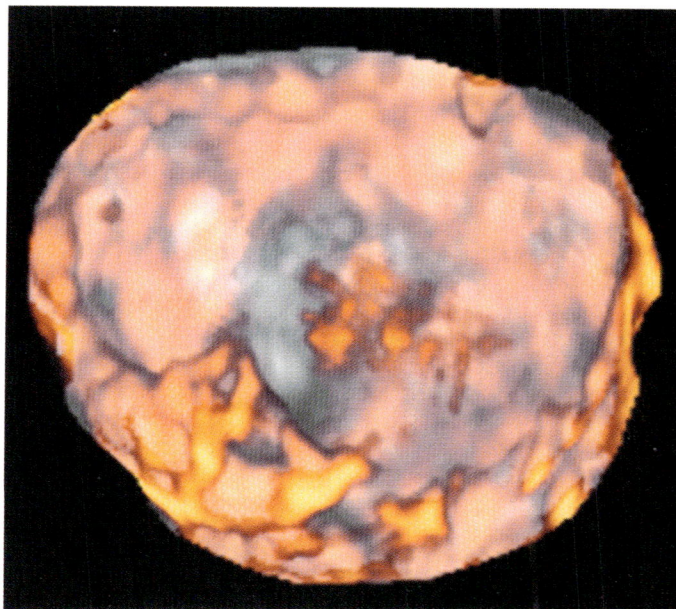

C

Figs 18.19A to C: Vascular network from several corpora lutea during early pregnancy with different 3D power Doppler rendering. A. Hypoechogenic corpus luteum; B. Corpus luteum in "layers"; C. Hyperechogenic corpus luteum

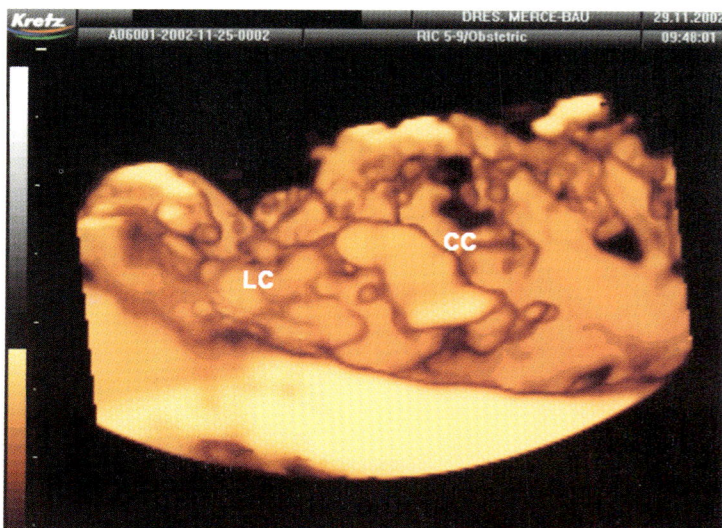

Fig. 18.20: Placental and corpus luteum vascular network in an ectopic pregnancy producing a "nest" image. LC: luteal circulation; CC: chorionic circulation

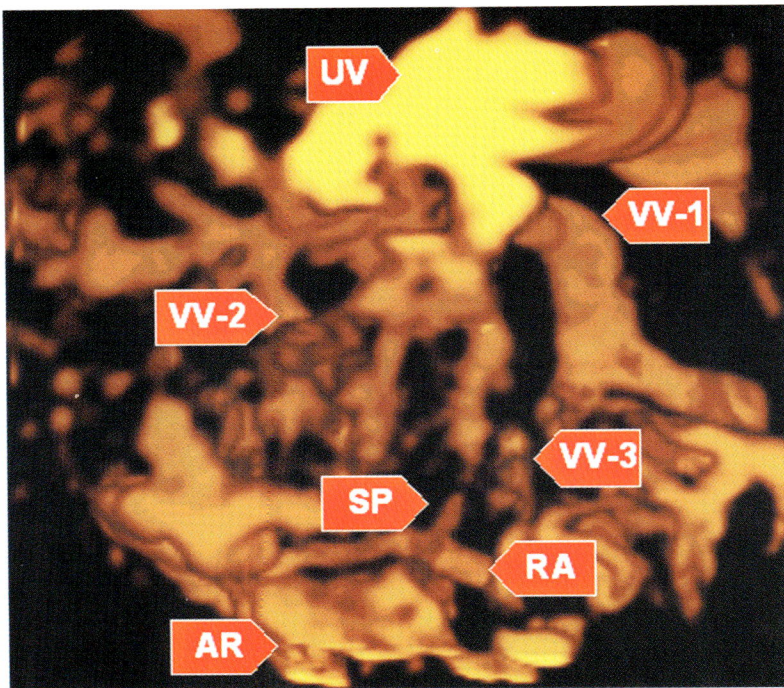

Fig. 18.21: 3D power Doppler angiography of the placental circulation during the normal third trimester pregnancy. UV: umbilical vessels; VV-1: 1st order villous vascular branch; VV-2: 2nd order villous vascular branch; VV-3: 3rd order villous vascular branch; SP: spiral vessels; RA: radial vessels; AR: arcuate vessels

indices with gestational age although there is no explanation from where the placental sample is obtained. 3D placental Doppler indices are positively related with fetal biometry and umbilical artery Doppler velocimetry, specially the flow index (Table 18.6).

The study of the placental circulation by 3D power Doppler has a great interest mainly for two reasons. An abnormal and deficient development of the placental vascular tree is closely associated to the fetal growth restriction.[48] Moreover, the decrease in the intraplacental blood flow may precede the umbilical resistance increase.[49] The blood flow through the intraplacental vascular tree could be affected in some cases with normal umbilical Doppler.[46] In fact, the intraplacental vascular resistance obtained by multigate spectral Doppler is more sensitive and its alteration precedes the umbilical Doppler changes to detect the fetal growth restriction.[49] It has been also proven that the number of villous arteries is significantly diminished in growth retarded gestations[46] (Figs 18.25A and B).

Finally, this technique should have an essential role in the assessment and prediction of the outcome of placental vascular tumors like chorioangiomas.[50]

Umbilical Circulation

3D power Doppler angiography can depict the whole umbilical cord from the placental to the fetal insertion. It is hampered by

gestation (Figs 18.24B and D). These results are slightly different from that of Yu et al.[47] These authors confirmed the progressive increase of the vascularization, flow and vascularization flow

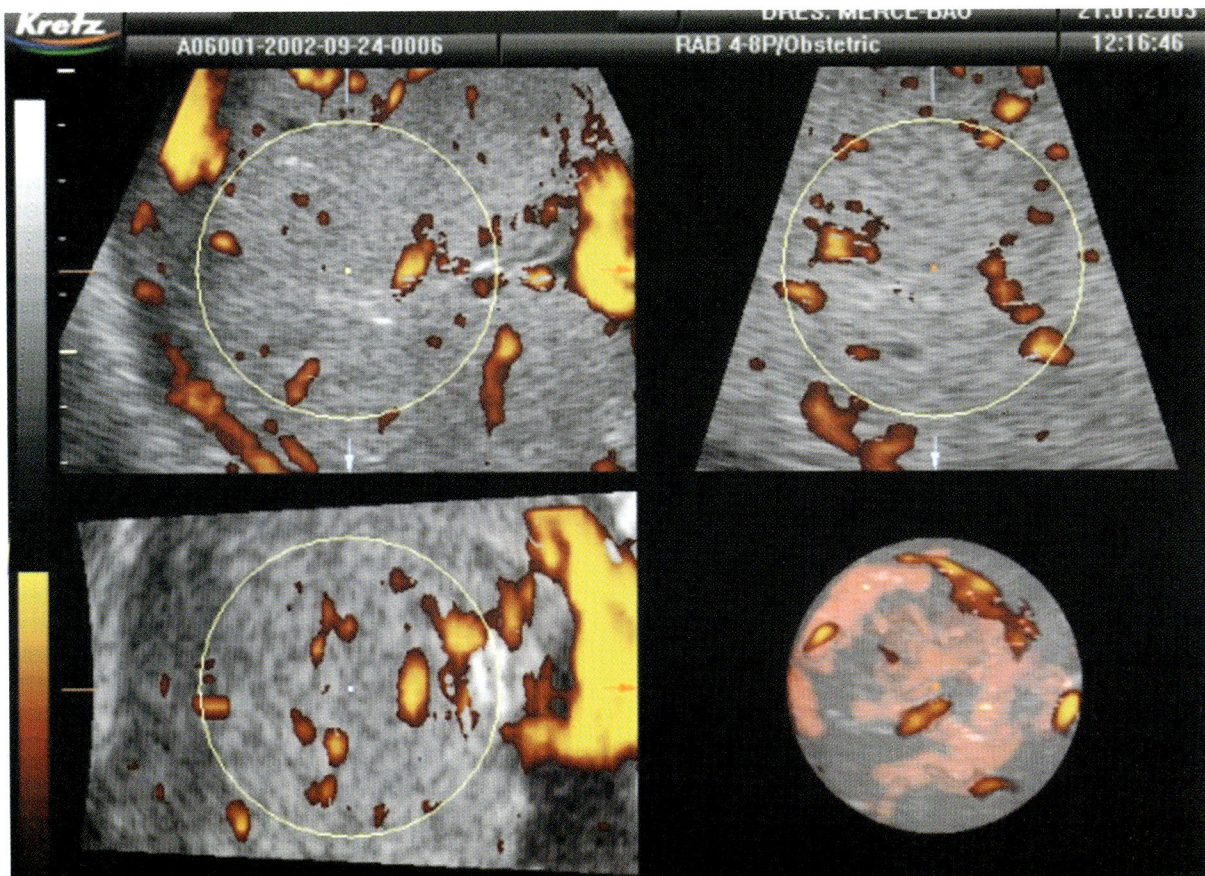

Fig. 18.22: Placental biopsy technique by 3D power Doppler. A sphere of placental tissue between the chorionic and basal plate is obtained

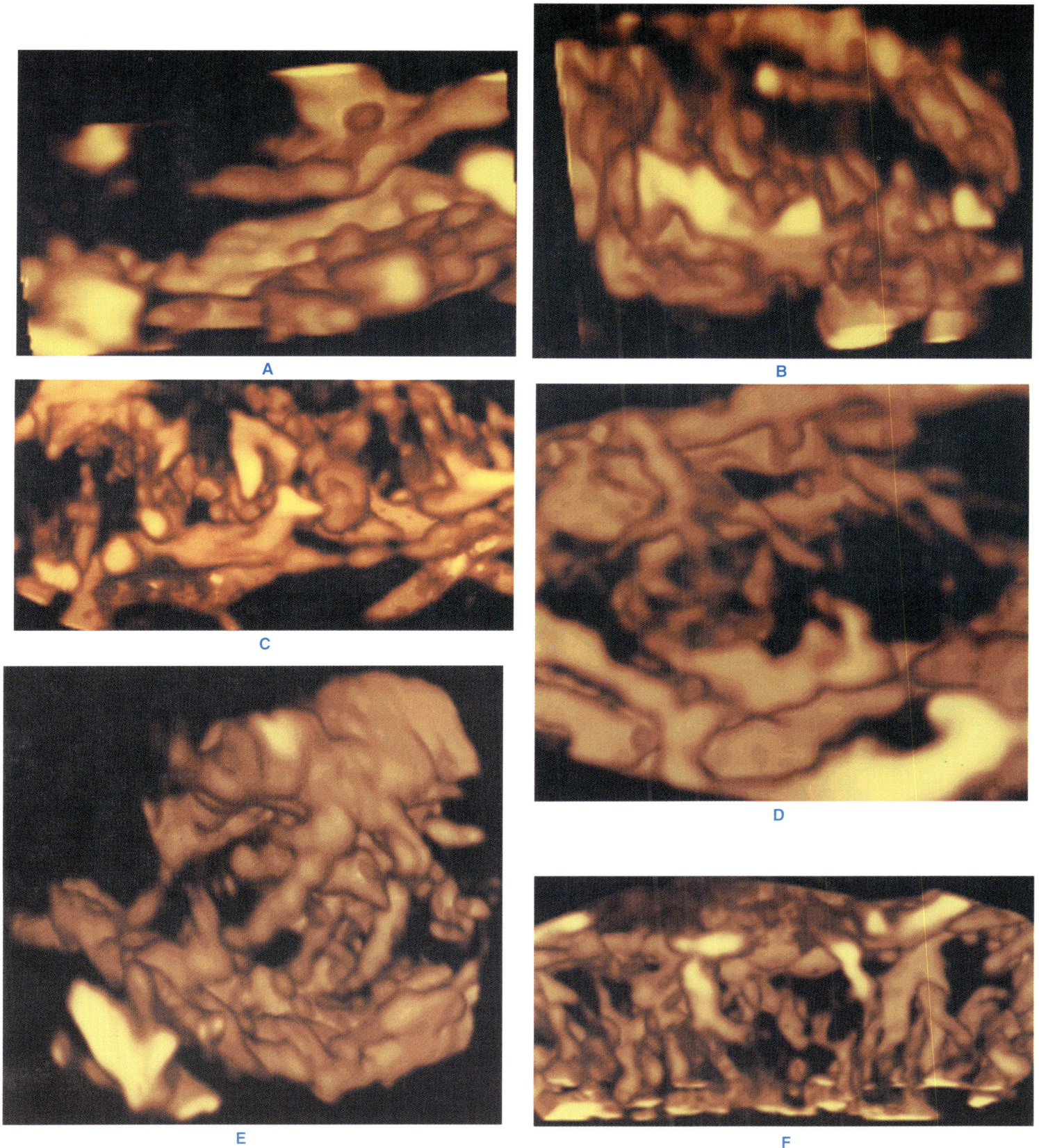

Figs 18.23A to F: Power Doppler angiography of the placental vascular tree throughout the normal gestation. A. 16th week; B. 20th week; C. 26th week; D. 32nd week; E. 36th week; F. 40th week

the same problems than conventional color Doppler, basically the cord location and its trajectory, usually hidden by the fetus.

It has been suggested that this technique provides more information than conventional ultrasound and color Doppler to detect the nuchal cord[51] (Figs 18.26A to C). Some authors give

it a small worth in the assessment of cord insertion[52] but it may help to diagnose some anomalies of insertion as vasa previa.[53]

Other anomalies of the umbilical vessels as the single umbilical artery (Figs 18.27A to C) can be visualized as well, although it does not seem to provide more information than conventional power Doppler.

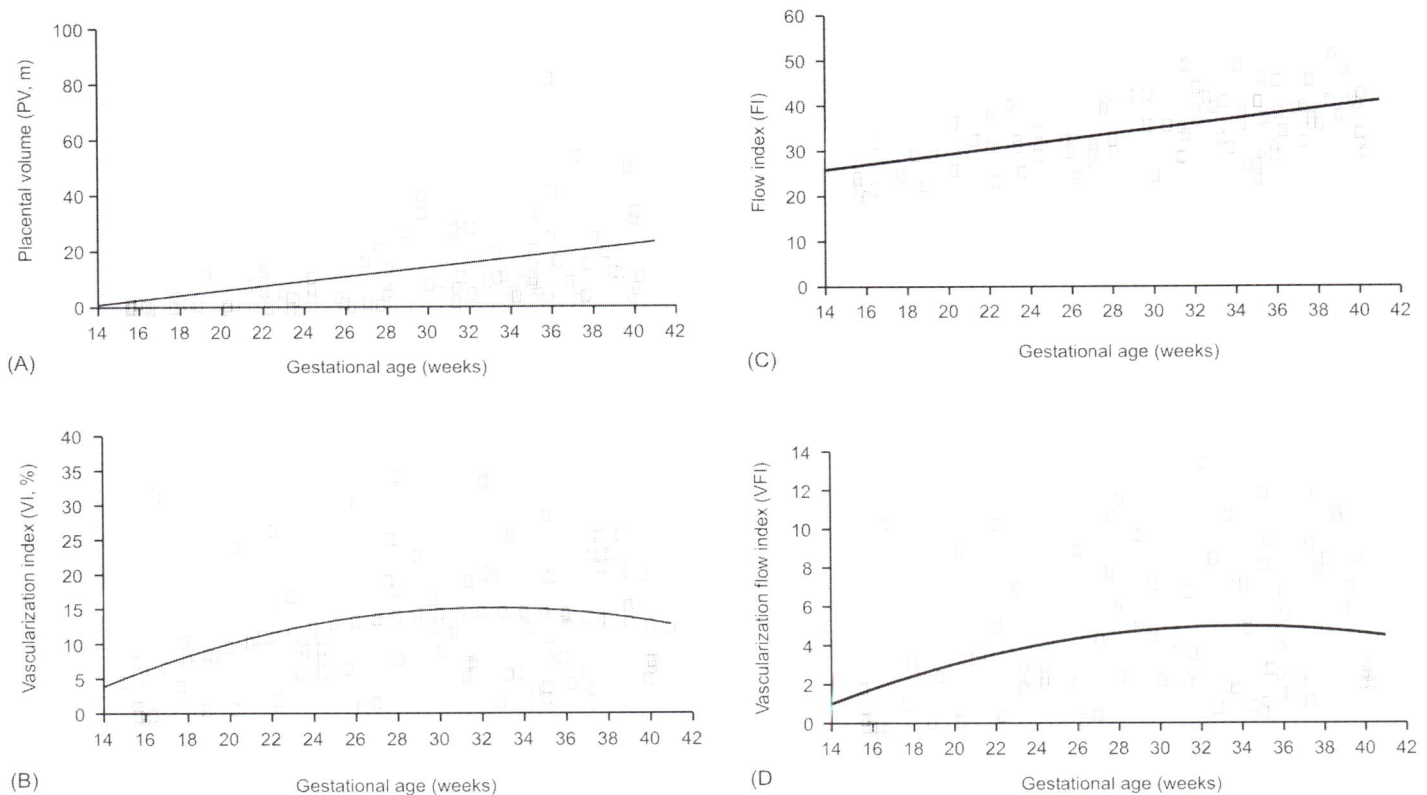

Figs 18.24A to D: Placental volume from "placental biopsy" and placental blood flow throughout the early normal pregnancy from 86 normal pregnancies: A. Chorionic volume; B. Vascularization index; C. Flow index and D. Vascularization flow index

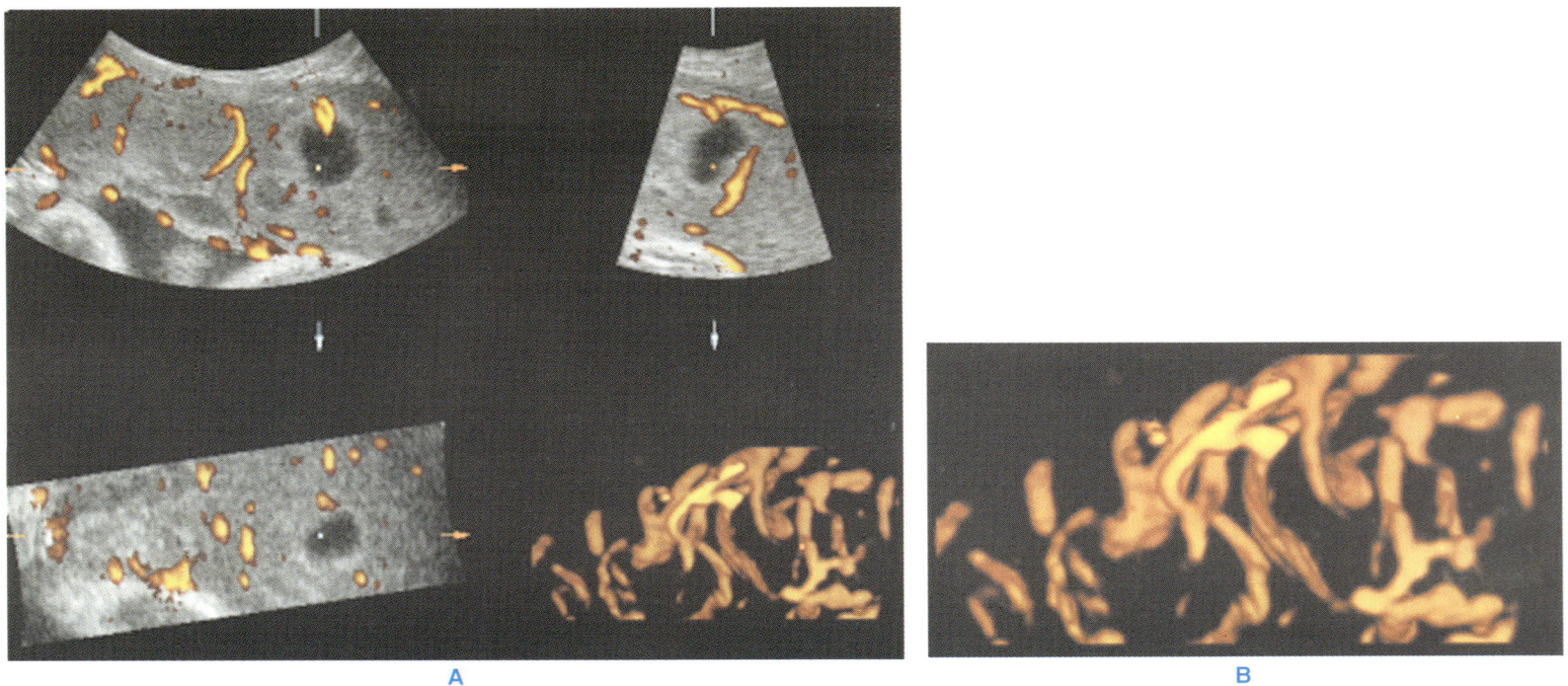

Figs 18.25A and B: Villous vascular tree in a growth restricted fetus confirmed after birth and normal umbilical artery Doppler. A. Multiplanar mode. Maternal blood can be seen entering the intervillous space. B. 3D power Doppler angiography. No 2nd and 3rd order villous vascular branches can be observed

Fetal Circulation

Every fetal vascular territory can be rendered by 3D power Doppler angiography but we will refer only to those focusing the attention of the investigators up to date.

From very early this technique was suggested as a very promising to the evaluation of cerebral circulation and its vascular malformations.[54] Pooh et al[55] point out that the multiplanar analysis and the potential to rotate the cerebral

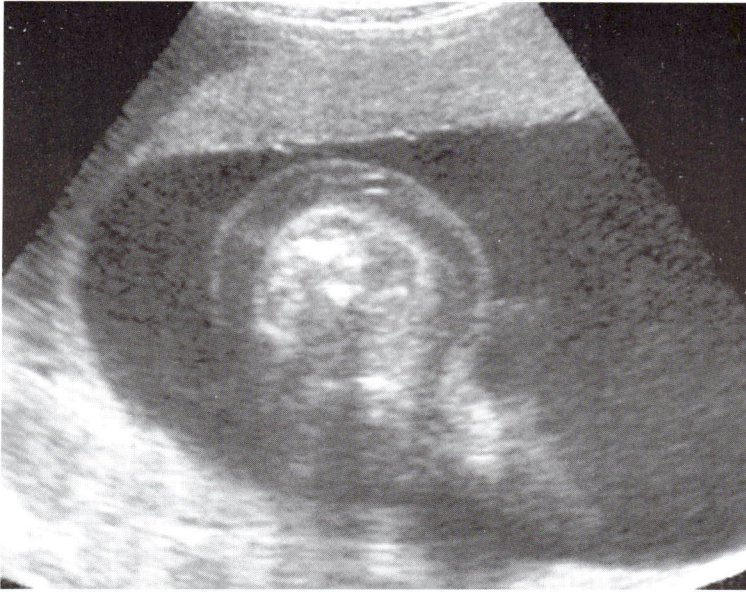

A

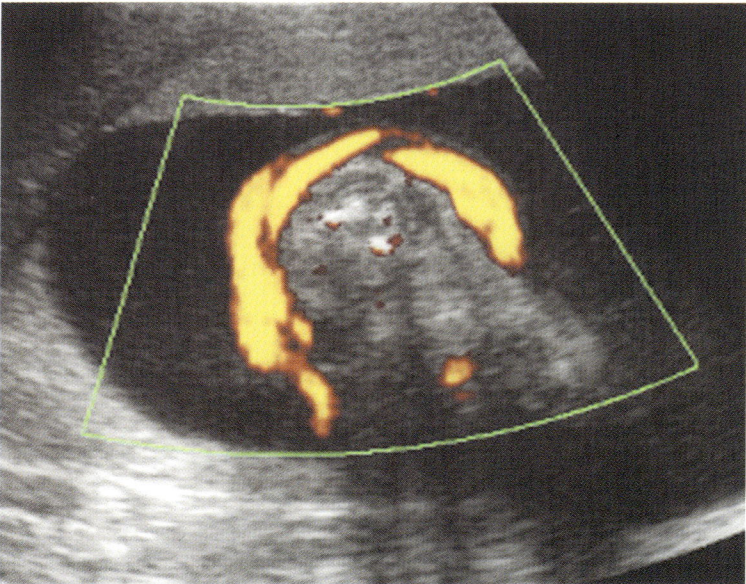

B

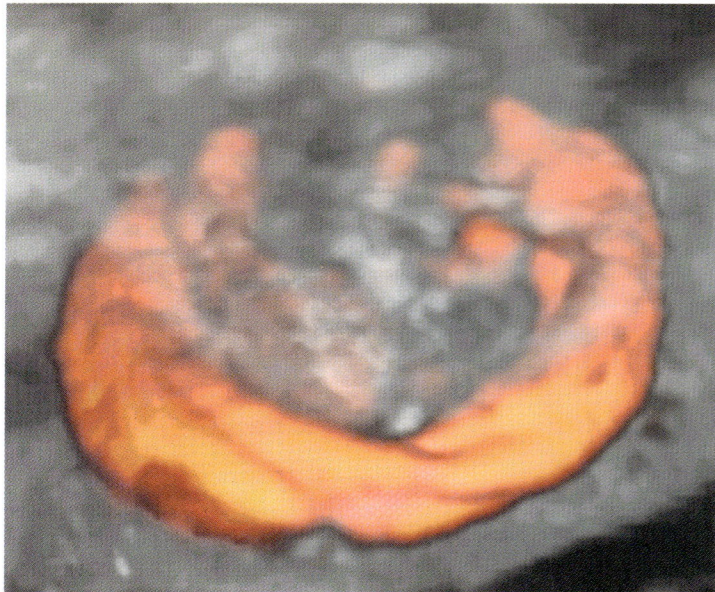

C

Figs 18.26A to C: Nuchal cord. A. Bi-dimensional ultrasonography;
B. Power Doppler; C. Three-dimensional power Doppler angiography

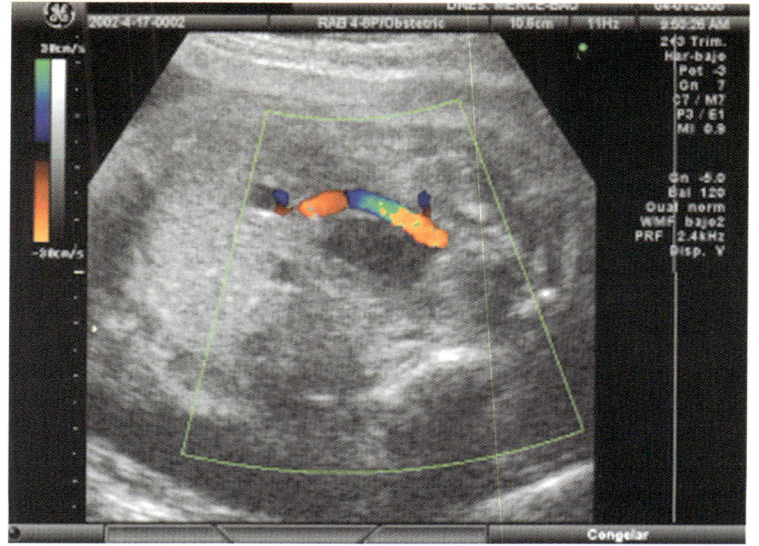

A

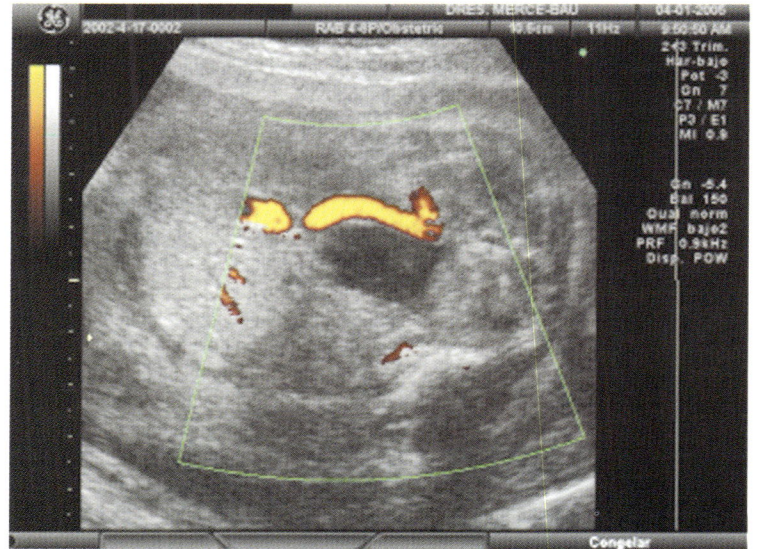

B

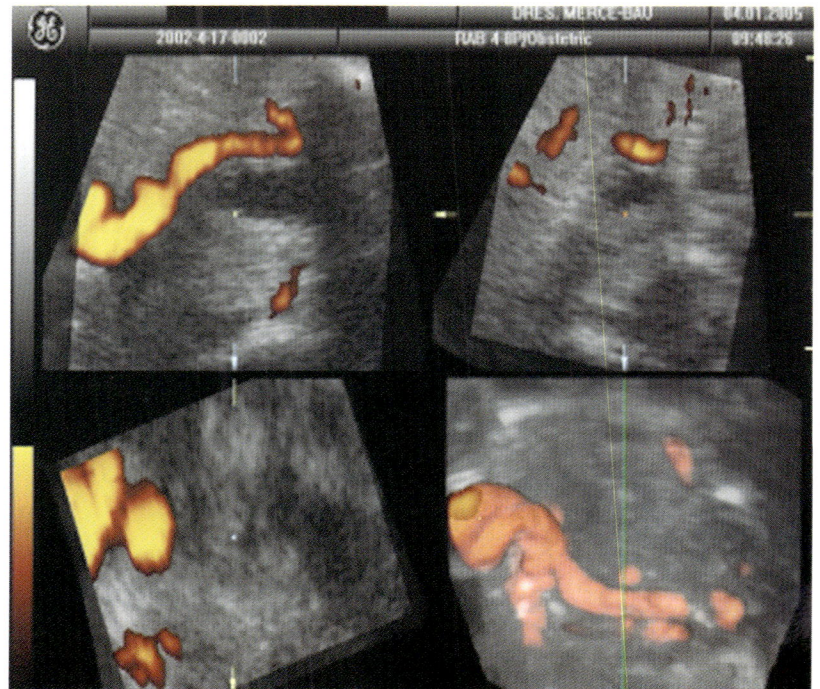

C

Figs 18.27A to C: Single umbilical artery at 27th week: A. Color Doppler;
B. Power Doppler; C. 3D power Doppler angiography

Table 18.5: Intraobserver reproducibility of the vascularization index, flow index and vascularization flow Index of "Placental Biopsy" by power Doppler three-dimensional (n=60)

Parameters	ICC	95%-CI ICC	Mean difference*	SD
VI (%)	0.88	0.76-0.94	−0.83	4.52
FI (units)	0.88	0.76-0.94	−0.52	2.82
VFI (units)	0.89	0.79-0.95	−0.31	1.71

* Mean of difference between both measurements. VI: Vascularization index; FI: Flow index; VFI: Vascularization flow index; ICC: intraclass correlation coefficient; 95%-IC: 95% confidence interval for ICC; SD: standard deviation

Table 18.6: Correlations between the placental volume (PV), vascularization index (VI), flow index (FI) and vascularization flow Index (VFI) of the placental vascular biopsy, and biometric parameters of fetal growth and umbilical Doppler velocimetry (n=52)

Parameters	BPD	HC	AC	FL	Weight	US	URI
PV	0.46**	0.51**	0.46**	0.48**	0.44**	029*	−0.34**
VI	0.28*	0.27*	0.25*	0.27*	0.20	0.29*	−0.24*
FI	0.64**	0.62**	0.64**	0.64**	0.60**	0.44**	−0.48**
VFI	0.33**	0.31**	0.31**	0.32**	0.27*	0.28*	−0.27*

BPD: biparietal diameter; HC: head circumference; AC: abdominal circumference; FL: femur length; US: umbilical systolic velocity; URI: umbilical resistance index. * $p < 0,05$; ** $p < 0,01$

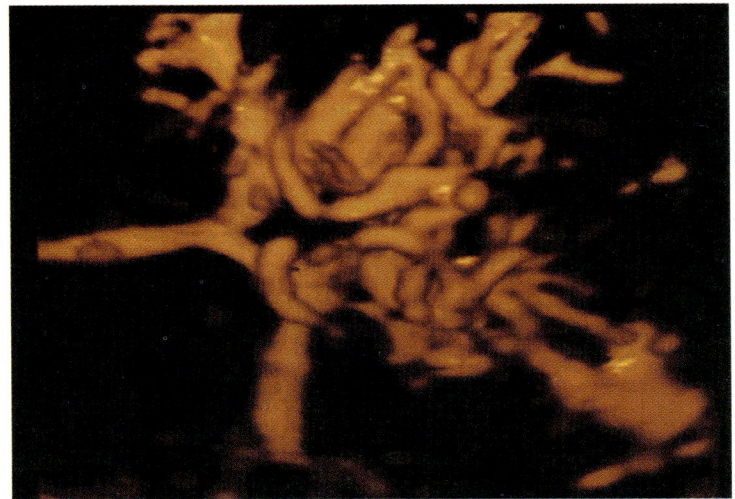

Fig. 18.28: Fetal cerebral circulation as seen by 3D power Doppler angiography: reconstruction of the circle of Willis

volume with the vessels included provide the same diagnostic possibilities than magnetic resonance imaging (Fig. 18.28).

More recently, it has been reported that the fetal cerebral vascularization and blood flow increase significantly during pregnancy[56] and that 3D power Doppler can detect optimally the aneurysms of the vein of Galen and its connexions.[57,58]

The fetal heart examination by 3D ultrasonography put initially the technical problem of being an organ constantly moving. This has been recently solved by the application of the STIC mode (Spatio-Temporal Image Correlation). Through this technology the cardiac volume is firstly achieved by automatic scanning. Afterwards, the image is analysed according to its spatial and temporal characteristics to achieve a 3D dynamic sequence on-line and a "surface" reconstruction of the heart.[59]

As advantages of the technique, a good resolution in B mode with an unlimited number of images, a shortage of the examination time and the three-dimensional reconstruction have been suggested.[59] The visualization of the outflow tracts and main connexions is easier achieved by the heart rotation around the X and Y axis from the four-chamber view as basal image[60,61] (Figs 18.29A and B). The only limitations pointed out are the big hearts in term gestations and the low discrimination of the signal in the early pregnancy.[62]

Another great advantage of this new technology is the storage of the volumes and the possibility to send them to a remote place to be analysed for other experts on the subject in a looped movie sequence.[59] This implies the STIC data could be acquired

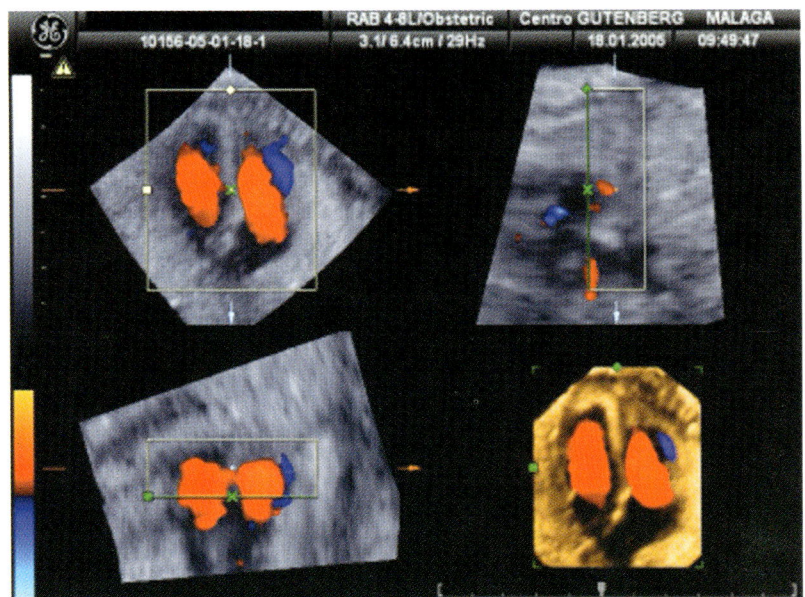

A

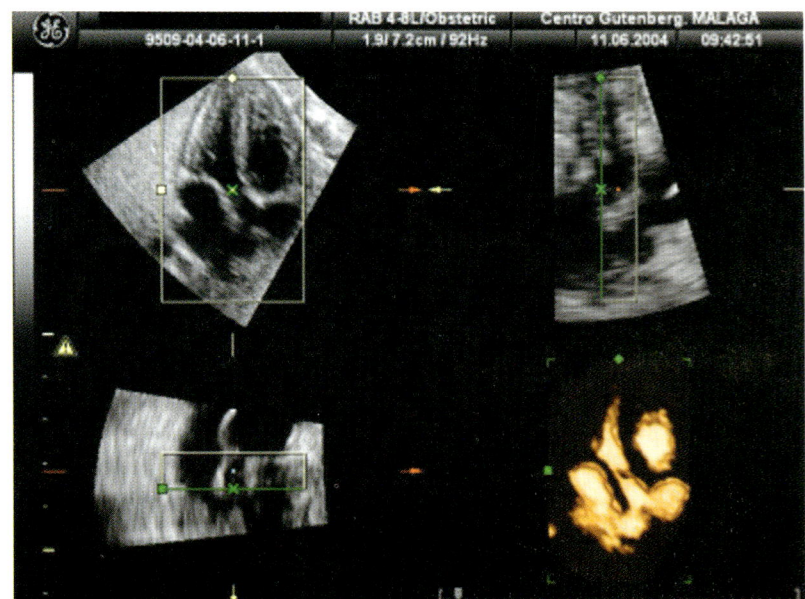

B

Figs 18.29A and B: Power Doppler angiography of the fetal heart. A. STIC color multiplanar; B. STIC multiplanar inverse mode. (By courtesy of Dr G Azumendi)

by a general obstetrician but be examined by a fetal echo-cardiologist in order to the prenatal confirmation of the normality of the cardiac structures or to rule out the major cardiac malformations.[60]

The percentage of 3D power Doppler representation of great vessels has increased considerably from the first publications.[63] According to the vessels, different detection rates have been reported: umbilical: 100 percent; abdominal and placental: 84 percent; pulmonary: 64 percent and renal ones: 51 percent. Failure in fetal vessels rendering are mainly due to a non-favorable fetal position and fetal movements.[64]

The 3D power Doppler is very useful to the visualization of fetal hepatic and portal circulations and to identify the vascular anomalies of umbilical and portosystemic venous systems (Fig. 18.30). These malformations reach the 2.6 percent prevalence and have been essentially described: the ductus venosus absence and the direct connexion between the umbilical and cava veins or the right atrium.[65] Through the calculation of 3D Doppler indices it has been proven that the hepatic vascularization and blood flow increase significantly during normal pregnancy.[66]

Even though it is not always easy to depict the fetal renal vascularization (Fig. 18.31)[64], by means of 3D power Doppler indices it has been demonstrated that the renal vascularization and blood flow increase significantly with gestational age during normal gestations.[67]

APPLICATIONS IN GYNECOLOGY

Three-dimensional power Doppler was initially applied to the diagnosis of uterine and ovarian tumoral diseases. Among its advantages are the possibility to assess the vascularization and blood flow from the whole tumor or the acquisition of a sample or "vascular biopsy" which seems more advantageous a priory than the signal from a single vessel.[68,69]

The "surface" mode reconstruction allows the evaluation of the morphology of the vascular network in the tumors or masses. A disorganized vascular architecture with scattered vessels and irregular branches suggest a malignant nature. On the contrary, a linear vascular network following a simple branching pattern is typical from benign lesions. Malignant tumors show microaneurysms, arteriovenous shunts, tumoral lakes, great diameter, spiralization and dichotomic branching too[70] (Fig. 18.32).

One of the main advantages is probably being a technique with similar possibilities to a magnetic resonance imaging portable unit. It is a less explorer-dependent examination because the volumes are automatically acquired and can be later revised for somebody different and even more experienced. The evaluation is made off-line, providing a more pondered and calm diagnostic and even the possibility to send it for an additional opinion. Therefore, three-dimensional diagnosis is more objective, reproducible and precise.

Uterine Pathology

Although three-dimensional ultrasound is the gold standard for the differential diagnosis of some uterine malformations, 3D power Doppler is scarcely applied to the assessment of benign conditions such as uterine myomas. In our opinion, this technology may be helpful to assess the growth potential and the response to conservative treatment in these cases. Besides its volume, uterine myomas are characterized by the importance of its vascular network which is probably the key of the success of the different non-surgical approaches currently in use (Figs 18.33A and B).

Along with conventional Doppler, the endometrial pathology is one of the main indications of this new technique. Kurjak et al[70] proved that ultrasound and 3D power Doppler, as compared with ultrasound and conventional color Doppler, increase the sensitivity to detect endometrial cancer from 67 to 89 percent by maintaining a false-positive rate of 3 percent. The endometrial volume was better than the endometrial thickness to diagnose endometrial cancer. In two cases of false-positive results for the volume, an organized and regular distribution of the vascular network suggested an endometrial hyperplasia.

In Table 18.7 are showed our preliminary results. We have not found significant differences between endometrial hyperplasia and cancer for the values of endometrial thickness, endometrial volume and average resistance index from both uterine arteries. On the contrary, endometrial cancer showed an endometrial resistance index significantly diminished with regard to hyperplasia. All the 3D vascular indices and specially the flow index were significantly increased in cases of endometrial cancer (Figs 18.34A and B).

The Table 18.8 shows the diagnostic competence of the different parameters from the ROC curve and the sensitivity and false-positive rate for the best cut-off value of the parameter studied. 3D vascular indices show the best results never forgetting the reduced number of cases.

3D vascular indices are also increased in cervical carcinoma. It has been demonstrated that they are related to the tumor size although the relationship between these indices and the clinicopathological characteristics or biological tumor factors has not yet been found[71] (Fig. 18.35).

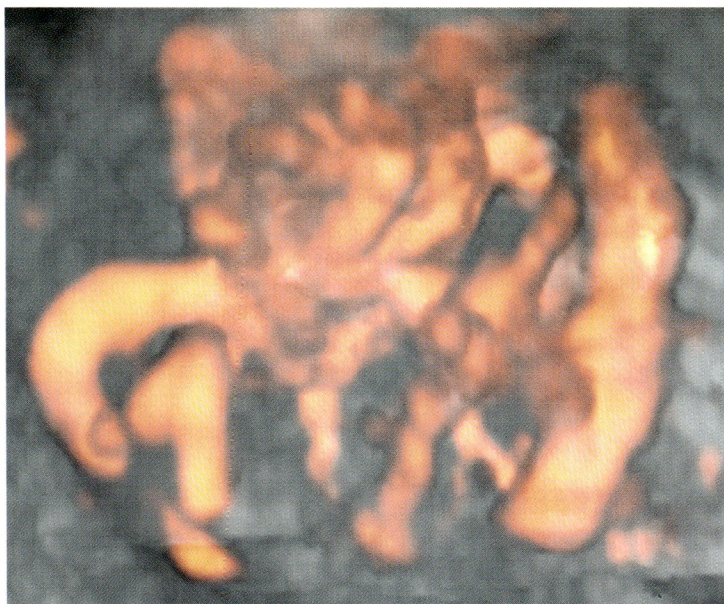

Fig. 18.30: 3D power Doppler angiography of the hepatic circulation

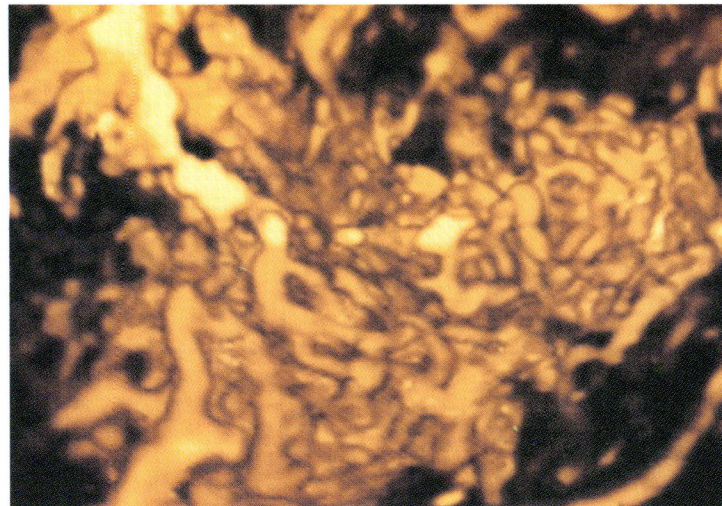

Fig. 18.32: Vascular architecture suggestive of malignity. It is characterized by a disarranged and scattered vascular disposition with irregular branching

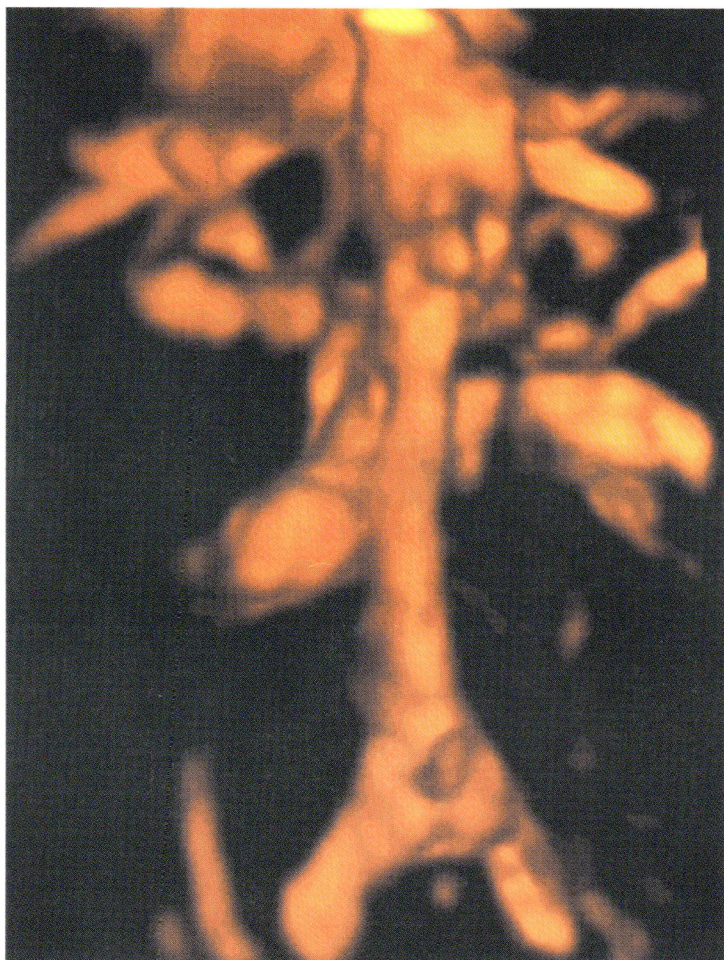

A

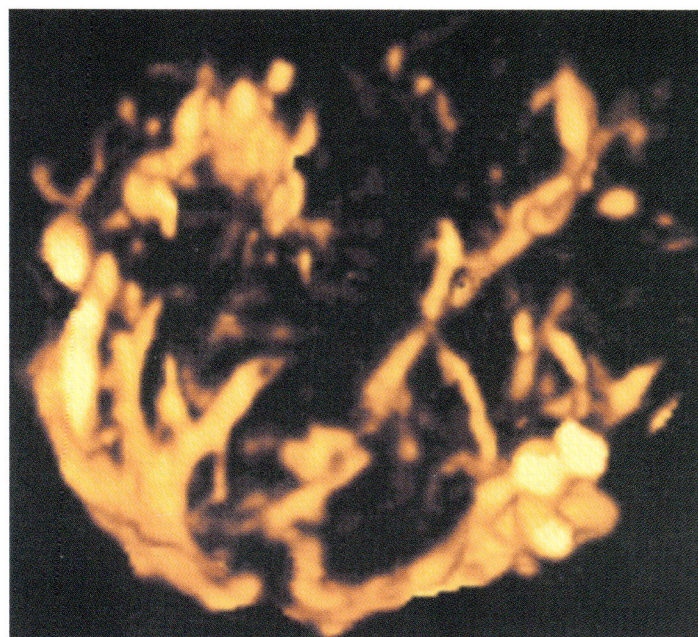

Fig. 18.31: 3D power Doppler angiography of the abdominal circulation: Iliac and renal vessels

Ovarian Pathology

Two hypotheses have been suggested in the application of 3D power Doppler angiography to the diagnosis of ovarian tumors.

Kurjak and his group[70] hold that the development of the vascular tree of the malignant tumors is a non-linear process following the chaos theory.[72] The vascular architecture of the

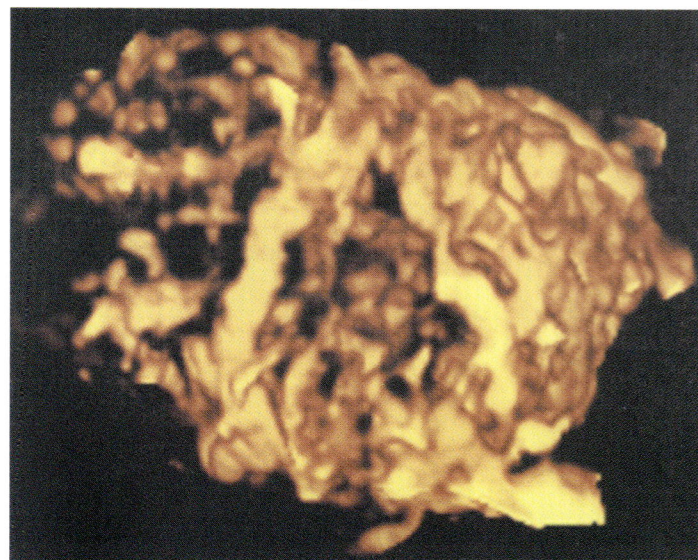

B

Figs 18.33A and B: 3D power Doppler angiography in two uterine myomas. The vascular network is greater in (B) with greater diameter vessels and (A) more irregular architecture

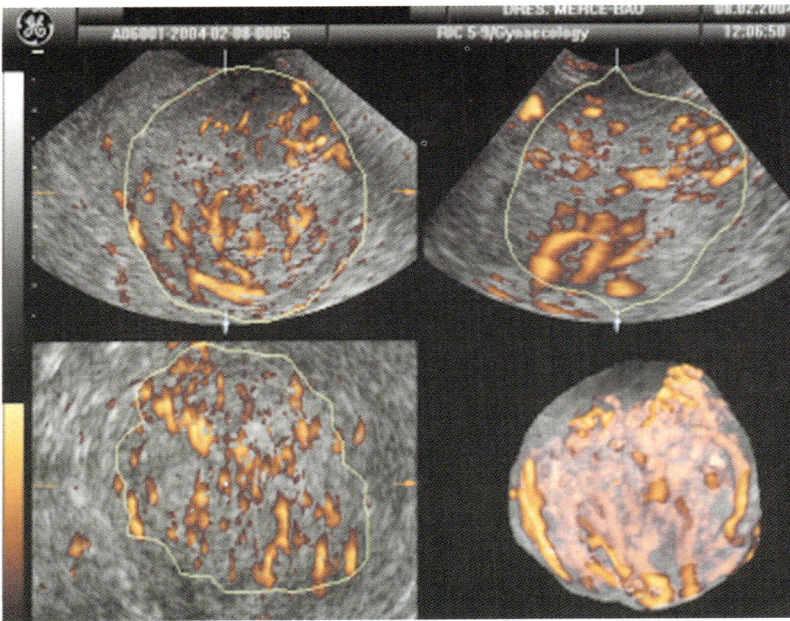

A

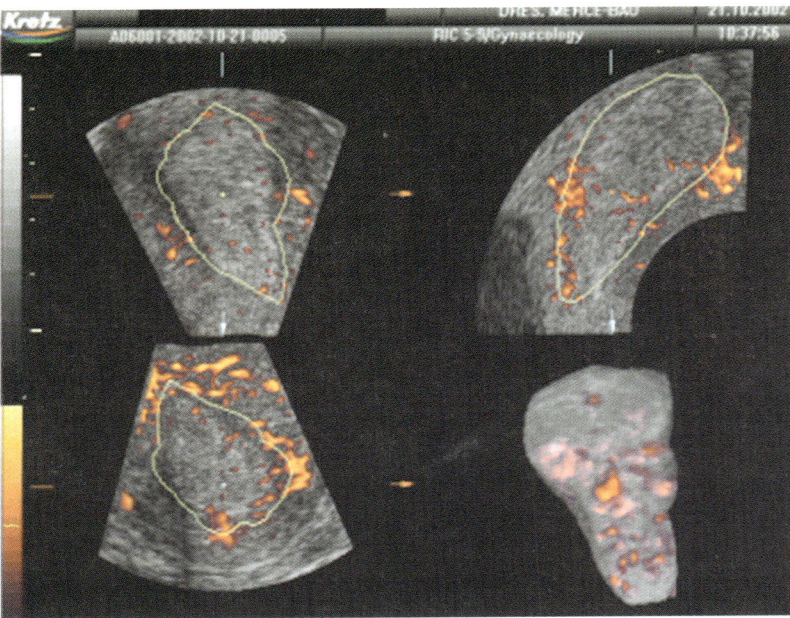

Fig. 18.35: 3D power Doppler in a cervical cancer.
(By courtesy of Dr JL Alcázar)

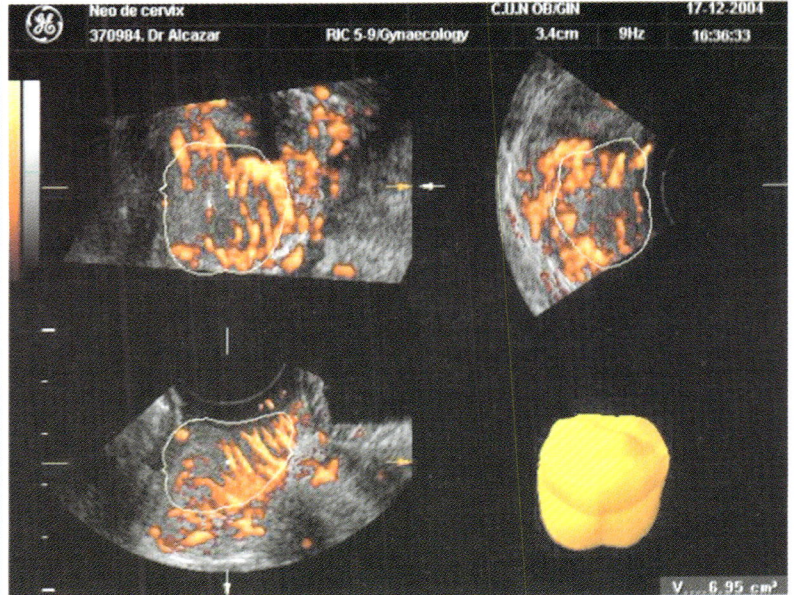

B

Figs 18.34A and B: 3D power Doppler angiography in an endometrial cancer (A) and an endometrial hyperplasia (B). In some cases, hyperplasias show an increased subendometrial flow

malignant tumors is characterised by a chaotic vascular distribution with irregular branching and disarranged vessels. That analysis has two main disadvantages. It is subjective, affecting reproducibility. The resolution limits of the technology hinder the small vessels recognition which is essential and characteristic of the tumoral growth.[73]

The large amount of publications of this group has proven the evaluation of the morphology of the vascular network by 3D power Doppler improves the diagnostic ability of Doppler to differentiate between benign and malignant conditions[70,74-76] (Figs 18.36A to F). Through the assessment of 251 adnexal masses (221 benign and 30 malignant) they confirm that ultrasonography and bidimensional power Doppler produce

three false-negatives (two-serous cystoadenocarcinomas and one mucinous cystoadenocarcinoma) and four false-positives (two ovarian fibromas, one dermoid cyst and one retroperitoneal fibromatosis). When ultrasonography and 3D power Doppler were used they found only one false-positive (retroperitoneal fibromatosis) and one false-negative (serous cystoadeno-carcinoma) (Table 18.9). Similar results have proven in the detection of stage I ovarian carcinoma. In 43 cases, 3D ultrasonography and 3D power Doppler reached a detection rate of 97.7 percent, significantly higher than the 86.5 percent found with bidimensional ultrasonography and power Doppler. Only one false-negative was registered due to a granulosa cells tumor with no vascularization[77] (Figs 18.37A to C).

The 3D power Doppler enhancement with contrast media provides a better visualization of the tumoral vascular network, increasing the diagnostic efficacy in complex adnexal masses.[78] These agents can help identify the blood flowing through small, deep or necrotic vessels by increasing the return signal (Table 18.9).

It has also been reported that 3D power Doppler, applying the same diagnostic criteria as bidimensional power Doppler, decreases the false-positive rate in complex adnexal masses.[79] Nevertheless, other authors do not find any difference between both examinations.[80]

Pairleitner et al[68] suggested that 3D power Doppler facilitates the blood flow and total vascularization analysis from an ovarian mass or tumor. The calculation of 3D vascular indices (vascularization index, flow index and vascularization flow index) through a histogram from a volume of interest is more precise than a single slice by bidimensional power Doppler or a single

Table 18.7: Endometrial thickness and volume, uterine and endometrial resistance index and endometrial vascular power Doppler indices in endometrial hyperplasia (n= 9) and endometrial carcinoma (n= 14)

	Hyperplasia	Carcinoma	p[(2)]
Endometrial thickness (mm)	13.7 ± 6.2	19.7 ± 10.1	NS
Endometrial volume (ml)	7.16 ± 7.10	15.02 ± 12.98	NS
Uterine resistance index [(1)]	0.78 ± 0.03	0.78 ± 0.12	NS
Endometrial resistance index	0.66 ± 0.15	0.45 ± 0.15	0.003
Vascularization index	5.65 ± 8.02	20.03 ± 15.89	0.009
Flow index	25.37 ± 3.59	32.01 ± 3.61	0.000
Vascularization flow index	1.61 ± 2.43	6.78 ± 6.11	0.004

All values indicate mean ± SD. [(1)] Average value from both uterine arteries. [(2)] Mann Whitney Test. NS: Not significant.

Table 18.8: Three-dimensional power Doppler angiography and endometrial cancer diagnosis

	Area under ROC curve	p	Cut-off value	S (%)	FPI
ET	0.71	NS	15.1 mm	71	11
EV	0.68	NS	5,78 ml	71	22
URI	0.47	NS	0.77	89	50
ERI	0.08	0.005	0.50	36	78
EVI	0.82	0.01	6.49	86	22
EFI	0.91	0.001	29.93	78	11
EVFII	0.85	0.006	1.12	93	22

ET: Endometrial thickness (mm); EV: Endometrial volume; URI: Uterine average resistance index; ERI: Endometrial resistance index; EVI: Endometrial vascularization index; EFI: Endometrial flow index; EVFI: Endometrial vascularization flow index. S: Sensitivity; FPI: Index of false-positives

Table 18.9: Predictive value of two-dimensional/transvaginal color Doppler sonography, three-dimensional/three-dimensional power Doppler sonography, and contrast-enhanced three-dimensional power Doppler sonography for detecting adnexal malignancies

Techniques	Sen %	Spe %	PPV %	NPV %
2DS/TVCDS	89	98	86	99
3DS/3DPDS	97	99	97	99
Contrast-enhanced 3DPS	100	99	93	100

Sen: Sensitivity; Spe: Specificity; PPV: Positive predictive value; NPV: Negative predictive value (Adapted from Kurjak and cols, 2001)

vessel by pulsed Doppler (Fig. 18.38). Recently, an acceptable reproducibility of 3D vascular indices has been demonstrated to assess gynecological solid tumors with intraclass correlation coefficients higher than 0.90 for all the parameters studied.[81]

The main limitation of the technique is the tumoral size. Three-dimensional as bidimensional probes have limited scanning fields and maximal volume acquired. To overcome this problem we have designed the "vascular biopsy" technique by 3D power Doppler.[69] It consists of the study of only the more suspicious tumoral area by vascular indices (Fig. 18.39). Preliminary results of the method after the evaluation of 56 complex adnexal masses show that the 3D vascular indices are significantly superior in the suspicious areas of malignant tumors (Table 18.10).

In summary, we have tried to review briefly the main applications of three-dimensional power Doppler angiography according to the previously reported in literature and our own

Table 18.10: Vascular and velocimetric indices in malignant and benign adnexal tumors

	VI	FI	VFI	RI	PI	PSV
Malignant (n=44)	15.0% (3.8-77%)	33.6 (16.2-51.9)	4,8 (1.1-40.1)	0,43 (0.23-0.74)	0.60 (0.27-1,48)	14.9 cm/s (7.0-40.0)
Benign (n= 12)	9.6% (0.2-37%	23.2 (12.6-36.9)	2.8 (0.04-12.6)	0.44 (0.30-0.60)	0.69 (0.44-1.03)	12 (7.5-31.7)

VI: Vascularization index; FI: Flow index; VFI: Vascularization flow index; RI: Resistance index; PI: Pulsatility index; PSV: Peak systolic velocity. Data expressed as median and range. Range in parentheses. VI.- p=0.043; FI.- p=0.009; VFI.- p=0.009; RI.- p=0.631. (Adapted from Alcazar and cols, 2005).

experience. As it is showed, this technology has many possibilities but for some future indications we have only preliminary results. We would like to point out that they are the characteristics of the technology itself, specially being less explorer-dependent and give more objective information, which produce the greater advantages of its application. Nevertheless, to reach this end we need a deep change of the specialist sonographer mentality. Only this way will it be possible to obtain all the diagnostic profit this new technology provides.

REFERENCES

1. Ritchie CJ, Edwards WS, Mack LA, Cyr DR, Kim Y. Three-dimensional ultrasonic angiography using power-mode Doppler. Ultrasound Med Biol 1996; 22: 277-86.
2. Rubin JM, Bude RO, Carson PL, Bree RL, Adler RS. Power Doppler US: a potentially useful alternative to mean frequency-based color Doppler US. Radiology 1994; 190: 853-6.
3. Maulik D. Sonographic color flow mapping: Basic principles. In Maulik D (Ed): Doppler Ultrasound in Obstetrics and Gynecology. New York: Springer-Verlag Inc, 1997; 68-87.
4. VOCAL (Virtual Organ Computer-aided Analysis. In VOLUSON 730. Operation Manual. Vienna: Kretztechnik AG, 2001; 10:98-109.
5. Mercé LT. Volumetría con VOCAL e índices de la angiografía power Doppler tridimensional. 1° Curso MISUS (Madrid Internacional School od 3D Ultrasonography). Madrid, 2 y 3 de junio de 2004.
6. Mercé LT, Bau S. Velocimetría Doppler del ciclo ovárico. En: Bajo Arenas JM, de. Ultrasonografía y reproducción. Barcelona: Prous Science 1996; pp 37-66.
7. Zaidi J, Barber J, Kyei-Mensah A, Bekir J, Campbell S, Tan SL. Relationship of ovarian stromal blood flow at the baseline ultrasound scan to subsequent follicular response in an in vitro fertilization program. Obstet Gynecol 1996; 88: 779-84.
8. Engmann L, Sladkevicius P, Agrawal R, Bekir JS, Campbell S, Tan SL. Value of ovarian stromal blood flow velocity measurement after pituitary suppression in the prediction of ovarian responsiveness and outcome of in vitro fertilization treatment. Fertil Steril 1999; 71: 22-9.
9. Pan HA, Cheng YC, Li CH, Wu MH, Chang FM. Ovarian stroma flow intensity decreases by age: a three-dimensional power Doppler ultrasonographic study. Ultrasound Med Biol 2002 ; 28: 425-30.
10. Wu MH, Tsai SJ, Pan HA, Hsiao KY, Chang FM. Three-dimensional power Doppler imaging of ovarian stromal blood flow in women with endometriosis undergoing in vitro fertilization. Ultrasound Obstet Gynecol 2003; 21: 480-5.
11. Pan HA, Wu MH, Cheng YC, Li CH, Chang FM. Quantification of Doppler signal in polycystic ovary syndrome using three-dimensional power Doppler ultrasonography: a possible new marker for diagnosis. Hum Reprod 2002; 17: 201-6.
12. Jarvela IY, Sladkevicius P, Kelly S, Ojha K, Campbell S, Nargund G. Effect of pituitary down-regulation on the ovary before in vitro fertilization as measured using three-dimensional power Doppler ultrasound. Fertil Steril 2003; 79: 1129-35.
13. Pan HA, Wu MH, Cheng YC, Wu LH, Chang FM. Quantification of ovarian Doppler signal in hyperresponders during in vitro fertilization treatment using three-dimensional power Doppler ultrasonography. Ultrasound Med Biol 2003; 29: 921-7.
14. Pan HA, Wu MH, Cheng YC, Wu LH, Chang FM. Quantification of ovarian stromal Doppler signals in poor responders undergoing in vitro fertilization with three-dimensional power Doppler ultrasonography. Am J Obstet Gynecol 2004; 190: 338-44.

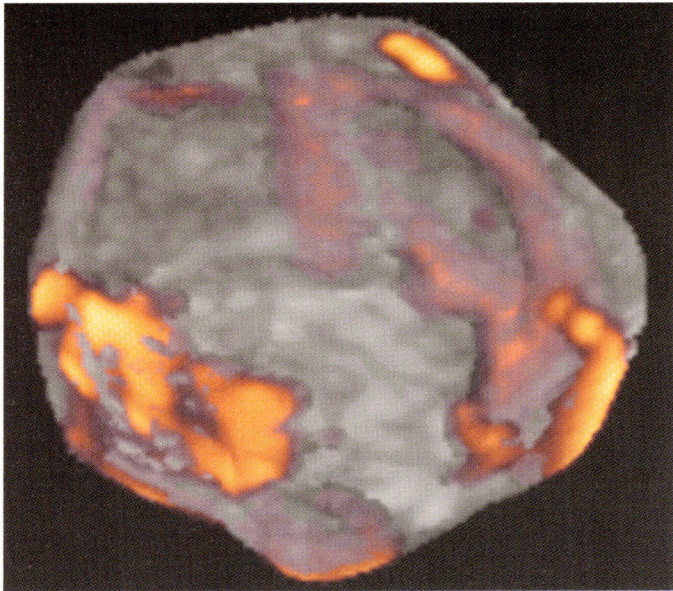

A

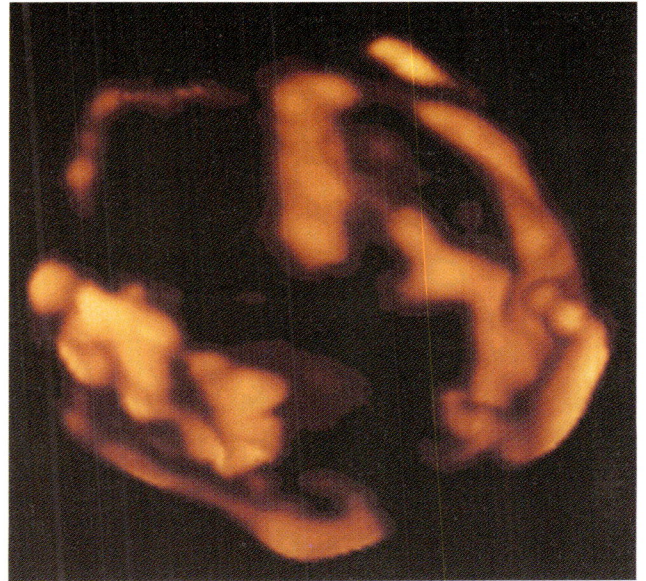

B

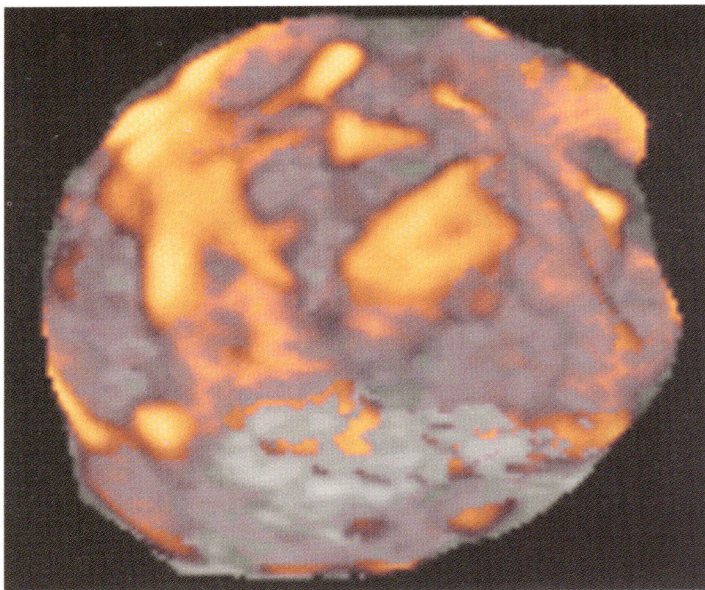

C

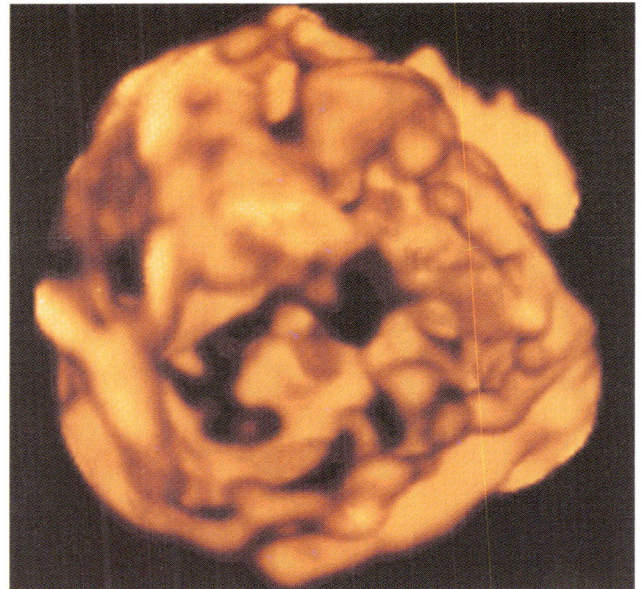

D

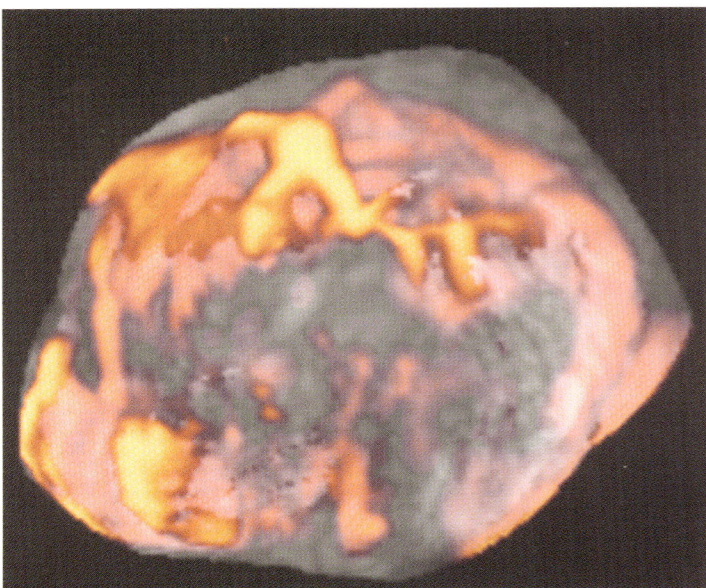

E

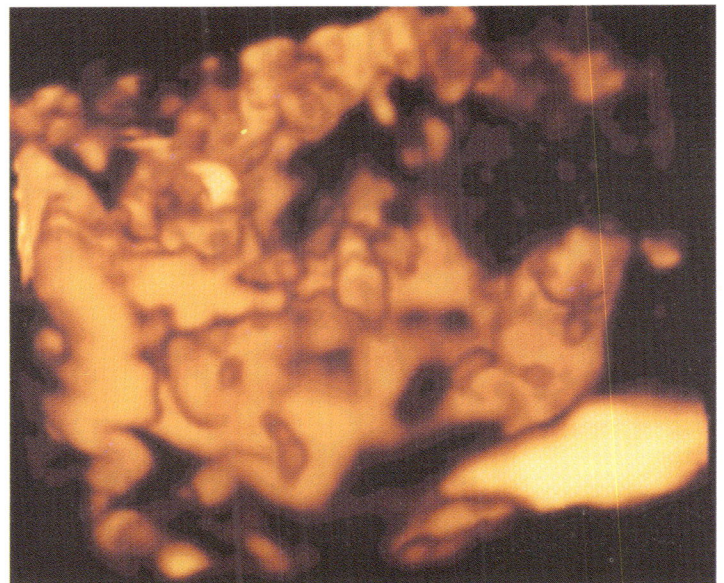

F

Figs 18.36A to F: 3D power Doppler in transparence and surface mode in different ovarian tumors according to diagnosis. A. and B. Endometrioma; C and D. Luteal cyst; E and F. Sero-papilar adenocarcinoma

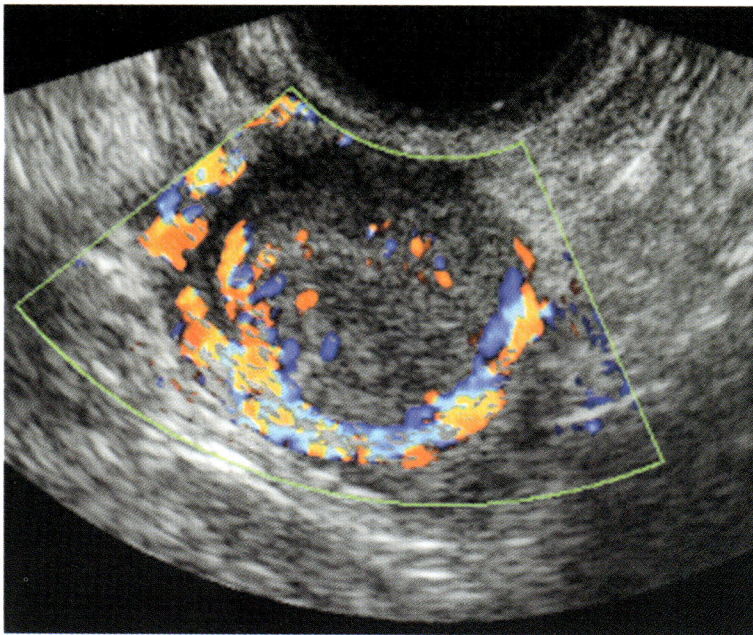

A

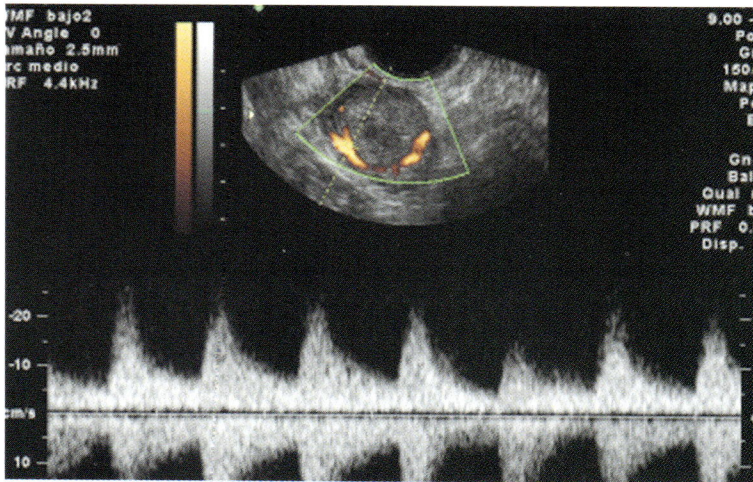

B

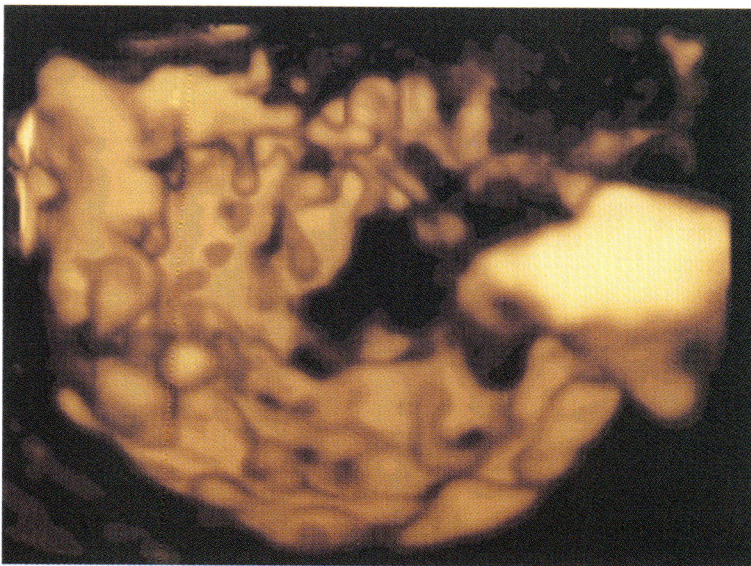

C

Figs 18.37A to C: Color map (A), power Doppler and FVW (B) and 3D power Doppler angiography in an ovarian endometrioid adenocarcinoma stage I

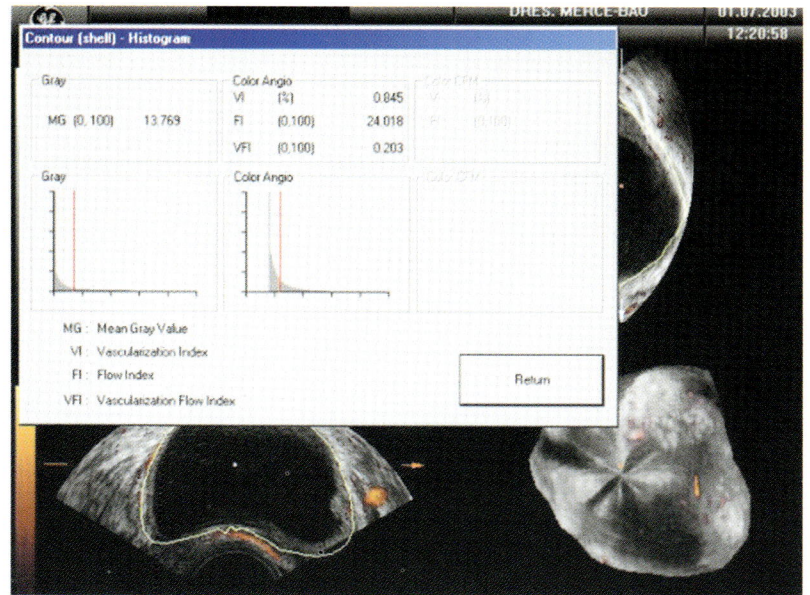

Fig. 18.38: Histogram from an ovarian teratoma where the power Doppler or color angioindices can be observed.

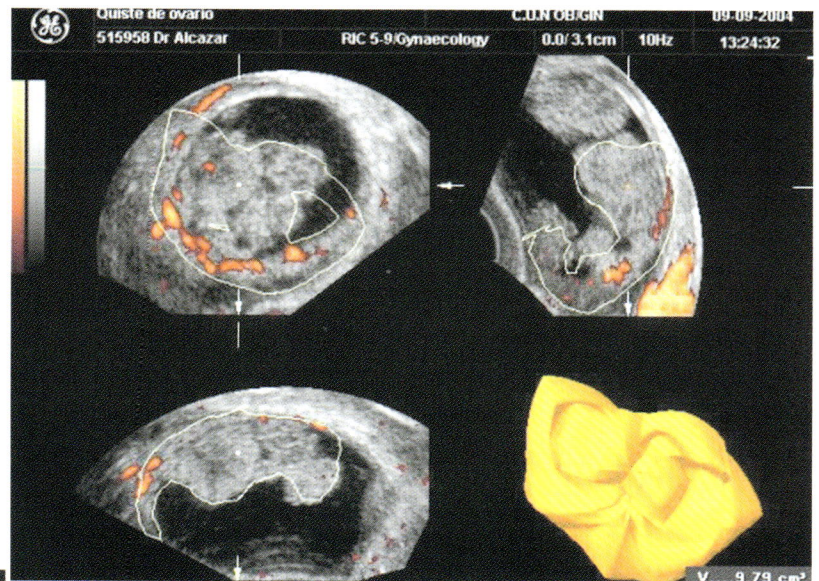

Fig. 18.39: Technique of the vascular biopsy with power Doppler over a suspicious area in a complex adnexal cyst (By courtesy of Dr JL Alcázar)

15. Jarvela IY, Sladkevicius P, Kellly S, Ojha K, Campbell S, Nargund G. Quantification of ovarian power Doppler signal with three-dimensional ultrasonography to predict response during in vitro fertilization. Obstet Gynecol 2003; 102: 816-22.
16. Raine-Fenning NJ, Campbell BK, Clewes JS, Kendall NR, Johnson IR. The reliability of virtual organ computer-aided analysis (VOCAL) for the semiquantification of ovarian, endometrial and subendometrial perfusion. Ultrasound Obstet Gynecol 2003; 22: 633-9.
17. Raine-Fenning NJ, Campbell BK, Clewes JS, Kendall NR, Johnson IR. The interobserver reliability of three-dimensional power Doppler data acquisition within the female pelvis. Ultrasound Obstet Gynecol 2004; 23: 501-8.
18. Van Blerkom J, Antczak M, Schrader R. The developmental potential of the human oocyte is related to the dissolved oxygen content of follicular fluid: association with vascular endothelial growth factor levels and perifollicular blood flow characteristics. Hum Reprod 1997; 12: 1047-55.
19. Mercé LT. Ultrasound markers of implantation. Ultrasound Rev Obstet Gynecol 2002; 2: 110-23.
20. Mercé LT, Barco MJ, Kupesic S, Kurjak A. 2D and 3D power Doppler ultrasound from ovulation to implantation. In Kurjak A, Chervenak F (Eds): Textbook of Perinatal Medicine. London: Parthenon Publishing, 2005; (in press).
21. Jarvela IY, Sladkevicius P, Kelly S, Ojha K, Nargund G, Campbell S. Three-dimensional sonographic and power Doppler characterization of ovaries in late follicular phase. Ultrasound Obstet Gynecol 2002; 20: 281-5.
22. Vlaisavljevic V, Reljic M, Gavric Lovrec V, Zazula D, Sergent N. Measurement of perifollicular blood flow of the dominant preovulatory follicle using three-dimensional power Doppler. Ultrasound Obstet Gynecol 2003; 22: 520-6.

23. Kupesic S, Kurjak A. Predictors of IVF outcome by three-dimensional ultrasound. Hum Reprod 2002 ;17:950-5.

24. Chien LW, Au HK, Chen PL, Xiao J, Tzeng CR. Assessment of uterine receptivity by the endometrial-subendometrial blood flow distribution pattern in women undergoing in vitro fertilization-embryo transfer. Fertil Steril 2002; 78: 245-51.

25. Maugey-Laulom B, Commenges-Ducos M, Jullien V, Papaxanthos-Roche A, Scotet V, Commenges D. Endometrial vascularity and ongoing pregnancy after IVF. Eur J Obstet Gynecol Reprod Biol 2002; 104: 137-43.

26. Zaidi J, Campbell S, Pittrof R, Tan SL. Endometrial thickness, morphology, vascular penetration and velocimetry in predicting implantation in an in vitro fertilization program. Ultrasound Obstet Gynecol 1995; 6:191-8.

27. Raine-Fenning NJ, Campbell BK, Kendall NR, Clewes JS, Johnson IR. Quantifying the changes in endometrial vascularity throughout the normal menstrual cycle with three-dimensional power Doppler angiography. Hum Reprod, 2004; 19:330-8.

28. Kupesic S, Bekavac I, Bjelos D, Kurjak A. Assessment of endometrial receptivity by transvaginal color Doppler and three-dimensional power Doppler ultrasonography in patients undergoing in vitro fertilization procedures. J Ultrasound Med 2001; 20: 125-34.

29. Wu HM, Chiang CH, Huang HY, Chao AS, Wang HS, Soong YK. Detection of the subendometrial vascularization flow index by three-dimensional ultrasound may be useful for predicting the pregnancy rate for patients undergoing in vitro fertilization-embryo transfer. Fertil Steril 2003; 79: 507-11.

30. Ng EH, Chan CC, Tang OS, Yeung WS, Ho PC. Endometrial and subendometrial blood flow measured during early luteal phase by three-dimensional power Doppler ultrasound in excessive ovarian responders. Hum Reprod 2004;19: 924-31.

31. Mercé LT, Barco MJ, de la Fuente F. Doppler velocimetry measured in retrochorionic space and uterine arteries during early human pregnancy. Acta Obstet Gynecol Scand 1989; 8: 603-7.

32. Mercé LT, Barco MJ, Bau S. Color Doppler sonographic assessment of placental circulation in the first trimester of normal pregnancy. J Ultrasound Med 1996; 15: 135-42.

33. Valentin L, Sladkevicius P, Laurini R, Söderberg H, Marsal K. Uteroplacental and luteal circulation in normal first-trimester pregnancies: Doppler ultrasonographic and morphologic study. Am J Obstet. Gynecol. 1996; 174: 768-75.

34. Kurjak A, Kupesic S. Doppler assessment of the intervillous blood flow in normal and abnormal early pregnancy. Obstet Gynecol 1997; 89: 252-6.

35. Jauniaux E, Jurkovic D, Campbell S, Hustin J. Doppler ultrasonographic features of the developing placental circulation: correlation with anatomic findings. Am J Obstet Gynecol 1992; 166: 585-7.

36. Jaffe R, Woods JR. Color Doppler imaging and in vivo assessment of the anatomy and physiology of the early uteroplacental circulation. Fertil Steril 1993; 60: 293-7.

37. Mercé LT, Barco MJ, Bau S. Color Doppler sonography of the retrochorionic and intervellous circulation: predictive value in small gestational sacs. Med Imag Internat 1997; 7: 16-9.

38. Jaffe R, Dorgan A, Abramowicz JS. Color Doppler imaging of the uteroplacental circulation in the first trimester: value in predicting pregnancy failure or complication. AJR 1995; 164: 1255-8.

39. Alcázar JL, Mercé LT, García-Manero M. Two-dimensional and three-dimensional Doppler assessment of abnormal early intrauterine pregnancy. In Kurjak A and Chervenak F, (Eds): Textbook of Perinatal Medicine. London: Parthenon Publishing, 2005; (in press).

40. Kurjak A, Kupesic S, Banovic I, Hafner T, Kos M. The study of morphology and circulation of early embryo by three-dimensional ultrasound and power Doppler. J Perinat Med 1999; 27: 145-57.

41. Pretorius DH, Nelson TR, Baergen RN, Pai E, Cantrell C. Imaging of placental vasculature using three-dimensional ultrasound and color power Doppler: a preliminary study. Ultrasound Obstet Gynecol 1998; 12: 45-9.

42. Matijevic R, Kurjak A. The assessment of placental blood vessels by three-dimensional power Doppler ultrasound. J Perinat Med 2002; 30: 26-32.

43. Konje JC, Huppertz B, Bell SC, Taylor DJ, Kaufmann P. 3-dimensional colour power angiography for staging human placental development. Lancet 2003; 362: 1199-1201.

44. Mercé LT, Bau, S. "Biopsia vascular placentaria" mediante mapa de amplitud tridimensional: Validación de la técnica. Rev Es Ultra Obs Gin 2003; 1: 0-5.

45. Mercé LT, Barco MJ, Bau S. Reproducibility of the study of placental vascularization by three-dimensional power Doppler. J Perinat Med 2004; 32: 228-33.

46. Mu J, Kanzaki T, Tomimatsu T, Fukuda H, Fujii E, Takeuchi H, et al. Investigation of intraplacental villous arteries by Doppler flow imaging in growth-restricted fetuses. Am J Obstet Gynecol 2002; 186: 297-302.

47. Yu CH, Chang CH, Ko HC, Chen WC, Chang FM. Assessment of placental fractional moving blood volume using quantitative three-dimensional power doppler ultrasound. Ultrasound Med Biol 2003; 29: 19-23.

48. Todros T, Sciarrone A, Piccoli E, Guiot C, Kaufmann P, Kingdom J. Umbilical Doppler waveforms and placental villous angiogenesis in pregnancies complicated by fetal growth restriction. Obstet Gynecol 1999; 93: 499-503.

49. Yagel S, Anteby EY, Shen O, Cohen SM, Friedman Z, Achiron R. Placental blood flow measured by simultaneous multigate spectral Doppler imaging in pregnancies complicate by placental vascular abnormalities. Ultrasound Obstet Gynecol 1999; 14: 262-6.

50. Shih JC, Ko TL, Lin MC, Shyu MK, Lee CN, Hsieh FJ. Quantitative three-dimensional power Doppler ultrasound predicts the outcome of placental chorioangioma. Ultrasound Obstet Gynecol 2004; 24: 202-6.

51. Hanaoka U, Yanagihara T, Tanaka H, Hata T. Comparison of three-dimensional, two-dimensional and color Doppler ultrasound in predicting the presence of a nuchal cord at birth. Ultrasound Obstet Gynecol 2002 ; 19: 471-4.

52. Sepulveda W, Rojas I, Robert JA, Schnapp C, Alcalde JL. Prenatal detection of velamentous insertion of the umbilical cord: a prospective color Doppler ultrasound study. Ultrasound Obstet Gynecol 2003; 21: 564-9.

53. Oyelese Y, Chavez MR, Yeo L, Giannina G, Kontopoulos EV, Smulian JC, Scorza WE. Three-dimensional sonographic diagnosis of vasa previa. Ultrasound Obstet Gynecol 2004; 24: 211-5.

54. Heling KS, Chaoui R, Bollmann R. Prenatal diagnosis of an aneurysm of the vein of Galen with three-dimensional color power angiography. Ultrasound Obstet Gynecol 2000; 15: 333-6.

55. Pooh RK, Pooh K. Transvaginal 3D and Doppler ultrasonography of the fetal brain. Semin Perinatol 2001; 25: 38-43.

56. Chang CH, Yu CH, Ko HC, Chen CL, Chang FM. Three-dimensional power Doppler ultrasound for the assessment of the fetal brain blood flow in normal gestation. Ultrasound Med Biol 2003;29: 1273-9.

57. Ruano R, Benachi A, Aubry MC, Brunelle F, Dumez Y, Dommergues M. Perinatal three-dimensional color power Doppler ultrasonography of vein of Galen aneurysms. J Ultrasound Med 2003; 22: 1357-62.

58. Gerards FA, Engels MA, Barkhof F, van den Dungen FA, Vermeulen RJ, van Vugt JM. Prenatal diagnosis of aneurysms of the vein of Galen (vena magna cerebri) with conventional sonography, three-dimensional sonography, and magnetic resonance imaging: report of 2 cases. J Ultrasound Med 2003; 22: 1363-8.

59. DeVore GR, Falkensammer P, Sklansky MS, Platt LD. Spatio-temporal image correlation (STIC): new technology for evaluation of the fetal heart. Ultrasound Obstet Gynecol 2003; 22: 380-7.

60. Vinals F, Poblete P, Giuliano A. Spatio-temporal image correlation (STIC): a new tool for the prenatal screening of congenital heart defects. Ultrasound Obstet Gynecol 2003; 22: 388-94.

61. DeVore GR, Polanco B, Sklansky MS, Platt LD. The 'spin' technique: a new method for examination of the fetal outflow tracts using three-dimensional ultrasound. Ultrasound Obstet Gynecol 2004; 24: 72-82.

62. Chaoui R, Hoffmann J, Heling KS. Three-dimensional (3D) and 4D color Doppler fetal echocardiography using spatio-temporal image correlation (STIC). Ultrasound Obstet Gynecol 2004; 23: 535-45.

63. Chaoui R, Kalache KD, Hartung J. Application of three-dimensional power Doppler ultrasound in prenatal diagnosis. Ultrasound Obstet Gynecol 2001; 17: 22-9.

64. Hartung J, Kalache KD, Chaoui R. Three-dimensional power Doppler ultrasonography (3D-PDU) in fetal diagnosis. Ultraschall Med 2004; 25: 200-5.

65. Kalache K, Romero R, Goncalves LF, Chaiworapongsa T, Espinoza J, Schoen ML, et al. Three-dimensional color power imaging of the fetal hepatic circulation. Am J Obstet Gynecol 2003;189: 1401-6.

66. Chang CH, Yu CH, Ko HC, Chang FM, Chen HY. Assessment of normal fetal liver blood flow using quantitative three-dimensional power Doppler ultrasound. Ultrasound Med Biol 2003; 29: 943-9.

67. Chang CH, Yu CH, Ko HC, Chen WC, Chang FM. Quantitative three-dimensional power Doppler sonography for assessment of the fetal renal blood flow in normal gestation. Ultrasound Med Biol. 2003 Jul;29(7):929-33.

68. Pairleitner H, Steiner H, Hasenoehrl G, Staudach A. Three-dimensional power Doppler sonography: imaging and quantifying blood flow and vascularization. Ultrasound Obstet Gynecol 1999; 14: 139-43.

69. Alcázar JL, Mercé LT, García-Manero M. 3D Power-Doppler vascular— a new method for predicting ovarian cancer in vascularized complex adnexal masses. J Ultrasound Med 2005; 24:689-96.

70. Kurjak A, Kupesic S, Sparac V, Bekavac I. Preoperative evaluation of pelvic tumors by Doppler and three-dimensional sonography. J Ultrasound Med 2001; 20: 829-40.

71. Testa AC, Ferrandina G, Distefano M, Fruscella E, Mansueto D, Basso D, Salutari V, Scambia G. Color Doppler velocimetry and three-dimensional color power angiography of cervical carcinoma. Ultrasound Obstet Gynecol 2004; 24: 445-52.

72. Breyer B, Kurjak A. Tumor vascularization Doppler measurements and chaos: what to do? Ultrasound Obstet Gynecol 1995; 5: 209.

73. Kurjak A, Kupesic S, Breyer B, Sparac V, Jukic S. The assessment of ovarian tumor angiogenesis: what does three-dimensional power Doppler add?. Ultrasound Obstet Gynecol 1998; 12: 136-46.

74. Kurjak A, Kupesic S, Jacobs I. Preoperative diagnosis of the primary fallopian tube carcinoma by three-dimensional static and power Doppler sonography. Ultrasound Obstet Gynecol 2000; 15: 246-51.

75. Kurjak A, Kupesic S, Sparac V, Kosuta D. Three-dimensional ultrasonographic and power Doppler characterization of ovarian lesions. Ultrasound Obstet Gynecol 2000; 16: 365-71.

76. Kurjak A, Kupesic S, Anic T, Kosuta D. Three-dimensional ultrasound and power Doppler improve the diagnosis of ovarian lesions. Gynecol Oncol 2000; 76: 28-32.

77. Kurjak A, Kupesic S, Sparac V, Prka M, Bekavac I. The detection of stage I ovarian cancer by three-dimensional sonography and power Doppler. Gynecol Oncol 2003; 90: 258-64.

78. Kupesic S, Kurjak A. Contrast-enhanced, three-dimensional power Doppler sonography for differentiation of adnexal masses. Obstet Gynecol 2000; 96: 452-8.

79. Cohen LS, Escobar PF, Scharm C, Glimco B, Fishman DA. Three-dimensional power Doppler ultrasound improves the diagnostic accuracy for ovarian cancer prediction. Gynecol Oncol 2001; 82: 40-8.

80. Alcázar JL, García-Manero M. Comparison of two-dimensional and three-dimensional Power-Doppler imaging in complex adnexal masses for predicting ovarian cancer. Am J Obstet Gynecl 2005; 192:807-12.

81. Testa AC, Mansueto D, Lorusso D, Fruscella E, Basso D, Scambia G, Ferrandina G. Angiographic power 3-dimensional quantitative analysis in gynecologic solid tumors: feasibility and reproducibility. J Ultrasound Med 2004 23: 821-8.

Section 2
Gynecology & Infertility

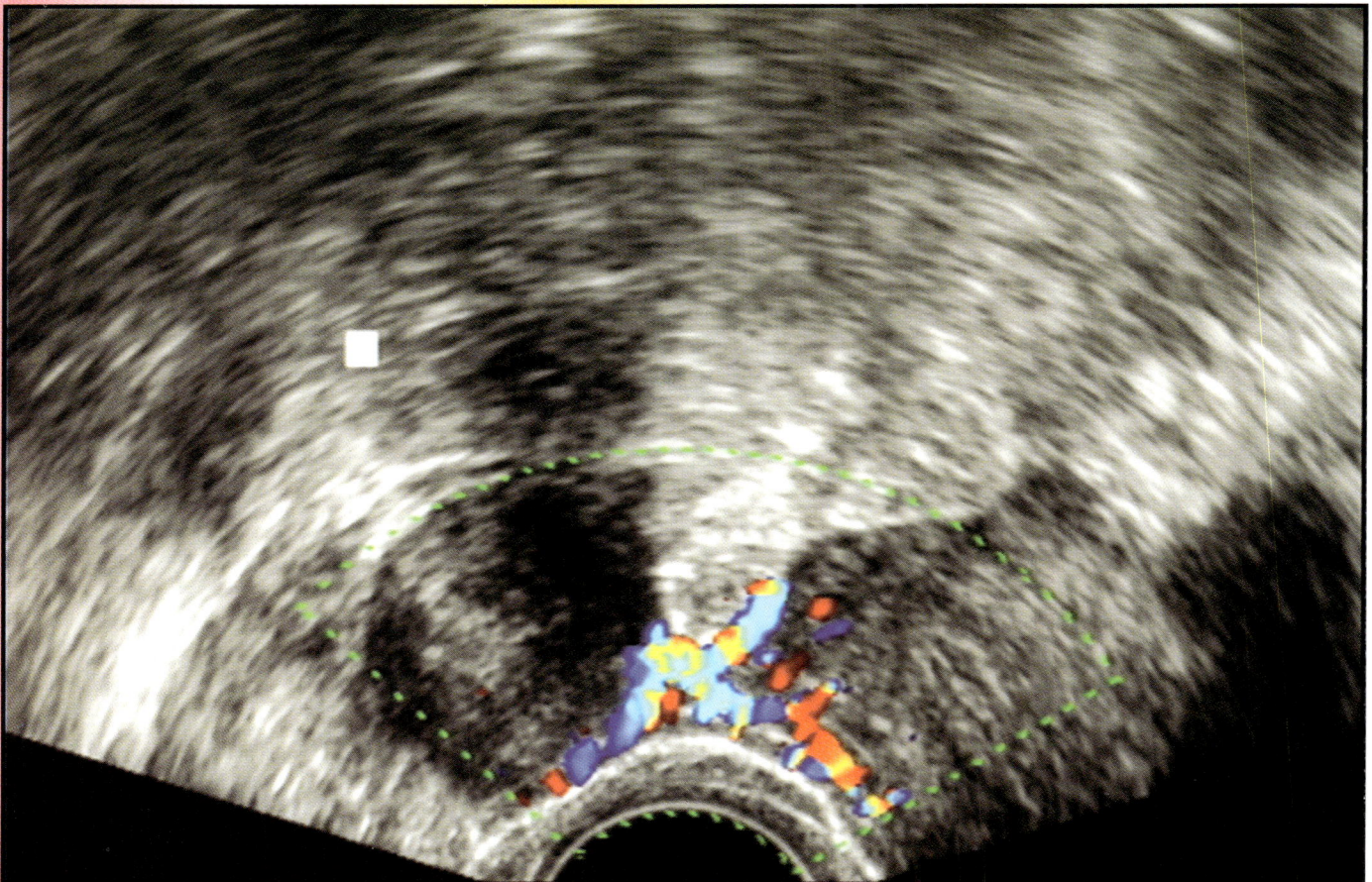

19

MA Pascual, S Kupesic, A Kurjak

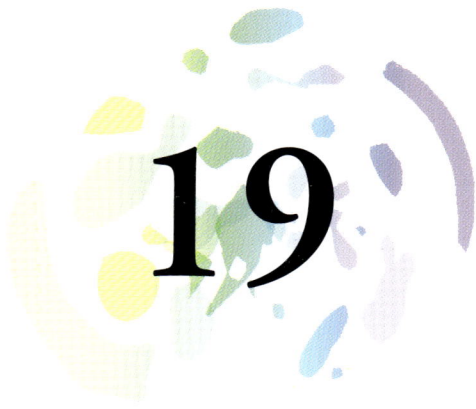

Normal and Abnormal Anatomy of Female Pelvis

SONOGRAPHY OF THE UTERUS

The ability of sonography to depict subtle changes in the myometrium and endometrium makes it the diagnostic modality for the evaluation of many uterine disorders. With sonography, the uterus can be imaged in several scanning planes; and with realtime, the sonographer can change the scanning plane and gain settings for optimal depiction of the endometrium and myometrium.

Sonographic evaluation of the uterus can be done by two different methods: abdominal, that should be done when the patient has a fully distended bladder (Figs 19.1 to 19.16), or transvaginal. At the present time, favored by the fast development and diffusion of vaginal probe, the best sonographic evaluation of the pelvic cavity should be performed by transvaginal sonography; this one does not require full bladder techniques.

The abdominal sonography is useful in patients in whom vaginal exploration is not possible, and the vagina is easily identified by this method (Figs 19.7, 19.15 and 19.16). It is also a complementary study when we diagnose big tumors.

Sonography can accurately depict the position, size, shape and texture of the uterus (Figs 19.17 to 19. 20). The size and shape of the uterus varies according to the patient's pubertal status, age and parity.

The texture of the normal myometrium is inconsistent throughout all age groups and is of a homogeneous, low to medium echogenicity. The innermost layers of the endometrium appear as a central linear echogenicity, most prominent during menses (Figs 19.21 to 19.28). The hypoechoic texture of the endometrium is most frequently seen in the proliferative phase.

The endometrium appears thickened and echogenic during the secretory phase.

The normal uterus has well-defined contours and a pear-shaped configuration. The uterine shape, contour and internal texture should be carefully evaluated in every patient because minor pathological alterations can change some of the characteristics of the normal uterus.

Foreign bodies and intrauterine or tubaric devices, and their placement, are easily demonstrated by ultrasound. The characteristic feature is the presence of high level echoes and posterior shadowing (Figs 19.29 to 19.45), but actually some type of intrauterine device is easily showed by three-dimensional sonography. Some physiological and pathologic changes can also be easily identified as a mucousmetra and hematometra (Figs 19.46 to 19.48) by sonography.

Congenital uterine anomalies can cause numerous clinical symptoms such as dysmenorrhea, metrorrhagia, repeated spontaneous abortions and infertility. Conventional B-mode sonography can detect all kinds of uterine anomalies (Figs 19.49 to 19.52), but accurate detection should be performed with three-dimensional sonography (Figs 19.53 to 19.60).

By conventional B-mode sonography, the diagnosis of uterine abnormalities is based on clear visualization of the uterine cavity echo in transverse section. In cases involving a suspected uterine anomaly the examination should be done in the secretory phase of the cycle when the endometrium is highly echogenic and clearly visualized. The uterine anomaly is then recognized as the presence of two separated uterine cavities (uterus bicornis, uterus duplex) or as the splitting of the single endometrial echo in the upper portions of the uterus in transverse section (uterus arcuatus).

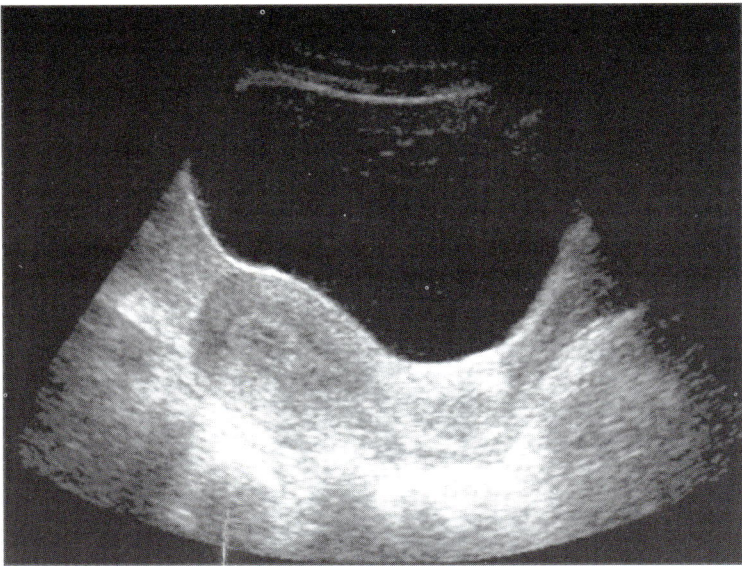

Fig. 19.1: The scan of a normal uterus and vagina. The uterus is anteverted. The corpus of the uterus is larger than the cervix

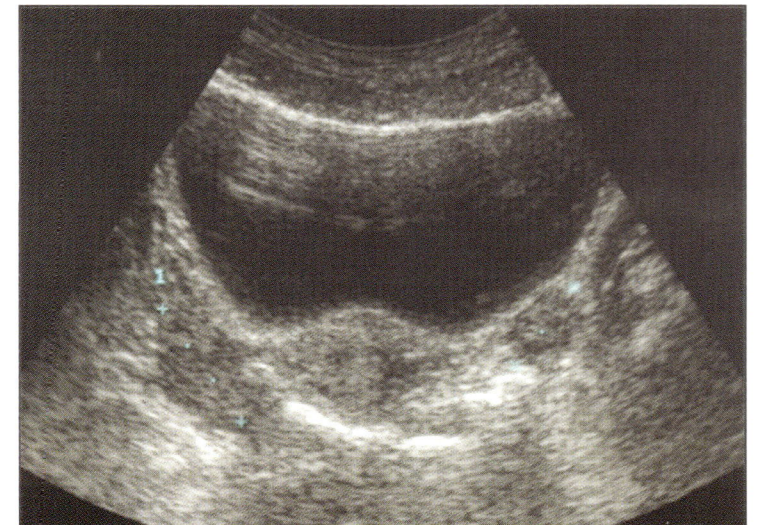

Fig. 19.2: The scan of a normal uterus and vagina. The uterus is in indifferent position

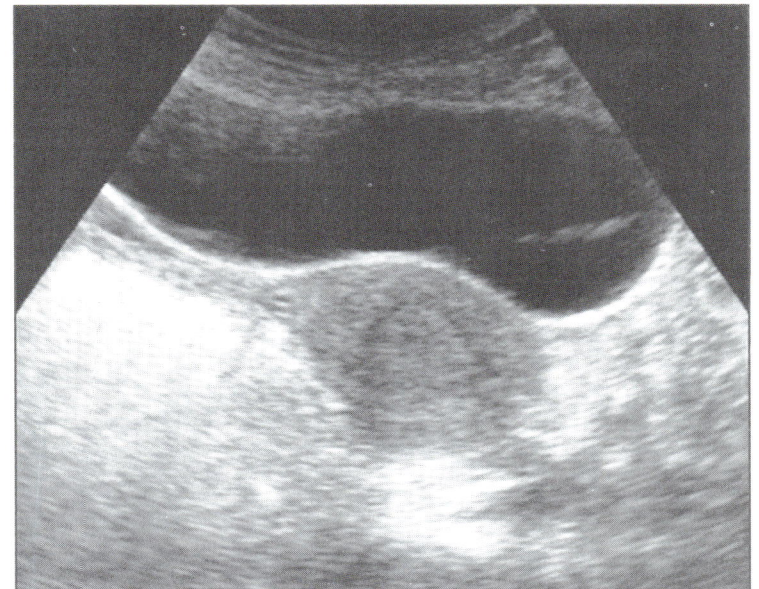

Fig. 19.3: The scan of a normal uterus and vagina. The uterus is retroverted. The corpus of the uterus is larger than the cervix

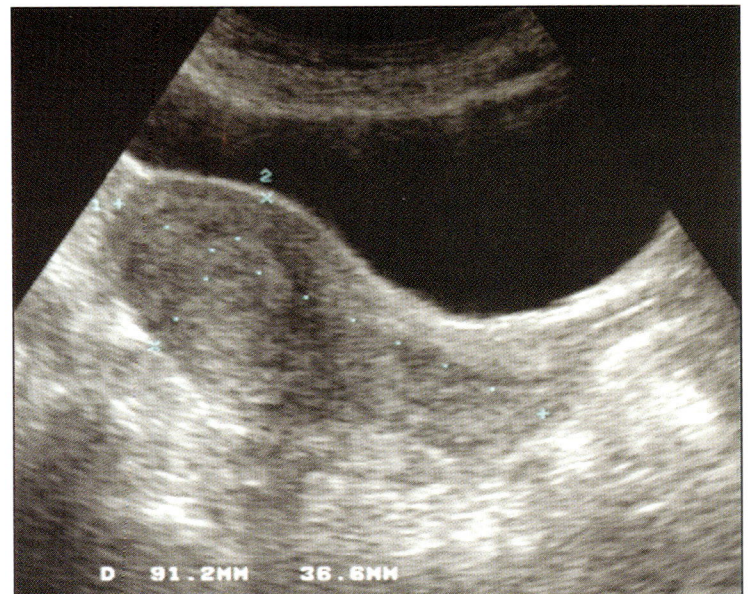

Fig. 19.4: Longitudinal sonogram of a normal uterus. The cavity and endocervical canal is clearly visible

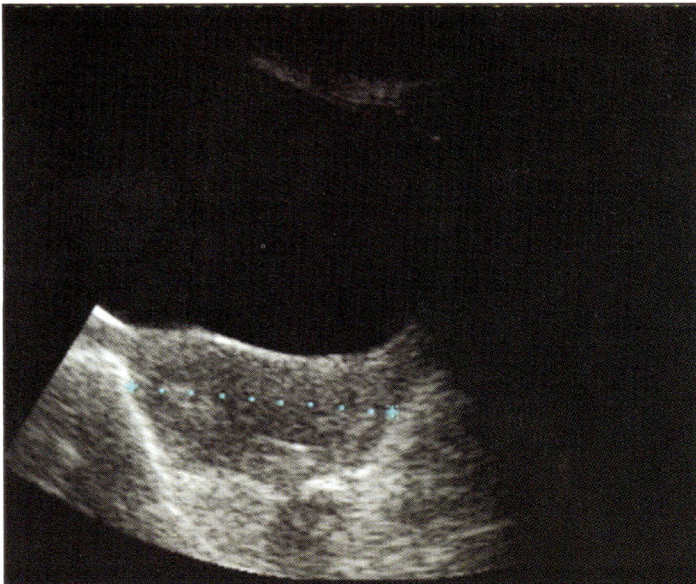

Fig. 19.5: Transverse sonogram of a normal uterus. The contour is clearly outlined and the pattern of myometrium displays homogeneous and moderate echogenicity. The central cavity is clearly visible

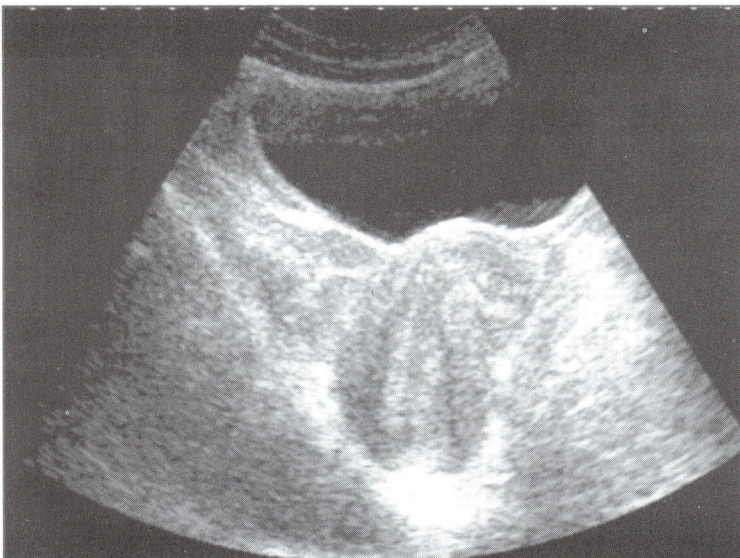

Fig. 19.6: Transverse sonogram of a normal uterus and ovaries. Both ovaries are seen in close proximity to the uterus

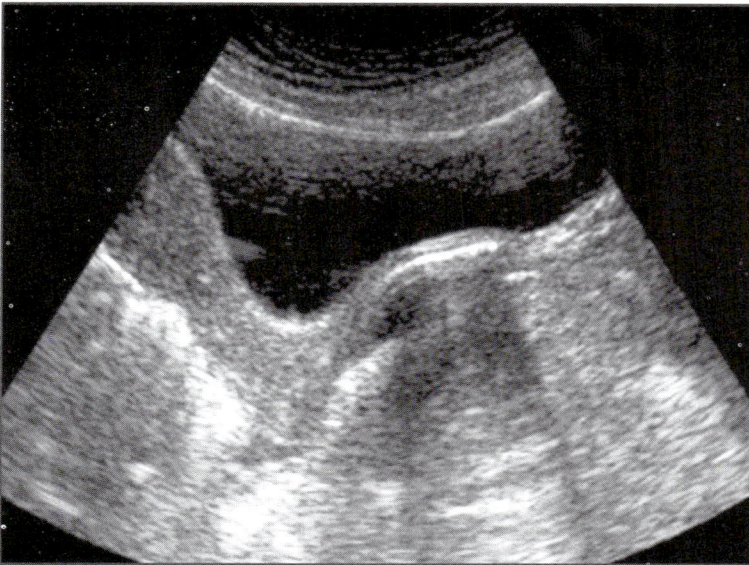

Fig. 19.7: Longitudinal scan of the uterus and vagina. We can see the vaginal tampon, note the shadowing below

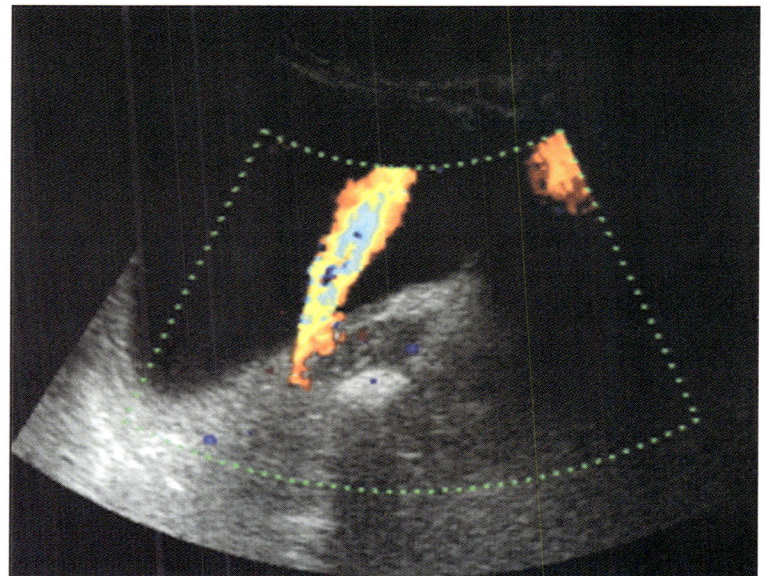

Fig. 19.8: Longitudinal scan of the ovaries. We can see the normal pattern and size of the ovaries

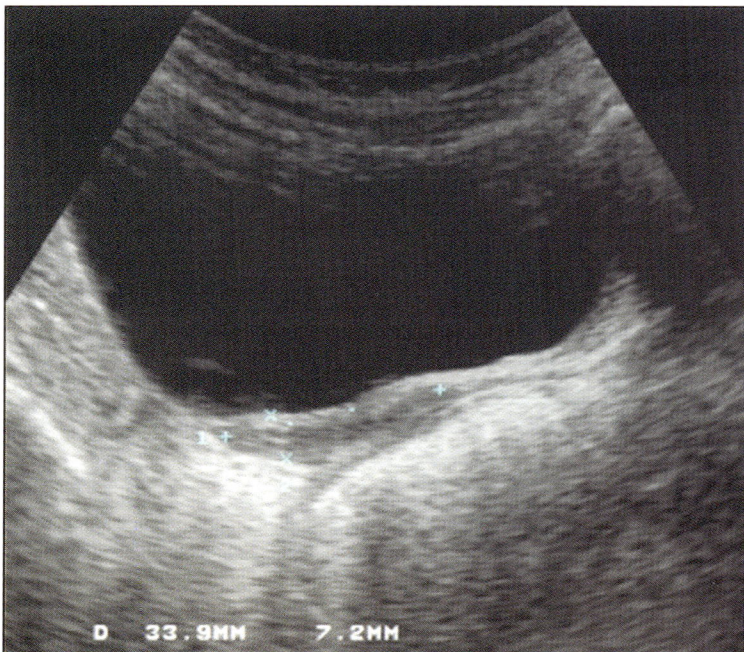

Fig. 19.9: Hypoplastic uterus. The endometrium is hardly recognizable

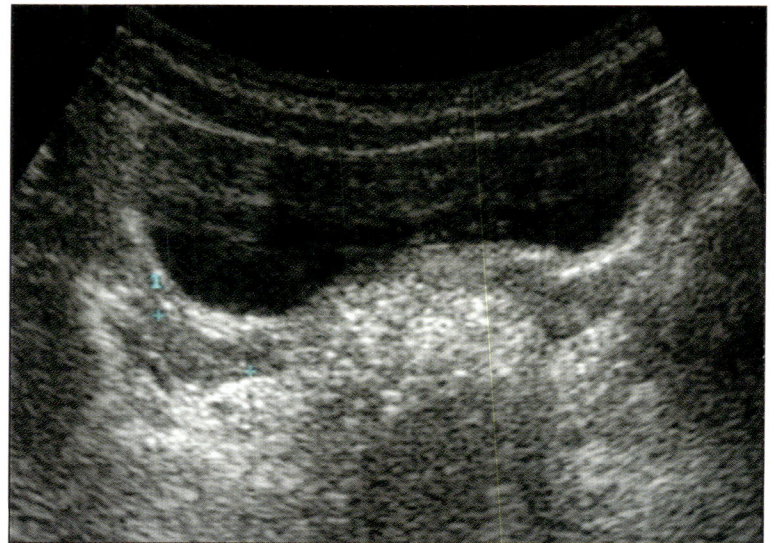

Fig. 19.10: Transverse sonogram of prepubertal patient. Both ovaries are visualized

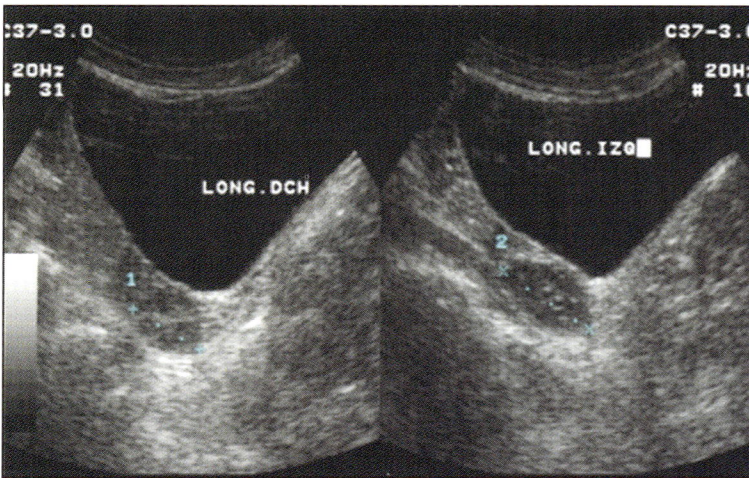

Fig. 19.11: Longitudinal scan with full bladder and color Doppler, we can see ureteral "jet"

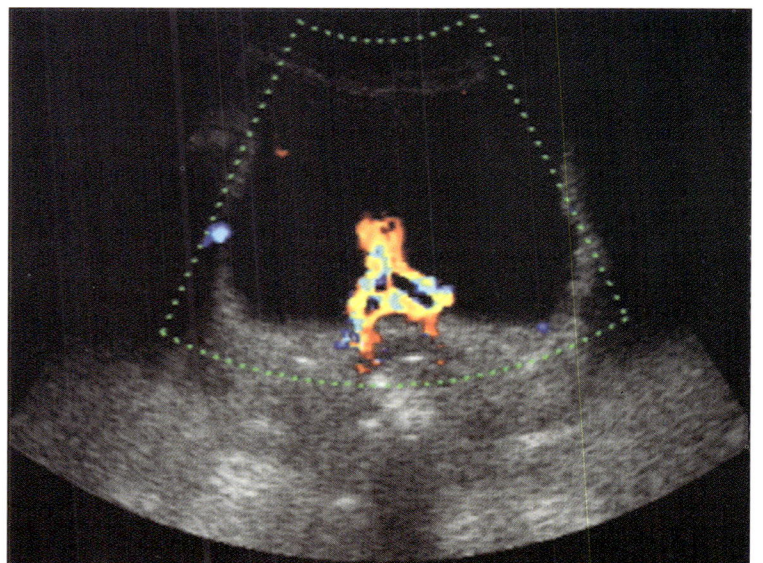

Fig. 19.12: Transversal scan with full bladder and color Doppler, that shows both right and left ureteral "jets"

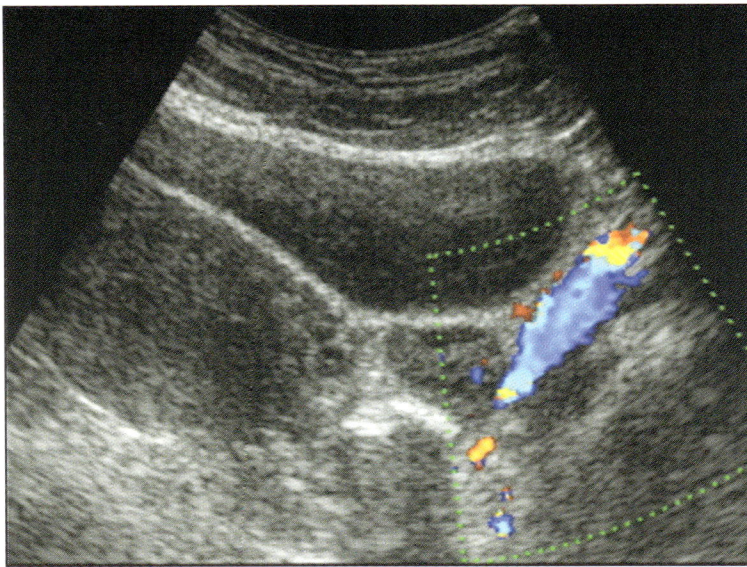

Fig. 19.13: Transversal scan with full bladder. Color Doppler shows left iliac artery behind ovary

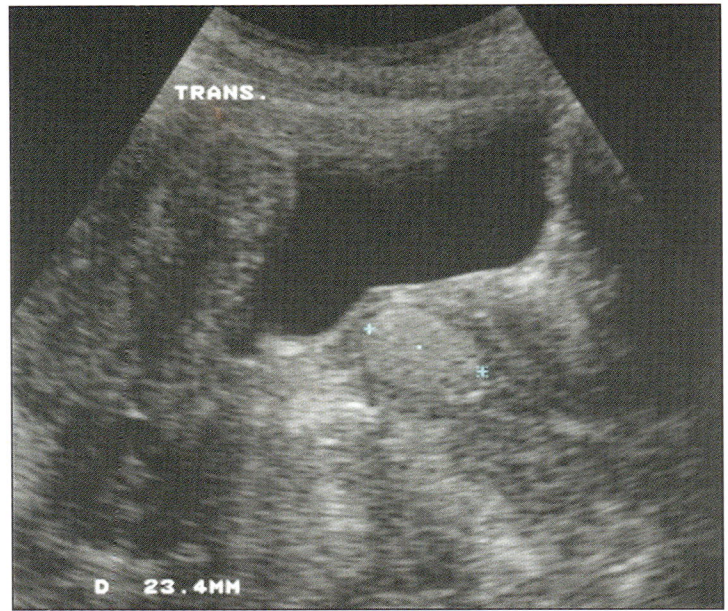

Fig. 19.16: Transversal scan with full bladder, that shows a echogenic vaginal nodule

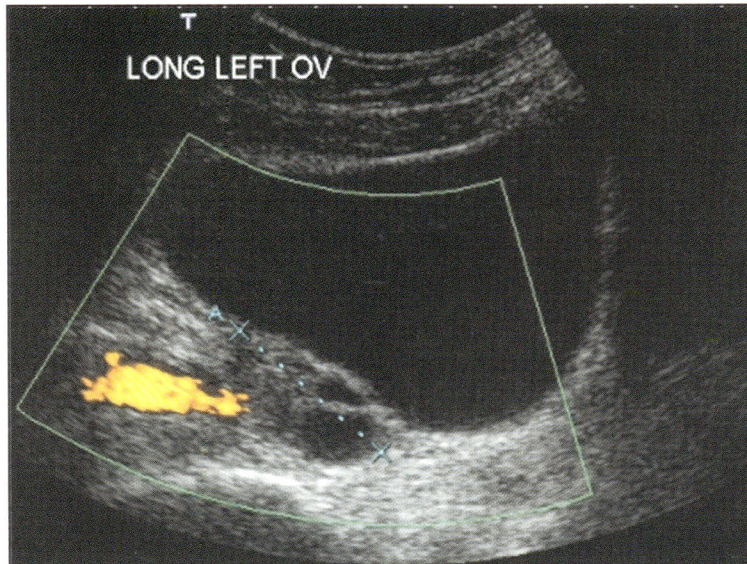

Fig. 19.14: Longitudinal scan with full bladder. We can see the left external iliac vessels, they are a good marker for the location of the ovaries

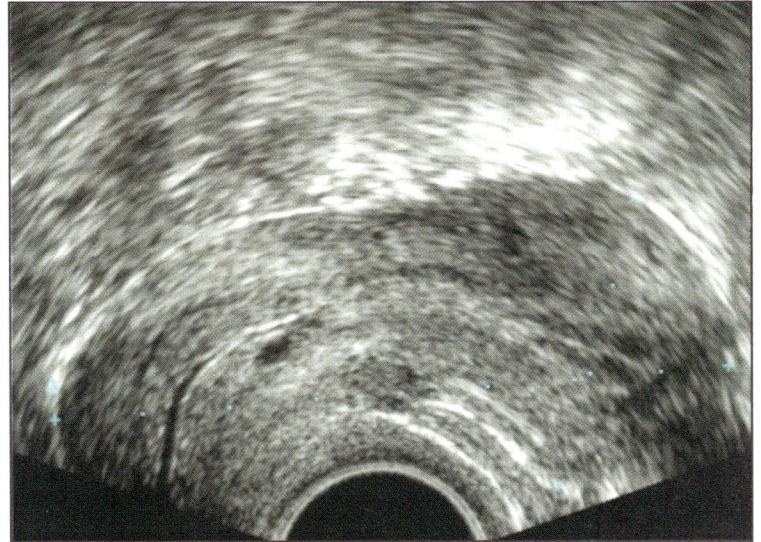

Fig. 19.17: Longitudinal scan of the uterus. Only examiner can interpret posititition of the uterus, depending on the level of rotation of transducer

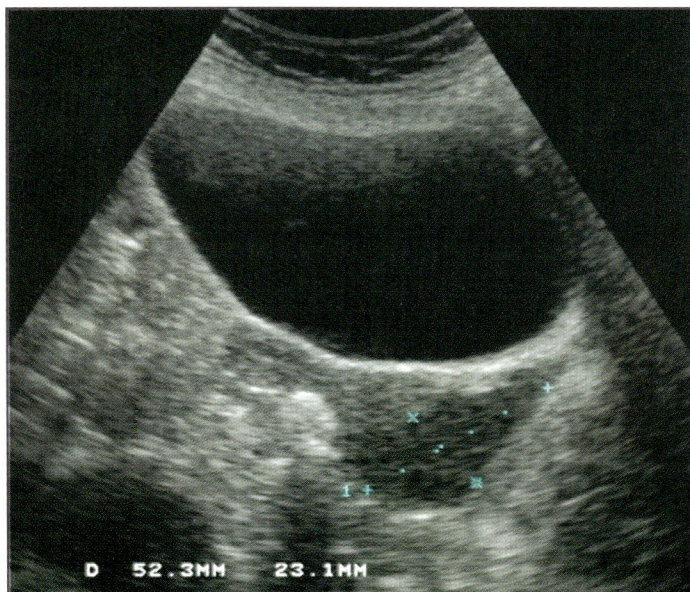

Fig. 19.15: Longitudinal sonogram with full bladder. We can show a vaginal cyst

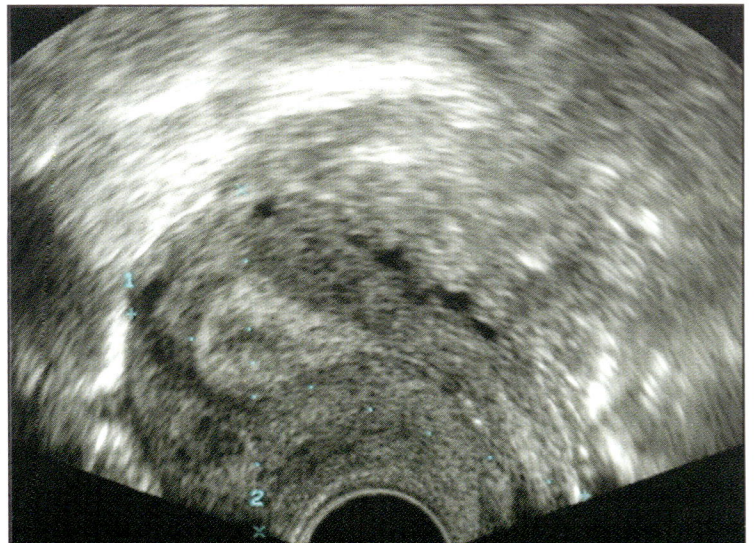

Fig. 19.18: Longitudinal sonogram that shows a retroverted uterus

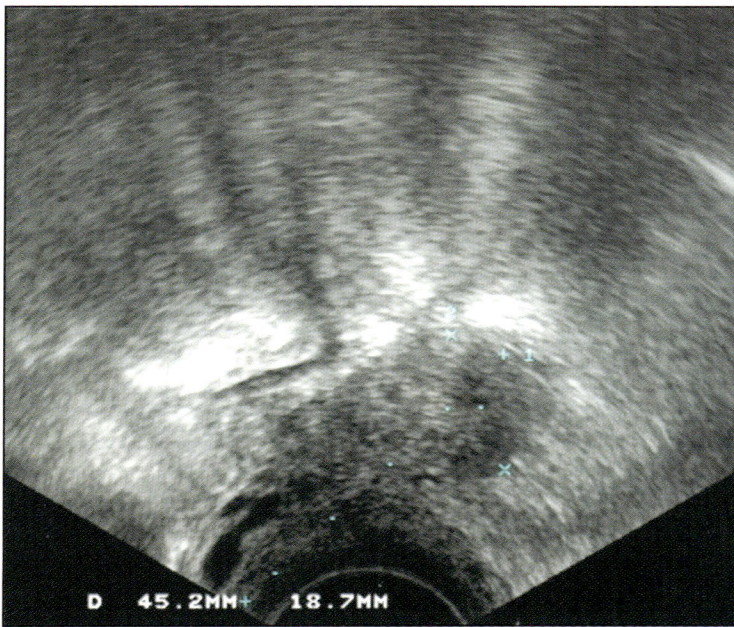

Fig. 19.19: Hypoplastic uterus

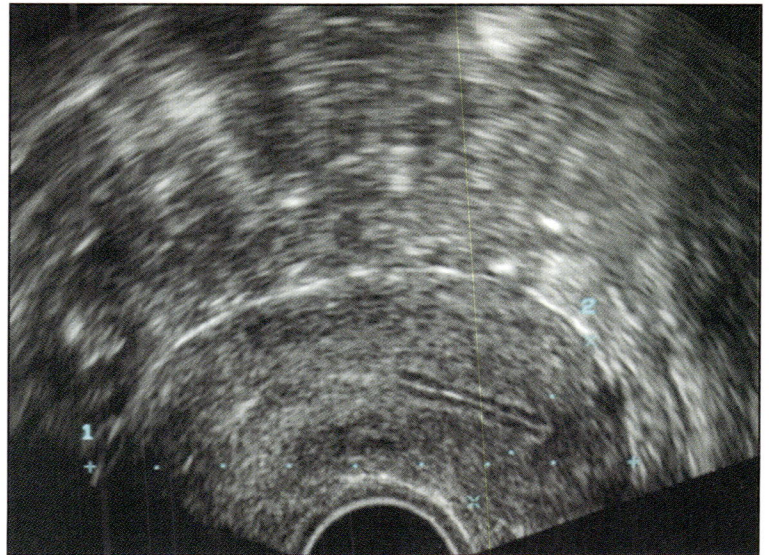

Fig. 19.22: Longitudinal sonogram of the folicullar endometrium

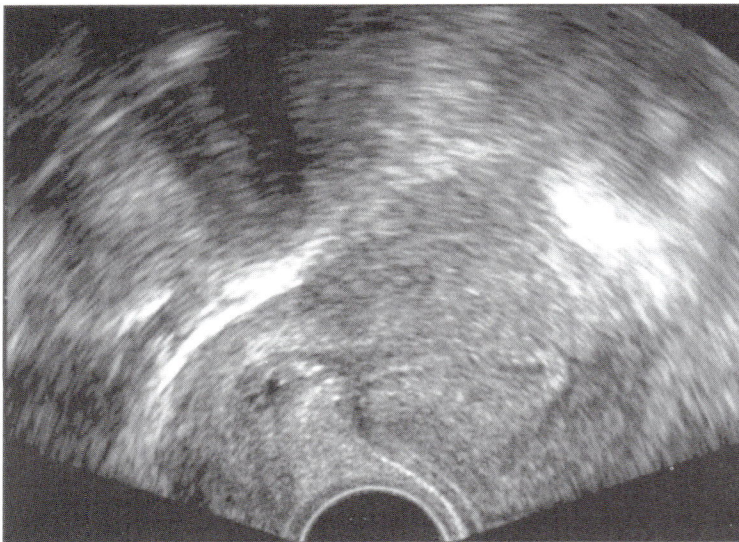

Fig. 19.20: Longitudinal scan of the uterus. We can see a scar after cesarean section

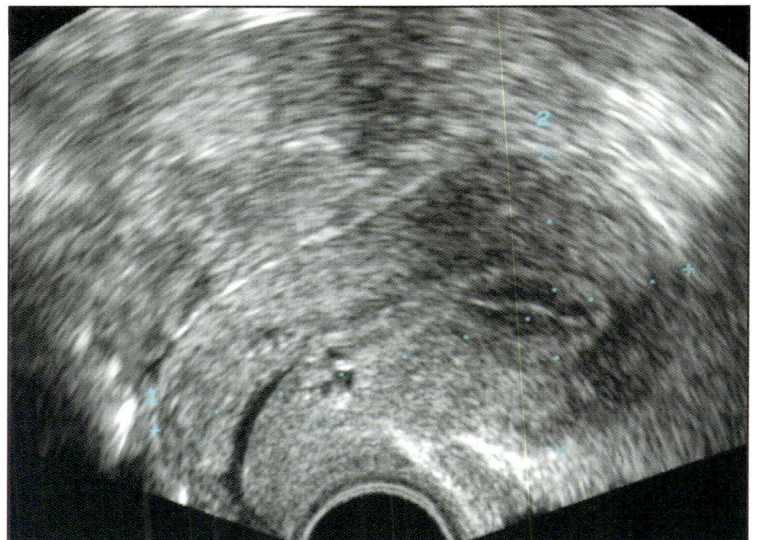

Fig. 19.23: Transvaginal scan of longitudinal uterus, demonstrating the triple-line endometrium

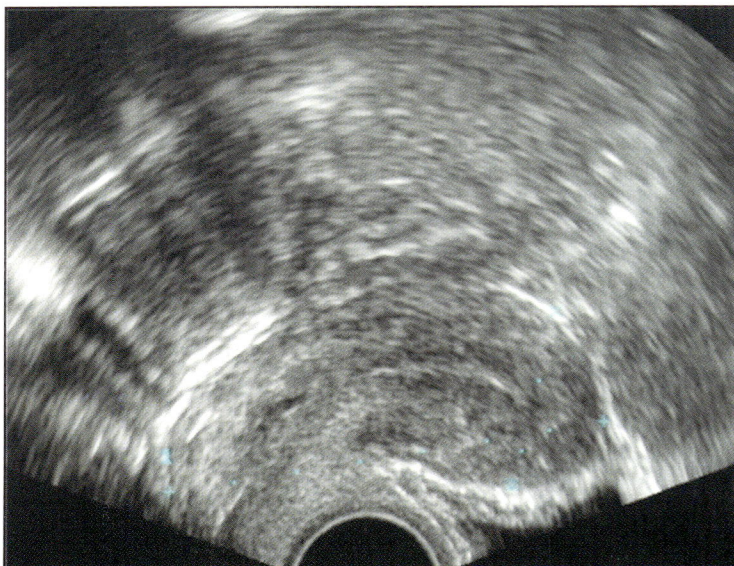

Fig. 19.21: Transvaginal longitudinal sonogram of the uterus shows a earlier follicular phase of the endometrium

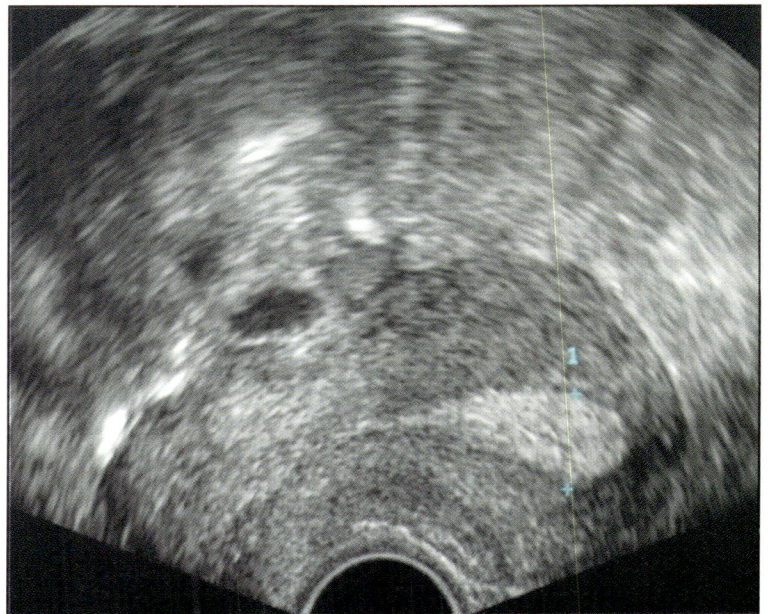

Fig. 19.24: Longitudinal scan of the secretory endometrium

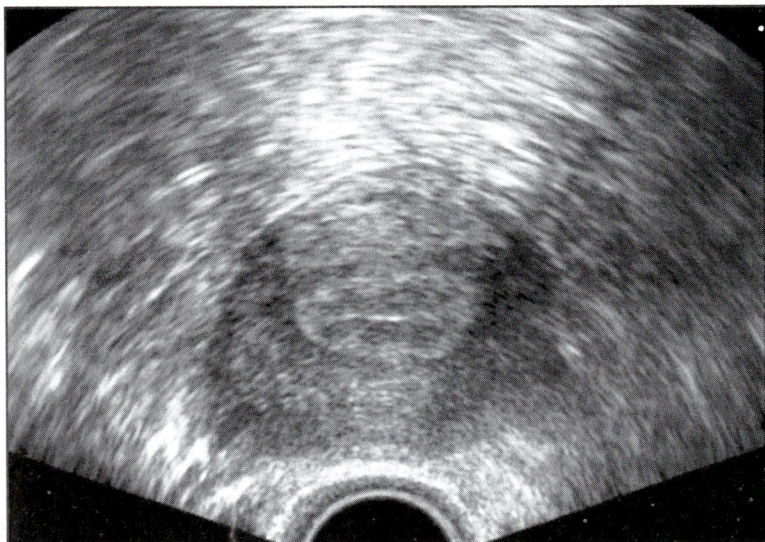

Fig. 19.25: Transversal scan of endometrium that shows preovulatory ring, typical sign of forthcoming ovulation

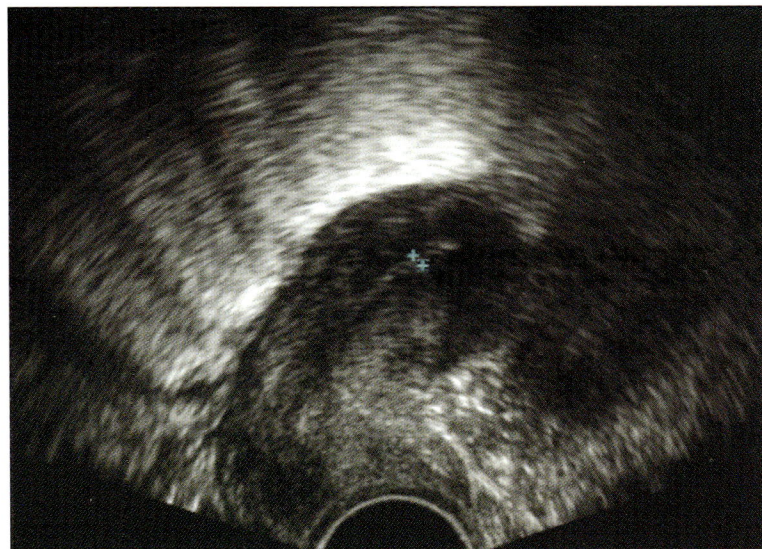

Fig. 19.28: Longitudinal sonogram of the uterus in postmenopausal patient. Note the thinness of the endometrium

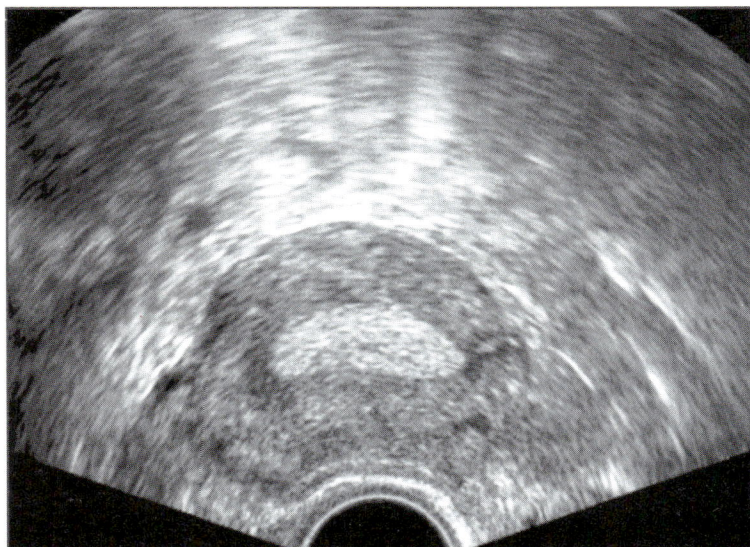

Fig. 19.26: Transversal sonogram of secretory endometrium

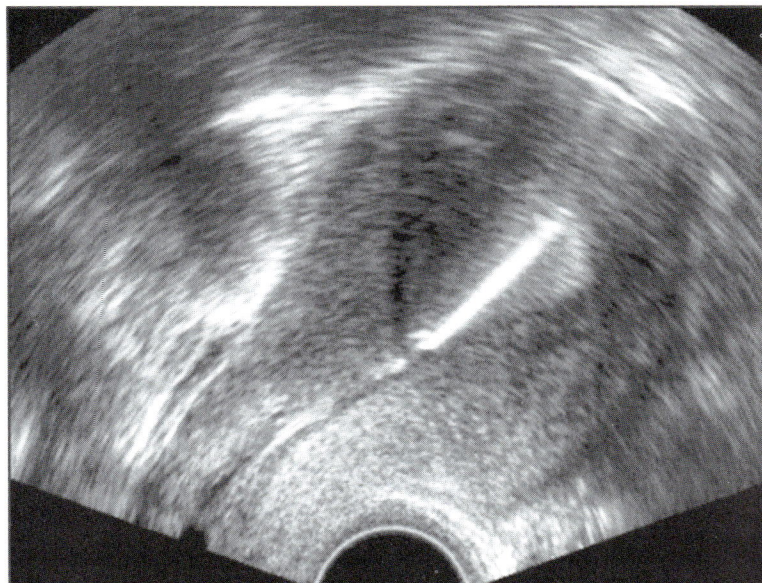

Fig. 19.29: Transvaginal scan of longitudinal uterus that shows a correct placed intrauterine device (IUD)

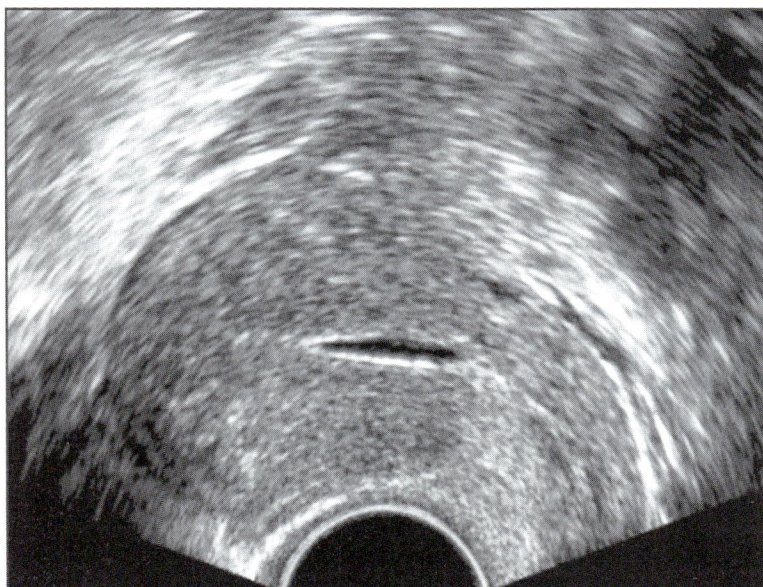

Fig. 19.27: Longitudinal scan of the menstrual endometrium

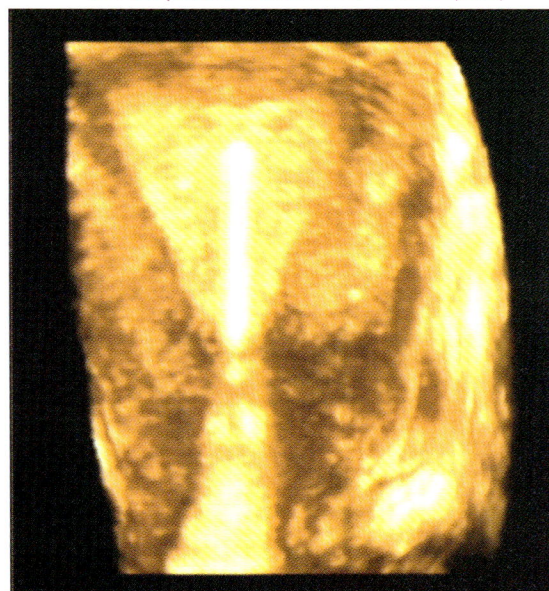

Fig. 19.30: Three-dimensional scan. We can see the endometrial cavity with the intrauterine device (IUD) correctly placed

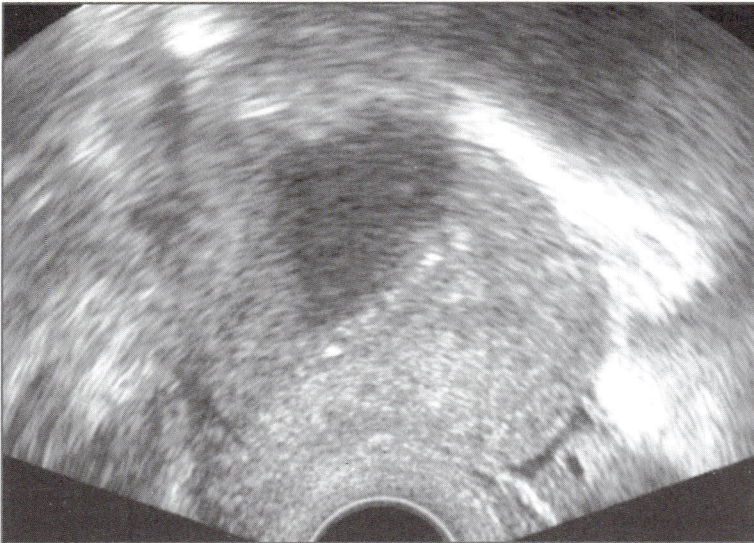

Fig. 19.31: Longitudinal sonogram of the uterus that shows a shadowing of Mirena™ possibililily for identification of IUD

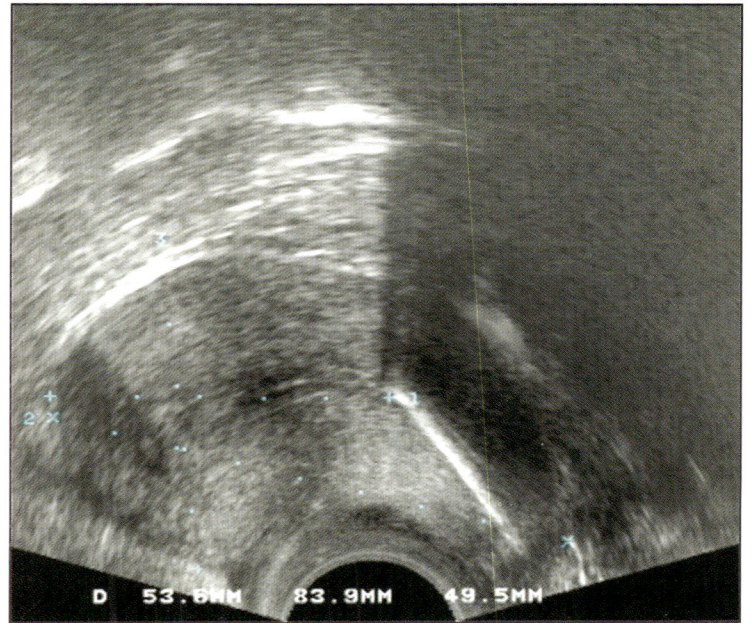

Fig. 19.34: Partially expelled intrauterine device (IUD)

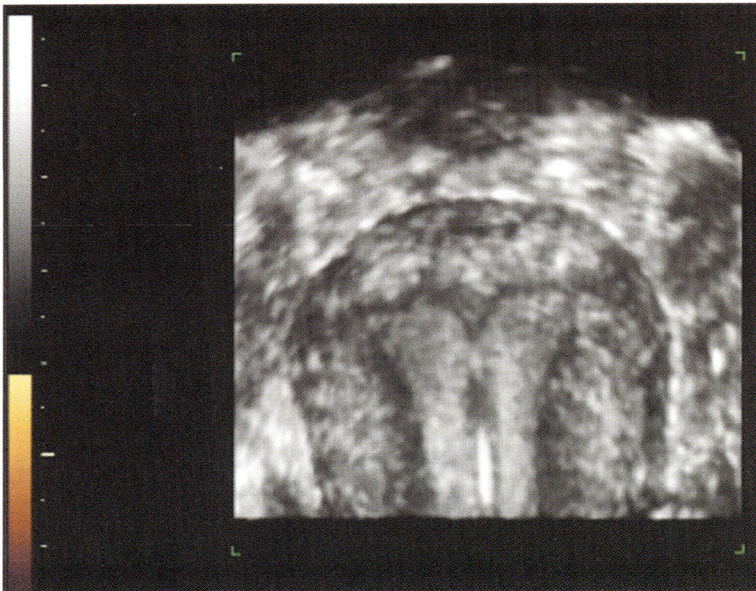

Fig. 19.32: Three-dimensional scan demonstrating Mirena™ intrauterine device correctly placed

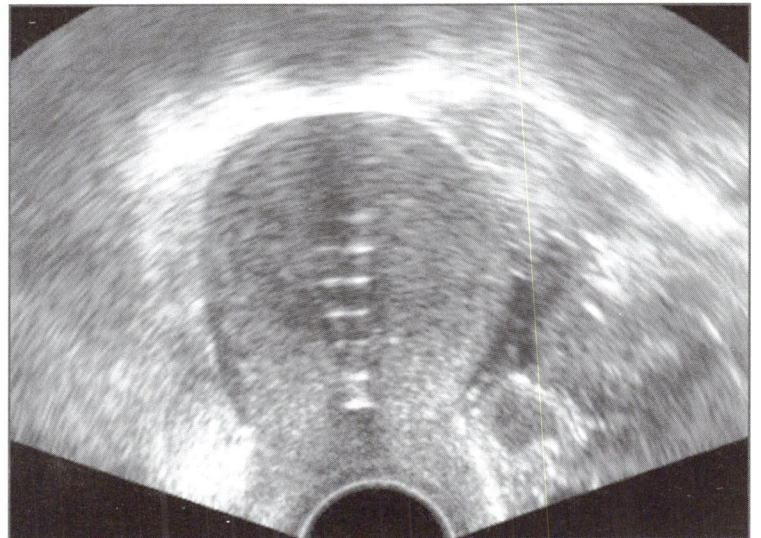

Fig. 19.35: Transvaginal sonogram demonstrating an intrauterine device Ginefix™ correctly placed. The rings one by one, can be calculated from the image

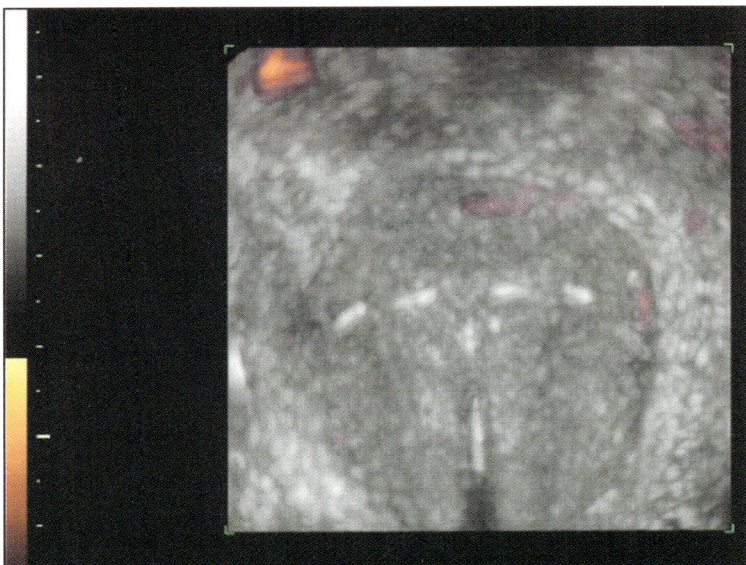

Fig. 19.33: Three-dimensional scan (Render Mode) shows a correct placed intrauterine Mirena™ device

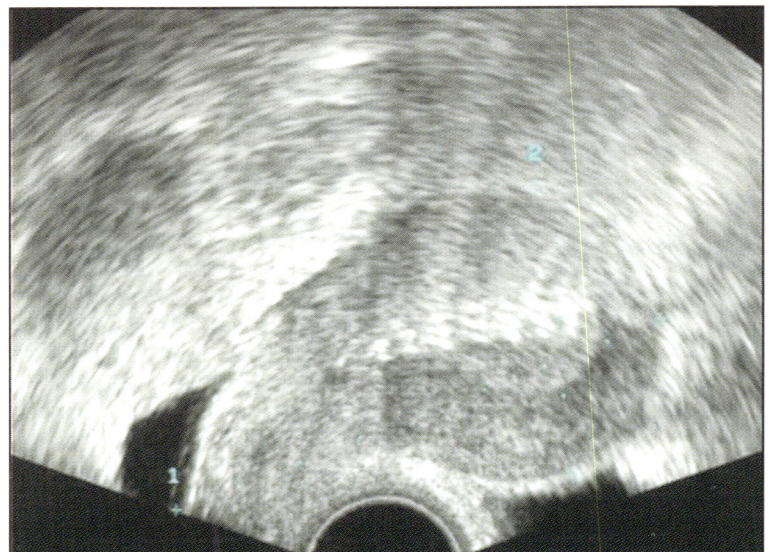

Fig. 19.36: Another transvaginal scan showing a correctly placed intrauterine device Ginefix™

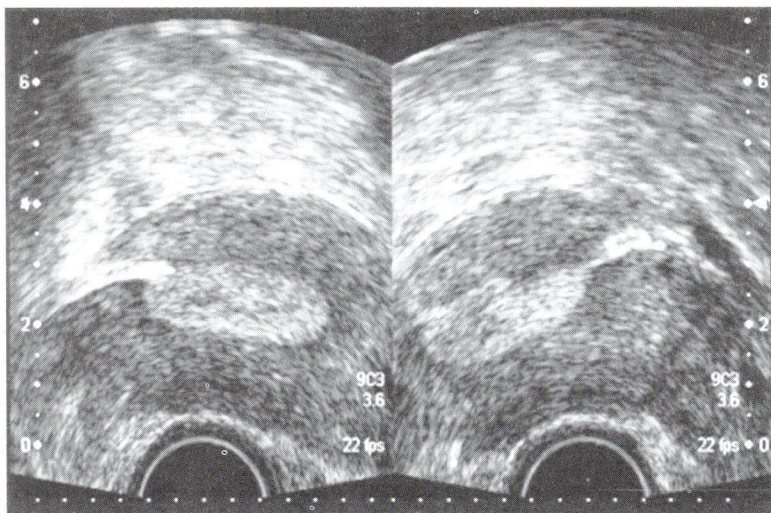

Fig. 19.37: Transversal sonogram showing correctly placed the tubarics device Essure™

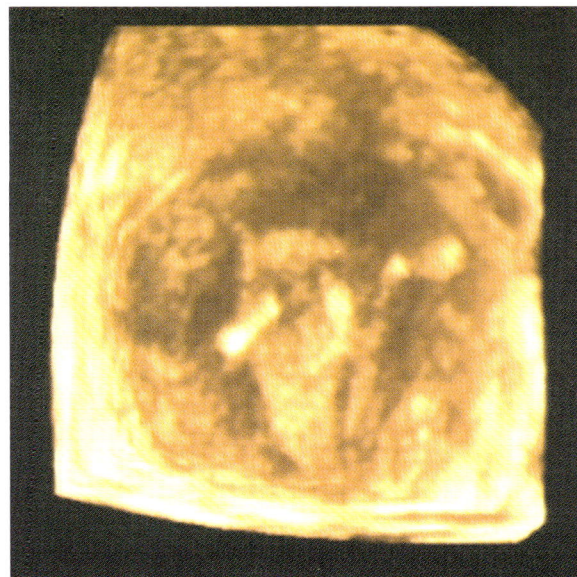

Fig. 19.38: Three-dimensional scan demonstrating very clear the correct position of tubarics device Essure™. We can see the detail of the rings that performed device

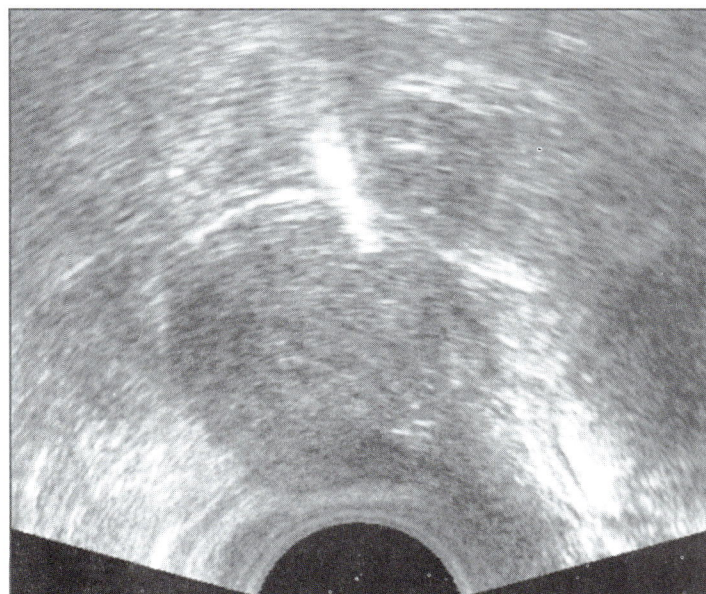

Fig. 19.39: Three-dimensional scan shows a detail of right tubaric device

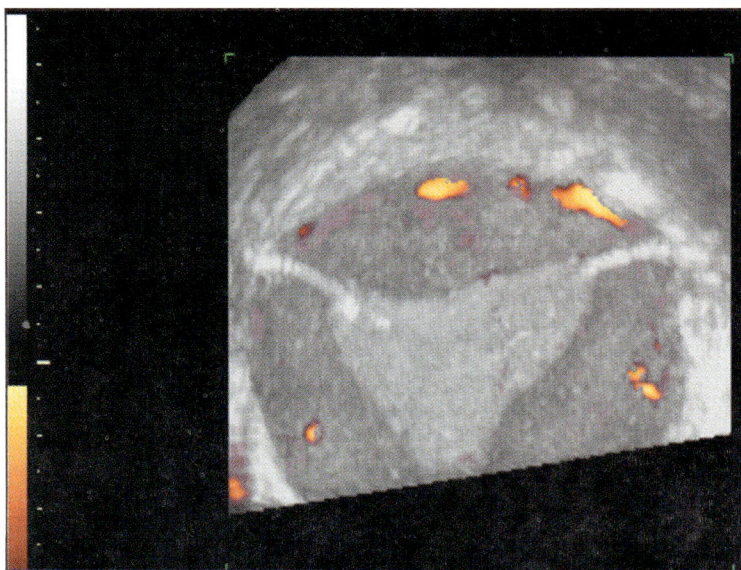

Fig. 19.40: Three-dimensional scan demonstrating conventional IUD piercing in the right myometrium

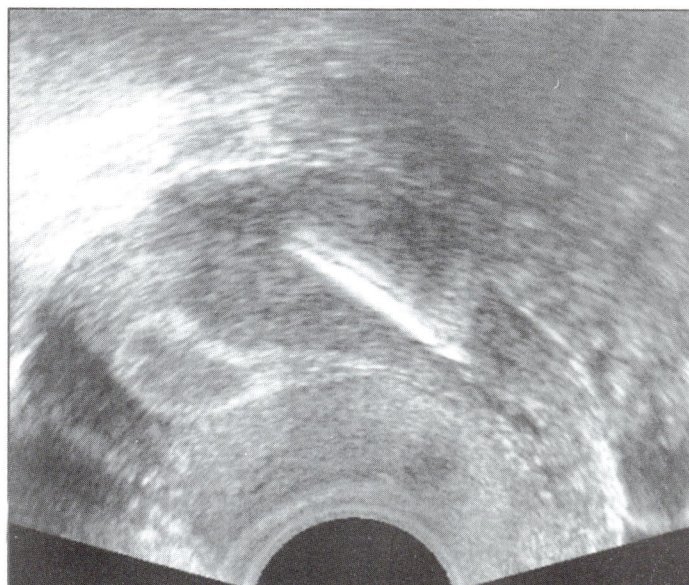

Fig. 19.41: Transvaginal sonogram of retroverted uterus that shows a IUD emigrated partially out of myometrium

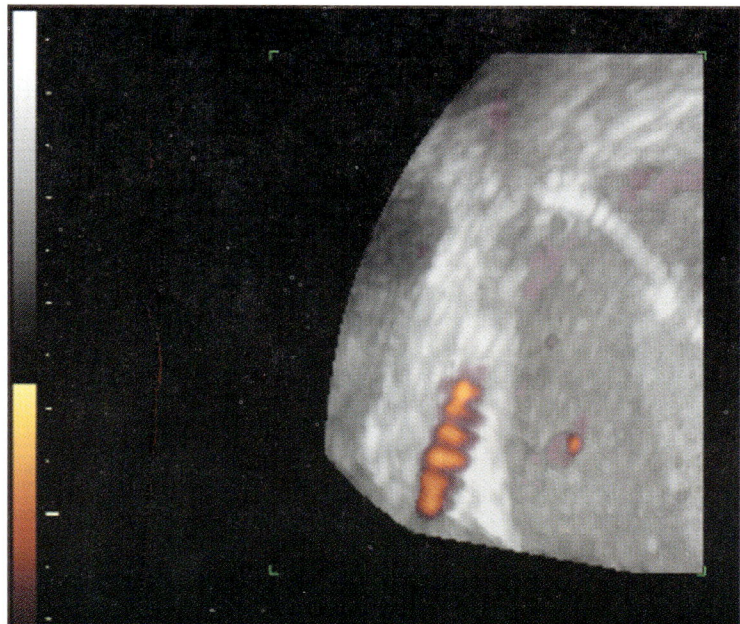

Fig. 19.42: Transvaginal sonogram of retroverted uterus. We can see IUD totally piercing into anterior wall of myometrium

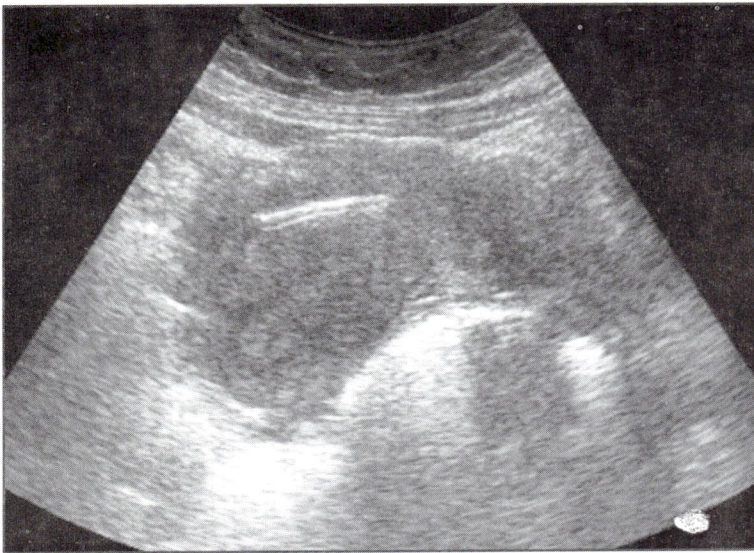

Fig. 19.43: Abdominal sonogram of the same case of Figure 19.15. that shows a IUD pierces into myometrium

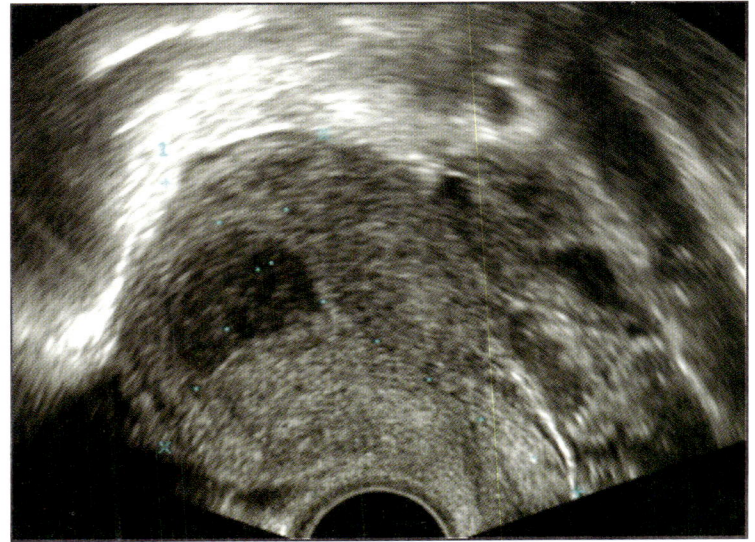

Fig. 19.46: Transvaginal sonogram shows a hematometra

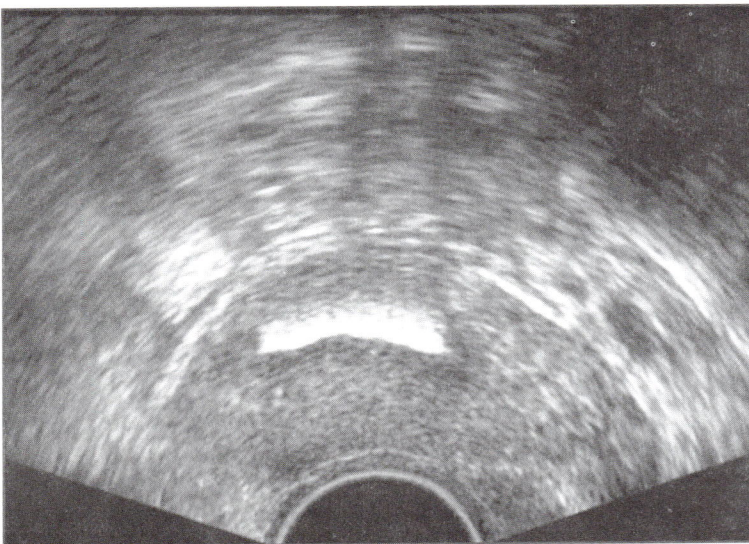

Fig. 19.44: Transvaginal sonogram that shows a high echogenicity lineal image into the endometrial cavity. Hysteroscopy reveals that is a bone metaplasia

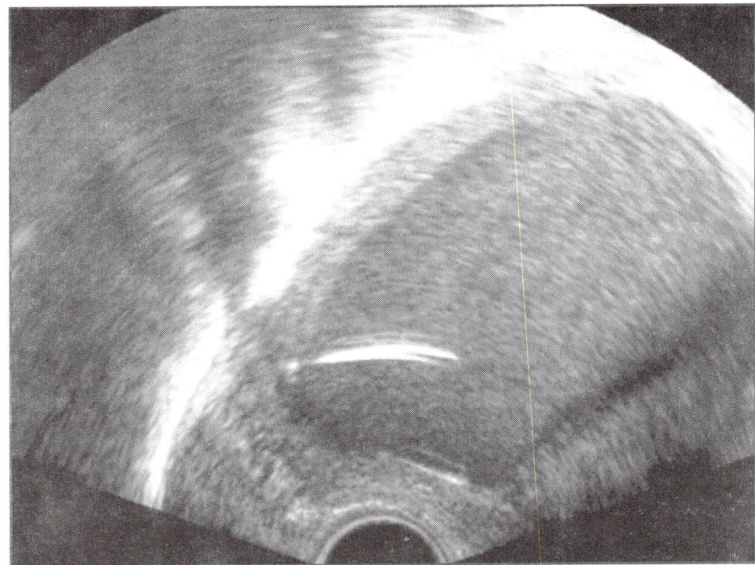

Fig. 19.47: Another case of hematometra, in these cases with an intrauterine device (IUD)

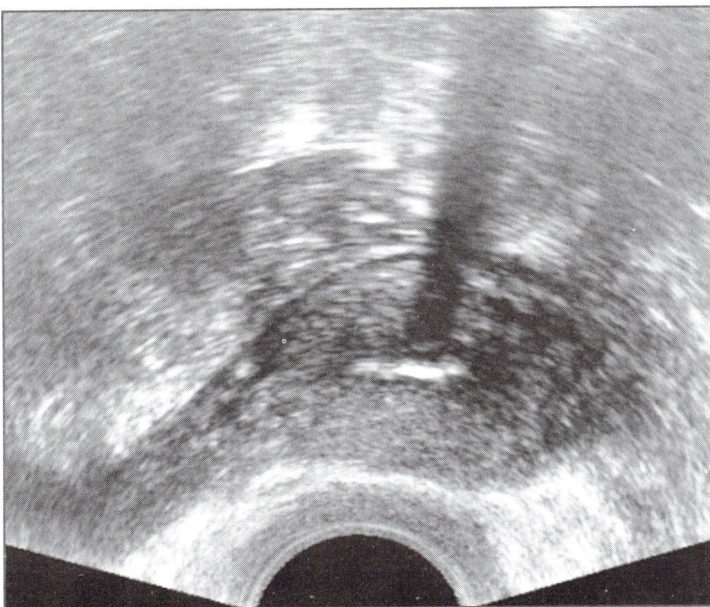

Fig. 19.45: Another example of bone metaplasia

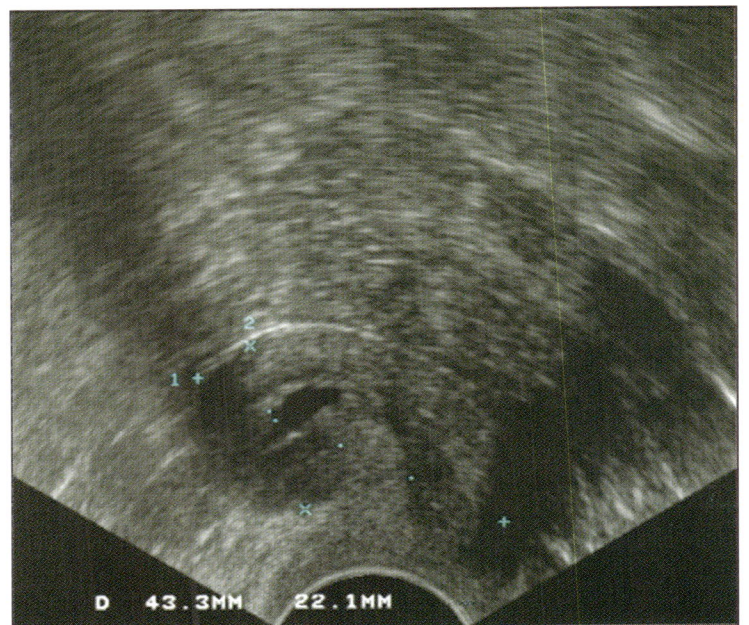

Fig. 19.48: Longitudinal scan of the uterus shows a mucous contents within the cavity. These findings are frequently in postmenopausal patients

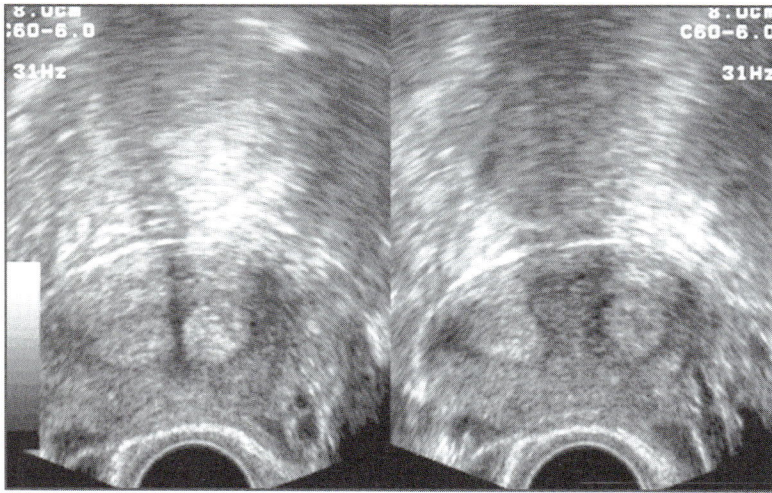

Fig. 19.49: Transvaginal scan showing a septate uterus

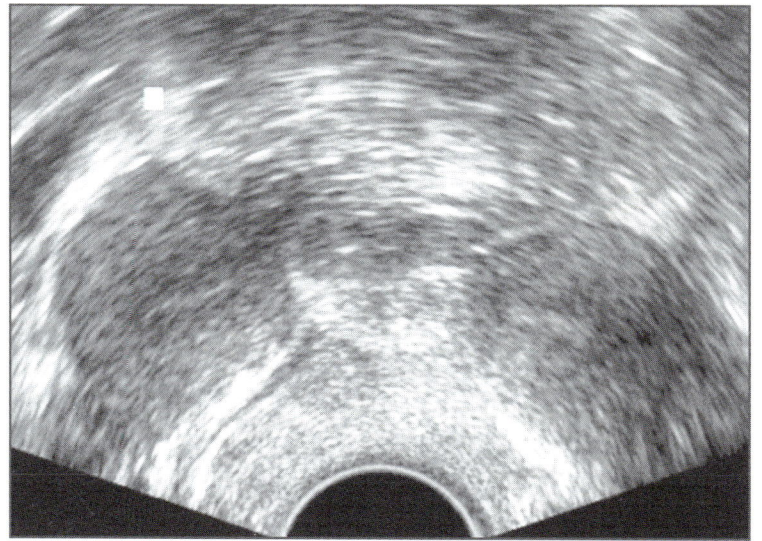

Fig. 19.50: Uterus bicornis unicollis: The transverse section displays two distinct cavities and two uterine horns

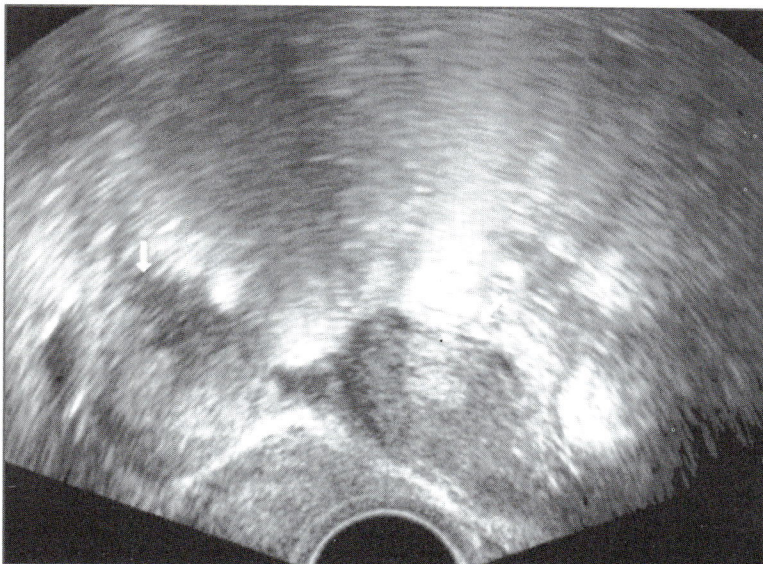

Fig. 19.51: Transverse sonogram of the uterus didelphis: Two uterine bodies and two separate uterine cavities are demonstrated

The diagnosis of Nabothian cysts which are demonstrated as a highly echogenic cysts close to the endocervical canal (Figs 19.61 to 19.62).

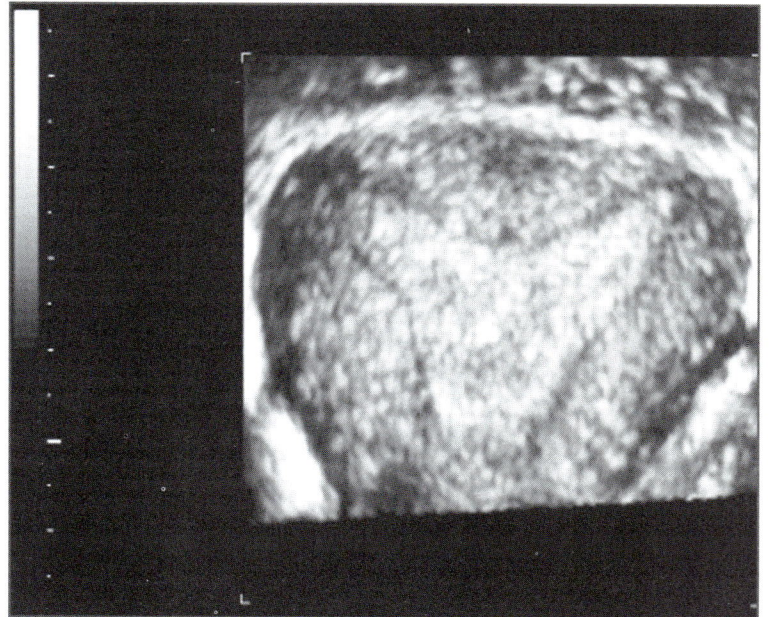

Fig. 19.52: Another example of the uterus didelphis, we can see two uterine bodies

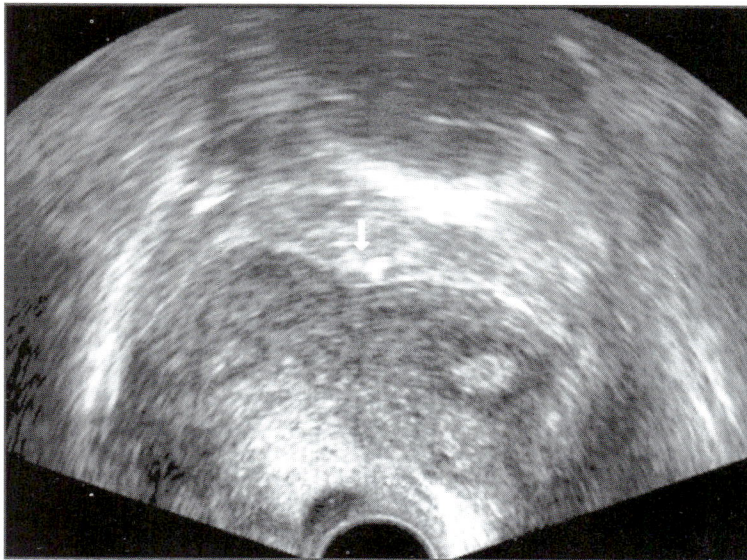

Fig. 19.53: Three-dimensional scan of arcuatus uterus

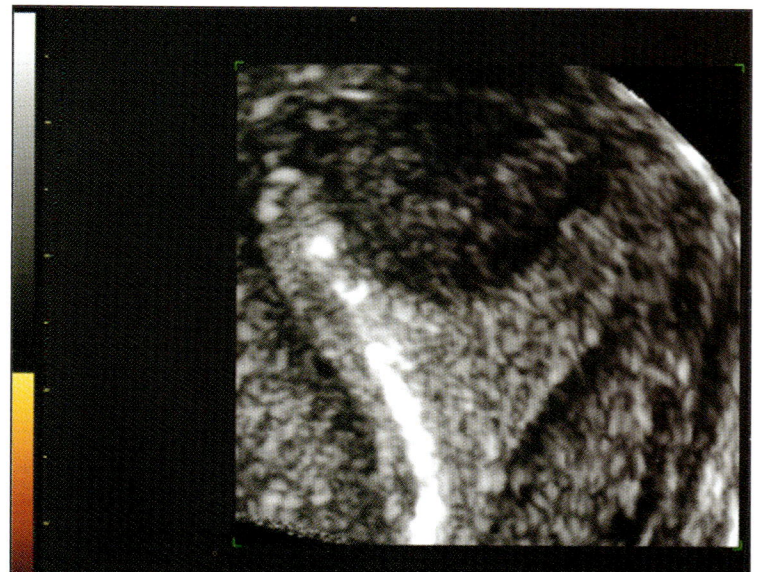

Fig. 19.54: Three-dimensional scan of arcuatus uterus. We can see correctly placed a intrauterine device (IUD) in the right horn

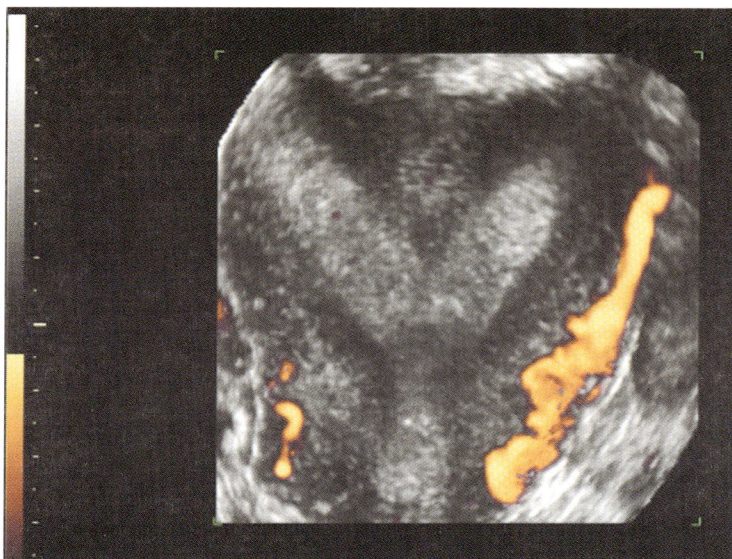

Fig. 19.55: Three-dimensional scan of subseptate uterus

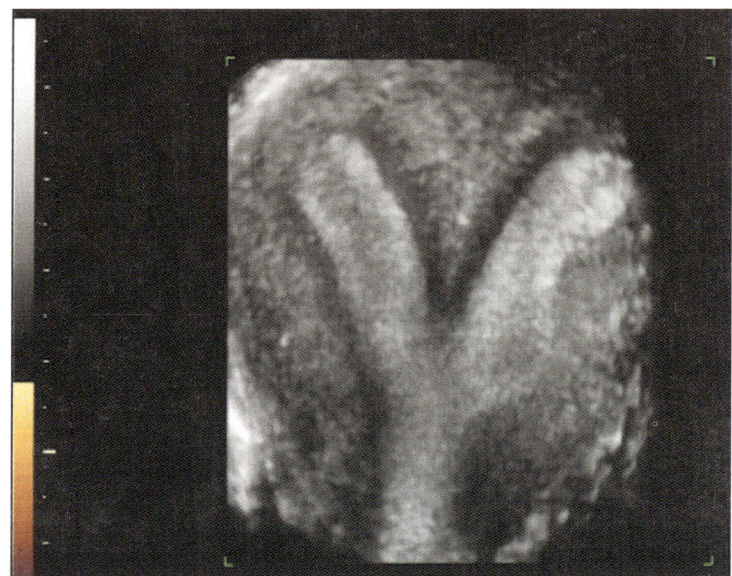

Fig. 19.58: The same case Figure 19.57. Volumen calculation (VOCAL™) with wire-mesh surface reconstruction

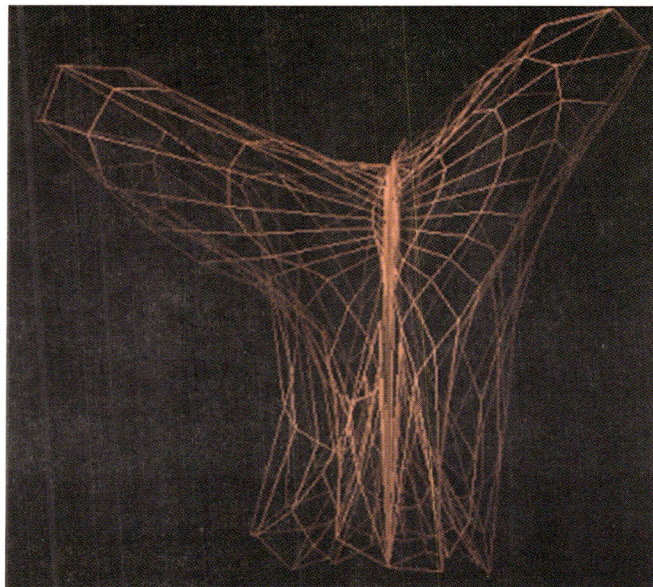

Fig. 19.56: Three-dimensional scan of septate uterus that shows two separate uterine cavities and one uterine body

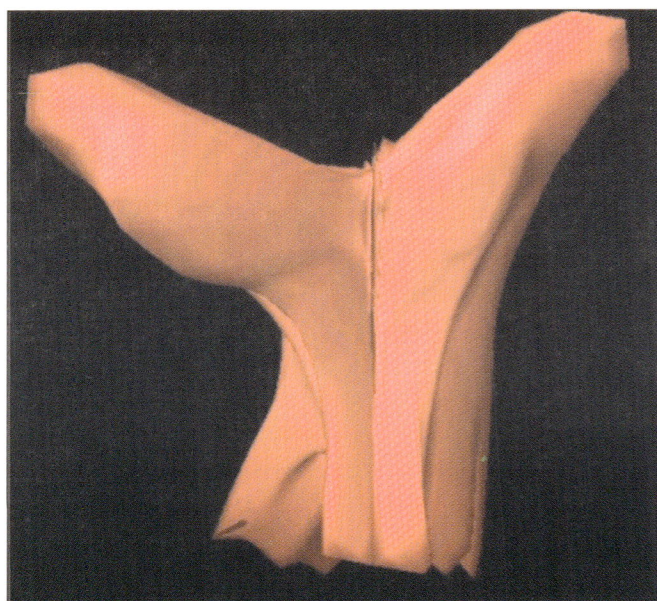

Fig. 19.59: Transversal scan shows a unicornis uterus

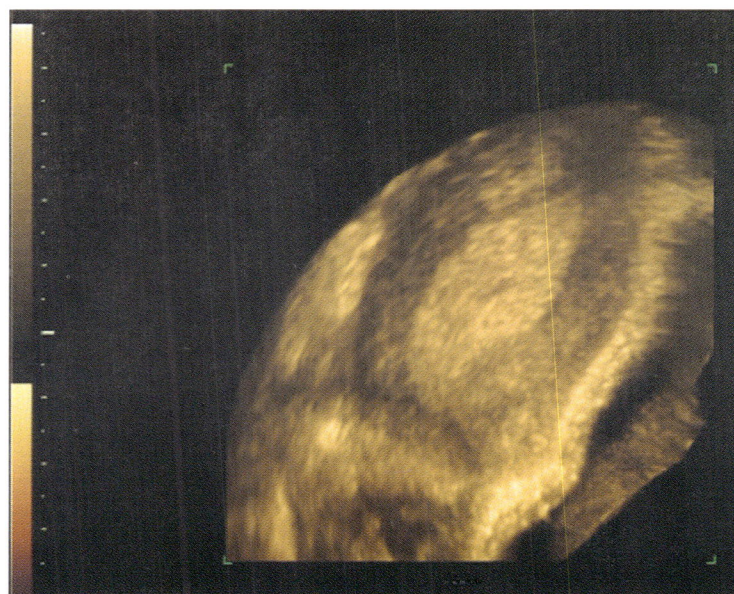

Fig. 19.57: Three-dimensional vaginal sonography. Volumen calculation (VOCAL™) of the subseptus uterus with skin surface reconstruction

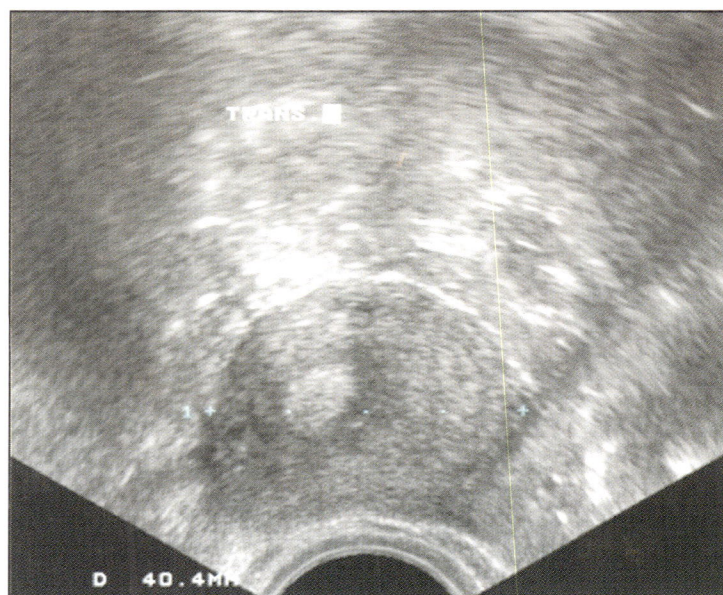

Fig. 19.60: Three-dimensional scan shows unicornis uterus

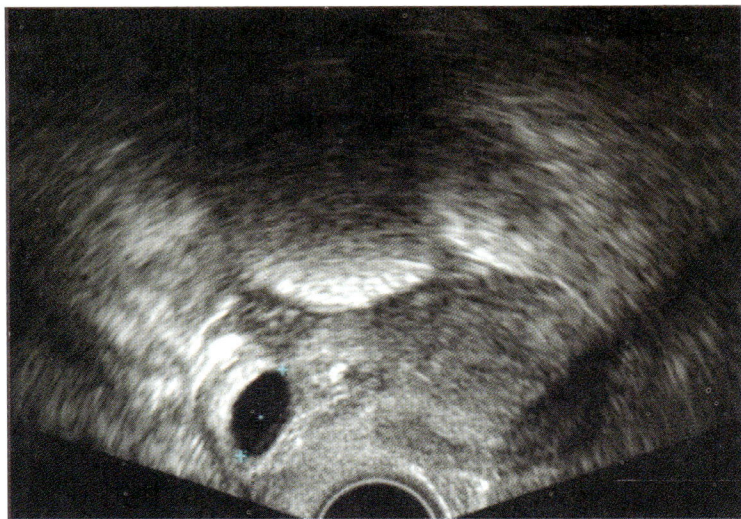

Fig. 19.61: Longitudinal section of the uterus shows the cervix with retention cyst (Nabothian cyst)

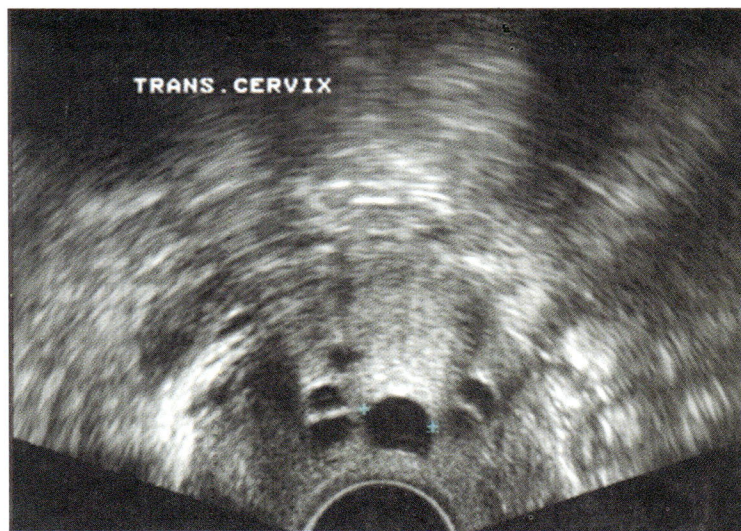

Fig. 19.62: Transversal scan with nabothian cysts in both the anterior and posterior labia

More information can be obtained using color or power Doppler ultrasound than can be gained from morphological study alone. Combination of high quality B-mode images, pulsed and color or power Doppler produces a simultaneous visualization of morphological and blood flow information from the female pelvic circulation.

Blood flow in the main pelvic vessels can be easily visualized and recognized (Figs 19.63 to 19.70). The artery and vein are distinguished according to the pulsation and brightness of color flow. The color Doppler signal from the main uterine vessels may be seen in all patients lateral to the cervix. The small branches of the uterine artery can be followed by searching the corpus uteri, ascending along the lateral wall. The resistance index depends on age, phase of menstrual cycle and any special conditions (e.g. pregnancy, tumor) and is usually very high.

The external iliac vessels are situated lateral to the ovary and present in prominent color due to high velocity blood flow. The

internal iliac vessels can be visualized easily in the entire population. They can be observed in the side wall of the pelvis, often lying deep close to the ovary. Both the internal and external iliac arteries produce prominent and pulsating color flow and very high impedance of flow.

Power Doppler three-dimensional ultrasound permits the visualization of vascular architecture (vessels and ramifications) (Fig. 19.71).

A small amount of free fluid can be observed in pouch of Douglas, specially during the ovulatory phase (Fig. 19.72).

Color Doppler sonography is very useful in distinguishing dilated pelvic veins shaping a pelvic congestion syndrom (Figs 19.73 and 19.74).

SONOGRAPHY OF THE ADNEXAL REGION

The adnexa consists of the broad ligament, fallopian tubes and ovaries. The broad ligament and fallopian tubes cannot be clearly distinguished by ultrasound under physiological conditions.

The normal ovary is relatively easy to detect by transvaginal sonography. Its appearance is characterized by the presence of the follicles or the corpus luteum in a premenopausal women. The ovary is usually located above and medially from the iliac vein (Figs 19.75 and 19.76). During the examination, the normal-sized ovary may change its location in the pelvis.

The vascularization of normally functioning ovaries can be detected by color Doppler sonography (Figs 19.77 to 19.84). Evaluation of follicular development by ultrasound is a well-established procedure in infertility treatment. Blood flow may be clearly visualized at the edge of the developing follicle. The appearance of the corpus luteum is well marked, and color flow is more easily obtainable from the ovarian tissue during the luteal phase. An abundant color pattern, displayed over the ovarian B-mode image, emphasizes the active corpus luteum even when the corpus luteum is not sonographically visible.

The most common type of cystic adnexal lesions are functional ovarian cysts (Figs 19.85 to 19.95). These are easily recognizable cysts structures with smooth thin walls and clear fluid content, usually unilateral. These cysts are originated from an unruptured follicle and are usually smaller than 10 cm. Pericystic vascularization shows moderate resistance to blood flow.

The corpus luteum cyst has numerous appearances when imaged transvaginally. Internal echoes created by the retracting clot make it difficult to distinguish from other benign and malignant ovarian tumors. The dimension of a persistent corpus luteum may exceeded 10 cm and its inner structure may appear liquid, solid, or both; it may contain septa or even papillae.

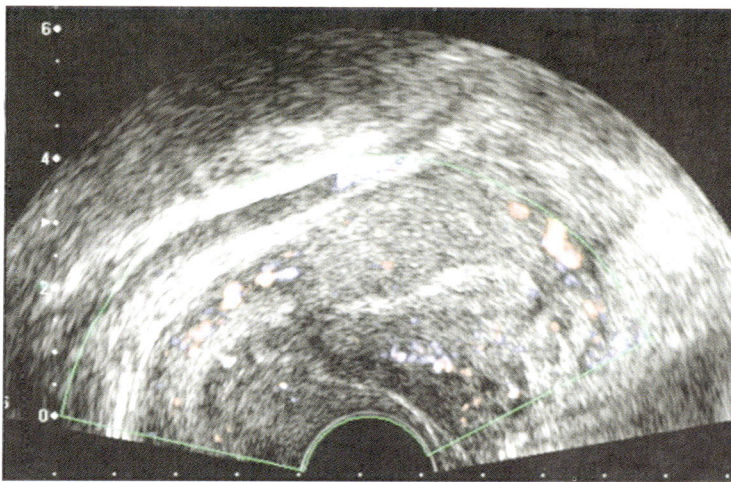

Fig. 19.63: Normal vascularization of non-pregnant uterus

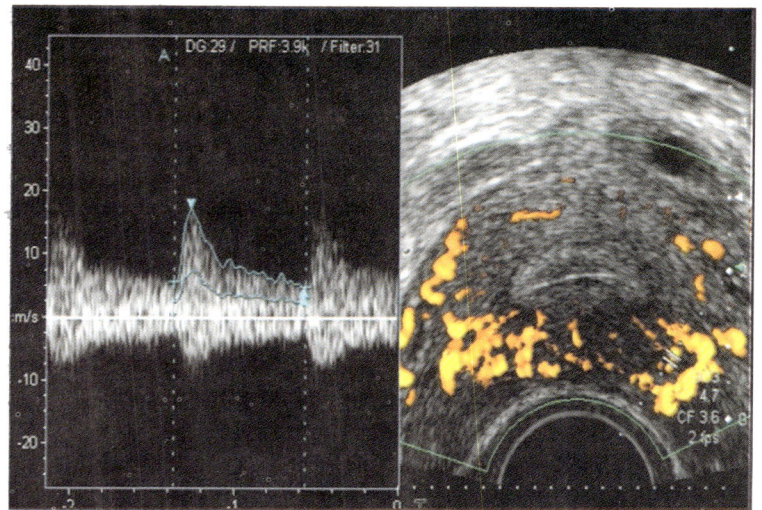

Fig. 19.64: Transversal scan that shows a uterine vascularization

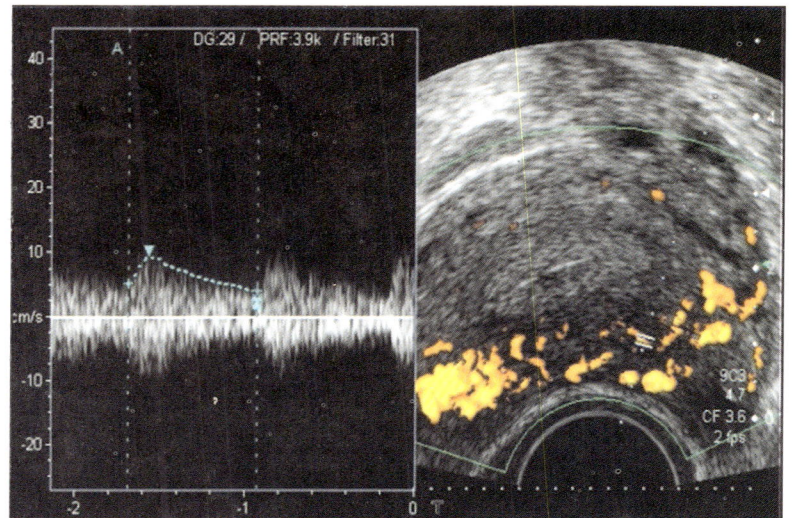

Fig. 19.65: Uterine artery demonstrated laterally to the cervix at the level of the cervicocorporeal junction (right). The blood flow velocity from the uterine artery in the secretory phase is characterized by increased end-diastolic velocity and decreased resistance index (RI = 0.74)

Unfortunately, a corpus luteum also shows rich angiogenic activity with abundant low-resistance vessels. Therefore, the main guideline for avoiding an incorrect diagnosis is to scan premenopausal patients at the beginning of the menstrual cycle.

In polycystic ovarian disease the ovaries become enlarged and the ovarian shape becomes more spherical. These ovaries

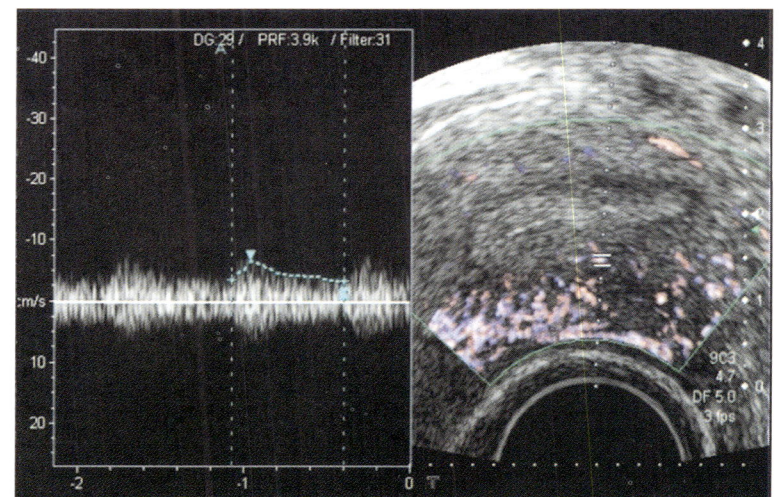

Fig. 19.66: Transvaginal color Doppler scan of the uterus shows the arcuate arteries in the outer third of the myometrium. The pulse Doppler waveform analysis obtained shows high-to-moderate resistance (RI = 0.72)

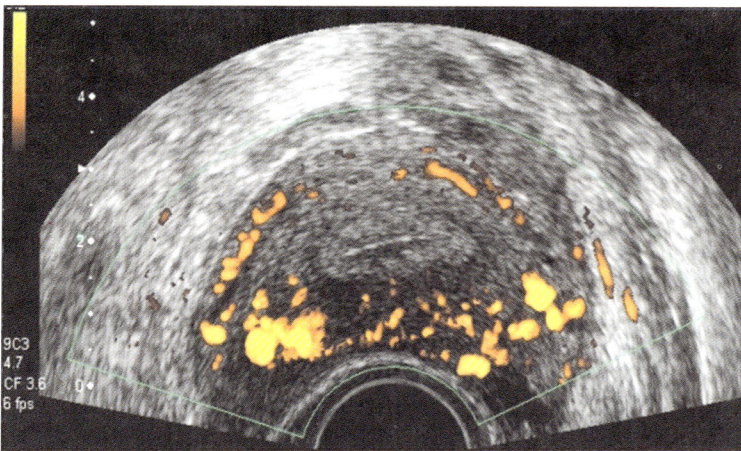

Fig. 19.67: Transvaginal color Doppler scan of the uterus. Note the radial arteries within the myometrial portion with moderate resistance (RI = 0.57)

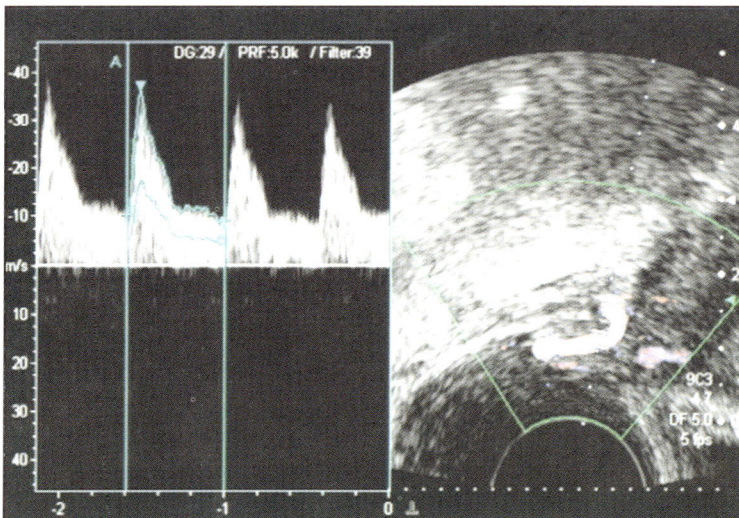

Fig. 19.68: Transvaginal dynamic flow scan of the uterus. We can see spiral arteries at the periphery of the secretory endometrium. The pulse Doppler waveform analysis obtained shows low-to-moderate resistance (RI = 0.50)

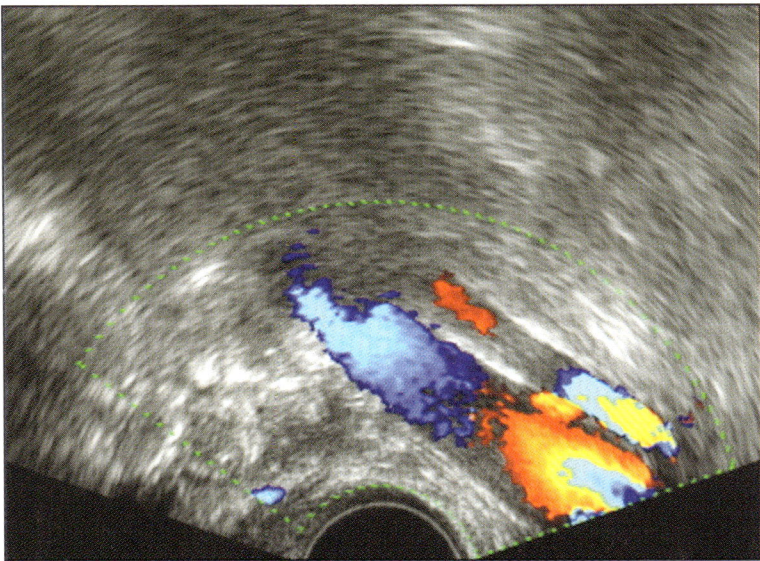

Fig. 19.69: Transvaginal scan shows the left internal iliac vein and artery (behind the vein)

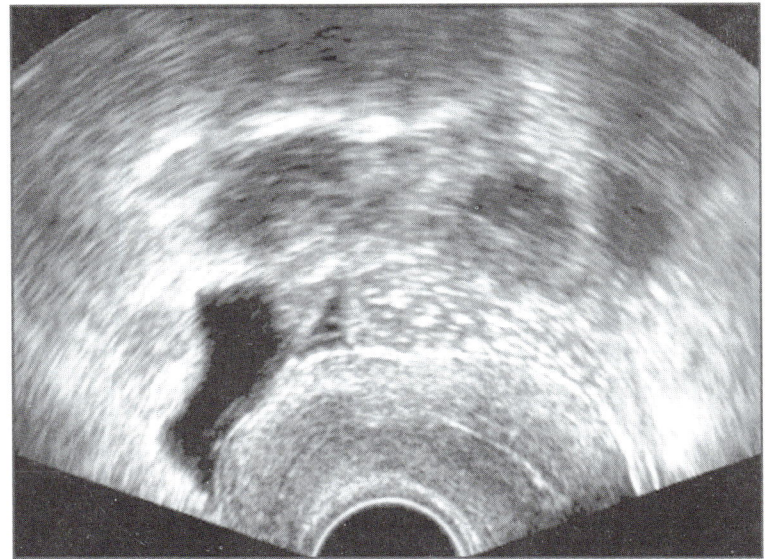

Fig. 19.72: Transvaginal sonogram that shows a moderate free fluid in pouch of Douglas

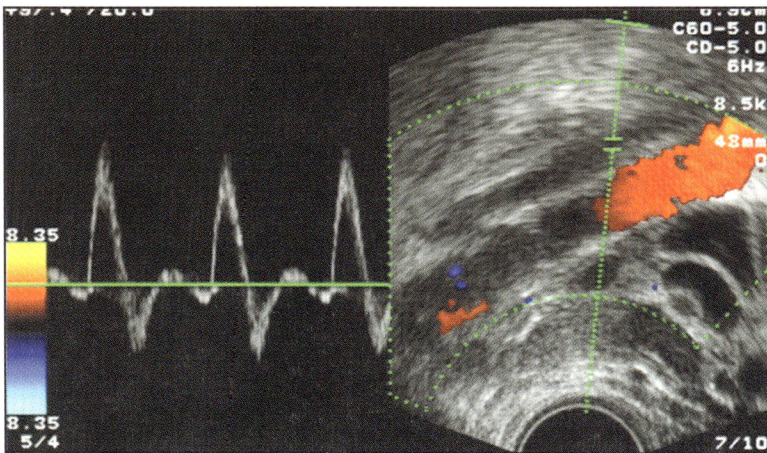

Fig. 19.70: The internal iliac artery. The pulsed Doppler waveform analysis (right) shows blood flow on high velocity and high resistance with the characteristic normal finding of reverse flow

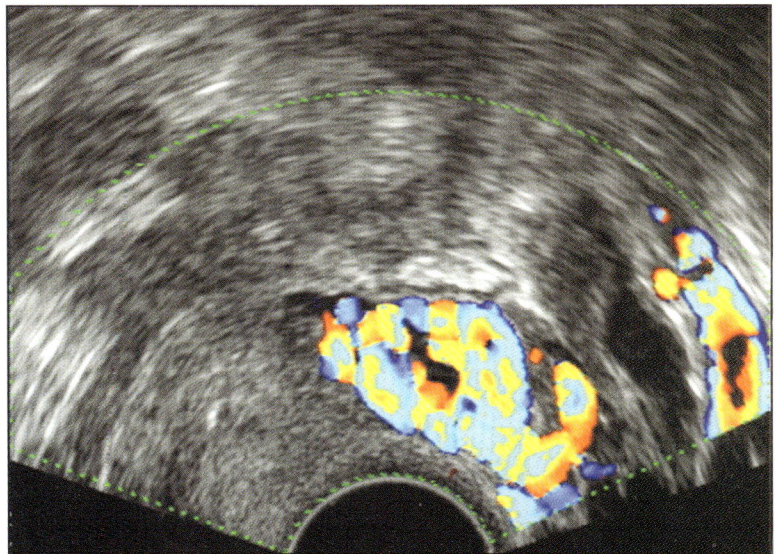

Fig. 19.73: Pelvic congestion syndrome. The picture shows dilated pelvic veins

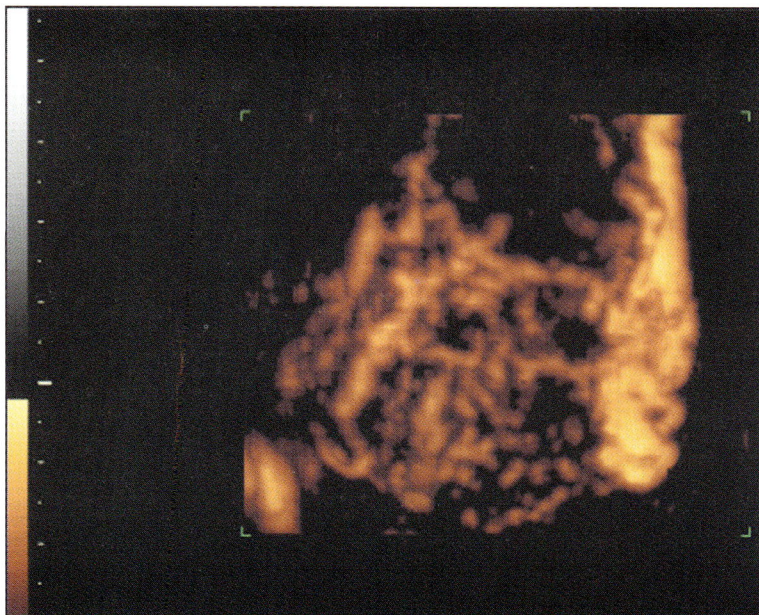

Fig. 19.71: Uterine vascularization shown by 3D power Doppler architecture of vessels

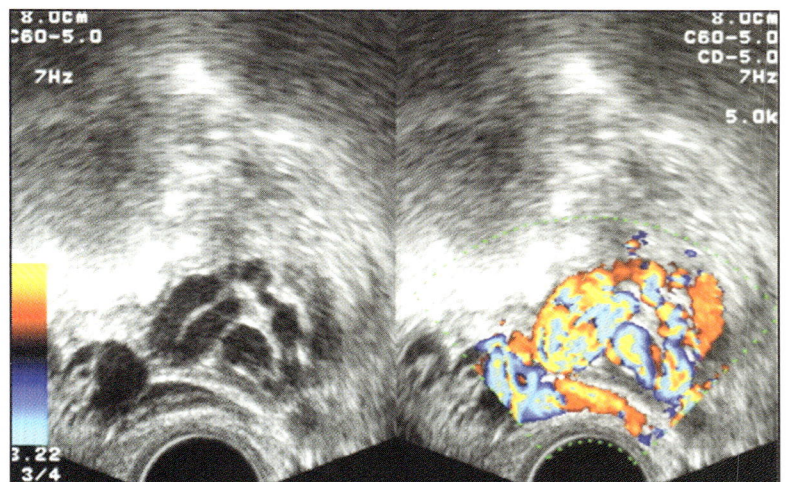

Fig. 19.74: Transvaginal sonogram of pelvic congestion syndrome

are characterized by the presence of multiple small cystic structures (<10 mm) and an increase in volume of the ovarian stroma. Cysts may be distributed predominantly around the

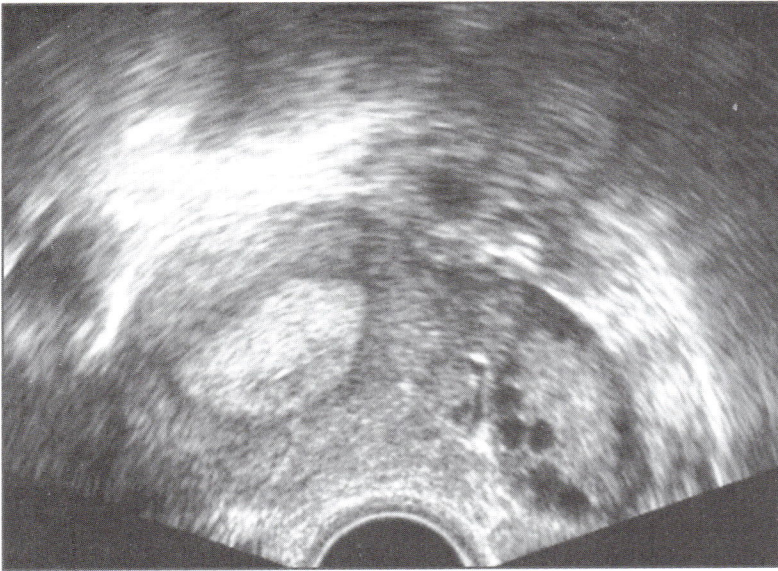

Fig. 19.75: Transversal sonogram normal left ovary. Uterus as on the left side of ovary

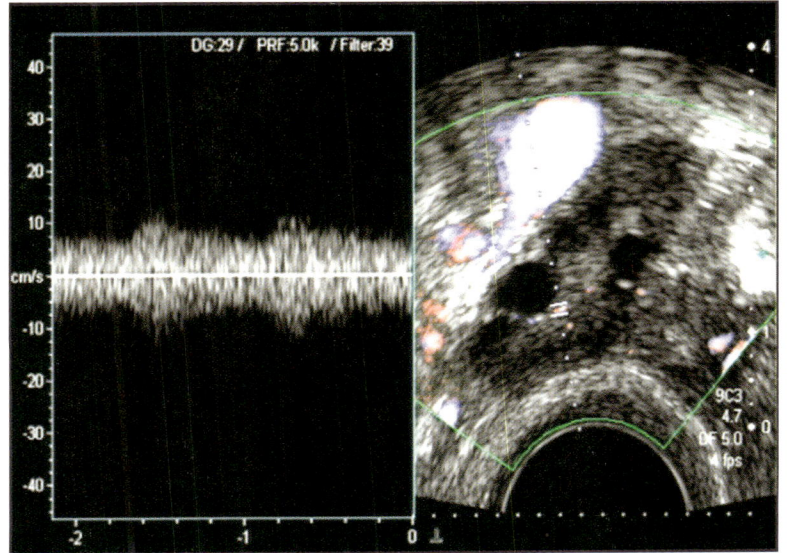

Fig. 19.78: Normal intraovarian blood flow

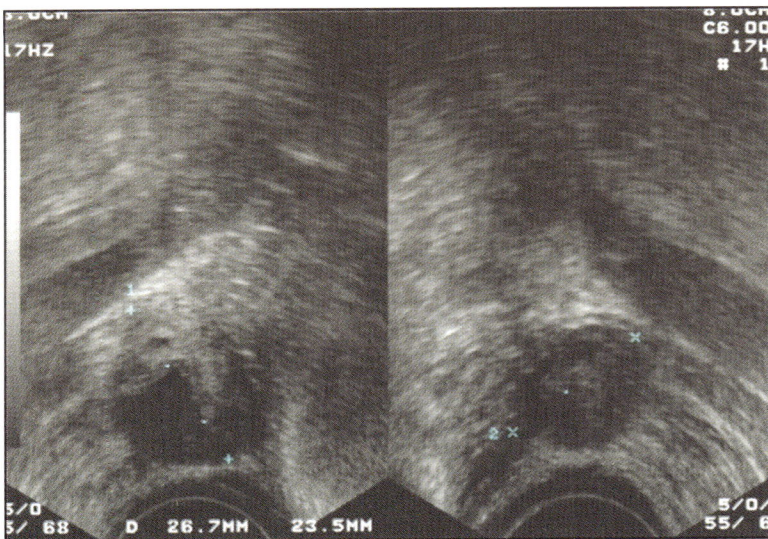

Fig. 19.76: Transversal scan that shows the iliac vessels are a good marker for to find the ovaries

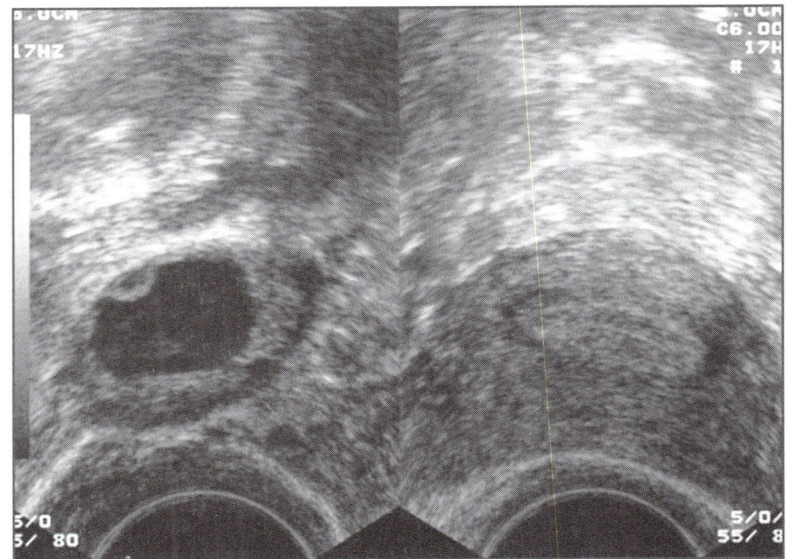

Fig. 19.79: Transvaginal sonogram of the ovary containing a preovulatory follicle with a cumulus oophorus during the moment of presumed ovulation. Note the triple-line endometrium

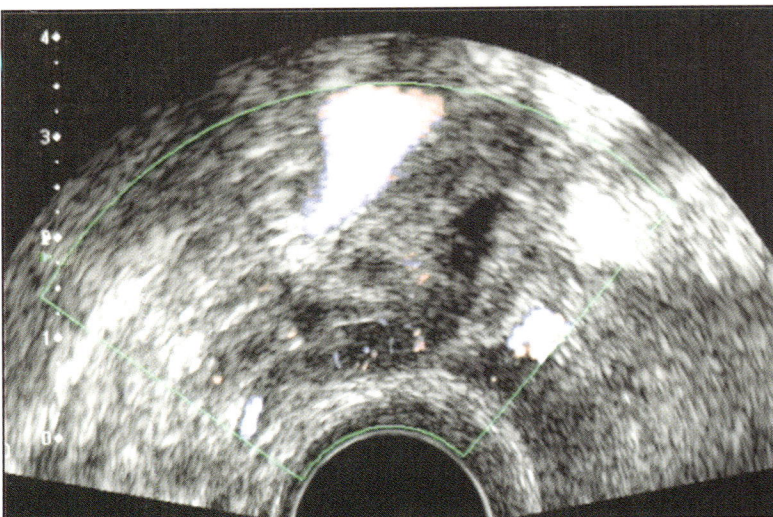

Fig. 19.77: Transvaginal scan of the right ovary that exhibits a normal shape and texture. Developing follicles are also demonstrated. Note internal iliac artery behind of the ovary

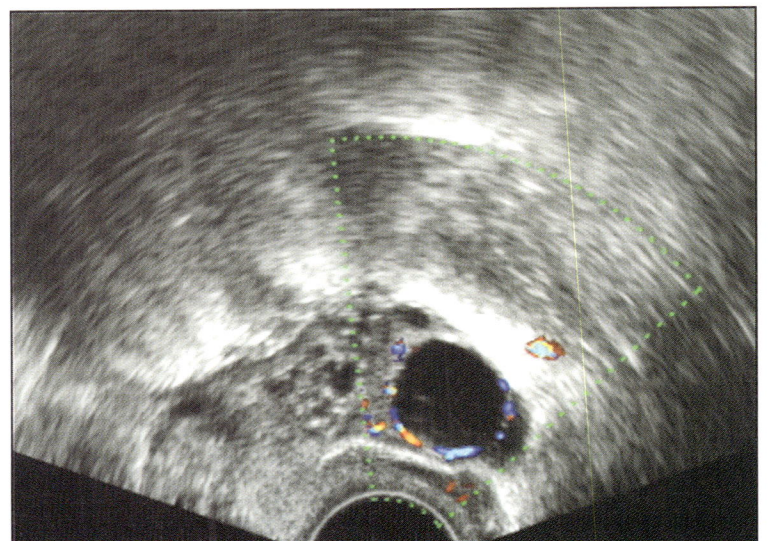

Fig. 19.80: Transvaginal color Doppler scan shows angiogenesis surrounding the follicle during the moment of presumed ovulation

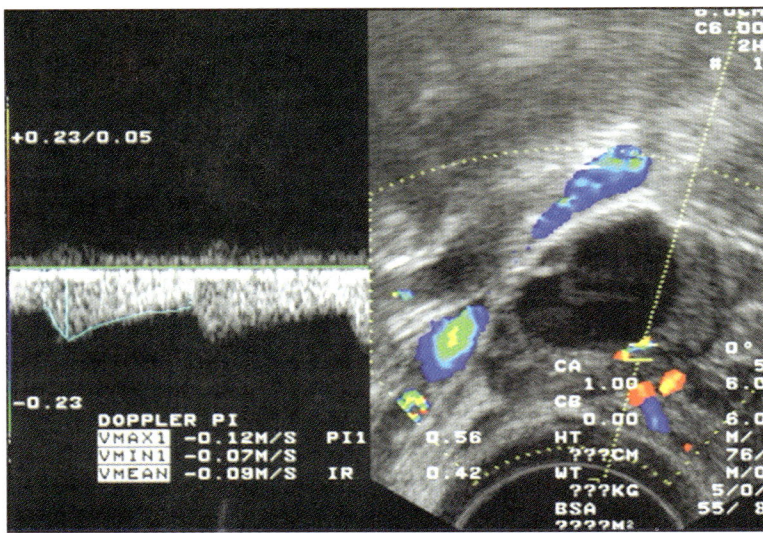

Fig. 19.81: Transvaginal sonogram of the dominant ovary containing a follicle with a cumulus oophorus. The pulsed Doppler waveform analysis of the follicular vessels as ovulation approaches shows a resistance index of 0.42

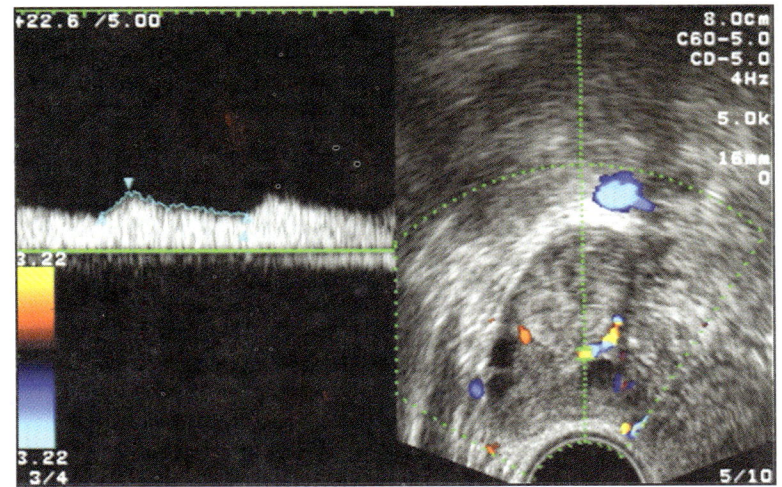

Fig. 19.84: Pulsed color Doppler of corpus luteum shows a high blood flow velocity and low resistance index (RI = 0.43) represent the typical flow pattern of the early corpus luteum

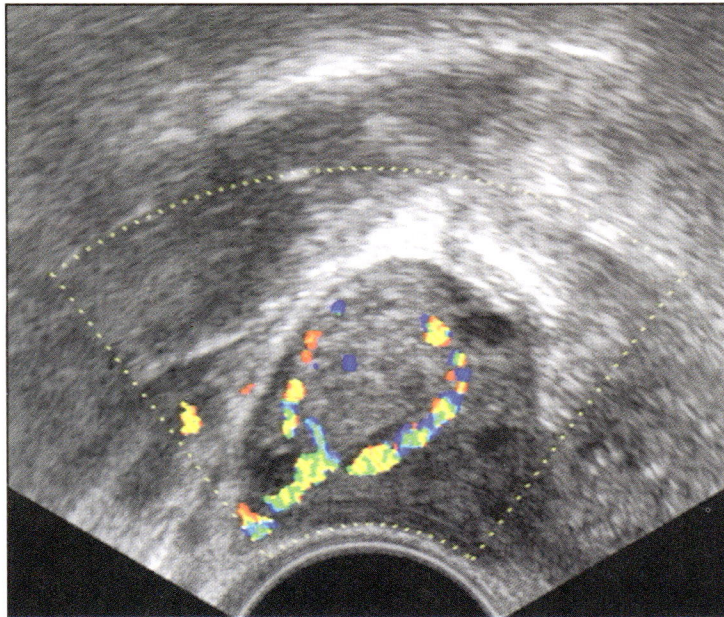

Fig. 19.82: Transvaginal color Doppler scan of the ovary in the midluteal phase. Increased vascularity of the corpus luteum is easily seen by color flow imaging

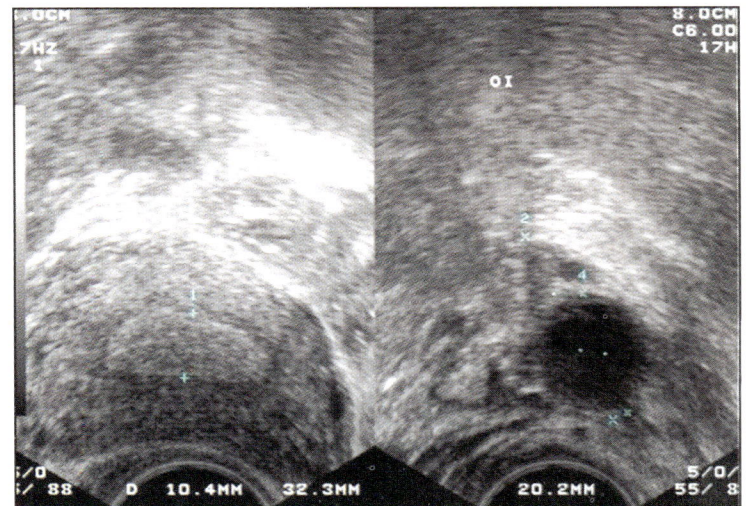

Fig. 19.85: Follicular persistence in the left ovary. Note in the left of picture transversal scan of secretory endometrium

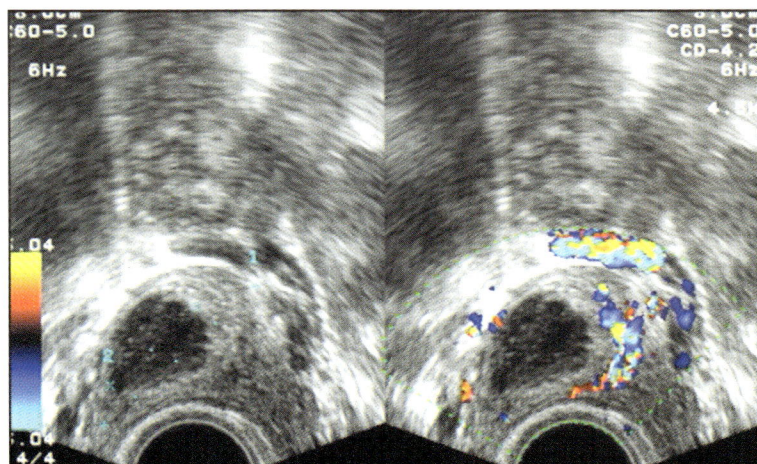

Fig. 19.83: Demonstration of increased vascularity in the corpus luteum during the stage of organization. Color-coded areas repesent the corpus luteum vascular network

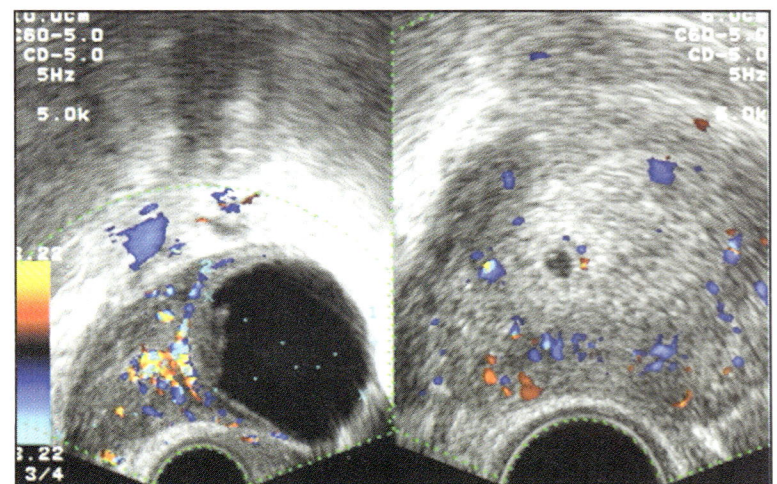

Fig. 19.86: The earliest gestational sac with corpus luteum graviditate being highly vascularized

periphery or scattered throughout the stroma (Figs 19.96 to 19.98). Increased stroma is the most important diagnostic sign that helps differentiate polycystic from multifollicular ovaries, which are a temporary feature of normal pubertal development.

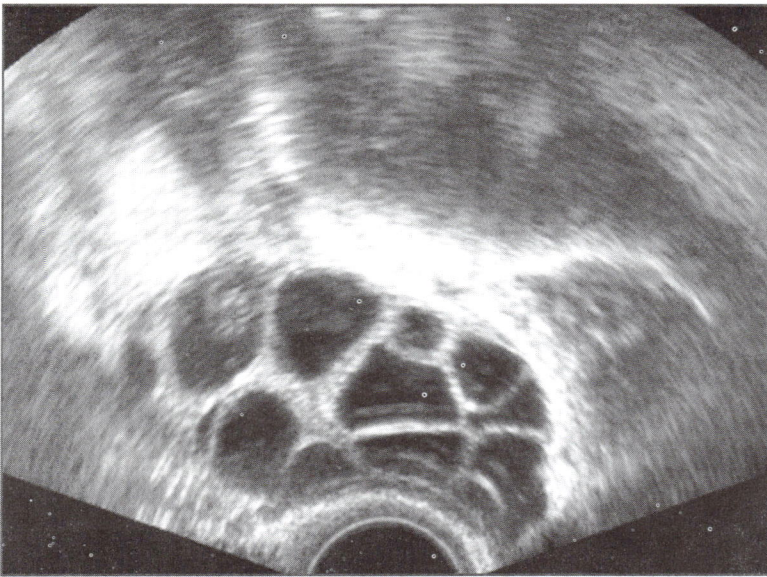
Fig. 19.87: Multifollicular development in left ovary

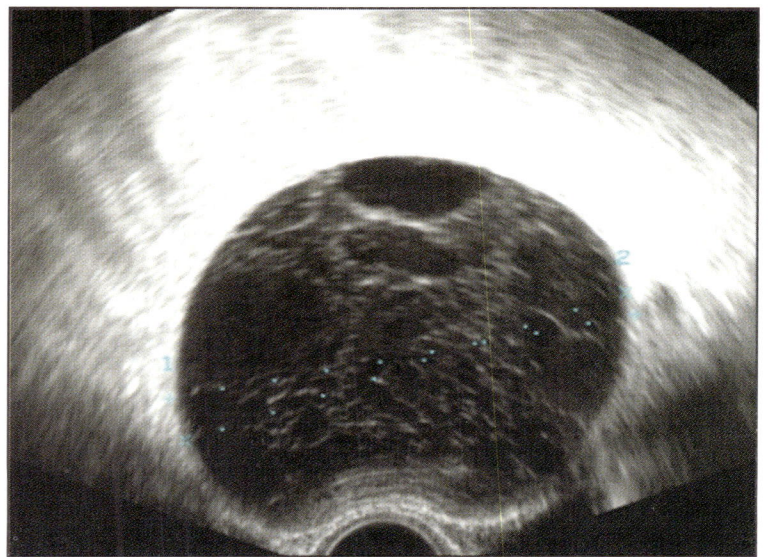
Fig. 19.90: Transvaginal sonogram shows a luteinized unruptured follicle (LUF) 89 mm larger. Note thin septas within the cyst cavity

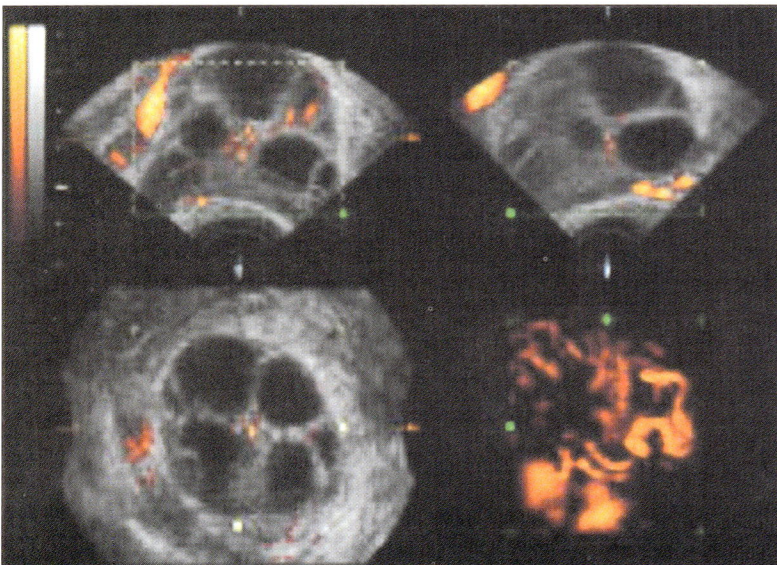
Fig. 19.88: Increased vascularization under gonadotropins therapy

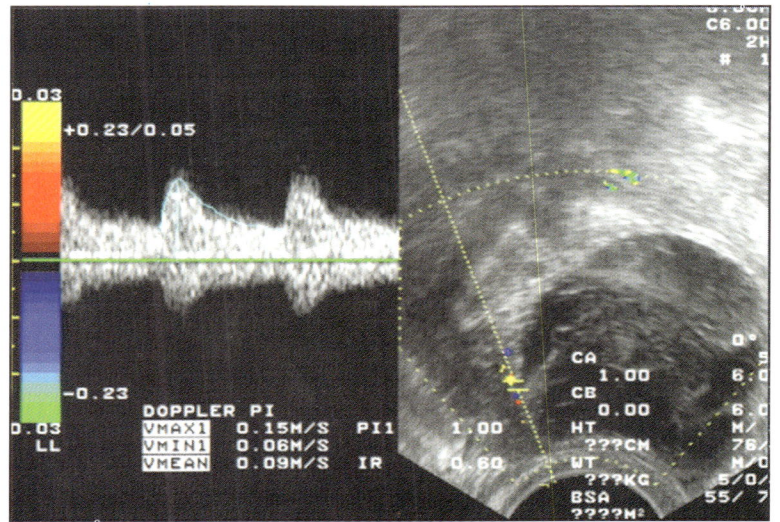
Fig. 19.91: Moderate vascular resistance (RI = 0.60) obtained after the luteinizing hormone peak from the perifollicular vessels is usual for luteinized unruptured follicle (LUF)

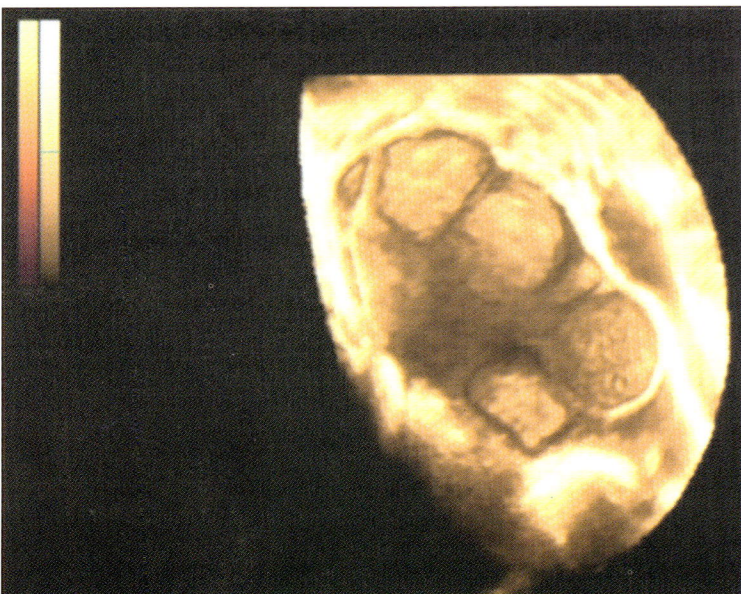
Fig. 19.89: Three-dimensional image of possible ovarian hyperstimulation

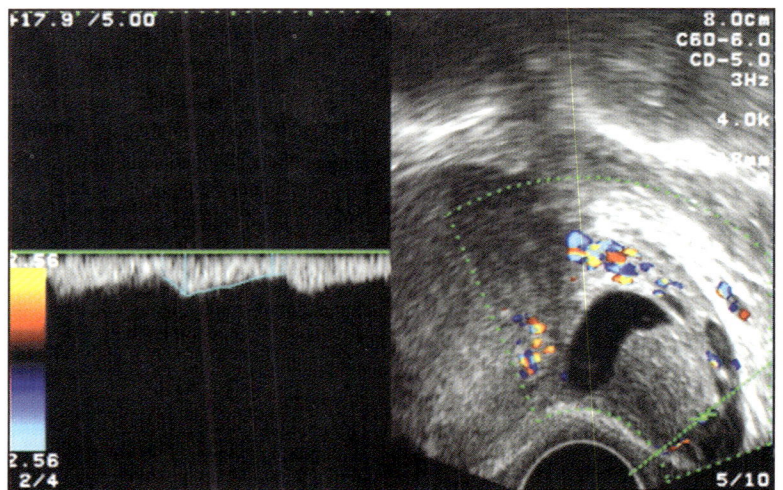
Fig. 19.92: Transvaginal scan of a luteinized unruptured follicle. Note the echogenic content representing a clot within the blood-filled cavity of the follicle. The pulsed color Doppler shows moderate vascular resistance (RI = 0.50)

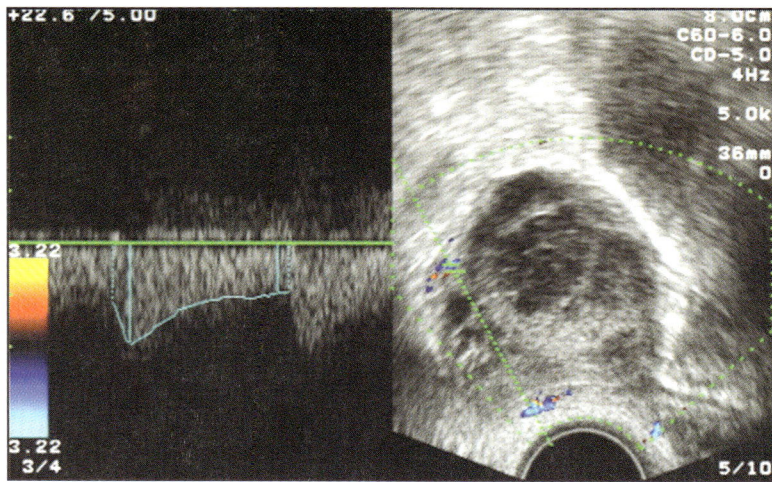

Fig. 19.93: Transvaginal scan of a luteinized unruptured follicle with hemorrhagic content. Pulsed color Doppler shows moderate vascular resistance (RI = 0.51)

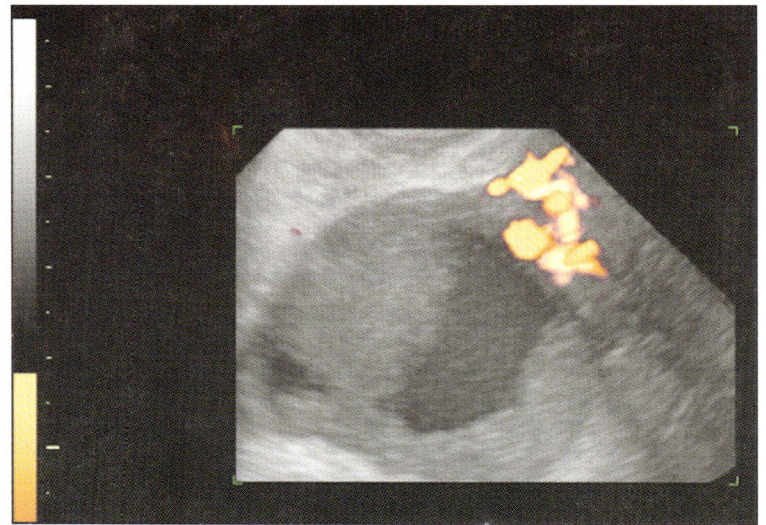

Fig. 19.96: 3D power Doppler image of luteinized unruptured follicle with hemorrhagic contents

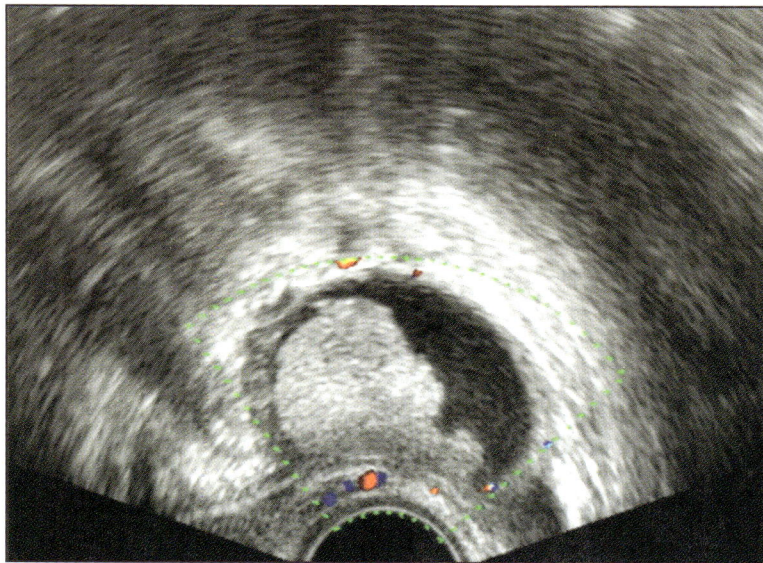

Fig. 19.94: Corpus luteum cyst. Imaged as a solid cystic ovarian structure. Color Doppler imaging detects absence os vascularity within the solid part

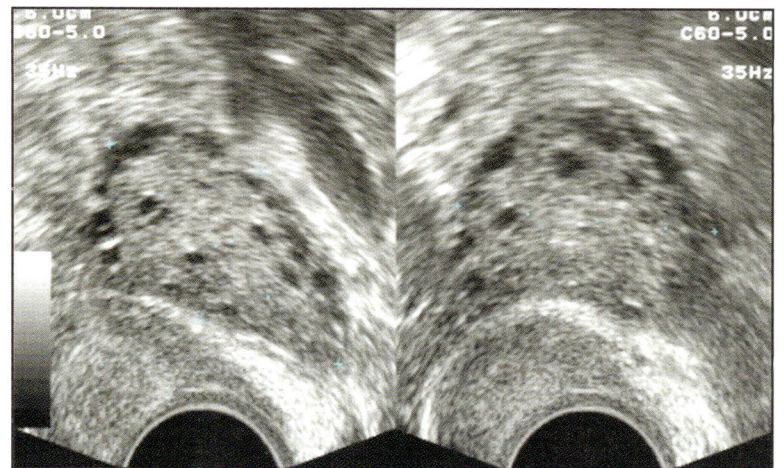

Fig. 19.97: Transvaginal sonogram of the polycystic ovary. A large number of small cystic structures are crowded together and stand out from the enlarged ovarian stroma (43 mm, 17.6 cc)

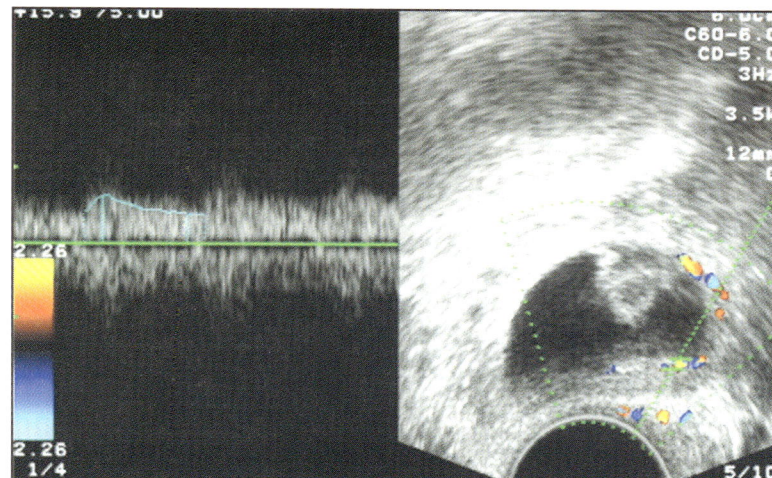

Fig. 19.95: Transvaginal color Doppler sonogram of a corpus luteum cyst containing a solid part that can imitate papillary protrusion

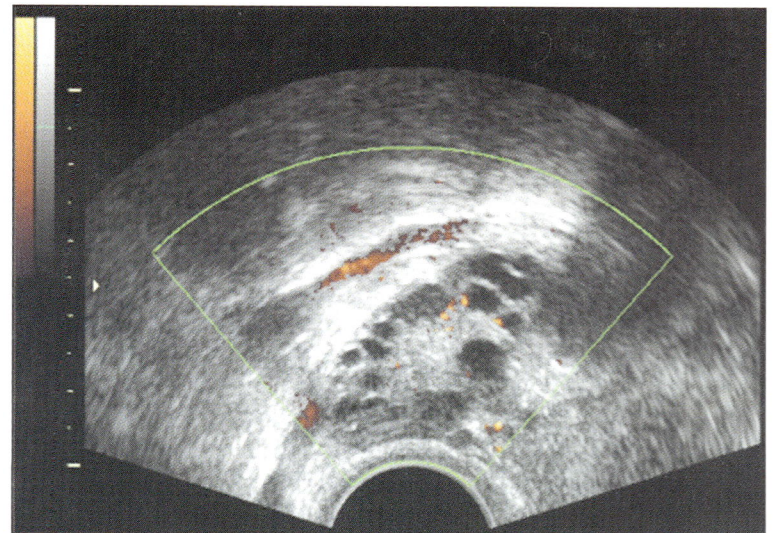

Fig. 19.98: Another example of the polycystic ovary. More than ten follicles can be calculated from the image

BIBLIOGRAPHY

1. Aleem F, Predanic M, Calame R, Moukhtar M, Pennisi J. Transvaginal color and pulsed Doppler sonography of the endometrium:a possible role in reducing the number of dilatation and curettage procedures. J Ultrasound Med 1995;14:139-45.
2. Aleem F, Predanic M. Transvaginal color Doppler determination of the ovarian and uterine blood flow characteristics in polycystic ovary disease. Fertil Steril 1996;65:510-6.
3. Balen AH, Laven JSE, Tan SL, Dewailly D. Ultrasound assessment of the polycystic

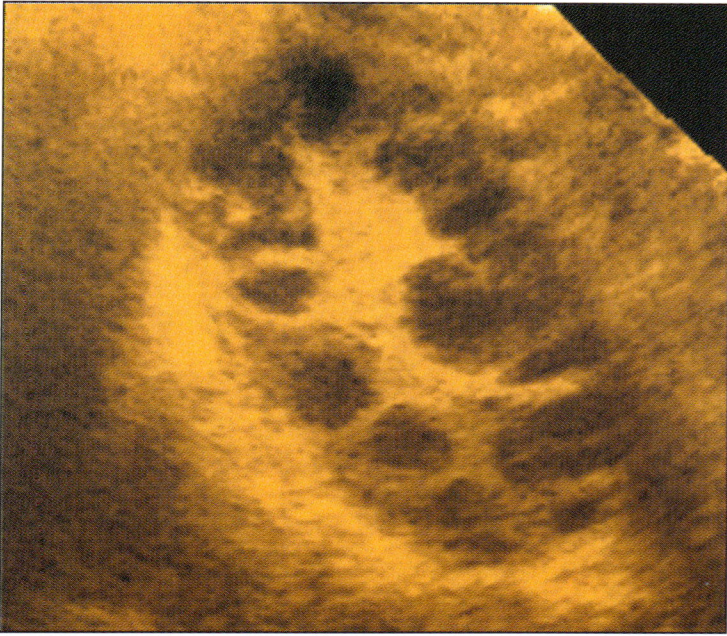

Fig. 19.99: Three-dimensional ultrasonography. The rendered view displays a unique cross-sectional view of the polycystic ovary

ovary: international consensus definitions. Hum Reprod 2003;9(6):505-14.

4. Bega G, Lev-Toaff A, O'Kane P, Becker E, Kurtz A. Three-dimensional ultrasonography in gynecology. J Ultrasound Med 2003;22:1249-69.
5. Bourne TH. Transvaginal color Doppler in gynecology. Ultrasound Obstet. Gynecol.1991; 359-73.
6. Cararach M, Penella J, Ubeda A, Labastida R. Hysteroscopic incisión of the septate uterus: scissors versus resectoscope. Hum Reprod. 1994;9(1):87-9
7. Demont F, Furquet F, Rogers M, Lansac J. Épidémiologie des kystes de l'ovaire apparemment bénins. J Gynecol Obstet Biol Reprod 2001;30:4S8-4S11.
8. Goldstein SR, Timor-Tritsch IE. Ultrasound in Gyneology. Churchill Livingstone Inc,1995.
9. Guerriero S, Ajossa S, Lai MP, Alcazar JL, Paoletti AM, Orrù M, Melis GB. The diagnosis of functional ovarian cysts using transvaginal ultrasound combined with clinical parameters, CA125 determinations, and color Doppler. Eu J Obstetrics and Gynecology and Reproductive Biology 2003;110:83-8.
10. Jones GL, Benes K, Clark TL, DENMA R, Holder MG, Haynes TJ, et al. The polycystic ovary syndrome health-related quality of life questionnaire (PCOSQ): a validation. Hum Reprod 2004;19(2):371-7.
11. Jurkovic D, Gruboeck K, Tailor A, Nicolaides KH. Ultrasound screening for congenital uterine anomalies. Br J Obstet Gynaecol. 1997;104(11):1320-1.
12. Kupesic S, Kurjak A, Babic MM. Uterine and ovarian perfusion changes from reproductive maturity to menopause. ACDS 1996;12:79-87.
13. Kurjak A, Fleischer AC. Doppler Ultrasound in Gynecology Parthenon Pubblishing Group. New York, London 1998.
14. Kurjak A, Kupesic S. Transvaginal color Doppler and pelvic tumor vascularity – lessons learned and future challenges. J Ultrasound Obstet Gynecol 1995;6:15-159.
15. Kurjak A. An Atlas of Transvaginal Color Doppler. Parthenon Publishing Group:. London,Casterton, Now York, 1994.
16. Marret H. Échographie et Doppler dans le diagnostic des kystes ovariens: indications, pertinence des critères diagnostiques. J Gynecol Obstet Biol Reprod 2001;30:4S20-4S33.
17. Maymon R, Herman A, Ariely S, Dreazn E, Buckovsky I, Weinraub Z. Three-dimensional vaginal sonography in obstetrics and gynaecology.Hum Reprod Update 2000;6:475-84.
18. Papp Z, Fekete T. The evolving role of ultrasound in obstetrics/gynecology practice. Int J Gynaecol Obstet. 2003;82:339-49.
19. Pascual MA, Hereter L, Tresserra F, Carreras O, Ubeda A, Dexeus S. Transvaginal sonographic appearance of functional ovarian cysts. Human Reproduction 1997;12(6):1246.
20. Raine-Fenning NJ, Campbell BK, Clewes JS, Kendall NR, Johson IR. The reliability of virtual organ computer-aided analysis (VOCAL) for the semiquantification of ovarian, endometrial and subendometrial perfusion. Ultrasound Obstet Gynecol 2003;22:633-9.
21. The Rotterdam ESHRE/ASRM-sponsored RCOS consensus workshop group. Revised 2003 consensus on diagnostic criteria and long-term health risks related to polycystic ovary syndrome (PCOS). Hum Reprod 2004;19(1):41-47.

MA Pascual, S Dexeus
A Kurjak, B Funduk

20

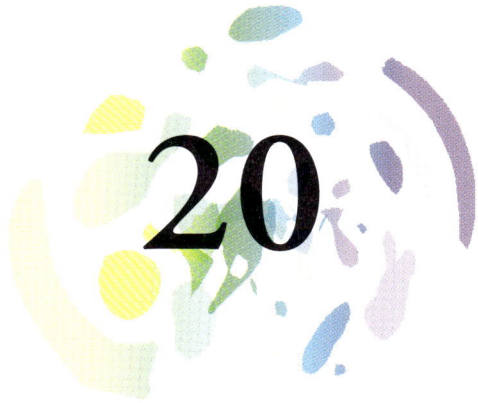

Uterine Tumors

SONOGRAPHY AND UTERINE DISORDERS

Transvaginal color Doppler ultrasound has improved the accuracy of clinical non-invasive diagnosis of uterine disorders and tumors.

The hypertrophia of the uterus is a frequent alteration in premenopausal women, that has a regular and homogeneous myometrium (Figs 20.1 and 20.2).

Uterine fibroids or leiomyoma are the more common acquired uterine disorders. These benign tumors are responsible for the wide spectrum of clinical complaints, e.g. menorrhagia, menstrual pain, acute pain if infarction occurs, pressure sensation, urinary retention or obstipation. Leiomyomas are frequently multiple (Figs 20.18 to 20.20) and they are all originated out of the myometrium of the uterine body and fundus. Very rarely myomas are located in the cervix (Figs 20.3 to 20.7).

Tumor growth can cause its displacement, and myomas are therefore classified subserous (Figs 20.8, 20.9 and 20.17), intramural (Figs 20.21 to 20.25), or submucous (Figs 20.26 to 20.37).

Leiomyomas that are pendunculated can be confused with other adnexal masses if their pedicle is not visualized (Figs 20.10 to 20.16). The color Doppler is very useful in detecting the pedicle of myoma.

With the conventional B-mode sonography, submucous leiomyomas may be difficult to differentiate from intramural leiomyomas, but the recent introduction of three-dimensional sonography has improved the accuracy in diagnosis of these type of myomas (Figs 20.38 and 20.39).

The diagnosis of uterine fibroma is based on texture changes, distortion of the uterine contour and uterine enlargement. The typical sonographic appearance of leiomyomas consists of mildly to moderately echogenic intrauterine masses that cause nodular distortion of the uterine outline. Small intramural or submucous leiomyomas may be recognized by their distortion of the normally linear central endometrial echoes.

The echogenicity of a fibroid depends upon the relative ratio of fibrous tissue to smooth muscle. With a more fibrous component, there is increased echogenicity of the nodule. The sonographic texture of fibroids also depends on the type and presence of degeneration and upon the vascular supply (Figs 20.40 to 20.46). Uterine enlargement is a constant but not pathognomonic sign of uterine fibroma. Color Doppler shows peripheral vascularization and facilitates delineation of the myoma from the surrounding myometrium.

In ultrasonic terms uterine malignancies can hardly be distinguished from fibromas. The uterine sarcomas (Figs 20.47 to 20.51) are less frequent, and demonstrate a similar echo pattern. The color Doppler in these types of malignant tumors shows areas of neovascularization with low resistance, but not specific findings.

Secondary tumoral changes are very common (necrosis, hemorrhage, calcification or degeneration) and cause a wide spectrum of ultrasonic images.

The most common cause of calcification within the uterus is calcific degeneration within a fibroid (Figs 20.52 and 20.53). There are other types of degeneration within leiomyomas that produce sonographically recognizable changes in uterine texture (Figs 20.54 to 20.56).

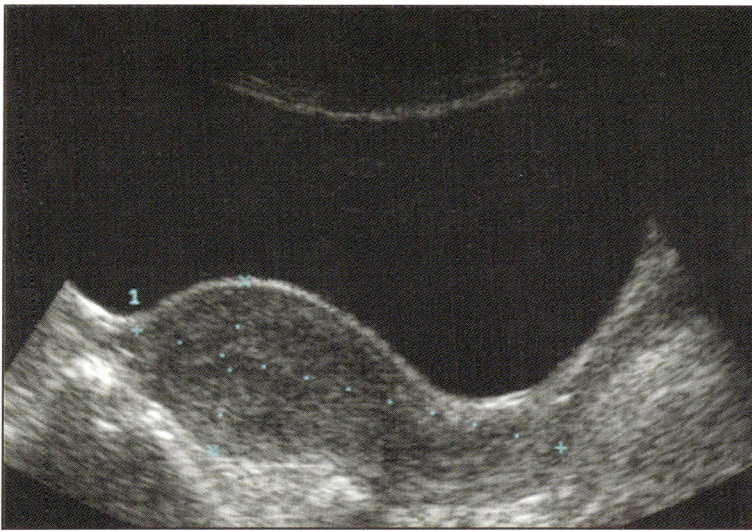

Fig. 20.1: Transabdominal scan showing a hypertrophic uterus (10.1 cm longitudinal diameter). Note the regular and homogeneous myometrium

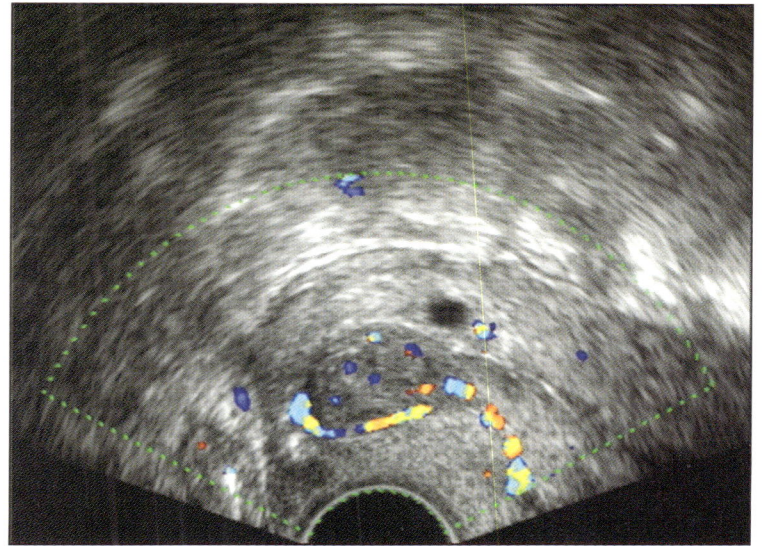

Fig. 20.4: The same patient as in Figure 20.3. Transvaginal color Doppler shows the pedicle and the peripheral vascularity of this benign lesion

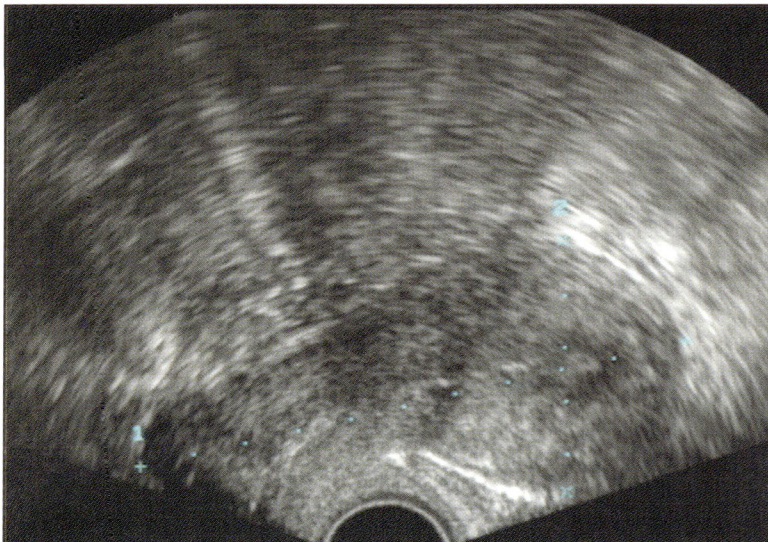

Fig. 20.2: Transvaginal sonogram of enlarged uterus (10.4 cm) with regular and homogeneous myometrial pattern. We can see the normal endometrial cavity

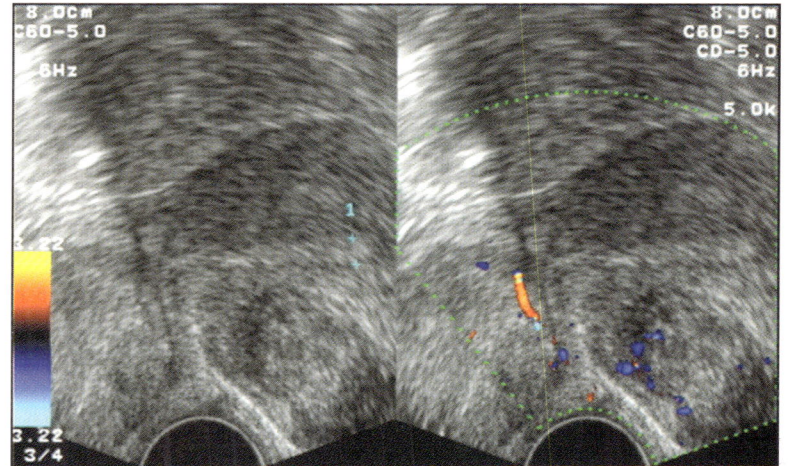

Fig. 20.5: Transvaginal color Doppler showing an intramural myoma and other tumor located in the cervix. Histopathology revealed a cervical malignant tumor (Glassycell type)

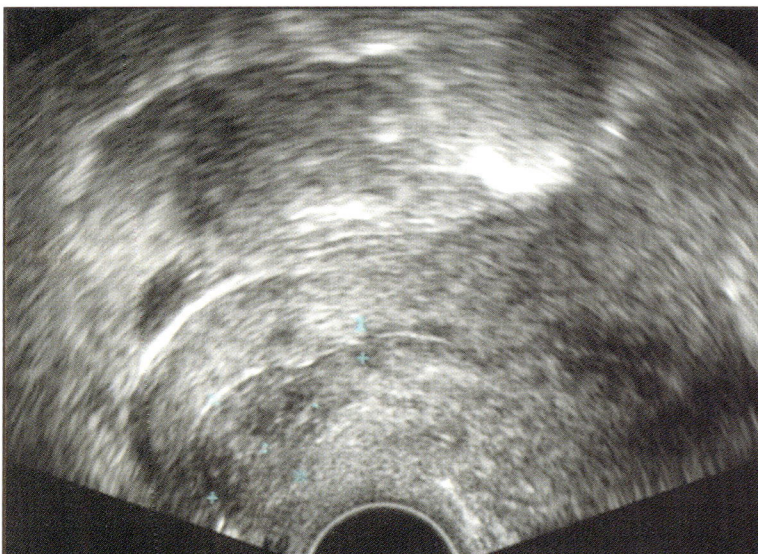

Fig. 20.3: Very rarely myomas are located in the cervix. This picture shows an intracervical myoma 3 cm larger

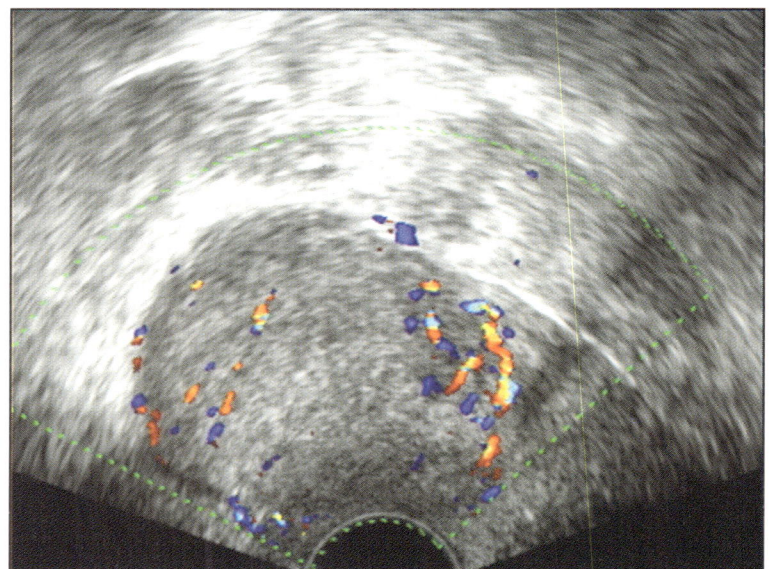

Fig. 20.6: The same patient as in Figure 20.5. Color Doppler demonstrates spread vessels within the tumor

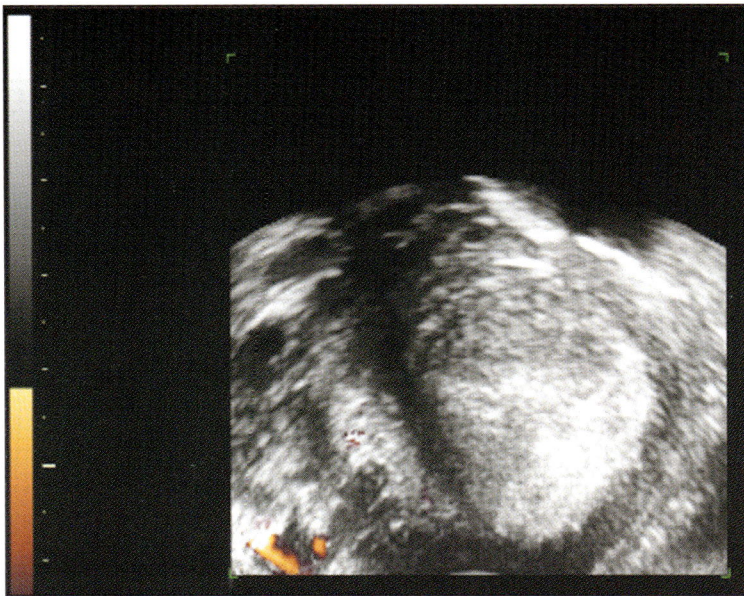

Fig. 20.7: Three-dimensional power Doppler sonogram of a benign cervical tumor. Note the absence of vascularization

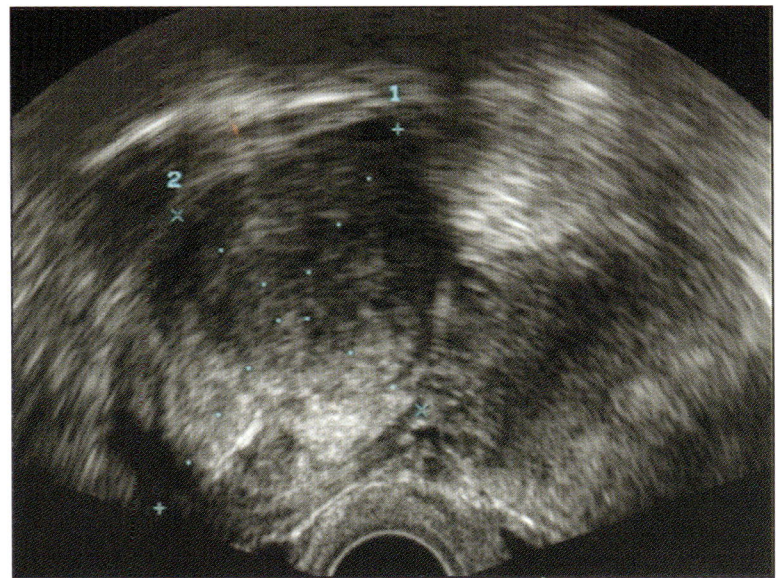

Fig. 20.10: Transvaginal sonogram of a subserous myoma mistaken for a solid adnexal mass

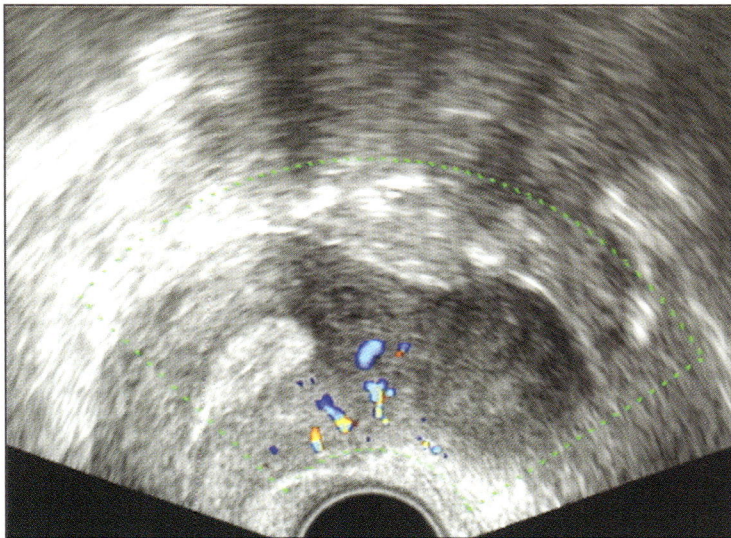

Fig. 20.8: Intramural/subserous myoma as seen by transvaginal color Doppler. Note the vascularity at the level of the pedicle

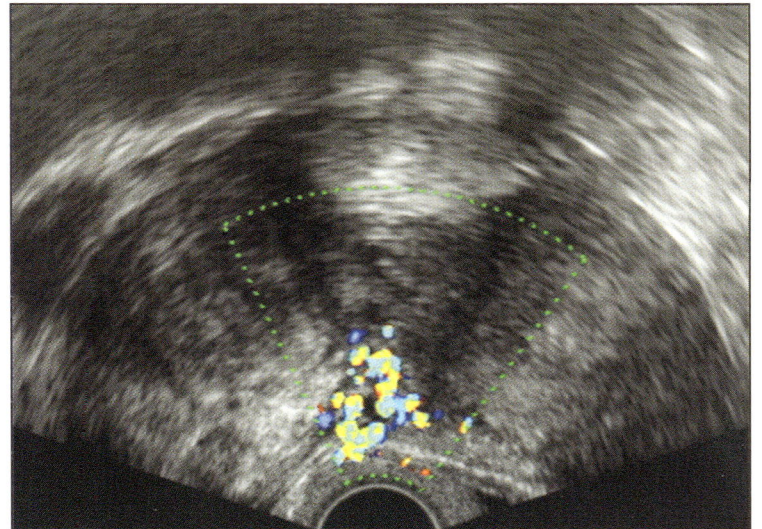

Fig. 20.11: The same patient as in Figure 20.10 showing clearly the vascular pedicle of union myoma with the corpus of the uterus

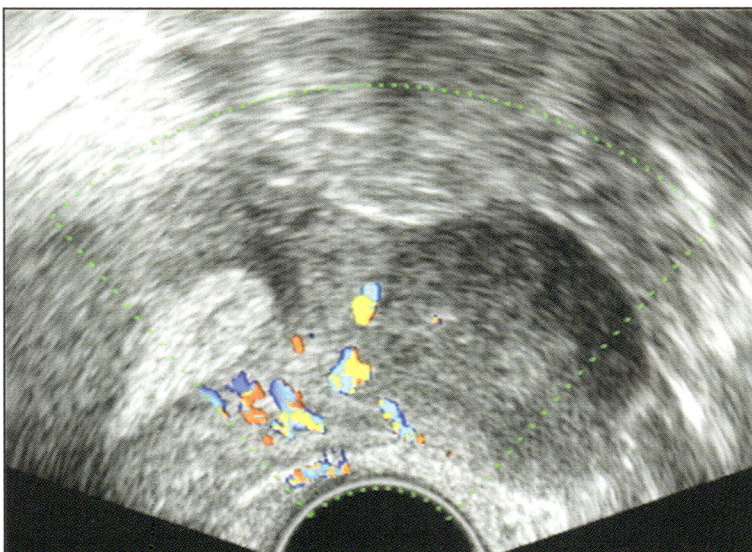

Fig. 20.9: Transvaginal color Doppler scan. Entirely subserous myoma with highly vascularized base

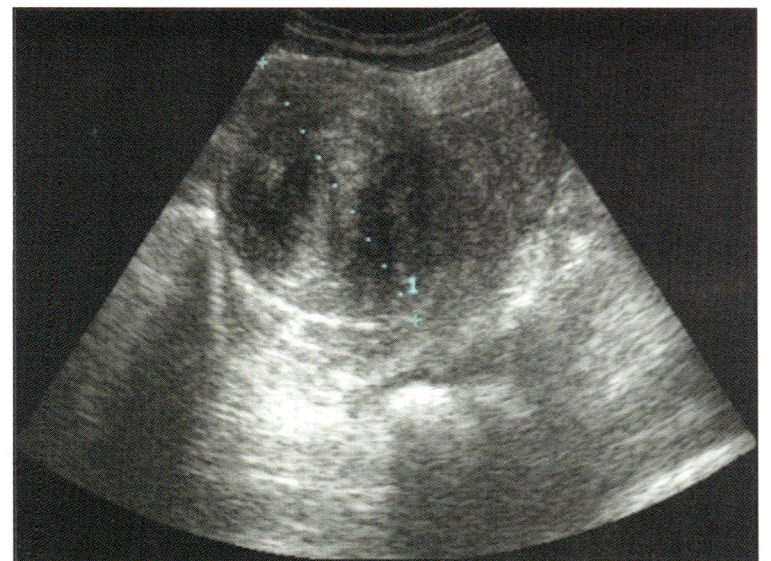

Fig. 20.12: Abdominal scan with a larger subserous myoma. Sometimes is necessary to complete the transvaginal sonographic exploration with the abdominal sonogram

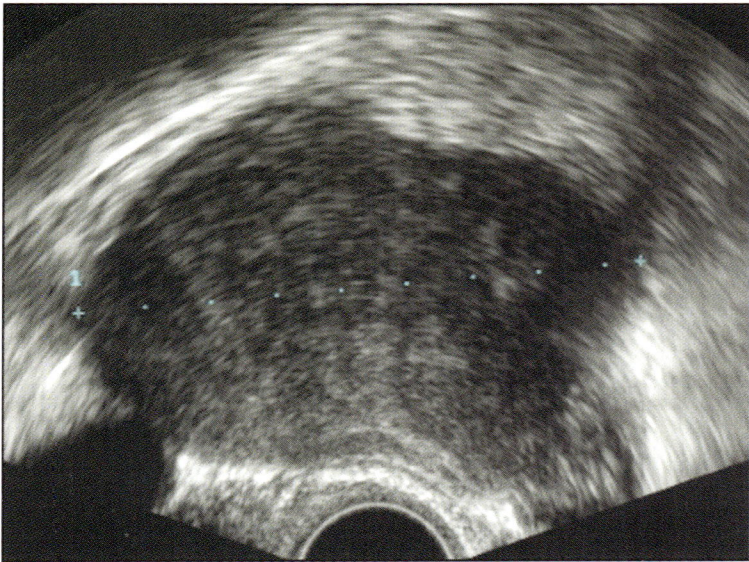

Fig. 20.13: Transvaginal scan of a larger subserous myoma (8.5 cm) mistaken for a solid adnexal mass

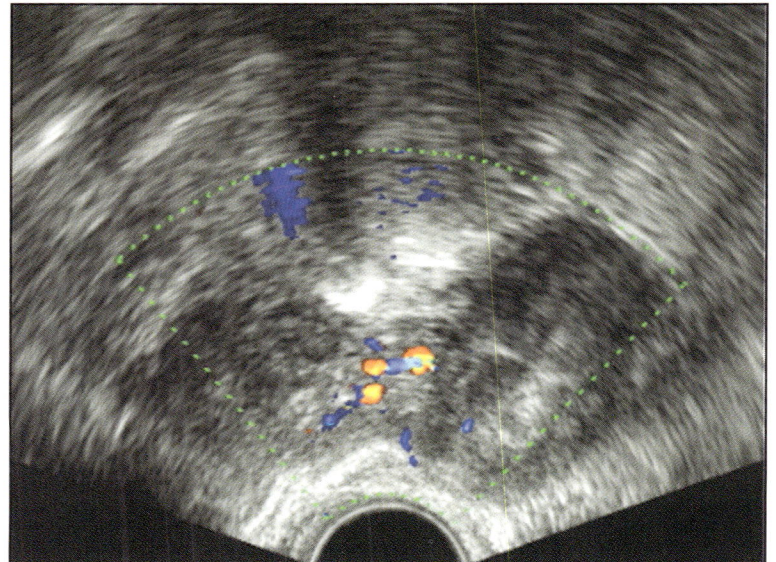

Fig. 20.16: Another example of the usufulness of color Doppler in distinguishing pedicle vessel of union myoma to the uterus

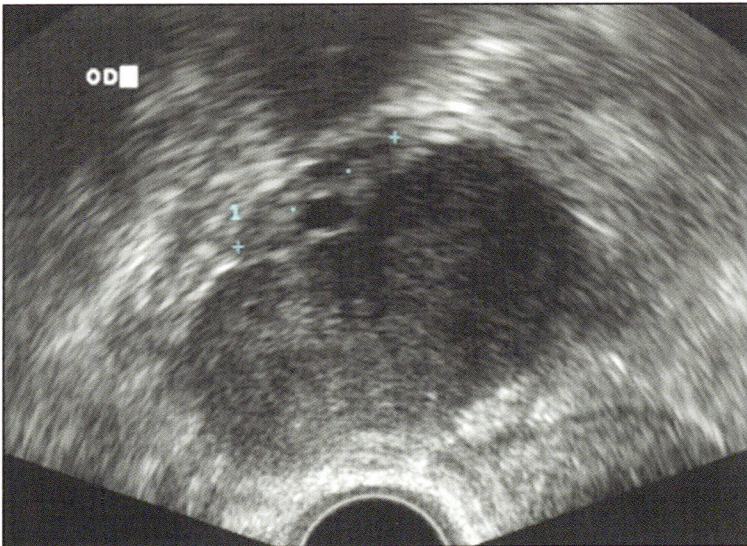

Fig. 20.14: The same patient as in Figure 20.13. Note the presence of the normal right ovary

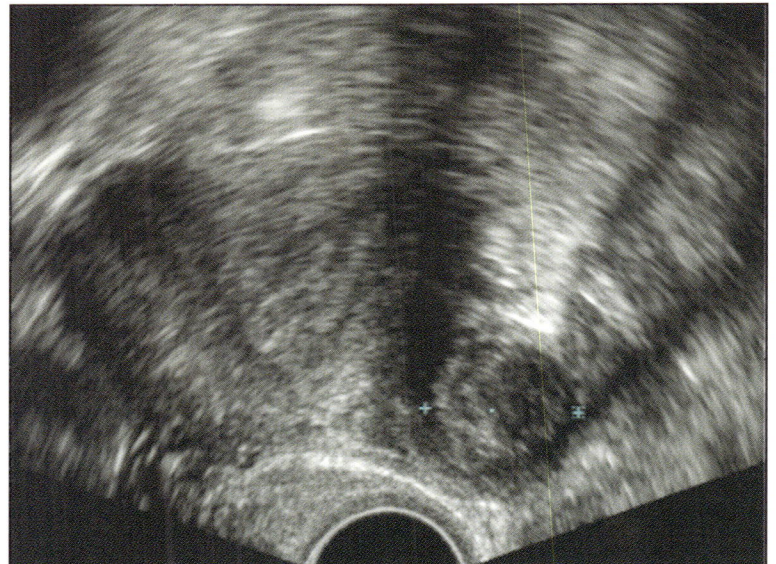

Fig. 20.17: Uterine sonogram demonstrating the uterine body with two subserous myomas

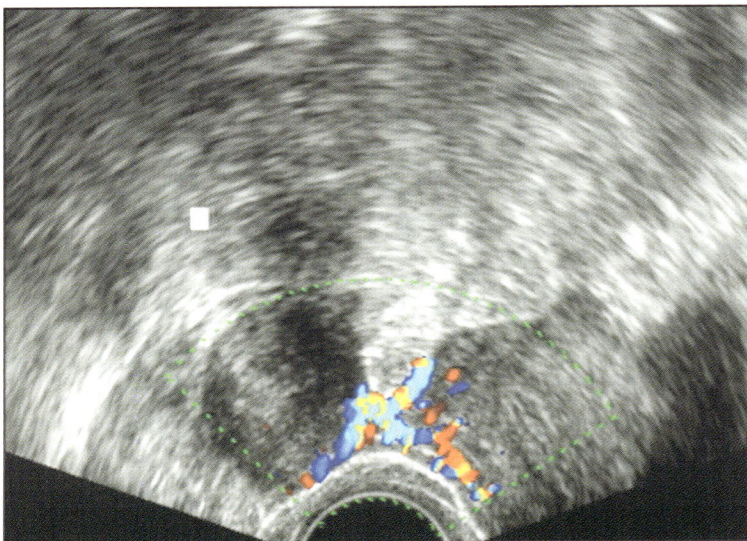

Fig. 20.15: Transvaginal color Doppler demonstrating the presence of union pedicle between myoma and uterus

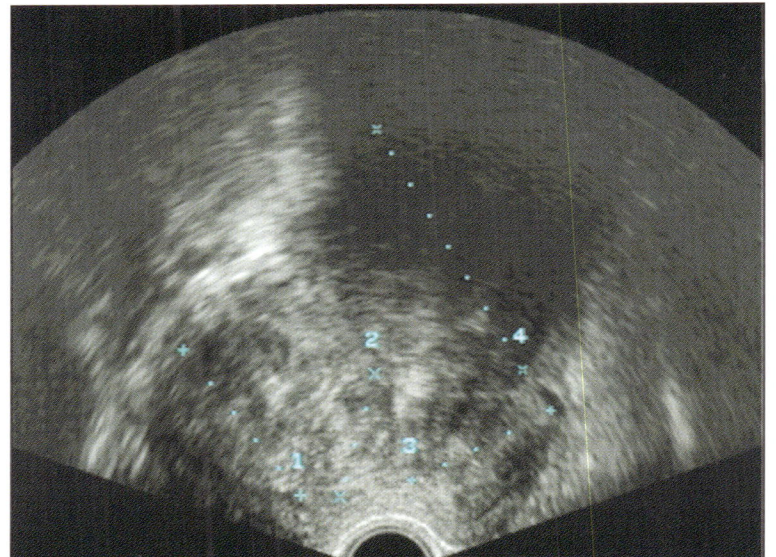

Fig. 20.18: Uterus with numerous small and large myomas which affected uterine tissue

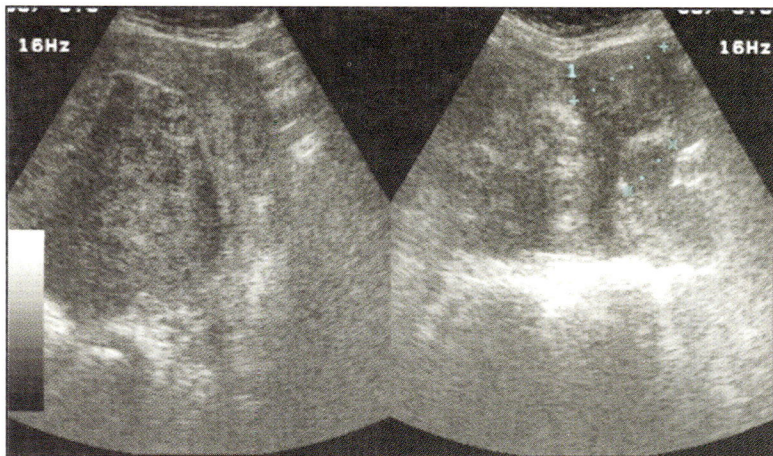

Fig. 20.19: Multiple myomas of the uterus affecting the normal shape and texture of the uterus: The uterus is of round shape and the uterine cavity is not recognizable

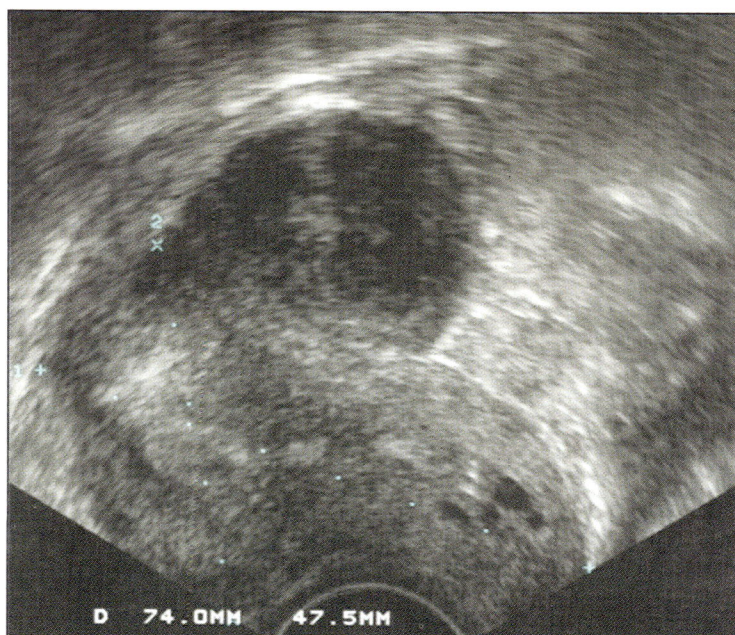

Fig. 20.20: Small intramural myoma detected on fundus and a larger subserous myoma on anterior uterine border in a retroverted uterus

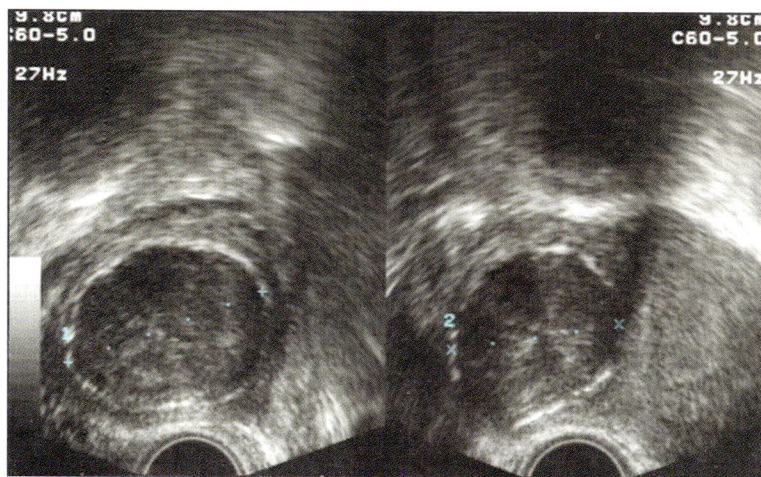

Fig. 20.21: Transvaginal sonogram of a patient with intramural myoma

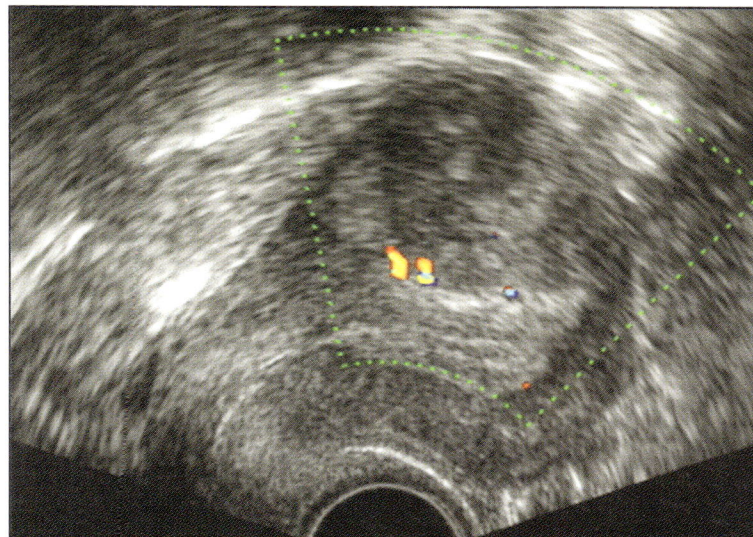

Fig. 20.22: The same patient as in Figure 20.21, examined by color Doppler imaging. Color Doppler facilitates delineation of the intramural myoma from the surrounding myometrium

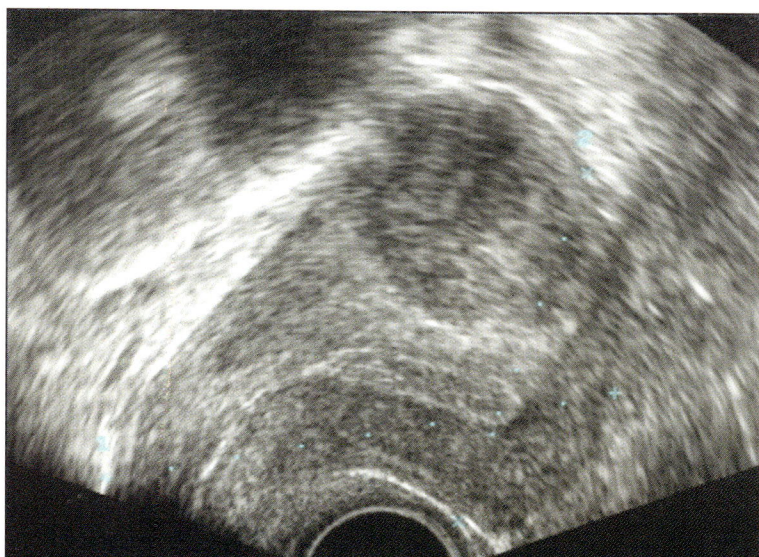

Fig. 20.23: Transvaginal sonogram demonstrating an another example of intramural myoma

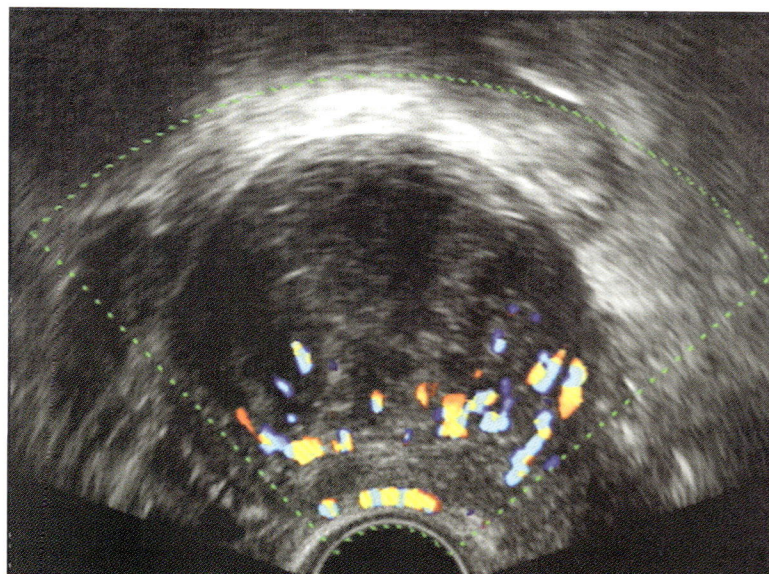

Fig. 20.24: Transvaginal color Doppler scan of a patient with intramural myoma. Color Doppler imaging demonstrates ring of angiogenesis at its periphery

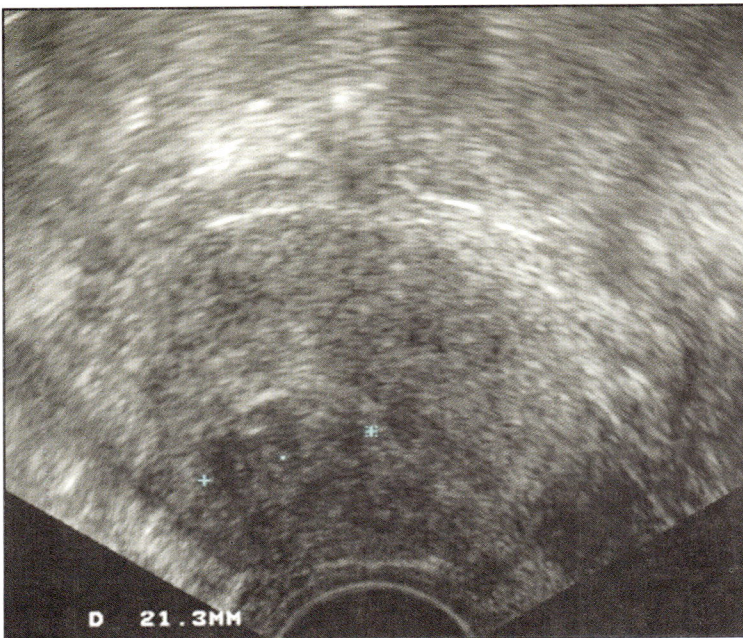

Fig. 20.25: Transvaginal sonogram with an isoechogenic intramural myoma

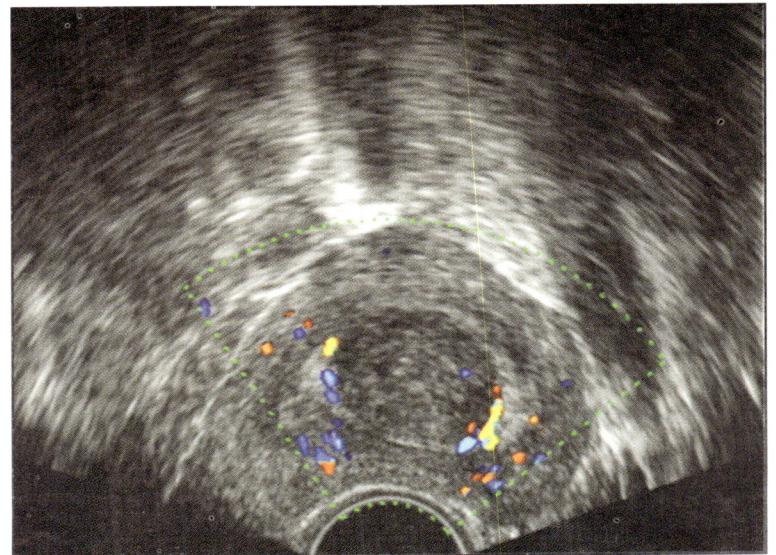

Fig. 20.28: The peripheral vascularity ("vascular ring") is characteristic of this type of tumor

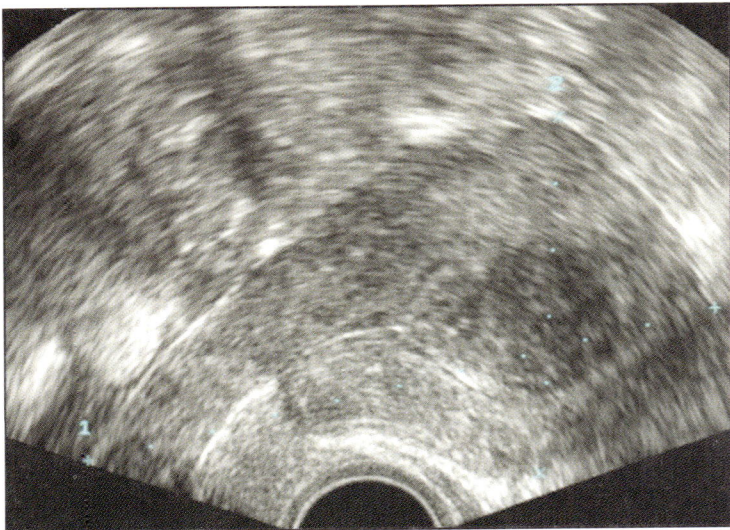

Fig. 20.26: Submucous myoma surrounded by endometrial layers

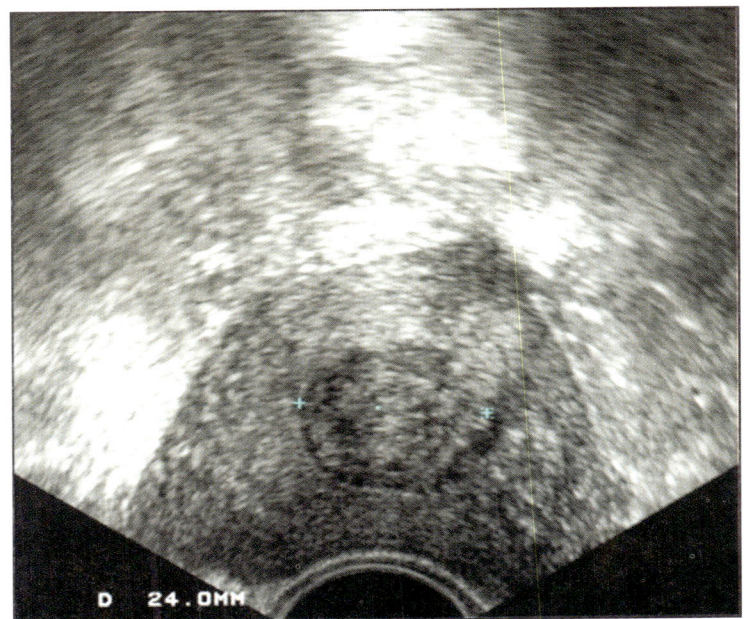

Fig. 20.29: Transversal scan of submucous myoma of 24 mm

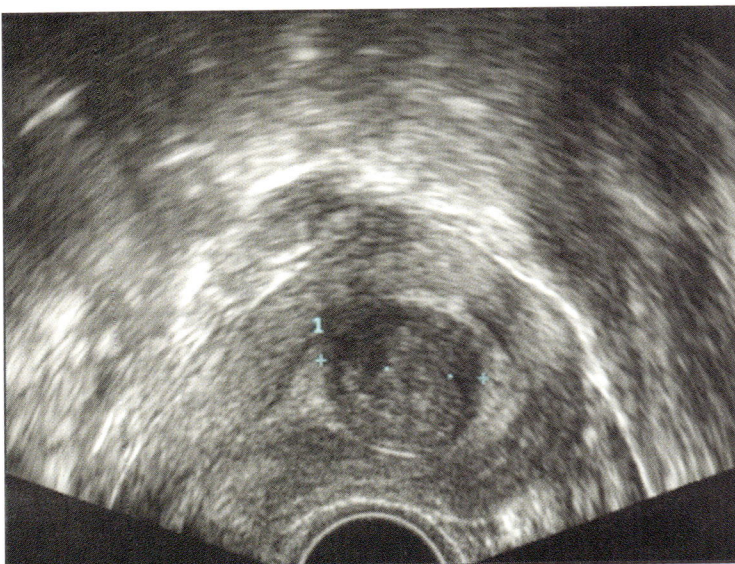

Fig. 20.27: Another example of a submucous myoma. We can see clearly the endometrium

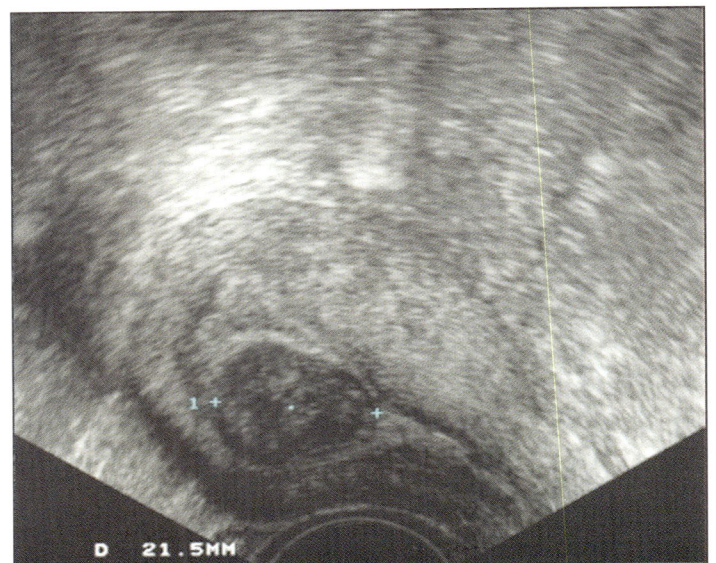

Fig. 20.30: Transvaginal sonogram shows a submucous myoma surrounded by endometrial layers

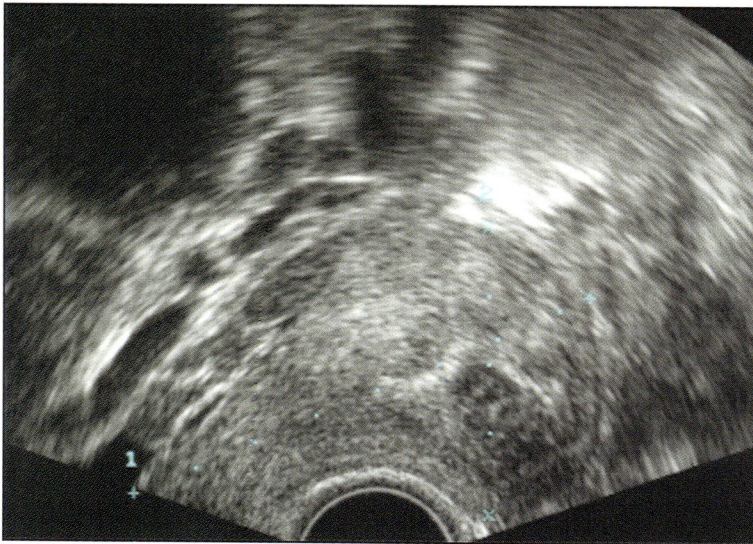

Fig. 20.31: Transvaginal scan of a small submucous myoma. The benign nature of the tumor was confirmed by hysteroscopy and histopathology

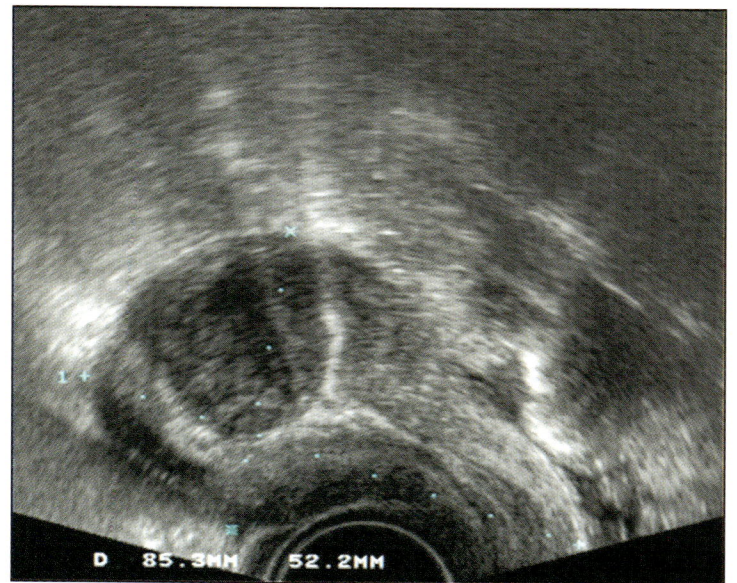

Fig. 20.34: Transvaginal sonogram showing a large submucous myoma

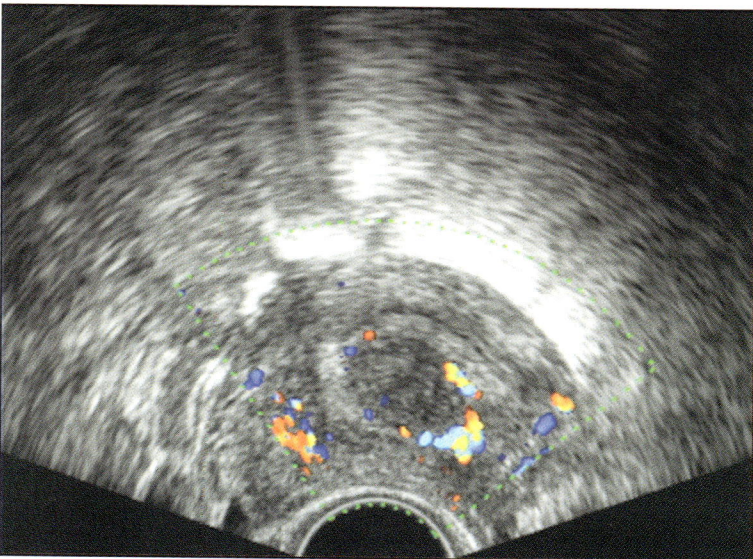

Fig. 20.32: Transvaginal color Doppler scan of a submucous myoma. Color Doppler imaging demonstrates regularly vessels in the border of the tumor

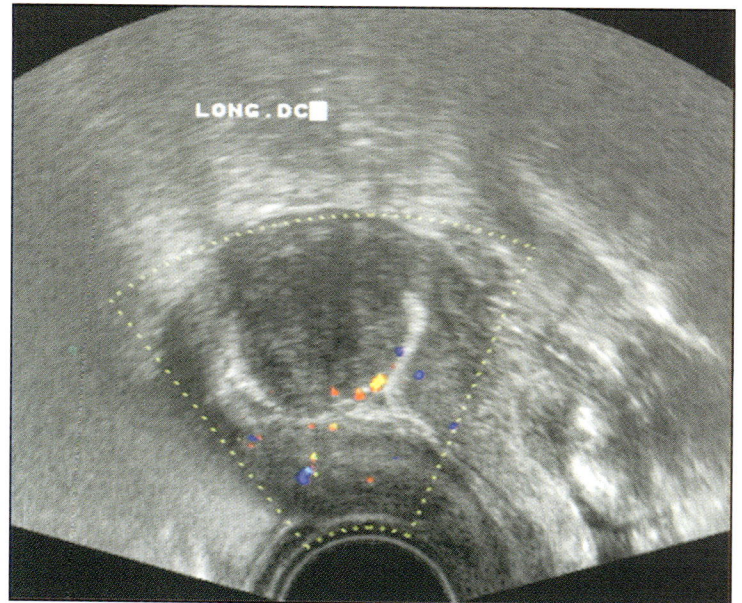

Fig. 20.35: The same patient as in Figure 20.34. Note the peripheral vascularity of this benign lesion

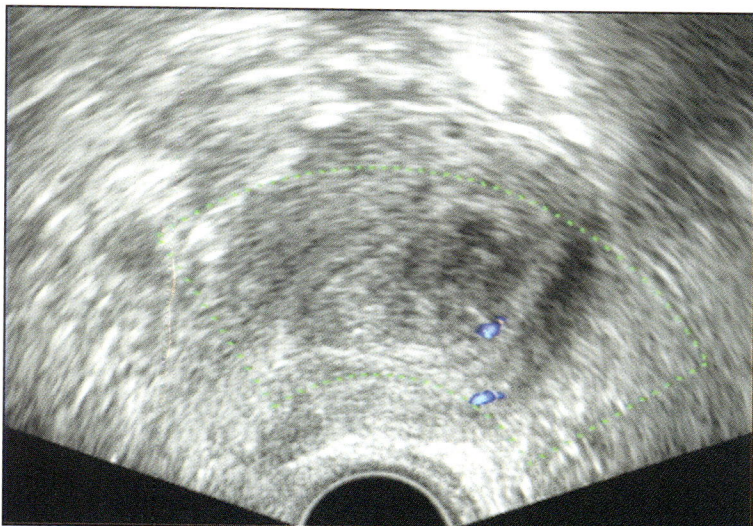

Fig. 20.33: Transvaginal sonogram demonstrating a large submucous myoma

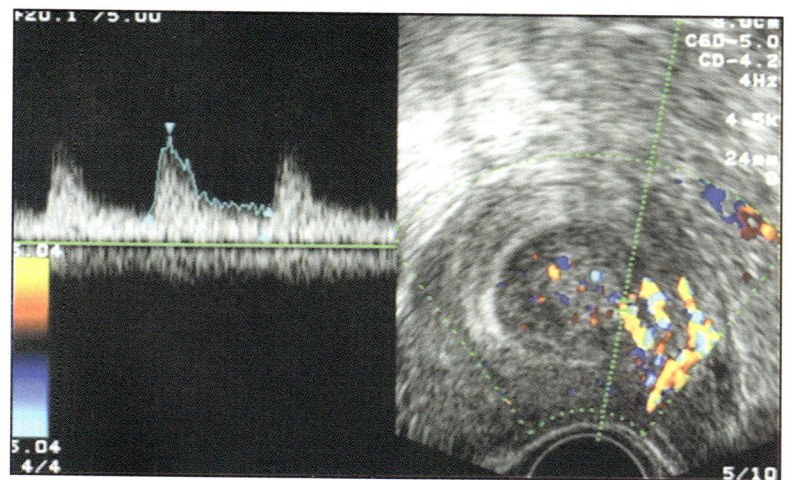

Fig. 20.36: Submucous myoma surrounded by endometrial layers. Color signals explored by pulsed Doppler waveform analysis show moderate resistance (RI = 0.62). The benign nature of the tumor was confirmed by hysteroscopy and histopathology

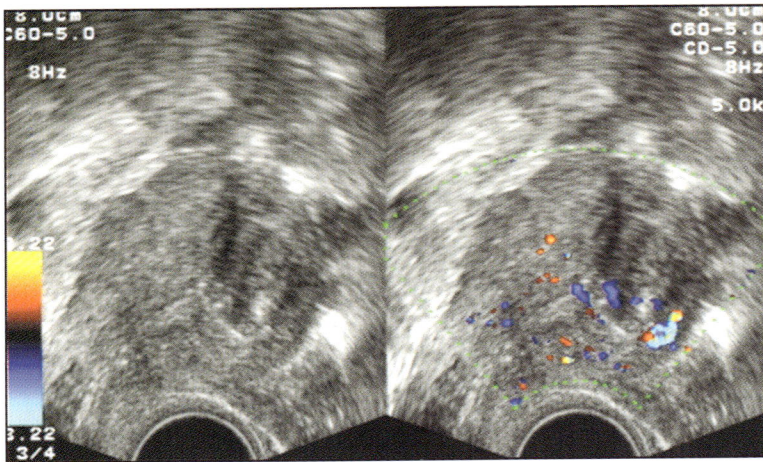

Fig. 20.37: Submucous leiomyoma may be difficult to differentiate from intramural leiomyomas

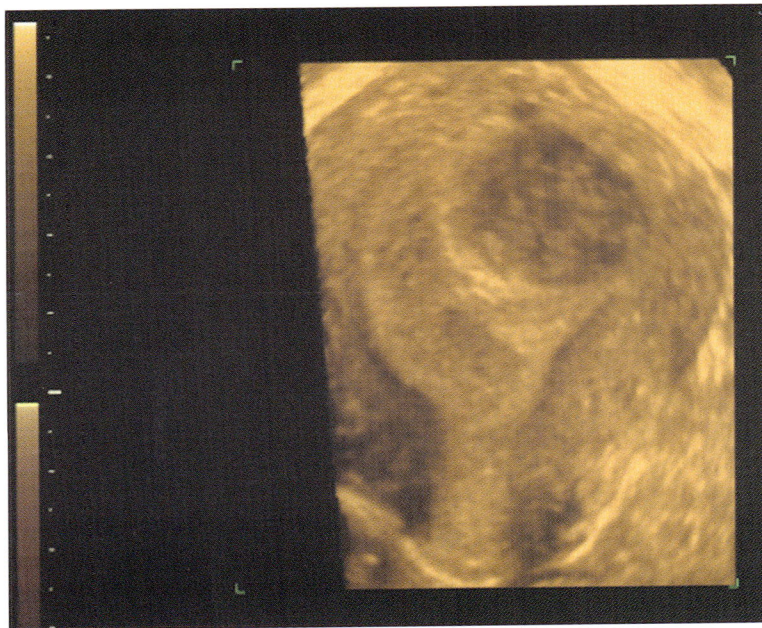

Fig. 20.40: Transabdominal scan of an subserous myoma mistaken of a solid heterogeneous mass

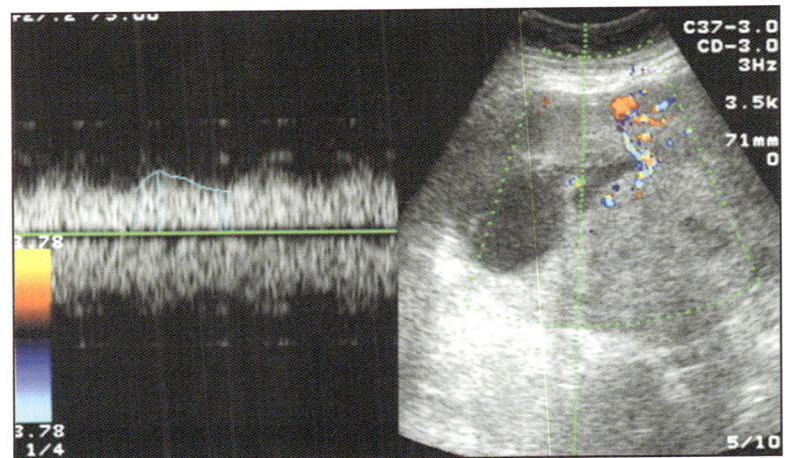

Fig. 20.38: Three-dimensional sonogram demonstrating the submucous myoma into the cavity

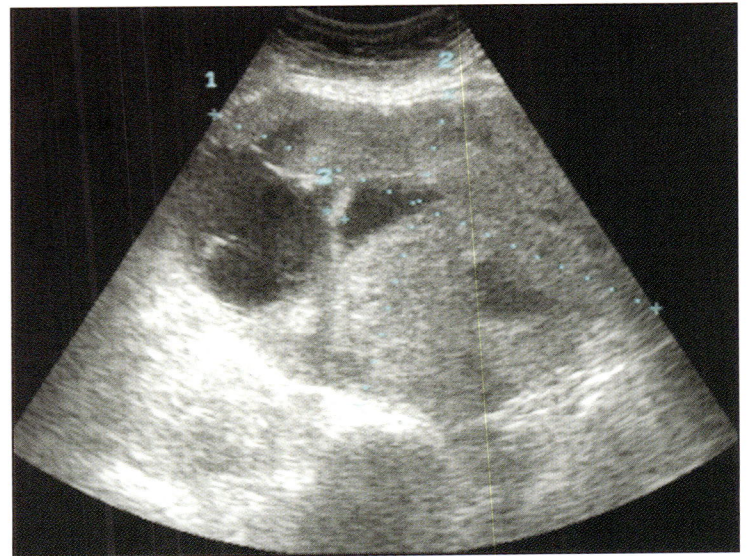

Fig. 20.41: The same patient as in Figure 20.40. Transvaginal color Doppler scan demonstrating myoma with areas of necrosis. Color Doppler depicts thick vessels at the periphery of the anechoic area, Pulsed Doppler analysis indicates low vascular resistance (RI = 0.34). Necrosis, degenerative and inflammatory changes within the myoma were confirmed by histopathology

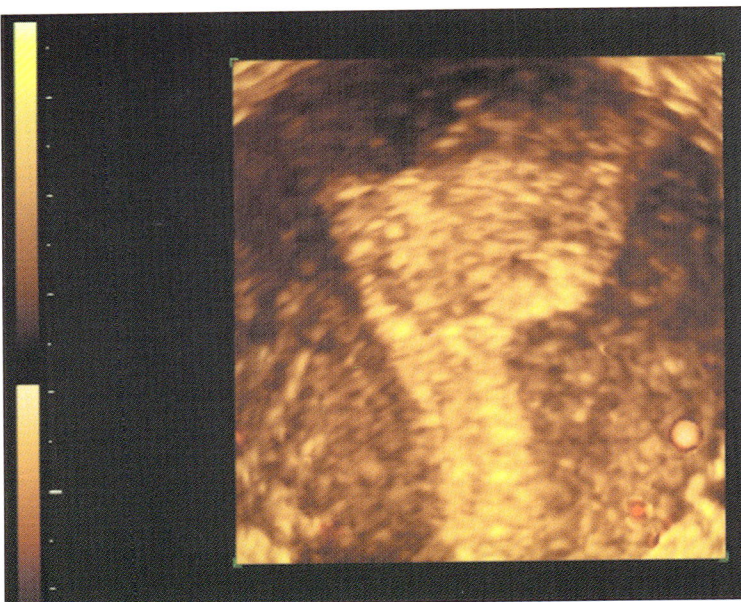

Fig. 20.39: Three-dimensional ultrasound (mode render) showing a submucous myomas surrounded by endometrium

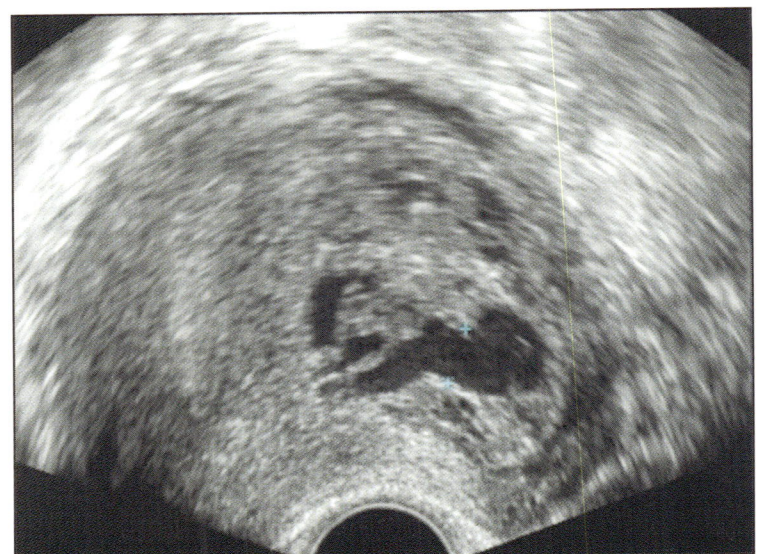

Fig. 20.42: Left myoma showing central and peripheral ischemia with consequent necrosis

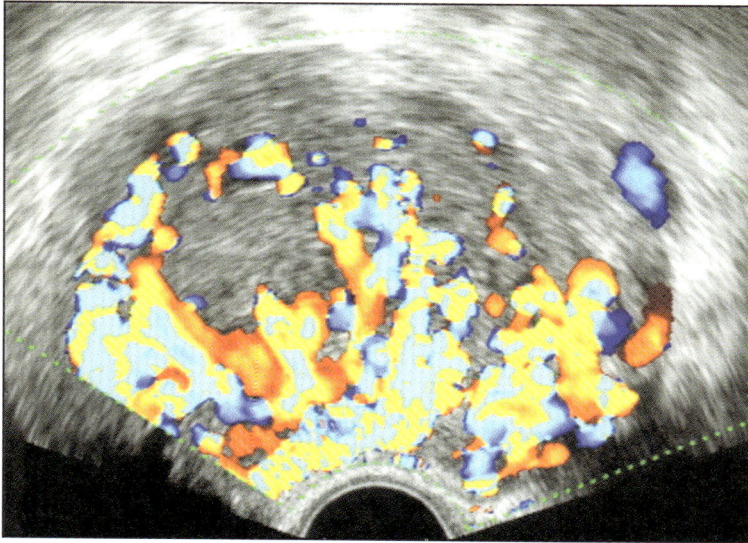

Fig. 20.43: The same patient as in Figure 20.42 Prominent color signals are detected in both central and peripheral parts of the tumor. Thick vessels displayed within the central part of the necrotic myoma represents dilated veins

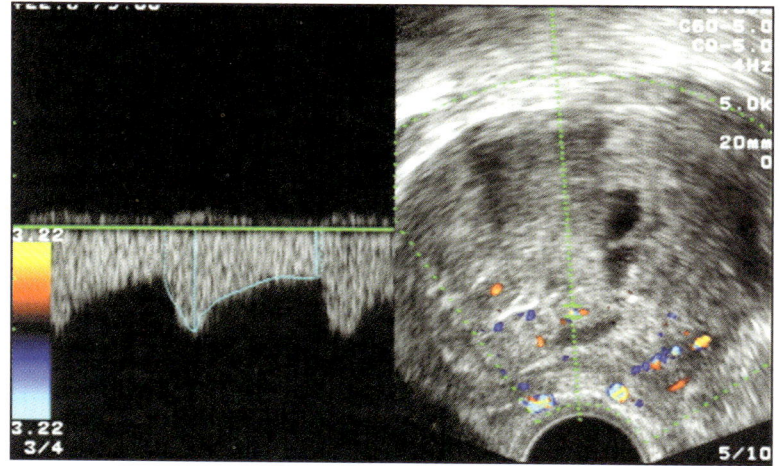

Fig. 20.44: Transvaginal color Doppler sonogram an intramural myoma with heterogeneous pattern. Color flow imaging demonstrating vessels encircling the myoma

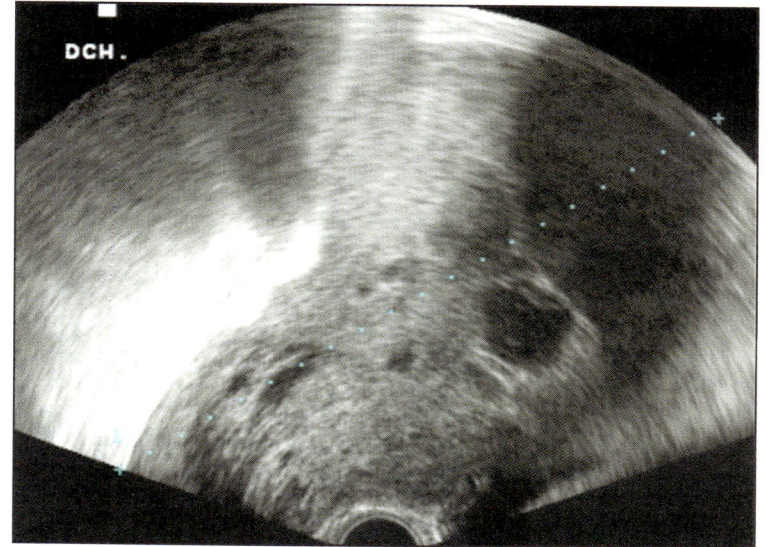

Fig. 20.45: Transvaginal scan of an ovarian fibroma mistaken a necrotic subserous myoma

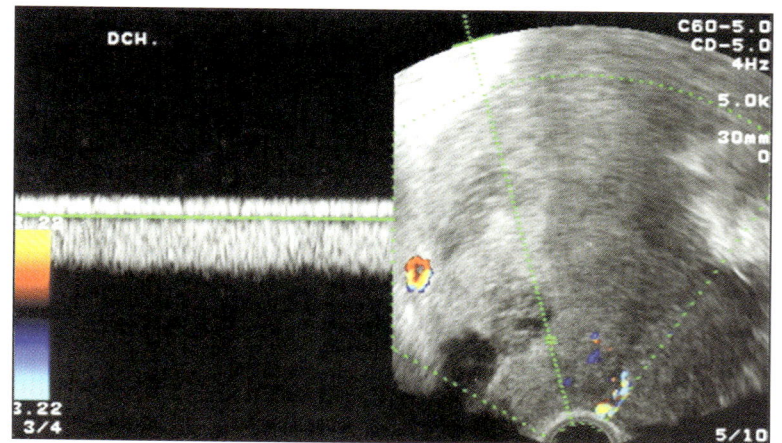

Fig. 20.46: The same patient as in Figure 20.45. Color Doppler shows a peripheral and central vessels with moderate-to-high resistance (RI = 0.56)

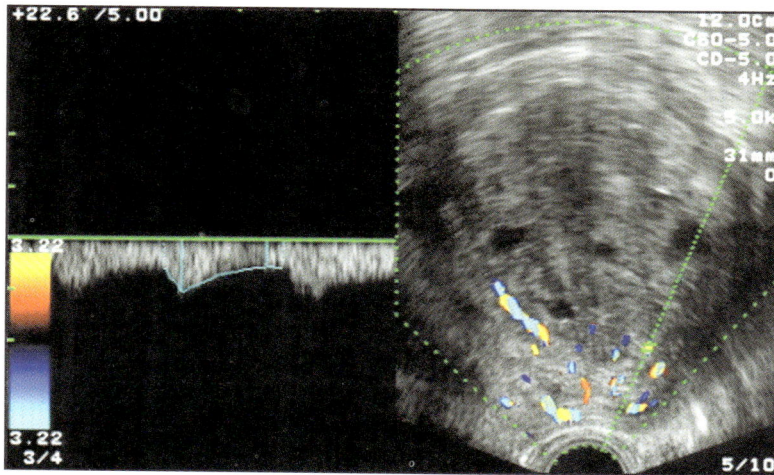

Fig. 20.47: Transvaginal scan of mixoid sarcoma . Note the heterogeneous pattern and partly cystic area of the solid tumor

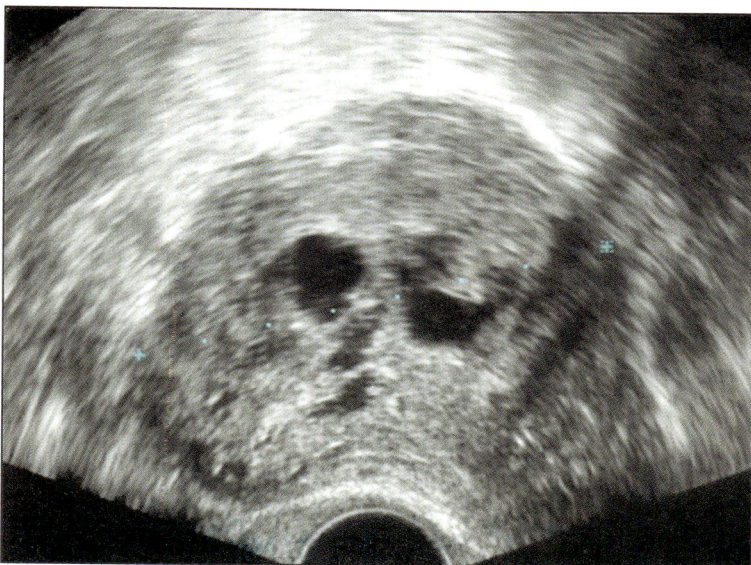

Fig. 20.48: The same patient as in Figure 20.47. Note the areas of tumor angicgenesis with shunts arterio-veneous

Serial sonographic evaluation of leiomyomas can be of significant value to the clinician. Follow-up scans of the fibroid uterus of a pregnant woman may help assess the growth and accelerated degeneration of this mass. Since fibroids should regress after menopause, serial sonograms can objectively document enlargement or regression of leiomyomas in the older woman.

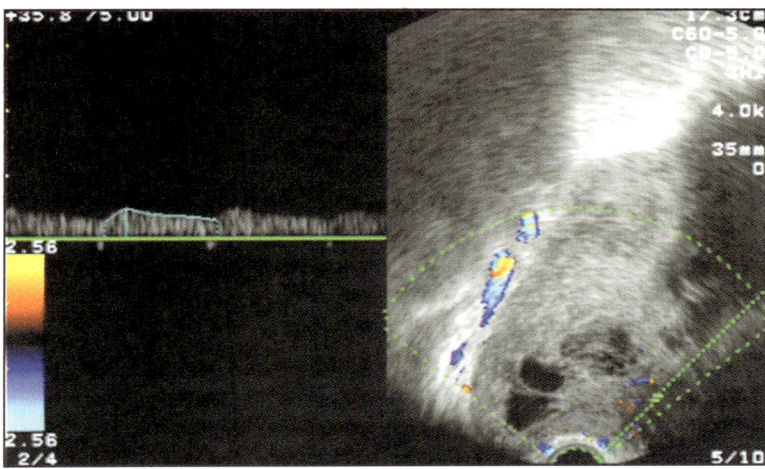

Fig. 20.49: The same patient as in Figures 20.47 and 20.48. Transvaginal color Doppler shows areas of neovascularization with low impedance to flow (RI = 0.43). Histopathology revealed uterine myxoid sarcoma

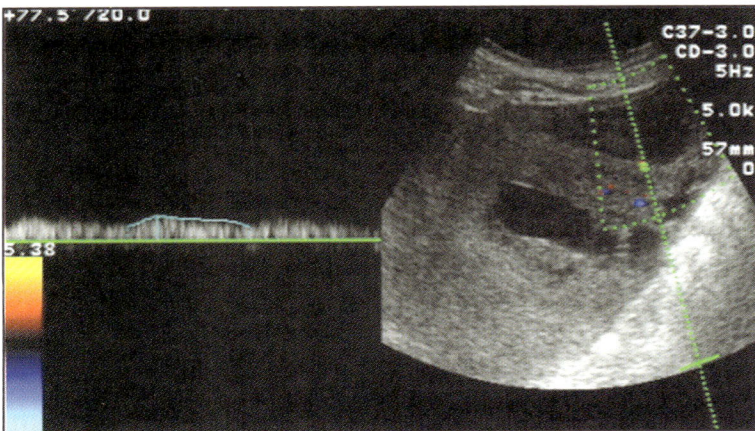

Fig. 20.50: The same case of as in Figures 20.47 to 20.49. Transabdominal color Doppler demonstrating vascularized areas with low resistance (RI = 0.42)

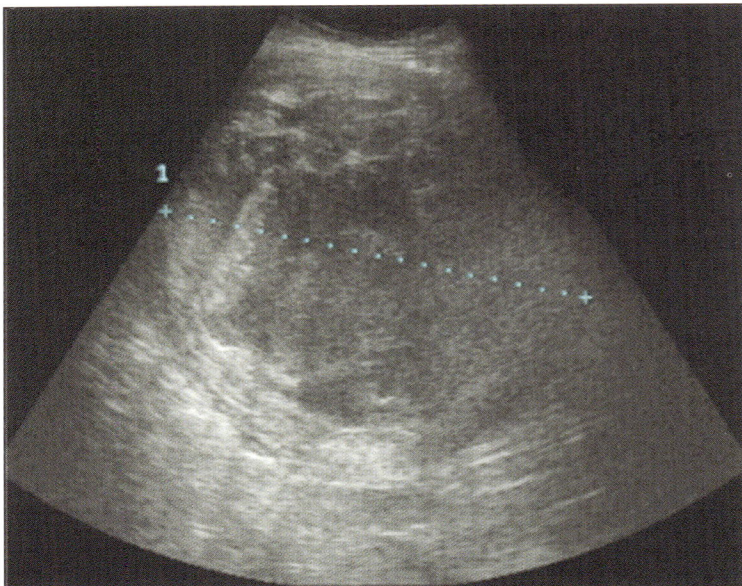

Fig. 20.51: Transabdominal scan of a large (17.9 cm) uterine sarcoma. Note the heterogeneous pattern and partly hyperechogenic texture of the solid tumor

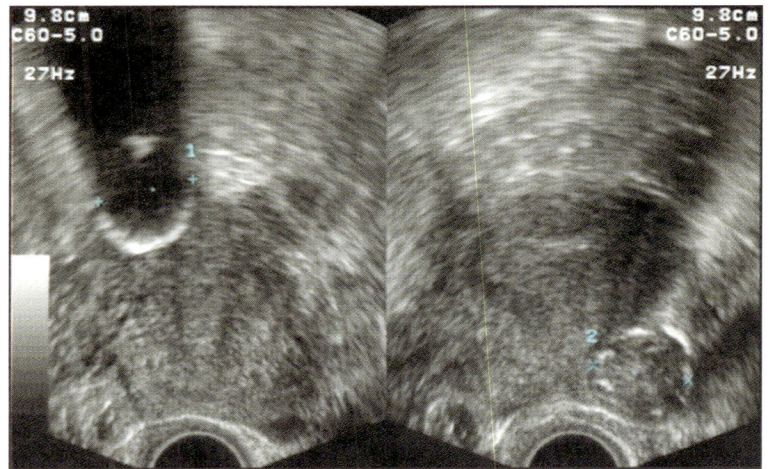

Fig. 20.52: Transvaginal sonogram of a calcified myomas. Note the shadowing behind the calcifications

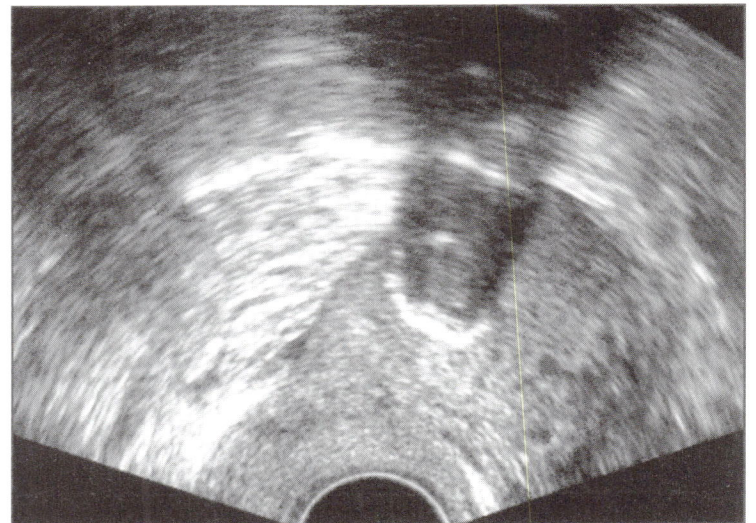

Fig. 20.53: Tranvaginal sonogram of a calcified myoma. Noted the shadowing after the myoma

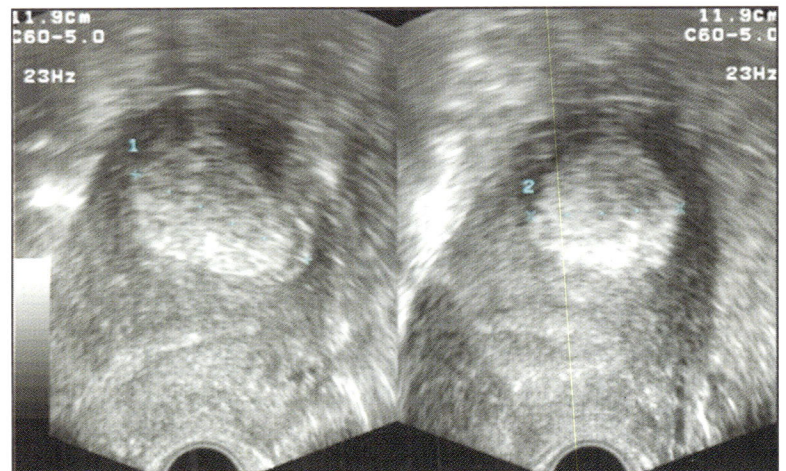

Fig. 20.54: Transvaginal sonogram showing a hyperechoic myoma. Histopathology reveals a fibromyolipoma

Adenomyosis or internal endometriosis is characterized by ingrowths of the endometrium into the myometrium (Figs 20.57 to 20.62). Adenomyosis is more often than not a diffuse process, but occasionally large adenomyomas can be seen. This condition can be diagnosed sonographically because of a thickened and "Swiss cheese" appearance of the myometrium due to areas of hemorrhage and clotting within the muscle. The uterus is slightly enlarged, with small cysts structures which affect uterine texture homogenicity.

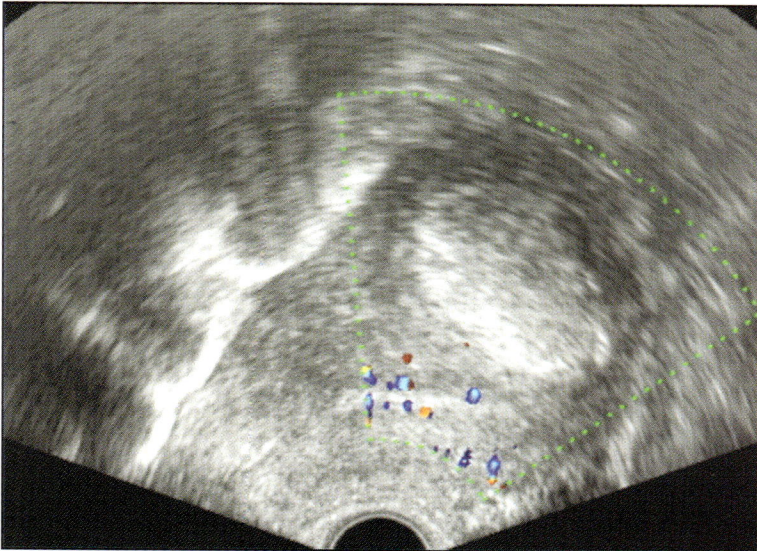

Fig. 20.55: The same patient as in Figure 20.54. Color Doppler shows no signal flow

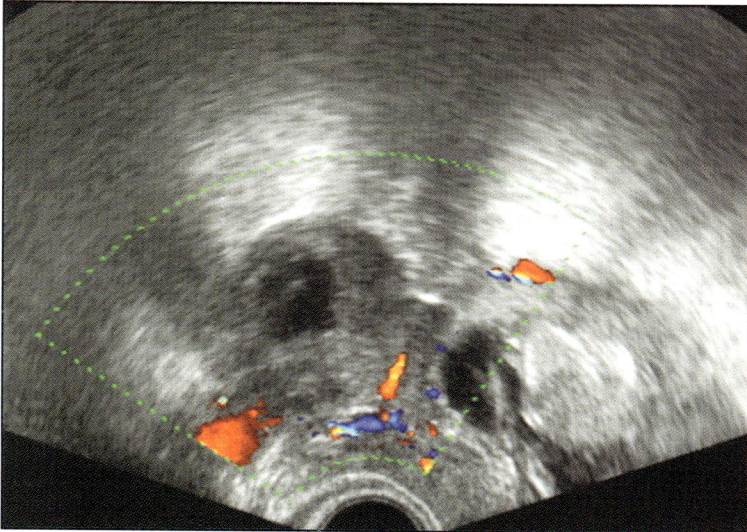

Fig. 20.58: Transvaginal sonogram of an adenomyosic uterus, the frequently findings are the asymmetric size of the myometrial walls, larger posterior than anterior (3.2 cm versus 2.1 cm)

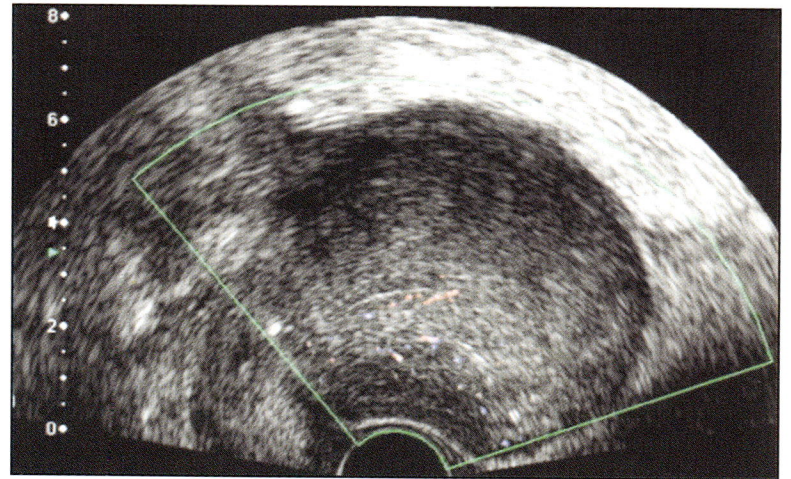

Fig. 20.56: Transvaginal sonogram showing a pregnant uterus with subserous myoma demonstrating necrotic phenomena

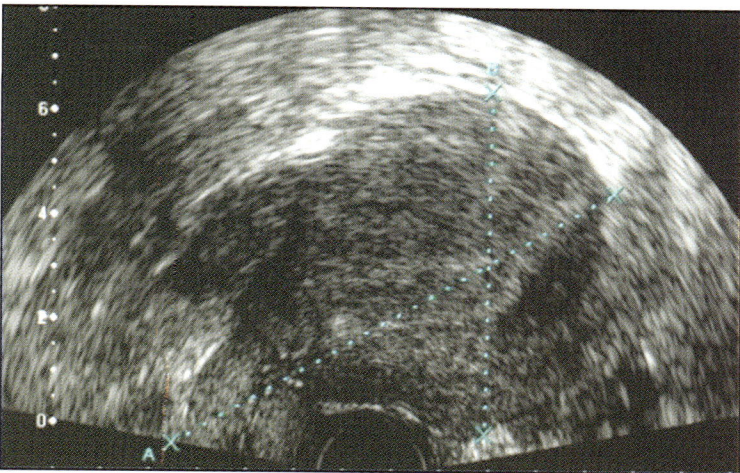

Fig. 20.59: Diffusely enlarged uterus with anechoic small cysts within the myometrial portion, in a patient suffering from dysmenorrhea and menometrorrhagia

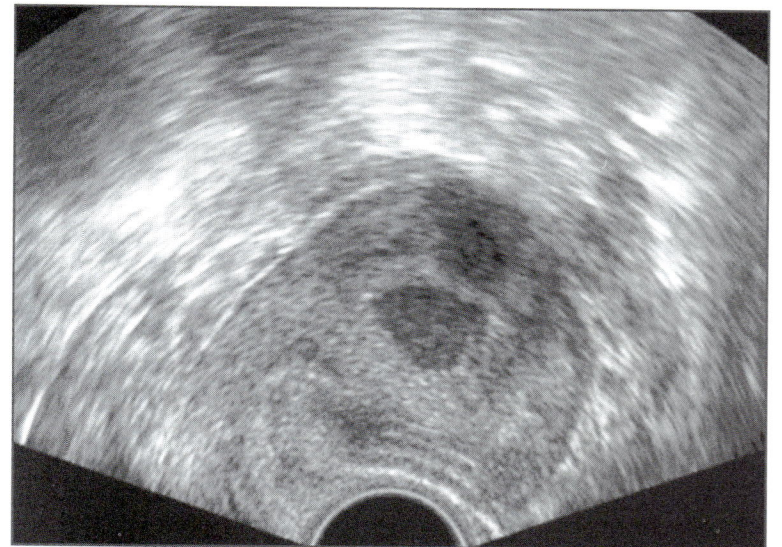

Fig. 20.57: Transvaginal sonogram showing an enlarged uterus affected by adenomyosis. The myometrial pattern is affected by small cystic structures contain blood

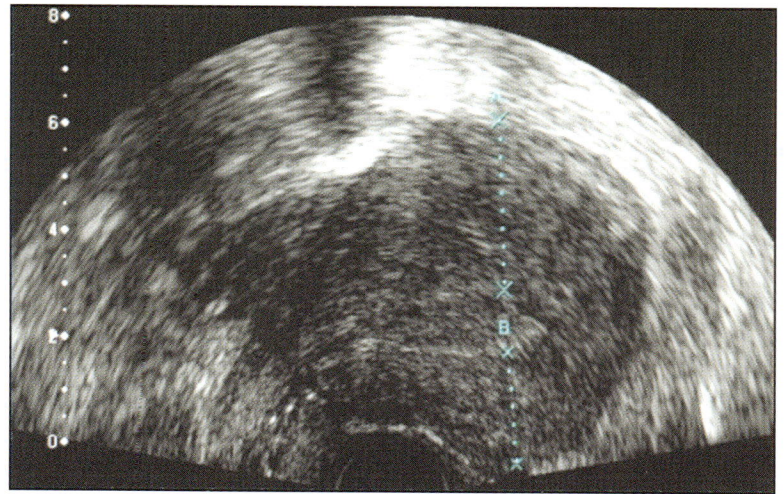

Fig. 20.60: Transvaginal sonogram of the uterus demonstrating endometrial clusters within the myometrium. This finding is suggestive of adenomyosis

Sonographically, some kinds of atrophy of endometrium (Figs 20.63 and 20.64) show confusing images similar to hypertrophy.

It is known that patients undertaken tamoxifen can change the endometrial pattern. In fact, the endometrium becomes

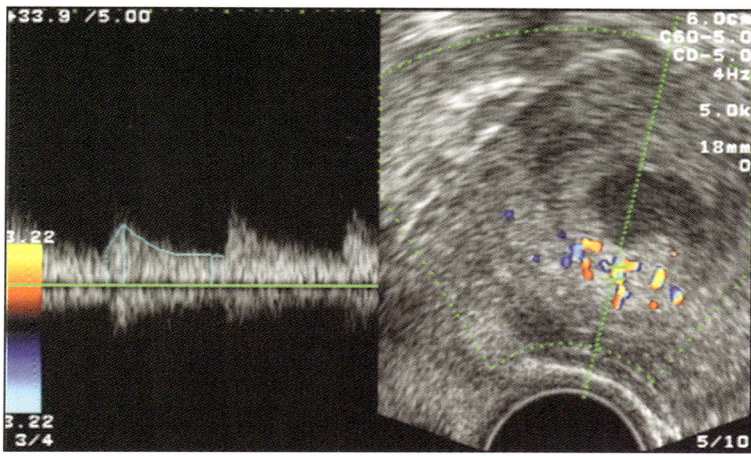

Fig. 20.61: The same patient as in Figure 20.60: Waveform analysis demonstrates blood flow of moderate resistance (RI = 0.51). Histopathology revealed adenomyosis

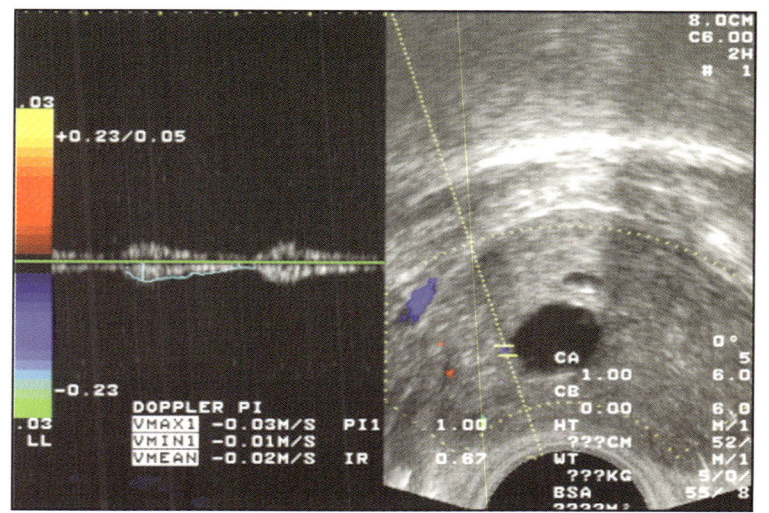

Fig. 20.64: The same patient as in Figure 20.63 Blood flow signals of high resistance (RI = 0.67) were obtained surrounding cyst structures

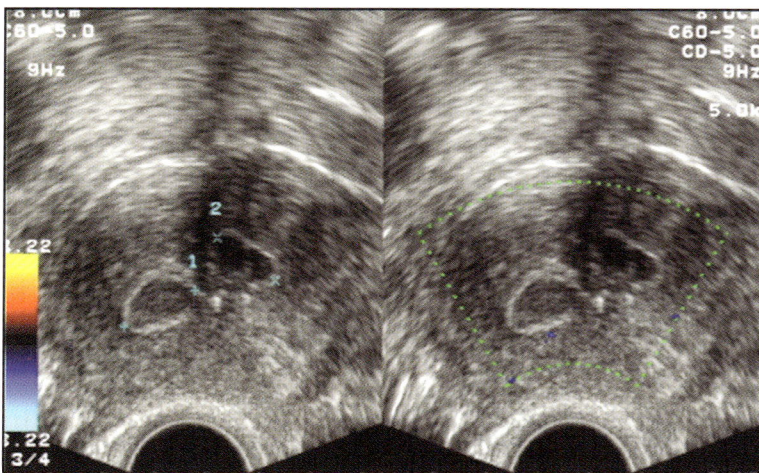

Fig. 20.62: Transvaginal color Doppler sonogram showing a focal adenomyosis after endometrial ablation

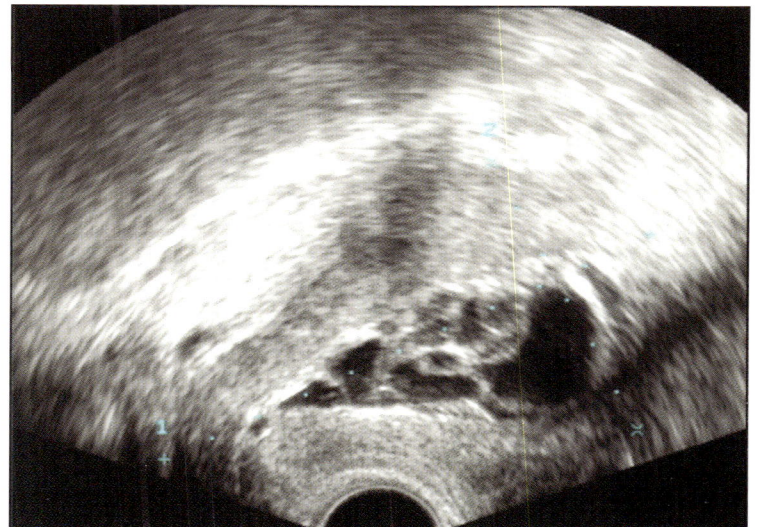

Fig. 20.65: Transvaginal sonogram of a patient receiving tamoxifen treatment. Note the intrauterine fluid collection and focal thickenings

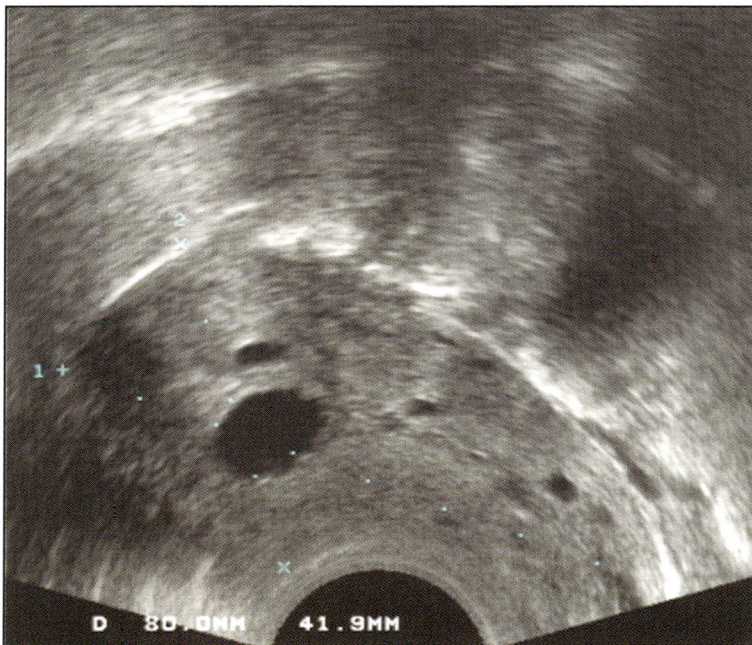

Fig. 20.63: Transvaginal sonogram of a postmenopausal patient showing periendometrial cyst. Hysteroscopy demonstrated an cystic atrophia of endometrium

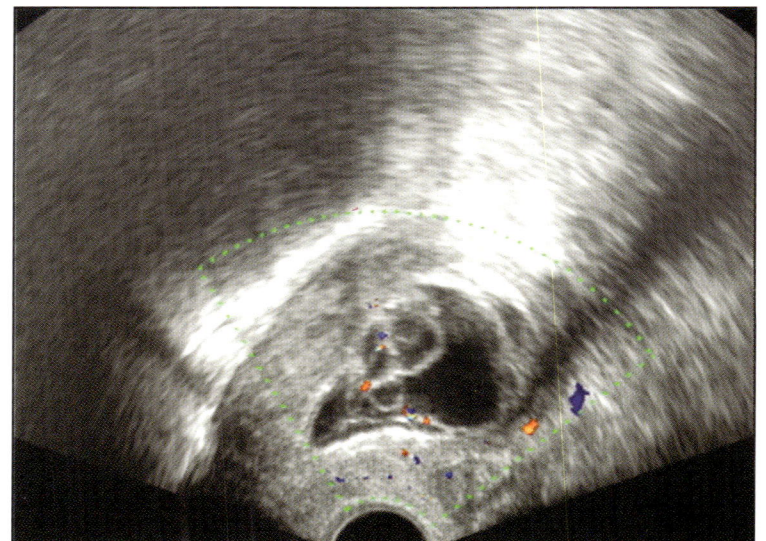

Fig. 20.66: The same patient as in Figure 20.65. Transvaginal color Doppler showing a few spots within the thick and cystic endometrium

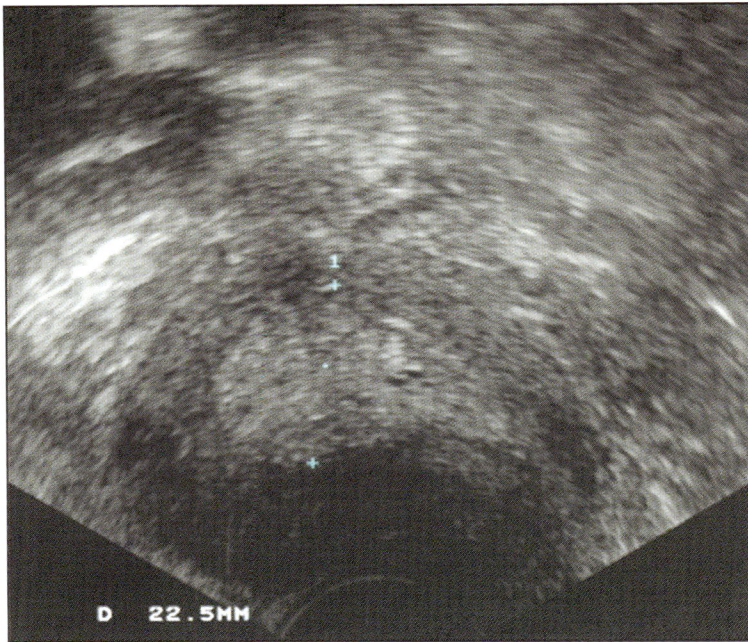

Fig. 20.67: Transvaginal sonogram of a patient receiving tamoxifen treatment. Note the thickened endometrium with a small cystic structures

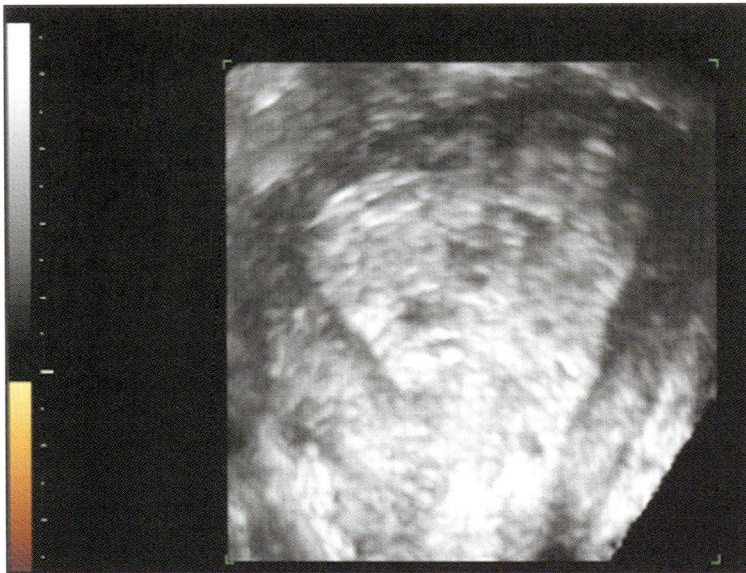

Fig. 20.68: Three-dimensional power Doppler sonogram of a postmenopausal patient on tamoxifen therapy. Note the increased endometrial thickening with multiple small cystic structures

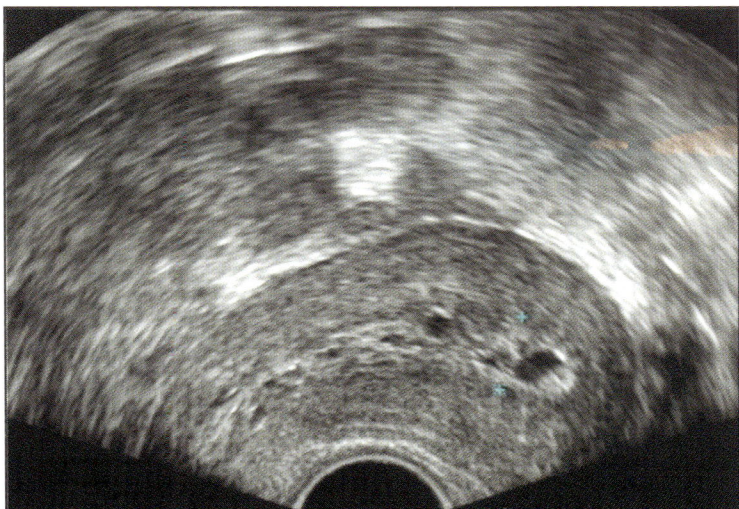

Fig. 20.69: Transvaginal sonogram of a patient receiving tamoxifen therapy. Note the irregular endometrial-myometrial border

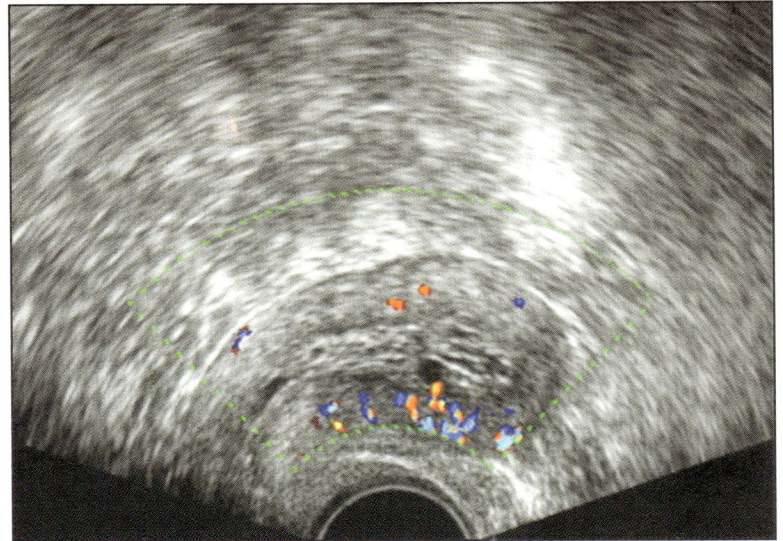

Fig. 20.70: Transvaginal sonogram of a patient receiving tamoxifen treatment. Note the thickened and irregular cystic endometrium

atrophic: it is an hypertrophy of the endometrial stroma. The sonography demonstrates cystic areas within the innermyometrium (Figs 20.65 to 20.70).

Hematometra occurs as a result of an obliteration and ultrasonically appears as low-level echoes within the distended uterine cavity (Figs 20.71 to 20.73).

Incomplete abortion demonstrates echogenic tissue within the uterine cavity arising from retained trophoblastic tissue. Color Doppler shows prominent blood flow signals with low resistance index (Figs 20.74 to 20.79).

Ultrasonically, endometritis (Fig. 20.80) is characterized with increased echogenicity, thickness and vascularity of the endometrium. In the acute stage of endometritis, the blood flow signals obtained from the periphery of the endometrium reveal low to moderate impedance. In the case of irreversible tissue damage, blood flow is usually absent.

Other uterine abnormalities include endometrial hyperplasia and polyps which are demonstrated as a thick and highly echogenic endometrium (Figs 20.81 to 20.101). Color Doppler demonstrates peripheral and regular vascularization with moderate resistance index in an hypertrophic endometrium. Vascular pedicle can be seen in polyps with moderate to high resistance index. Since three-dimensional transvaginal ultrasound allows frontal reformatted section through the uterus, it can give more precise information on the endometrial polyps' location and size.

The transvaginal color Doppler applied to molar pregnancy depicts prominent zones of vascularization inside the uterine cavity as well as in the peritrophoblastic area. Inside the uterine cavity the color-coded zones can be visualized, superimposed on the characteristic "snow storm" ultrasonic appearance. In cases of invasive mole uterine circulation undergoes significant changes as a result of the proliferation of the trophoblastic tissue

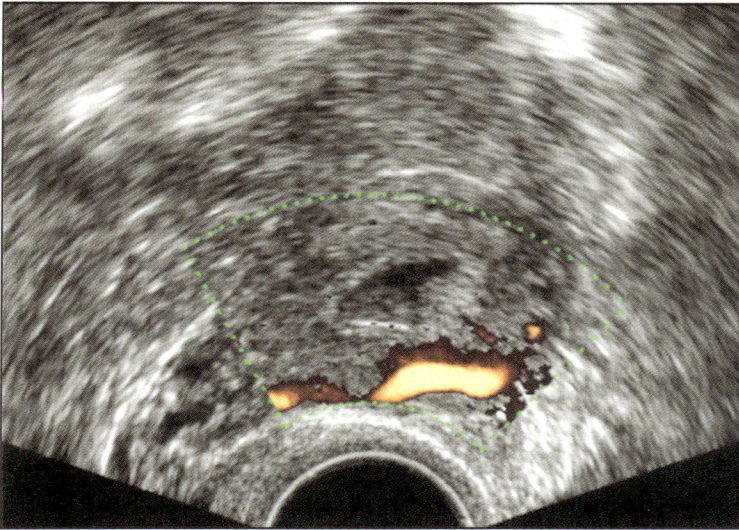

Fig. 20.71: Transvaginal power Doppler scan of a patient with partial obliteration of the endometrial cavity. The menstrual pattern in this particular patient is characterized by hypomenorrhea. Note the presence the endometrial echoes within the cavity

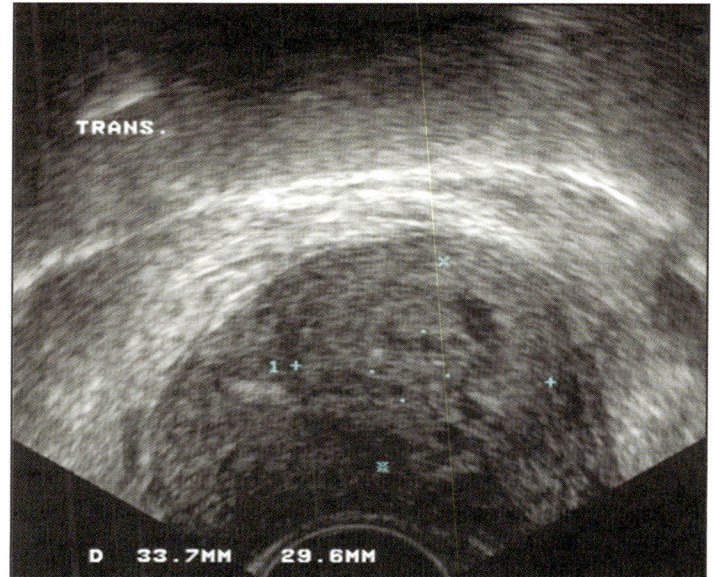

Fig. 20.74: Transvaginal scan demonstrating disorganized echogenic contens and fluid, indicative of residual trophoblastic tissue

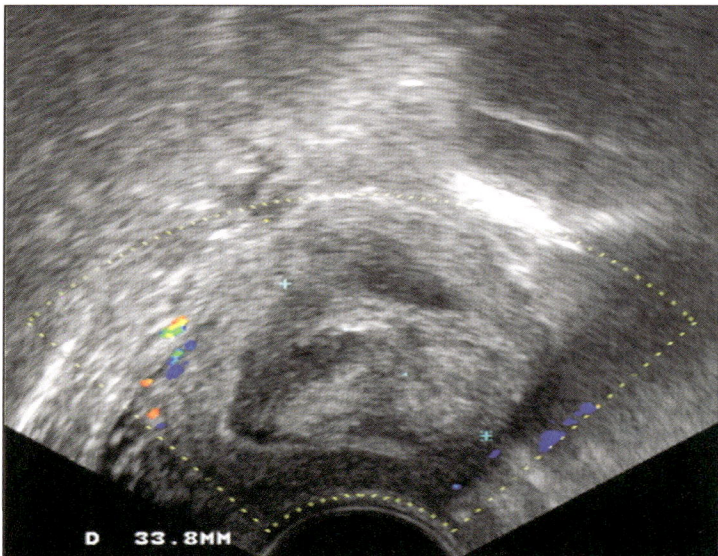

Fig. 20.72: Transvaginal sonogram showing full cavity of clot blood. This finding is indicative of intrauterine adhesions occurring in a patient after vigorous curettage

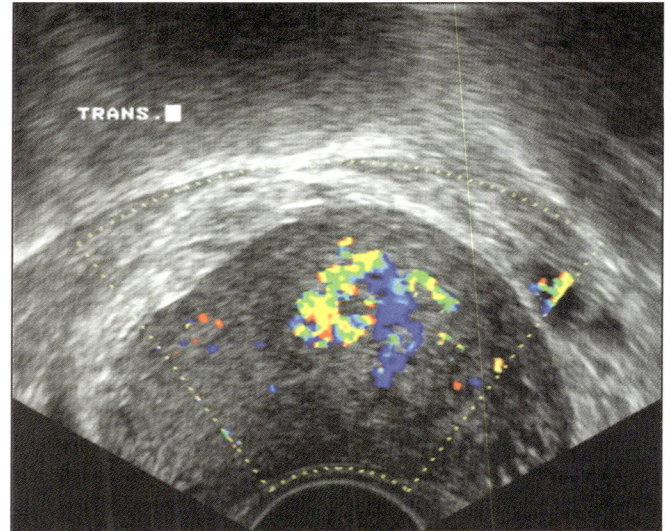

Fig. 20.75: The same patient as in Figure 20.74. Abundant color Doppler flow is easily detected by color Doppler and represents the response of the dilated spiral arteries and venous system to the active trophoblastic tissue

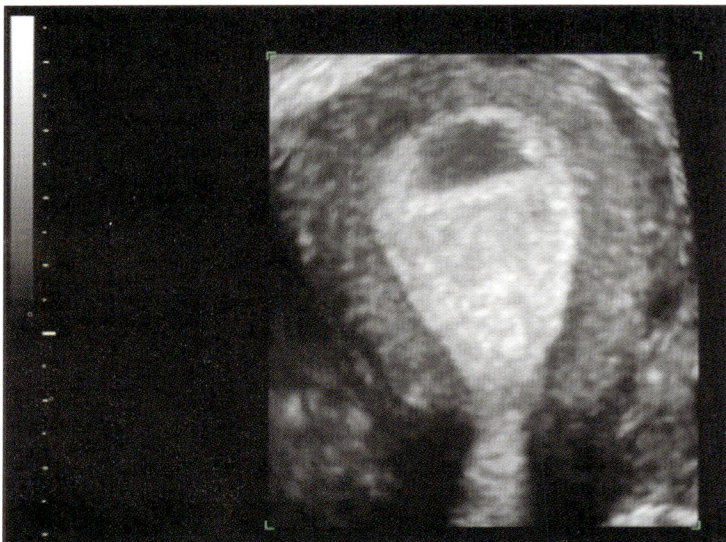

Fig. 20.73: Three-dimensional sonogram showing clot blood full endometrial cavity. Note the level up the cavity

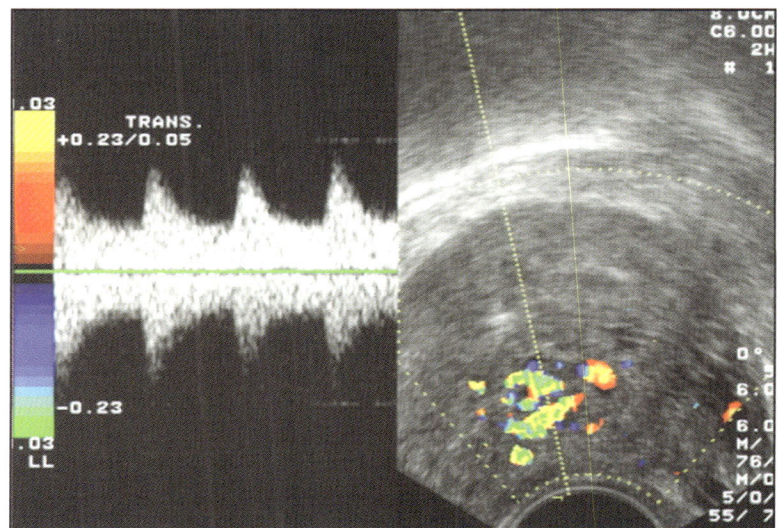

Fig. 20.76: Pulsed Doppler color showing arterial vessels in a patient with active trophoblastic tissue

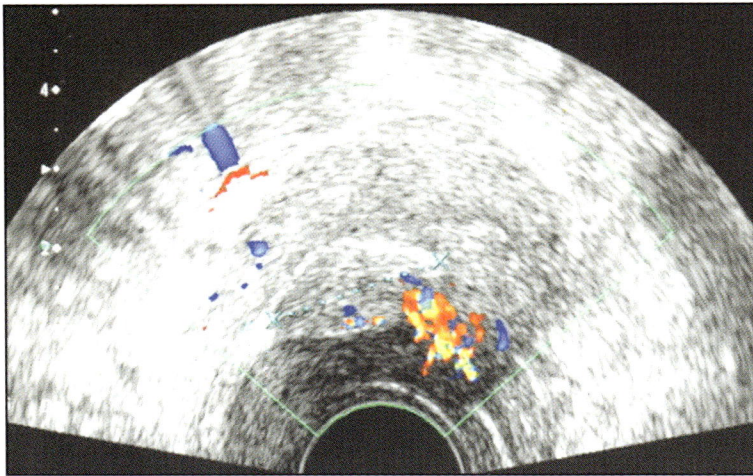

Fig. 20.77: Transvaginal color Doppler scan of a patient with signs of residua. Color Doppler reveals prominent blood flow signals at the periphery of endometrial echo

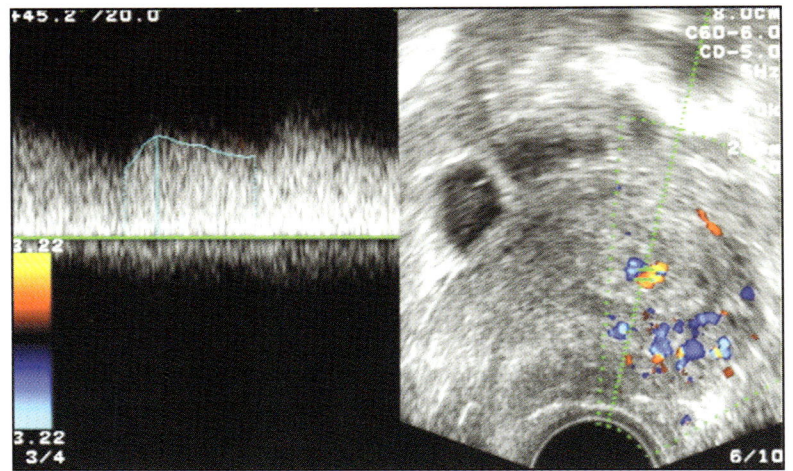

Fig. 20.79: Transvaginal scan of patient with residua demonstrating mixed endometrial pattern. Low vascular resistance (RI = 0.32) is easily observed in the hyperechogenic area

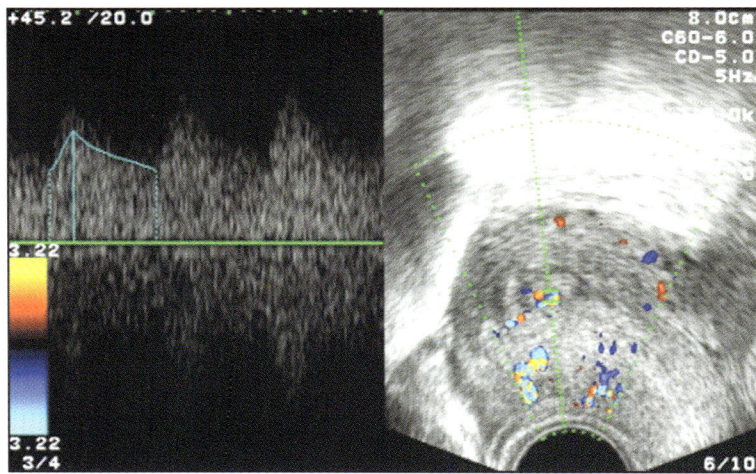

Fig. 20.78: Transvaginal color Doppler scan of a patient with atypical sign of residua. Color Doppler reveals flow signals at the periphery of endometrial echo. Low vascular resistance (RI = 0.35) signals easily obtained from the remaining products of conception

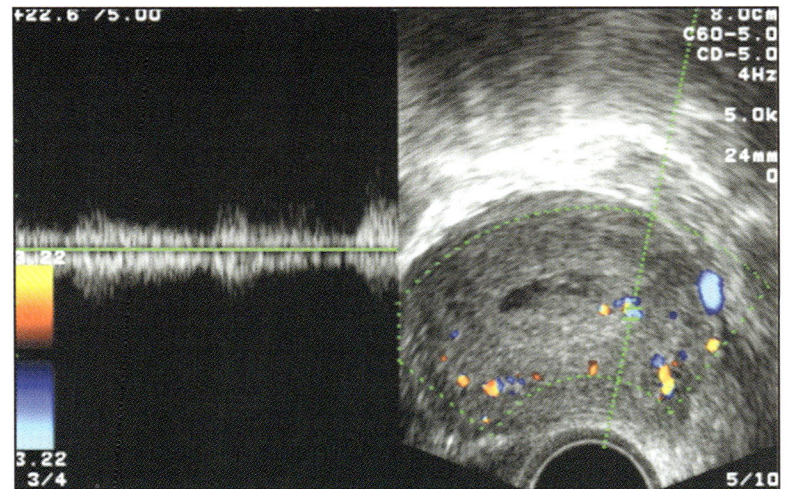

Fig. 20.80: Transvaginal sonogram of the uterus with irregular echogenic contens within the uterine cavity. This finding is suggestive of endometritis. Doppler color does not reveal increased vascularity in the subendometrial space

and its invasion into the myometrium. The hypervascularity transforms the uterus into a low-impedance organ with significant changes in the flow patterns of the uterine artery and its branches (Figs 20.102 and 20.103). By color Doppler technique, other conditions such as postabortal uterus and other endometrial pathologies can be recognized, differentiating these pathological conditions from gestational trophoblastic disease.

The more common uterine malignancy is endometrial carcinoma. Postmenopausal bleeding associated with an ultrasound finding of uterine enlargement, thick endometrium and hypoechoic and non-homogeneous texture is highly suggestive of this malignancy (Figs 20.104 to 20.113). Color Doppler demonstrates intratumoral blood flow with irregular vessels and very low resistance index.

Power Doppler three-dimensional ultrasound greatly improves the accuracy in the diagnosis of endometrial carcinoma (Figs 20.114 to 20.123).

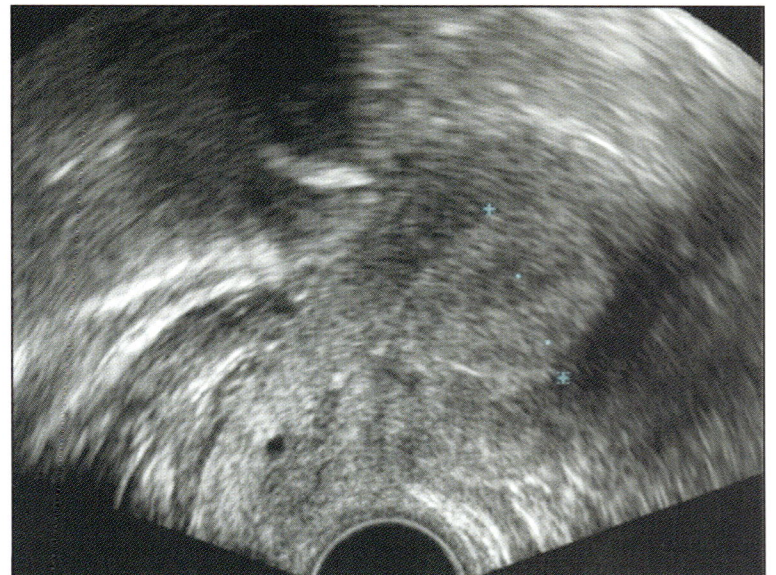

Fig. 20.81: Transvaginal sonogram of an asymptomatic postmenopausal patient with thickened endometrium (2.5 cm). Histopathology demonstrated endometrial hyperplasia

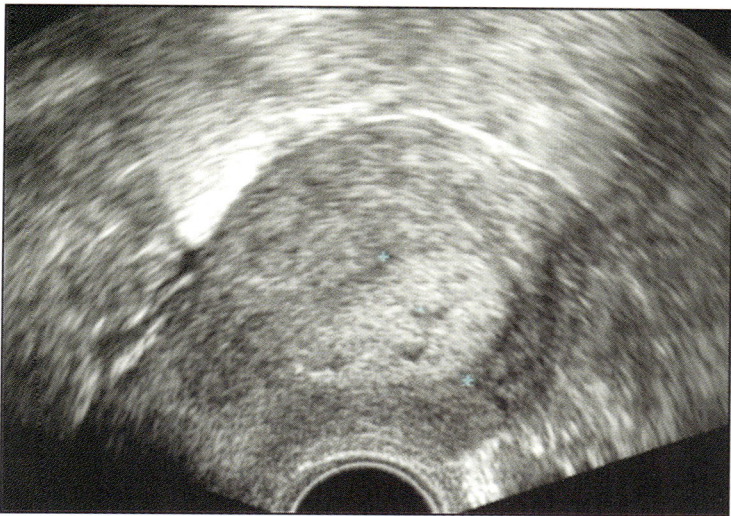

Fig. 20.82: Another example of thickened nodular endometrium (2.3 cm). Note the preserved integrity of the subendometrial halo

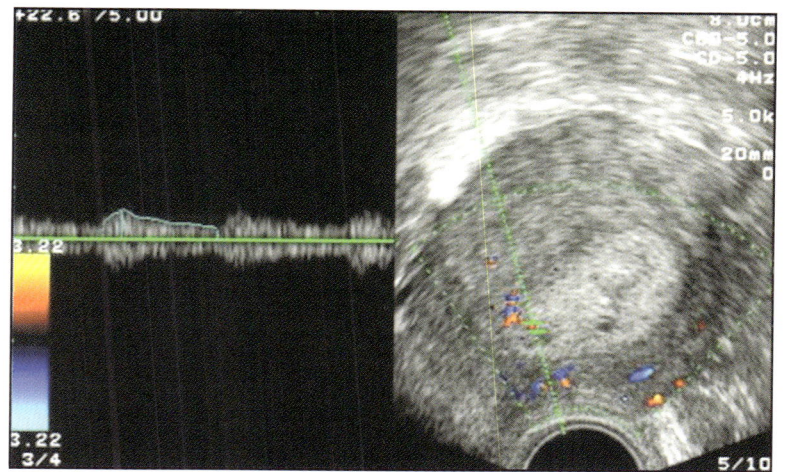

Fig. 20.85: Transvaginal color Doppler scan of thickened nodular endometrium. Peripheral distribution of the vessels and moderate-to-high vascular resistance (RI = 0.64) indicates a benign endometrial lesion

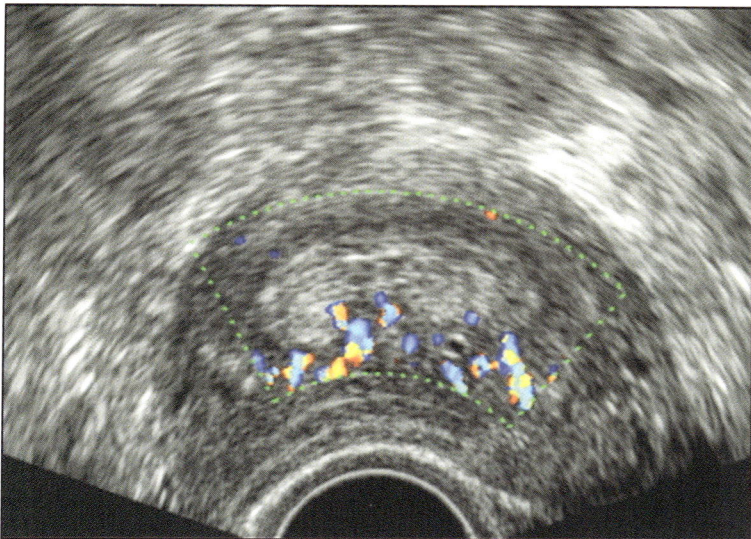

Fig. 20.83: Transvaginal color Doppler scan of thickened endometrium in a perimenopausal patient with bleeding. Peripheral distribution of the regularly separated vessels indicates a benign endometrial lesion. Histopathology confirmed an endometrial hyperplasia

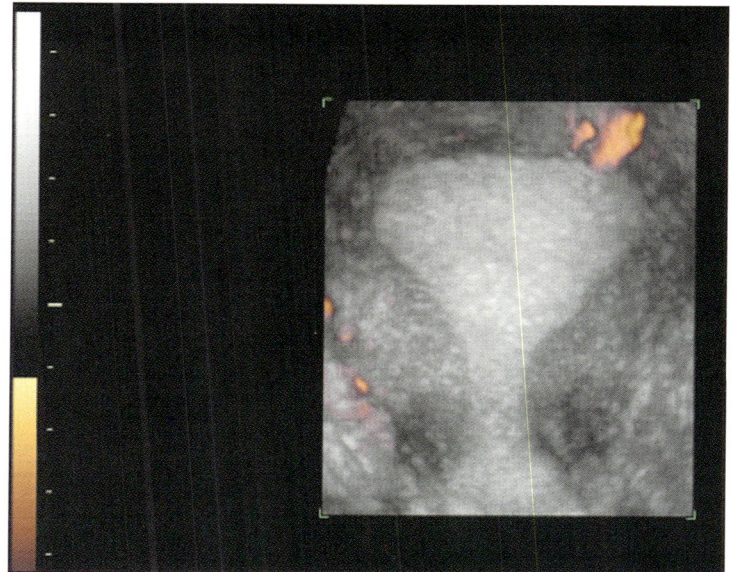

Fig. 20.86: Three-dimensional scan with abnormal endometrial thickening. Note a vessel penetrating within the cavity

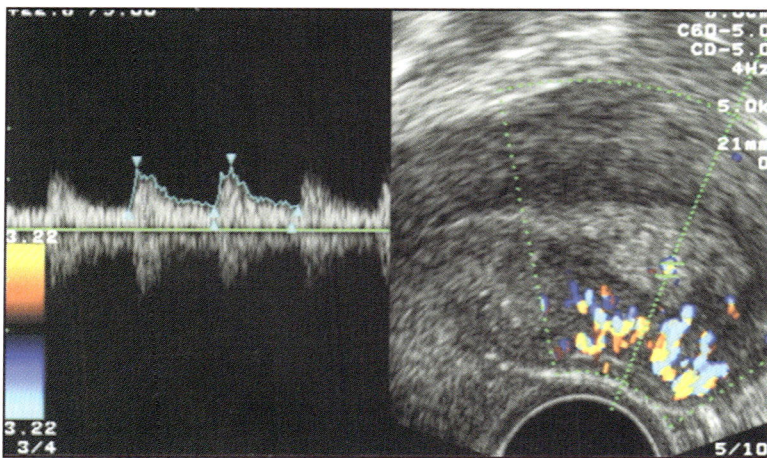

Fig. 20.84: Transvaginal color Doppler scan of a postmenopausal patient with thickened endometrium and vaginal bleeding. Blood flow signals were obtained from the central part of the lesion. Moderate-to-high vascular resistance (RI = 0.60) was detected in the area of angiogenesis within the endometrium. Histopathology revealed endometrial hyperplasia

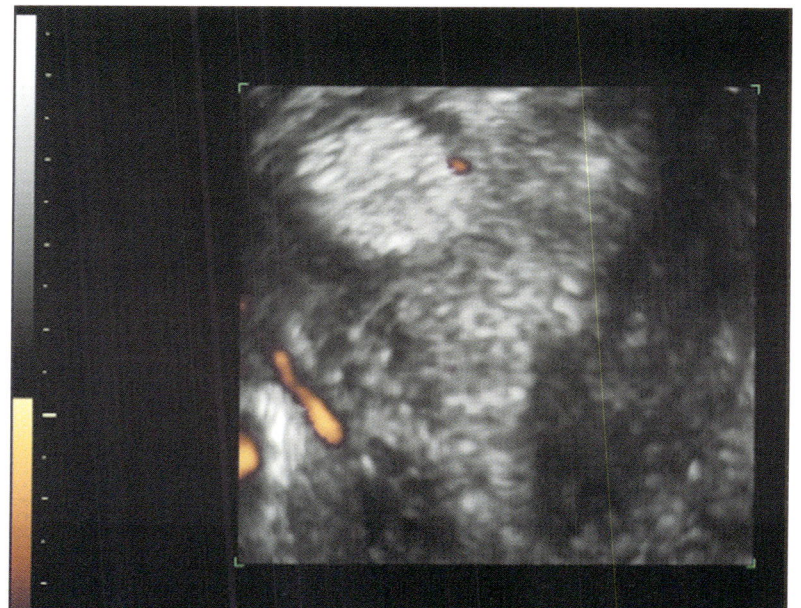

Fig. 20.87: The same case as in Figure 20.86: Transvaginal scan shows an endometrial polyp in the right uterine horn

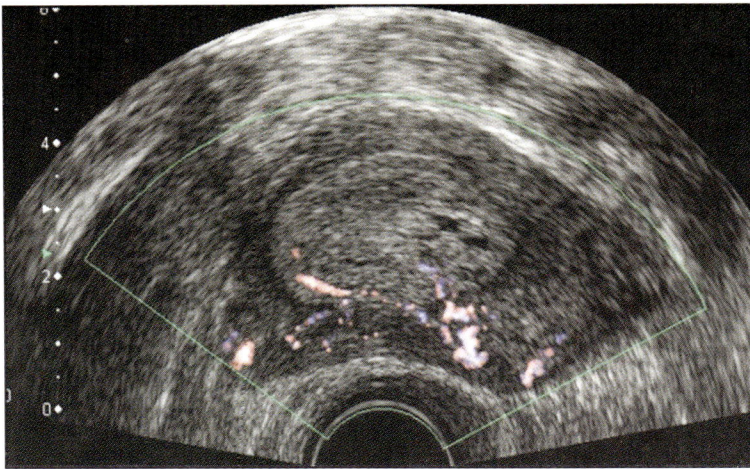

Fig. 20.88: Transvaginal color Doppler scan demonstrating a focal area of increased echogenicity and peripheral distribution of regulary separated vessels, typical of and endometrial polyp

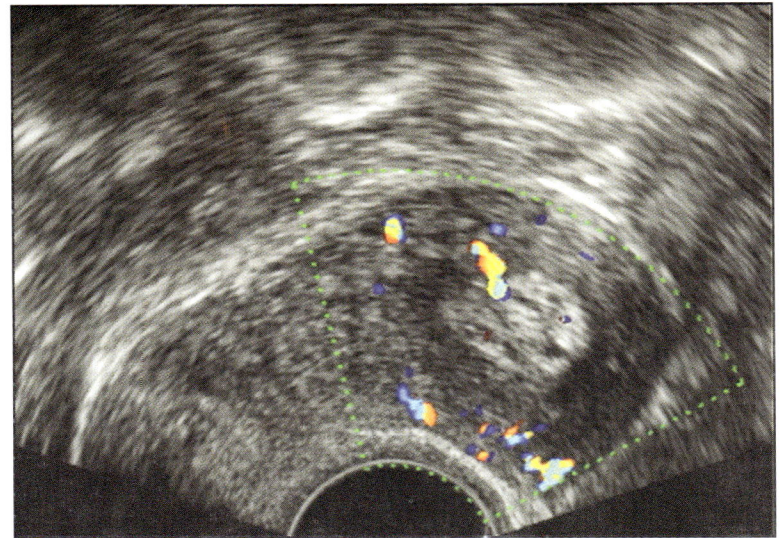

Fig. 20.91: Another picture showing an endometrial polyp with pedicle vessel

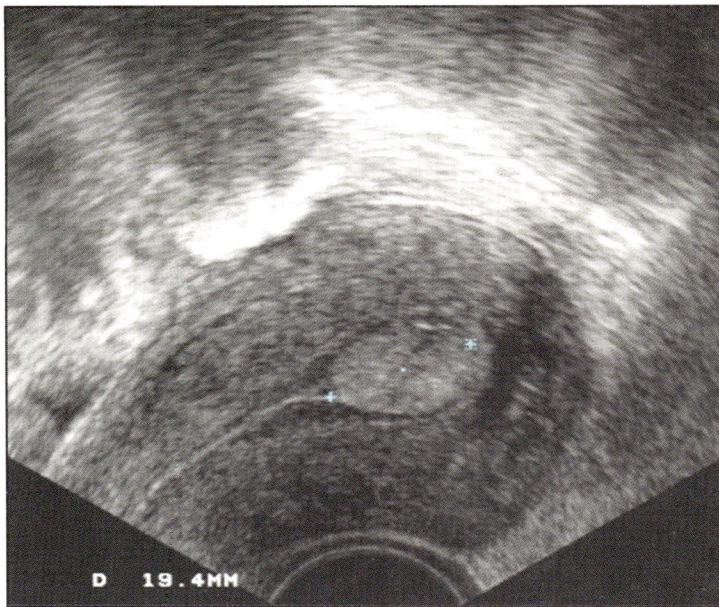

Fig. 20.89: B-mode tansvaginal scan showing a nodular echogenic lesion within the endometrium suspected to be an endometrial polyp. Histeroscopy confirmed a polyp

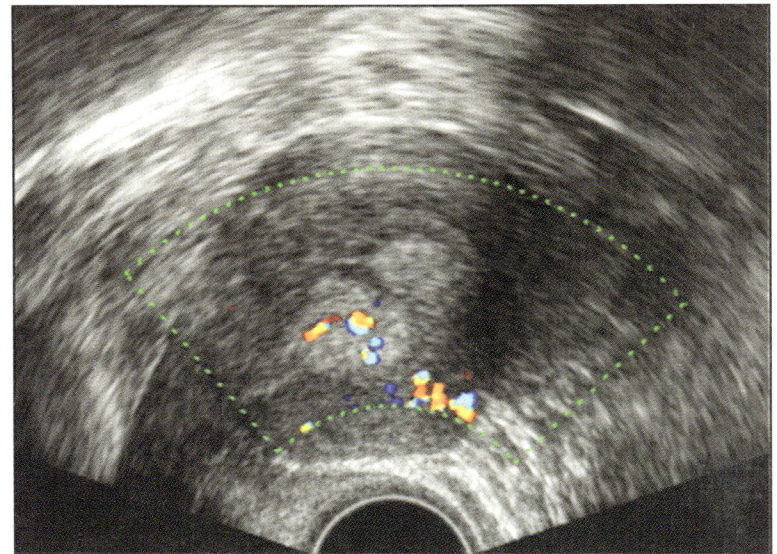

Fig. 20.92: Transvaginal color Doppler scan showing two polyps and its pedicles vessels respectively

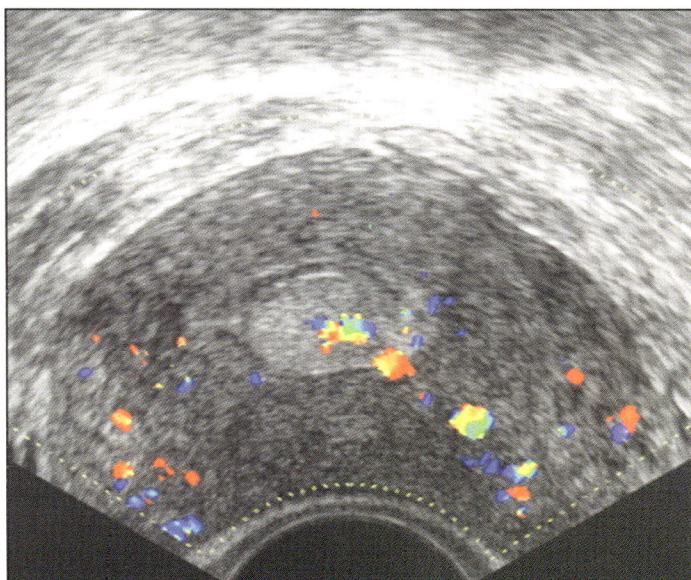

Fig. 20.90: Transvaginal color Doppler sonogram showing a single vessel penetrating to the endometrial polyp. This vessel corresponds to the polyps´ pedicle

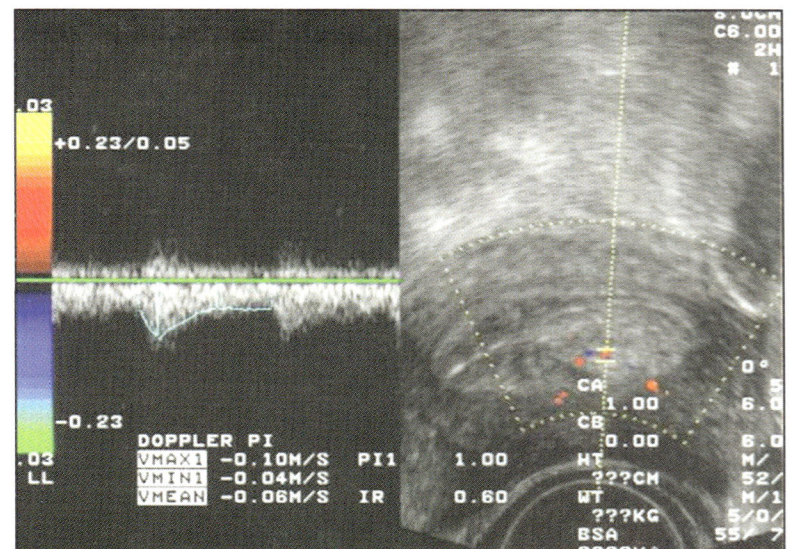

Fig. 20.93: Pulsed Doppler color from polyp's pedicle showing an arterial vessel. Moderate vascular impedance is observed in the endometrial polyp. Demonstrating a resistance index of 0.60

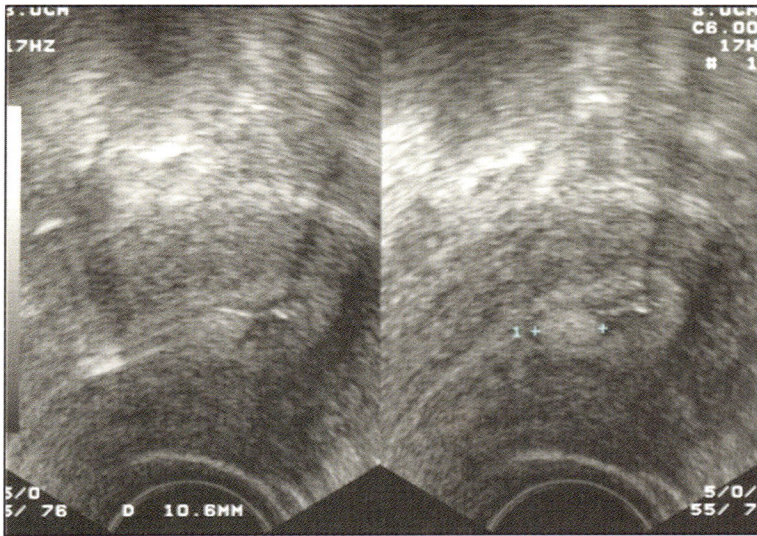

Fig. 20.94: Transvaginal sonogram showing an endometrial polyp 10 mm larger and intrauterine device correctly placed

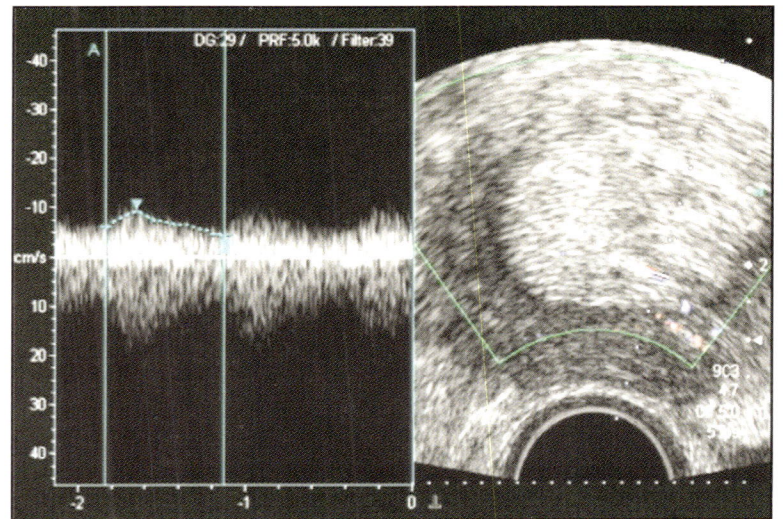

Fig. 20.97: The same case of Figures 20.95 and 20.96. Pulsed Doppler showing an arterial signal with moderate resistance index (RI = 0.54)

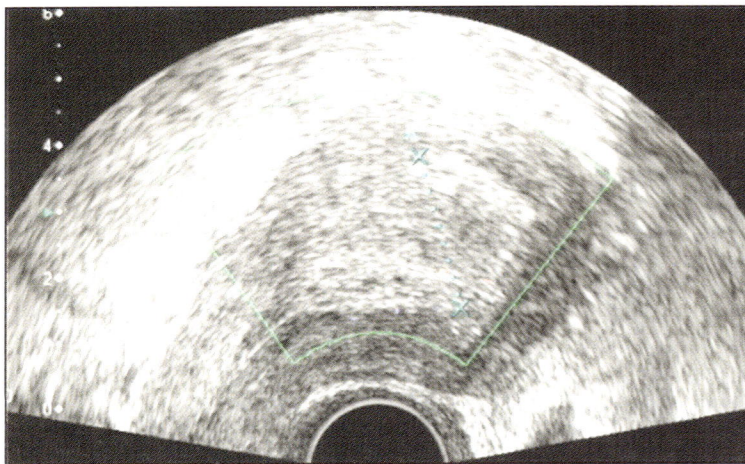

Fig. 20.95: Transvaginal color Doppler scan of the uterus showing a larger endometrial polyp (2.4 cm)

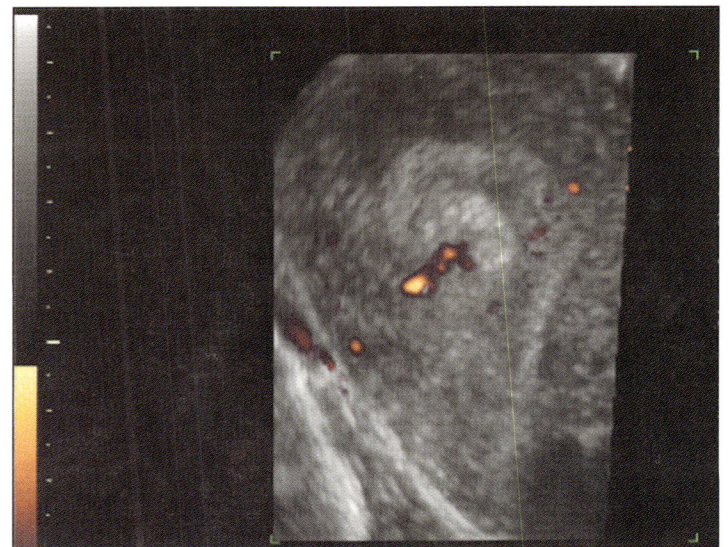

Fig. 20.98: Three-dimensional power Doppler sonogram showing an endometrial polyp into the cavity and its vascular pedicle penetrating

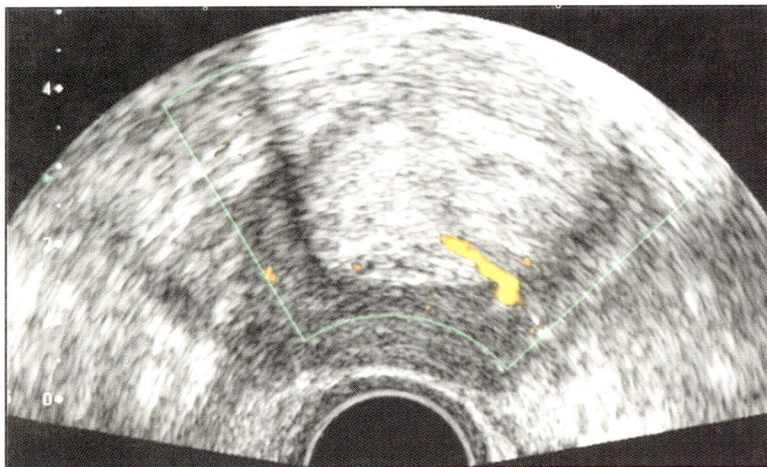

Fig. 20.96: The same case as in Figure 20.95. We can see a vascular pedicle

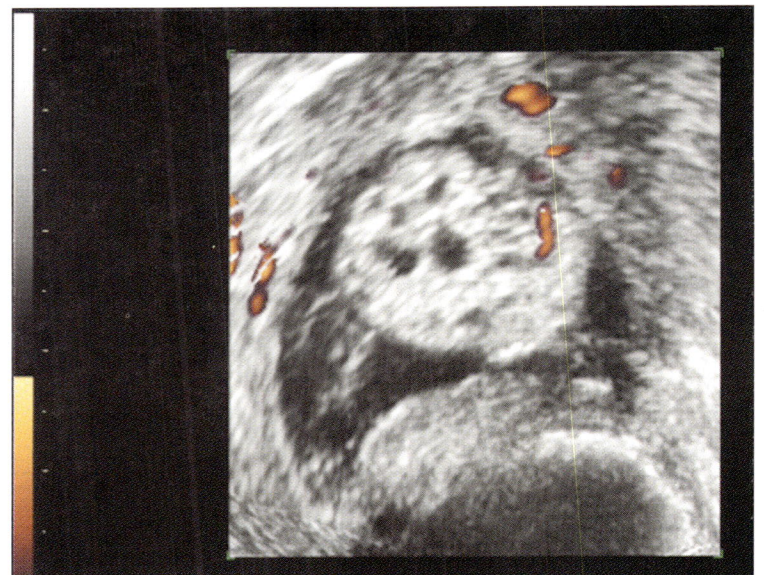

Fig. 20.99: Three-dimensional power Doppler sonogram showing a filling deffect within the uterine cavity after instillation of the isotonic saline solution. The area of increased endometrial thickening representing a polyp with small cysts is clearly outlined

BIBLIOGRAPHY

1. Alcazar JL, Castillo G, Minguez JA, Galan MJ. Endometrial blood flow mapping using transvaginal power Doppler sonography in women with postmenopausal bleeding and thickened endometrium. Ultrasound Obstet Gynecol 2003;21:583-8.

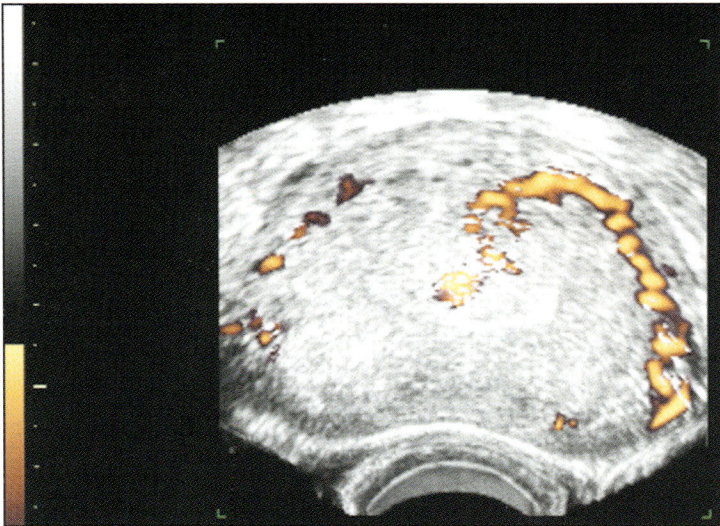

Fig. 20.100: Transvaginal three-dimensional scan of the pedicle vessel penetrating within endometrial polyp

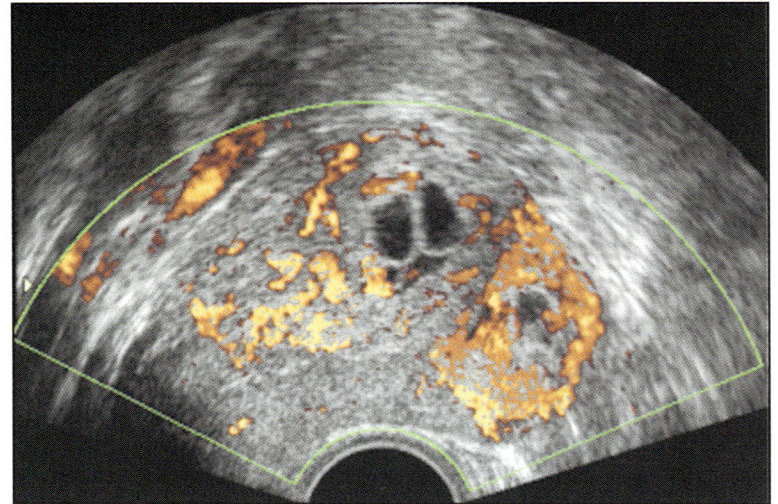

Fig. 20.101: Three-dimensional sonogram: A frontal reformatted section of uterus cavity. Note a focal area of increased echogenicity within the endometrial portion. An endometrial polyp with pedicle vessel penetrating is easily visualized

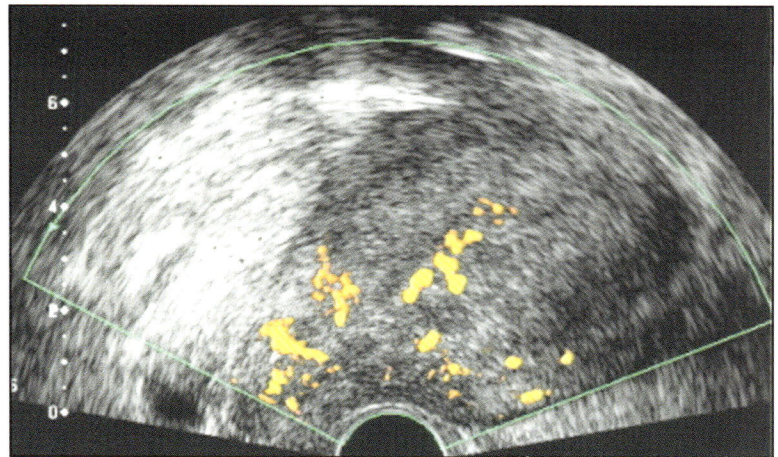

Fig. 20.102: Tranvaginal tranversal scan showing a cysts structures typical of molar process

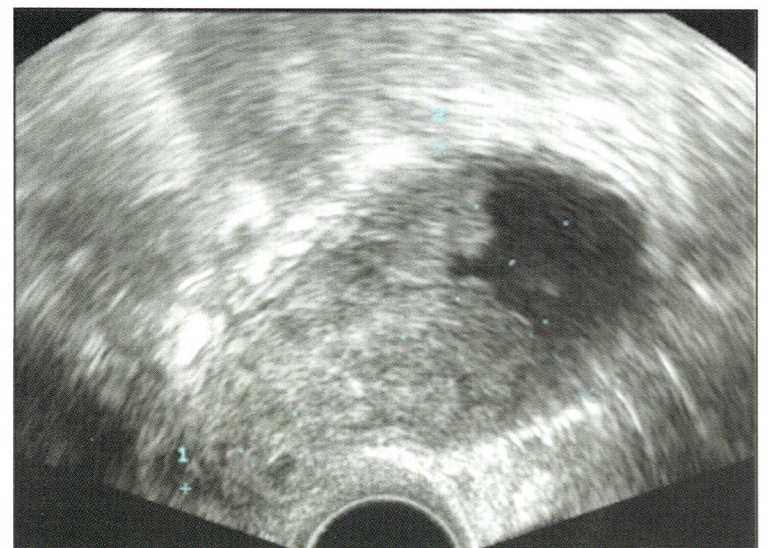

Fig. 20.103: Transvaginal power Doppler sonogram showing a cysts structures within the posterior myometrium and important increased vascularization. Histopathology revelead a molar process

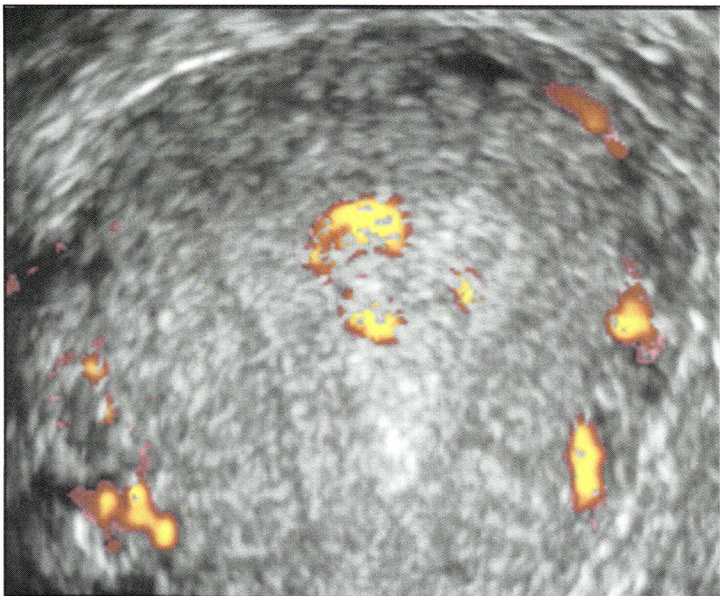

Fig. 20.104: Transvaginal power Doppler scan of a premenopausal patient with vaginal bleeding. Interruption of the subendometrial halo, stellate peripheral and intratumoral neovascularization seen by power flow imaging was suggestive of endometrial malignancy. Histopathology revealed endometrial cancer

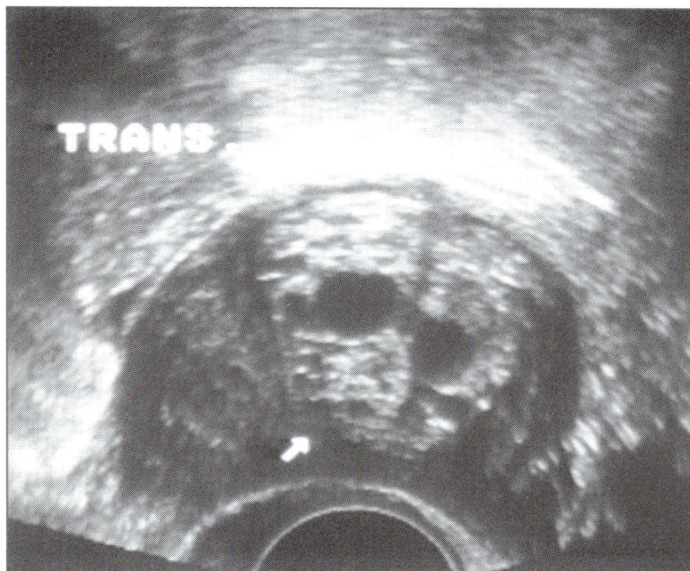

Fig. 20.105: Transvaginal scan of a postmenopausal patient with enlarged and heterogeneous uterus. Using conventional transvaginal ultrasound it was impossible to delineate an endometrial echo. Note the presence of intracavitary fluid

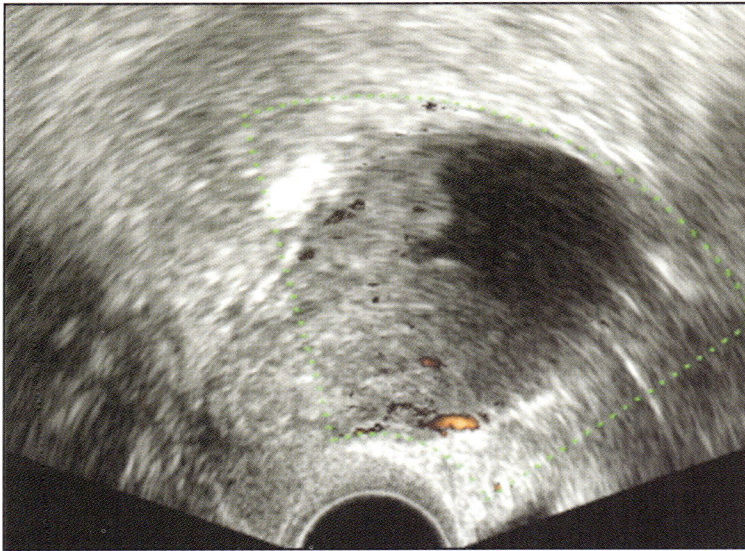

Fig. 20.106: The same patient as in Figure 20.105. Power Doppler facilitates detection a few vessels within the extremely thin myometrial portion of the uterus. Histopathology reveals a invasive endometrial cancer

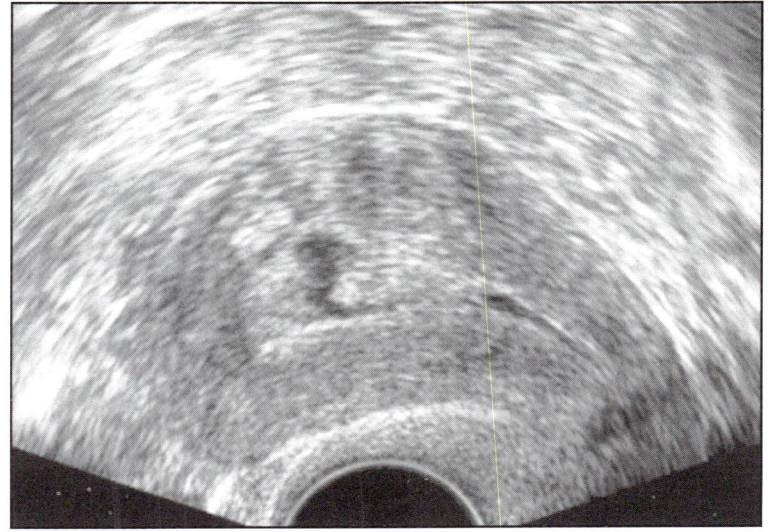

Fig. 20.109: Transvaginal scan of the uterus in a postmenopausal patient with uterine bleeding. We can see two focal areas of increased echogenicity within the endometrial cavity

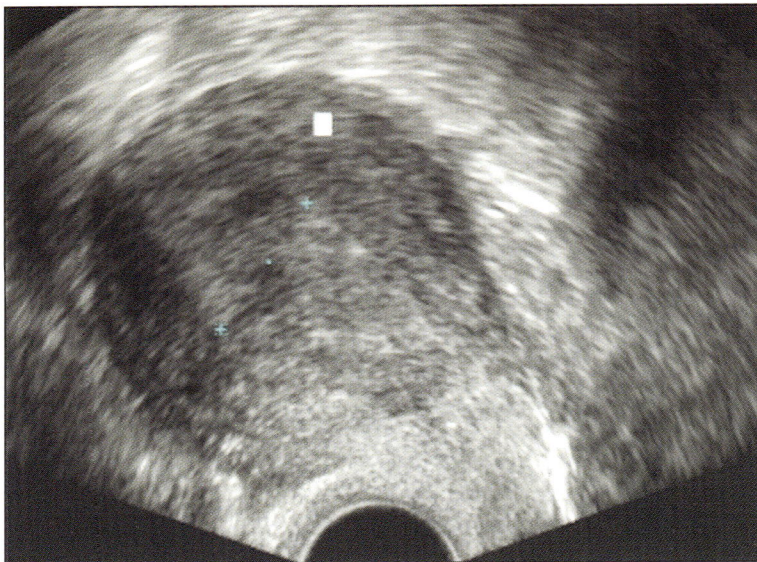

Fig. 20.107: Enlarged heterogeneous uterus as seen by transvaginal sonography. The endometrial portion is not clearly distinguished

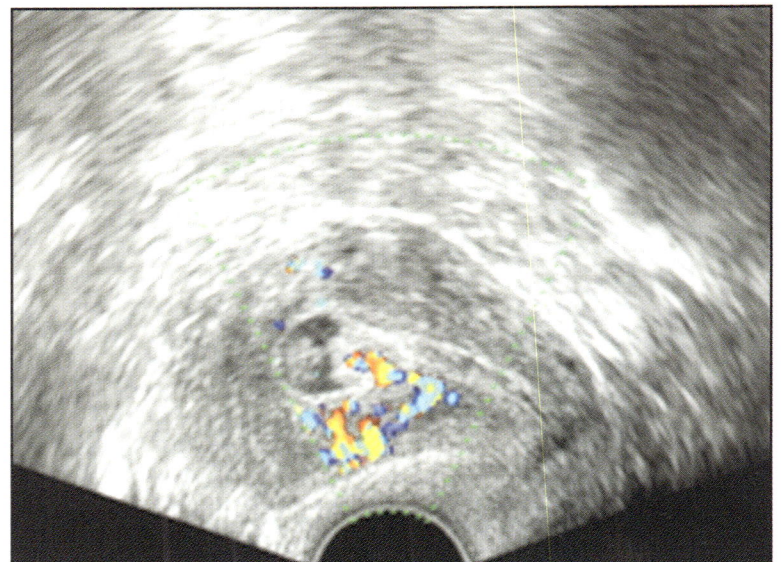

Fig. 20.110: The same patient as in Figure 20.109. The area of neovascularization is easily depicted by transvaginal color Doppler

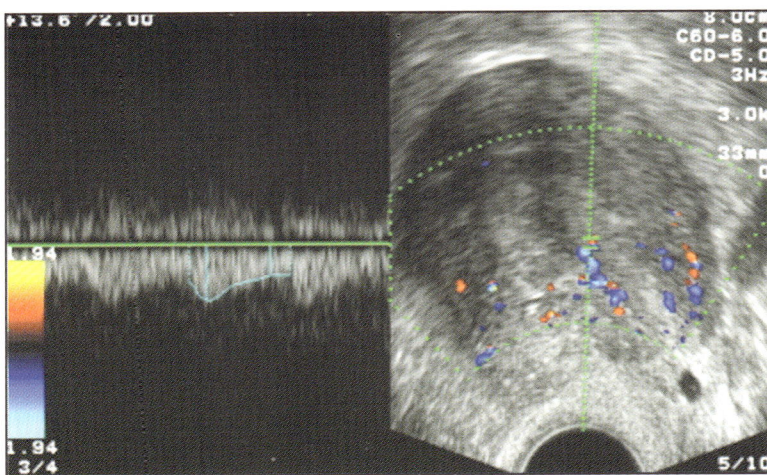

Fig. 20.108: The same patient as in Figure 20.107. Color Doppler demonstrates randomly dispersed vessels within the myometrial portion of the uterus, suggestive of myometrial invasion and intratumoral vessels with low resistance (RI = 0.45). Histopathology revealed deep myometrial invasion of endometrial carcinoma

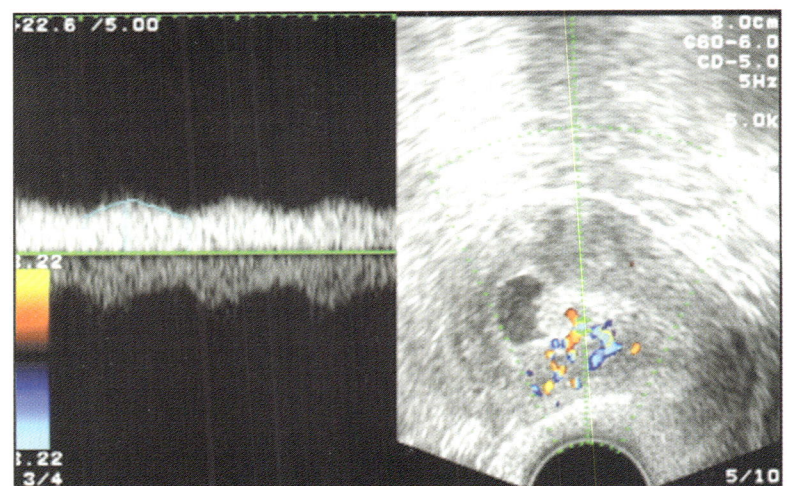

Fig. 20.111: The same case as in Figures 20.109 and 20.110. Blood flow obtained from intratumoral vessels demonstrate low resistance (RI = 0.34). Histopatholohy revealed endometrial cancer

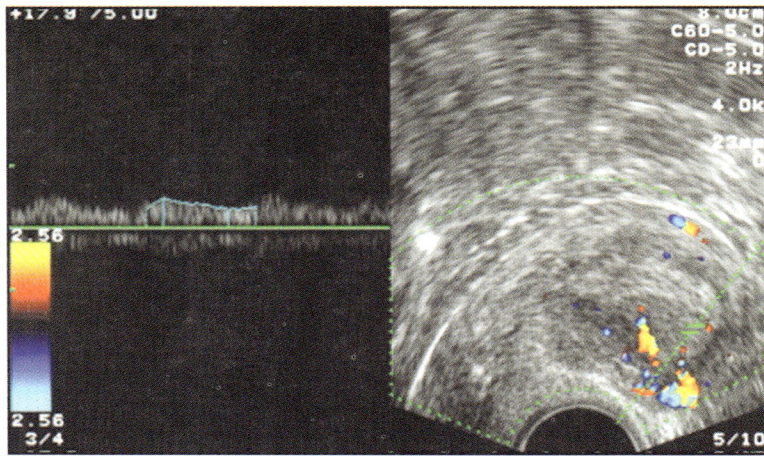

Fig. 20.112: Transvaginal color Doppler scan of endometrial carcinoma vessels. Blood flow velocity waveforms obtained from intratumoral vessels demonstrate low resistance (RI = 0.39)

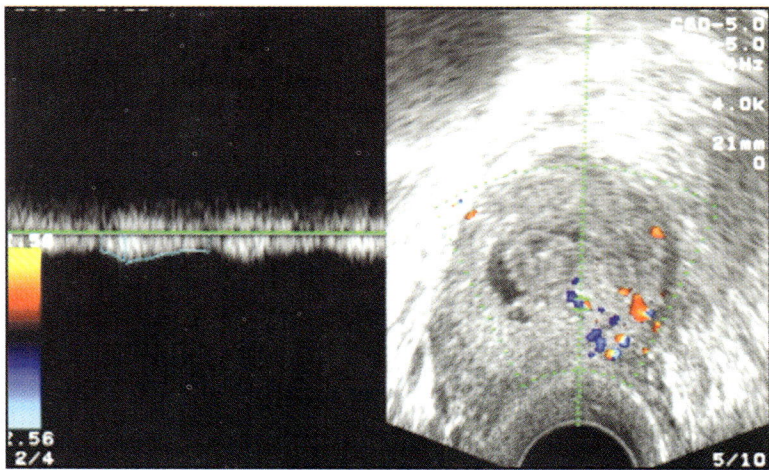

Fig. 20.113: Transvaginal sonogram of postmenopausal patient. Note the tumor, presence of intracavitary fluid and interruption of the subendometrial halo, suggestive of myometrial invasion. Intratumoral vessels demonstrate low resistance (RI = 0.43). Endometrial malignancy was confirmed by histopathology

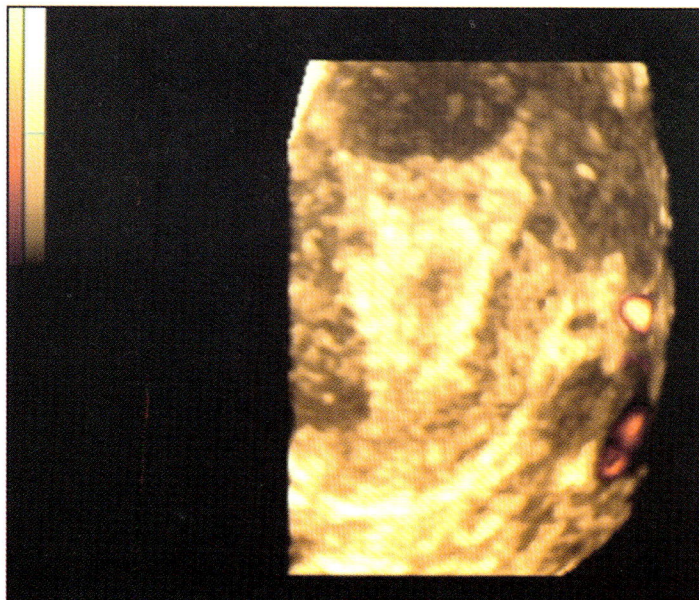

Fig. 20.114: Three-dimensional sonogram. Note the right interface endometrial-myometrial was not clearly defined, suggestive of myometrial invasion. Histopathology confirmed invasive endometrial carcinoma

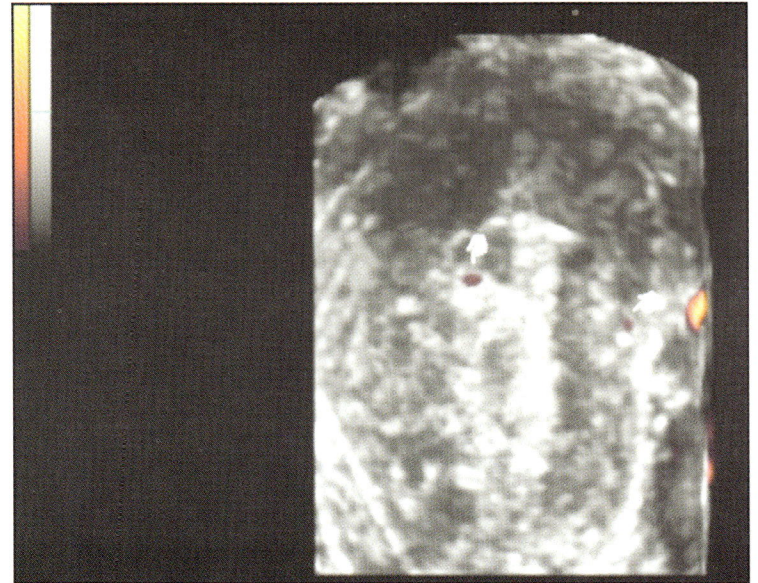

Fig. 20.115: Three-dimensional sonogram shows the interruption of the subendometrial halo specially in the right side and the intratumoral blood flow signals suggestive of endometrial malignancy

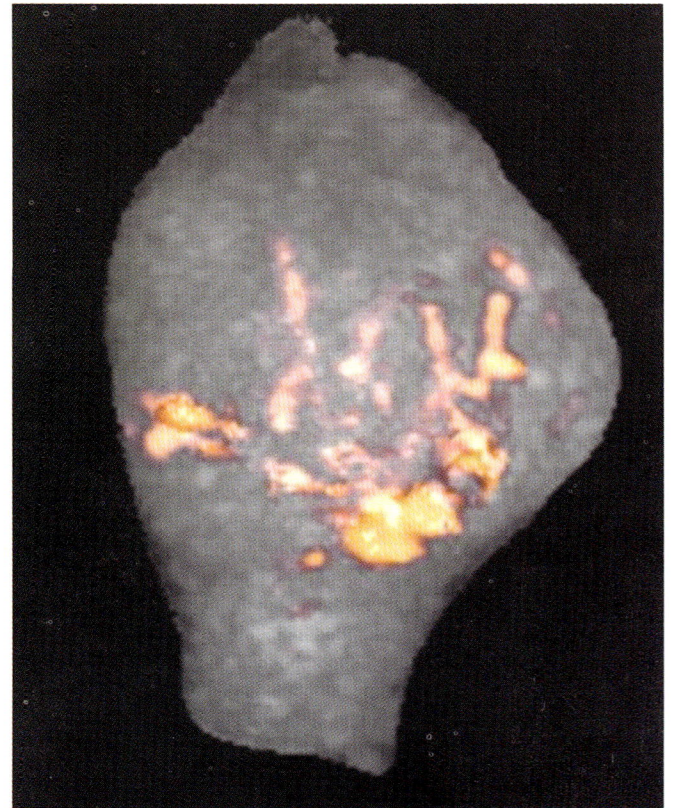

Fig. 20.116: Three-dimensional power Doppler sonogram with Render mode™ demonstrating a localizated increased vascularization within the endometrium. Note the irregular architecture of the vessels. Histopathology reveals endometrial carcinoma stage Ia

2. Alcazar JL, Galan MJ, Jurado M, Lopez-Garcia G. Intratumoral blood flow análisis in endometrial carcinoma: correlation with tumor characteristics and risk for recurrence. Gynecol Oncol 2002;84:258-62.
3. Alcazar JL, Jurado M, Lopez-Garcia G. Comparative study of transvaginal ultrasonography and CA 125 in the preoperative evaluation of myometrial invasión in endometrial carcinoma. Ultrasound Obstet Gynecol 1999;14:210-4.
4. Doubilet PM. Consensus Conference statement on postmenopausal bleeding. J Ultrasound Med 2001;20:1037-1042.
5. Dueholm M, Lundorf E, Sorensen JS, Ledertoug S, Olesen F, Laursen H. Reproducibility of evaluation of the uterus by transvaginal sonography, hysterosonographic examination, hyseroscopy and magnetic resonance imaging. Hum Reprod 2002;17:195-200.

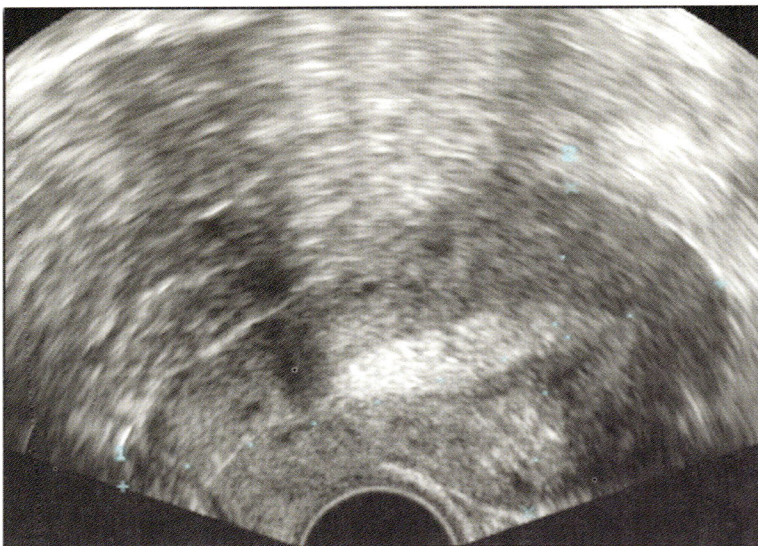

Fig. 20.117: Transvaginal sonogram of a thickened homogeneous endometrium in a perimenopausal patient

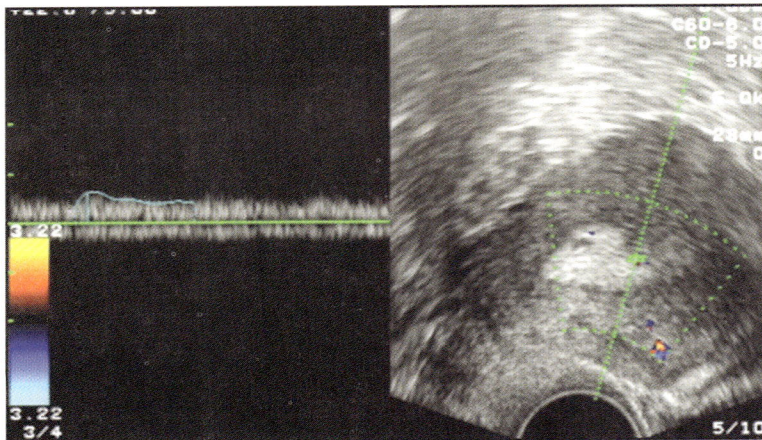

Fig. 20.118: The same patient as in Figure 20.117. Color pulsed Doppler study shows intratumoral vessels with moderate resistance (RI = 0.50)

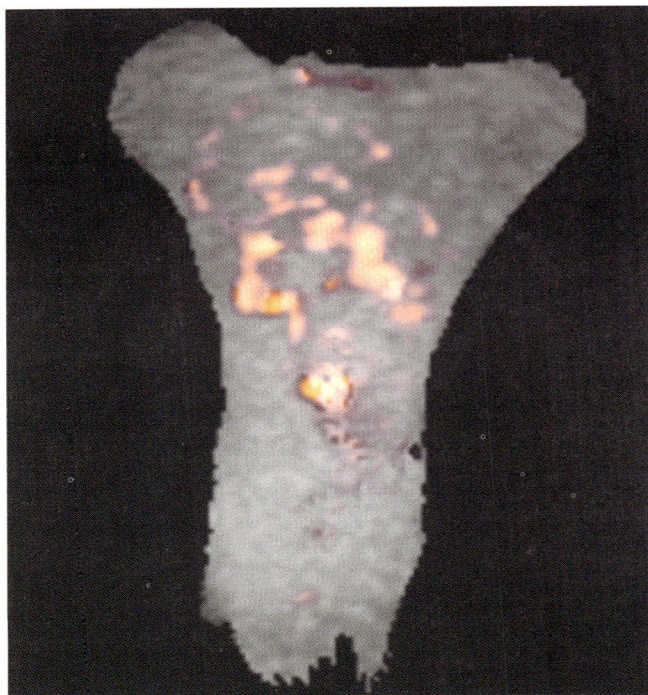

Fig. 20.119: The same patient as in Figures 20.117 and 20.118. Three-dimensional sonogram (Render mode™) demonstrating a localized neovascularization. Note the irregular course of the vessels within the endometrium. Histopathology confirmed localized endometrial carcinoma

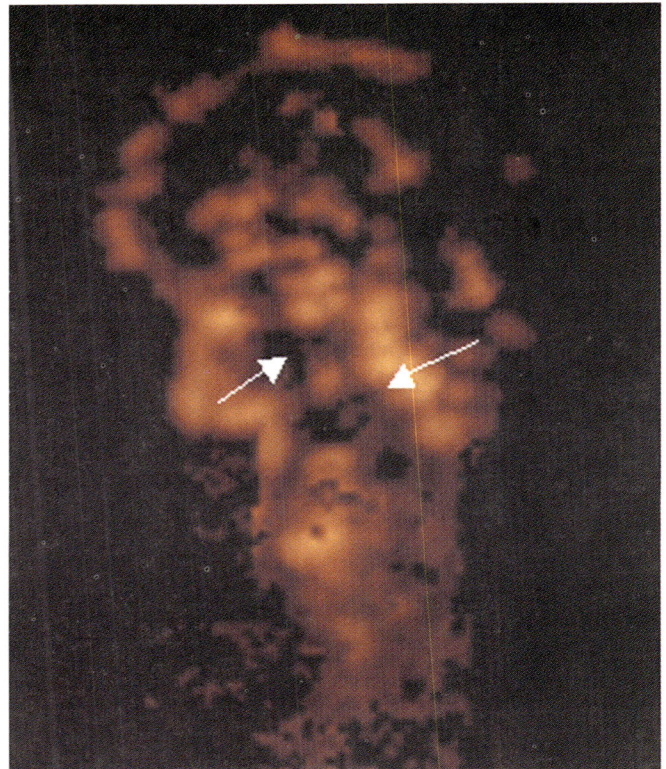

Fig. 20.120: The same patient as in Figures 20.117 to 20.119. Vascular Render mode™ demonstrating details of irregular architecture of the intratumoral vessels

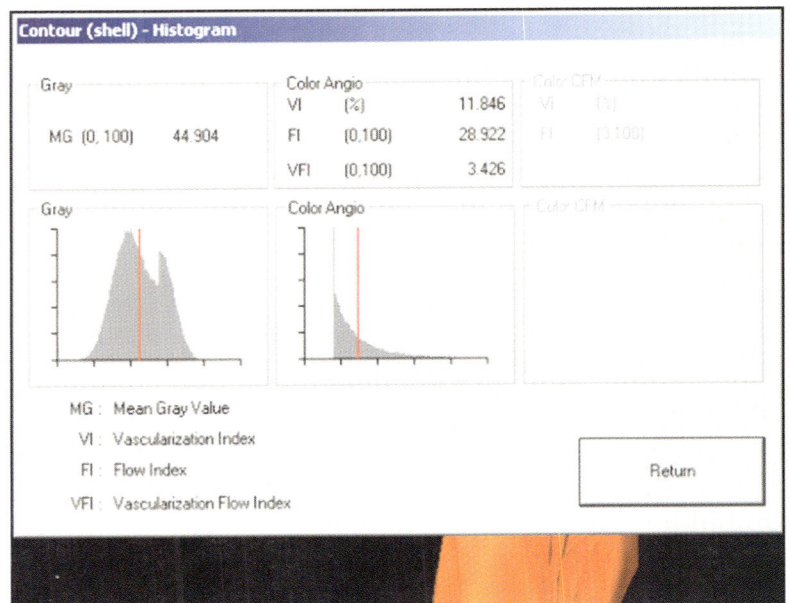

Fig. 20.121: The same patient as in Figures 20.117 to 20.120. Three-dimensional ultrasound permits to calculate migh be Histogram™ increased blood flow within the malignant tumor

6. Epstein E, Skoog L, Isberg PE, De Smet F, De Moor B, Olofsson PA, et al. An algorithm including results of gray-scale and power Doppler ultrasound examination to pedict endometrial malignancy in women with postmenopausal bleeding. Ultrasound Obstet Gynecol 2002;20:370-6.
7. Ferenczy A. Pathophysiology of endometrial bleeding. Maturitas 2003;45:1-14.
8. Fernandez-Cid A, Lopez-Marin L. Citopatología Ginecológica y Mamaria 2ª Ed. Masson-Salvat Medicina. Barcelona, 1993.
9. Fleischer AC, Shappell HW, Parker LP, Hanemann CW. Color Doppler sonography of endometrial masses. J Ultrasound Med 2002;21:861-5.
10. Fleischer AC. Sonographic assessment of endometrial disorders. Semin Ultrasound CT MR 1999;20:259-60.
11. Fleischer AC.Color Doppler sonography of uterine disorders. Ultrasound Q 2003;19:179-89.

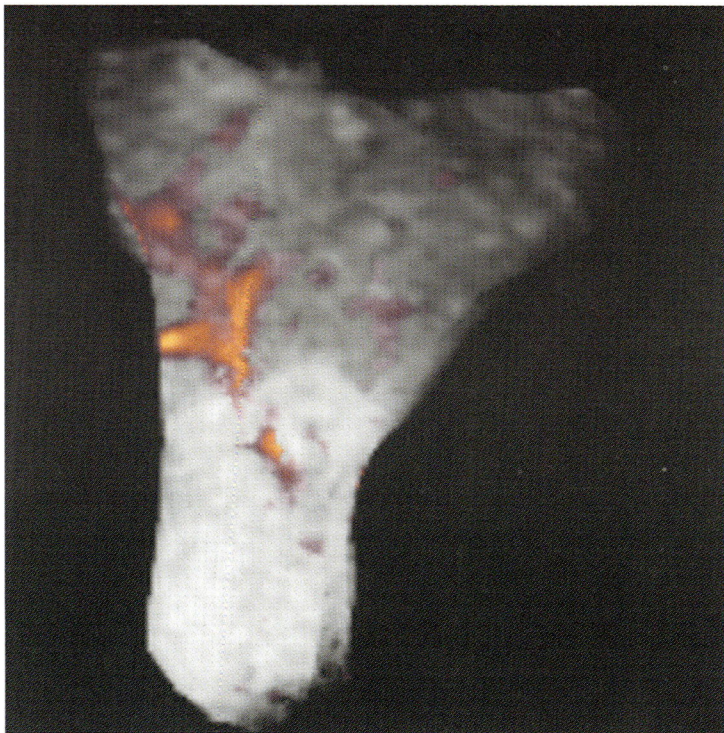

Fig. 20.122: Three-dimensional sonogram by Render mode™ showing another example of localized malignant endometrial tumor. Note the irregular branching pattern of the tumoral vessels

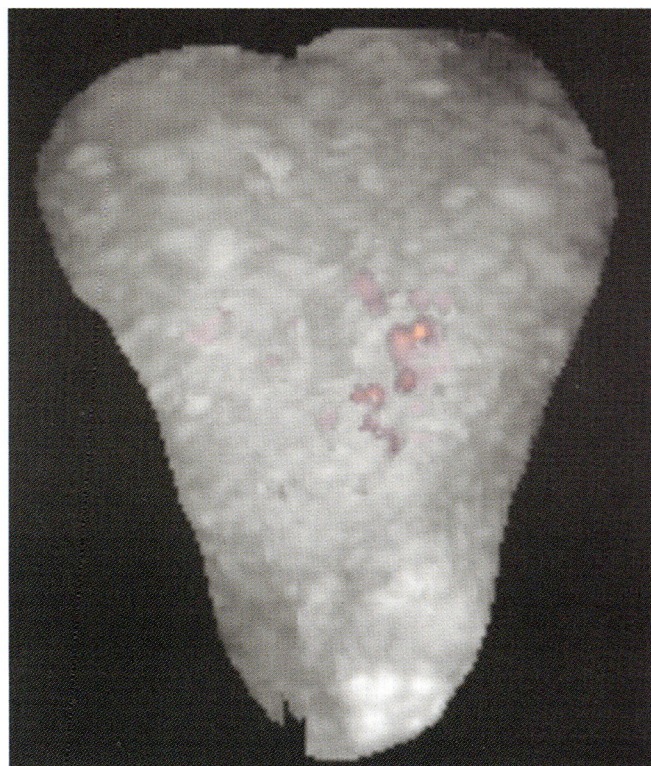

Fig. 20.123: Three-dimensional sonogram by Render mode™. Note the difference of vascularization in this patient we can see a few regular vessels. Histopathology confirmed the benign lesion

12. Goldstein SR, Monteagudo A, Popiolek D, Mayberry P, Timor-Tritsch I. Evaluation of endometrial polyps. Am J Obstet Gynecol 2002;186:669-74.

13. Gull B, Carlsson SA, Karlsson B, Ylöstalo P, Milsom I, Granberg S. Transvaginal ultrasonography of the endometrium in women with postmenopausal bleeding: Is it always necessary to perform an endometrial biopsy? Am J Obstet Gynecol 2000;182:509-15.

14. Kupesic S, Kurjak A, Hajder E. Ultrasonic assessment of the postmenopausal uterus. Maturitas 2002;41:255-67.

15. Kurjak A, Kupesic S. Miric D. The assessment of benign uterine tumor vascularization by transvaginal color Doppler. Ultrasound Med Biol 1992;18:645-9.

16. Kurjak A, Kupesic S, Sparac V, Bekavak I. Preoperative evaluation of pelvic tumors by Doppler and three-dimensional sonography. J Ultrasound Med 2001;20:829-40.

17. Kurjak A, Shlan H, Sosic A, Benic S, Zudenigo D, Kupesic S, Predanic M. Endometrial carcinoma in postmenopausal women:evaluation by transvaginal color Doppler ultrasonography. Am J Obstet Gynecol 1993;169:1597-1603.

18. Kurjak A, Zalud I. The characterization of uterine tumors by transvaginal color Doppler. Ultrasound Obstet Gynecol 1991;1:50-2

19. Perez-Medina T, Bajo J, Huertas MA, Rubio A. Predicting atypia incide endometrial polyps. J Ultrasound Med 2002;21:125-8.

20. Raine-Fenning NJ, Campbell BK, Clewes JS, Kendall NR, Johnson IR. The reliability of virtual organ computer-aided analysis (VOCAL) for the semiquantification of ovarian, endometrial and subendometrial perfusion. Ultrasound Obstet Gynecol 2003;22:633-9.

21. Sladkevicius P, Valentin L, Marsal K. Transvaginal Doppler examination of uteri with myomas. J Clin Ultrasound 1996;24:135-40.

22. Timmerman D, Verguts J, Konstantinovic L, Moerman P, Van Schoubroeck D, Deprest J, Van Huffel . The pedicle artery sign based on sonography with color Doppler imaging can replace second-stage tests in women with abnormal vaginal bleeding. Ultrasound Obstet Gynecol 2003;22:166-71.

23. Wu HH, Harshbarger KE, Berner HW, Elsheikh TM. Endometrial brush biopsy (Tao brush). Histologic diagnosis of 200 cases with complementary cytology: an acurate sampling technique for the detection of endometrial abnormalities. Am J Clin Pathol 2000;114:412-8.

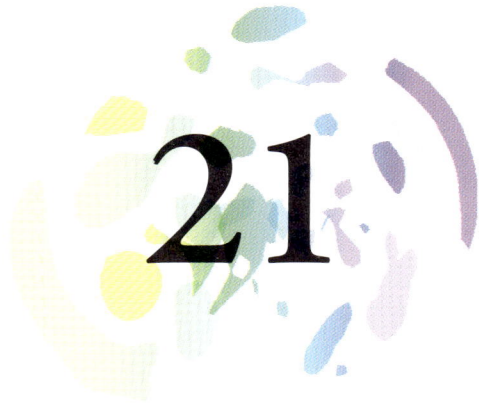

MA Pascual, A Kurjak,
M Prka, PN Barri

21

Ultrasonic Assessment of Adnexal Masses

BASIC ASPECTS

Ovarian lesions are a cause of great concern because of their malignant potential and the limited ability to distinguish accurately between benign and malignant tumors prior to surgery. This particularly concerns complex structures such a dermoid cysts, large endometriomas, complex corpus luteum cysts and cystadenomas. Sonography has an important role in the evaluation of these ovarian lesions.

The frequent anomaly of the ovaries recognized by ultrasound is the polycystic ovary (Figs 21.1 and 21.2). In polycystic ovarian disease the ovaries become enlarged and the ovarian shape becomes more spherical. These ovaries are characterized by the presence of multiple small cystic structures (<10 mm) and an increase in volume of the ovarian stroma. Cysts may be distributed predominantly around the periphery or scattered throughout the stroma. The intraovarian vascularity is localized within the ovarian stroma without cyclic changes.

The most common type of cystic adnexal lesions are functional ovarian cysts. These are easily recognizable cystic structures with smooth thin walls and clear fluid content, usually unilateral (Figs 21.3 to 21.6). These cysts are originated from an unruptured follicle and are usually smaller than 10 cm. Pericystic vascularization shows moderate resistance to blood flow.

Hydrosalpinx and tubo-ovarian abscesses (Figs 21.7 to 21.24) often appear as cystic mass. A smaller hydrosalpinx usually assumes a fusiform shape, but if large it is of rather round shape. A tubo-ovarian abscess can be differentiated from hydrosalpinx by the demonstration of ovarian tissue incorporated within the abscess wall. Tubo-ovarian abscesses are usually extremely well perfused. An increased vascularization is probably caused by the blood vessel dilatation due to degrading products of an inflammation. Vascular impedance to blood flow varies from very low to moderate high.

Paraovarian cysts (Figs 21.25 to 21.27) develop from Gartners's duct and have the same appearance as functional cysts. Only occasionally are they distinguishable from them. A thin and smooth wall, lack of septation within the cystic cavity, sonolucent fluid and preserved ovarian tissue are indicators of paraovarian cysts. These lesions usually do not reveal increased vascularity.

Serous and mucinous cystoadenomas are also common lesions. Serous cystoadenomas (Figs 21.28 to 21.38) may be unilocular but are mostly multilocular, with or without papillary growth into the cavity. Mucinous cystoadenomas (Figs 21.39 to 21.45) may attain a huge size. Grossly, they present as rounded or ovoid masses with a smooth capsule that is usually translucent or bluish-whitish gray. Mucinous cystoadenomas are thin-walled and mostly multilocular. Papillary formations may be present but they are less common than are serous cystoadenomas. In this group of ovarian tumors moderate vascular resistance is usually observed in peripheral and regularly separated vessels. It can be difficult to distinguish a benign ovarian tumor from a malignant or borderline tumor in this group of ovarian cysts.

Dermoid cysts appear extremely variable, but some of them have a specific ultrasonic appearance, and a prominent acoustic shadowing observed behind the echogenic focus (Figs 21.46 to 21.55). Indeed, overlapping with ovarian endometriosis is possible, owing to its complex texture, thick walls and solid echogenic appearance of hemorrhagic clots within the cystic cavity. Pelvic inflammatory disease is another entity that may

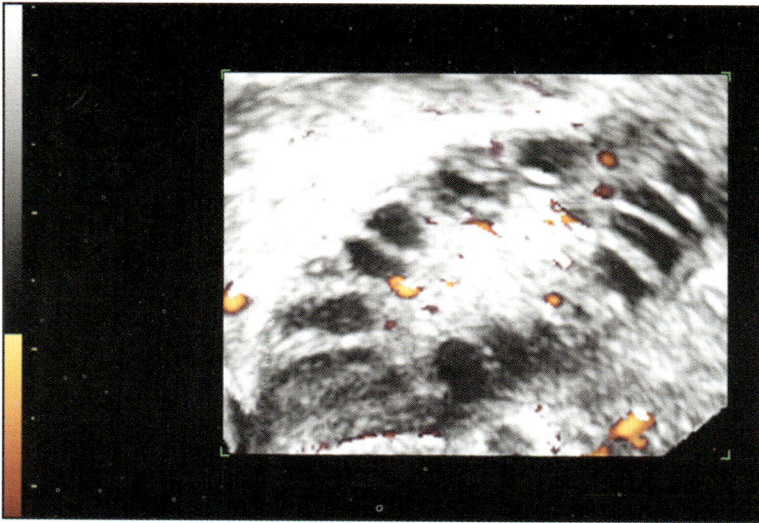

Fig. 21.1: Three-dimensional ultrasound with power Doppler of the polycystic ovary. Note the small cysts distributed in the subcapsular region of the ovary. Power Doppler depicts blood flow signals from the enlarged ovarian stroma

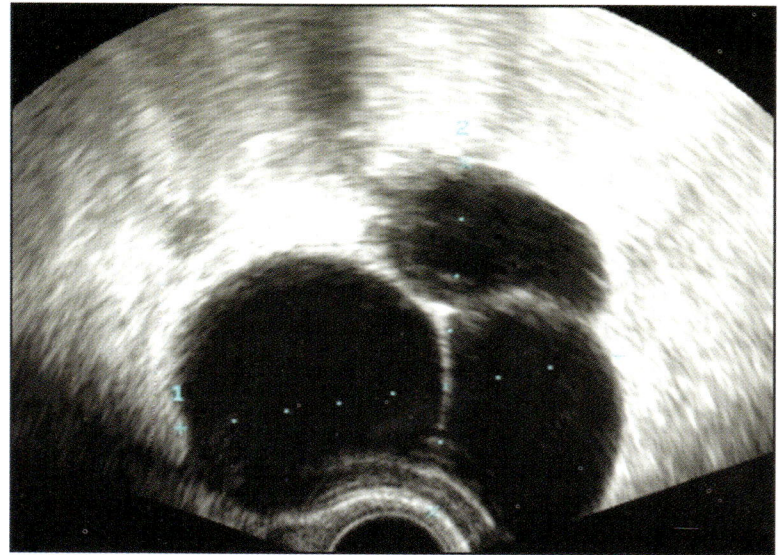

Fig. 21.4: Large cyst in the ovary: The cyst simple, trilocular with thin and well-defined borders and no internal echoes. A case of physiological ovarian cyst

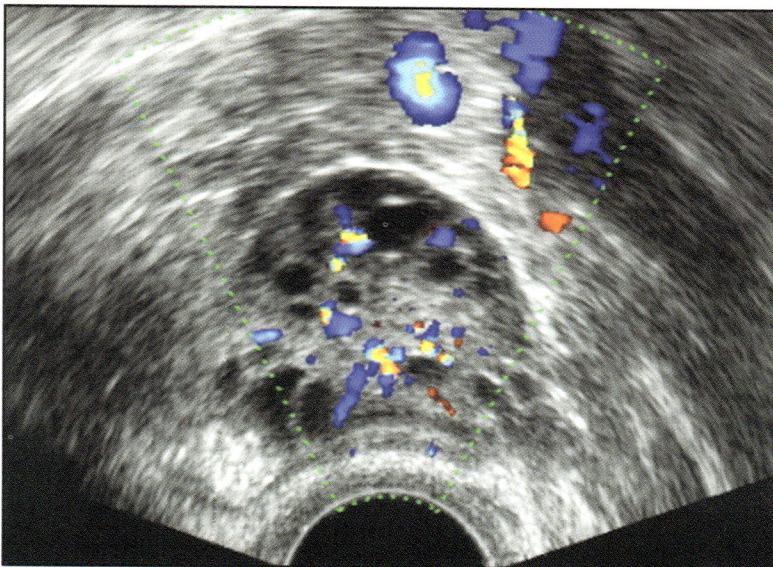

Fig. 21.2: Transvaginal color Doppler sonogram of the polycystic ovary. Note the small cysts scattered throughout the entire ovarian parenchyma

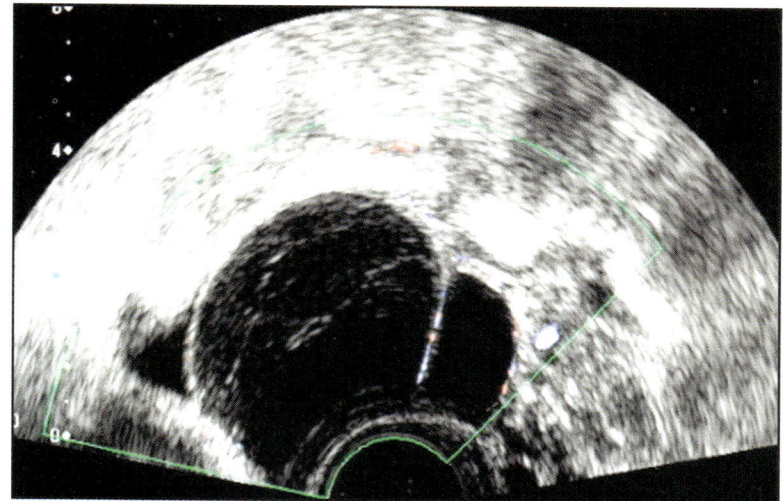

Fig. 21.5: Transvaginal color Doppler scan of a cyst. Note the thin walls, clear fluid content and pericystic flow

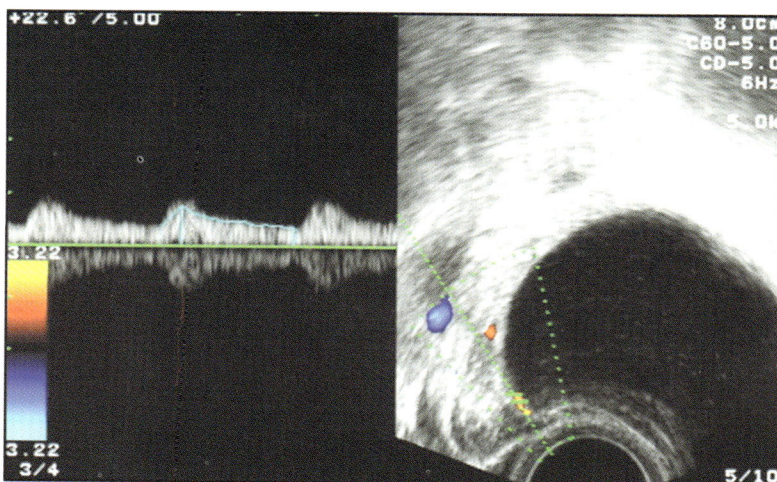

Fig. 21.3: Functional ovarian cyst. Unilocular cystic structure with peripheral type of vascularization, showing moderate-to-high vascular resistance (RI = 0.55)

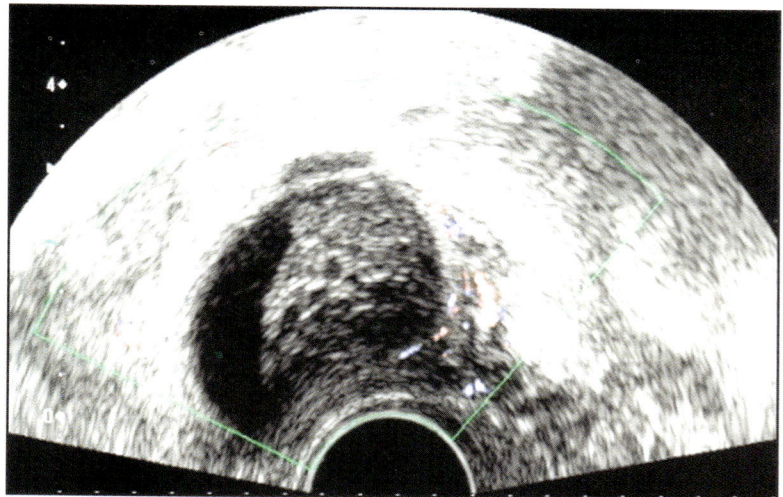

Fig. 21.6: Appearance of luteinized unruptured follicle with hemorrhagic phenomenon. Peripheral vessels are easily depicted by dynamic flow imaging

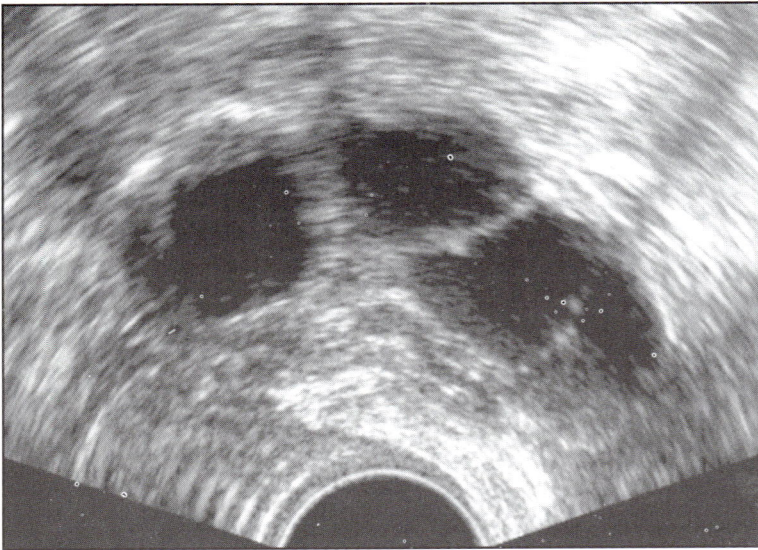

Fig. 21.7: Complex adnexal mass containing a fluid-filled distended tube, with pseudosepta

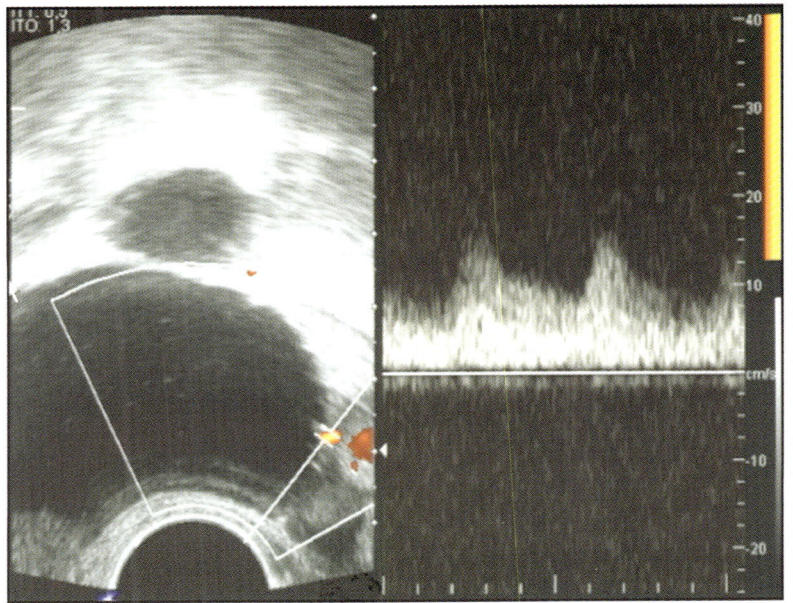

Fig. 21.10: Increased vascularity is a response to various bacterial antigens and inflammatory products and is easily detectable using color Doppler

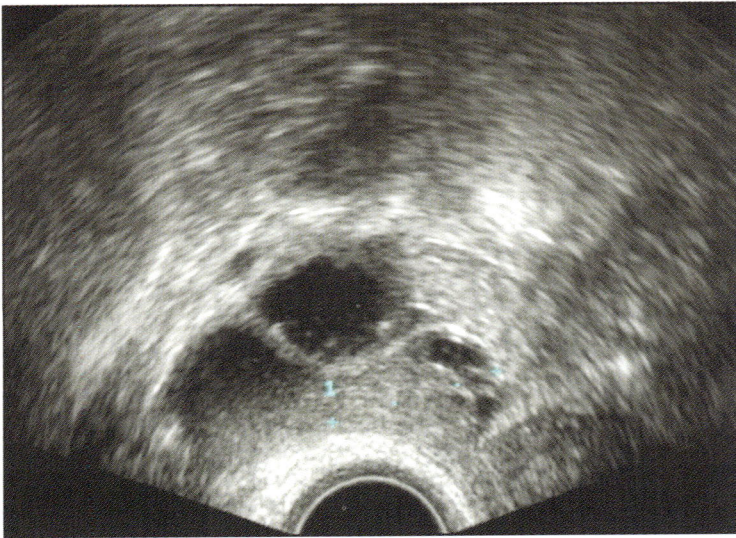

Fig. 21.8: Transvaginal sonogram of a complex adnexal mass containing a folded dilated tube and attached ovary

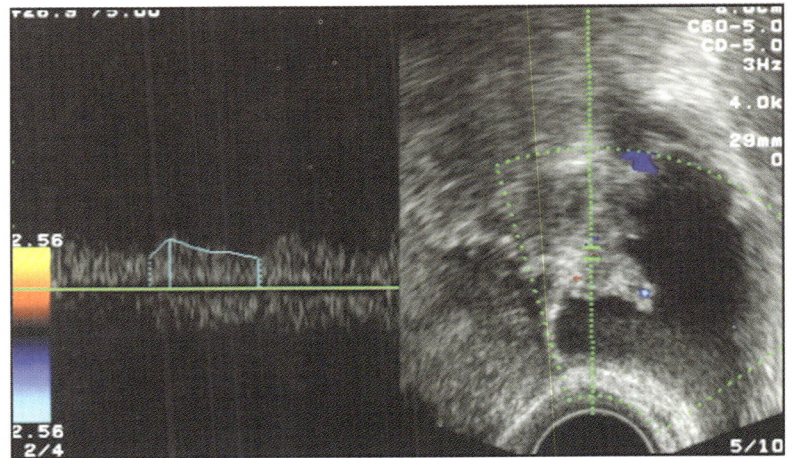

Fig. 21.11: Complex adnexal mass containing a fluid-filled dilated tube in a patient with acute pelvic inflammation, low-impedance signals (RI = 0.42) are obtained from tiny tubal arteries

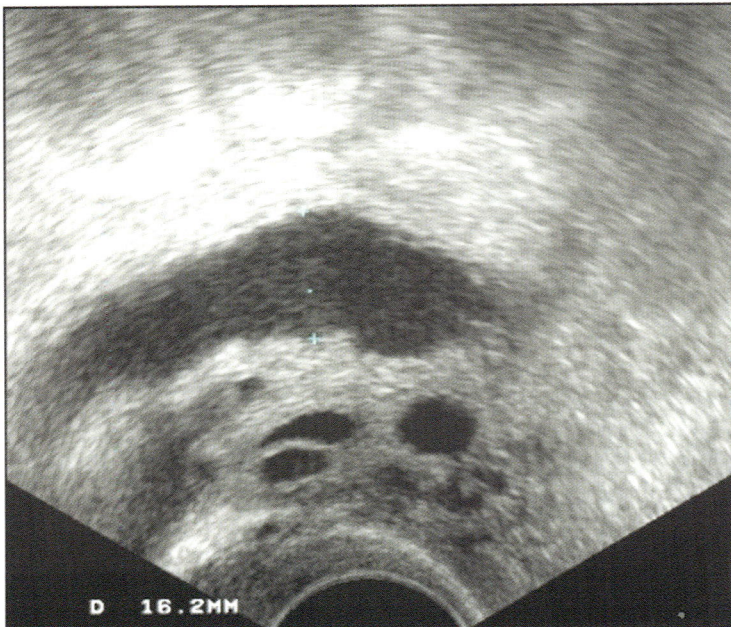

Fig. 21.9: Hydrosalpinx involving right ovary, presenting a fusiform shape. Note the increased tubal diameter (16 mm) and thickened tubal mucosa

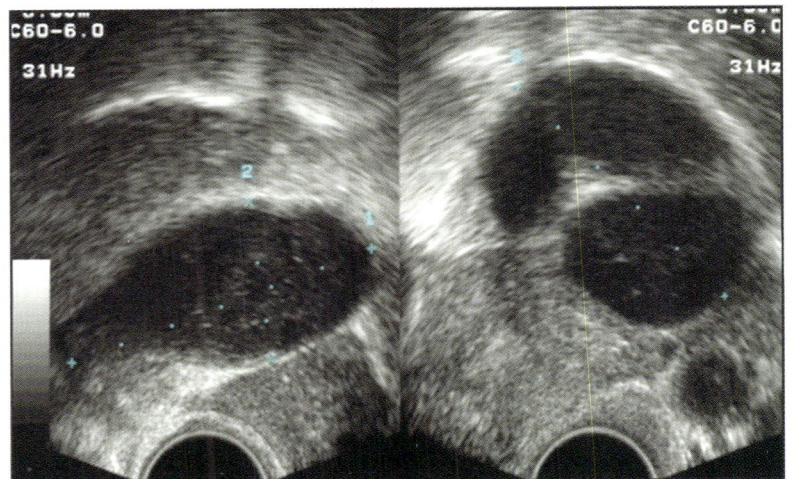

Fig. 21.12: Bilateral complex adnexal mass occupying the pouch of Douglas in a patient with acute pelvic inflammation. Note the increased tubal diameter; thickened tubal mucosa and echogenic fluid within the tubal lumen

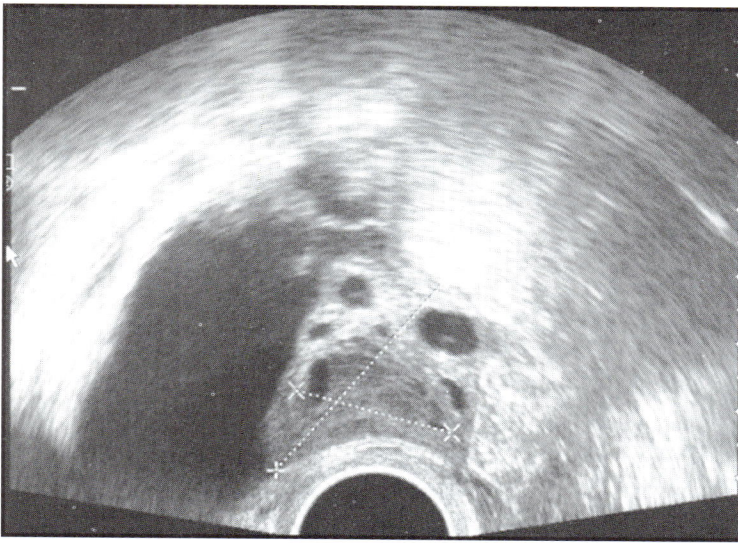

Fig. 21.13: Transvaginal scan of a complex adnexal mass containing a sausage-like structure (dilated tube) and enlarged ovary with indistinct border and fluid-filled cystic cavities

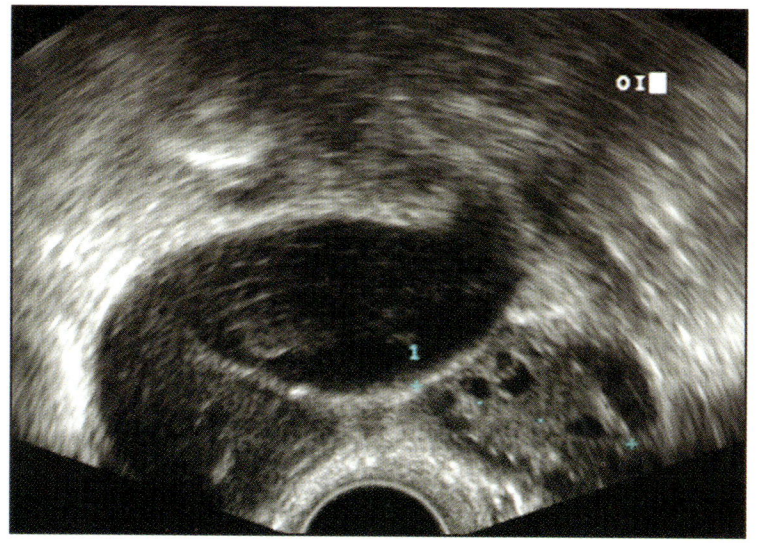

Fig. 21.16: Transvaginal scan of a pseudoseptate adnexal mass containing a tubular fluid-filled structure (dilated tube) and normal ovary

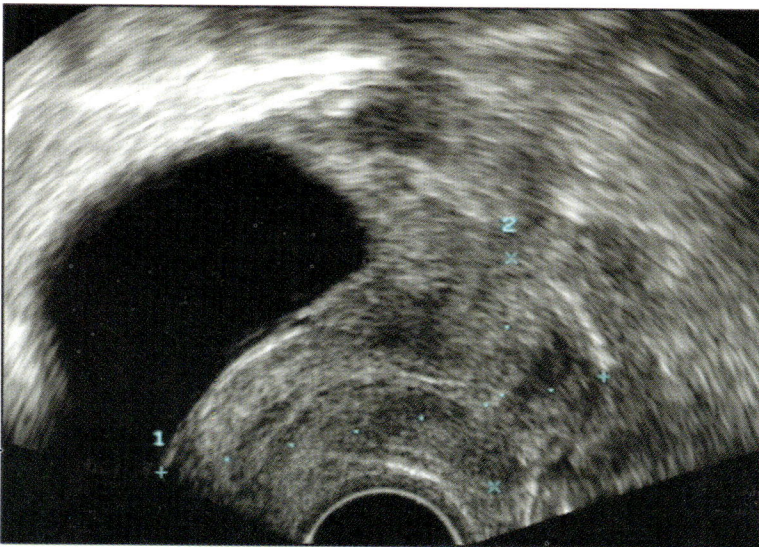

Fig. 21.14: A case of hydrosalpinx as seen by transvaginal echography. Note the enormously dilated thin-walled fallopian tube

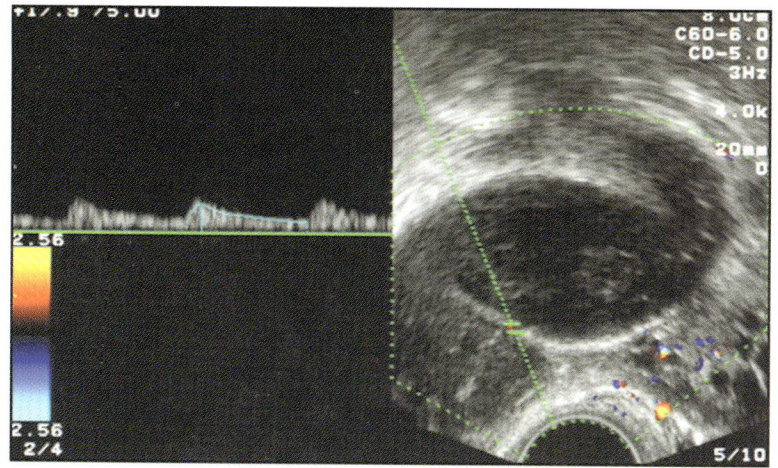

Fig. 21.17: The same case patient as in Figure 21.16: Color Doppler imaging facilitates visualization of the intraovarian and tubal artery blood flow. Moderate-to-high resistance blood flow signals (RI = 0.65) are shown from the walls of the fallopian tube

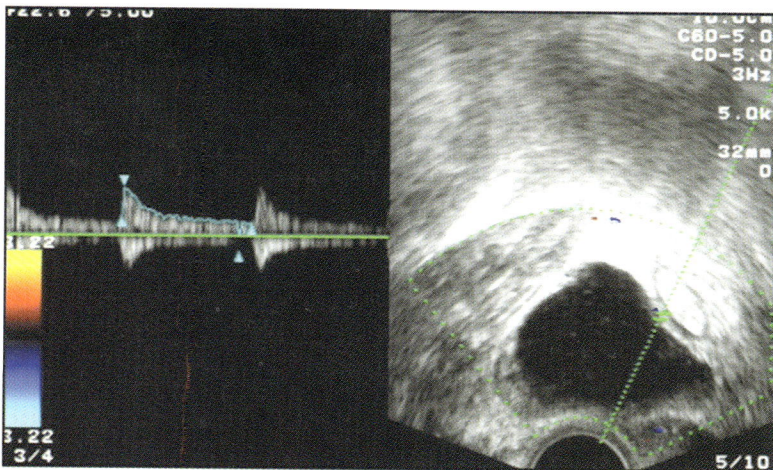

Fig. 21.15: Moderate-to-high vascular resistance (RI = 0.71) provides additional information in the diagnosis of chronic pelvic inflammatory disease

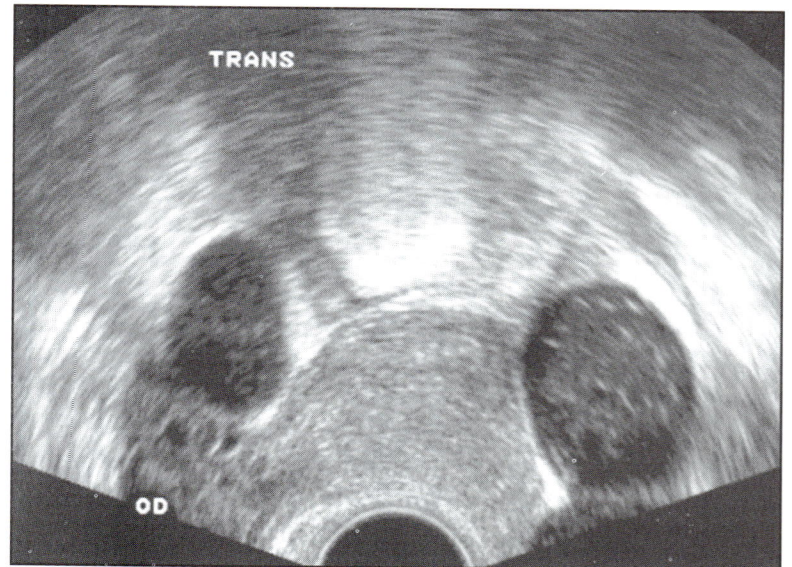

Fig. 21.18: Transverse transvaginal scan shows a bilateral hydrosalpinx

mimic a wide variety of findings, such as a dermoid cyst, and sometimes even malignancy. Dermoid cyst is usually poorly vascularized; therefore color Doppler is helpful when a bizarre solid-cystic dermoid mass is encountered. Even if a blood flow is visualized, blood flow resistance is high to moderate. Usually, color Doppler will fail to demonstrate blood flow within the "solid"

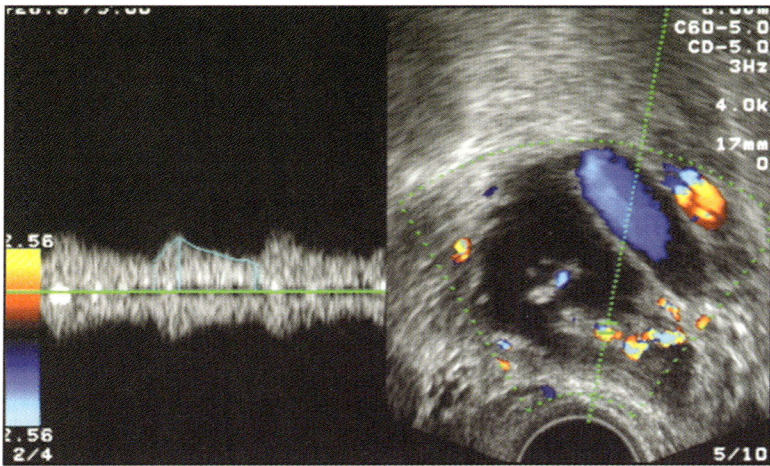

Fig. 21.19: Moderate-to-high resistance blood flow signals are obtained from a pseudopapillomatous structure protruding into the tubal lumen (RI = 0.50). This finding suggests chronic pelvic inflammatory disease

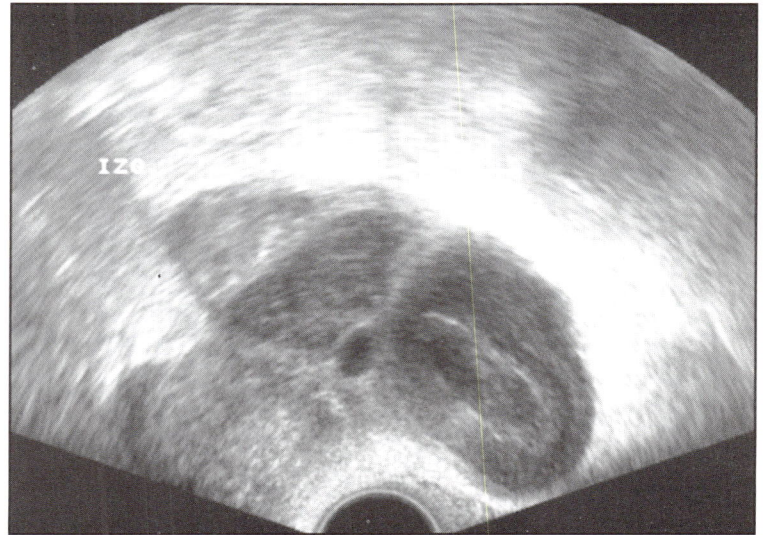

Fig. 21.22: Transvaginal sonogram of a complex adnexal mass that could be interpreted as a tubo-ovarian abscess

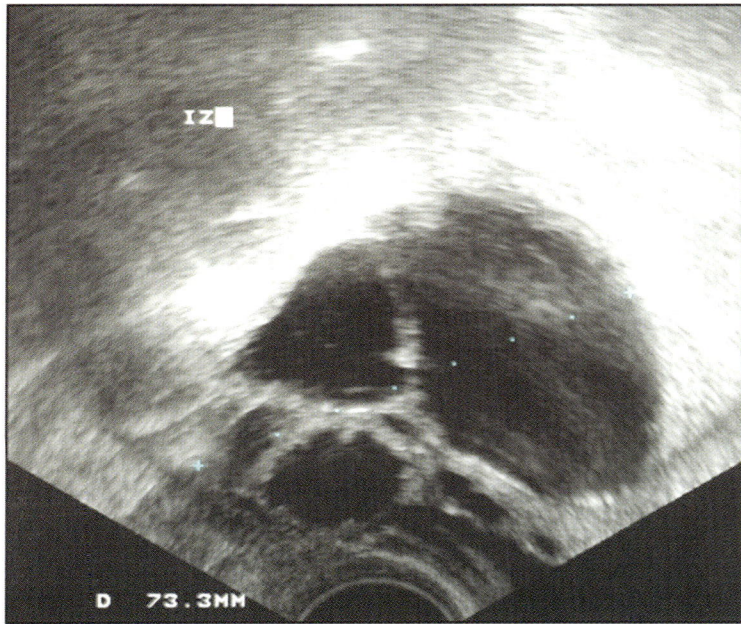

Fig. 21.20: Transvaginal scan shows a chronic salpingitis. Note the "cogwheel sign" produced by hyperechogenic "knots" visualizad every few millimeters in a traverse section of the inflamed fallopian tube

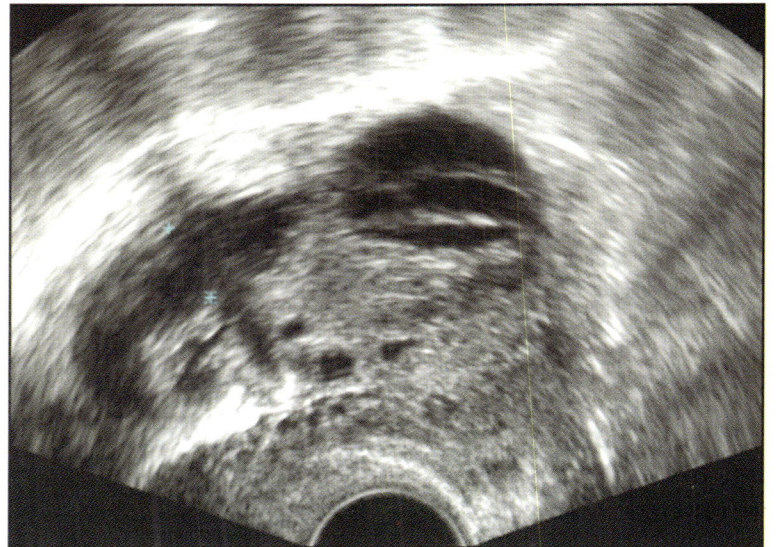

Fig. 21.23: Transvaginal scan of a tubo-ovarian abscess. Note the thickened and irregular margins and echogenic fluid

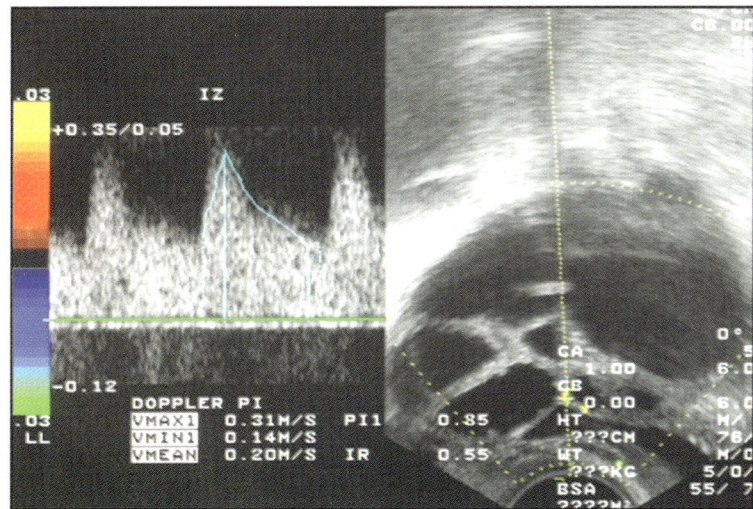

Fig. 21.21: The same patient as in Figure 21.20. Moderate-to-high resistance blood flow signals (RI = 0.55) are depicted from the walls of the fallopian tube

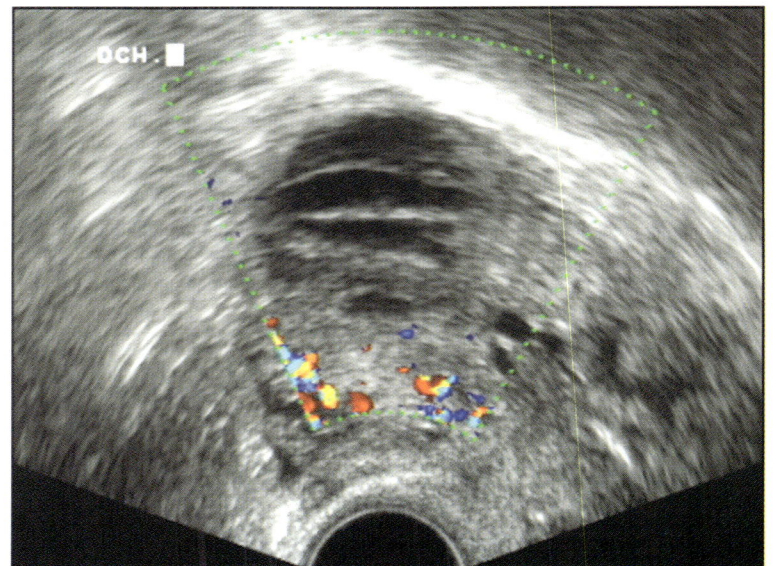

Fig. 21.24: The same patient as in Figure 21.23. Color Doppler detects vessels within the tubal walls and ovarian parenchyma

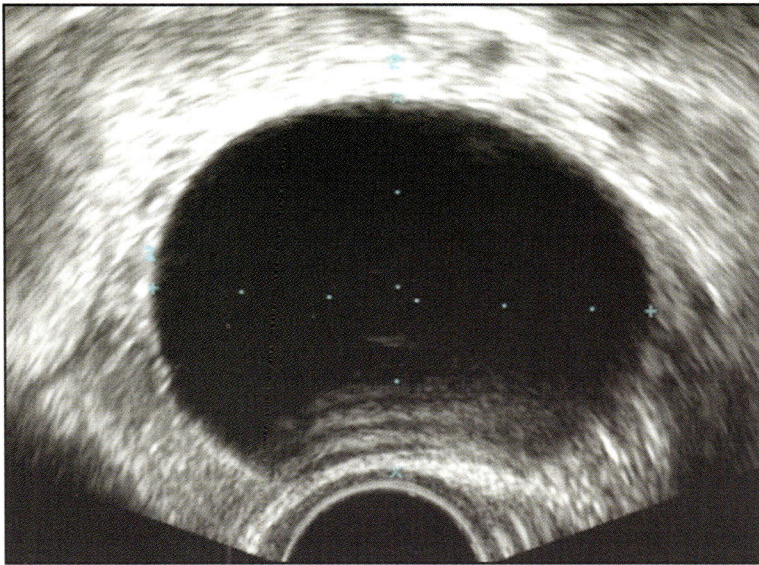

Fig. 21.25: Simple benign paraovarian cyst. Note smooth walls of paraovarian cyst

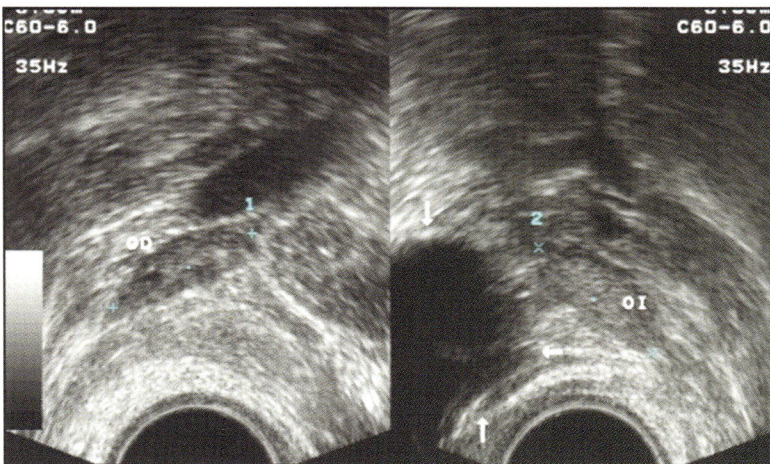

Fig. 21.26: Other example of paraovarian cyst. We can see both ovaries (right and left) independent of the paraovarian cyst (near left ovary)

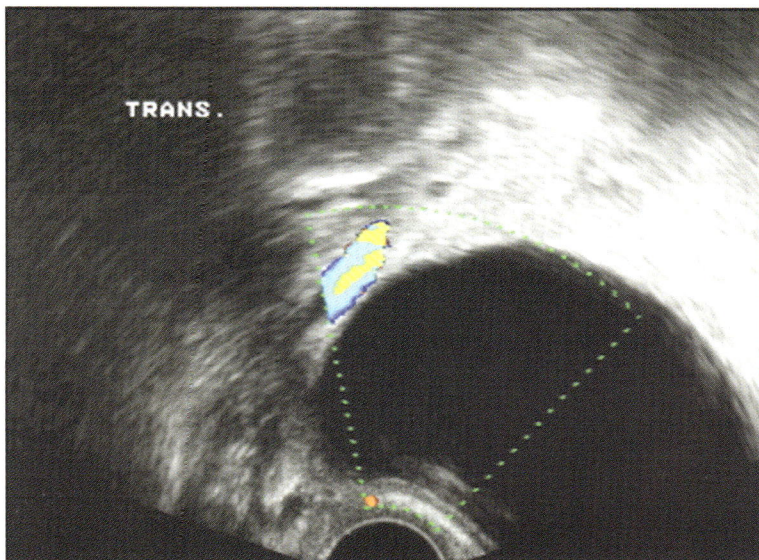

Fig. 21.27: Simple benign paraovarian cyst. Note smooth walls and absence of cyst vascularization

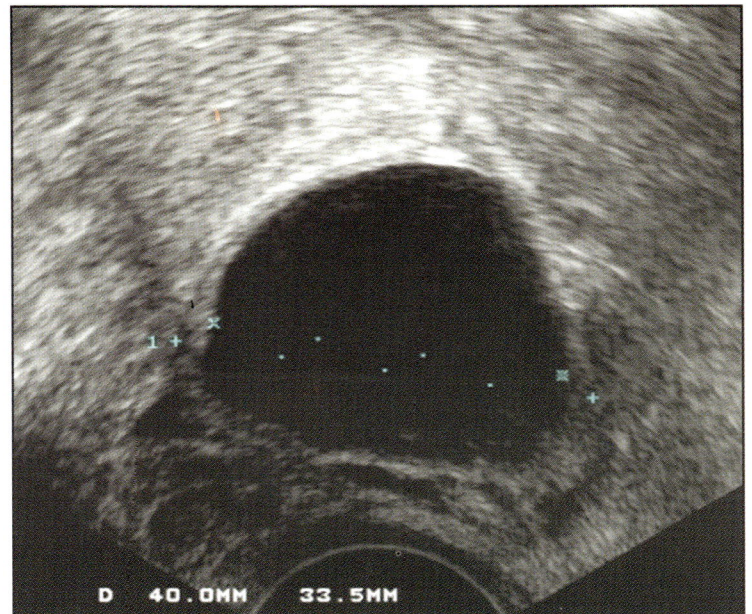

Fig. 21.28: Transvaginal sonogram of a simple serous cyst. Note the regular borders and anechoic fluid

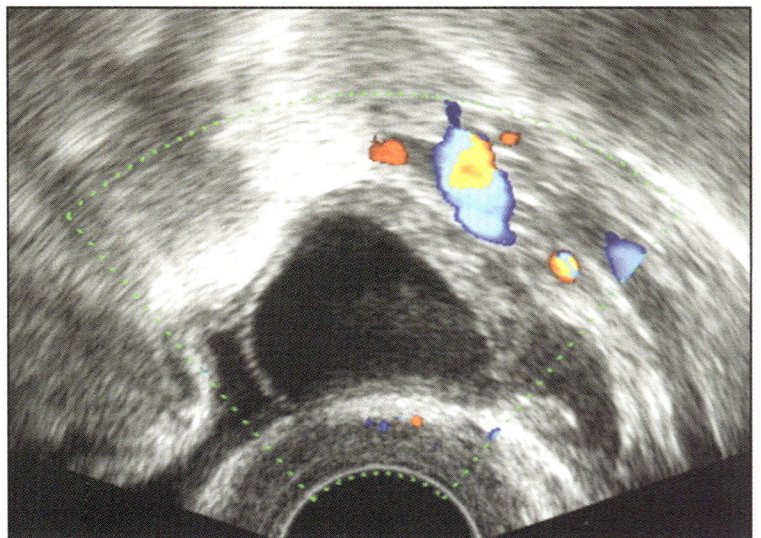

Fig. 21.29: Another example of a simple cyst with normal parenchyma peripheral. Color Doppler shows absence of vascularization

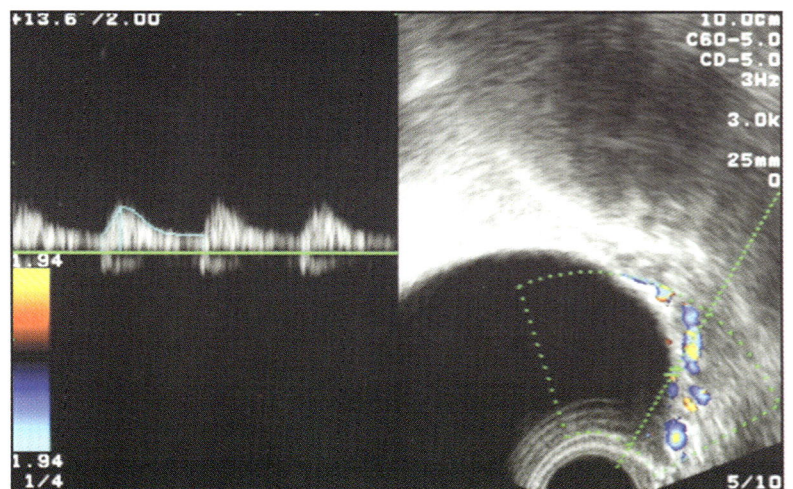

Fig. 21.30: Simple ovarian cyst, appearing completely sonolucent with a thin, smooth wall without internal excresence. Moderate peripheral vascular resistance (RI = 0.64) indicates the benign nature of the lesion. A serous cystoadenoma was confirmed by histopathology

component because it is not a really solid tissue, rather a very dense cystic component.

Endometriosis is one of the most often encountered benign gynecological conditions. Endometriosis is defined as a disease

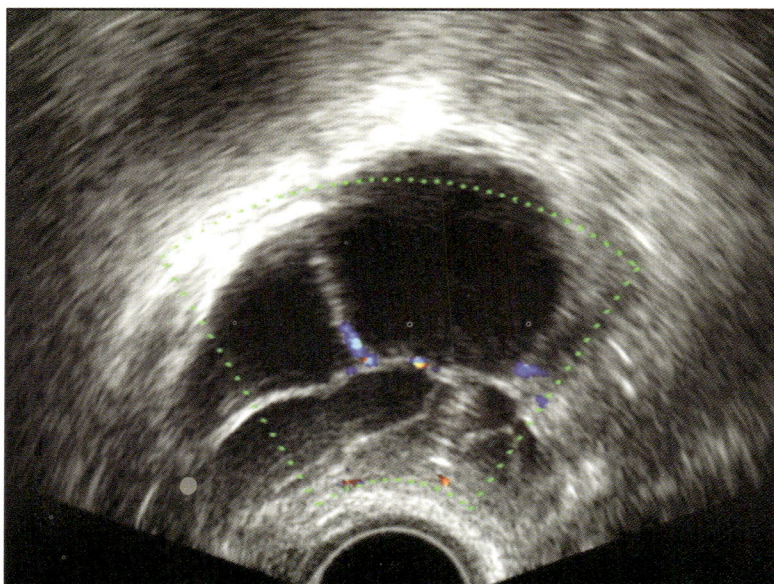

Fig. 21.31: Complex ovarian mass demonstrate by color flow imaging. Note the presence of thin septa. A serous cystoadenoma was confirmed by histopathology

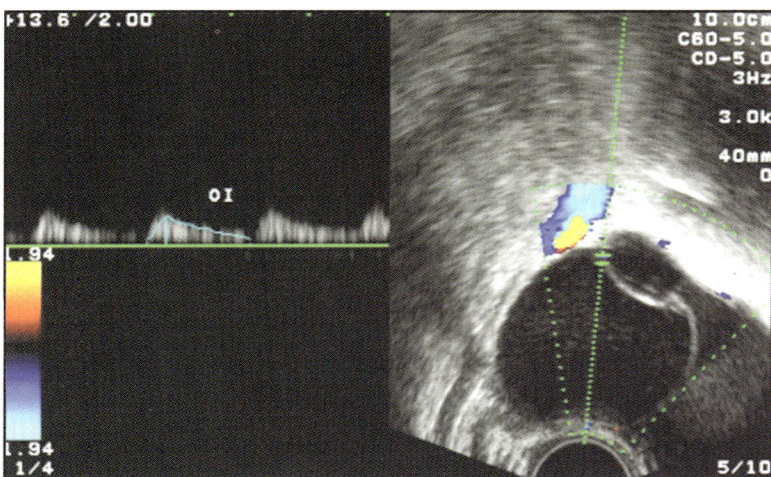

Fig. 21.32: Ovarian tumor containing thin septa. Color Doppler facilitates detection of blood flow within the septa. High-resistance signals (RI = 0.77) depicted from color-code areas. The benign nature of the tumor was confirmed by histopathology

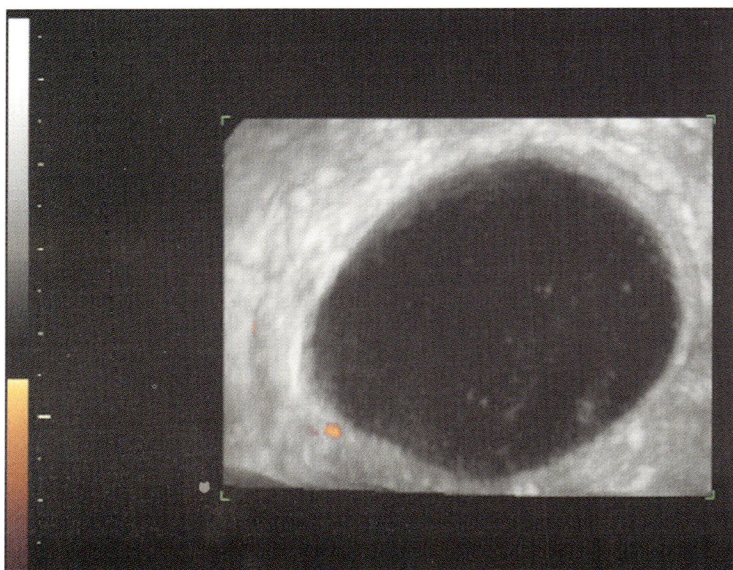

Fig. 21.33: Three-dimensional color Doppler scan of a serous cyst, shows absence of vascularization

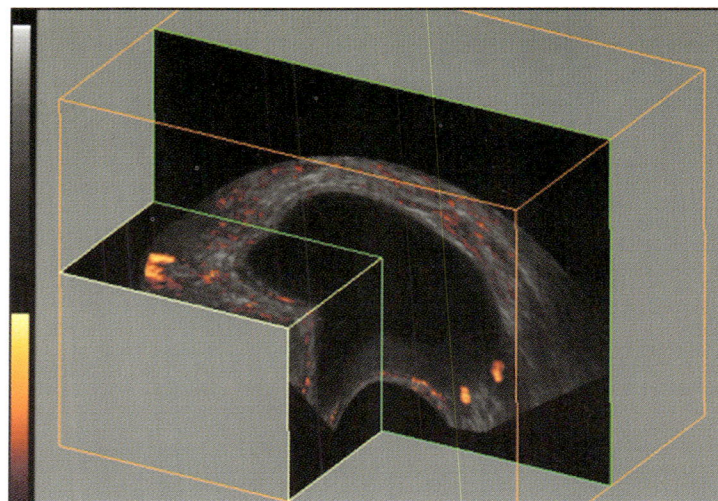

Fig. 21.34: Reformatted section ("niche" imaging) allows more precise estimation of the few vessels in the peripheral wall in a simple serous cyst confirmed by laparoscopy

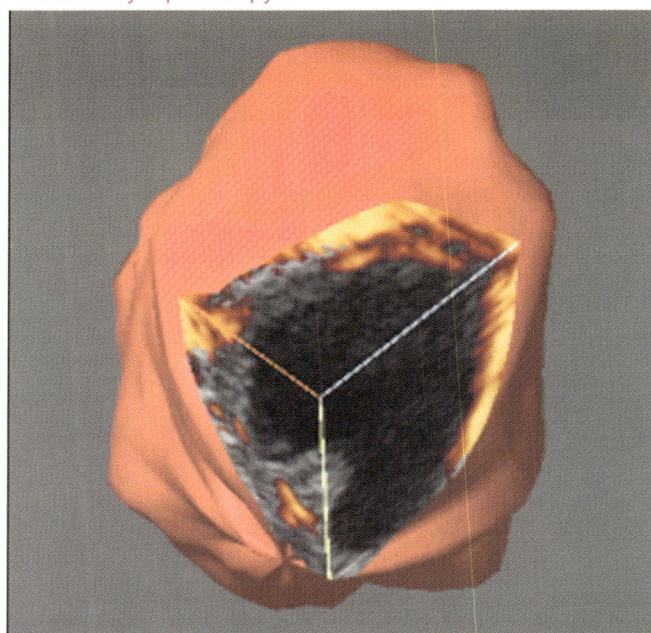

Fig. 21.35: A case of benign papillar serous cystoadenoma that shows in reformatted section ("vocal" imaging) a papillar structures into the lumen of the cyst. Power Doppler does not demonstrate any blood flow signals into the papillae

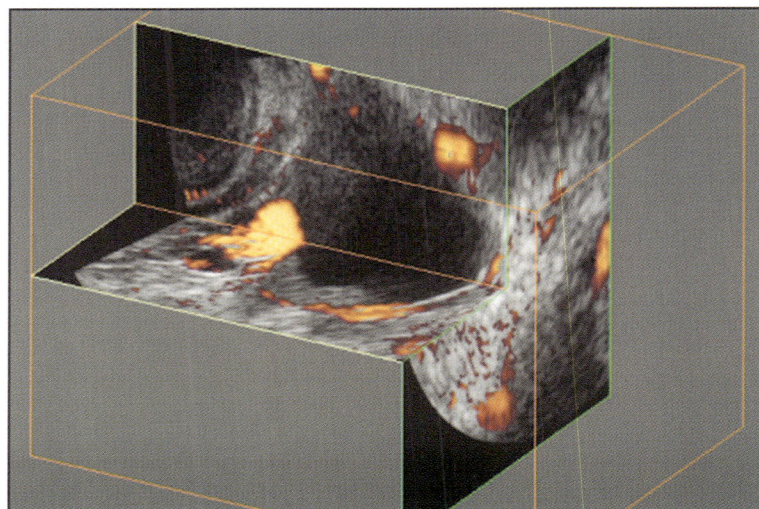

Fig. 21.36: A same case of Figure 21.35: Reformatted section ("niche" imaging) allows into the lumen of the cyst a papillary projections without vascularization

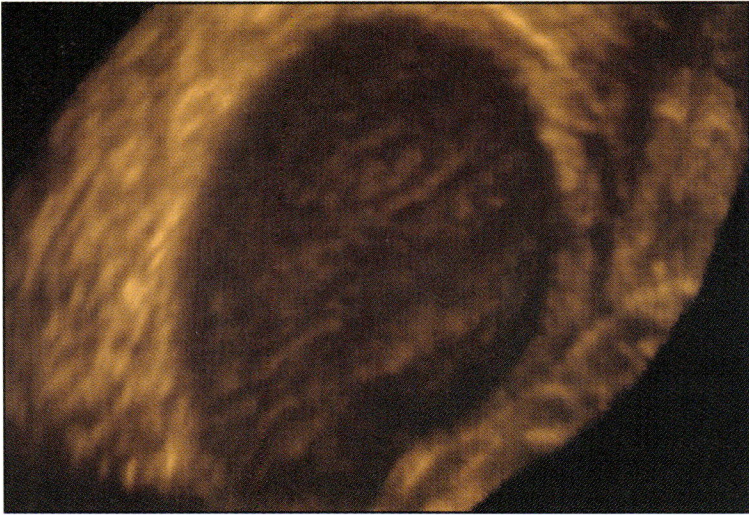

Fig. 21.37: Three-dimensional scan of a serous ovarian cyst. The regular thin wall is clearly demonstrated

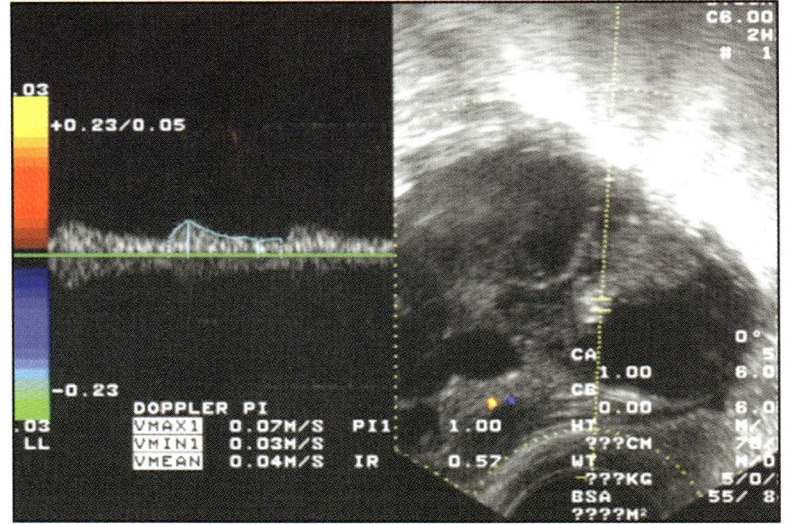

Fig. 21.40: Transvaginal color Doppler scan of a cystic tumor. Color Doppler imaging demonstrates vascularity within the thick septa. Moderate-high-resistance signals (RI = 0.57) depicted from a thick septa suggest the benign nature of the lesion. The tumor was diagnosed as a mucinous cystoadenoma

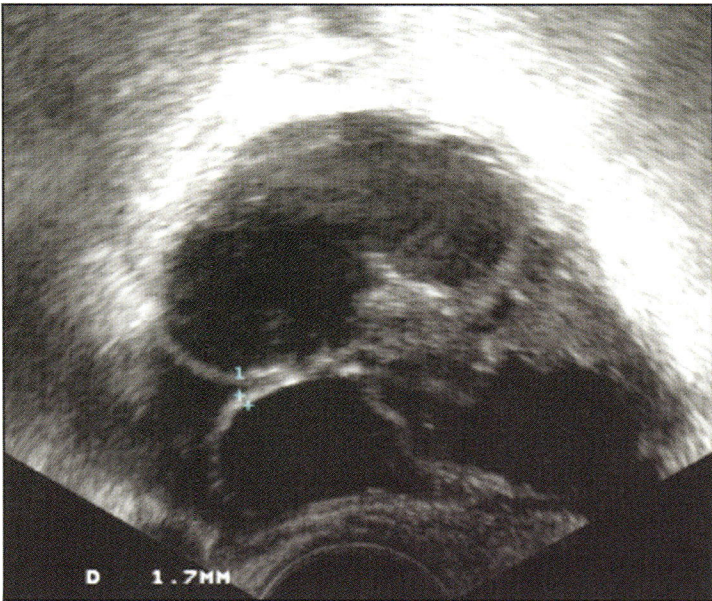

Fig. 21.38: Multilocular ovarian tumor presenting thick septa and echogenic content. Histopathology confirmed mucinous cystoadenoma

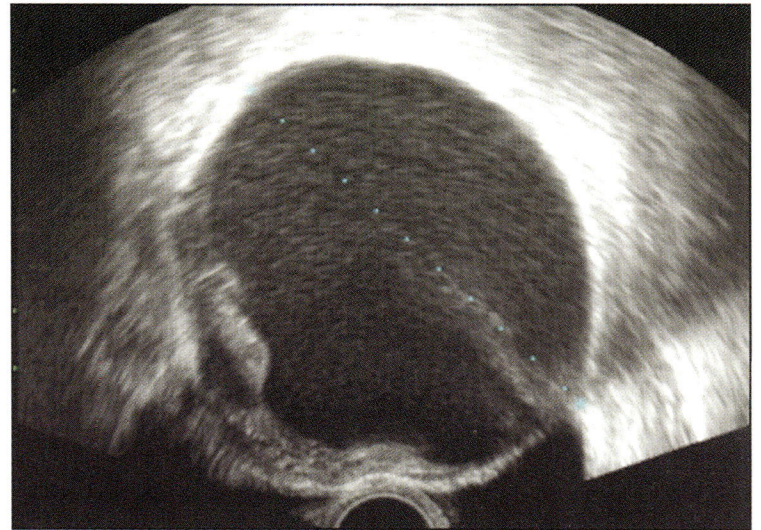

Fig. 21.41: Transvaginal sonogram shows a big cyst with thick septa and diffuse echoes. Histopathology reveals a moucinous cistoadenoma

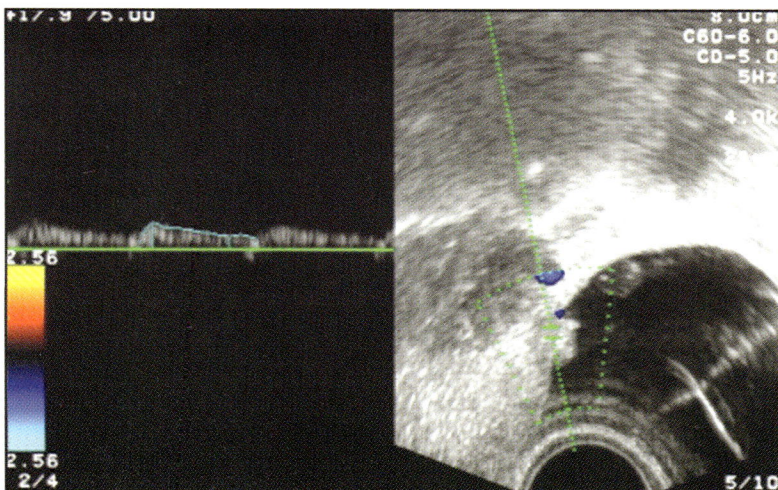

Fig. 21.39: Another example of ovarian tumor containing thick ovarian septa and papillary formations. Color Doppler imaging demonstrates vascularity in the basis of papillary projection (RI = 0.53). Mucinous cystoadenoma was confirmed by histopathology

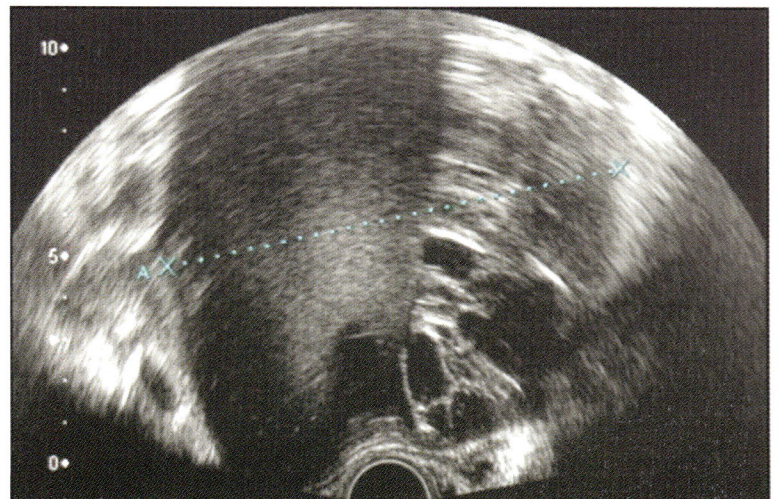

Fig. 21.42: Multilocular ovarian tumor presenting thick septa and echogenic content. Histopathology confirmed mucinous cystoadenoma

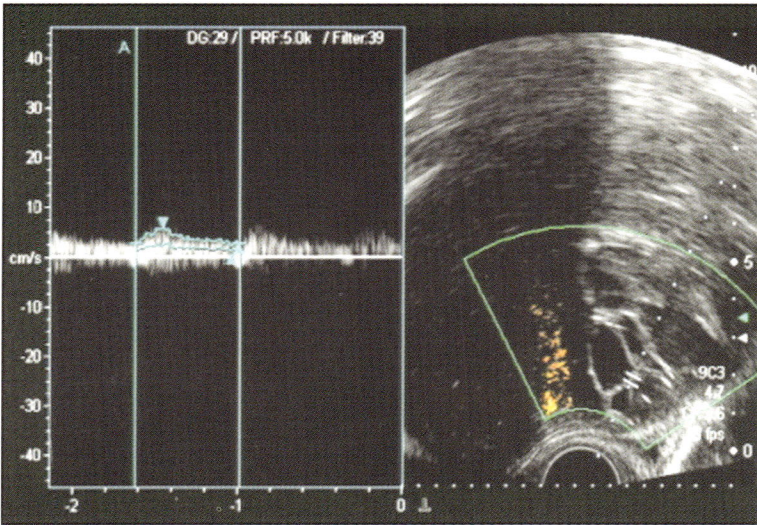

Fig. 21.43: The same patient as in Figure 21.42: Power Doppler shows a moderate-high-resistance signals (RI = 0.53). The benign nature of the tumor was confirmed by histopathology

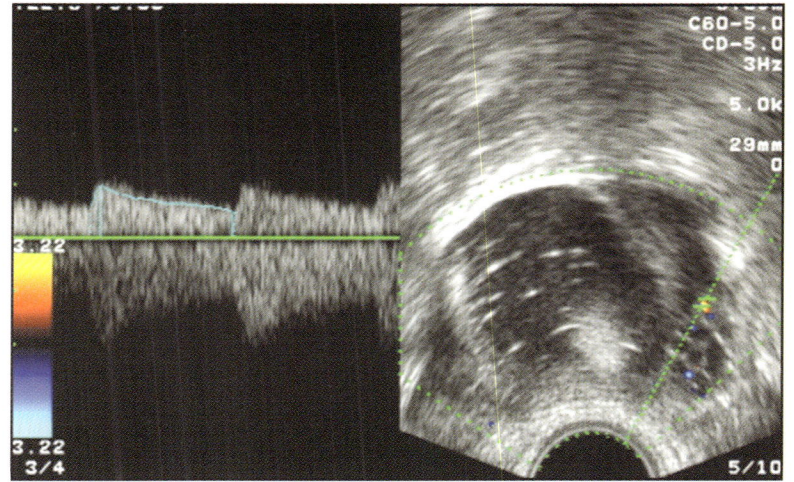

Fig. 21.46: Transvaginal color Doppler scan of a complex ovarian tumor with echogenic tubercle and scattered internal echoes. Color Doppler shows moderate-high resistance (RI = 0.51). The lesion was histopathologically diagnosed as a cystic teratoma

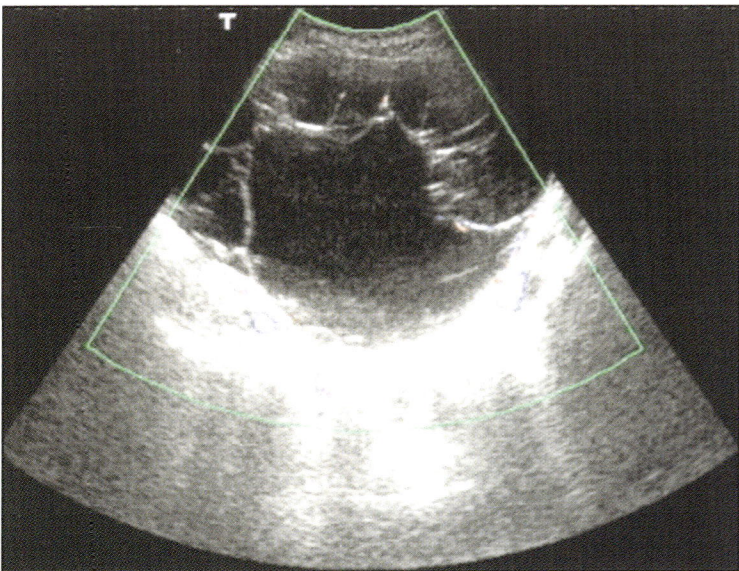

Fig. 21.44: Abdominal sonogram of the same cases of Figures 21.42 and 21.43. Note the typical septa of mucinous cyst

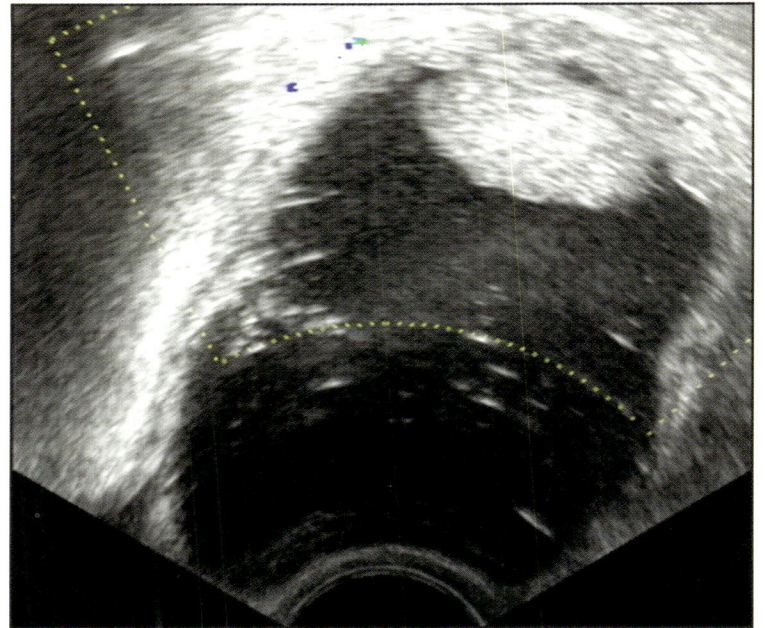

Fig. 21.47: Another case of an avascular dermoid cyst. Note the prominent echogenicity of the solid tumor part, scattered internal echoes and absence of intratumoral vascularity

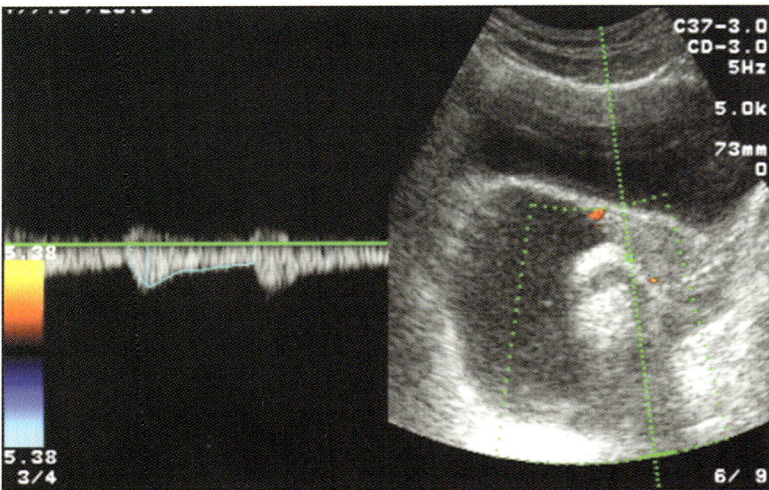

Fig. 21.45: Transabdominal scan of a cystic-solid ovarian lesion. Note the prominent echogenicity and fat-fluid, both suggestive of a cystic teratoma. Moderate vascular resistance (RI = 0.59) obtained from the periphery of the ovarian lesion suggest inflammatory changes. This was confirmed by laparoscopy and histopathology

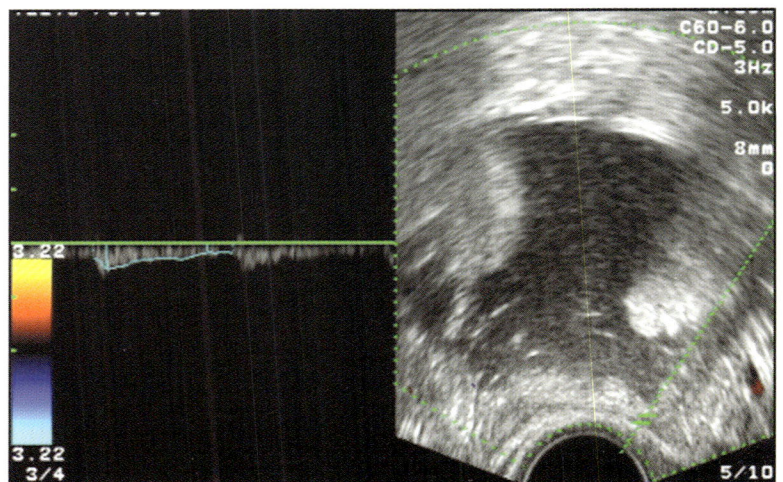

Fig. 21.48: Transvaginal sonogram of a bizarre ovarian lesion. Echogenic tubercle and dense echo pattern are sonographic criteria for the diagnosis of cystic teratoma. Color Doppler shows a high resistance flow (RI = 0.67)

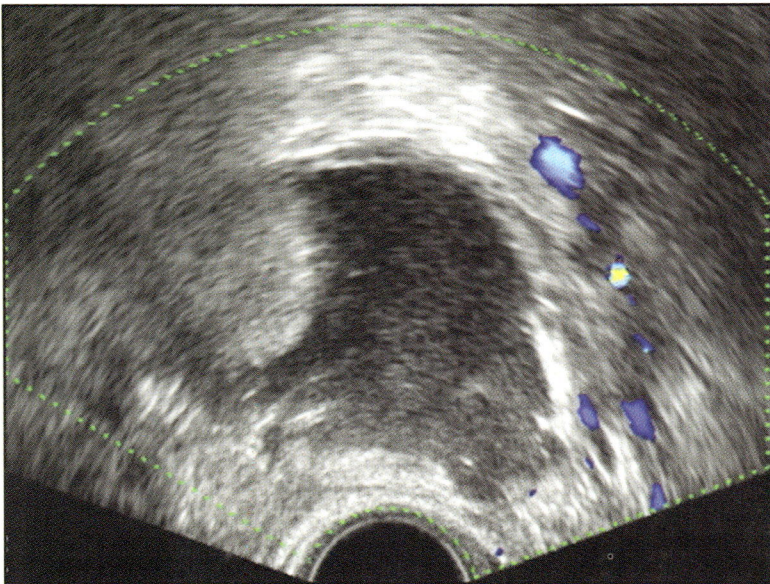

Fig. 21.49: Another case of an vascular dermoid cyst. Note the echogenic tubercle and scattered internal echoes

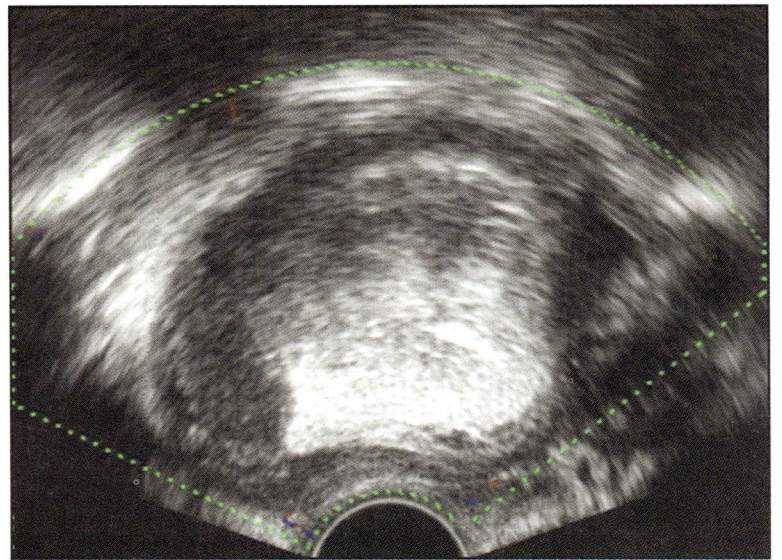

Fig. 21.52: Transvaginal color Doppler scan of a bizarre adnexal mass. Color Doppler does not reveal intratumoral vascularization. A dermoid cyst was confirmed by histopathology

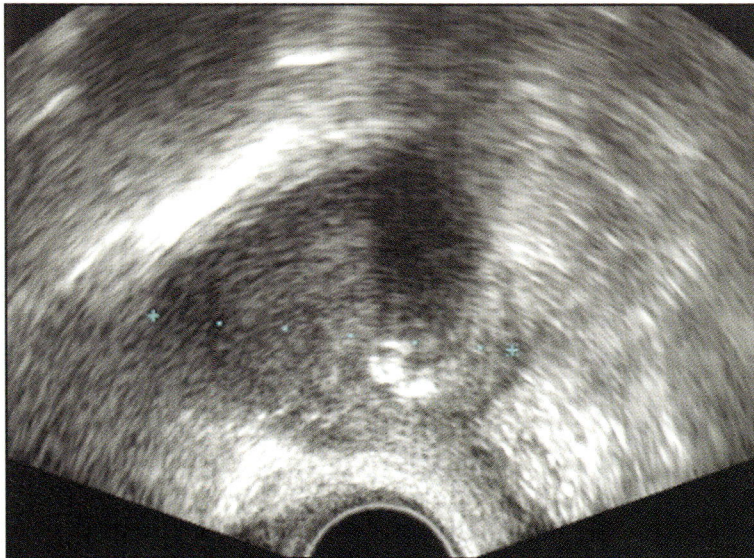

Fig. 21.50: Echoic pattern of dermoid mass, fat-fluid contents and acoustic shadowing assisted in performing the diagnosis of cystic teratoma

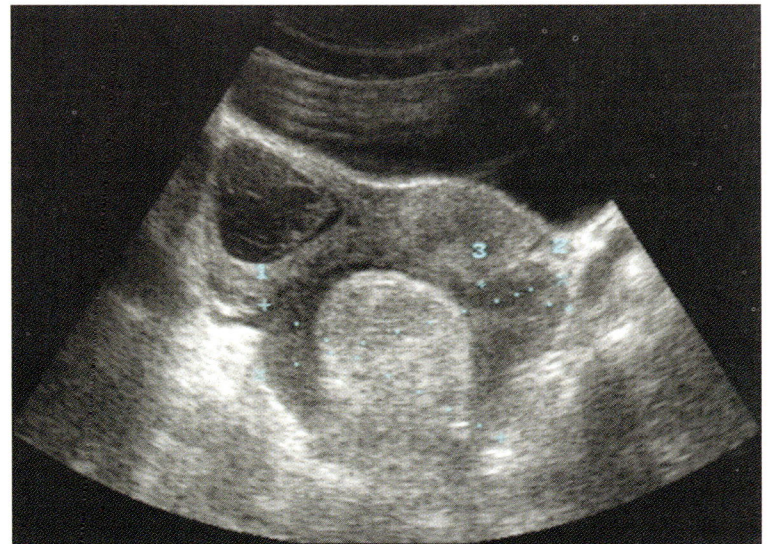

Fig. 21.53: The same case of Figure 21.53 by abdominal full bladder. We can see the echogenic tubercle and dense echo pattern

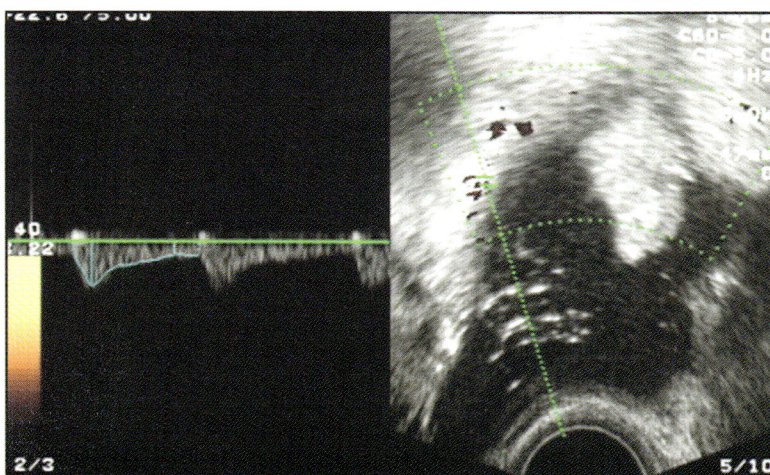

Fig. 21.51: Vascularized cystic-solid ovarian lesion. Note the prominent echogenicity of the solid tumor part and absence of intratumoral vascularity

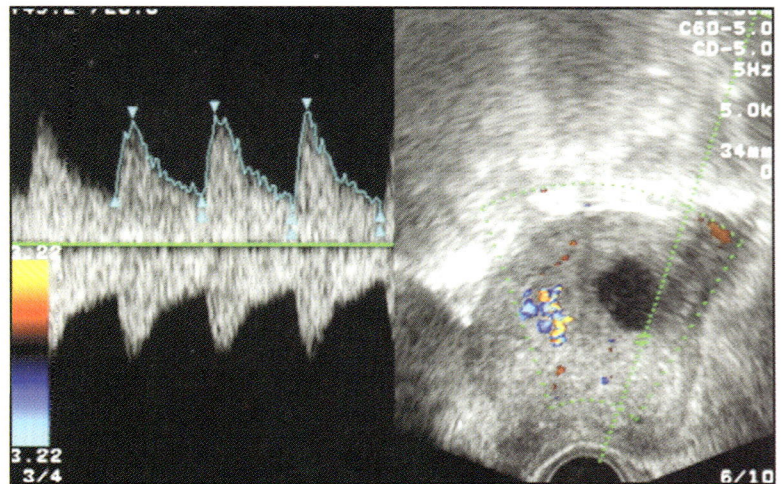

Fig. 21.54: Complex ovarian lesion as seen by transvaginal ultrasound. High vascular resistance (RI = 0.69) is detected in a patient with laparoscopically proven chronical tubo-ovarian abscess

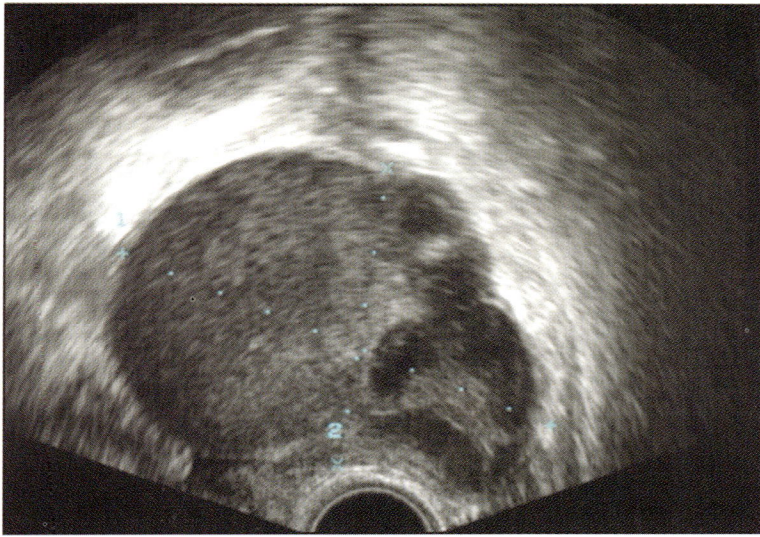

Fig. 21.55: Large endometrioma with pronounced internal echos: Such a finding be distinguished from a tubo-ovarian abscess and the diagnosis was made on laparotomy

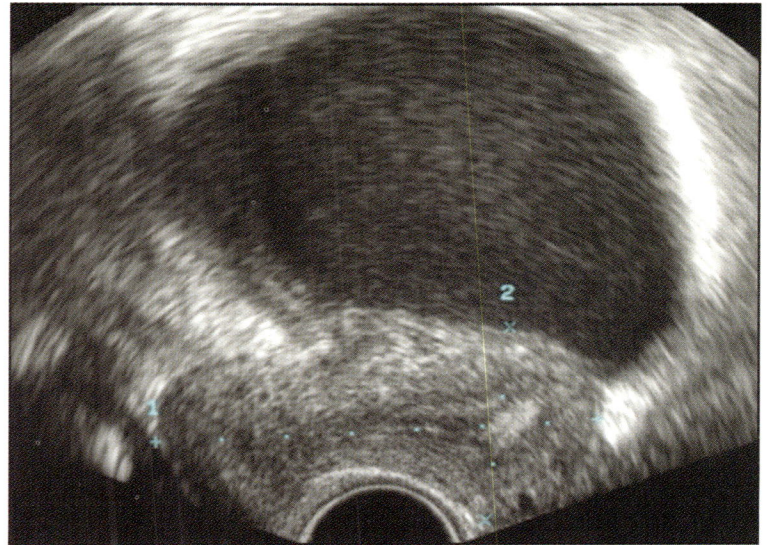

Fig. 21.56: Large endometriotic cyst with clearly visible intracystic echoes

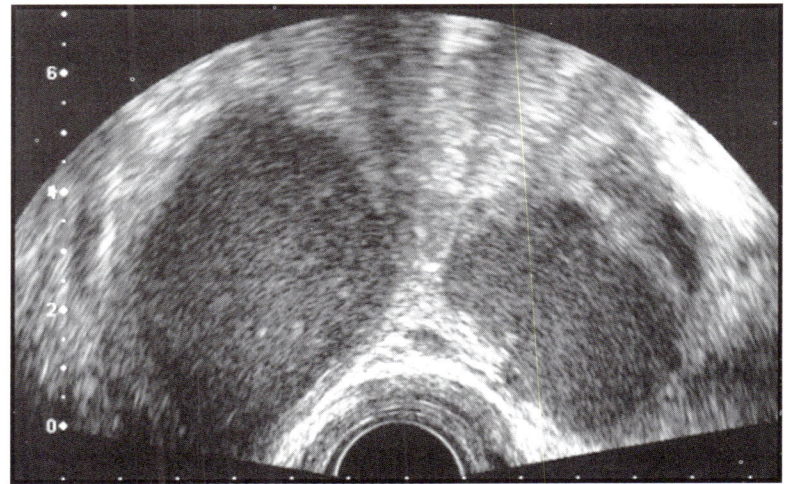

Fig. 21.57: Two endometriotic cysts with high-level internal echoes

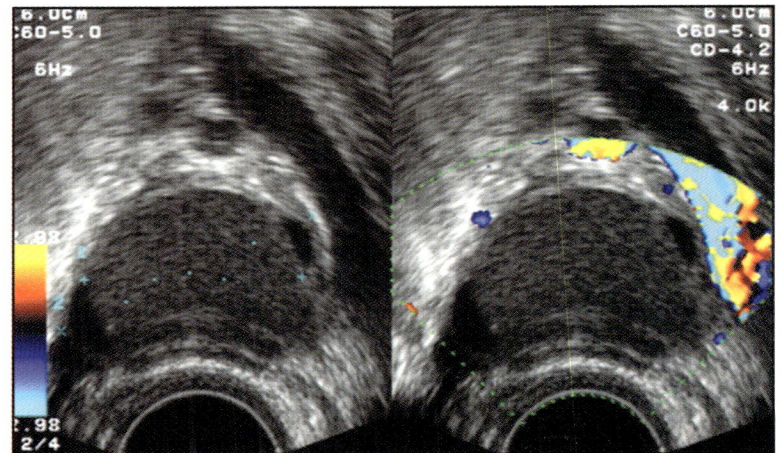

Fig. 21.58: Transvaginal sonogram of an ovarian endometrioma. Note the homogeneous "carpet-like" echoes of the cystic lesion

characterized by the presence of functional endometrial glands and stroma in ectopic location outside the uterine cavity. Endometrial tissue within the myometrium, adenomyosis, is a separate pathological entity with a different patient population etiology and clinical course.

An endometriotic cyst, also called an endometrioma or "chocolate cyst", is a special kind of endometriotic lesion within the ovary (Figs 21.56 to 21.69).

Sonography is an accurate method for determining the type (cystic, mixed or solid), shape and location of endometriosis. Cystic lesions are seen as irregular cysts with some evidence of septation. The sonographic appearance of the mixed-type cysts could be interpreted as pelvic inflammatory disease from an infectious cause , while a solid pattern may suggest ovarian malignancy. Sometimes it is difficult to differentiate an endometrioma from a hemorrhagic ovarian cyst or a corpus luteum cyst. Fibrinolysis of the hemolytic content of a hemorrhagic ovarian cyst may change its pattern. Endometriomas usually remain constant as non-echogenic cysts with a semisolid content of a "parenchymatous" texture representing "chocolate" paste-like fluid within the cyst. The experienced ultrasonographer can distinguish them accurately on the basis of low-level echoes, irregular shape and persistence over several menstrual cycles. Color Doppler demonstrates a pericystic vascular location at the level of the ovarian hilus which is typical of endometrioma. In the initial phases, when extensive angiogenic activity important for further outgrowth and progression of the endometrial implants occurs, low-to-moderate vascular impedance is obtained.

Torsions of ovarian cyst (Fig. 21.70) can occur in all type of cyst, but it is more frequent in dermoid cyst. Occasionally the tumors may rupture, producing acute peritonitis. The most usual

benign ovarian tumors are ovarian fibromas. These are usually round, with a well-delineated hyperechogenic appearance (Figs 21.71 and 21.72). If a solid lesion is observed in the adnexa of a premenopausal woman, it is more likely to be a pedunculated or broad-ligament leiomyoma than a solid ovarian neoplasm.

Transvaginal color Doppler is useful in differentiating fibroids from solid ovarian masses on the basis of their vascularity. Within

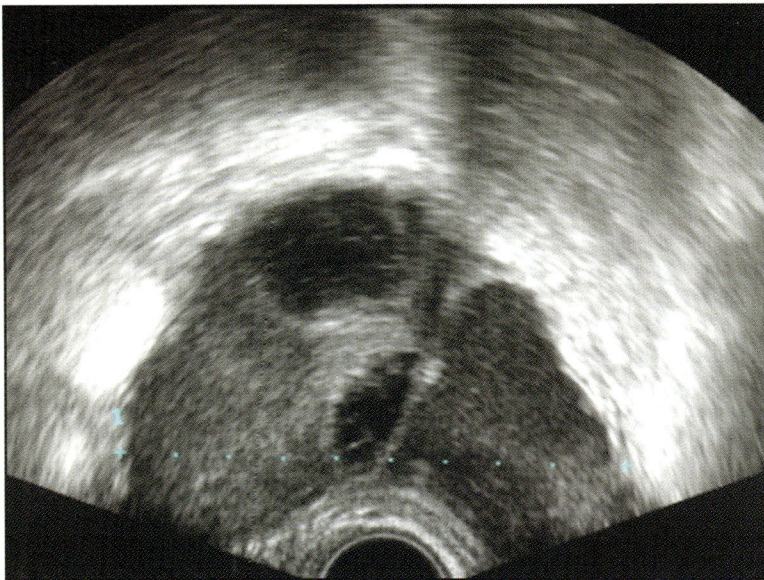

Fig. 21.59: Transvaginal scan demonstrating a multilocular endometriotic cyst

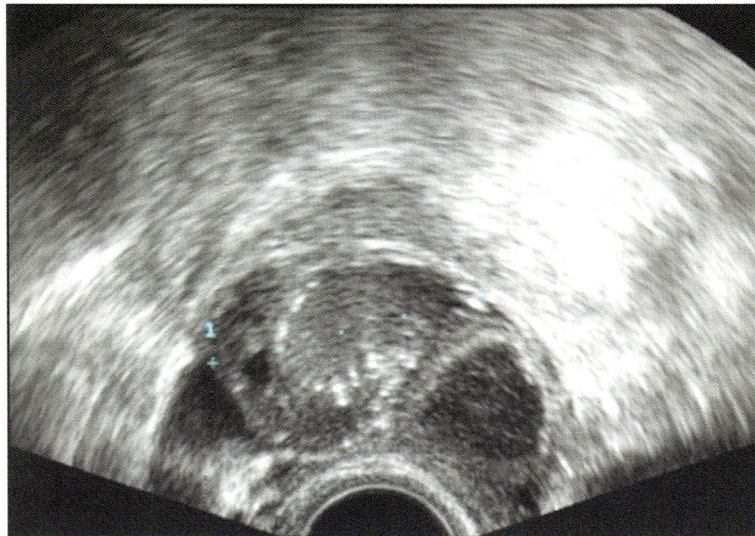

Fig. 21.60: Transvaginal color Doppler scan of multilocular ovarian endometrioma. Note the different areas of echogenicity within the septated structure due to fibrinolysis of the hemolytic content

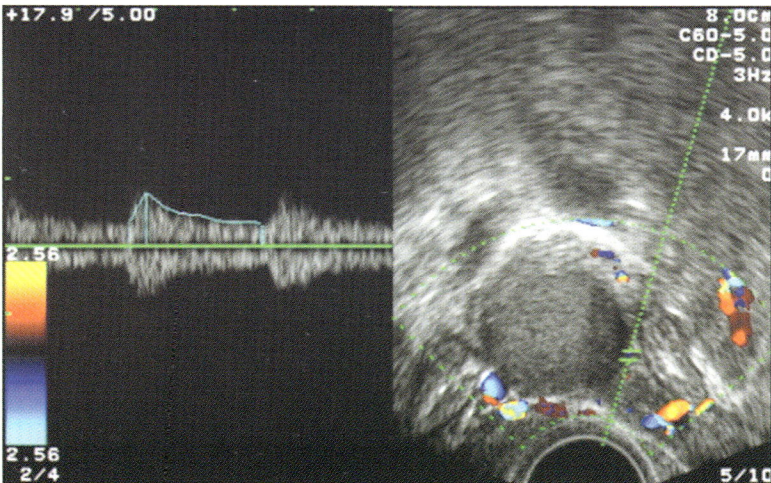

Fig. 21.61: Transvaginal color Doppler ultrasound shows an ovarian cysts with homogeneous echogenic content and hilar vascularization. Pulsed Doppler signals shows moderate vascular impedance (RI = 0.61)

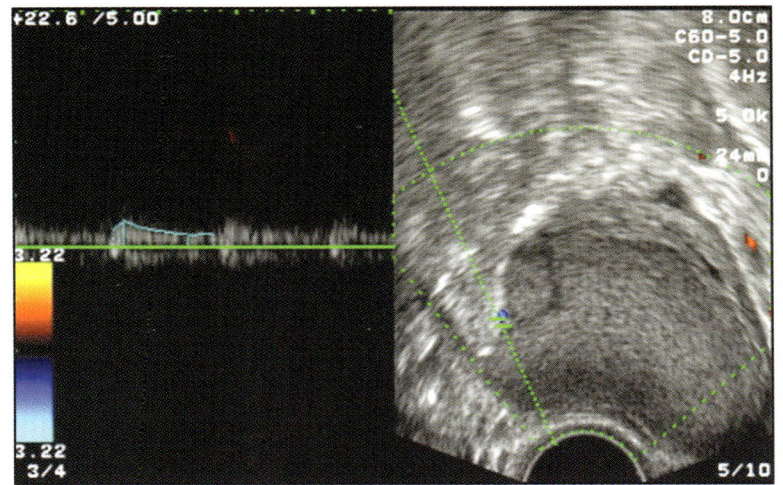

Fig. 21.62: Transvaginal color Doppler scan shows an ovarian endometrioma. Note the homogeneous "chocolate" fluid within the cyst and vascularization at the level of the ovarian hilus

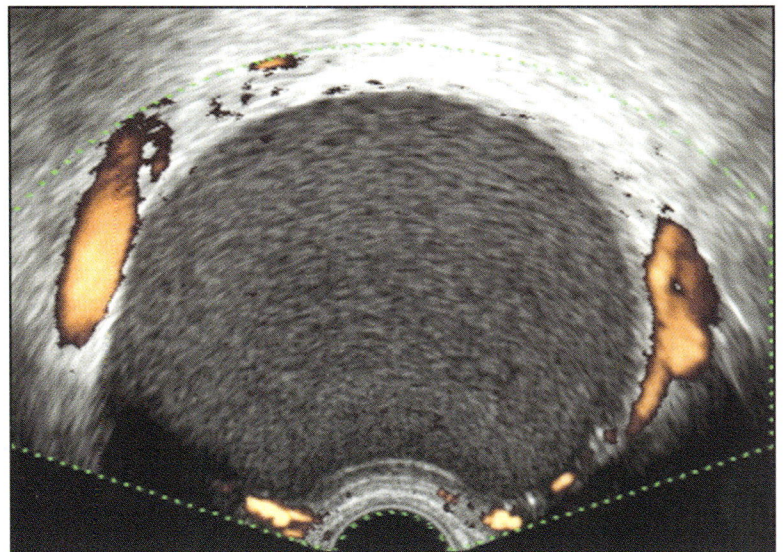

Fig. 21.63: Avascular ovarian endometrioma. Color Doppler does not reveal endometrioma vascularity, but surrounding vessels are easily depicted

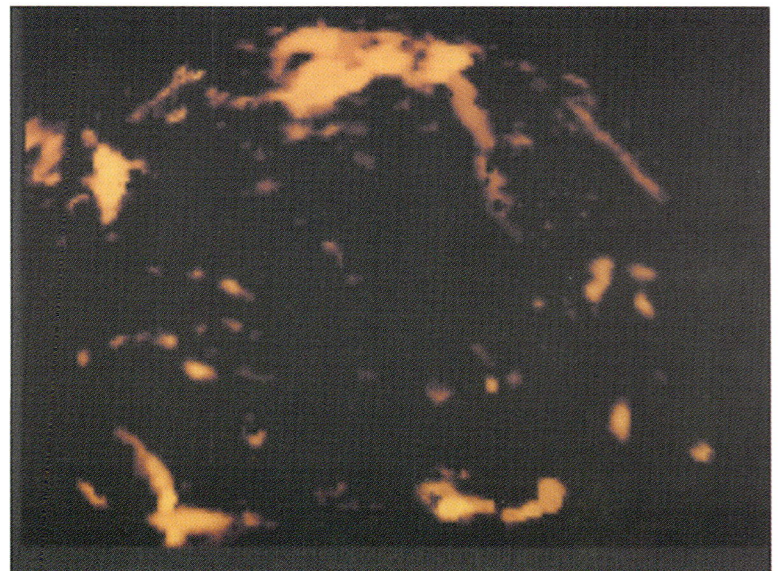

Fig. 21.64: Three-dimensional power Doppler of an endometriotic cyst, we can see the vascularization surrounding wall cyst

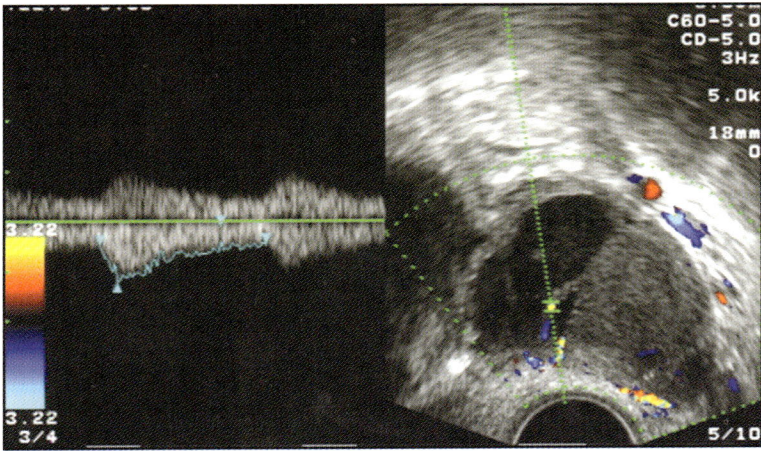

Fig. 21.65: Transvaginal color Doppler sonogram of a "chocolate" cyst during the luteal phase of the menstrual cycle. Moderate vascular impedance (RI = 0.59) is easily observed during the late follicular phase

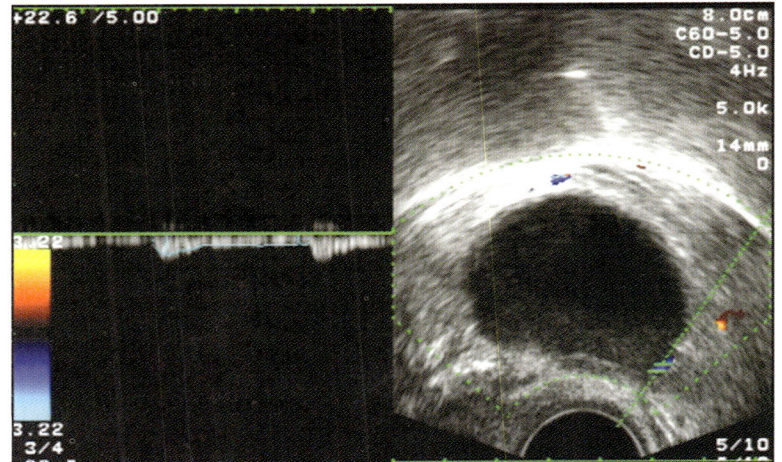

Fig. 21.68: Another example of endometriotic cyst : Sometimes the pattern seems a simple cyst. Pulsed Doppler color shows a moderate-high-resistance (RI = 0.56)

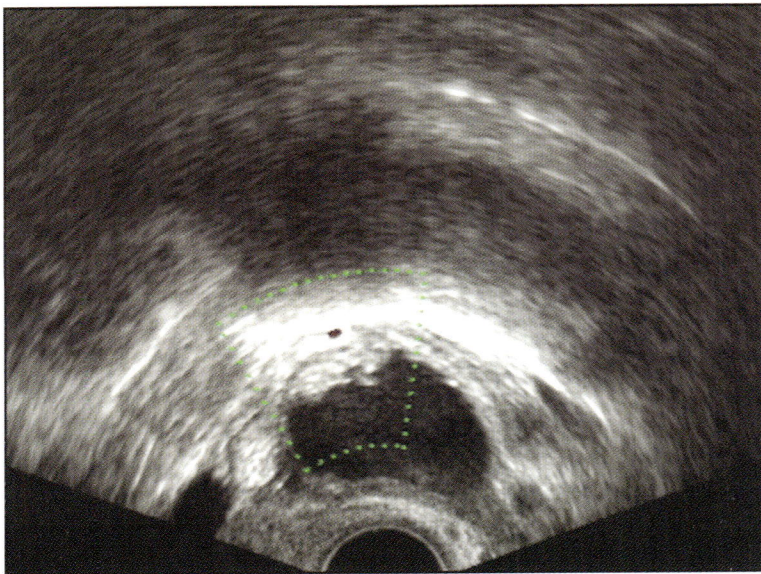

Fig. 21.66: Transvaginal scan of a complex adnexal mass containing a papillary protrusion. Power Doppler does not reveal areas of vascularity. Despite the suspicious morphology, histopathology confirmed that the lesion was an endometriotic cyst

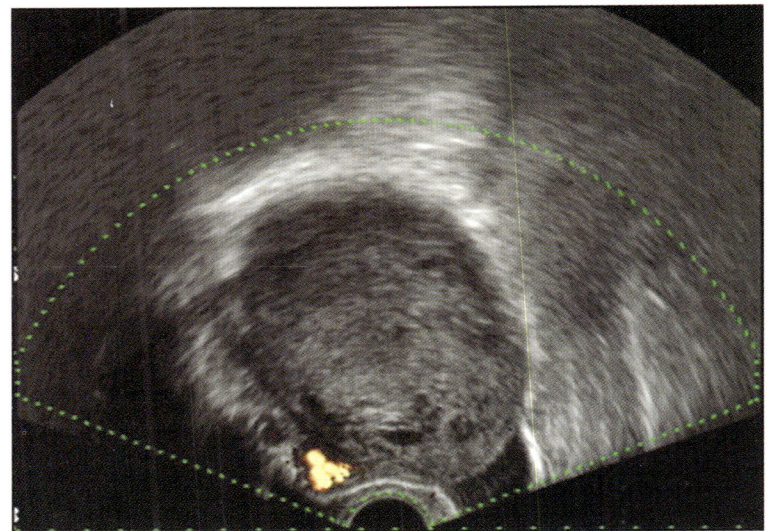

Fig. 21.69: Transvaginal power Doppler scan shows a vascular tumor. Patient presents acute pain. We can suspect an ovarian torsion

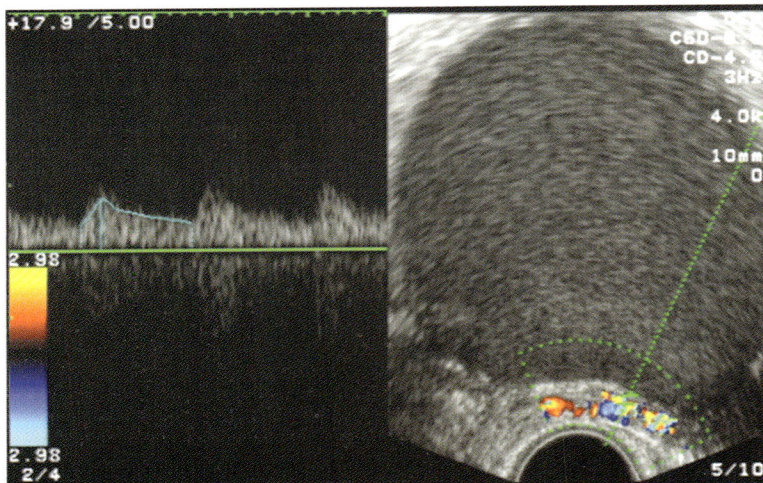

Fig. 21.67: Transvaginal color Doppler ultrasound shows an ovarian cyst with homogeneous echogenic content and hilar vascularization. Pulsed Doppler signals shows moderate vascular impedance (RI = 0.53). Histopathology confirmed that the lesion was an endometriotic cyst

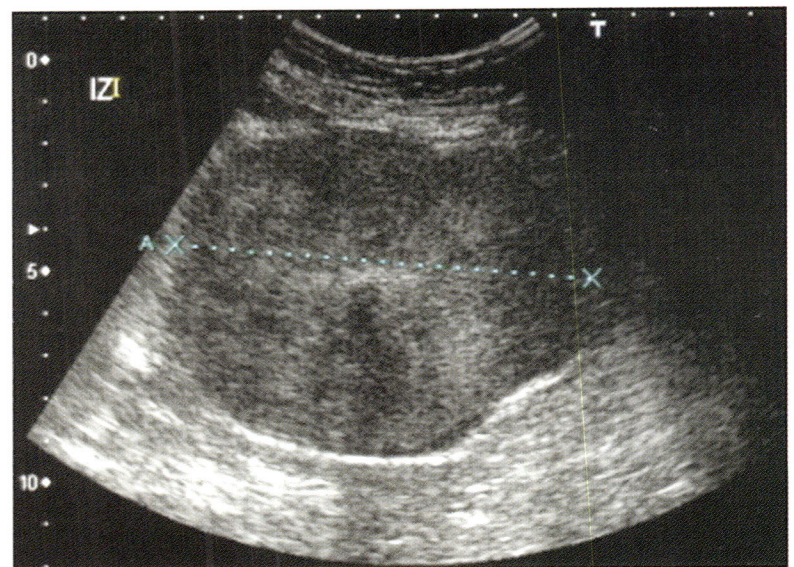

Fig. 21.70: Another case of solid ovarian tumor as seen by transabdominal ultrasound. A large solid ovarian mass can be confused with a pedunculated myoma because of a similar echo pattern. Absence or a few vessels detected by color Doppler permits it to distinguish from a malignant ovarian tumor

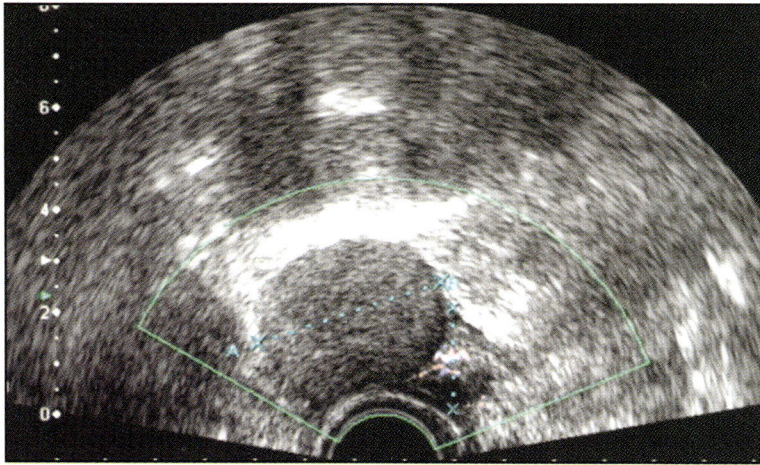

Fig. 21.71: Transvaginal color Doppler scan demonstrating a case of avascular, solid ovarian tumor. The diagnosis of ovarian fibroma was confirmed after surgery

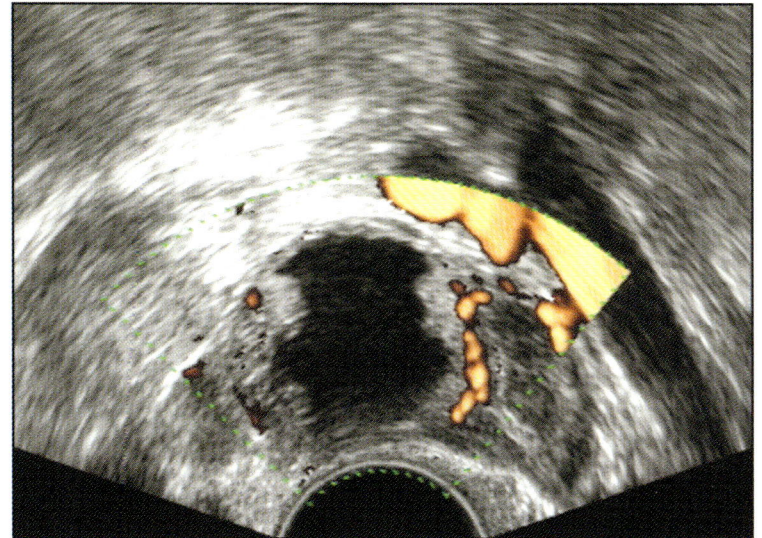

Fig. 21.73: The same case of Figure 21.72 power Doppler used to locate the blood flow

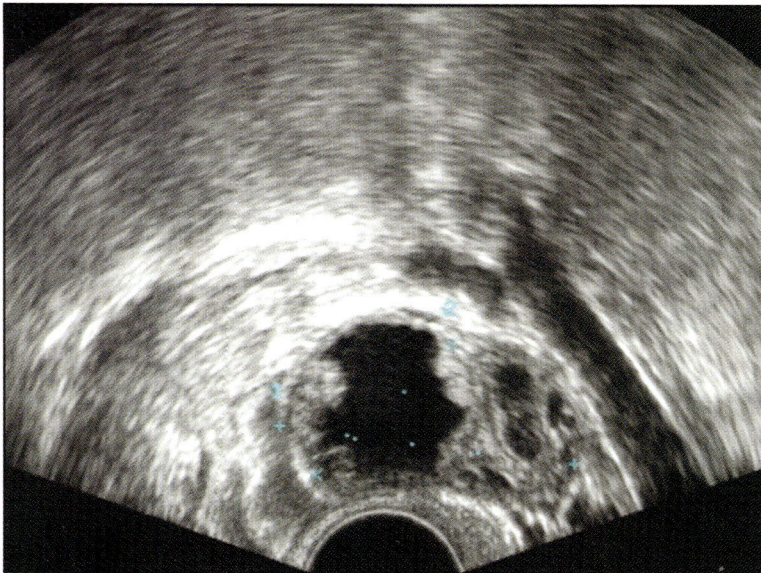

Fig. 21.72: B-mode ultrasound scan of a little cyst (27 mm). Note a papillary projection into the cyst

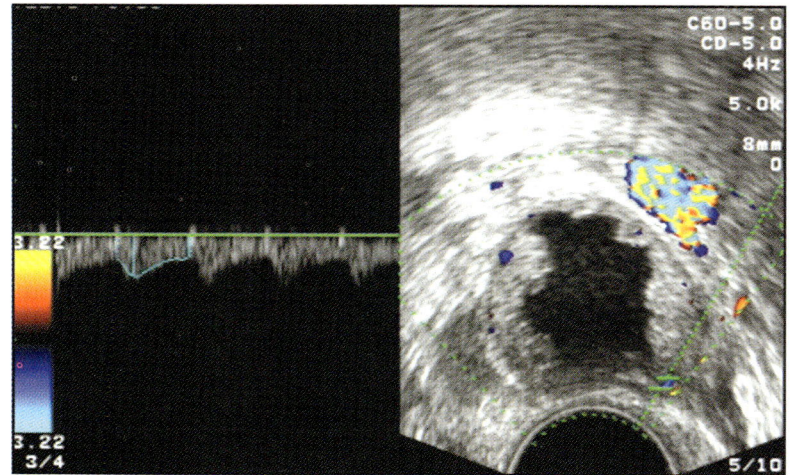

Fig. 21.74: The same cases of Figures 21.72 and 21.73. Note the pulsed Doppler shows low resistance (RI = 0.48)

or on the periphery of the uterine mass, even when it is out of the contour of the uterus, it is possible to detect waveform signals that are typical of the uterine vascular network. In such cases, blood flow is usually similar to normal myometrial perfusion, originating from terminal branches of the uterine artery. On the other hand, small vessels that feed a growing ovarian tumor are derived from ovarian vasculature.

Although complex tumors with solid or cystic component include most of the benign ovarian masses described above, malignant ovarian lesions such as cystoadenocarcinomas, endometrioid carcinomas, clear cell carcinomas and borderline tumors also exhibit a similar ultrasonic appearance (Figs 21.73 to 21.100). Among the several findings of ovarian tumors, it is possible to encounter three of them that have a statistically significant correlation between ovarian malignancy and the presence of sonographic ovarian lesions such as papillae, solid components and thick septa.

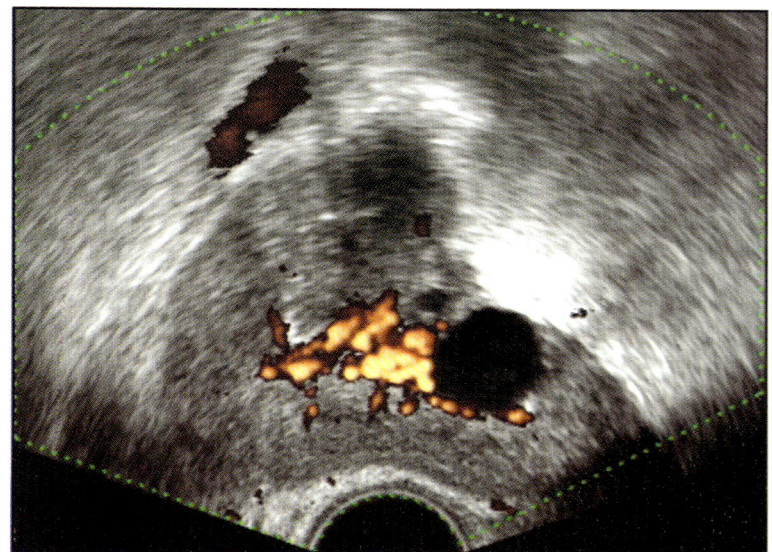

Fig. 21.75: Transvaginal power Doppler scan of a complex adnexal mass demonstrating predominantly central vascularity. Histology reveals a tumor

Vascularization of malignant ovarian masses is present in all three ultrasonic findings. Blood flow can be seen at the base of

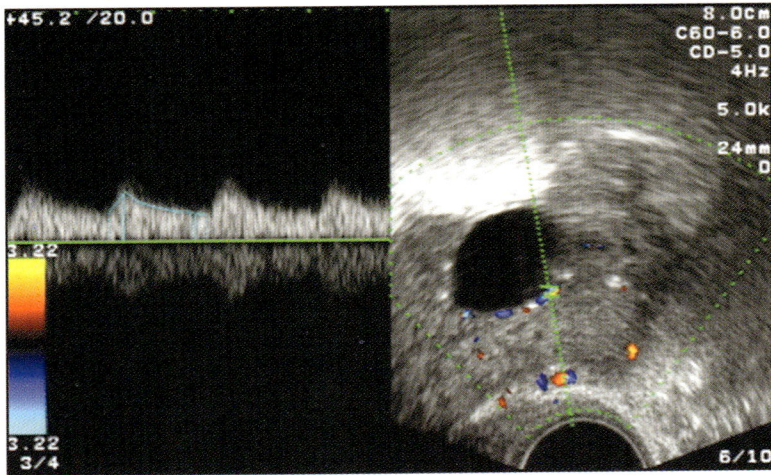

Fig. 21.76: Low-impedance signals (RI = 0.46) obtained from the central part of the malignant tumor. Borderline tumor was confirmed by histopathology

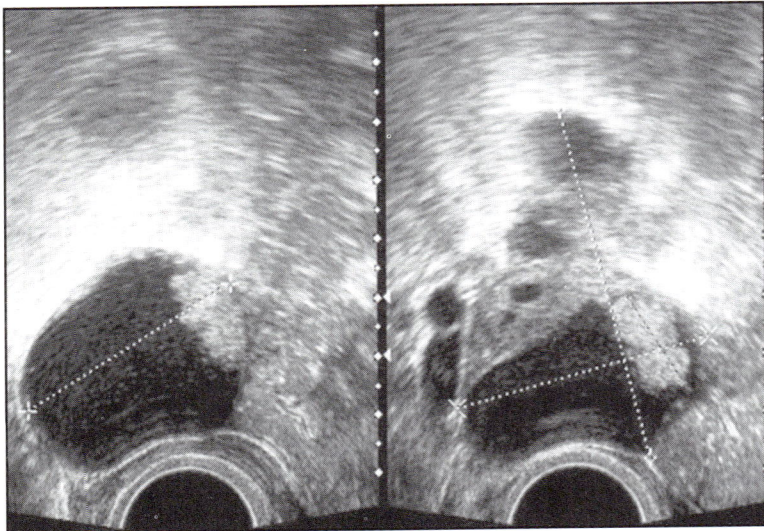

Fig. 21.77: Transvaginal sonogram showing a 46 mm intraovarian cyst containing papillae

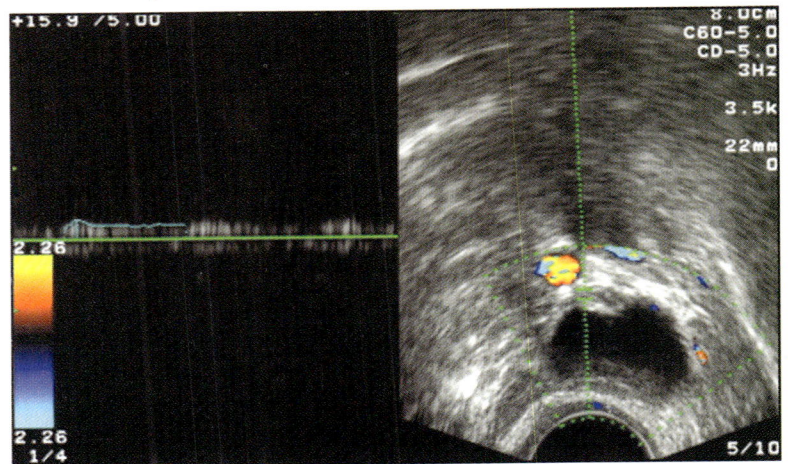

Fig. 21.78: The same case as in Figure 21.77: Color Doppler shows neovascularization into the papillae

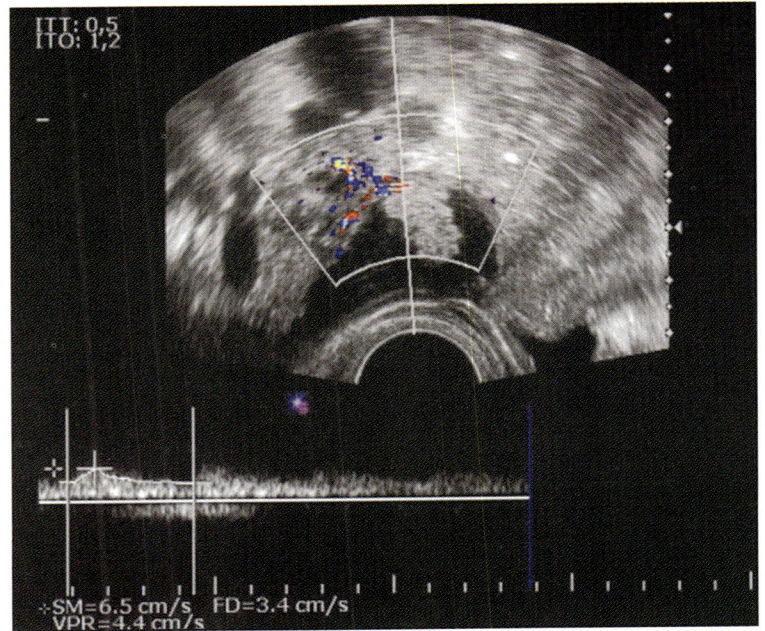

Fig. 21.79: The same cases of Figures 21.77 and 21.78. Pulsed Doppler showing low resistance (RI = 0.48). Histopathologic examination revealed a borderline cystic tumor

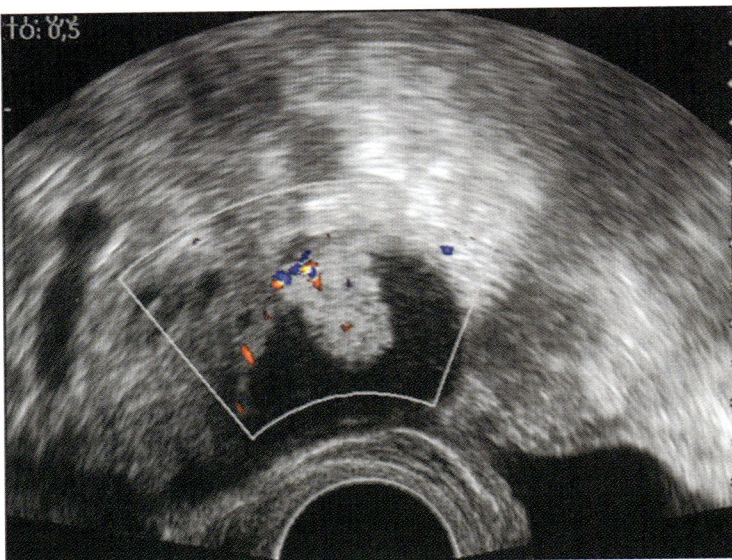

Fig. 21.80: Transvaginal color Doppler duplex sonogram of lesion with papillae. Pulsed Doppler shows vascularization in the capsule a low resistance (RI = 0.44). Histopathology reveals a corpus albicans

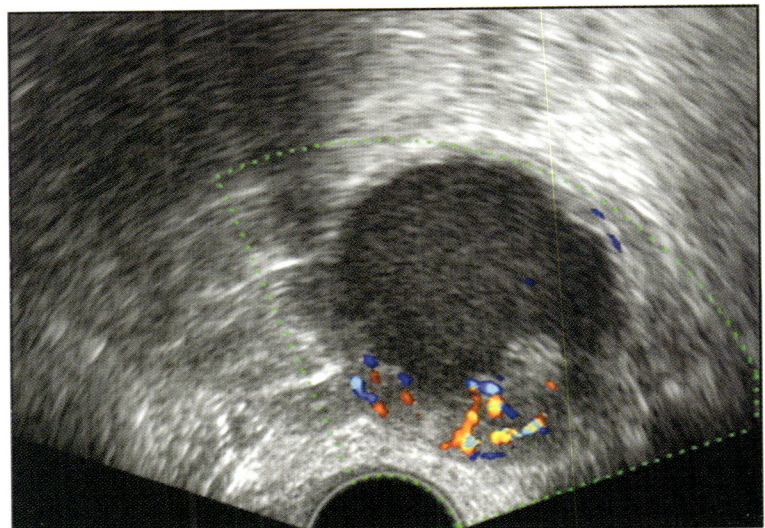

Fig. 21.81: Doppler color transvaginal sonography of a cystic mass containing papillae. Color Doppler shows neovascularization into the papillae. This was a papillary serous cystoadenocarcinoma

the papillae, within the septa and in the solid part of an ovarian mass. Although the main characteristics of the malignant ovarian tumor are high velocity and low vascular resistance due to

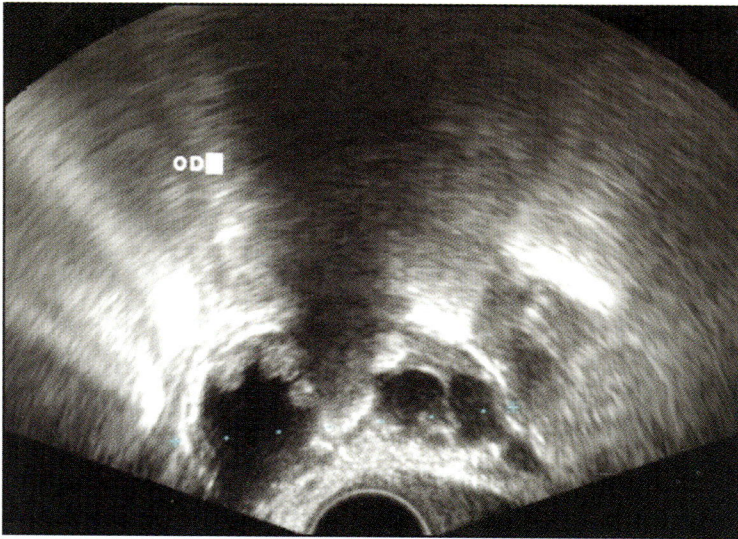

Fig. 21.82: Malignant tumor of the right ovary appearing as a complex mass, more than 80 percent was solid tumor

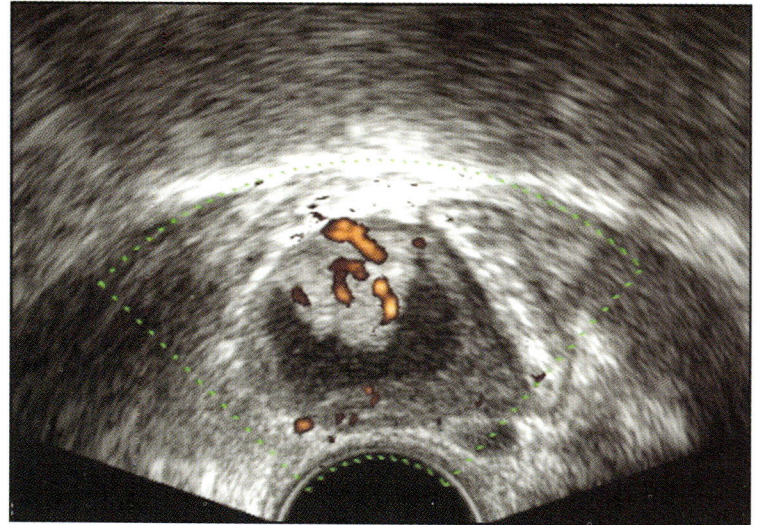

Fig. 21.85: Ovary normal sized, with a small cysts with papillae. Power Doppler shows vessels penetrating into the papilla

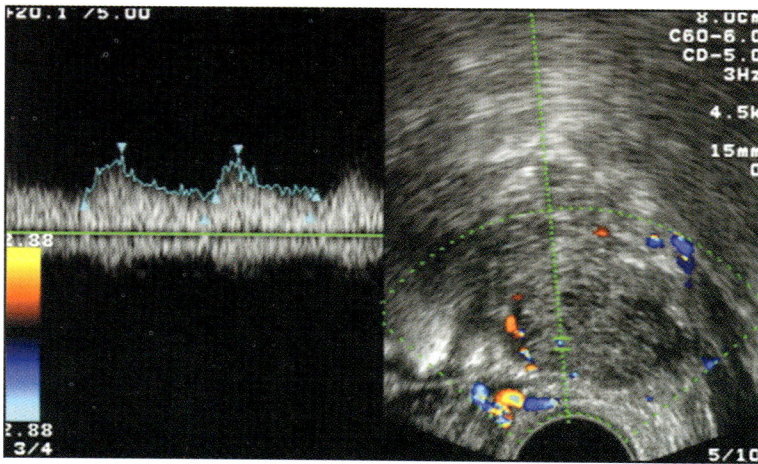

Fig. 21.83: The same case of Figure 21.82 in other part of the tumor shows low resistance (RI = 0.43). Histology reveals a malignant tumor

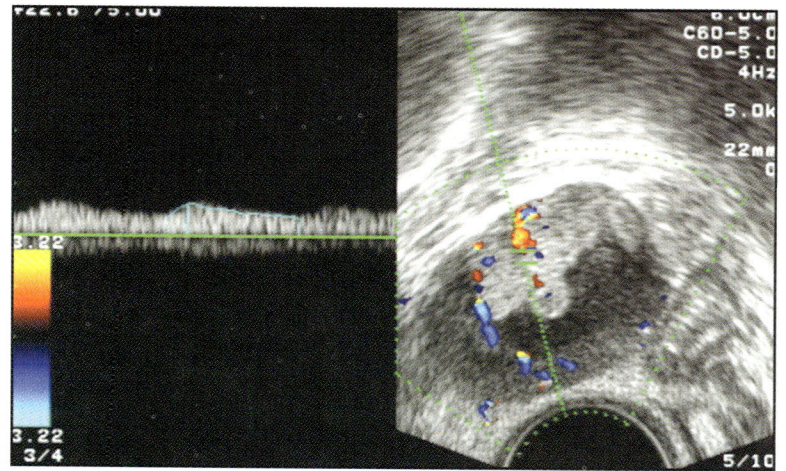

Fig. 21.86: The same case of Figure 21.85: Pulsed Doppler shows neovascularization with low resistance (RI = 0.42). Early-stage ovarian carcinoma was confirmed by histopathology

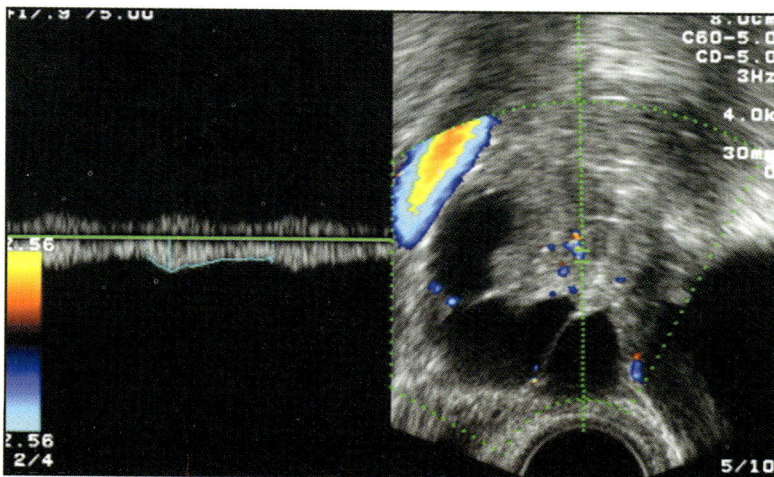

Fig. 21.84: Solid cystic adnexal mass with marked heterogeneous pattern. Color Doppler demonstrating neovascularization with low resistance (RI = 0.46). Histopathology confirmed the malignancy

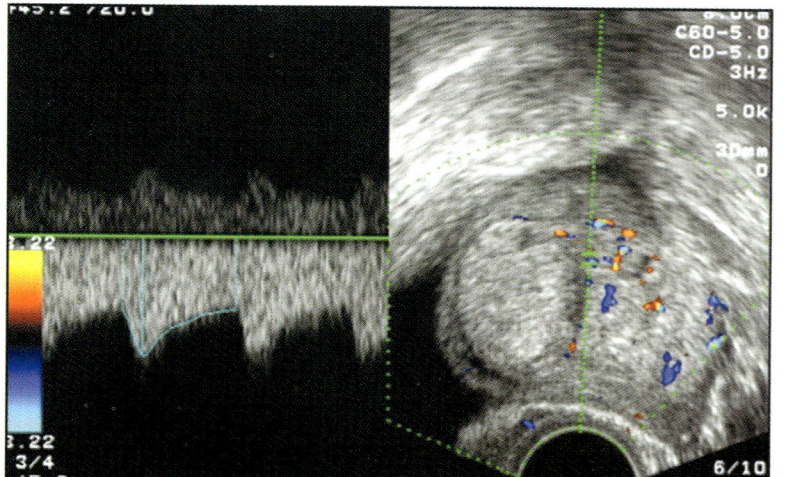

Fig. 21.87: Transvaginal sonogram of a complex solid adnexal mass. Randomly dispersed vessels are clearly visualizad using color Doppler imaging and the low vascular resistance (RI = 0.40) is observed, indicative of neovascularization. The malignant nature of the tumor was confirmed by histopathology

neovascularization, a large scale of blood flow resistance, from very low to moderate and high, can be found. This fact emphasizes the importance of recognizing tumor neovascularization as a pathognomonic finding of malignant lesions by means of color and pulsed Doppler assessment.

RECENT ADVANCES

Sonography is the diagnostic method of choice for evaluation of pelvic masses, particularly for those thought, on basis of

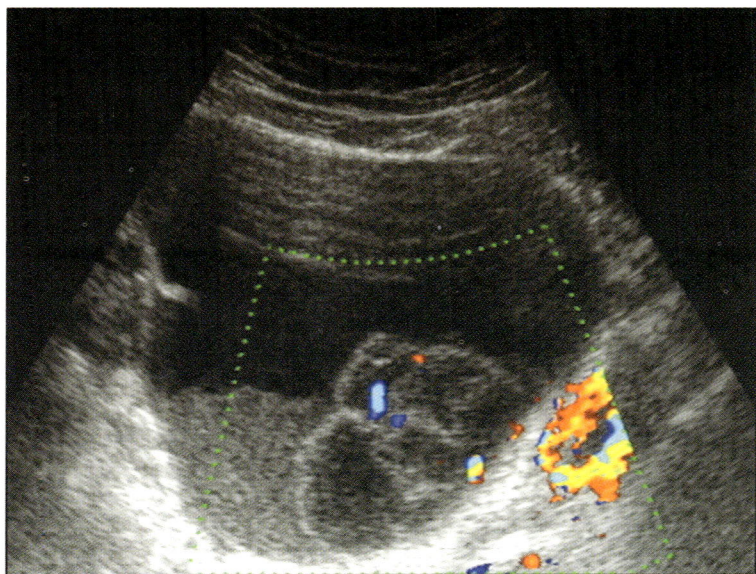

Fig. 21.88: Complex ovarian mass with thick septa and diffuse echoes, these type of septas are common in mucinous cyst

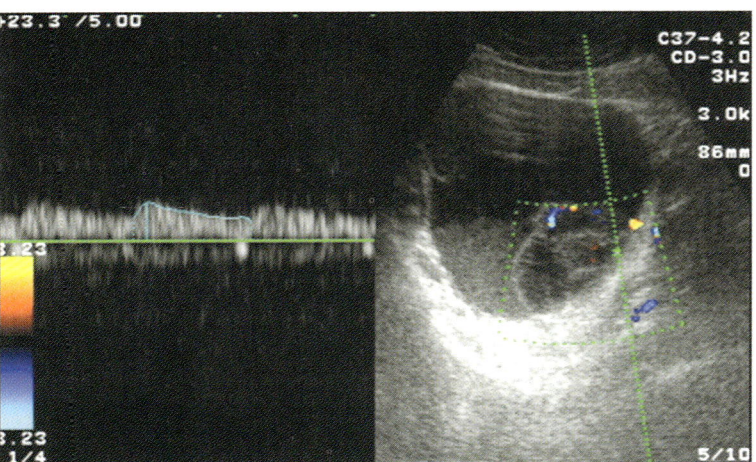

Fig. 21.91: Thick vascularized septa in a noncomplicated cyst. The pulsed Doppler shows low resistance (RI = 0.44). Histopathology revealed a cystoadenocarcinoma

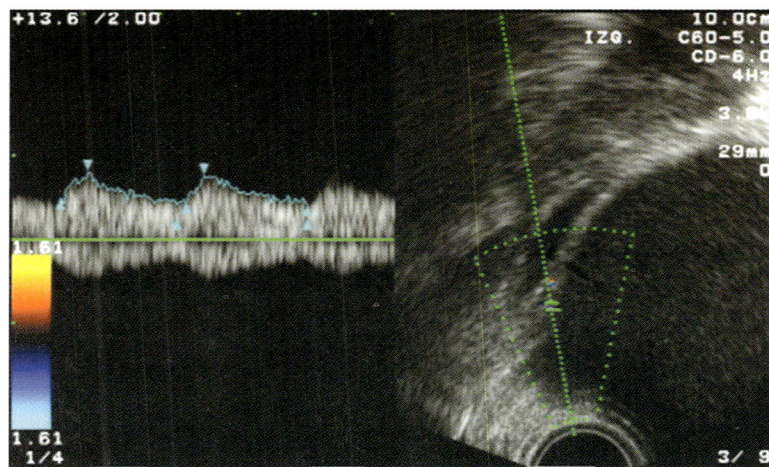

Fig. 21.89: The same case of Figure 21.89. Pulsed color Doppler shows low resistance (RI = 0.48). The histopathology reveals a mucinous cistoadenocarcinoma

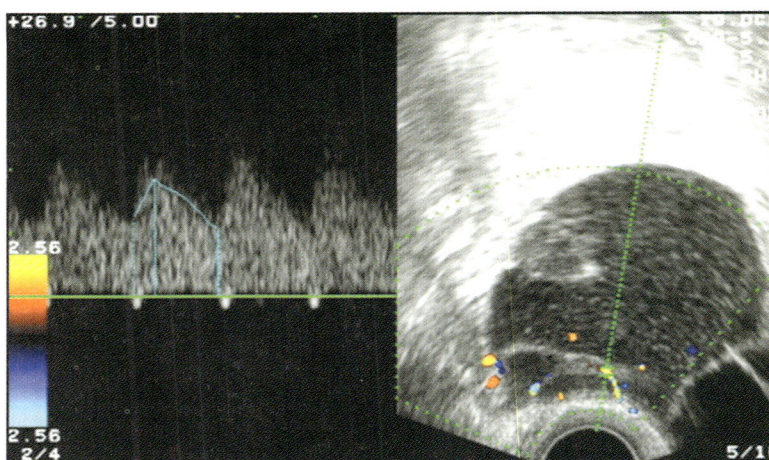

Fig. 21.92: Complex adnexal mass with thick septa. Low vascular resistance (RI = 0.43) in the thick septum indicates ovarian malignancy, which was confirmed by histopathology

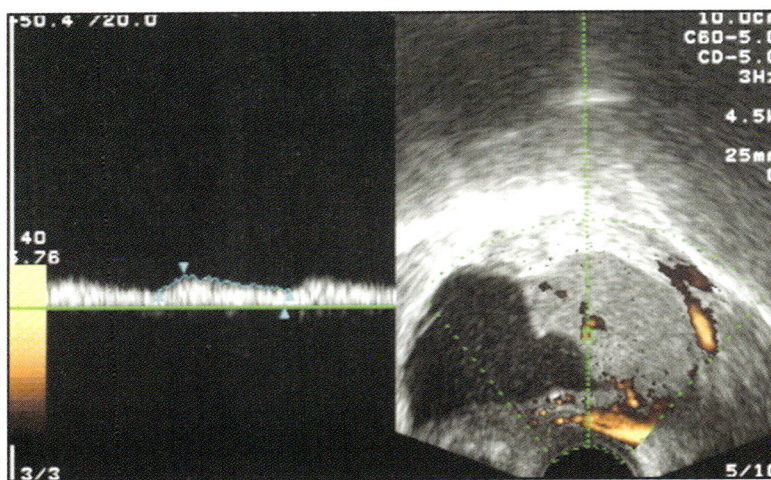

Fig. 21.90: Complex mass with extensive solid component. Power Doppler demonstrating extensive areas neovascularized, and low resistance (RI = 0.43) raises a suspicion of ovarian malignancy. Carcinoma was confirmed by histopathology

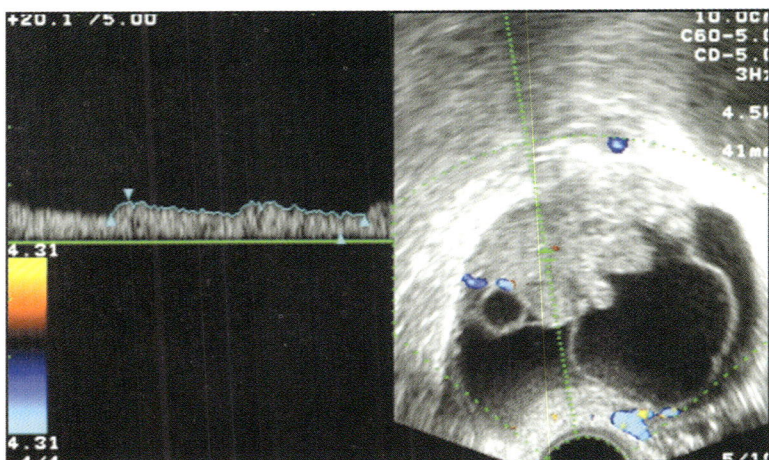

Fig. 21.93: Complex adnexal mass with solid component involving more than a half of the lesional area. Low resistance (RI = 0.33) are detected within the central part of the tumor. Malignant ovarian tumor was confirmed by histopathology

histopathologic diagnosis, sonography usually provides clinically important parameters for the pelvic mass.[1]

A number of studies proved superiority of the transvaginal approach to transabdominal ultrasonography.[2-4] The resolution clinical exam, to be benign. Although the sonographic features of a pelvic mass frequently do not permit a specific

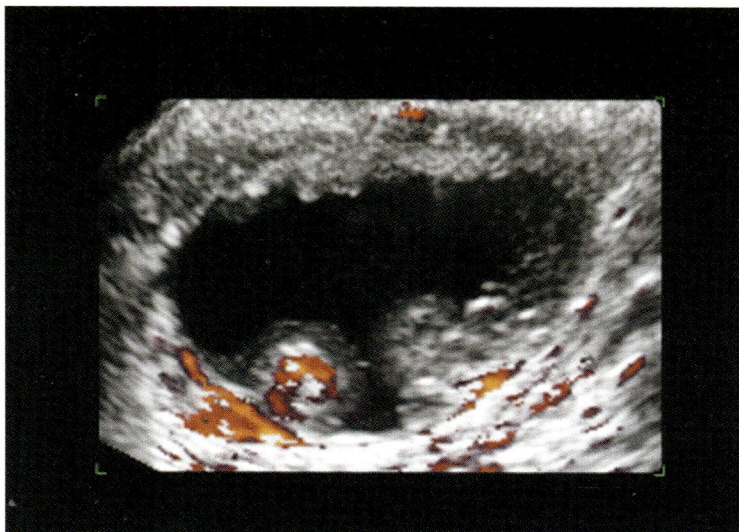

Fig. 21.94: Three-dimensional ultrasound shows a cysts with papillae. Power Doppler demonstrating vascularization in papilla's core

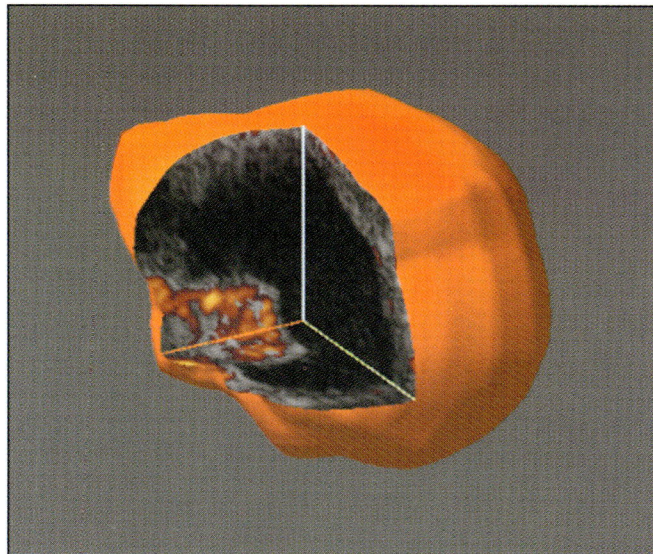

Fig. 21.96: Reformatted section shows ("vocal" imaging) a papillar structures into the lumen of the cyst by power Doppler. We can see clearly the neovascularization within the papilla

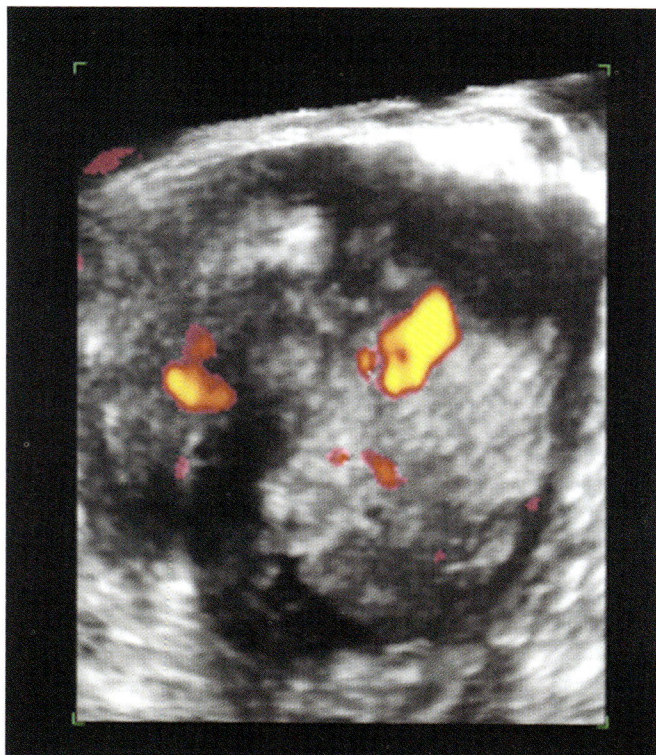

Fig. 21.95: Three-dimensional ultrasound showing a malignant tumor. Sacular vessels are clearly depicted

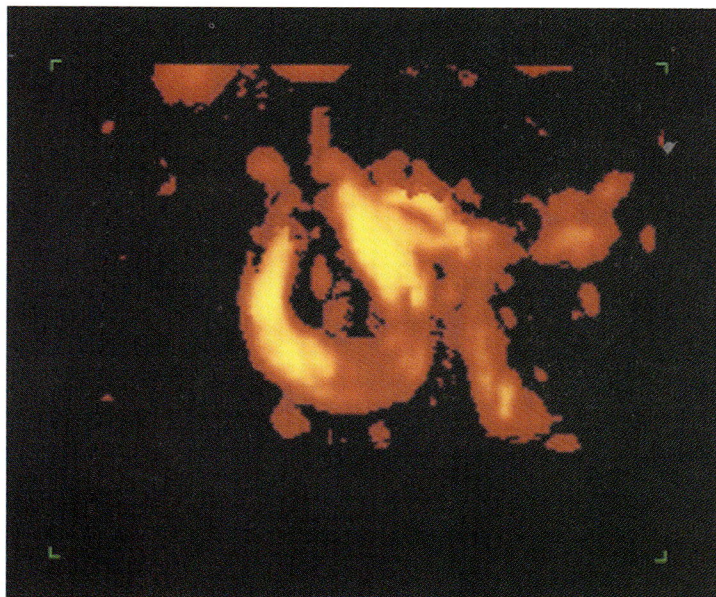

Fig. 21.97: Three-dimensional power Doppler scan of an ovarian carcinoma. Malignant neovascularization arises from vessels. Note irregular, thorn-like vessels, shunting and tumoral lakes, all suggestive of ovarian malignancy

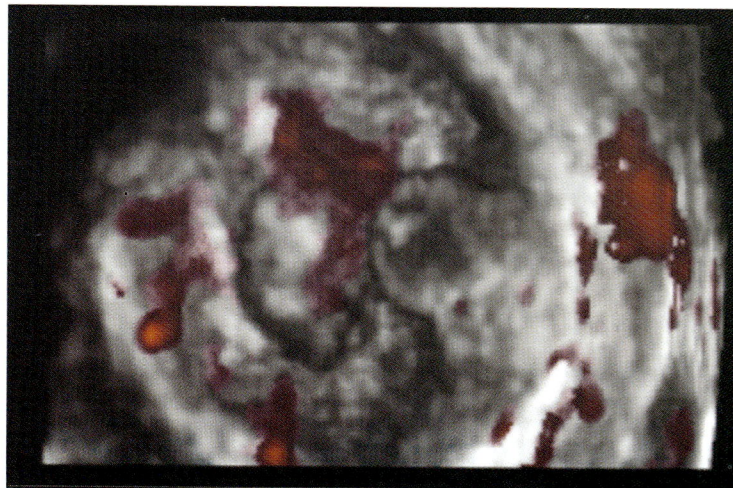

Fig. 21.98: Three-dimensional scan (render mode) showing a papillae protruding within the cyst cavity with neovascularization

as well as the specificity of information about sonographic findings of specific diseases depend on the proximity at which the transvaginal probe can be placed to the pelvic contents, as well as the transducer frequencies used (optimally >5 MHz).

Information gained by tranavaginal gray scale sonography, taken into account with other diagnostic modalities, is useful in guiding the gynecologic surgeon through decisions regarding surgical intervention (Table 21.1). Generally, the consensus is that a surgical treatment is required in cases when masses that are over 10 cm in average dimension, contain irregular solid components, or are associated with significant (over 20 ml) of intraperitoneal fluid.[5] Similarly, pelvic masses that are associated

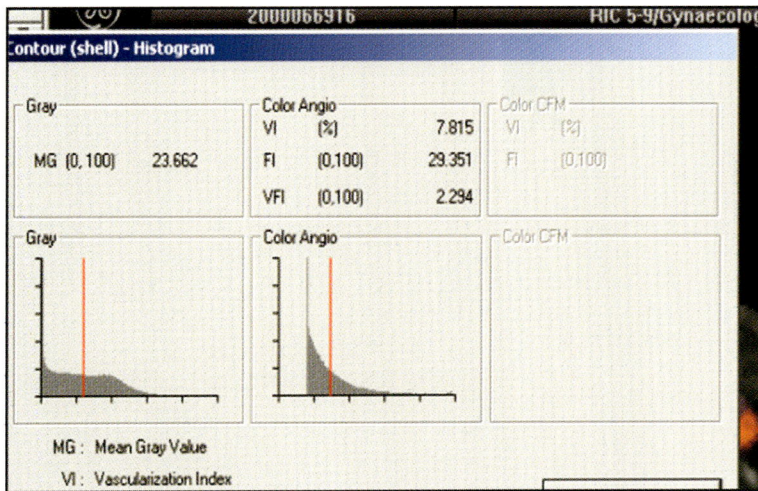

Fig. 21.99: Three-dimensional power Doppler ultrasound permits to calculate with the histogram exactly relation between tissue and vessels

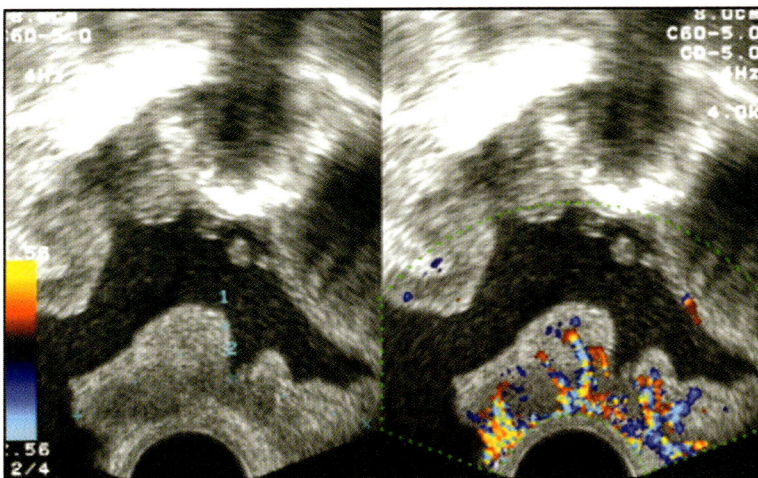

Fig. 21.100: Aditional findings like ascites or implant nodules in the peritoneum, are suggestive of malignancy

with acute pelvic pain may require immediate surgical intervention because they may be associated with adnexal torsion.[6] On the other hand, masses that are completely cystic and smaller than 5 cm may only be observed over a few months with repeated sonograms, to document any change in size. In postmenopausal women, only a low percentage (approximately 3%) of small (less than 5 cm) adnexal masses will represent a malignant neoplasm.[7]

This chapter brings up certain differential points that are clinically important when evaluating a patient with a pelvic mass via transvaginal sonography.

SONOGRAPHIC PARAMETERS

Pelvic sonography has an important role in examining a pelvic mass that may have been palpated or suspected on pelvic examination. It is particularly useful in patients in whom an adequate pelvic examination cannot be performed, or in whom a poorly defined pelvic mass is found on examination.

Table 21.1: Sonographic differential dignoses of pelvic masses[a,b]

Cystic	Complex	Solid
Completely cystic	Predominantly cystic	Ovarian origin
Physiologic ovarian cysts	Cystoadenomas	Fibroma
Cystoadenomas	Tubo-ovarian abscess	Thecoma
Hydrosalpinx	Dermoid cyst	Uterine origin
Endometrioma	Predominantly solid	Pedunculated
Paraovarian cyst	Cystoadenoma (carcinoma)	subserosal fibroid
Hydatid cyst of Morgagni	Germ cell tumor	
Multiple		
Endometriomas		
Multiple follicular cysts		
Septated		
Cystoadenoma (carcinoma):		
- serous		
- mucinous		

(Adapted from Fleischer AC, Manning FA, Jeanty P, Romero R (Eds). Sonography in Obstetrics & Gynecology, 6th ed, New York, McGraw-Hill, 2001, pages 883-912)
[a]Based on most common appearance.
[b]Pelvic masses with a spectrum of sonographic appearances are mentioned in more than one category.

Since some masses may be outside the range of the examiner's finger, sonography may occasionally detect masses that cannot be palpated adequately. In this situation, a realtime sonographic examination during pelvic examination can be used to demonstrate the presence or absence of a mass.[8] Transvaginal sonography can be used to particular advantage in the delineation of the uterus and ovaries in obese patients. In fact, sonography has been found to be more reliable than palpation in the identification of normal-sized ovaries — even in the postmenopausal women.[9]

Origin and Size

Transvaginal sonography can provide detailed delineation of a pelvic mass smaller than 10 cm, and determine its origin.[2,10,11] The uterus serves as a central landmark for identifying the location of a mass within the pelvis. An additional landmark for delineation of its borders is the echogenic endometrial interface within the uterus.[12] Masses within the ovary can usually be identified by the rim of compressed parenchyma ("beak") that is present between the mass and the remaining portion of the ovary. This feature is particularly well depicted with transvaginal scanning.

Abnormally distended tubes originate from the lateral aspect of the uterine "cornu" and their fusiform enlargement as they extend from the uterus into the pelvis. This is particularly helpful when differentiating between inflammatory disease that may involve the tube or ovary, such as a tuboovarian abscess, and simple hydrosalpinx.

Applying gentle pressure between the mass and the uterus may further elucidate the origin of a mass. For example, pedunculated subserosal fibroids are attached to the uterus by a pedicle, in contrast to an adnexal mass, which are separable from the uterus. This serves as a differentiating factor between the two.

Occasionally, the size of a pelvic mass can help in differential diagnosis. Physiologic cysts, for example, are rarely larger than between 3 and 5 cm average dimension, while symptomatic ovarian tumors are generally about 10 cm. Exceptions to this may be encountered in acute hemorrhage or torsion of the ovary, when it can quickly enlarge over 24 to 48 hours. Size alone, however, is not a specific criterion because it depends on when the patient presents for an examination relative to the growth pattern of the mass.

Internal Architecture

In over three-fourths of women studied, transvaginal sonography allows for a detailed delineation of the internal consistency of a pelvic mass, adding diagnostically specific information.[13] The mass that has no internal echoes, has smooth borders, and is enhanced through transmission, can be inferred. Occasionally, low-level echoes may be present within a cyst arising from proteinaceous fluid, blood, or cellular debris. A truly solid mass typically contains internal echoes, whereas a complex mass contains both solid and cystic components.

Generally, ovarian masses are more often cystic, whereas nonovarian masses solid. Thin and echogenic internal septations suggest the diagnosis of an epithelial ovarian neoplasm, usually a cystoadenoma. However, the internal interfaces can also be found in hemorrhagic cysts resulting from partial coagulation of an internal clot. Hyperechoic material within an area can be seen in some dermoid cysts that contain sebaceous material, bone tissue, or teeth. Homogenous echogenic internal contents, such as endometriomas that contain clotted blood, may also be encounterd in a mass. Areas of hemorrhagic necrosis present as irregular anechoic regions within a mass. The more solid and irregular components that are present within a mass suggest it is more likely to be malignant.[5,14] Papillary excrescences also usually mean the possibility of malignancy. Irregularities and disruption in the borders of the mass suggest that malignant spread or rupture through the capsule has occurred.

Associated Lesions

Sonography is very accurate in detecting the amount of intraperitoneal fluid sometimes associated with adnexal masses. Although a small amount (3 to 5 ml) of fluid may be present due to physiologic processes, it is uncommon to have more than 10 ml of fluid in the cul-de-sac or peritoneal cavity of a healthy woman. Intraperitoneal fluid associated with pelvic masses increases the likelihood of a lesion to be neoplastic, and the possibility of malignant spread or rupture. In some cases, such as ovarian torsion, however, the fluid can represent a transudate related to obstructed venous and lymphatic return.[6] Rarely, intraperitoneal fluid can be associated with an ovarian fibroma or other benign adnexal masses.

SONOGRAPHIC DIFFERENTIAL DIAGNOSIS OF PELVIC MASSES

This discussion on the transvaginal sonographic differential diagnoses of pelvic masses is organized according to the most frequently seen sonographic appearance of particular types of a pelvic mass (Table 21.1). If a particular pelvic mass has a spectrum of sonographic appearances, it is mentioned in more than one category.

This differentiating scheme should be used only as a general approach to the sonographic characterization of a pelvic mass. Sonographic findings must be correlated with the clinical ones. The sonographic depiction of morphology is helpful in determining the chance that a mass is malignant. The presences of wall or septal irregularity, or papillary excrescences, correlate with the chance of malignancy.

Cystic Masses

Pelvic masses appearing as cystic adnexal masses on transvaginal sonography most often include physiologic (follicular or luteal) ovarian cysts, hydrosalpinges, endometriomas, and paraovarian cysts. Even with the similar sonographic appearance of several types of cystic adnexal masses, the diagnostic possibilities can usually be narrowed to one or two entities based on clinical presentation and evaluation. In general, most cystic masses that arise within the pelvis are of ovarian origin. Depending on the referral population, physiologic ovarian cysts or hydrosalpinges will be the most common cystic pelvic masses encountered by the sonologist.

Physiologic Ovarian Cysts

Since functional cysts are usually asymptomatic, their precise incidence is unknown. They are most common during the reproductive years, but may occur at any age. Several types of cystic masses can result from abnormalities that occur at different stages of folliculogenesis. In general, follicular cysts occur either due to failure of a mature follicle to rupture at the time of ovulation, or following the collection of blood within the follicle after ovulation occurs (corpus luteum cyst). In most women, a mature follicle average size ranges from 15 to 20 mm.[7,15] Follicular cysts of the ovary are usually larger than a mature follicle, ranging from 3 to 8 cm in size. Luteal cysts, compared to follicular cysts, usually have a thicker wall and tend to contain hemorrhagic areas. Patients with hemorrhagic cysts may experience the abrupt onset of lower abdominal or pelvic pain.[16,17] Because this history can also pertain to cases of ruptured ectopic pregnancy, it is important to obatain an accurate pregnancy test in these patients.

Sonography has an important role in documenting any change in size of the cyst during and after clinical observation or treatment. At transvaginal sonography, a typical follicular cyst is clear, unilocular, and has a smooth, thin wall. A corpus luteum cyst most commonly has a thick hyperechoic, occasionally "crenulated" wall, and usually has echogenic content. The increased echogenicity of the cyst wall is probably the result of its higher fat content.[18] The corpus luteum may appear predominantly solid after complete collapse of the cyst. This appearance may range from an echogenic slit surrounded by a hypoechoic halo to a large, solid mass. These masses tend to be very vascular and show low-impedance flow.

Hemorrhagic ovarian cysts can present as a variety of sonographic findings, depending on the size and organization of internal clot. Because of the presence of hemorrhage, the complicated functional cyst can have an appearance suggestive of that of a malignant tumor.[18] Although fibrinolyzed clot is typically hypoechoic, acute hemorrhage frequently appears as an irregular echogenic area, and may mimic a solid mass. As the clot begins to hemolyze, a reticular network of low-amplitude net-like strands is often demonstrated. Color Doppler can help support the diagnosis of hemorrhage by demonstrating absence of vascularity within solid portions consisting of organized clot.

It is important to point out that 53 to 89 percent of all functional cysts will undergo spontaneous regression; therefore, unless it is clinically unwise to delay surgical exploration (e.g. the presence of a very large mass,[19] a follow-up scan after 4 to 6 weeks is recommended.[20]

Hydrosalpinx/Tubo-ovarian Complex or Abscess

Hydrosalpinges occur as a result of an inflammatory process, which produces adhesions of the fimbriated end of the tube, trapping intraluminal secretions. The secreted fluid distends the tube, resulting in a fusiform anechoic adnexal mass. The tapered fusiform shape and lack of peristalsis of a hydrosalpinx usually allows it to be differentiated from fluid-filled small bowel loops.

In addition, the typical configuration of a hydrosalpinx (tapering as it enters the uterus and enlarging distally) is helpful in its sonographic recognition.

A tubo-ovarian complex may arise if the inflammatory process involves the ovary, almost always secondary to salpingitis caused by pelvic inflammatory disease of bacterial origin.[21] It usually appears as a unilateral inflammatory conglomerate within which the ovary and tube are still recognizable. This may or may not progress to a tubo-ovarian abscess, in which there is a total breakdown of the adnexal structures on one or both sides.[22] With resolution, the only sequelae may be tubo-ovarian fibrous adhesions, but a healed abscess occasionally becomes a tubo-ovarian cyst, which may ultrasonographically resemble a cystic ovarian neoplasm. The typical symptoms are abdominal or pelvic pain and, less consistently, fever, vaginal discharge or bleeding, and urinary symptoms. A history of pelvic inflammatory disease is present in only one-third to one-half of patients, suggesting common subclinical infections. Sonographic markers for tubal inflammatory disease have been described by Timor-Tritsch et al.[22] The following findings were considered helpful:

- Thickening of the tube wall of 5 mm (100% of acute and 3% of chronic cases)
- "Cogwheel" sign,[23] defined as a sonolucent cogwheel-shaped structure visible in cross-section of a tube with thick walls (86% of acute and 3% of chronic cases)
- Incomplete septa, correlating with folds or kinks in the dilated tube, which may be sonolucent or contain low-level echoes. These were seen in 92 percent of all cases; however, they were not discriminatory between acute and chronic cases
- "Beads-on-a-string" sign, defined as hyperechoic mural nodules, measuring about 2 to 3 mm and seen on the cross-section of a fluid-filled distended structure. This is considred to represent flattened and fibrotic endosalpingeal folds (0% of acute, 57% of chronic cases)
- Tubo-ovarian complex, defined in the setting of pelvic inflammatory disease in which the ovaries and tubes are recognized but the ovary cannot be separated from the tube by pushing with the vaginal probe (36% of acute and 2% of chronic cases)
- Tubo-ovarian abscess, in which an acutely ill patient with marked tenderness at the touch of the ultrasonic probe demonstrates a total breakdown of the normal architecture of one or both adnexa, with formation of a conglomerate mass or fluid collection
- Cul-de-sac fluid (50% of acute and 10% of chronic cases).

Although the true sensitivity and specificity of transvaginal sonography findings are not known, demonstration of sonographic markers as outlined previously, in the appropriate clinical setting, can assist in establishing the correct diagnosis. This will lower the frequency of more invasive diagnostic procedures. In the absence of a clinical history or findings in keeping with pelvic inflammatory disease, differentiation of a tubo-ovarian complex or tubo-ovarian abscess from a neoplastic process may be difficult sonographically.

Endometriosis

Endometriosis is defined as the presence of endometrial tissue outside of the endometrium and myometrium. It can involve a wide variety of locations, most commonly ovaries, uterine ligaments, rectovaginal septum, cul-de-sac, and pelvic peritoneum.[21] The true prevalence of endometriosis is unknown because most cases are asymptomatic. Estimates for the prevalence of the disease in women of reproductive age (80% of patients) range up to 15 percent.[21] Endometriosis has been documented in 15 percent of infertile women.[24]

Typical symptoms attributed to pelvic endometriosis are acquired dysmenorrhea, lower abdominal, pelvic, and back pain, dyspareunia, irregular bleeding, and infertility.[21] The recurrent cyclic menstrual, inflammatory, and fibrotic changes within endometriotic lesions are likely responsible for most of the symptoms, although there is often no direct relationship between the extent of the disease and severity of symptoms.

Endometriotic foci may appear as punctate spots or patches of variable color, with a slightly raised or puckered surface, forming nodules, cysts, or both. In one-third to one-half of cases, ovarian endometriotic cysts are bilateral. They can partially or almost completely replace the normal tissue. The cysts rarely exceed 15 cm in diameter. They are commonly covered by dense fibrous adhesions, which may result in fixation to adjacent structures. The cyst walls are usually thick and fibrotic, with a smooth or shaggy, brown- to yellow-colored lining. The cyst content is typically altered, semifluid, or inspissated, chocolate-colored material.[21]

Transvaginal sonography does not detect endometriotic implants.[25,26] Endometriomas have a variety of appearances, ranging from an anechoic cyst to a cyst containing diffuse low-level echoes with or without solid components to a solid-appearing mass. Kupfer et al[26] described a typical sonographic pattern of a "cystic pelvic mass with homogeneous hypoechoic low-level echoes" in 82 percent of 38 surgically proven endometriomas. Further studies confirmed these findings and showed that transvaginal sonography had a sensitivity of 82.4 to 88.9 percent, with a specificity of 89 to 97.7 percent.[27-31] False-positive diagnoses were mostly hemorrhagic cysts.[27,28]

Although the ultrasonographic findings are sometimes nonspecific, generally, differentiation from functional hemorrhage cysts or other echogenic cysts is possible by demonstrating multiple thick walls, homogeneity of the echogeniccontent, and multiplicity of the lesions.[19,32] In addition, unlike endometriomas, hemorrhagic cysts will usually demonstrate regression over subsequent cycles. Also, the presence of punctate or linear bright echogenic foci in the wall of the cyst favors the diagnosis of an endometrioma.

The use of color velocity imaging, pulsed Doppler,[27] or tumor markers (CA-125, CA 19-9)[30] do not improve the diagnostic accuracy of transvaginal sonography.

Paraovarian Cysts

Adnexal cystic masses that do not arise directly from the ovaries include paraovarian cyst, peritoneal inclusion cyst, and cyst of Morgagni, which arises from the fimbriated end of the tube.

The most common type is the paraovarian cyst, which arises from wolffian duct remnants in the mesovarium. It usually measures 3 to 5 cm, but can be as large as a pelvoabdominal cystoadenoma. Occasionally, these cysts contain hemorrhage, and rarely they can contain internal septations.[33,34] Paraovarian cysts and tumors can usually be distinguished from the ovarian ones by their location. As in ovarian tumors, paraovarian ones that contain solid areas or septation should be considered as potentially malignant.[35].

Complex Masses

Complex masses contain both fluid and solid areas. They can be predominantly cystic, or predominantly solid. Ovarian tumors that contain solid components or irregular septations, e.g. dermoid cysts, and most common surface epithelial-stromal ovarian tumors of a serous, mucinous, and endometrioid subtype, are usually classified into this complex mass category.

Ovarian Dermoid Cyst

Mature cystic teratomas of the ovary, or dermoid cysts, are the most common benign germ cell tumor, and the most common ovarian neoplasm,[36] constituting 5 to 25 percent of all ovarian neoplasms. They occur most commonly during the reproductive years. Unlike other germ cell tumors of the ovary, however, they have a wider age distribution and may be encountered from infancy to old age.[21]

A dermoid cyst is composed of well-differentiated derivatives of the three germ layers: ectoderm, mesoderm, and endoderm, with ectodermal elements predominating. In its pure form it is benign, but a malignant transformation in one of its elements can occur in approximately 2 percent of the cases.

In 8 to 15 percent of the cases, the ovarian dermoid cysts are bilateral, with the possibility of several tumors being present in the same ovary. Grossly, the tumors vary in size from 0.5 cm to more than 40 cm. Approximately 60 percent measure 5 to 10 cm in diameter, and more than 90 percent measure less than 15 cm in diameter. The cut surface of the tumor reveals a cavity filled with fatty material, similar to normal sebum, and hair surrounded by a firm capsule of varying thickness. It is usually unilocular, but may also be multilocular.[21]

Usually a single, but possibly a multiple protuberance (Rokitansky protuberance) arises from the cyst wall and projects into the lumen. The protuberance is most commonly solid (although it can be partly cystic) and consists of a variety of different tissues. The hair present in the tumor arises from this protuberance, and bone or teeth, when present, tend to be located within this area.

Dermoid cysts are often discovered as an incidental finding. When symptomatic, they usually present with abdominal pain, abdominal mass or swelling, and abnormal uterine bleeding.

Sonographic features ascribed to dermoid masses include the presence of regional diffuse bright echoes with or without posterior acoustic shadowing, hyperechoic lines and dots, shadowing echodensity, and a fluid-fluid level.[18,37]

The feature that most commonly defines an ovarian mass as a cystic teratoma is regional diffuse hyperechoic solid components that attenuate the acoustic beam. Two types of tissue can produce this finding: clumps of hair in a cystic cavity or fat in a Rokitansky protuberance.[38] Hyperechoic lines and dots in a dermoid mass are attributed to the presence of hair.[39,40] Regional diffuse bright echoes and hyperechoic lines and dots are highly specific features of ovarian dermoids. Calcified structures, such as bone or teeth, result in shadowing echodensity, which is nonspecific. Fluid-fluid levels are presumably a result of sebum layered on serous fluid.[41]

In an evaluation of 252 adnexal masses, 74 of which were cystic teratomas, the positive predictive value for individual sonographic features associated with dermoid masses was 80 percent for shadowing echodensity, 75 percent for regionally bright echoes, 50 percent for hyperechoic lines and dots, and 20 percent for a fluid-fluid level. Fifty-five (74%) of the dermoids had two or more dermoid features, whereas none of the nondermoid masses had more than one feature, giving a positive predictive value for two or more ultrasonic dermoid features of 100 percent.[37]

Kurjak et al[42] using a morphologic scoring system for dermoid cysts, achieved a sensitivity and specificity of 93.1 and 99.4 percent, respectively, in a study of 887 adnexal masses. When the presence of vascularity was assessed using color Doppler, 72 percent of cystic teratomas were mostly avascular, which, when combined with the scoring system, produced a sensitivity and specificity of 99.02 percent and 99.75 percent, respectively.

Ovarian Tumors Originating from the Surface Epithelium

Surface epithelial-stromal ovarian tumors account for about 60 percent of all ovarian neoplasms, and 80 to 90 percent of primary ovarian malignancies. Three broad epithelial categories, on the basis of epithelial differentiation, predominantly occur in this group: serous, mucinous, and endometroid, with frequencies of 46 percent, 36.5 percent, and 7.5 percent, respectively.

The spectrum of proliferative change these tumors exhibit is divided arbitrarily into three categories: benign, atypically proliferating ("of low malignant potential", "borderline"), and malignant. The intermediate group of atypically proliferating tumors is defined as exhibiting greater cellular proliferation than that encountered in the benign form of the same type of tumor but showing no destructive invasion of the stromal component.[21,43]

The mean age of patients with benign epithelial tumors is 45 years, and 50 years for those with atypically proliferating neoplasms. Invasive epithelial tumors are uncommon before 40 years of age. These tumors do not produce specific symptoms (Table 21.2).

Serous tumors. Benign serous tumors are common, accounting for about one-quarter of all benign ovarian neoplasms, and 50-70 percent of all ovarian serous tumors. Although reported at all ages, they show a peak incidence in the fourth and fifth decade of life.[21]

Between 10 and 15 percent of ovarian serous tumors are categorized as atypically proliferating serous tumors. Their peak incidence is between 45 and 50 years of age.[21] Malignant serous tumors account for approximately 40 to 50 percent of malignant ovarian neoplasms. They occur most frequently between 45 and 65 years of age, and in 80 to 85 percent of the cases they are widely disseminated at diagnosis.[21] Between 12 and 20 percent of the benign serous tumors are bilateral (more often in the elderly women), while about 66 percent of malignant serous tumors are bilateral.[21]

Variations in gross appearances of benign serous tumors are due to the relative prominence in a given lesion between the three growth patterns: cystic, papillary, and adenofibromatous.

Table 21.2: Preoperative investigation and malignancy risk assessment in the diagnosis of ovarian tumors

Standard investigation	Risk for malignancy	Advanced investigation
Anamnesis		
• reproductive data (parity,abortions), menstrual history, oral contraceptive use, infertility treatment, hormonal replacement therapy, earlier operations (ovary)		
Age		
• premenopausal	Low	
• postmenopausal	High	
Family history of ovarian and/or breast cancer		
• negative	Low	Genetic counseling
• positive	High	
Symptoms (if occur)		
• abdominal distention, fullness or pressure in the abdomen or pelvis, abdominal or lower back pain, frequent urination or urgency,constipation, lack of energy, lack of appetite, weight loss	High	Exclude an extraovarian abdominal disease (X-rays, CT, MRI)
Bimanual palpation		
• smooth, round, mobile, unilateral, < 10 cm	Low	
• uneven, non-mobile, bilateral, hard, with adhesions, > 10 cm	High	
Transvaginal gray scale sonography		
Volume		
• < 20 cm^3 – premenopausal < 10 cm^3 – postmenopausal	Low	*Calculating ovarian volume* Three-dimensional sonography
• > 20 cm^3 – premenopausal > 10 cm^3 – postmenopausal	High	In comparison to 2D US superior in: - showing characteristics of internal cyst walls - identifying the extent of capsular infiltration
Morphology		
• smooth cystic wall, thin septa, no solid parts, anechoic	Low	of tumors
• intracystic growth, papillary projections, thick septa, solid parts, mixed echogenicity	High	
Transvaginal color/power Doppler		
Blood flow parameters		
• PI > 1.0, RI > 0.42	Low	Three-dimensional power Doppler
• PI < 1.0, RI = 0.42	High	Qualitative analysis of tumor blood vessels:
Location of blood flow		
• peripheral	Low	- position
• central	High	- structure - branching pattern
Tumor markers		
• CA 125 < 35 U/ml	Low	Second generation CA 125, CA 15-3, CA 19-9
• CA 125 = 35 U/ml	High	

Most cystic tumors are unilocular, but multilocular forms occur and vary in size up to 30 cm diameter. The cysts are usually filled with serous fluid. The linings of the cysts are either entirely flat or have focal, grossly visible, coarse papillary projections. Such papillary excrescences rarely cover the entire inner surface of the benign serous cysts. The third (adenofibromatous) variant is a solid neoplasm.[21]

Atypically proliferating serous tumors have gross features similar to those of benign serous tumors, but tend to have finer, more friable and exuberant papillary projections.[21] Well-differentiated carcinomas are mostly cystic, multilocular tumors with soft, friable papillae, partly or mostly filling the cavities, and containing usually turbid or bloody fluid. External surfaces may be smooth or bosselated, and sometimes include surface papillae. Tumor adhesions to surrounding organs are common.[21]

Psamomatous calcifications are present in 15 percent of benign tumors and 60 percent of malignant tumors, and may occasionally be very prominent, producing macroscopic calcification.[21]

Sonographically, benign serous cystoadenomas appear as sharply marginated, anechoic masses that may be large and are usually unilocular. Internal thin-walled septations and, occasionally, papillary projections may be seen, the later often more florid in borderline tumors.[21]

Serous cystoadenocarcinomas are usually multilocular, containing multiple papillary projections and septations; echogenic material is occasionally present within loculi. Cystoadenofibroma tends to have a solid component and is the most likely to mimic a malignant lesion. Ascites is common in serous cystoadenocarcinomas but quite uncommon in cystadenomas.[44]

Mucinous tumors. Benign mucinous cysts and cystadenomas comprise 20 to 25 percent of all benign ovarian neoplasms, and 75 to 85 percent of all ovarian mucinous tumors. They occur most often during the third to fifth decade of life, and are bilateral in only about 2 to 3 percent of the cases.[21]

Atypically proliferating mucinous tumors comprise 14 percent of all mucinous tumors. They have peak prevalence in women in the 30s, and are bilateral in 6 to 8 percent of tumors with intestinal-type epithelium, and 40 percent of tumors with endocervical-like epithelium.[21]

Malignant mucinous tumors comprise 5 to 10 percent of malignant primary ovarian neoplasms and a similar percentage of all ovarian mucinous tumors. They occur most commonly between the fourth and the seventh decades of life. Although in 15 to 20 percent of the cases they are bilateral, only 5 percent show extension beyond the ovaries at the time of laparotomy.[21]

Grossly, benign mucinous tumors and atypical proliferating mucinous tumors are typically multiloculated, cystic tumors measuring up to 50 cm in diameter. The serosal surface of the usually thick outer wall is smooth and opaque. The cysts contain a thick, tenacious mucinous material, occasionally somewhat more watery in consistency. Loculi are usually small and multiple, but tumors may be parvilocular or even a large simple cyst. The frank mucinous carcinomas tend to be cystic, multiloculated neoplasms, usually measuring 15 to 30 cm in diameter.

Sonographically, mucinous cystoadenomas have thicker and more numerous septations and frequently contain fine, gravity-dependent echoes produced by the thick contents.[45] The presence of debris may cause them to mimic solid components; however, gentle tapping on the cyst wall with the probe may result in movement, confirming the diagnosis of a pseudomass.

Mucinous cystadenocarcinomas usually appear as large multiloculated cystic lesions containing echogenic material and papillary excrescences. They have papillary projections less frequently than the serous type.[44]

Endometrioid tumors. Approximately 80 percent of ovarian endometrioid tumors are malignant. Endometrioid carcinomas are the second most frequently encountered malignant ovarian epithelial tumor, accounting for 20 to 25 percent of all ovarian carcinomas. They are bilateral in 28 percent of cases, and occur most frequently in the fifth and sixth decade of life. About 20 to 25 percent of these carcinomas are associated with a histologically similar lesion of the endometrium. Endometrioid carcinoma accounts for 70 percent of the tumors arising from endometriosis. Direct origin of endometrioid carcinoma from endometriotic tissue has been reported in up to 24 percent of the cases in some series.[21]

Grossly, endometrioid carcinomas are primarily cystic, most measuring 12 to 20 cm in diameter. On section, cysts contain friable, soft masses or papillae, as well as bloodstained fluid. Less commonly, neoplasms are solid, with widespread necrosis and hemorrhage.[21]

Ovarian endometrioid tumors are defined by "the presence of epithelial elements, stromal elements, or a combination of the two, that resemble closely the components of typical tumors of the endometrium".[21] Endometrioid ovarian carcinomas generally are regarded as having an overall better prognosis than either serous or mucinous carcinomas.[21]

Sonographically, endometrioid tumors usually present as a cystic mass containing papillary projections, although in some cases they are a predominantly solid mass.[46]

Solid Masses

Sex cord-stromal ovarian tumors (i.e, fibromas, thecomas, granulosa cell, and Sertoli-Leydig cell tumors) account for approximately 8 percent of all ovarian tumors. They are mostly solid; fibromas account for approximately one-half of cases, thus representing the most common ovarian lesion to appear on transvaginal sonography as a solid mass.

Fibroma

Fibromas account for 4 percent of all ovarian tumors. They occur at all ages but are most frequent in middle aged women (mean, 48 years).[21] Ovarian fibromas may also be part of basal cell nevus syndrome, a hereditary disease, when they are typically bilateral, multinodular, and calcified. Meigs' syndrome (ascites and pleural effusion accompanying a fibrous ovarian tumor, usually a fibroma, and disappearing after the removal of the tumor) complicates about 1 percent of ovarian fibromas. Ascites alone is present 10 to 15 percent of ovarian fibromas larger than 10 cm in diameter.[21]

Fibromas range in size from microscopic to very large. Sectioning typically reveals hard, flat, chalky-white surfaces that have a whorled appearance. Focal or diffuse calcification and bilaterality are each observed in fewer than 10 percent of the cases. Microscopy reveals intersecting bundles of spindle cells producing collagen. The absence of fat differentiates a fibroma from a thecoma. Differentiation from a fibrosed thecoma, however, is not always possible.[21]

Sonographically, two typical appearances have been described. The first has fetures similar to that of a uterine fibroid, with variable attenuation and multiple-edge shadows, occurring because of the whorl gross appearance of these tumors. This type of fibroma may be difficult to differentiate from a pedunculated fibroid if it completely replaces normal ovarian tissue and reaches large dimensions.[19] The second appearance is that of a hypoechoic mass with substantial attenuation.[19,47] Atypically, fibromas may be hyperechoic or may demonstrate a mixed heterogeneous pattern. Calcification may be identified.[48]

EVALUATION OF AN OVARIAN MASS

During preoperative evaluation of an ovarian mass, transvaginal gray scale sonography is a "golden standard" for sonographic orientation in a female pelvis, localization of suspected ovarian lesion, and collecting of basic morphologic findings (Table 21.3). Further blood flow analysis obtained by transvaginal color Doppler provide clinically useful information about ovarian tumor nature. Recent technological advances such as 3D volume acquisition and 3D power Doppler imaging have an important role in accurate diagnosis of ovarian cancer, and especially in the early identification of abnormal ovarian vascularity and architecture (Table 21.3).

Table 21.3: Two- and three-dimensional sonographic and Doppler criteria for diagnosis of the ovarian malignancy

Diagnostic criteria		2D	3D
Volume			
Premenopausal	< 20 cm^3	0	0
	> 20 cm^3	2	2
Postmenopausal	< 10 cm^3	0	0
	> 10 cm^3	2	2
Cyst wall	smooth < 3 mm	0	0
thickness/structure	smooth > 3 mm	1	1
	papillarities < 3 mm	1	1
	papillarities > 3 mm	2	2
Shadowing	present	0	0
	absent	1	1
Septa	no septa	0	0
	thin septa < 3 mm	1	1
	thick septa > 3 mm	2	2
Solid parts	solid area < 1 cm	1	1
	solid area > 1 cm	2	2
Echogenicity	sonolucency/low level echo	0	0
	mixed/high level echo	2	2
Relationship with	normal	–	0
surrounding structures (3D)	disturbed	–	1
Tumoral blood flow (2D)	RI > 0.42	0	–
	RI ≤ 0.42	2	–
Vessels¢ architecture (3D)	linear	–	0
	chaotic	–	2
Branching pattern (3D)	simple	–	0
	complex	–	2

Total score (2D) = sum of individual scores. Cut-off score greater or equal to 4 for morphology index and greater or equal to 6 for combined (2D morphology and color Doppler score) index was associated with high risk of ovarian malignancy.
Total score (3D) = sum of individual scores. Cut-off score greater or equal to 5 for morphology index and greater or equal to 7 for combined (3D morphology and power Doppler score) index was associated with high risk of ovarian malignancy.

Morphologic Assessment

Transvaginal gray scale sonography plays an important role in the assessment of adnexal masses; however, the significant number of false-positive results produced limits the accuracy of the technique. Ultrasonic signs of malignant ovarian tumors include multilocular or multiple cysts, thick or irregular septa or walls, poorly defined borders, papillary projections, solid components, and echogenic elements.[49,50] In an attempt to improve specificity, different morphologic criteria, many of which are given a numeric value to produce a summated score,

have been examined.[45-53] Depending on the value of the score, investigators hope to distinguish between benign and malignant masses using a cutoff value.

In a prospective comparison of four previously published morphologic scoring systems and a new "multicenter score", Ferrazzi et al[54] demonstrated a significant improvement in diagnostic accuracy with the multicenter system. This was accounted for mainly by the introduction of two criteria that allowed correction for typical dermoids and endohemorrhagic corpora lutea. Even so, although the scores were sensitive, they were not specific, with the best diagnostic accuracy of 72 percent obtained with a sensitivity of 87 percent and specificity of 67 percent. By lowering the cut-off score by 1 point from 9 to 8, a sensitivity of 93 percent was achieved; the specificity fell to 56 percent.

Several investigators examined adnexal masses with three-dimensional ultrasound (3D US) and found the simultaneous, multiplanar display of perpendicular planes advantageous for examining the structure of masses or cystic collections and for assessing papillary projections or irregularities in the walls of otherwise benign appearing cysts. Bonilla-Musoles et al[55] reported on 76 women with ovarian masses studied with both 2D US and 3D US and found that 3D US was superior in (i) evaluating for papillary projections, (ii) showing characteristics of cystic walls, (iii) identifying the extent of capsular infiltration of tumors, and (iv) calculating ovarian volume. In one patient, papillary projections were identified on 3D US that were not seen on 2D US. In a series of 45 patients with ovarian tumors, Weber et al[56] found that it was the multiplanar capability that was the most advantageous in examining these tumors. It was particularly helpful in grading the tumors that were cystic.

Doppler Parameters

Transvaginal color Doppler sonography has been shown to be a clinically useful adjunct to gray scale sonography for the evaluation of patients with pelvic masses.[47,58] Color Doppler evaluation of the presence or absence of flow, the distribution of flow and the flow velocity waveforms seems to be helpful in distinguishing benign from malignant ovarian lesions.

The advantages of color Doppler in evaluation of the adnexal masses were demonstrated and used for the first time in the late 1990s by groups in Zagreb and London.[59,60] The Zagreb group has studied pelvic masses, and observed low impedance intratumoral blood flow (RI < 0.41) in malignant ovarian lesions. Both groups agreed that color Doppler can detect ovarian cancer as early as FIGO stage IA, and can be used as a screening technique for the disease. From those days one, nothing has essentially changed. A lot of research has been done to prove or dispute the use of color Doppler, but the final verdict was never reached.[61-68] It is a fact that a difference in vascularity exists, and blood vessels in malignant adnexal lesions show lower resistance to blood flow than to those in benign adnexal masses.

Tumor blood vessels have a paucity or lack of muscular media of normal vessels and are more distensible. This combined with arteriovenous shunts seen in the tumor vascular network results in low impedance flow. However, because of focal areas of narrowing and dilatation within tumor vessels, focal areas of high systolic velocity can also be found. Another factor that confounds this is the fact that most tumors have areas of variable perfusion. Our study reported on pre-existing vessels with normal wall structure in 60 percent of malignant ovarian tumors.[69] This contributes to uneven tumor blood flow that makes it difficult to generalize a "characteristic" flow of ovarian tumors.[70]

Diagnostic accuracy of values of flow indices in differentiating benign from malignant ovarian lesions has varied considerably, from over 96 percent to less than 40 percent.[71] More than 15 years of experience in multiple centers has shown that overlap in the specific impedance values obtained from vessels surrounding the ovary by color Doppler imaging precludes differentiation of benign versus malignant ovarian masses on the basis of impedance values alone.[72] Other limiting factors for this type of imaging represent slow flow and vessels of small diameter which are barely detectable.[73] Also, part of the problem with this technique is that only those vessels that are depicted can be adequately studied. More specifically, it seems more important to provide information involving the vascular network rather than particular vessels.

A solution to this problem has been offered by the introduction of three-dimensional power Doppler imaging.[74] While 2D color Doppler is useful in detecting vascularized structures, 3D power Doppler is superior in the study of vascular morphology. Microscopically, ovarian tumor vasculature is highly heterogeneous and does not conform to normal vascular organization.[75] In a recently published work, we presented results of 3D power Doppler imaging in the interactive analysis of ovarian tumor microcirculation anatomy; irregular and randomly dispersed vessels with complex branching were suggestive of ovarian malignancy.[76]

One year after, Cohen et al. reported that 3D power Doppler ultrasound improves the diagnostic accuracy for ovarian cancer prediction.[77] In their study, 71 women with a known complex pelvic mass were referred for a preoperative ultrasound evaluation with both 2D gray scale and 3D sonography with power Doppler facilities. They correctly identified all 14 ovarian malignancies (2 FIGO stage I, 2 stage II, 7 stage III, and 3

metastatic colon) by both 2D grays cale and 3D power Doppler imaging (sensitivity of 100%), and moreover, 3D power Doppler significantly improved the specificity, from 54 to 75 percent, as compared with 2D gray scale sonography.

Very recently, retrospective analysis on preoperative sonographic assessment of 43 referred patients with suspected stage I ovarian cancer was published by our group.[78] Despite initial studies reported improved morphological evaluation of ovarian tumors by using 3D sonography alone[55,79] in our analysis 3D sonography reached unsatisfactory detection rate of 74.4 percent, while combined 3D sonography and power Doppler imaging achieved the highest detection rate of 97.7 percent in preoperative sonographic assessment of suspected ovarian lesions ($p \leq 0.002$).

As a result, we proved that 3D sonography with power Doppler facilities allows accurate detection of the earliest appearance of ovarian malignancy, i.e. FIGO stage I ovarian cancer.

PERSISTENT VS. REGRESSING MASSES

In the pre- or perimenopausal women, a follow-up examination may be indicated 6 to 8 weeks after the initial sonographic finding, in those masses thought to be benign, even though some may persist up to 2 to 3 months. About 70 percent of cysts in premenopausal women will demonstrate regression in 2 to 3 months.[80] If regression does not take place, one should consider other etiologies. Acute enlargement can result from intraluminal hemorrhage and/or torsion.

In postmenopausal women there is an increased risk of a pelvic mass malignancy. However, one study showed that up to 15 percent of asymptomatic postmenopausal women had cystic masses up to 3 cm in size.[81] If followed for 6 months, over half regress and approximately one-fourth enlarge, and one-fourth stay the same in size.[82] Clinical judgement in these cases is needed to determine which patients may benefit from surgery, aspiration and cytology, or observation. Serum CA-125 has only a limited role because of its poor sensitivity and specificity. Signs indicating the possibility of malignancy are enlargement, development of irregular solid areas, and ascites.

CONCLUSIONS

Evaluation of adnexal masses is of particular importance in gynecological practice. Two main problems need answers: discrimination of benign and malignant ovarian tumors and choice of the appropriate surgical treatment, if necessary. Because ultrasound depicts the mass, characterization of the mass is typically performed during the same examination. Thus, de facto, ultrasound becomes the main triage method prior treatment. In most institutions, the type of surgery performed (laparotomy vs. laparoscopy) depends on the probability of malignancy. The optimal ultrasound technique and diagnostic criteria to use when characterising a suspected ovarian neoplasm remains controversial.

It is now well established that transvaginal gray scale sonography is accepted as the "golden standard" in the preoperative evaluation of ovarian masses. Papillary formations on the inside of the cyst wall and non-hyperechoic solid components protruding into the cystic cavity are the most important morphologic predictors of a malignant ovarian tumor. Transvaginal color Doppler demonstrates the vascularity of an ovarian mass, revealing the tumor histology and metabolism. Therefore, blood flow data should be considered to indicate the angiogenic intensity of a tumor, rather than indicating malignancy itself. It is a fact that sonographic estimation of ovarian masses should include color Doppler analysis, but there is still no consensus which Doppler parameter and what cut-off value are the most predictive of malignancy. Three-dimensional power Doppler provides a new tool for measuring the quality of tumor vascularity, and its clinical value is being evaluated. Improved detection and classification of ovarian tumor angiogenesis contributes to better diagnostic accuracy and consequently reduction of false-positive findings and invasive procedures, which might lead to a significant reduction of morbidity and mortality from ovarian cancer.

REFERENCES

1. Fleischer AC, James AE Jr, Millis JB, Julian C. Differential diagnosis of pelvic masses by gray scale sonography. AJR Am J Roentgenol 1978; 11: 469-76.
2. Mendelson EB, Bohm-Velez M, Joseph N, Neiman HL. Gynecologic imaging: comparison of transabdominal and transvaginal sonography. Radiology 1988; 166: 321-4.
3. Leibman AJ, Kruse B, McSweeney MB. Transvaginal sonography: comparison with transabdominal sonography in the diagnosis of pelvic masses. AJR Am J Roentgenol 1988; 151: 89-92.
4. Tessler FN, Schiller VL, Perrella RR, Sutherland ML, Grant EG. Transabdominal versus endovaginal pelvic sonography: prospective study. Radiology 1989; 170: 553-6.
5. Moyle JW, Rochester D, Sider L, Shrock K, Krause P. Sonography of ovarian tumors: predictability of tumor type. AJR Am J Roentgenol 1983; 141: 985-91.
6. Warner MA, Fleischer AC, Edell SL, Thieme GA, Bundy AL, Kurtz AB, James AE Jr. Uterine adnexal torsion: sonographic findings. Radiology 1985; 154: 773-5.
7. Fleischer AC, Daniell JF, Rodier J, Lindsay AM, James AE Jr. Sonographic monitoring of ovarian follicular development. J Clin Ultrasound 1981; 9: 275-80.
8. Bluth EI, Ferrari BT, Sullivan MA. Real-time pelvic ultrasonography as an adjunct to digital examination. Radiology 1984; 153: 789-90.
9. Granberg S, Wikland M. A comparison between ultrasound and gynecologic examination for detection of enlarged ovaries in a group of women at risk for ovarian carcinoma. J Ultrasound Med 1988; 7: 59-64.
10. Lande IM, Hill MC, Cosco FE, Kator NN. Adnexal and cul-de-sac abnormalities: transvaginal sonography. Radiology 1988; 166: 325-32.
11. Vilaro MM, Rifkin MD, Pennell RG, Baltarovich OH, Needleman L, Kurtz AB, Goldberg BB. Endovaginal ultrasound: a technique for evaluation of nonfollicular pelvic masses. J Ultrasound Med 1987; 6: 697-701.
12. Callen PW, DeMartini WJ, Filly RA. The central uterine cavity echo: a useful anatomic sign in ultrasonographic evaluation of the female pelvis. Radiology 1979; 131: 187-90.
13. Fleischer AC, Gordon AN, Entman SS. Transabdominal and transvaginal sonography of pelvic masses. Ultrasound Med Biol 1989; 15: 529-33.
14. Meire HB, Farrant P, Guha T. Distinction of benign from malignant ovarian cysts by ultrasound. Br J Obstet Gynaecol 1978; 85: 893-9.
15. Hall DA, Hann LE, Ferrucci JT Jr, Black EB, Braitman BS, Crowley WF, Nikrul N, Kelley JA. Sonographic morphology of the normal menstrual cycle. Radiology 1979; 133: 185-8.
16. Baltarovich OH, Kurtz AB, Pasto ME, Rifkin MD, Needleman L, Goldberg BB. The spectrum of sonographic findings in hemorrhagic ovarian cysts. AJR Am J Roentgenol 1987; 148: 901-5.
17. Reynolds T, Hill MC, Glassman LM. Sonography of hemorrhagic ovarian cysts. J Clin Ultrasound 1986; 14: 449-53.
18. Atri M, Nazarnia S, Bret PM, Aldis AE, Kintzen G, Reinhold C. Endovaginal sonographic appearance of benign ovarian masses. Radiographics 1994; 14: 747-60.
19. Osmers R. Sonographic evaluation of ovarian masses and its therapeutical implications. Ultrasound Obstet Gynecol 1996; 8: 217-22.
20. Pascual MA, Hereter L, Tresserra F, Carreras O, Ubeda A, Dexeus S. Transvaginal sonographic appearance of functional ovarian cysts. Hum Reproduction 1997; 12(6): 1246-9.
21. Kurman RJ (Ed). Blaustein's Pathology of the Female Genital Tract, 4th ed. New York, Springer-Verlag, 1994.
22. Timor-Tritsch IE, Lerner JP, Monteagudo A, Murphy KE, Heller DS. Transvaginal sonographic markers of tubal inflammatory disease. Ultrasound Obstet Gynecol 1998; 12: 56-66.
23. Bellah RD, Rosenberg HK. Transvaginal ultrasound in a children's hospital: is it worthwhile? Pediatr Radiol 1991; 21: 570-4.
24. Strathy JH, Molgaard CA, Coulam CB, Melton LJ 3rd. Endometriosis and infertility: a laparoscopic study of endometriosis among fertile and infertile women. Fertil Steril 1982; 38: 667-72.
25. Friedman H, Vogelzang RL, Mendelson EB, Neiman HL, Cohen M. Endometriosis detection by US with laparoscopic correlation. Radiology 1985; 157: 217-20.
26. Kupfer MC, Schwimer SR, Lebovic J. Transvaginal sonographic appearance of endometriomata: spectrum of findings. J Ultrasound Med 1992; 11: 129-33.
27. Alcazar JL, Laparte C, Jurado M, Lopez-Garcia G. The role of transvaginal ultrasonography combined with color velocity imaging and pulsed Doppler in the diagnosis of endometrioma. Fertil Steril 1997; 67: 487-91.
28. Mais V, Guerriero S, Ajossa S, Angiolucci M, Paoletti AM, Mellis GB. The efficiency of transvaginal ultrasonography in the diagnosis of endometrioma. Fertil Steril 1993; 60: 776-80.
29. Volpi E, De Grandis T, Zuccaro G, La Vista A, Sismondi P. Role of transvaginal sonography in the detection of endometriomata. J Clin Ultrasound 1995; 23: 163-7.
30. Guerriero S, Ajossa S, Paoletti AM, Mais V, Angiolucci M, Mellis GB. Tumor markers and transvaginal ultrasonography in the diagnosis of endometrioma. Obstet Gynecol 1996; 88: 403-7.
31. Guerriero S, Mais V, Ajossa S, Paoletti AM, Angiolucci M, Labate F, Mellis GB. The role of endovaginal ultrasound in differentiating endometriomas from other ovarian cysts. Clin Exp Obstet Gynecol 1995; 22: 20-2.
32. Pascual MA, Tresserra F, Lopez-Marin L, Ubeda A, Grases PJ, Dexeus S. Role of color Doppler ultrasonography in the diagnosis of endometriotic cyst. J Ultrasound Med 2000; 19: 695-9.
33. Alpern MB, Sandler MA, Madrazo BL. Sonographic features of paraovarian cysts and their complications. AJR Am J Roentgenol 1984; 143: 157-60.
34. Athey PA, Cooper NB. Sonographic features of paraovarian cysts. AJR Am J Roentgenol 1985; 144: 83-6.
35. Korbin CD, Brown DL, Welch WR. Paraovarian cystodenomas and cystadenofibromas: sonographic characteristics in 14 cases. Radiology 1998; 208: 459-62.
36. Koonings PP, Campbell K, Mishell DR Jr, Grimes DA. Relative frequency of primary ovarian neoplasms: a 10-year review. Obstet Gynecol 1989; 74: 921-6.
37. Patel MD, Feldstein VA, Lipson SD, Chen DC, Filly RA. Cystic teratomas of the ovary: diagnostic value of sonography. AJR Am J Roentgenol 1998; 171: 1061-5.
38. Quinn SF, Erickson S, Black WC. Cystic ovarian teratomas: the sonographic appearance of the dermoid plug. Radiology 1985; 155: 477-8.
39. Malde HM, Kedar RP, Chadha D, Nayak S. Dermoid mesh: a sonographic sign of ovarian teratoma. AJR Am J Roentgenol 1992; 159: 1349-50.
40. Bronshtein M, Yoffe N, Brandes JM, Blumenfeld Z. Hair as a sonographic marker of ovarian teratomas: improved identification using transvaginal sonography and simulation model. J Clin Ultrasound 1991; 19: 351-5.
41. Sheth S, Fishman EK, Buck JL, Hamper UM, Sanders RC. The variable sonographic appearances of ovarian teratomas: correlation with CT. AJR Am J Roentgenol 1988; 151: 331-4.

42. Kurjak A, Kupesic S, Babic MM, Goldenberg M, Ilijas M, Kosuta D. Preoperative evaluation of cystic teratoma: what does color Doppler add? J Clin Ultrasound 1997; 25: 309-16.

43. Pascual MA, Tresserra F, Grases PJ, Labastida R, Dexeus S. Borderline cystic tumors of the ovary: gray-scale and color Doppler sonographic findings. J Clin Ultrasound 2002; 30(2): 76-82.

44. Sutton CL, McKinney CD, Jones JE, Gay SB. Ovarian masses revisited: radiologic and pathologic correlation. Radiographics 1992; 12: 853-77.

45. Fried AM, Kenney CM 3rd, Stigers KB, Kacki MH, Buckley SL. Benign pelvic masses: sonographic spectrum. Radiographics 1996; 16: 321-34.

46. Wagner BJ, Buck JL, Seidman JD, McCabe KM. From the archives of the AFIP. Ovarian epithelial neoplasms: radiologic-pathologic correlation. Radiographics 1994; 14: 1351-74.

47. Stephenson WM, Laing FC. Sonography of ovarian fibromas. AJR Am J Roentgenol 1985; 144: 1239-40.

48. Athey PA, Malone RS. Sonography of ovarian fibromas/thecomas. J Ultrasound Med 1987; 6: 431-6.

49. Granberg S, Norstrom A, Wikland M. Tumors in the lower pelvis as imaged by vaginal sonography. Gynecol Oncol 1990; 37: 224-9.

50. Rottem S, Levit N, Thaler I, Yoffe N, Bronshtein M, Manor D, Brandes JM. Classification of ovarian lesions by high-frequency transvaginal sonography. J Clin Ultrasound 1990; 18: 359-63.

51. Sassone AM, Timor-Tritsch IE, Artner A, Westhoff C, Warren WB. Transvaginal sonographic characterization of ovarian disease: evaluation of a new scoring system to predict ovarian malignancy. Obstet Gynecol 1991; 78: 70-6.

52. DePriest PD, Shenson D, Fried A, Hunter JE, Andrews SJ, Gallion HH, Pavlik EJ, Kryscio RJ, van Nagell JR Jr. A morphology index based on sonographic findings in ovarian cancer. Gynecol Oncol 1993; 51: 7-11.

53. Lerner JP, Timor-Tritsch IE, Federman A, Abramovich G. Transvaginal ultrasonographic characterization of ovarian masses with an improved, weighted scoring system. Am J Obstet Gynecol 1994; 170: 81-5.

54. Ferrazzi E, Zanetta G, Dordoni D, Berlanda N, Mezzopane R, Lissoni AA, Lissoni G. Transvaginal ultrasonographic characterization of ovarian masses: comparison of five scoring systems in a multicenter study. Ultrasound Obstet Gynecol 1997; 10: 192-7.

55. Bonilla Musoles F, Raga F, Osborne NG. Three-dimensional ultrasound evaluation of ovarian masses. Gynecol Oncol 1995; 59: 129-35.

56. Weber G, Merz E, Bahlmann F, Macchiella D. Ultrasound assessment of ovarian tumors: comparison between transvaginal 3D technique and conventional 2-dimensional vaginal ultrasonography. Ultraschall Med 1997; 18: 26-30.

57. Fleischer AC, Rodgers WH, Kepple DM, Williams LL, Jones HW 3rd, Gross PR. Color Doppler sonography of benign and malignant ovarian masses. Radiographics 1992; 12: 879-85.

58. Kurjak A, Shalan H, Kupesic S, Predanic M, Zalud I, Breyer B, Jukic S. Transvaginal color Doppler sonography in the assessment of pelvic tumor vascularity. Ultrasound Obstet Gynecol 1993; 3: 137-54.

59. Kurjak A, Zalud I, Jurkovic D, Alfirevic Z, Miljan M. Transvaginal color Doppler for the assessment of pelvic circulation. Acta Obstet Gynecol Scand 1989; 68: 131-7.

60. Bourne T, Campbell S, Steer C, Whitehead MI, Collins WP. Transvaginal color flow imaging: a possible new screening technique for ovarian cancer. BMJ 1989; 299: 1367-70.

61. Kurjak A, Zalud I, Alfirevic Z. Evaluation of adnexal masses with transvaginal color ultrasound. J Ultrasound Med 1991; 10: 295-7.

62. Fleisher AC, Rodgers WH, Rao BJ, Keppler DM, Worrel JA, Williams L, Jones HW 3rd. Assessment of ovarian tumor vascularity with transvaginal color Doppler sonography. J Ultrasound Med 1991; 10: 563-8.

63. Weiner Z, Thaler I, Beck D, Rottem S, Deutsch M, Brandes JM. Differentiating malignant from benign ovarian tumors with transvaginal color flow imaging. Obstet Gynecol 1992; 79: 159-62.

64. Kurjak A, Schulman H, Sosic A, Zalud I, Shalan H. Transvaginal ultrasound, color flow, and Doppler waveform of the postmenopausal adnexal mass. Obstet Gynecol 1992; 80: 917-21.

65. Hamper UM, Sheth S, Abbas FM, Rosenshein BN, Aronson D, Kurman JR. Transvaginal color Doppler sonography of adnexal masses: differences in blood flow impedance in benign and malignant lesions. AJR Am J Roentgenol 1993; 160: 1225-8.

66. Carter J, Saltzman A, Hartenbach E, Fowler J, Carlson L, Twiggs LB. Flow characteristics in benign and malignant gynecologic tumors using transvaginal color flow Doppler. Obstet Gynecol 1994; 83: 125-30.

67. Sawicki W, Spiewankiewicz B, Cendrowski K, Stelmachow J. Preoperative discrimination between malignant and benign adnexal masses with transvaginal ultrasonography and colour blood flow imaging. Eur J Gynaecol Oncol 2001; 22: 137-42.

68. Guerriero S, Alcazar JL, Coccia ME, Ajossa S, Scarselli G, Boi M, Gerada M, Mellis GB. Complex pelvic mass as a target of evaluation of vessel distribution by color Doppler sonography for the diagnosis of adnexal malignancies: results of a multicenter European study. J Ultrasound Med 2002; 21: 1105-11.

69. Kurjak A, Jukic S, Kupesic S, Babic D. A combined Doppler and morphopathological study of ovarian tumors. Eur J Obstet Gynecol Reprod Biol 1997; 71: 147-50.

70. Levine D, Feldstein VA, Babcook CJ, Filly RA. Sonography of ovarian masses: poor sensitivity of resistive index for identifying malignant lesions. AJR Am J Roentgenol 1994; 162: 1355-9.

71. Kurjak A, Kupesic S. Transvaginal color Doppler and pelvic tumor angiogenesis: lessons learned and future challenges. Ultrasound Obstet Gynecol 1995; 6: 145-59.

72. Brown DL, Frates MC, Laing FC, DiSalvo DN, Doubilet PM, Benson CB, Waitzkin ED, Muto MG. Ovarian masses: can benign and malignant lesions be differentiated with color and pulsed Doppler US? Radiology 1994; 190: 333-6.

73. Stein SM, Laifer-Narin S, Johnson MB, Roman LD, Muderspach LI, Tyszka JM, Ralls PW. Differentiation of benign and malignant adnexal masses: relative value of gray-scale, color Doppler, and spectral Doppler sonography. AJR Am J Roentgenol 1995; 164: 381-6.

74. Downey BD, Fenster A. Vascular imaging with a three-dimensional power Doppler system. AJR Am J Roentgenol 1995; 165: 665-8.

75. Kurjak A, Kupesic S, Breyer B, Sparac V, Jukic S. The assessment of ovarian tumor angiogenesis: what does three-dimensional power Doppler add? Ultrasound Obstet Gynecol 1998; 12: 136-46.

76. Kurjak A, Kupesic S, Anic T, Kosuta D. Three-dimensional ultrasound and power Doppler improve the diagnosis of ovarian lesions. Gynecol Oncol 2000; 76: 28-32.

77. Cohen LS, Escobar PF, Scharm C, Glimco B, Fishman DA. Three-dimensional power Doppler ultrasound improves the diagnostic accuracy for ovarian cancer prediction. Gynecol Oncol 2001; 82: 40-8.

78. Kurjak A, Kupesic S, Sparac V, Prka M, Bekavac I. The detection of stage I ovarian cancer by three-dimensional sonography and power Doppler. Gynecol Oncol 2003; 90: 258-64.

79. Chan L, Lin WM, Uerpairojkit B, Hartman D, Reece EA, Helm W. Evaluation of adnexal masses using three-dimensional ultrasonographic technology: preliminary report. J Ultrasound Med 1997; 16: 349-54.

80. Pinotti JA, de Franzin CM, Marussi EF, Zeferino LC. Evolution of cystic and adnexal tumors identified by ecography. Int J Gynaecol Obstet 1988; 26: 109-14.

81. Wolf SI, Gosink BB, Feldesman MR, Lin MC, Stuenkel CA, Braly PS, Pretorius DH. Prevalence of simple adnexal cysts in postmenopausal women. Radiology 1991; 180: 65-71.

82. Levine D, Gosink BB, Wolf SI, Feldesman MR, Pretorius DH. Simple adnexal cysts: the natural history in postmenopausal women. Radiology 1992; 184: 653-9.

BIBLIOGRAPHY

1. Alcazar JL, Errasti T, Laparte C, Jurado M, Lopez-Garcia G. Assessment of a new logistic model in the preoperative evaluation of adnexal masses. J Ultrasound Med 2001;20:841-8.

2. Alcazar JL, Galan MJ, Ceamanos C, Garcia-Manero M. Transvaginal gray sale and color Doppler sonography in primary ovarian cancer and metastatic tumors to the ovary. J Ultrasound Med 2003;22:243-7.

3. Alcazar JL, Galan MJ, Garcia-Manero M, Guerriero S. Three-dimensional sonographic morphologic assessment in complex adnexal masses: preliminary experience. J Ultrasound Med 2003;22:249-54.

4. Alcazar JL, Jurado M. Prospective evaluation of a logistic model based on sonographic morphology and color Doppler findings developed to predict adnexal malignancy. J Ultrasound Med 1999;18:837-42.

5. Alcazar JL, Laparte C, Jurado M, Lopez-Garcia G. The role of transvaginal ultrasonography combined with color velocity imaging and pulsed Doppler in the diagnosis of endometrioma. Fertil Steril 1997;67:487-91.

6. Beck RP, Latour JPA. Review of 1019 benign ovarian neoplasms. Obstet Gynecol 1960;16:479-82.

7. Castillo G, Alcazar JL, Jurado M. Natural history of sonographically detected simple unilocular adnexal cysts in asymptomatic postmenopausal women. Obstet Gynecol Surv 2004;59:511-3.

8. Cohen LS, Escobar PF, Scharm C, Glimco B, Fishman DA. Three-dimensional power Doppler ulrasound improves the diagnostic accuracy for ovarian cancer prediction. Gynecol Oncol 2001;82:40-8.

9. D'Arcy TJ, Jayaram V, Lynch M, Soutter WP, Cosrove DO, Harvey CJ, Patel N. Ovarian cancer detected non-invasively by contrast-enhanced power Doppler ultrasound. BJOG 2004;111:619-23.

10. Emoto M, Iwasaki H, Mimura K, Kawarabayashi T, Kikuchi M. Differences in the angiogenesis of benign and malignant ovarian tumors, demonstrated by analyses of color Doppler ultrasound, immunohistochemistry, and microvessel density. Cancer 1997;80:899-907.

11. Fleischer AC, Rodgers WH, Rao BJ, Keppler DM, Worrell JA, Williams L, Jones III HW. Assessment of ovarian tumor vascularity with transvaginal color Doppler sonography. J Ultrasound Med 1991;10:563-8.

12. Fleischer AC, Cullinan JA, Peri CV, Jones III JW. Early detection of ovarian carcinoma with transvaginal color Doppler ultrasound. Am J Obstet Gynecol 1996;174:101-6.

13. Folkman J, Klaysburn M. Angiogenic factors. Science 1987;235:442-7.

14. Folkman J, Watson K, Ingber D, Hanahan D. Induction of angiogenesis during the transition from hyperplasia to neoplasia. Nature 1989;339:58-61.

15. Folkman J. tumor angiogenesis. Adv Cancer Res 1985;48:2641-5.

16. Guerriero S, Alcazar JL. Ajossa S, Lai MP, Errasti T, Mallarini G, Melis GB. Comparison of conventicnal color Doppler imaging and power doppler imaging for the diagnosis of ovarian cancer: results of European study. Gynecol Oncol. 2002;84:299-304.

17. Guerriero S, Alcazar JL, Ajossa S, Lai MP, Errasti T, Mallarini G, Melis GB. Comparison of conventional color Doppler imaging and power Doppler imagng for the diagnosis of ovarian cancer: results of a European study. Gynecol Oncol 2001;83:299-304.

18. Guerriero S, Alcazar JL, Coccia ME, Ajossa S, Scarselli G, Boi M, et al. Complex pelvic mass as a target of evaluation of vessel distribution by color Doppler sonography for the diagnosis of adnexal malignancies: results of a multicenter European study. J Ultrasound Med 2002;21:1105-11.

19. Jain RK. Transport of molecules across tumor vasculature. Cancer Metastasis Rev 1987;6:559-61.

20. Kurjak A, Jukic S, Kupesic S, Babic D. A combined Doppler and morphopathological study of ovarian tumors. Eur J Obstet Gynecol 1997;71:147-50.

21. Kurjak A, Kupesic S, Breyer B, Sparac V, Jukic S. The assessment of ovarian tumor angiogenesis: what does 3D power DOppler add? Ultrasound Obstet Gynecol 1998;12:1-11.

22. Kurjak A, Kupesic S, Sparac V, Kosuta D. Three-dimensional ultrasonographic and power Doppler characterization of ovarian lesions. Ultrasound Obstet Gynecol 2000;16:365-371.

23. Kurjak A, Kupesic S, Sparac V, Prka M, Bekavac I. The detection of stage I ovarian cancer by three-dimensional sonography and power Doppler. Gynecologic Oncology 2003;90:258-64.

24. Kurjak A, Kupesic S, Sparac V, Prka M, Bekavac I. The detection of stage I ovarian cancer by three-dimensional sonograpy and power Doppler. Gynecol Oncol 2003;90:258-64.

25. Kurjak A, Predanic M, Kupesic-Urek S, Jukic S. Transvaginal color and pulsed Doppler assessment of adnexal tumor vascularity. Gynecologic Oncol 1993;50:3-9.

26. Kurjak A, Predanic M. New scoring system for prediction of ovarian malignancy based on transvaginal color Doppler sonography. J Ultrasound Med 1992;11:631-8.

27. Kurjak A, Prka M. New developments in ovarian cancer screening. Ultrasound Rev Obstet Gynecol 2002;2:167-77.

28. Kurjak A, Shalan H, Matijevic R, Predanic M, Kupesic-Urek S. Stage I ovarian cancer by transvaginal color Doppler sonography: a report of 18 cases. Ultrasound Obstet Gynecol 1993;3:195-8.

29. Luxman D, Bergman A, Sagi J, David M. The postmenopausal adnexal mass:correlation between ultrasonic and pathologic findings. Obstet Gynecol 1991;77:726-9.

30. Merce LT, Caballero RA, Barco MJ, Bau S, Lopez G. B-mode, utero-ovarian and intratumoural transvaginal color Doppler ultrasonography for differential diagnosis of ovarian tumours. Eur J Obstet Gynecol Reprod Biol1998;76:97-107.

31. Merce LT, Garces D, Barco MJ, de la Fuente F. Intraovarian Doppler velocimetry in ovulatory, dysovulatory and anovulatory cycles.Ultrasound Obstet Gynecol 1992;2:197-202.

32. Obeidat BR, Amarin ZO, Latimer JA, Crawfrd RA. Risk of malignancy index in the preoperative evaluation of pelvic masses. Int J Gynecol Obstet 2004;85:255-8.

33. Pascual MA, Tresserra F, Grases PJ, Labastida R, Dexeus S. Borderline cystic tumors of the ovary: gray-scale and color Doppler sonographic findings. J Clin Ultrasound 2002;30:76-82.

34. Pascual MA, Tresserra F, Lopez-Marin L, Ubeda A, Grases PJ. Role of color Doppler ultrasonography in the diagnosis of endometriotic cysts. J Ultrasound Med 2000;19:695-9.

35. Prompeler HJ, Sauerbrei WM, Latternann U, Pfleiderer A. Quantitative flow measurements for classification of ovarian tumors by transvaginal color Doppler sonography in postmenopausal patients. Ultrasound Obstet Gynecol 1994;4:406-13.

36. Rottem S, Levit N, Thaler I, Yoffe N, Bronshtein M, Manor D, Brandes JM. Classification of ovarian lesions by high frequency transvaginal sonography. J Clin Ultrasound 1990;18:359-63.

37. Rottem S, Timor-Tritsch IE. Ovarian pathology. In Timor-Tritsch IE, Rottem S (Eds) Transvaginal Sonography, 2nd ed. New York-Amsterdam-London: Elsevier), 1991; pp 145-73

38. Sassone M, Timor-Tritsch I, Artner A, Caroly W, Warren WB. Transvaginal sonographic characterization of ovarian disease: evaluation of new scoring system to predict ovarian malignancy. Obstet Gynecol 1991;78:70-6.

39. Suren A, Osmers R, Kuhn W. 3D color power angio imaging: a new method to assess intracervical vascularization in benign and pathological conditions. Ultrasound Obstet Gynecol 1998;11:133-37.

40. Timmerman D, Valentin L, Bourne T, Collins WP, Verrelst H, Vergote I; International Ovarian Tumor Analysis (IOTA) Group. Terms, definitions and measurements to describe the sonographic feature adnexal tumors: a consensus opinion from the Inernational Ovarian Tumor Analysis (IOTA) Group. Ultrasound Obstet Gynecol

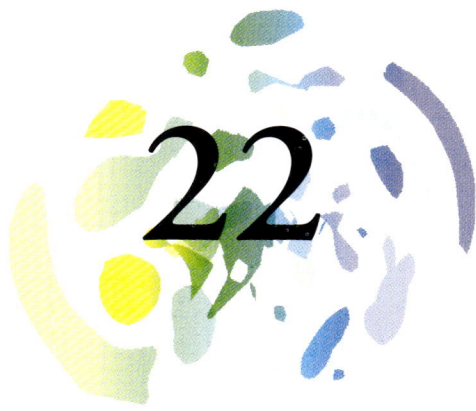

22

Sonographic Imaging in Infertility

S Kupesic

INTRODUCTION

Infertility is defined as the failure to conceive a desired pregnancy after 12 months of unprotected intercourse, and affects 10 percent of married couples. With recent technological development and proper use of medically assisted reproduction techniques, one-half of these couples will become pregnant.

More than any other new method, ultrasound has made significant improvements in the modern management of female infertility. Transvaginal sonography provides the reproductive endocrinologist with a tool that cannot only evaluate normal and stimulated cycles but also assists in follicle aspiration and subsequent transfer of the embryo. The addition of color Doppler capabilities to transvaginal probes permits visualization of small intraovarian and endometrial vessels, allowing depiction of normal and abnormal physiologic changes in the ovary and uterus. It may help in prediction of ovulation and detection of certain ovulatory disorders and the luteal phase defect. Doppler investigation of ovarian blood flow may improve the early diagnosis of ovarian hyperstimulation syndrome in patients with ovulation induction. Initial impressions concerning the usefulness of blood flow studies in infertile patients have been confirmed by numerous studies during the last decade. This chapter reviews on the assessment of ovarian, uterine and tubal causes of infertility and on the current and future role of color Doppler and three-dimensional ultrasound in the field of reproductive endocrinology.

UTERINE CAUSES OF INFERTILITY

The uterine cavity must provide an environment for successful sperm migration from the cervix to the fallopian tube. The normality of the mucosal lining, glandular secretion and vascularity are necessary to support implantation and placentation. Uterine anomalies, polyps, leiomyomas, neoplasia, infections and intrauterine scar tissue can lead to poor reproductive performance. Attempts have been made to correlate the sonographic parameters (such as thickness and reflectivity) and endometrial receptivity.

Perfusion in Infertile Patients

Transvaginal color and pulsed Doppler sonography has been established as an additional tool in the management of infertile patients. In anovulatory cycles, a continuous increase of the uterine artery RI has been detected (Fig. 22.1).[1,2] Moreover, in some infertile patients, an end-diastolic flow is absent.[3] The results of some research indicate that absent diastolic flow might be associated with infertility and poor reproductive performance.

Therefore, the uterine artery blood flow could be potentially used to predict a hostile uterine environment prior to embryo transfer (Figs 22.2A to C). Steer and coworkers[4] calculated the probability of pregnancy by using PI values obtained from the uterine artery on the day of embryo transfer. With the use of these measurements, the highest probability of becoming pregnant was obtained in those patients with the medium values of PI for uterine arteries. A mean PI of more than 3.0 before the transfer can predict up to 35 percent of pregnancy failures. Tsai and colleagues[5] evaluated the prognostic value of uterine perfusion on the day of human chorionic gonadotropin (hCG) administration in patients who were undergoing intrauterine insemination. They calculated pulsatility index of the ascending branch of the uterine arteries on the day of administration of hCG, and compared the uterine artery vascular resistance to

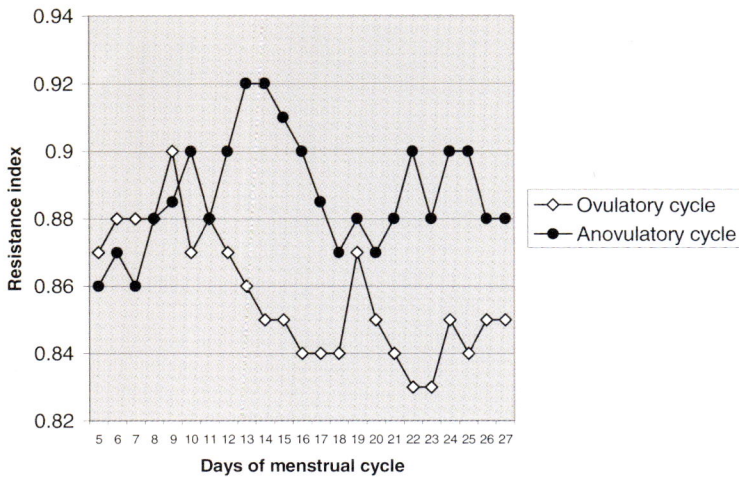

Fig. 22.1: Changes in the uterine artery blood flow in ovulatory and anovulatory cycles (from Reference 1 with permission)

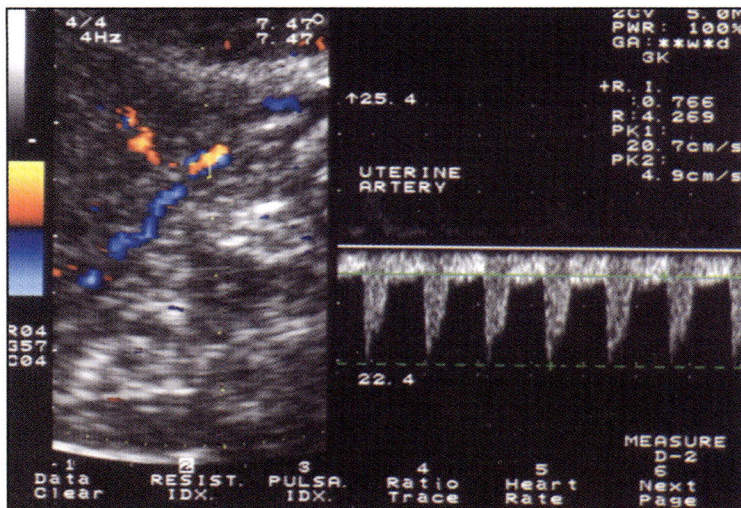

Fig. 22.2A: Uterine artery demonstrated laterally to the cervix at the level of the cervicocorporeal junction (left). The blood flow velocity from the uterine artery in the secretory phase is characterized by increased end-diastolic velocity and decreased resistance index (RI=0.76)

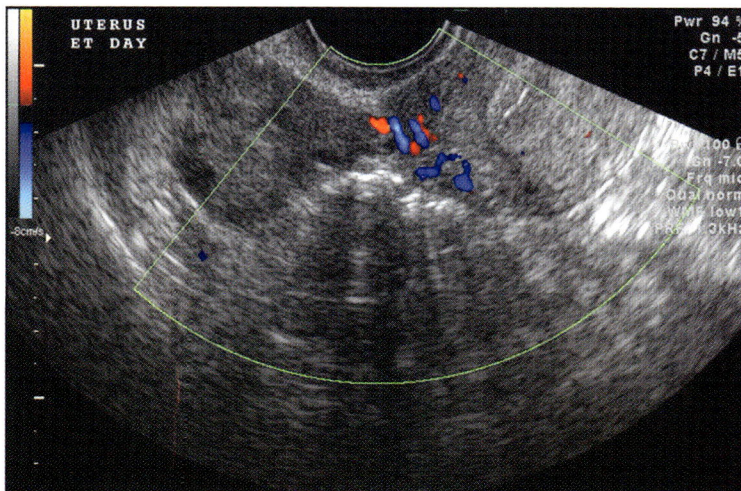

Fig. 22.2B: Uterine artery can be easily found. Note the ovary on the left and the uterus with early secretory endometrium on the right side of the image

the outcome of intrauterine insemination. No pregnancy occurred when the pulsatility index of the ascending branch of

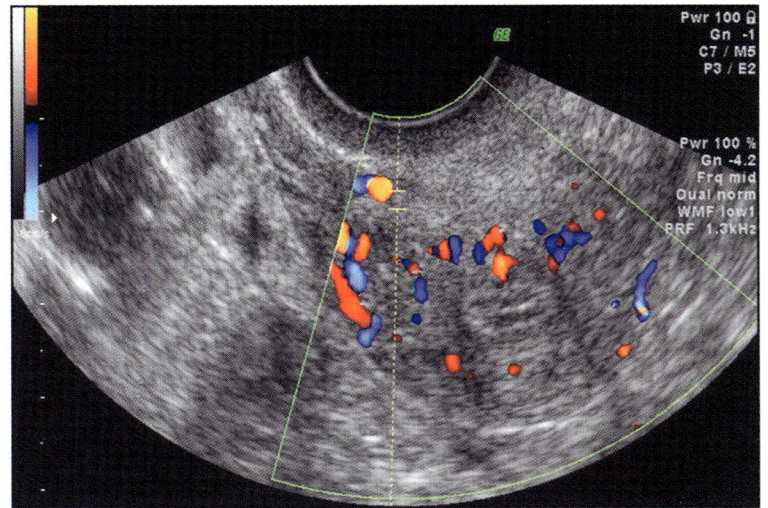

Fig. 22.2C: Transvaginal color Doppler of the uterine circulation. Note the uterine, arcuate, radial and spiral arteries

the uterine arteries was more than 3 (Fig. 22.3). The fecundity rate was 18 percent when the pulsatility was less than 2 and was 19.8 percent when the pulsatility index was between 2 and 3. Their data suggest that the measurement of uterine perfusion on the day of hCG administration may have predictive value regarding fecundity in patients undergoing intrauterine insemination.

In infertile women uterine artery pulsatility indices measured in midluteal phase of unstimulated cycles correlate inversely with endometrial thickness[6] suggesting a direct effect of uterine perfusion on endometrial growth.[7] Furthermore, pulsatility index correlates directly with the age of the patients[3], suggesting a detrimental effect of age on uterine perfusion. Cacciatore et al[8] did not find any correlation between uterine artery pulsatility index measured at the time of ET and endometrial thickness or the age of the patients. These findings could be explained also by the hormonal environment of the superovulated cycles, where the high E_2 levels achieved in almost all subjects are likely to reduce differences between individuals.

A high prevalence of increased uterine artery impedance among infertile patients with the diagnosis of endometriosis has been reported by Steer and coworkers.[6] In the present study women with a history of endometriosis have significantly higher pulsatility index and resistance index values than the others even after hormonal stimulation. These evidences, although gained in different settings, seem to suggest an adverse effect of endometriosis on uterine perfusion. That could be another way endometriosis compromises a woman fertility potential. Whether this is due to mechanical effects on the pelvic vessels as a result of adhesions or is mediated by production of agents with vasoactive properties remains to be explained.

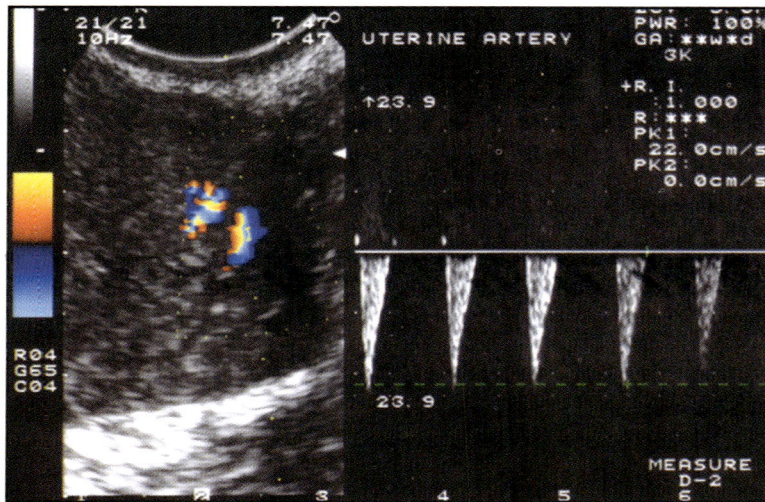

Fig. 22.3: Absent diastolic flow of the uterine artery may be associated with infertility or poor reproductive performance

Endometrial Thickness, Endometrial Volume and Vascularity

The question of a correlation between endometrial thickness and the likelihood of conception, in the context of assisted conception, remains a contentious issue. However, a very thin endometrium (below 7 mm) seems to be accepted as a reliable sign of suboptimal implantation potential.

Recently, Freidler and colleagues[9] reviewed 2,665 assisted conception cycles from 25 reports. Eight reports found that the difference in the mean endometrial thickness of conception and non-conception cycles was statistically significant, while 17 reports found no significant difference. They concluded that results from various trials are conflicting and that insufficient data exist describing a linear correlation between endometrial thickness and the probability of conception. The main advantage of measuring endometrial thickness lies in its high negative predictive value in cases where there is minimal endometrial thickness. Gonen and colleagues[10] reported an absence of pregnancies in donor insemination cycles where the endometrium thickness did not reach at least 6 mm. Similarly, in a group of oocyte recipients, no pregnancies were reported in women who had an endometrial thickness of less than 5 mm, whereas several pregnancies occurred in patients with an endometrium thinner than 7.5 mm.[11] Finally, in IVF cycles, Khalifa and colleagues reported a minimal endometrial thickness of 7 mm to be compatible with pregnancy.[12]

Endometrial pattern is defined as the relative echogenicity of the endometrium and the adjacent myometrium as demonstrated on a longitudinal ultrasound scan.

In a prospective study, Serafini and colleagues[13] found the multilayered pattern to be more predictive of implantation than any other parameter measured. Sher and colleagues[14] correlated a non-multilayered echo pattern with advanced age and the

presence of uterine abnormalities. In the literature, of 13 studies which examined the value of endometrial pattern in predicting pregnancy, only four failed to confirm its predictive value. The endometrial pattern does not appear to be influenced by the type of ovarian stimulation and it is of prognostic value in both fresh IVF, as well as frozen embryo transfer cycles.

Zaidi et al[15] reported that if subendometrial blood flow is detectable, the endometrial morphology may be less important than previously described and it may be that the absence of blood flow is more significant.

The authors evaluated 96 women undergoing in vitro fertilization (IVF) treatment on the day of human chorionic gonadotropin (hCG) administration. They assessed endometrial thickness, endometrial morphology, presence or absence of subendometrial or intraendometrial color flow, intraendometrial vascular penetration and subendometrial blood flow velocimetry on the day of hCG administration and related the results to pregnancy rates (Figs 22.4A and B). The overall pregnancy rate was 32.3 percent (31/96) and there was no significant difference between the pregnant and non-pregnant groups with regard to endometrial thickness, subendometrial peak systolic blood flow velocity (V_{max}) or subendometrial pulsatility index (PI). The pregnancy rates based on endometrial morphology were not significantly different, being 17.6 percent (3/17), 33.3 percent (2/6) and 35.6 percent (26/73) for types A (hyperechoic), B (isoechoic) and C (triple-line) endometria, respectively. In eight (8.3%) patients, subendometrial color flow and intraendometrial vascularization were not detected. This absence of blood flow was associated with failure of implantation (p<0.05). The pregnancy rates related to the zones of vascular penetration into the subendometrial and endometrial regions were: 26.7 percent (4/15) for zone 1 (subendometrial zone), 36.4 percent (16/44) for zone 2 (outer hyperechogenic zone) and 37.9 percent (11/29) for zone 3 (inner hypoechogenic zone), and were not significantly different.

Endometrial thickness obtained by two-dimensional sonography is considered the most important parameter of endometrial growth. However, this parameter does not include the total volume of the endometrium. For certain diagnostic information on endometrium endometrial volume measurement can be important. Furthermore, retarded endometrial development can be associated with primary infertility. The ability to quantify the volume of the endometrium using 3D ultrasound may help correlate cycle outcome with a quantitative parameter rather than endometrial thickness, which is prone to greater subjective variation in measurement.[16] By stepping through the volume in plane mode, the outer limits of

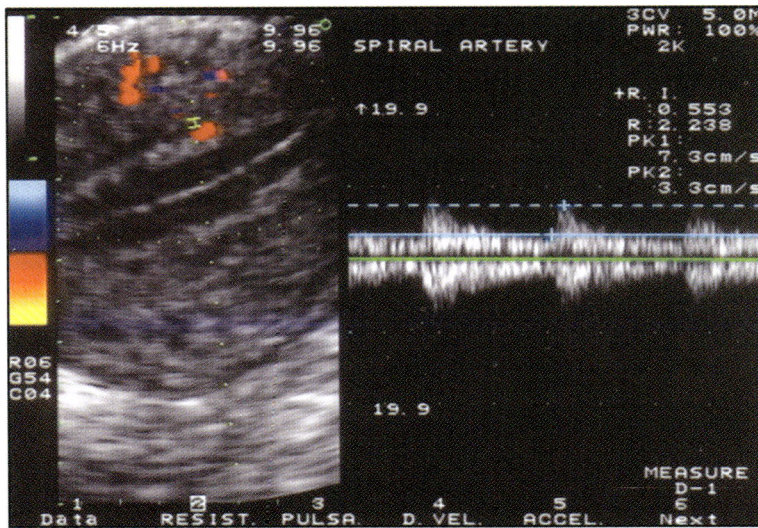

Fig. 22.4A: Blood flow velocity waveforms of the spiral arteries during the follicular phase. Note the triple-line endometrium (left) and the moderate resistance index (RI=0.55) (right) obtained from spiral arteries

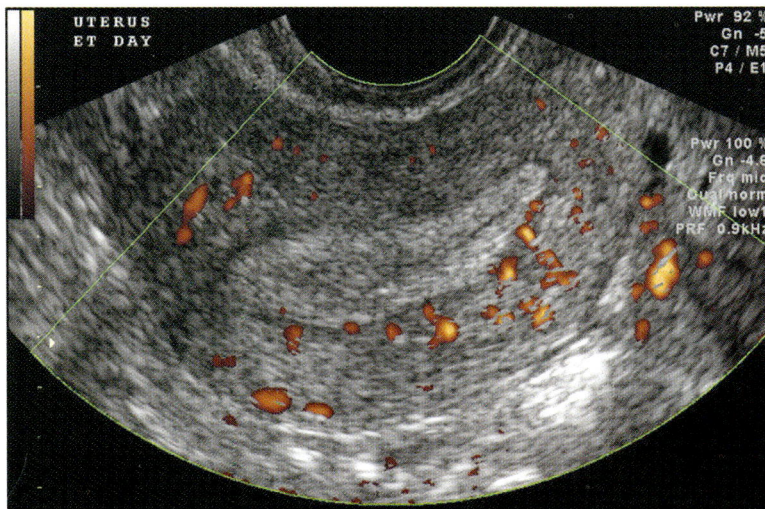

Fig. 22.4B: Transvaginal power Doppler of spiral arteries on day of embryo transfer shows optimal vascularization end endometrial receptivity

endometrium are traced and stepping through the volume in plane mode can perform volume calculations performed immediately. The accurateness of this method has already been described.[17,18] To obtain the best results, stepping through the volume should be performed in small units. In each new plane the area tracing has to be corrected to its new extent. Low contrast in ultrasound data can increase the error of volume estimation. In general, the endometrium shows a good contrast to the surrounding myometrial tissue and therefore, in most cases volume estimation can be performed. Measurements could best be reproduced in longitudinal and transverse viewing planes. Other sources of measuring error may derive from the low contrast of the caudal end of the endometrium and the uterus. Endometrial fluid may also increase measuring error because the fluid volume may be too small to be measured accurately by three-dimensional ultrasound.

Lee et al[19] were first to demonstrate volume estimation of the endometrium by three-dimensional ultrasound. Using the same method Kyei-Mensah et al[20] assessed the reliability of 3D ultrasound in measuring endometrial volume on twenty patients undergoing ovarian stimulation. Endometrial volumes of these patients were obtained on the day of hCG administration. The intraobserver and interobserver coefficient of variation were 8 and 11 percent, respectively. Repeatability within and between investigators was also expressed as the intra-CC and inter-CC. The coefficients describe the proportion of variation in a measurement, which is caused by true biological subject differences. For a single measurement of endometrial volume, the intra-CC was 0.90 and Inter-CC was 0.82. These results clearly demonstrate that 3D ultrasound volume measurements are highly reliable, with a small measurement error. However, one could expect higher interobserver differences in accurate locating the internal os and endometrial margins, which may explain the greater interobserver variability for endometrial volume than for ovarian volume. Since it is applied in the same manner as two-dimensional vaginal ultrasound it does not cause additional discomfort.

It is expected that three-dimensional endometrial volumetry studies will increase diagnostic potential and give additional information to two-dimensional ultrasound. Furthermore, quantification of endometrial volume by 3D ultrasound in combination with blood flow studies may be the best way to predict pregnancy rates.

Kupesic et al[21] investigated the usefulness of transvaginal color Doppler and three-dimensional power Doppler ultrasonography for the assessment of endometrial receptivity in patients undergoing in vitro fertilization procedures. The patients were evaluated for endometrial thickness and volume, endometrial morphology and subendometrial perfusion on the day of embryo transfer. Neither the volume nor the thickness of the endometrium on the day of embryo transfer had a predictive value for conception during in vitro fertilization cycles. Patients who became pregnant were characterized by a significantly lower resistance index (0.53+/–0.04 versus 0.64+/–0.04), obtained from subendometrial vessels by transvaginal color Doppler ultrasonography and a significantly higher flow index (13.2+/–2.2 versus 11.9+/–2.4), as measured by a 3D power Doppler histogram. No difference was found in the predictive value of scoring systems analyzing endometrial thickness and volume, endometrial morphology and subendometrial perfusion by color Doppler and 3D power Doppler ultrasonography. The high degree of endometrial perfusion shown by both techniques on the day of embryo transfer can indicate a more favorable endometrial milieu for successful in vitro fertilization.

Congenital Anomalies

Congenital uterine malformations are variable in frequency and are usually estimated to represent 3 to 4 percent, although less than half have clinical symptoms.[22-24]

The respective frequency of symptomatic malformations is dominated by septate uterus.[24,25] During the first trimester of pregnancy, the risk of spontaneous abortion in this group is between 28 and 45 percent, while during the second trimester the frequency of late spontaneous abortions is approximately 5 percent.[24] Premature deliveries, abnormal fetal presentations, irregular uterine activity and dystocia at delivery are likely to prevail in cases of septate uterus.[26] Poor vascularization of the septum was proposed as a potential cause of miscarriages.[25] Electron microscopy study of Fedele et al[21] indicated a decrease in the sensitivity of the endometrium covering the septa of malformed uteri to preovulatory changes. This could play a role in the pathogenesis of primary infertility in patients with septate uterus.

It is clear that unfavorable obstetric prognosis can be transformed by surgical correction of the intrauterine septum. Hysteroscopic treatment was currently proposed as the procedure of choice for the management of these disorders. This simple and effective treatment has an obvious advantage that uterus is not weakened by a myometrial scar. Cararach et al[28] and Goldenberg et al[29] reported 75 and 88.7 percent pregnancy rates after operative hysteroscopy.

Clearly, simplicity and effectiveness of the hysteroscopy have faced the clinician with need of an early and correct diagnosis of the uterine anomalies. When used as a screening test for detection of congenital uterine anomalies transvaginal ultrasound had a sensitivity of almost 100 percent.[30,31] However, clear distinction between different types of abnormalities was impossible and operator dependent.[32,33]

X-ray hysterosalpingography (X-ray HSG) is an invasive test, which requires the use of contrast medium and exposure to radiation. Although HSG provides a good outline of the uterine cavity, the visualization of minor anomalies and clear distinction between different types of lateral fusion disorders is sometimes impossible. Fifteen years ago hysterosonography has been introduced.[34] This method implies transvaginal ultrasound after distention of the uterine cavity by instillation of a saline solution. This simple and minimally invasive approach allows anatomical images of endometrium and myometrium, accurate depiction of the septate uterus and even the measurement of the thickness and height of the septum.[35]

Although some reports have indicated a high diagnostic accuracy of magnetic resonance imaging[36,37] in the diagnosis of congenital uterine anomalies, this technique is rarely routinely used for this indication. More recently, three-dimensional ultrasound showed high diagnostic accuracy in detection of the septate uterus[38] suggesting that invasive procedures such as CO_2 diagnostic hysteroscopy are not needed in patients scheduled for corrective surgery.[39]

Kupesic and Kurjak attempted to evaluate the combined use of transvaginal ultrasound, transvaginal color and pulsed Doppler sonography, hysterosonography and three-dimensional ultrasound in the preoperative diagnosis of septate uterus.[40]

A total of 420 infertile patients undergoing operative hysteroscopy were included in this study. With the use of B mode transvaginal sonography, the morphology of uterus was carefully explored with emphasis to endometrial lining in both sagittal and transverse sections. The septum was visualized as an echogenic portion separating the uterine cavity into two parts. Once experienced sonographer completed B mode examination, another skilled operator who was unaware of the previous finding performed transvaginal color Doppler examination.

Color and pulsed Doppler was superimposed to visualize intraseptal and myometrial vascularity. Flow velocity waveforms were obtained from all the interrogated vessels. For each recording, at least five waveform signals of good quality were obtained. During each procedure the resistance index (RI) was automatically calculated. The RI was calculated from the maximum frequency envelope and was peak systolic velocity minus end-diastolic velocity divided by peak systolic velocity. Instillation of isotonic saline (hysterosonography) was carried out on a gynecological examination table. Transverse and sagittal sections were carefully explored, and septum was visualized as an echogenic portion separating the uterine cavity into two parts.

Eighty-six women undergoing hysteroscopy were examined by three-dimensional ultrasound. When the patients were evaluated on 3D ultrasound, three perpendicular planes of the uterus were simultaneously displayed on the screen, allowing a detailed analysis of the uterine morphology. Frontal reformatted sections were particularly useful for detection of the uterine abnormalities.

Table 22.1 summarizes the sensitivity, specificity, positive and negative predictive values of transvaginal sonography, transvaginal color and pulsed Doppler ultrasound, hysterosalpingography and three-dimensional ultrasound for the diagnosis of the septate uterus. The sensitivity of transvaginal sonography in the diagnosis of septate uteri was 95.21 percent. Transvaginal color and pulsed Doppler enabled the diagnosis of septate uterus in 276 cases, reaching the sensitivity of 99.29 percent. In one patient with endometrial polyp and one with intrauterine synechiae, septate uteri were not correctly diagnosed. Therefore, the reliability of color and pulsed Doppler examination was reduced if other intracavitary structures (such as endometrial polyp or submucous leiomyoma) were present.

Table 22.1: Sensitivity, specificity, positive (PPV) and negative predictive (NPV) values of various imaging modalities for the diagnosis of septate uterus in 420 patients with history of infertility and recurrent abortions

Imaging modality	Sensitivity (%)	Specificity (%)	PPV (%)	NPV (%)
Transvaginal sonography	95.21	92.21	95.86	91.03
Transvaginal color Doppler	99.29	97.93	98.03	98.61
Hysterosonography	98.18	100.00	100.00	95.45
Three-dimensional ultrasound	98.38	100.00	100.00	96.00

From reference 34, with permission

Color and pulsed Doppler studies of the septal area revealed vascularity in 198 (71.22%) patients. The RI values obtained from the septum ranged from 0.68 to 1.0 (mean RI=0.84±0.16) (Figs 22.5 and 22.6). Hysterosonography reached 100 percent specificity and positive predictive value. In one patient with extensive intrauterine synechiae, hysterosonography did not detect an intrauterine septum.

The sensitivity and specificity of three-dimensional ultrasonography were 98.38 percent and 100 percent, respectively. A false-negative result in one patient was caused by a fundal fibroid distorting the uterine cavity. Interestingly, in our study septate uterus was not mistaken for bicornuate uterus. The transvaginal color Doppler sonography, hysterosonography, and three-dimensional ultrasonography were performed. However, in one patient with bicornuate uterus transvaginal ultrasonography misinterpreted septate uterus.

One hundred eighty-eight patients underwent X-ray HSG within 12 months prior to our examination. The sensitivity of X-ray HSG in the diagnosis of septate uteri was only 26.06 percent.

Fedele et al[27] recently indicated that intrauterine septum may be a cause of primary infertility. The ultrastructural morphological alterations of the septal area were indicative of irregular differentiation and estrogenic maturation of septal endometrial mucosa. Since the hormonal levels of the patients enrolled in this study were normal for the cycle phase, the most convincing hypothesis was that endometrial mucosa covering the septum was poorly responsive to estrogens probably due to scanty vascularization of septal connective tissue.

Dabirashrafi et al[41] performed histologic study of the uterine septa from 16 patients undergoing abdominal metroplasty. Statistical analysis confirmed less connective tissue in the septum compared to the amount of muscle tissue, amount of muscle interlacing and vessels with a muscle wall, which was contradictory to the classic view about the histologic features of

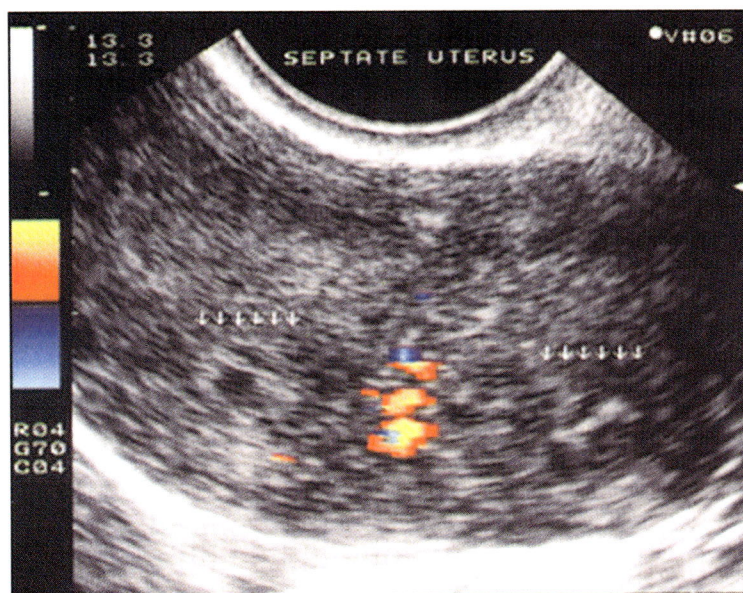

Fig. 22.5: Septate uterus demonstrated by color Doppler imaging. Vascularity within the septal area is easily observed by this technique

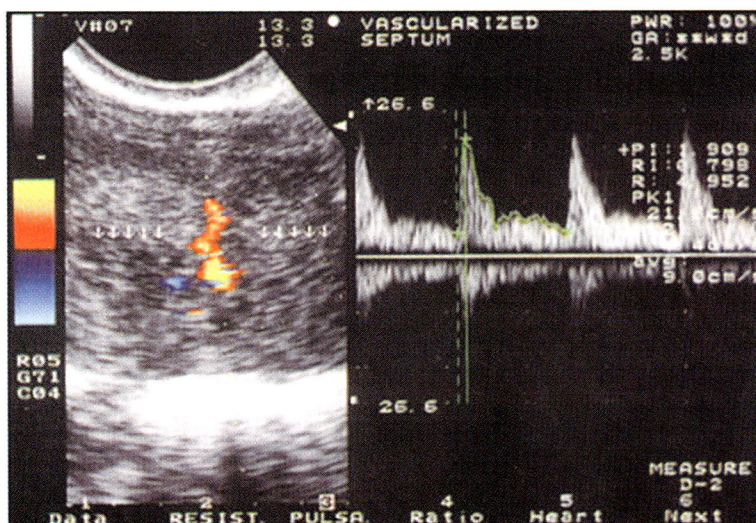

Fig. 22.6: Pulsed Doppler waveform analysis (right) reveals moderate to high vascular resistance (RI=0.79) of the vessels involved in the septum

the uterine septum. Less connective tissue in the septum can be the reason for poor decidualization and placentation in the area of implantation.[35] Increased amounts of muscle tissue and muscle interlacing in the septum can cause an abortion by the higher and uncoordinated contractility of these muscles.

Recent study from our Department[40] found no correlation between septal height and thickness and occurrence of obstetrical complications (p>0.05). Pregnancy loss correlated significantly with septal vascularity. Patients with vascularized septa had significantly higher incidence of early pregnancy failure and late pregnancy complications than those with avascularized septa (p<0.05).

Three dimensional ultrasound enables planar reformatted sections through the uterus which allow precise evaluation of the fundal indentation and the length of the septum (Figs 22.7A and B). Based on our experience, this technique may give a

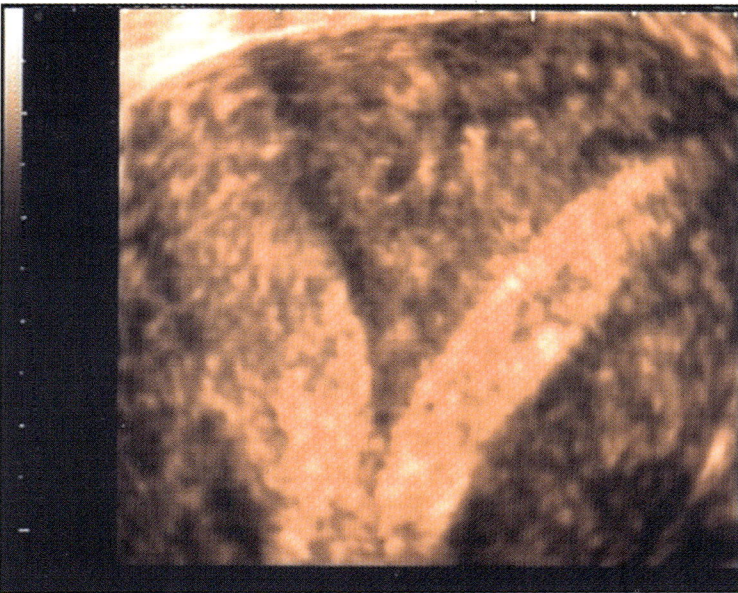

Fig. 22.7A: Frontal reformatted section of the septate uterus. Note the complete division of the uterine cavity and the concave shape of the uterine muscle. Since the fundal cleft is less than 1 cm this uterine anomaly is defined as a septate uterus. This was confirmed by a hysterolaparoscopic procedure

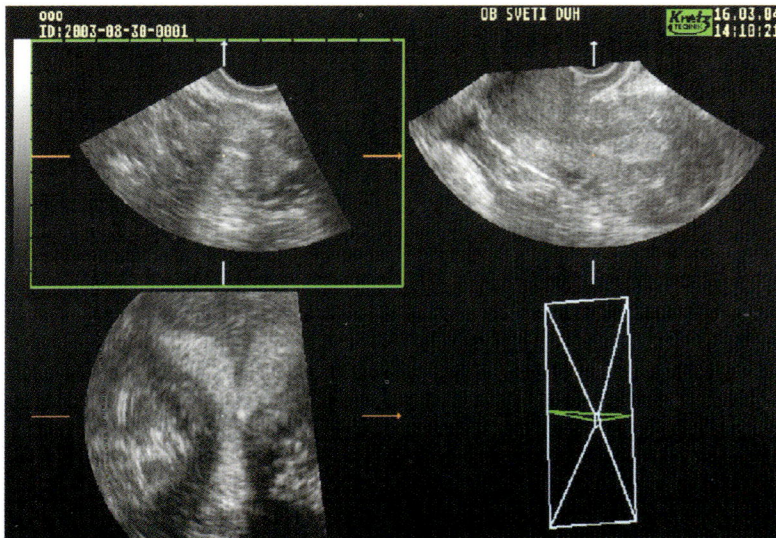

Fig. 22.7B: Three-dimensional ultrasound is a method of choice for detection of uterine abnormalities. Frontal section of the uterus gives us the precise information about the size of the septu

wrong impression of an arcuate uterus in patients with fundal location of the leiomyoma. In these cases uterine cavity has a concave shape, while fundal indentation is shallower. Furthermore, shadowing caused by the uterine fibroids, irregular endometrial lining and decreased volume of the uterine cavity (in cases of intrauterine adhesions) are obvious limitations of 3D ultrasound. More recently three-dimensional power Doppler was used to detect vascularization of the uterine septa in a combined angio and gray rendering mode. This approach allows simultaneous analysis of the morphology, texture and vascularization.

Balen et al[42] described a technique of three-dimensional reconstruction of the uterine cavity using a positive contrast medium (Echovist). The main problem that was encountered with Echovist was an acoustic shadowing artifact owing to its highly reflective properties. Despite this, Echovist proved to be superior to saline as an intrauterine contrast agent for 3D reconstruction while testing 10 patient with both methods.

Weinraub et al[43] applied 3D saline contrast hysterosonography to 32 volunteers 22 to 65 years of age, all in good health and with no evidence of active infections disease.

It seems that contrast 3D hysterosonography offers a more comprehensive overview of the uterine cavity and surrounding myometrium, and gives access to planes unobtainable by conventional 2D ultrasound examination. Further research is required to document whether contrast instillation contributes to better diagnosis of uterine cavity pathology when compared to unenhanced frontal reformatted section.

Kupesic et al[44] studied the incidence of surgically correctable uterine abnormalities (congenital uterine anomalies, submucous leiomyoma, endometrial polyps and intrauterine synechiae) in the infertile population attending tertiary infertility clinic. All of the infertile patients enrolled in the study were evaluated by 3D ultrasound. Another objective was to assess pregnancy rates before and after operative hysteroscopy in patients affected by uterine causes of infertility. They found the incidence of uterine septum in their general infertile population of 17.9 percent. Uterine septum was the most common uterine abnormality accounting for 77.1 percent of the intrauterine lesions. Out of 310 patients that were followed up, 225 (72.6%) patients achieved pregnancy after hysteroscopic metroplasty for intrauterine septum.

Endometrial Polyp

Endometrial polyp is the anatomic defect that is implicated in the etiology of a recurrent pregnancy loss and infertility. Polyps appear as diffuse or focal thickening of the endometrium. Using sonohysterography an intracavitary polyp is seen surrounded by anechoic fluid, with the point of the attachment. If the examination is performed in the follicular phase, use of the distending medium is not necessary to detect abnormal endometrial thickening. However, during the periovulatory and secretory phase, polyps are better visualized when outlined by fluid.

By using transvaginal color and pulsed Doppler we can study minor arteries supplying the growth of the endometrial polyp. Three-dimensional ultrasound allows a detailed analysis of the uterine cavity in frontal reformatted sections, which enables clear demarcation of the polyps (Fig. 22.8).

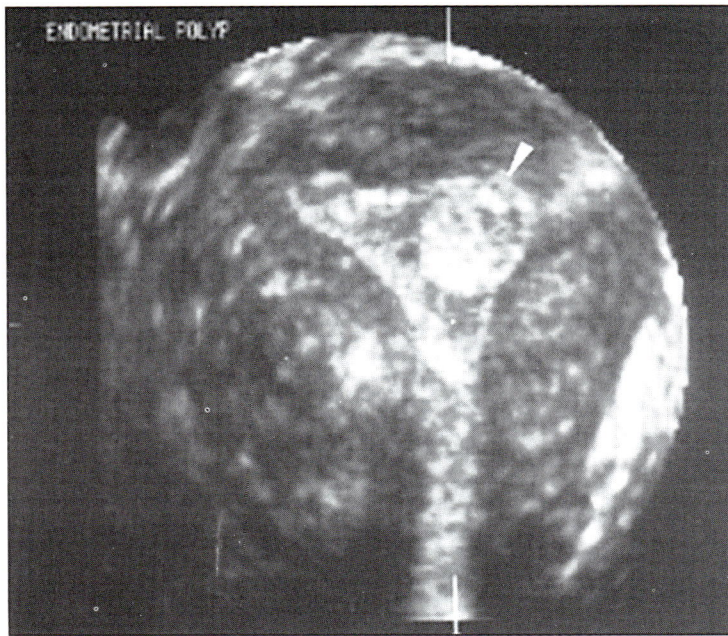

Fig. 22.8: Transvaginal three-dimensional ultrasound of the endometrial polyp located in the left uterine horn

Submucous Leiomyomas

The diagnosis of a submucous leiomyoma is based on distortion of the uterine contour, uterine enlargement and textural changes. Since leiomyomas have a varying amount of smooth muscle and connective tissue, these benign tumors also have a variety of sonographic features. Sonographic texture ranges from hypoechoic to echogenic, depending on the amount of smooth muscle and connective tissue. Central ischemia, which is a consequence of tumor enlargement and inadequate blood supply, is usually followed by various stages of degeneration. The most common cause of calcification within the uterus is calcific degeneration within a fibroid. Other types of degeneration include cystic, myxomatous, and hyaline degeneration. Sometimes, because of the variety of appearances, submucous leiomyomas may be mistaken for endometrial polyps, endometrial carcinoma, blood or mucus. Patients with submucous fibroids have the uterine environment not conducive to nidation of a fertilized ovum and blood supply might be inadequate. Leiomyoma grows centripetally as proliferations of smooth muscle cells and fibrous connective tissue, creating pseudocapsule of compressed muscle fibers. Therefore, color Doppler demonstrates most of the myometrial blood vessels at its periphery (Figs 22.9A and B). Presence of blood vessels in the central portion of the leiomyomas is usually correlated with necrotic, degenerative and inflammatory changes. These vessels display lower RI values than peripherally located vessels, and sometimes can be misinterpreted for malignant neovascular pulsed Doppler signal.[45] Vascular impedance to blood flow in myometrial supplying vessels depends not only on size but

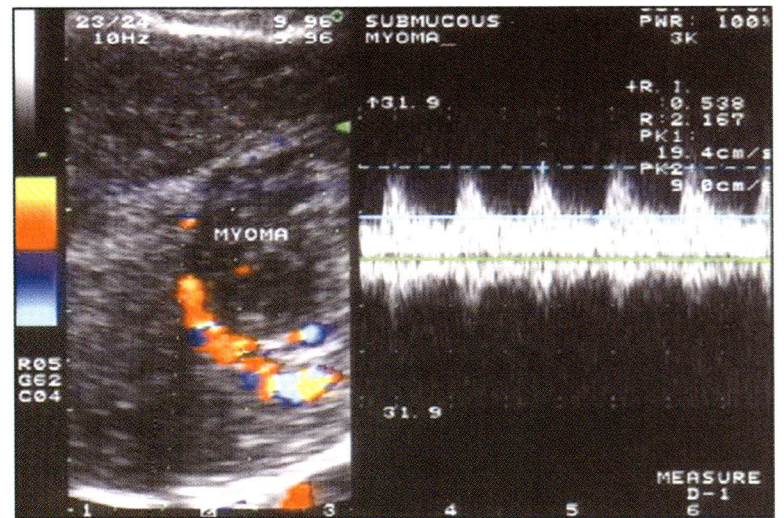

Fig. 22.9A: Transvaginal color Doppler scan of the uterus with submucous leiomyoma. Waveform analysis (right) indicates moderate resistance of the tumor blood flow (RI=0.53)

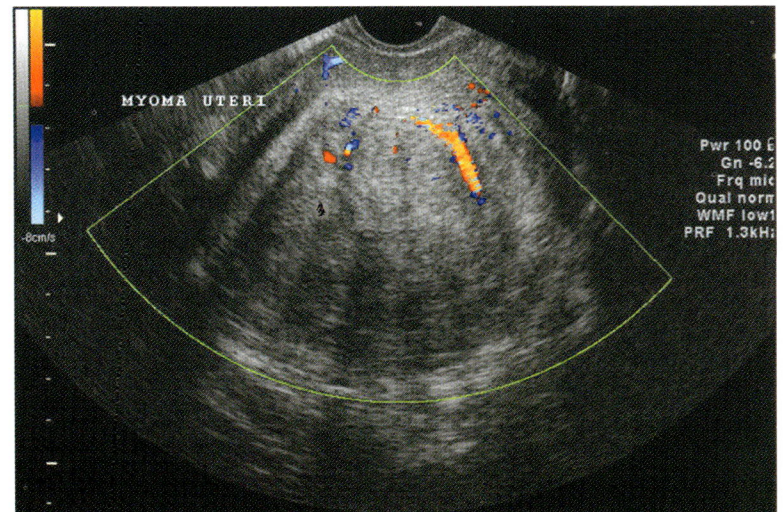

Fig. 22.9B: Transvaginal color Doppler image of intramural myoma with typical periferal circulation

location within the uterus. A significant difference was shown in blood flow characteristics for leiomyoma supplying vessels between entirely subserosal versus intramural and submucous leiomyomas. Lower impedance value for subserosal leiomyomas can be explained by the fact that these leiomyomas are supplied with blood vessels through a very small contact area. These blood vessels are surrounded with loose connective tissue and therefore dilated with very low vascular impedance to blood flow. In contrast, submucous leiomyomas and those located within the myometrium are supplied by blood vessels with higher vascular impedance. High basal tonus of myometrial tissue surrounding intramural or submucous leiomyomas could cause a difference in hemodynamic parameters. Three-dimensional ultrasound precisely estimates the relationship between submucous leiomyoma and uterine cavity.

Kurjak et al[45] performed transvaginal color flow evaluation in 101 patients with palpable uterine fibroids and 60 healthy volunteers. The mean resistance index from the periphery of leiomyoma covered the value of 0.54. Mean PI value was 0.89. The pathohistological finding was benign uterine tumor in all the cases, even when RI was very low. Lowered resistance indices were present in cases with necrosis and secondary degenerative and inflammatory changes within the fibroid. Increased blood flow velocity and decreased RI (mean RI=0.74) in both uterine arteries occurred in patients with uterine fibroids.

Adenomyosis

Adenomyosis, characterized by ingrowing of the endometrium into the myometrium is usually asymptomatic, but may be presented by uterine bleeding, pain and infertility. A diffusely enlarged uterus without discrete fibroids, an intact endometrium and multiple small cysts in the myometrium have been reported as a suggestive appearance of adenomyosis.[46] Disordered echogenicity of the middle layer of the myometrium is present in some severe cases. Reported sensitivity and specificity of transvaginal ultrasound in detection of this benign entity is 86 and 50 percent, respectively.[46] Color Doppler may reveal increased vascularity mainly characterized by moderate vascular resistance.

Endometritis

Chronic endometritis is characterized by increased echogenicity, thickness and vascularity of the endometrium. The most common cause of chronic endometrial infection is *Mycobacterium tuberculosis*. During the activation of infection, pregnancy often terminates ectopically or as an abortion. Transvaginal sonographic findings may include calcified pelvic lymph nodes or smaller irregular calcifications in the adnexa, and deformity of the endometrial cavity suggestive of adhesions in the absence of a history of prior curettage or abortion. In the acute stage of the endometritis low to moderate impedance blood flow signals are easily obtained on the periphery of the endometrium. On the contrary, blood flow is usually absent in cases with irreversible tissue damage. Transvaginal sonography allows elucidation of the abnormal endometrial morphology, after which appropriate cultures should be taken and broad-spectrum antibiotic therapy administered. In order to prevent the development of intrauterine adhesions (especially after D&C) administration of conjugated estrogen for one to two months is recommended. This therapy allows regeneration of the healthy endometrium, which is paralleled by sharp increase in end-diastolic velocities of the spiral arteries at the time of color flow and pulsed Doppler analysis.

Asherman's Syndrome

Destruction of the endometrium may result in scarring and the development of bands of scar tissue, or synechia, within the uterine cavity. This destruction may occur as a result of a vigorous curettage of the uterus following an abortion or, more often, after curettage of an advanced pregnancy. Tuberculosis may also cause uterine synechiae, but only in rare cases. This may result in formation of adhesive bands of different size with a subsequent partial or total obliteration of the endometrial cavity. Amenorrhea or hypomenorrhea characterizes menstrual pattern.

Patients with endometrial adhesion, such as Asherman's syndrome, may have a distorted endometrial pattern with areas where no endometrium can be imaged mixed with areas that appear normal. Adhesions are observed as endometrial irregularities or hyperechoic bridges within the endometrial cavity.

Schlaff and Hurst[47] analyzed seven amenorrheic patients with severe Asherman's syndrome. Transvaginal sonography demonstrated a well-developed endometrial stripe in three of seven women, while three others had virtually no endometrium seen. All the patients with well-developed endometrium were found to have adhesions excluding the lower uterine segment and had resumption of normal menses and normalization of the cavity after hysteroscopy. The women with minimal endometrium had no cavity identified and derived no benefit from surgery. The conclusion of that study was that endometrial pattern on transvaginal sonography is highly predictive of both surgical and clinical outcome in patients with severe Asherman's syndrome characterized by complete obstruction of the cavity at hysterosalpingogram.

Intrauterine synechiae do not present increased vascularity on color Doppler examination. They are better visualized during menstruation when intracavitary fluid outlines them or following the hysterosonography. Three-dimensional ultrasound demonstrates a significant reduction of the endometrial cavity volume in all reformatted sections.

OVARIAN CAUSES OF INFERTILITY

Transvaginal sonography is considered the most reliable method for monitoring the follicular growth. It enables accurate prediction of ovulation and detection of the ovulation abnormalities.

The success of IVF treatment is dependent on the ability of the ovary to respond to controlled stimulation by gonadotropins and to develop a reasonable number of mature follicles and oocytes simultaneously. Failure to respond is associated with cancellation of the cycle or poor outcome of treatment. Prior prediction of the likelihood of optimal ovarian response is therefore essential in identifying patients who are most likely to benefit from IVF treatment.

Zaidi et al[48] were the first to show that there was a relation between ovarian stromal blood flow velocity and ovarian follicular response. They measured the ovarian stromal PSV in the early follicular phase and showed that poor responders had low ovarian blood flow PSV. Increased ovarian stromal blood flow velocity was detected in polycystic ovaries, in combination with relatively unchanged impedance to blood flow. This may reflect increased intraovarian perfusion and thus a greater delivery of gonadotropins to the granulosa-thecal cell complex with a resultant greater number of follicles being produced. This mechanism may help explain why patients with polycystic ovaries tend to respond excessively to the administration of gonadotropins,[56] and may possibly explain their increased risk of ovarian hyperstimulation syndrome.

Documentation of ovarian stromal vascularity at the initial baseline scan may be important and may provide useful information for assisted reproduction techniques. Furthermore, it seems that measurement of ovarian stromal blood flow in the early follicular phase is related to subsequent ovarian responsiveness in IVF treatment.[48] This is particularly useful since the ability to predict ovarian response to stimulation by exogenous gonadotropins is still central to success in any IVF program. Most units determine the dose of gonadotropins used for the first attempt based on the chronological age of the patient, with adjustments being made in subsequent attempts depending on their initial response. Unfortunately the ovarian age (capacity of the ovary to produce fertilizable oocytes) and chronological age are not always synchronous, leading to a degree of unpredictability of the number of developing follicles and collected oocytes. Certainly, if an inadequate dose of gonadotropins is used then there may be a relatively poor response, which reduces the number of oocytes retrieved, whereas if an excessive dose is used, there may be an increased risk of ovarian hyperstimulation syndrome (Figs 22.10A and B).

Engman et al[49] speculated that the ovarian stromal blood flow velocity after 2 to 3 weeks of pituitary suppression is a true representative of baseline ovarian blood flow because the ovaries are in a quiescent state. The primordial follicles in the ovary have no independent capillary network, lying simply among vessels of the stroma, and therefore depend on their proximity to the stromal vessels for the delivery of nutrients and hormones. The subsequent growth of primary follicles leads to the acquisition of a vascular sheath through the process of angiogenesis. The administration of a GnRH agonist suppresses

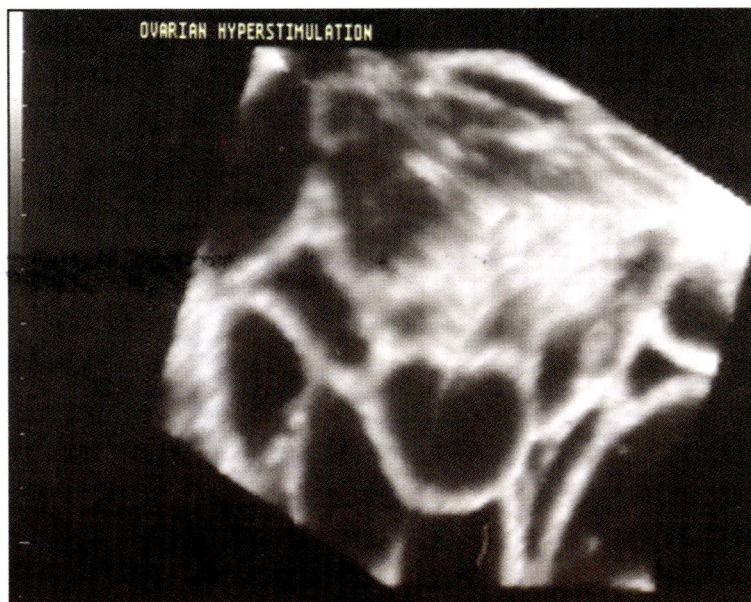

Fig. 22.10A: Three-dimensional ultrasound image of the hyperstimulated ovary. The ovary is enlarged and filled with numerous follicles

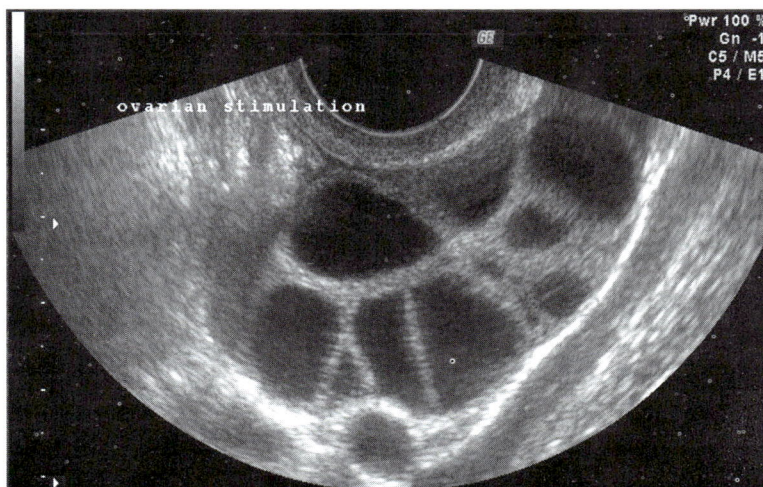

Fig. 22.10B: Two-dimensional image of ovarian stimulation

follicular activity and consequently the ovaries become inactive; ovarian stromal blood flow at this time might be at its lowest and may truly reflect the baseline ovarian blood flow.

Therefore, ovarian stromal blood flow velocity after pituitary suppression is predictive of ovarian responsiveness and the outcome of IVF treatment.

One might speculate that by improving the ovarian stromal blood flow velocity, the delivery of gonadotropins to the follicles will be improved and as a result, the number and quality of mature oocytes produced and the implantation rate will improve.

The accuracy of diagnosis and monitoring of infertility treatments such as ovulation-induction has increased greatly because of the availability of sophisticated ultrasound technology and equipment.[20] Accurate follicular assessment is essential for safe and effective infertility treatment. In IVF-ET cycles, follicles with a mean follicular diameter of 12 to 24 mm are associated with optimal rates of oocyte recovery, fertilization, and cleavage.[50]

This corresponds to follicular volumes of between 3 and 7 ml. In the hands of experienced operators, ultrasound alone suffices for cycle monitoring, with no necessity for additional hormonal estimations.[51-53]

The basic structural information provided by conventional scans in the longitudinal and transverse planes now can be augmented by new three-dimensional 3D ultrasound systems that provide an additional view of the coronal or C-plane, which is parallel to the transducer face.[20] The computer-generated scan is displayed in three perpendicular planes. Translation or rotation can be carried out in one plane, while maintaining the perpendicular orientation of all three so that serial translation will result in an ultrasound tomogram from which volumetric data can be captured.[54] Kyei-Mensah et al[20] evaluated the accuracy of 3D ultrasound measurement of follicular volume compared with current standard techniques by comparing the volume of individual follicles estimated by both methods with the corresponding follicular aspirates. The volume of follicular fluid aspirated was compared with the corresponding volume of the follicle measured by 3D ultrasound and with the conventional 2D ultrasound volume measurement calculated using the formula $0.52 \times (D_1 \times D_2 \times D_3)$. Limits of agreement and 95 percent confidence intervals were calculated and systematic bias between the methods was analyzed. The limits of agreement between the volume of follicular aspirate and follicular volume determined by ultrasound were $+0.96$ to -0.43 ml for 3D measurements and $+3.47$ to -2.42 ml for 2D measurements. The high accuracy of 3D measurement of follicular volume is demonstrated clearly in this study by the limits of agreement, which are within 1 ml of the true volume. These limits encompass 95 percent of the volume measurements. On the other hand, the 2D method produced limits of agreement that was up to 3.5 ml above or 2.5 ml below the true volume within the most important clinical range.

Therefore, the shape and numbers of the follicles influence the reliability of the standard 2D ultrasound technique of follicular volume measurement. There may be technical difficulty in measuring the diameters of a follicle when its shape is distorted because of compression by adjacent follicles. Penzias et al[55] showed that mean follicular diameter accurately predicted volume in round and polygonal follicles but not in those that were ellipsoid. Rounded follicles were most prevalent in patients with the fewest follicles. The patients selected for this study had produced fewer follicles than normal and therefore represent the group in which the conventional technique was likely to be most accurate. Kyei-Mensah et al[20] found that 3D assessment of follicular volume produced a more accurate reflection of the true volume. This is because 3D measurement is not affected by

follicular shape since the changing contours are outlined serially to obtain the specific volume measurement. The disparity in accuracy between 3D assessment of follicular volume and the conventional approach therefore is likely to increase significantly if there is a florid multifollicular ovarian response because the conventional formula is less precise with ellipsoid follicles, which are likely to predominate in these cases. One limitation of 3D volume assessment is that follicles with a mean diameter of <10 mm cannot be assessed accurately because the limits of agreement are too wide in this range.

Feichtinger et al[56] found that three-dimensional ultrasound may be useful for distinction of the ovarian cysts from the ovarian follicles. Since both the ovarian cysts and follicles demonstrate an elevation of the serum estradiol levels, it is difficult to distinguish between them by E2 assay alone. For the purpose of the prospective observational study the authors evaluated 50 IVF patients after ovulation induction. Three-dimensional ultrasound was used to search for the presence of cumuli in follicles greater than 15 mm. Only cumuli demonstrable in all three planes by multiplanar imaging predicted mature oocytes recovery. Follicles without visualization of the cumulus in all three planes were not likely to contain mature fertilizable oocytes.

Lass et al[57] tested the hypothesis that small ovaries measured on transvaginal sonography are associated with a poor response to ovulation induction by human menopausal gonadotropin (hMG) for in vitro fertilization (IVF). A total of 140 infertile patients with morphologically normal ovaries undergoing IVF was studied and represented. The mean ovarian volume of each patient was measured on transvaginal sonography before starting hMG. Subsequent routine IVF management was conducted without knowledge of the results of transvaginal sonography. The mean ovarian volume was 6.3 cm^3 (range 0.5–18.9, SD=3.1). Patients (n=17; group A) with small ovaries of or=3 cm^3 represented group B. Both groups were of similar age (mean 35.8 versus 34.4 years). Early basal FSH concentrations were increased in group A (9.5 versus 7.0 mIU/ml, P=0.025). The cycle was abandoned before planned oocyte recovery in nine patients (52.8%) from group A and in 11 patients (8.9%) from group B because of poor response to ovulation induction.

Oyesanya et al[58] measured total ovarian volumes before the administration of hCG in 42 women undergoing treatment for infertility by in vitro fertilization and embryo transfer and considered to have an exaggerated response to stimulation (>20 follicles). Seven women who subsequently developed moderate or severe ovarian hyperstimulation syndrome (OHSS) (n=7; group 1) were compared with 35 matched controls (five matched controls per case; n=35; group 2) of similar age, number of follicles and duration of infertility who underwent follicular stimulation, oocyte recovery, in vitro fertilization and embryo transfer during the same period but did not develop moderate or severe OHSS. The mean age, duration of infertility and total number of follicles were similar, but the mean total ovarian volume was significantly higher in the group of women who developed moderate or severe OHSS compared with controls (271.00±87.00 versus 157.30±54.20 ml).

Kupesic and Kurjak[59] designed a study to evaluate whether ovarian antral follicle number, ovarian volume, stromal area and ovarian stromal blood flow are predictive of ovarian response and in vitro fertilization (IVF) outcome. Total ovarian antral follicle number, total ovarian volume, total stromal area and mean flow index (FI) of the ovarian stromal blood flow were determined by three dimensional (3D) and power Doppler ultrasound after pituitary suppression. Pre-treatment 3D ultrasound ovarian measurements were compared with subsequent ovulation induction parameters (peak estradiol on hCG administration day and number of oocytes) and cycle outcome (fertilization and pregnancy rates). The total number of antral follicles achieved the best predictive value for favorable IVF outcome, followed by ovarian stromal FI, total ovarian stromal area and total ovarian volume.

Recent study from Kupesic et al[60] evaluated whether ovarian antral follicle number, ovarian volume and ovarian stromal blood flow change with women age and if they are predictive of ovarian response and in vitro fertilization (IVF) outcome. Total ovarian antral follicle number, total ovarian volume and mean flow index (FI) of the ovarian stromal blood flow were determined by three dimensional (3D) and power Doppler ultrasound after pituitary suppression. Patients were separated into three groups based upon age and in each group median values of 3D ultrasound parameters (total ovarian antral follicle number, total ovarian volume and mean ovarian stromal vascularity) were measured and presented. Pre-treatment 3D ultrasound ovarian measurements were compared with subsequent ovulation induction parameter (number of oocytes) and cycle outcome (fertilization and pregnancy rate). Increasing age is associated with poor ovarian response, smaller ovarian volume, and lower antral follicle count and poor stromal vascularity.

Clearly, there is a place for three-dimensional ultrasound in the assessment of the ovaries prior to ovulation induction and medically assisted reproduction.

Polycystic Ovarian Syndrome

Polycystic ovarian syndrome (PCOS) is one of the causes of anovulation and amenorrhea. In its classic form it is characterized by infertility, oligo- and amenorrhea, hirsutism, acne or seborrhea, and obesity. Adams et al defined in 1986 the criteria for ultrasonographic diagnosis of polycystic ovaries: multiple (n>10), small (2 to 8 mm) peripheral cysts around a dense core of stroma in enlarged (≥8 ml) ovaries.[61] However, ovaries which are normal in volume can be polycystic, as demonstrated by histological and biochemical studies. Anatomic structure of the ovaries cannot adequately be assessed with the transabdominal approach in about 42 percent of cases. Underlying causes are obesity, limited resolution of low-frequency transducers, a full bladder distorting pelvic anatomy, and bowel loops covering the adjacent ovary. More recently, the transvaginal approach for ultrasound scanning of pelvic organs has been used. The high frequency of the transvaginal probe avoids the need for a full bladder and bypasses the problems of attenuation and artifacts associated with obesity. Furthermore, transvaginal ultrasonography has the advantage of improved resolution, better visualization of pelvic organs, and greater acceptance among patients.

The number of follicles necessary to establish the diagnosis of polycystic ovaries by ultrasonography has been reported to vary between five and fifteen. However, in many reports the highest number of atretic follicles obtained in normal control patients was five per ovary, so it may conventionally be established that in polycystic ovaries the number of atretic follicles per ovary would be at least six. Matsunaga and colleagues identified two types of polycystic ovary on the basis of ultrasonographic follicular distribution: the peripheral cystic pattern (PCP) and the general cystic pattern (GCP).[62] In the PCP, small cysts are distributed in the subcapsular region of the ovary, whereas in the GCP they are scattered through the entire ovarian parenchyma. Recently, Takahashi and colleagues showed that these two different ovarian morphologies reflect histopathological differences, and that the PCP and GCP appearances reflect specific endocrine PCOS patterns.[63]

Another parameter considered in the diagnosis of polycystic ovaries is the ovarian volume. However, the wide volume overlap between normal and PCOS patients suggests that the discriminative capacity of ovarian volume alone is not sufficient for ultrasound diagnosis of PCOS.[64] The role of a hyperechogenic ovarian stroma has been emphasized, but appraisal of the ovarian stroma echodensity,[65] although comparable with computerized quantification,[66] is absolutely subjective and may be differently interpreted by the operator.

Color Doppler studies showed that in patients with polycystic ovarian syndrome important changes in ovarian vascularization occur at the level of the intraovarian arteries (Fig. 22.11). Although intraovarian arteries are usually not seen before days

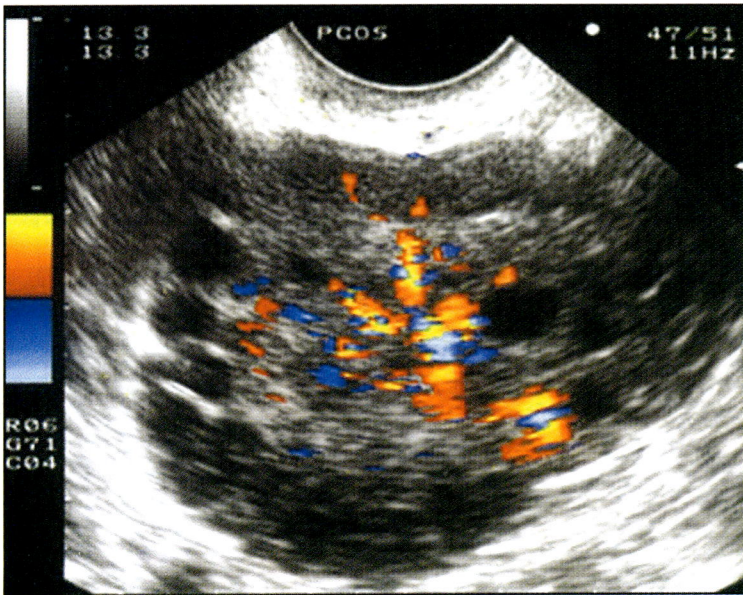

Fig. 22.11: This is a case of a polycystic ovary. A large number of small cystic structures are crowded together and stand out from the enlarged ovarian stroma. Stromal vessels are easily visualized by color Doppler imaging

8 to 10 of the 28-day cycle,[67] Battaglia and colleagues detected distinct arteries with characteristic low vascular impedance as early as cycle days 3 to 5.[68] In the studied population the results were associated with typical PCOS hormonal parameters and were inversely correlated with the LH/FSH ratio. Tonic hypersecretion of LH during the follicular phase of the menstrual cycle occurs in PCOS and is associated with theca cells and stromal hyperplasia with consequent androgen overproduction.[68] Elevated LH levels may be responsible for increased stromal vascularization by different mechanisms that may act individually or in a cumulative way: neoangiogenesis, catecholaminergic stimulation, and leukocyte and cytokine activation. In the same study the PCOS patients showed higher uterine pulsatility index (PI) values than non-hirsute normally menstruating women. This finding was correlated with androstenedione levels, confirming a possible direct androgen vasoconstrictive effect due to activation of specific receptors present in the arterial vessel walls and collagen and elastin deposition in smooth muscle cells. The above condition, by reducing the uterine perfusion, has been supposed to be the cause that prevents blastocyst implantation, increasing the incidence of miscarriages in PCOS patients. Zaidi and colleagues[48] and Aleem and Predanic,[70] confirming that the Doppler analysis of stromal arteries in PCOS may be useful to improve the diagnosis and to provide further information about the pathophysiology and evolution of the syndrome obtained similar results.

Doppler evaluation showed that PCP patients, in comparison with GCP patients, present significantly lower resistance index (RI) values at the level of the ovarian stromal arteries and that in

22 percent of GCP patients the intraovarian vessels are not recognized.[71] In addition, the GCP appearance of the ovary is more common in the early phase of the disease[62,63] during the peripubertal period. Thus, the ovarian morphology may evolve from a normal multicystic to polycystic PCP pattern, passing through an ovarian GCP aspect and untreated PCOS may be regarded as a progressive syndrome. Furthermore, by comparing oligo-vs. amenorrheic PCOS patients, it has recently been shown that amenorrheic patients are older and present higher PI values in uterine arteries and lower RI values in intraovarian vessels than oligomenorrheic patients.[72] This finding is associated with higher plasma LH and androstenedione levels and with a more elevated LH/FSH ratio. Furthermore, significantly higher ovarian volumes and subcapsular small-sized follicles are observed in amenorrheic PCOS patients. These data show that as the number of ovarian microcysts increases, ovarian volume enlarges and Doppler indices worsen, the clinical and endocrine abnormalities become more remarkable and the menstrual disturbances become more severe.[71]

Recently, it has been demonstrated that obese PCOS women show higher PI values within the uterine arteries than do lean patients.[73] This is associated with higher hematocrit values, hyperinsulinemia, higher triglyceride levels and lower high-density lipid (HDL) concentrations.

In overweight patients, hyperinsulinemia may be proposed as the uniting factor between increased vascular resistance, obesity, lipid abnormalities and cardiovascular disease.[73,74] Thus, assuming that PCOS patients are at increased risk for cardiovascular disease, it is possible to affirm that obesity may further increase the risk. Unopposed estrogen stimulation is an important contributing factor of endometrial carcinoma and this helps explain the increased risk in patients with obesity and chronic anovulation.

Recent advances in three-dimensional ultrasound have made accurate noninvasive assessment of the pelvic organs feasible. The ability to visualize the oblique or coronal plane allows accurate volume measurements, especially of irregularly shaped objects.[17,20] Due to accurate track of the individual variations in structure during the measurement process measurements are considered reliable and highly reproducible.[16]

Wu et al[75] studied 44 women who presented with a history of irregular menstrual periods; the conditions of most of the women had been diagnosed as polycystic ovary disease (PCOD). The diagnosis of PCOD was based on the clinical symptoms (e.g. menstrual problems, obesity, acne, hirsutism), endocrinologic data (all with reversed serum LH/FSH ratio), and ultrasonographic features (increased ovarian stroma and volume, subcapsular cysts, and thickened capsule). Another 22 women with regular ovulatory cycles were recruited as normal controls. There was no statistically significant difference in age (range, 17 to 35 years) between the patient groups. Three-dimensional ultrasonography was performed to store and document whole volumes of the ovaries for evaluation. Three perpendicular planes of bilateral ovaries were rotatable to obtain the largest dimensions. The three-dimensional volume was measured using the trapezoid formula. The ovaries of the patients with PCOD were larger in size, area, and volume than those of normal controls. The mean ovarian volumes (three dimensions; mean $\pm$ SD) were 11.3 ± 3.5 cm^3 in patients with PCOD and 5.5 ± 1.4 cm^3 in the normal controls (P<0.0001). The volumes of the right ovary were 12.2 ± 4.7 cm^3 and 5.3 ± 2.0 cm^3 and the left ones were 10.5 ± 3.6 cm^3 and 5.7 ± 1.6 cm^3 in the PCOD and normal groups, respectively. The right ovary demonstrated a larger volume than the left ovary in women with PCOD (P<0.0001); however, the left ovary was significantly larger than the right one in the normal controls (P<0.0001).

The ovaries in PCOD were significantly increased in size, stroma, and volume (P<0.0001) compared with those of the normal controls. Cut-off values for ovarian area, stroma, and volume in PCOD were 5.2 cm^2 (sensitivity 93%, specificity 91%), 4.6 cm^2 (sensitivity 91%, specificity 86%), and 6.6 cm^3 (sensitivity 91%, specificity 91%), respectively. The stroma, total ovarian areas, and volume detected by careful rotation and outlining of the longitudinal ovarian cut were increased in 84 percent (37 of 44), 89 percent (39 of 44), and 80 percent (35 of 44) of the patients with PCOD, respectively, in comparison with normal controls. The total ovarian area was highly correlated with the stromal area (r^2=0.66).

Undoubtedly, three-dimensional ultrasonography facilitates noninvasive retrospective evaluation and volume calculation. The examination time is short, without increasing patient discomfort. Three maximal dimensions of the ovaries can be measured easily once the digital volume is documented from either transvaginal or transabdominal three-dimensional ultrasonography, and superior volume determination can be obtained from three-dimensional images. The volume measurement in three-dimensional ultrasonography is accurate and highly reproducible. The volume of follicles can be determined precisely, and the volume of the ovary from three-dimensional sonography correlates better with direct measurement of the surgical specimen than that from two-dimensional ultrasonography.[20] The ability of reconstruction increases the diagnostic potential for PCOD. The ovaries in PCOD are usually enlarged bilaterally, but they may be about normal size (up to

20% in our study). The stroma areas in PCOD are hypertrophic, and provide yet another subjective ultrasonographic criterion that could differentiate PCOD from the multifollicular ovary. The multifollicular ovary demonstrates a normal or slightly increased size, but an increased number of follicles is noted without an increased amount of stroma. However, the results are usually subjective and not quantitative. Using the computerized quantification measurement, an increased total ovarian area of more than 5.5 cm^2 highly correlates with increased ovarian stroma at a strict longitudinal ovarian section in the diagnosis of PCOD.[76]

Three-dimensional ultrasonography allows careful and objective evaluation of the ovaries and can repeatedly follow the outline of the ovarian area even after the examination. The value of ovarian stroma can be obtained after subtracting the sum area of ovarian cysts from the total area. The three-dimensional scanning can obtain more accurate volume data by outlining the contour of the target organ, which is better than traditional two-dimensional ultrasonographic scanning calculated by the ellipsoid formula (height $\times$ width $\times$ thickness $\times$ 0.523).

In conclusion, three-dimensional ultrasonography can complement two-dimensional ultrasonography for the diagnosis of PCOD. It allows excellent spatial evaluation of PCOD with direct quantitative computations from the data.

Apart from morphological and volume measurements assessment of ovarian and uterine vessels can be added to the traditional endocrinologic and ultrasonographic parameters clinically used for diagnosis of the PCOD.

Patients with PCOD undergoing ovulation induction for IVF are more likely to develop a greater number of follicles and generate more oocytes compared with women with normal ovaries even though they require less gonadotropin stimulation.[77] Furthermore, since they develop more follicles of all sizes and, in particular small and medium sized follicles, women with PCOD are at greater risk of OHSS.[78] This suggests that the PCOD is more sensitive to gonadotropin stimulation. The exact mechanism is unknown although it is possible that the increased ovarian stromal blood flow velocity, in combination with a relatively unchanged impedance to blood flow, may reflect increased intraovarian perfusion and thus a greater delivery of gonadotropins to the granulosa cells of the developing follicles. This theory may help to explain the greater likelihood of a multifollicular response. In conclusion, women with PCOD have significantly greater stromal blood flow velocity as detected by transvaginal color Doppler ultrasound. The implication of this in ovulation induction treatment is unknown but may help explain the excessive response often seen in women with PCOD when they are administered gonadotropins. The presence of increased stromal blood flow velocity in both the PCOD and PCOS groups compared to women with normal ovaries supports the notion that the PCOD is a primary disorder of the ovary. The detection of increased ovarian stromal blood flow velocity by color and pulsed Doppler ultrasound may be a marker in the diagnosis of PCOD. It seems that evaluation of the ovarian stromal vascularity by 3D power Doppler will further increase our knowledge on this enigmatic syndrome.

Luteinized Unruptured Follicle Syndrome

Luteinized unruptured follicle (LUF) syndrome is characterized by regular menses and presumptive ovulation as suggested by a cyclic hormonal profile, similar to that seen in normal ovulatory women but without release of the ovum. Although LUF was first diagnosed at laparoscopy by the absence of an ovulation stigma and the demonstration of lower concentrations of estradiol and progesterone in peritoneal fluid compared with normal ovulatory cycles, diagnosis is most commonly made on ultrasound examination, in which there is persistence of the ovarian follicle with progressive loss of its typical echo-free cystic appearance and accumulation of internal echogenicity. The precise etiology of LUF remains uncertain, but impairment of the mid-cycle luteinizing hormone (LH) surge, the absence of the preovulatory progesterone rise, abnormalities of prostaglandin synthesis and a primary abnormality of the oocyte have all been suggested as possible causes. There is a possible association between LUF syndrome and unexplained infertility, chronic pelvic infection and endometriosis. The estimated frequency of this syndrome is between 6 and 47 percent.

Kupesic and coworkers[79] tried to evaluate intraovarian resistance index RI in 47 healthy volunteers with ovulatory cycles and compare them to 28 patients with luteal phase defect (LPD), and four patients with luteinized unruptured follicle (LUF Sy). Serial sonography allowed daily measurement of the mean follicular diameter and observation of LUF syndrome development: the follicular collapse, demarcation of the hypoechoic structure with an irregular wall, formation of solid or complex structure representing the corpus luteum, and the extraovarian signs, such as the thickened endometrium and the lack of the free fluid in the cul-de-sac. All these findings were suggestive of ovulation. Doubtful cases (non-visualization of the corpus luteum and/or lack of the serial measurement) were excluded from the current study. LUF syndrome was documented by daily ultrasound observations and endocrinological measurement. During the period of expected ovulation the follicle remained the same size and maintained tense appearance. Luteinization of the unruptured follicle was seen as a progressive accumulation of the strong echoes located on its periphery.

In the group with regular ovulatory cycles, moderate to high RI (0.56+/–0.06) was obtained at the rim of the follicle. Significant decline of the RI occurred on the day of LH peak (RI 0.44+/–0.04). The lowest RI values were obtained during the mid-luteal phase (RI 0.42+/–0.06), with a return to higher vascular resistance of 0.50+/–0.04 during the late luteal phase. In 15 patients, endometrial biopsy was performed, and normal endometrial dating was detected. In the patients with LUF Sy, no difference in terms of intraovarian RI was obtained after the LH peak. Similar RI values were obtained during the follicular and luteal phase (0.55+/–0.04 vs. 0.54+/–0.06). Furthermore, there was no difference between the sides in terms of intraovarian vascular resistance. The mean progesterone value in this group was 14.1±6.2 ng/ml, and normal endometrial dating was obtained in all patients with LUF Sy.

Similar results were reported by Merce and colleagues[80] who did not observe any drop in perifollicular intraovarian resistance after the LH peak. Interestingly, the so called "luteal conversion" did not take place, indicating that the intraovarian and perifollicular neovascularization were either not produced, or were altered in LUF, probably because follicle failed to rupture.

Indeed, the rise in perifollicular blood flow during the periovulatory period appears to be primarily regulated by LH. Zaidi et al[69] reported decreased blood flow velocity of the peripheral vessels in a patient with LUF Sy after the LH surge to values comparable with those seen in the early follicular phase of the cycle. The reduction in perifollicular blood flow velocity has also been reported in a patient with drug-associated LUF.[81]

Extensive Doppler measurement, biochemical research and three-dimensional ultrasound studies still have to be done to fully clarify the causes and consequences of this syndrome.

Luteal Phase Defect

The formation of corpus luteum is an important event in reproductive cycle and one of the crucial factors in early pregnancy support. After ovulation, blood vessels of the theca layer invade the cavity of the ruptured follicle starting the formation of the corpus luteum.

Small luteal cells produce more and more LH receptors and thus amplify the production of progesterone. This chain reaction goes till the so called mid-luteal phase which is characterized by peak values of blood LH, progesterone, and the lowest resistance index (RI) in corpus luteum blood vessels as proven by transvaginal color and pulsed Doppler by Kupesic et al.[82]

Consequently progesterone suppresses the secretion of gonadotropins, LH and progesterone levels decrease, and RI in the vessels of corpus luteum increases. Whether because of "intrinsic error of mechanism," or because of the interference with external factors (e.g. strenuous exercise, ovulation stimulating drugs), a condition called luteal phase defect (LPD) occurs. Various names have been assigned to the disorder: short luteal phase, luteal insufficiency, inadequate luteal phase, luteal defect and luteal phase deficiency (LPD). All these names describe the same condition: lack of progesterone, luteal phase of the cycle shorter than 11 days and, when related to endometrium, an out-of-phase endometrium by 2 or more days. The new method to detect corpus luteum abnormality is ultrasonography. For a better visualization of the corpus luteum transvaginal approach is used. As an addition to B-mode and realtime image, sophisticated ultrasound equipment includes color and pulsed Doppler sonography. The research into the corpus luteum, LPD, early pregnancy and early pregnancy failures has already taken a whole new direction. Until recently, research in this field was carried out mainly using B mode and realtime imaging. Glock et al[83] tried to determine whether the ultrasound appearance size, or change in size of the corpus luteum of early pregnancy correlated with serum progesterone, estradiol E_2, or 17-hydroxyprogesterone or were even predictive of pregnancy outcome. Their hypothesis was: corpus luteum volumes of early human pregnancy would correlate with the serum concentration of steroids produced in the corpus luteum; appearance of the corpus luteum, based on the amount of cystic component, would correlate with serum hormone concentration or pregnancy outcome; and a decrease in corpus luteum volume would be associated with pregnancy loss. Disappointingly, the acquired data showed a lack of correlation between corpus luteum size and steroid products and no correlation between changes in volume and changes in steroid products in early human pregnancy. However, a decreasing corpus luteum volume before 8th week of gestation is associated with a higher probability of pregnancy loss. Color flow pulsed Doppler was only used to determine dominant ovary with corpus luteum and the contralateral one. Dominant ovary showed low impedance waveform with RI 0.39 to 0.49, characteristic of the blood flow in early pregnancy. The contralateral ovary in each patient demonstrated a high impedance flow RI 0.69 to 1.0, characteristic of nondominant ovary. One patient had an RI value of 0.74 in the ovary identified as having a corpus luteum, and RI of 0.79 in the opposite ovary; this high RI in both ovaries was associated with a nonviable outcome.

Kupesic et al[82] tried to evaluate intraovarian resistance index RI in 47 healthy fertile volunteers with ovulatory cycles and compare them to 28 patients with luteal phase defect (LPD)

and four patients with luteinized unruptured follicle (LUF Sy). Serial sonography allowed daily measurement of the mean follicular diameter, visualization of the follicular collapse and demarcation of the hypoechoic structure with an irregular wall, solid or complex structure representing the corpus luteum, as well as observation of the thickened endometrium, and presence of the free fluid in the cul-de-sac. All these findings were suggestive of ovulation. Doubtful cases (non-visualization of the corpus luteum and/or lack of the serial measurements) were excluded from the current study. LPD was diagnosed by measuring the progesterone levels and performing the endometrial biopsy during the mid-luteal phase of the menstrual cycle. Sonographic and Doppler findings were correlated to hormonal and histopathological data.

In the group with regular ovulatory cycles (n=47) different ovarian RI values have been observed. During the stage of the follicular growth and development, moderate to high RI (mean 0.56 ± 0.06) was obtained at the rim of the follicle. Significant decline of the RI occurred for the day of LH peak (RI 0.44 ± 0.04). The lowest RI values were obtained during the mid-luteal phase (RI 0.42 ± 0.06), with a return to higher vascular resistance of 0.50 ± 0.04 during the late luteal phase. In the LPD group (n=28) no difference was obtained in terms of intraovarian RI during the follicular phase. However, the mean RI throughout the luteal phase (RI 0.56 ± 0.04) was significantly higher compared to the normals. Furthermore, it did not show any difference between the early, middle and late luteal phase in LPD group.

In the control group, both follicular and luteal RI was significantly lower on the dominant side. However, in the LPD group no difference occurred in terms of intraovarian RI between the sides. Mean progesterone levels were significantly lower in the LPD group (6.9 ± 2.3 ng/ml) than in the controls (24.1 ± 11.4 ng/ml), while histopathology revealed delayed endometrial pattern in all the patients with LPD. The correlation was observed between progesterone and RI during the mid-luteal phase.

Merce et al[80] elaborated on all aspects of transvaginal color and pulsed Doppler ultrasonography: its advantages, disadvantages, current possibilities and future directions. In their study of luteal ovarian blood flow they introduced the term "luteal conversion" to describe Doppler findings during the luteal phase: easily obtained Doppler signals, increase in intensity of frequency spectrum, increase in turbulence of the blood flow with extensive dispersion of the maximum frequencies and superposition of multiple waveforms presenting variable maximum systolic velocities and, finally, an increase in the surface and intensity that the color signal occupies in the ovary. The same authors, in their study of LPD, observed that the resistance index (RI) of the dominant ovary drops during the luteal phase with respect to the follicular phase, as also occurs in normal cycles and no differences were noted in this aspect when comparing with any phase of the normal cycle. No significant correlation was demonstrated between the index values and serum progesterone levels either.

Glock and Brumsted[84] correlated ovarian blood flow to values of progesterone throughout the cycle. Mean progesterone levels were significantly lower for LPD patients than for normal women throughout the luteal phase. Mean resistance index in LPD patients was significantly higher compared with normal women throughout the follicular and luteal phases. Although systolic and diastolic velocities were observed to be lower in LPD patients compared with normal women, these differences were not statistically different. High correlations were observed between progesterone and resistance index within each of the luteal time points, achieving its highest value during the mid-luteal phase luteal. The mean resistance index in the dominant ovary was significantly lower than in the nondominant ovary throughout the cycle in normal women (0.50 versus 0.65), but not in those with LPD (0.60 versus 0.66 P=0.37). In single patient with anovulatory cycle, intraovarian resistance index values remained high (mean 0.76, range 0.70 to 0.82).

This study[84] showed a clear correlation between the resistance index of corpus luteum blood flow and plasma progesterone in the natural cycle. The strongest correlation was seen in the mid-luteal phase, the period that corresponds to peak neovascularization of the corpus luteum. Consistent to this finding, the authors showed an increase in blood flow impedance in the late luteal phase, the period associated with the onset of corpus luteum regression. These findings suggest the possibility of using the resistance index of corpus luteum blood flow as an adjunct to plasma progesterone assay, as an index of luteal function.

Tinkanen,[85] on the other hand found no difference between the blood flow in the corpus luteum in controls with normal luteal phase and infertility patients with abnormal luteal phase. Short luteal phase, claims the author, is not due to premature vascular regression of the corpus luteum as evaluated by measurement of the vascular resistance.

Strigini et al.[86] observed the change of impedance during the luteal phase of FSH-treated cycles. The uterine pulsatility index during stimulated cycles, both before and after ovulation, was significantly reduced compared with spontaneous cycles. That was explained by the increase of plasma E$_2$. Furthermore, Strigini advocates administration of exogenous progesterone as a

supplementation to FSH treated cycles, stating that uterine pulsatility index after administration of progesterone drops even more than in spontaneous or only with FSH treated cycles.

Kupesic et al[82] correlated Doppler velocimetry, histological and hormonal markers. They presumed that when combined together, ultrasound results, measurement of hormone values and endometrial biopsy could explain more about LPD. They found out that mean progesterone levels were significantly lower in the group with luteal phase defect (10.2 ± 4.3 ng/ml) than in controls (21 ± 4.2 ng/ml). The FSH/LH ratio was significantly lower in the group with a delayed endometrial pattern compared to normal subjects during follicular and periovulatory phases (0.70 vs. 1.24; 0.58 vs. 0.75, respectively). There was a close correlation between estradiol levels and the mean diameter of the dominant follicle from days –5 to –1 relative to the days of sonographically observed ovulation. An increase in follicular diameter and endometrial thickness was noted for both normal and luteal phase defect groups.

Intraovarian blood flow resistance showed no difference between the groups during the proliferative phase. A significant decline of the RI occurred in the control group for the day of the LH peak (RI=0.45 ± 0.04), with a return to the follicular phase level of 0.49 ± 0.02 during the second phase of the menstrual cycle (Figs 22.12A to F). The mean intraovarian RI for the luteal phase defect group (RI=0.58 ± 0.04) was significantly higher than in the control group throughout the luteal phase (Fig. 22.13). Patients in control group had a significantly lower RI in dominant than in nondominant ovary, whereas LPD patients had the almost same RI in both ovaries. The authors measured blood flow in spiral arteries as well. Spiral arteries in the control group demonstrated an RI of 0.53 ± 0.04 during the periovulatory phase, and RI values of 0.50 ± 0.02 and 0.51 ± 0.04 were obtained during the mid-luteal and late luteal phase, respectively. Higher impedance values during the periovulatory phase (RI=0.70 ± 0.06, p<0.001), mid-luteal phase (RI=0.72 ± 0.06, p<0.001) and late luteal phase (RI=0.72 ± 0.04, p<0.001) were obtained from the spiral arteries in the luteal phase defect group. A close correlation has been found between plasma levels of estradiol and the mean diameter of the follicle. The study clearly demonstrated that patients with normal endometrial development show a similar trend of regression for uterine, radial and spiral artery impedance from the follicular to the luteal phase. In contrast, patients with a delayed endometrial pattern are characterized by increased uterine vascular resistance during the luteal phase. Since the most significant difference in terms of RI is obtained for spiral arteries, it might be expected that endometrial blood flow changes could be used to predict the development of the endometrium and likelihood of pregnancy.

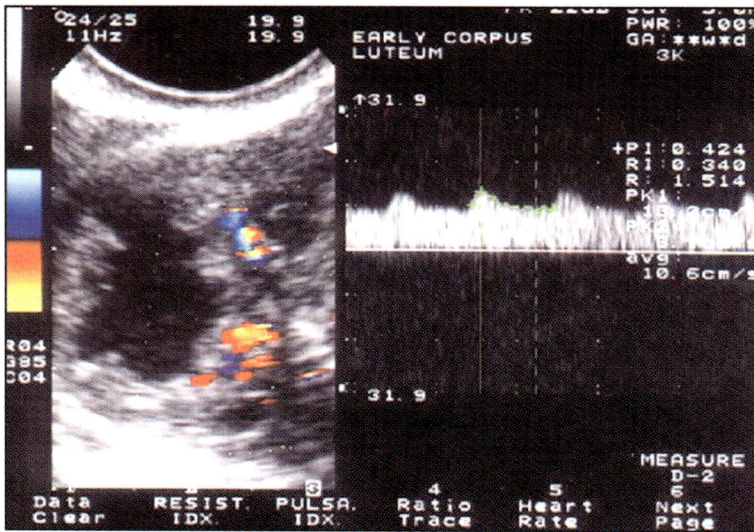

Fig. 22.12A: Pulsed Doppler waveform analysis shows high velocity and low resistance index (RI=0.34), both indicative of normal corpus luteum function

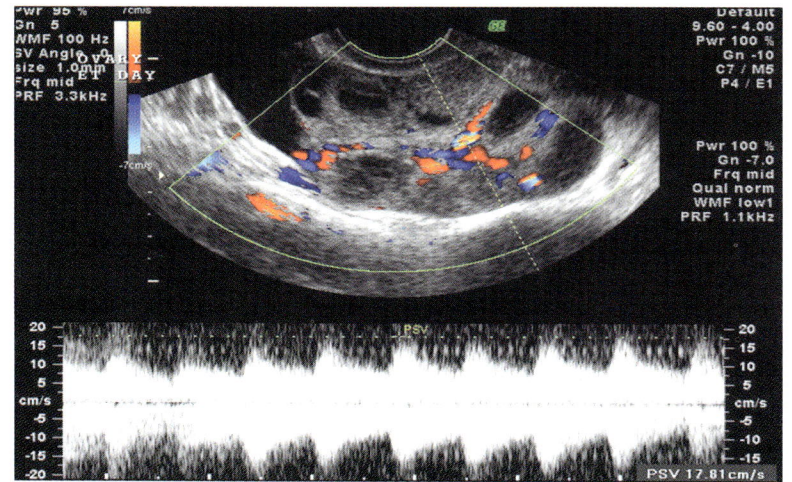

Fig. 22.12B: Transvaginal image of corpus luteum, present retrouterine fluid is another sign of ovulation

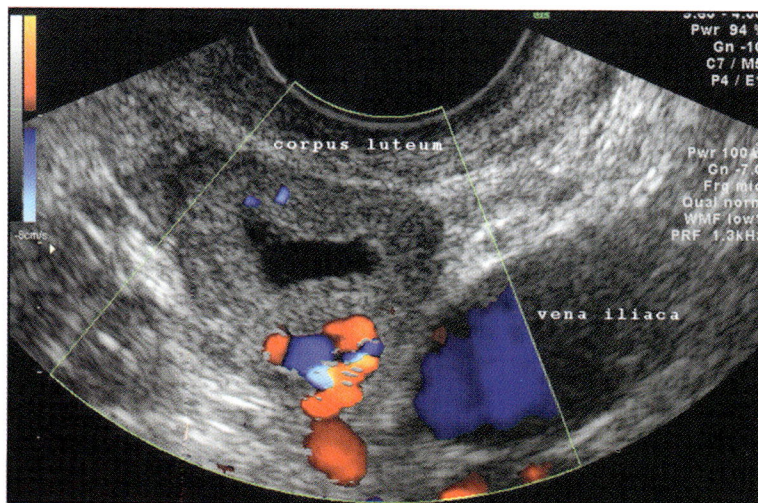

Fig. 22.12C: Color Doppler image of corpus luteum, note the peripheral vascularization

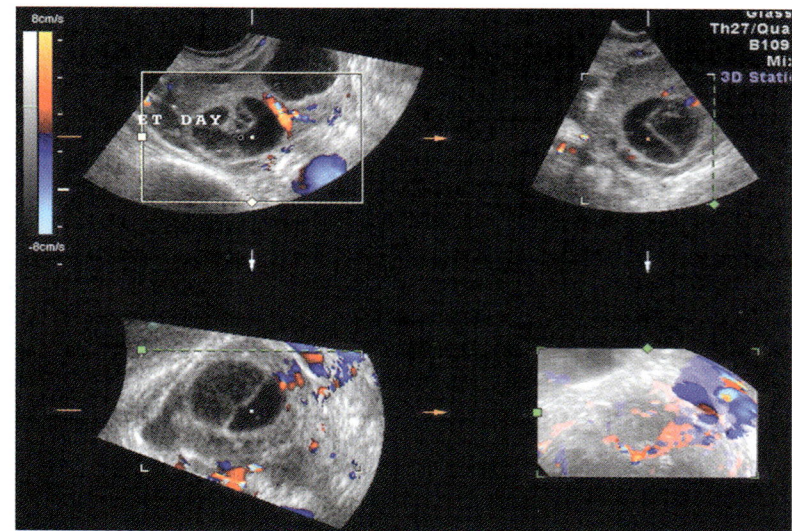

Fig. 22.12D: Hyperstimulated ovary prior to embryo transfer procedure. Color Doppler flow analysis can predict luteal function

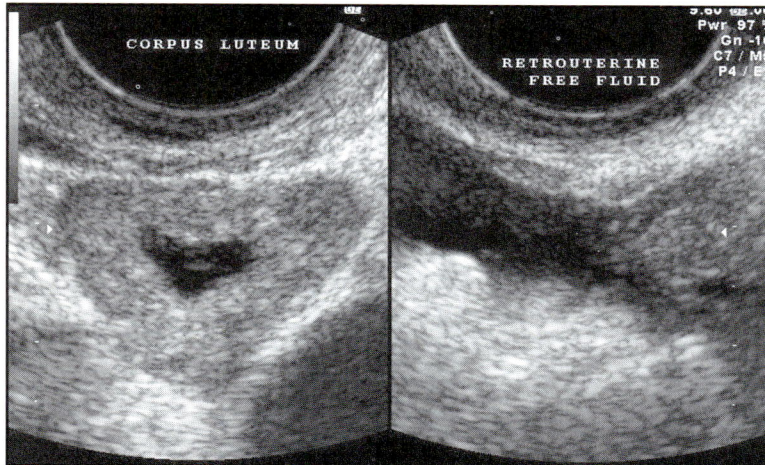

Fig. 22.12E: Three-dimensional color Doppler image of corpus luteum prior to embryo transfer procedure

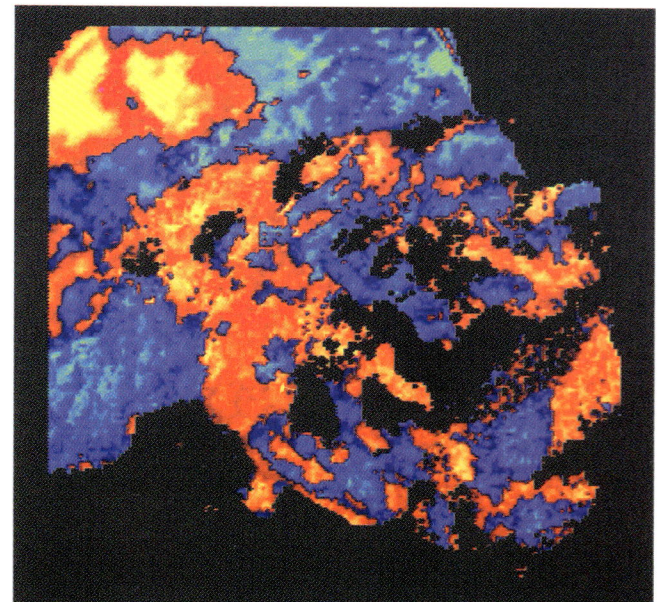

Fig. 22.12F: Three-dimensional color Doppler image of corpus luteum vascularization

Salim et al[87] correlated luteal blood in normal pregnancies to the flow in abnormal pregnancies. Their study proved the hypothesis that an absence of luteal flow cannot coexist with normal pregnancy. Impedance to intraovarian blood flow was significantly higher in patients with abnormal early pregnancy (missed, incomplete, and threatened abortion) than in women

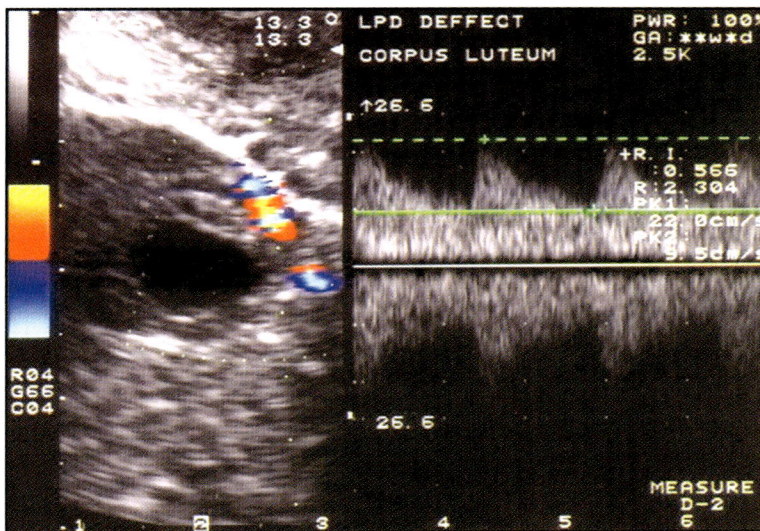

Fig. 22.13: This is a case of luteal phase defect. The increased intraovarian resistance index (RI=0.56) obtained during the midluteal phase indicates luteal phase defect

with normal pregnancy. However, this was not confirmed in patients with blighted ovum, molar, and ectopic pregnancy. The impedance to luteal blood flow was almost the same as in normal pregnancy. This difference among subgroups of abnormal early pregnancy may relate to a different natural history of the disease. Missed and incomplete abortions are manifested as failed early pregnancy with no prospects for further development. Threatened abortion is a potentially similar condition. Whether decreased corpus luteum blood flow is a potential cause or a consequence of the disease remains unclear. Anembryonic pregnancies, molar or ectopic pregnancies are somewhat different. These pathologic conditions usually are progressive and not self-limited. This can explain why is impedance to luteal blood flow in these women similar to that in women with normally progressing pregnancies.

Alcazar et al.[88] agree only partially on the results Salim et al Obtained.[87] Alcazar's grop found out that mean RI in missed abortion was higher than in controls. This increased vascular resistance could be explained by the fact that missed abortion consists of a failure of early pregnancy to develop, in which the production of human chorionic gonadotropin is impaired, which in turn could have a negative effect on luteal function. On the other hand, they found no statistically significant difference in RI of patients with threatened abortion.

TUBAL CAUSES OF INFERTILITY

The tubal mucosa responds to the hormonal changes during the menstrual cycle in order to facilitate the transport of sperm and fertilized ova in the process of fertilization. During the luteal phase, decreased tube secretion and more prominent ciliary activity propel the ova into the uterine fundus. If conception

does not occur, the secretory and ciliary cells are significantly reduced in number due to withdrawal of endocrine support.

The normal fallopian tubes are narrow and usually not seen by transabdominal or transvaginal ultrasound unless they contain fluid within their lumina or are surrounded by fluid. The motility and transport function of the oviducts are impaired during all stages of pelvic inflammatory disease. First, in the acute phase, the tube becomes thick and edematous and a large amount of purulent exudates fill the lumen. Later on, the inflammatory process may be organized to form tuboovarian abscess, which will, in most cases lead to scarring and occlusion of the tube. Chronic hydrosalpinx is the ultimate remnant of the PID: the tube is occluded, thin-walled and filled with fluid. (Figs 22.14A and B).

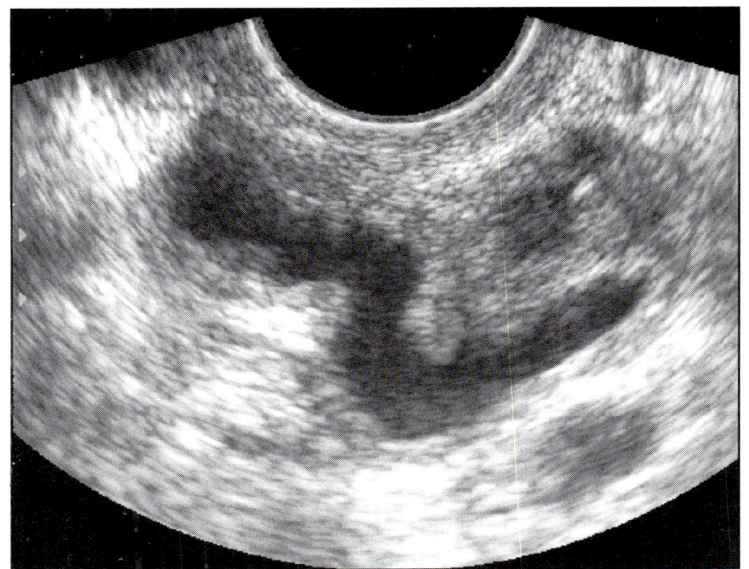

Fig. 22.14A: Unilateral sactosalpinx visualized by transvaginal ultrasound

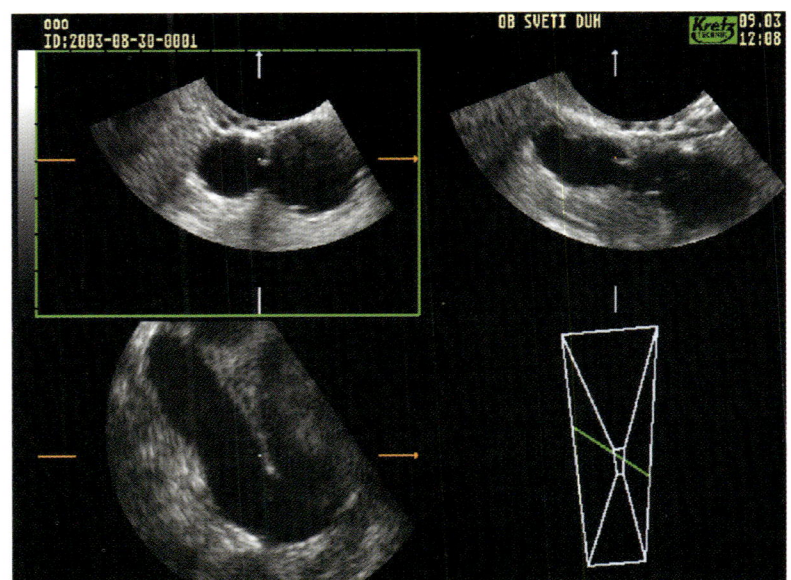

Fig. 22.14B: Three-dimensional image of sactosalpinx

Infertility caused by tubal dysfunction is found in approximately 35 percent of patients. A history of pelvic inflammatory disease, septic abortion, intrauterine contraceptive device, ruptured appendix, tubal surgery or ectopic pregnancy should alert the physician to the possibility of tubal damage. Amorphous acellular plugs have been identified as the probable cause of obstruction in the proximal tube in nearly 50 percent of women whose tubes did not opacify on hysterosalpingography. The improved pregnancy rate after uterotubal insufflation and hysterosalpingography suggests that their therapeutic effect may partially result from dislodgment of fallopian tube debris. Reversible spasm at the uterotubal junction is another cause of apparent obstruction on conventional hysterosalpingography. In 100 patients with nonfilling on an initial hysterosalpingogram, Lang[89] found that only 39 had persistent occlusion after pharmacologic manipulation and selective tubal salpingography. In the remaining 61 patients the apparent cause of tubal nonfilling was spasm and debris in 49 patients, submucous fibroids in six, synechiae in three, salpingitis isthmica nodosa in two, and septated uterus in one.

Until a few years ago the assessment of the uterine cavity and the fallopian tube lumen relied on complicated, painful and invasive procedures. The major problem was how to visualize the hollow space within these organs and how to describe the contours of uterine and oviduct walls. The functions of the uterus and the fallopian tubes depend on their cavities: a uterus filled with endometrial polyp or distorted by a myoma is an obstacle to implantation, while a tortuous and narrow tube with the PID changes does not permit oocytes to descend.

Hysterosalpingography, using radiopaque dye for X-ray assessment of tubal and uterine anatomy, has been the standard form of investigation for several decades. The disadvantage of this type of investigation is that ionizing radiation presents a risk to the oocyte: if the conception takes place in the investigation cycle, congenital fetal anomalies may occur. Furthermore, iodine-containing dyes used in X-ray hysterosalpingography can cause allergic reaction.

In the last two decades, laparoscopy has been the usual procedure for the assessment of tubal status. However, it requires general anesthesia and carries the risk of anesthetic and surgical complications, such as bowel or vascular injury, false pneumoperitoneum and postoperative discomfort.

Together with the development of ultrasound technique, a totally new concept of diagnostic procedures has been developed. We have already described in the chapter on hysterosonosalpingography benefits and limitations of the sonographic evaluation of the tubal patency.

CONCLUSIONS

Transvaginal sonography, color Doppler and three-dimensional ultrasound with power Doppler facilities have made a significant improvement in the assessment of infertility. They may help in prediction of ovulation and detection of ovulatory disorders. Measurements of uterine perfusion have a predictive value regarding fecundity in patients undergoing different methods of medically-assisted reproduction. Absent subendometrial and intraendometrial vascularization on the day of hCG administration appears to be a useful predictor of failure of implantation in IVF cycles, irrespective of the morphological appearance of the endometrium. Studies on spiral artery perfusion might produce a non-invasive assay of uterine receptivity, giving us more information on the pathophysiology of infertility, especially in the group of patients with unexplained causes.

REFERENCES

1. Kurjak A, Kupesic-Urek S, Schulman H, Zalud I. Transvaginal color Doppler in the assessment of ovarian and uterine blood flow in infertile women. Fertil. Steril., 1991;56: 870.
2. Kurjak A, Kupesic-Urek S. Normal and abnormal uterine perfusion. In Jaffe R, Warsof LS (Eds) : Color Doppler Imaging in Obstetrics and Gynecology, New York: McGraw Hill. 1992; pp 255-63.
3. Goswamy RK, Silliams G, Steptoe PC. Decreased uterine perfusion a cause of infertility. Hum Reprod 1988; 3:955-8.
4. Steer CV, Mills CV, Campbell S. Vaginal color Doppler assessment on the day of embryo transfer (ET) accurately predicts patients in an in vitro fertilization programme with suboptimal uterine perfusion who fail to become pregnant. Ultrasound Obstet Gynaecol 1991;1:79-82.
5. Tsai YC, Chang JC, Tai MJ, Kung FT, Yang LC, Chang SY. Relationship of uterine perfusion to outcome of intrauterine insemination. J. Ultrasound Med., 1996; 5:633-6.
6. Steer CV, Tan SL, Mason BA, Campbell S. Midluteal phase vaginal color Doppler assessment of uterine artery impedance in a subfertile population. Fertil. Steril, 1994;61:53-8.
7. Kupesic S. The first three weeks assessed by transvaginal color Doppler. J. Perinat Med 1996;24:301-17.
8. Cacciatore B, Simberg N, Fusaro P, Tiitinen A. Transvaginal Doppler study of uterine artery blood flow in in vitro fertilization - embryo transfer cycles. Fertil. Steril 1996;66(1):130-4.
9. Freidler S, Schenker JG, Herman A, Lewin A. The role of ultrasonography in the evaluation of endometrial receptivity following assisted reproductive treatments: a critical review. Hum Reprod Update, 1996;2:323-35.
10. Gonen Y, Calderon M, Direnfeld M, Abramovici H. The impact of sonographic assessment of the endometrium and meticulous hormonal monitoring during natural cycles in patients with failed donor artificial insemination. Ultrasound Obstet Gynecol 1991;1:122-6.
11. Abdalla HI, Brooks AA, Johnson MR, Kirkland A, Thomas A, Studd JW. Endometrial thickness: a predictor of implantation in ovum recipients? Hum Reprod 1994;9:363-5.
12. Khalifa E, Brzyski RG, Oehninger S, Acosta AA, Muasher SJ. Sonographic appearance of the endometrium: the predictive value for the outcome of in vitro fertilization in stimulated cycles. Hum Reprod 1992;7:677-80.
13. Serafini P, Batzofin J, Nelson J, Olive D. Sonographic uterine predictors of pregnancy in women undergoing ovulation induction for assisted reproductive treatments. Fertil Steril 1994;62:815-22.
14. Sher G, Herbert C, Maassarani G, Jacobs MH. Assessment of the late proliferative phase endometrium by ultrasonography in patients undergoing in vitro fertilization and embryo transfer (IVF/ET). Hum Reprod 1991;6:232-7.
15. Zaidi J, Campbell S, Pitroff R, Tan SL. Endometrial thickness, morphology, vascular penetration and velocimetry in predicting implantation in an in vitro fertilization program. Ultrasound Obstet 1995.
16. Kyei-Mensah A, Maconochie N, Zaidi J, Pittrof R, Campbell S, Tan SL. Transvaginal three-dimensional ultrasound: reproducibility of ovarian and endometrial volume measurements. Fertil Steril 1996;66:718-22.
17. Riccabona M, Nelson TR, Pretorius DH. Three-dimensional ultrasound: accuracy of distance and volume measurements. Ultrasound Obstet Gynecol., 1996;4:29-34.
18. Gilja OH, Smievoll I, Thune N, Matre K, Hausken T, Odegaard S. In vivo comparison of 3D ultrasonography and magnetic resonance imaging in volume estimation of human kidney. Ultrasound Med Biol 1995;21:25-32.

19. Lee A, Sator M, Kratochwil A, Deutinger J, Vytiska-Binsdorfer E, Bernaschek G. Endometrial volume change during spontaneous menstrual cycles: volumetry by transvaginal three-dimensional ultrasound. Fertil Steril 1997;68:831-5.

20. Kyei-Mensah A, Zaidi J, Pittrof R, Shaker A, Campbell S, Tan SL. Transvaginal three-dimensional ultrasound: accuracy of follicular volume measurements. Fertil Steril 1996;65:371-6.

21. Kupesic S, Bekavac I, Bjelos D, Kurjak A. Assessment of endometrial receptivity by transvaginal color Doppler and three-dimensional power Doppler ultrasonography in patients undergoing in vitro fertilization procedures. J Ultrasound Med 2001;20:125-34.

22. Ashton D, Amin HK, Richart RM, Neuwirth R. S. The incidence of asymptomatic uterine anomalies in women undergoing transcervical tubal sterilization. Obstet Gynecol 1988;72:28-30.

23. Sorensen S. Estimated prevalence of mulerian anomalies. Acta Obstet Gynecol Scand 1988;67:441-5.

24. Gaucherand P, Awada A, Rudigoz RC, Dargent D. Obstetrical prognosis of septate uterus: a plea for treatment of the septum. Eur. J. Obstet Gynecol Reprod Biol 1994;54:109-12.

25. Fedele L, Arcaini L, Parazzini F, Vercellini P, Nola GD. Metroplastic hysteroscopy and fertility Fertil Steril, 1993;59:768-70.

26. Heinonen PK, Saarikoski S, Pystynen P. Reproductive performance of women with uterine anomalies. An evaluation of 182 cases. Acta Obstet Gynecol Scand 1982;61:157-62.

27. Fedele L, Bianchi S, Marchini M, Franchi D, Tozzi L, Dorta M. Ultrastructural aspects of endometrium in infertile women with septate uterus. Fertil Steril 1996;65:750-2.

28. Cararach M, Penella J, Ubeda, J, Iabastida R. Hysteroscopic incision of the septate uterus: scissors versus resectoscope. Hum Reprod 1994;9:87-9.

29. Goldenberg M, Sivan E, Sharabi Z. Reproductive outcome following hysteroscopic management of intrauterine septum and adhesions. Hum Reprod 1995;10:2663-5.

30. Valdes C, Malini S, Malinak LR. Ultrasound evaluation of female genital tract anomalies: a review of 64 cases. Am J Obstet Gynecol 1984;149:285-90.

31. Nicolini U, Bellotti B, Bonazzi D, Zamberleti G, Battista C. Can ultrasound be used to screen uterine malformation? Fertil Steril 1987;47:89-93.

32. Reuter KL, Daly DC, Cohen SM. Septate versus bicornuate uteri: errors in imaging diagnosis. Radiology. 1989;172:749-52.

33. Randolph J, Ying Y, Maier D, Schmidt C, Riddick D. Comparison of realtime ultrasonography, hysterosalpingography, and laparoscopy/hysteroscopy in the evaluation of uterine abnormalities and tubal patency. Fertil. Steril. 1986;5:828-32.

34. Richman TS, Viscomi GN, Cherney AD, Polan A. Fallopian tubal patency assessment by ultrasound following fluid injection. Radiology, 1984;152:507-10.

35. Salle B, Sergeant P, Galcherand P, Guimont I, De Saint Hilaire P, Rudigoz RC. Transvaginal hysterosonographic evaluation of septate uteri: a preliminary report. Hum. Reprod. 1996;11:1004-7.

36. Marshall C, Mintz DI, Thickman D, Gussman H, Kressel Y. MR evaluation of uterine anomalies. Radiology, 1987;148:287-9.

37. Carrington BM, Hricak M, Naruddin RN. Mullerian duct anomalies: MR evaluation. Radiology, 1990;170:715-20.

38. Jurkovic D, Giepel A, Gurboeck K, Jauniaux E, Natucci M. Campbell S. Three dimensional ultrasound for the assessment of uterine anatomy and detection of congenital anomalies: a comparison with hysterosalpingography and two-dimensional sonography. Ultrasound Obstet. Gynecol. 1995;5:233-7.

39. Taylor PJ, Cumming DC. Hysteroscopy in 100 patients. Fertil Steril 1979;31:301-4.

40. Kupesic S, Kurjak A. Septate uterus: detection and prediction of obstetrical complications by different forms of ultrasonography. J. Ultrasound Med. 1998;17:631-6.

41. Dabrashrafi H, Bahadori M, Mohammad K, Alavi M, Moghadami-Tabrizi N, Zandinejad R. Septate uterus: new idea on the histologic features of the septum in this abnormal uterus. Am J Obstet Gynecol 1995;172:105-7.

42. Balen FG, Allen CM, Gardener JE, Siddle NC, Lees WR. 3-dimensional reconstruction of ultrasound images of the uterine cavity. The British Journal of Radiology. 1993;66;588-91.

43. Weinraub Z, Maymon R, Shulman A, Bukovsky J, Kratochwil A, Lee A, Herman A. Three-dimensional saline contrast rendering of uterine cavity pathology. Ultrasound Obstet. Gynecol. 1996;277-82.

44. Kupesic S, Kurjak A, Skenderovic S, Bjelos D. Screening for uterine abnormalities by three-dimensional ultrasound improves perinatal outcome. J. Preinat. Med. 2002;30:9-17.

45. Kurjak A, Kupesic S, Miric D. The assessment of benign uterine tumor vascularization by transvaginal color Doppler. Ultrasound Med. Biol. 1992;18:645-9.

46. Brosens JJ, deSouza NM, Barker FG, Paraschos T, Winston RM. Endovaginal ultrasonography in the diagnosis of adenomyosis uteri: identifying the predictive characteristics. Br. J. Obstet Gynaecol 1995;102(6); 471.

47. Schlaff WD, Hurst BS. Preoperative sonographic measurement of endometrial pattern predicts outcome of surgical repair in patients with severe Asherman's syndrome. Fertil Steril 1995;63:410-3.

48. Zaidi J, Barber J, Kyei-Mensah A, Pittrof R, Campbell S, Tan SL. Relationship of ovarian stromal blood flow at baseline ultrasound to subsequent follicular response in an in vitro fertilization program. Obstet Gynecol 1996;88:779-84.

49. Engmann L, Sladkevicius P, Agrawal R, Bekir JS, Campbell S, Tan SL. Value of ovarian stromal blood flow velocity measurement after pituitary suppression in the prediction of ovarian responsiveness and outcome of in vitro fertilization treatment. Fertil. Steril. 1999;71(1):22-9.

50. Wittmack FM, Kreger DO, Blasco L, Tureck RW, Mastroianni L Jr, Lessey BA. Effect of follicular size on oocyte retrieval, fertilization, cleavage, and embryo quality in vitro fertilization cycles: a 6-year data collection. Fertil. Steril. 1994;62:1205-10.

51. Golan A, Herman A, Soffer, Y, Bukovsky, I. Ron-El, R. Ultrasonic control without hormone determination for ovulation induction in in-vitro fertilization/embryo-transfer with gonadotropin-releasing hormone analogue and human menopausal gonadotrophin. Hum Reprod, 1994;9:1631-3.

52. Shoham Z, DiCarlo C, Pater A, Conway GS, Jacobs HS. Is it possible to run a successful ovulation induction program based solely on ultrasound monitoring? The importance of endometrial measurements. Fertil Steril 1991;56:836-41.

53. Tan SL. Simplification of IVF therapy. Curr Opin Obstet Gynecol 1994;6:111-4.

54. Steiner H, Staudach A, Spitzer D, Schaffer H. Three-dimensional US in obstetrics and gynaecology: technique, possibilities and limitations. Hum. Reprod. 1994;9;1773-8.

55. Penzias AS, Emmi AM, Dubey AK, Layman LC, DeCherney AH, Reindollar RH. Ultrasound prediction of follicle volume: is the mean diameter reflective? Fertil. Steril, 1994;62:1274-6.

56. Feichtinger W. Transvaginal three-dimensional imaging for evaluation and treatment of infertility. In Merz E (Ed). 3-D Ultrasound in Obstetrics and Gynecology. Philadelphia: Lipincott Williams & Wilkins, 1998;pp 37-43.

57. Lass A, Skull J, McVeigh E, Margara R, Winston RM. Measurement of ovarian volume by transvaginal sonography before ovulation induction with human menopausal gonadotropin for in vitro fertilization can predict poor response. Hum Reprod 1997;12:294-7.

58. Oyesanya OA, Parsons JH, Collins WP, Campbell S. Total ovarian volume before human chorionic gonadotrophin administration for ovulation induction may predict the hyperstimulation syndrome. Hum Reprod 1995;10;3211-2.

59. Kupesic S, Kurjak A. Predictors of in vitro fertilization outcome by three-dimensional ultrasound. Hum Reprod 2002;17(4):950-5.

60. Kupesic S. The present and future role of three-dimesional ultrsound in assisted conception. Ultrsound Obstet Gynecol 2001;18:191-4.

61. Adams J, Franks S, Polson DW, Mason HD, Abdulwahid N, Tucker M, Morris DV, Price J, Jacobs HS. Multifollicular ovaries: clinical and endocrine features and response to pulsatile gonadotropin-releasing hormone. Lancet. 1985;2;1375-8.

62. Matsunaga I, Hata T, Kitao M. Ultrasonographic identification of polycystic ovary. Asia-Oceania J Obstet Gynecol 1985;11:227-32.

63. Takahashi K, Ozaki T, Okada M, Uchida A, Kitao M. Relationship between ultrasonography and histopathological changes in polycystic ovarian syndrome. Hum Reprod 1994;9:2255-8.

64. Battaglia C, Artini PG, D'Ambrogio G, Galli PA, Genazzani AR. Uterine and ovarian blood flow measurement. Does the full bladder modify the flow resistance? Acta Obstet Gynecol Scand 1994;73:716-8.

65. Ardaens Y, Robert Y, Lemaitre L, Fossati P, Dewailly D. Polycystic ovarian disease: contribution of vaginal endosonography and reassessment of ultrasonic diagnosis. Fertil Steril 1991;55:1062-8.

66. Robert Y, Dubrulle F, Gaillandre L, Ardaens Y, Thomas-Desrousseaux P, Lemaitre L, Dewailly D. Ultrasound assessment of ovarian stroma hypertrophy in hyperandrogenism and ovulation disorders: visual analysis versus computerized quantification. Fertil Steril 1995;64:307-12.

67. Merce LT, Garces D, Barco MJ, De la Fuente P. Intraovarian Doppler velocimetry in ovulatory, dysovulatory and anovulatory cycles. Ultrasound Obstet Gynecol 1992;2:197-202.

68. Battaglia C, Artini PG, D'Ambrogio G, Genazzani AD, Genazzani AR. The role of color Doppler imaging in the diagnosis of polycystic ovary syndrome. Am J Obstet Gynecol 1995;172:108-13.

69. Zaidi J, Campbell S, Pittrof R, Kyei-Mensah A, Shaker A, Jacobs HS, Tan SL. Ovarian stromal blood flow in women with polycystic ovaries— a possible new marker for diagnosis? Hum Reprod 1995;10:1992-5.

70. Aleem FA, Predanic M. Transvaginal color Doppler determination of the ovarian and uterine blood flow characteristics in polycystic ovary disease. Fertil Steril 1996;65:510-6.

71. Battaglia C, Artini PG, Salvatori M, Giulini S, Petraglia F, Maxia N, Volpe A. Ultrasonographic patterns of polycystic ovaries; color Doppler and hormonal correlations. Ultrasound Obstet Gynecol. 1998;11:332-6.

72. Battaglia C, Artini PG, Genazzani AD, Florio P, Salvatori M, Sgherzi MR, Giulini S, Lombardo M, Volpe A. Color Doppler analysis in oligo- and amenorrheic women with polycystic ovary syndrome. Gynecol Endocrinol 1997;11:105-10.

73. Battaglia C, Artini PG, Genazzani AD, Sgherzi MR, Salvatori M, Giulini S, Volpe A. Color Doppler analysis in lean and obese women with polycystic ovary syndrome. Ultrasound Obstet Gynecol 1996;7:342-6.

74. Wild RA, Van Nort JJ, Grubb B, Bachman W, Hartz A, Bartholomew M. Clinical signs of androgen excess as risk factors for coronary artery disease. Fertil Steril 1990;54:255-9.

75. Wu MH, Tang HH, Hsu CC, Wang ST, Huang KE. The role of three-dimensional ultrasonographic images in ovarian measurement. Fertil Steril 1998;69:1152-5.

76. Robert Y, Dubrulle F, Gaillandre L, Ardaens Y, Thomas-Desrousseaux P, Lemaitre L. Ultrasound assessment of ovarian stroma hypertrophy in hyperandrogenism and ovulation disorders: visual analysis versus computerized quantification. Fertil. Steril 1995;64:307-12.

77. MacDougall MJ, Tan SL, Balen A, Jacobs HS. A controlled study comparing patients with and without polycystic ovaries undergoing in-vitro fertilization. Hum Reprod. 1993;8:233-7.

78. MacDougall MJ, Tan SL, Jacobs HS. In-vitro fertilization and the ovarian hyperstimulation syndrome. Hum Reprod 1992;7:597-600.

79. Kupesic S, Kurjak A. The assessment of normal and abnormal luteal function by transvaginal color Doppler sonography Eur J Obstet Gynecol Reprod Biol 1997;72:83-87.

80. Merce LT, Garces D, De la Fuente F Conversion lutea de la onda de velocidad de fluio ovarica: nuevo parametro ecografico de ovulacion y funcion lutea. Acta. Obstet. Gynecol. Scand (ed. Esp) 1989;2:113-4.

81. Bourne TH, Reynolds K, Waterstone J, Okokon E, Jurkovic D, Campbell S, Collins WP. Paracetamol-associated luteinized unruptured follicle syndrome: effect on intrafollicular blood flow. Ultrasound Obstet Gynecol 1991;1:420-5.

82. Kupesic S, Kurjak A, Vujisic S, Petrovic Z. Luteal phase defect: comparison between Doppler velocimetry, histological and hormonal markers. Ultrasound Obstet Gynaecol, 1997;9:1-8.

83. Glock JL, Blackman JA, Badger GJ, Brumsted JR. Prognostic significance of morphologic changes of the corpus luteum by transvaginal ultrasound in early pregnancy monitoring Obstet Gynecol 1995;85:37-41.

84. Glock JL, Brumsted JR. Color flow pulsed Doppler ultrasound in diagnosing luteal phase defect Fertil Steril 1995;64:500-4.

85. Tinkanen H. The role of vascularization of the corpus luteum in the short luteal phase studied by Doppler ultrasound. Acta Obstet Gynecol Scand 1994;73: 321-3.

86. Strigini FAL, Scida PAM, Parri C, Visconti A, Susini S, Genazzani AR. Modifications in uterine and intraovarian artery impedance in cycles of treatment with exogenous gonadotropins: effects of luteal phase support. Fertil Steril 1995;64:76-80.

87. Salim A, •alud I, Farmakides G, Schulman H, Kurjak A, Latin V. Corpus luteum blood flow in normal and abnormal early pregnancy: Evaluation with transvaginal color and pulsed Doppler sonography. J Ultrasound Med 1994;13:971-95.

88. Alcazar JL, Laparte C, Lopez-Garcia G. Corpus luteum blood flow in abnormal early pregnancy. J Ultrasound Med 1996;15:645-69.

89. Lang, E K Organic vs. functional obstruction of the fallopian tubes: differentiation with prostaglandin antagonist-and B2-mediated hysterosalpingography and selective ostial salpingography. AJR, 1991;157, 77-80

S Kupesic, A Kurjak, D Bjelos

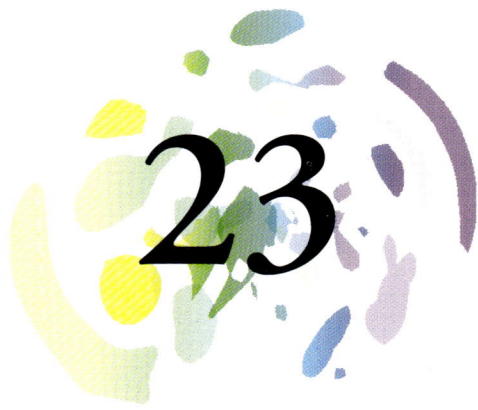

23
Sonohysterography and Sonohysterosalpingography: A Text-atlas of Normal and Abnormal Findings

INTRODUCTION

The number of cases of tubal sterility is increasing and tubal factors, such as tubal dysfunction or obstruction, account for approximately 35 percent of the causes of infertility.[1,2] A history of pelvic inflammatory disease (PID), septic abortion, intrauterine contraceptive device use, ruptured appendix, tubal surgery, or ectopic pregnancy should alter the physician to the possibility of tubal damage. One aspect of the infertility investigation, which has changed little over the last 20 years, is that of the assessment of fallopian tube patency. Until now, the most frequently used procedures to demonstrate tubal patency have been X-ray hysterosalpingography (HSG) and chromopertubation during laparoscopy.[3]

Hysteroscopy is a technique, which complements hysterosalpingography. It can accurately differentiate between endometrial polyps and submucous leiomyomas and can be used for their treatment. The same method is useful in establishing the definitive diagnosis and treatment of intrauterine adhesions and some congenital anomalies of the uterus. Risk factors include perforation of the uterus, hemorrhage, infection and eventually anesthetic risk if anesthesia is required.

Hysteroscopy-directed falloposcopy can detect obstruction of the tubal ostium, and can be utilized to examine the entire length of the tubal lumen.[4] Treatment of the proximal tubal obstruction can immediately follow the diagnosis. Transcervical tubal cannulation or balloon tuboplasty performed by hysteroscopic approach are the methods of choice.[5]

Laparoscopy has been used as the gold standard for investigation of the luteal status in the last two decades, but it requires a general anesthesia and carries the risk of surgical complications, such as bowel or vascular injury, hemorrhage, infection, anesthetic risk, false pneumoperitoneum and postoperative discomfort. With a Jarcho-type of cannula placed in the uterine cavity, one can manipulate the uterus, and by instilling indigo-carmine saline, or other tinted saline, can test for tubal competence. Through laparoscopy one is equally able to visualize the total pelvic anatomy and the upper abdominal cavity. It is also useful for evaluation of the ovarian disease, genital anomalies, tubal and adnexal competence and to differentiate between pelvic distortions. Furthermore, it is valuable to reach an accurate classification of endometriosis of the pelvis. Laparoscopy can be used as an adjunct in assessing possible causes of pelvic pain, the extent of pelvic neoplasia, as well as for a prognostic review of the previous infertility surgical procedure. It has also been helpful in obtaining peritoneal washings and cultures in patients with positive history of PID.

Ultrasound imaging of the pelvic organs has improved significantly with the use of high-frequency vaginal ultrasound probes where the need for bladder filling can be avoided. The normal fallopian tube is usually not seen by vaginal sonography unless some fluid surrounds it. The contrasting fluid may be one of the following: the normal serous fluid, follicular fluid during or after ovulation, blood, ascitic fluid, or products of an exudative or infectious process. If the fallopian tube is not filled with fluid its lumen cannot be detected.

Sonohysterography (SHG) of the uterine cavity and sonohysterosalpingography (sono-HSG) of the tubes are informataive variations of hysterosalpingography (HSG), a standard radiographic technique for studying the reproductive lumina outlined by transcervical infusion of the iodinated contrast under fluoroscopic observation. When sonographic evaluation of the uterine lumen with contrast is combined with evaluation of the tubes, this procedure can be termed sonohysterosalpingography, or sono-HSG. Sonohysterography has also been called hysterosonography and saline infusion sonohysterography.

Benefits of sonohysterosalpingography (sono-HSG) are: avoidance of the ionization or idiosyncrasy to contrast media, method is easily repeatable, requires intraprocedural active participation of the patient (increases her knowledge of tubal status), is a dynamic procedure analyzing tubal motility, the procedure course may be stored, reviewed, analyzed and interpreted to the infertile couple using video-recorder, anesthesia is not required and also collaboration with the Radiology Department.

The accuracy of sono-HSG compared to X-ray HSG varies from 70.37 to 92.20 percent according to Peters et al.[6] and Volpi et al[7] (Table 23.1). The accuracy of sono-HSG compared to chromopertubation is from 81.82 percent according to Stern et al[8], 91.48 percent Kupesic et al[9] to 100.00 percent according to Deichert et al[10] (Table 23.2).

Table 23.1: The accuracy of sonohysterosalpingography (sono-HSG) compared to X-ray HSG

Authors (year)	Total number	Accuracy N (%)	Sensitivity (%)	Specificity (%)
Richman et al (1984)[13]	36	–	100	96
Peters and Coulam (1991)[6]	27	19 (70,37)	–	–
Volpi et al (1991)[7]	21	19 (92,20)	–	–
Stern et al (1992)[8]	89	72 (80,90)	–	–
Battaglia et al (1996)[31]	60	52 (86,66)	–	–

Table 23.2: The accuracy of sono-HSG compared to chromopertubation

Authors (year)	Total number	Accuracy (percent)
Allahbadia et al (1993) [33]	27	25 (92,59)
Tüfekci et al (1992) [20]	38	37 (97,37)
Peters and Coulam (1991) [6]	58	50 (86,20)
Kupesic et al (1994) [9]	47	43 (91,48)
Stern et al (1992) [8]	121	99 (81,82)
Deichert et al (1992) [10]	16	16 (100,00)
Volpi et al (1996) [7]	29	24 (82.7)
Battaglia (1996)[31]	60	56 (93.33)
Raga (1996)[36*]	42	39 (92)
Sladkevicius (2000)[39*]	67	–
Jeanty (2000)[30]	115	91 (79.4)
Kiyokawa (2000)[42*]	25	–

* three-dimensional hysterosonosalpingography

HISTORICAL DEVELOPMENT OF THE ULTRASONIC ASSESSMENT OF THE FALLOPIAN TUBE

In 1954, Rubin[11] the first attempt by insufflating the fallopian tubes.

Ultrasound visualization of the internal genital tract using exogenous contrast media was first described by Nanini et al, Richman et al and Randolph et al[12-14] who performed abdominal sonography after intracervical injection of the fluid.

Richman and colleagues[13] were the first to report on the transabdominal sonographic evaluation of tubal patency. In their studies they used a special intrauterine catheter, Harris uterine injector (Unimar, Canoga Park, CA). After injection of at least 20 ml of the ultrasonic contrast medium Hyskon (dextron in dextrose; Pharmacia Laboratories, Piscataway, NJ), the accumulation of the fluid in the cul-de-sac has been accepted as an indicator of tubal patency.

Randolph and coworkers[14] used transabdominal ultrasound for observation of the cul-de-sac after the injection of 200 ml isotonic saline through the Rubin cannula. The presence of retrouterine fluid was accepted as a criterion for patency of one or both tubes. Tubal patency was deduced indirectly from the presence of increasing fluid in the pouch of Douglas, without differentiation of the sides.

Following instillation of dextran or saline solution into the uterine cavity it was possible to visualize lesions such as submucous myomas and polyps by sonography and subsequently to confirm their presence by hysteroscopy. Although lesions of this type, which project into the uterine cavity, are clearly delineated by poorly echogenic or anechoic media, very small hollow cavities, such as the lumen of normal tubes, are rarely visualizable using these techniques.[13,15] Their demonstration requires visualization of the movement of a fluid, which in turn requires the use of a highly echogenic medium.[16-18]

A new transvaginal ultrasonographic technique was developed in 1989 by Deichert and colleagues.[19] They visualized the patent tube directly and hence showed tubal patency by transcervical injection of an echogenic and ultrasonic contrast fluid SHU 454 (Echovist; Schering, Berlin, Germany). The method has been called Hy-Co-Sy: transvaginal hysterosalpingo-contrast-sonography. They used Rubin cannula or a bladder catheter no.8.

Tüfekci and coworkers[20] have developed an easier technique in which the patient does not require hospitalization. By intrauterine injection of isotonic saline, they evaluated tubal patency directly and called this method transvaginal sonosalpingography.

Transvaginal sonosalpingography performed by using isotonic saline without anesthesia is physiological, easy to perform, safe, cost-effective, noninvasive and more convenient when compared with other conventional methods. Idiosyncrasy to the contrast agent cannot be expected.

ULTRASOUND CONTRAST AGENTS

All media having a different echogenicity from that of the human body can be used as contrast media. Contrast media are divided into two groups: hypoechogenic and hyperechogenic media.

Isotonic saline, Ringer or dextran solutions belong to the first group. Instillation of these media facilitates the detection of echogenic border surfaces. The main disadvantage is that it is not possible to visualize the phenomena of motion and flow.

Hyperechogenic contrast media enhances echo signals, allowing detection of the flow by both B-mode and Doppler ultrasound. Gramiak and Shah[21] and Meltzer and coworkers[22] found that small gas bubbles effectively reflect ultrasonic waves. Therefore, all the commercial echo contrast media contain microbubbles. Commercial products Echovist and Levovist (Schering AG, Berlin) represent suspension of microbubbles made of special galactose microparticles. Galactose microparticle granules are suspended either in galactose solution (Echovist) or in a sterile water (Levovist).[23]

Echovist (SHU 454) is an ultrasound contrast medium consisting of a suspension of only monosaccharide microparticles (50% galactose, diameter 2 mm), in a 20 percent aqueous solution of galactose (w/v). The echogenic suspension is reconstituted immediately before the use from granules and a vehicle solution (200 mg microparticles in 1 ml of suspension).[24] This contrast medium has been licensed for gynecological applications on the market in 1995.

Levovist (SHU 508) microparticle granules contain in addition a very low concentration of physiological palmitic acid.

A few minutes before use, the granules have to be shaken vigorously for 5 to 10 seconds to be dissolved by an appropriate volume of aqueous galactose solution (Echovist) or sterile water (Levovist). A milky suspension of galactose microparticles in a solution is created after disaggregation of the microparticle "snowball." The suspension of Echovist is stable for about 5 min after preparation. Due to its extended stability, Levovist may be administered up to 10 min after the suspension procedure. Depending on the indication and the imaging modality (B-mode or Doppler), clinically adequate suspension of Echovist are with concentrations of 200 and 300 mg/ml. For Levovist, the maximum concentration is 400 mg/ml. The predominant limitation at concentrations lower than 200 mg/ml is the decreasing suspension stability. Concentrations exceeding 400 mg/ml are limited by a rapid increase of viscosity.

After intrauterine administration and emergence of Echovist from the fimbriae into the pelvis, the galactose microparticles dissolve. Warming to body temperature and dilution by the peritoneal fluid increases this progress. In vitro, a rise in temperature of the Echovist suspension to 37°C leads to complete dissolution within 30 min. The dissolved galactose is subsequently absorbed and metabolized.

Numerous clinical studies in the field of echocardiography, venous vascular system analysis and HSG showed no evidence of serious side effects.

Absolute contraindication for instillation of these fluids is galactosemia (autosomal recessive disease in which, due to deficiency of galactose-1-phosphate uridyltransferase, galactose cannot be metabolized into glucose).

In addition, ultrasound contrast agents are media which when administered via the vascular system or into body cavities, change the acoustic properties of the body region under investigation. The acoustic parameters, which contribute to tissue imaging by conventional sonographic units, are backscatter, attenuation and velocity of sound. Enhancement of backscatter is the most important contrast effect, since contrast agents introduce acoustic inhomogenities caused by microstructures (scatterers).

TECHNIQUE OF HY-CO-SY

Requirements

A case history must be obtained from a woman considered for examination using this technique, to rule out the possibility of the rare condition of galactosemia, which is the only absolute contraindication, apart from acute inflammatory disease of the genital organs. A gynecological and ultrasound examination prior to the procedure is necessary to define uterine position and anomalies if present, as well as both adnexal regions. Before any intervention, we perform a pregnancy test for legal reasons. The possibility of local or systemic infections is excluded by clinical examination (absence of elevated temperature), inspection of the genital tract and cervical smears. The procedure should not be performed on patients with active pelvic infections, and antibiotic prophylaxis (doxycycline and metronidazole) should be used in patients with a history of Hy-Co-Sy should be performed during the early follicular phase of the menstrual cycle, after complete cessation of menses. This avoids dispersion of menstrual debris into the peritoneal cavity. Procedures done in this period allow absorption of the media prior to ovulation, thus avoiding the presence of a foreign substance around the time of an imminent corpus luteum. This decreases any theoretic effect the media may have on tubal transport. Hysterosalpingography performed during the immediate premenstrual phase of the cycle has been advocated in the evolution of possible cervical incompetence, as that is the point in the cycle at which there is the maximum uterine constriction. Therefore, in order to maximize the information obtained, the indication for the study has an influence on timing.

Patients are informed of the benefits and the possible risks of the procedure and the procedure itself is described to them in detail.

Anesthesia is generally not required for Hy-Co-Sy, and the patient can follow the results of the examination by herself on the monitor. If Hy-Co-Sy is performed without anesthesia, patients occasionally report discomfort, especially if the tubes are occluded. The degree of discomfort depends on the individual response of the patient. Premedication or sedation is routinely used: 5 to 10 mg of diazepam intravenously is beneficial, especially in anxious patients. Pain signifies the obstruction and potential intravasation or tubal rupture, and should not be masked by anesthesia. However, tubal spasm may occur if Hy-Co-Sy is performed without or even with anesthesia. This could mimic a tubal occlusion. Pretreatment with atropine (0.5 mg) may prevent this complication. The parenteral administration of 1 mg glucagon may relieve the spasm and allow the flow of the contrast.

Benefits and limitations of hysterosonosalpingography are represented in Table 23.3

Table 23.3: Benefits and limitations of sono-HSG

Benefits	*Limitations*
■ Reproducible and reliable assessment of tubal patency if used by a trained physician	■ Tubal spasm may lead to misdiagnosis of tubal occlusion (spasm also seen with other methods)
■ Avoids exposure to X-rays	■ In hydrosalpinx, tubal flow may give a false impression of tubal patency
■ Avoids allergic reactions	■ Cannot visualize intrapelvic pathology and bowel
■ Avoids general anesthesia	■ Requires a degree of technical competence
■ Can be performed as outpatient procedure	■ 10 to 20 investigations needed to acquire the new technique
■ Rapid	
■ Well tolerated: little discomfort and few adverse events	
■ Shows tubal patency to the patient in "realtime"	

Procedure

The patient voids and is positioned supine on the gynecological table. With the patient's legs flexed, a speculum is inserted into the vagina and positioned such that the entire cervix is visualized and the os is easily accessible. The cervix and the vagina are then thoroughly scrubbed with betadine solution. A tenaculum is placed on the anterior lip of the cervix, and the cannula is gently guided into the endocervical canal. Application of the contrast medium is performed via a small and very thin uterine catheter fitted with a balloon for stabilization and occlusion of the internal cervical os. The first observation to be made is of the uterine cavity, with verification of the catheter placement. After removal of the tenaculum, the transvaginal probe is gently introduced into the posterior fornix of the vagina. The contrast (sterile saline) is then injected slowly, under control of the ultrasound. Usually, no more then 5 to 10 ml of contrast is instilled into the uterine cavity. At this stage one can observe the morphology of the uterus and its endometrial lining and detect duplication anomalies of the uterus or existence of endometrial polyps or submucous fibroids that are protruding into the uterine cavity which is marked with anechoic contrast.

Benefits of sono-HSG include: reproducible and reliable assessment of tubal patency if used by a trained physician, avoids exposure to X-rays, allergic reactions and general anesthesia, it can be performed as outpatient procedure, is well tolerated, rapid and shows tubal patency to the patient in "realtime." Limitations include: tubal spasm may lead to misdiagnosis of tubal occlusion (spasm also seen with other methods), tubal flow may give a false impression of tubal patency in hydrosalpinx, cannot visualize intrapelvic pathology and bowel, requires a degree of technical competence and 10 to 20 investigations are needed to acquire the new technique.

Gray Scale Hy-Co-Sy (B-Mode)

Deichert and colleagues[10,25] evaluated transvaginal Hy-Co-Sy for the assessment of tubal patency with gray scale imaging (B-mode) and additional use of pulsed wave Doppler. During the last stages of the examination the ultrasound contrast medium, Echovist is prepared. The uterine cavity, which in most cases will still be dilated by the Ringer's solution instilled previously, is slowly filled with the echogenic ultrasound contrast medium. If the tube is patent, constant flow in a pattern resembling a point, spot or streak is seen. Further intermittent injections of volumes of 1 to 2 ml, given slowly and continuously, with further lateral sweeps of the US probe, allow visualization of intraluminal or intratubal flow under normal anatomical conditions via the pars intramuralis into the medial and distal segments of the tubes. For the diagnosis of tubal patency, two or three observation phases per tube are needed, with an observation period of continuous flow of about 10 seconds (while contrast medium is slowly injected). Although visualization of a longer segment of the tube beyond the pars intramuralis is convincing for tubal patency, one should carefully examine the adnexal regions for filling of the distal segments of the tube to exclude sactosalpinx. Examination of the pouch of Douglas for any increase in retrouterine fluid, compared with the picture at the start of the examination, completes the examination procedure.

PULSED DOPPLER ANALYSIS OF TUBAL PATENCY

Deichert and colleagues advise to confirm the findings using pulsed wave Doppler scanning, if the examination in B-mode reveals evidence suggesting tubal occlusion or if it is only possible to visualize a segment of tube of less than 2 cm in length.[10, 25]

After the Doppler gate has been positioned over the area to be examined, the gate width is reduced to measure only the flow noise from the pertubation and not vascular or other noise. Brief injections (about 5 sec) of contrast medium are made again. The sounds heard, which are long, drawn-out and initially hissing, and the simultaneous visualization of a broad noise band on the monitor, the width of the band that slowly decreases after injection, indicate that the tube is patent. Thus unobstructed flow is characterized by a short filling phase with a rapid, steep increase in Doppler shift and a slow, uniform fall in Doppler shift along the time axis, indicating unobstructed free distal outflow. The absence of these acoustic signals or optical tracings indicates obstruction of tubal flow or tubal occlusion. In this case there is only a short, steep Doppler shift with no subsequent noise signals. This indicates an absence of outflow of contrast medium distal to the Doppler gate. A sonographic finding of unobstructed tubes on the basis of noise band in pulsed wave Doppler sonography is more impressive than that of a shorter segment of tube in standing B-mode.

Deichert and colleagues tried to determine whether the additional use of pulsed wave Doppler can improve the tubal diagnosis reached with gray scale imaging in doubtful cases.[10] They studied 17 patients with diagnosed sterility problems. Hysterosalpingo-contrast sonography by gray scale and by pulsed wave Doppler and follow-up chromolaparoscopy (n = 16) or HSG (n = 1) were performed. The diagnostic efficacies of gray scale and pulsed wave Doppler were compared with each other and with a conventional control procedure (chromolaparoscopy or HSG). The gray scale findings were confirmed by pulsed wave Doppler in five cases on one side; confirmed by pulsed wave Doppler in seven cases on both sides; corrected by pulsed wave Doppler in one case on one side and confirmed on the other side by pulsed wave Doppler. In all 17 cases, the tubal findings after pulsed wave Doppler were confirmed by chromolaparoscopy or HSG. The additional use of pulsed wave Doppler in Hy-Co-Sy is recommended as a supplement to gray scale imaging in cases of suspected tubal occlusion and in the event of intratubal flow demonstrable only over a short distance.

Deichert assessed tubal patency, using Hy-Co-Sy, conventional HSG or laparoscopy with dye, in 76 women and visualized 152 fallopian tubes.[25] In this study, Hy-Co-Sy showed 87.5 percent concordance with other techniques, predicted 100 percent of tubal occlusions and detected 86 percent of patent tubes.

According to Ayida and colleagues[26] saline contrast sonohysterography as a screening test for any cavity abnormality, had 87.5 percent sensitivity, 100 percent specificity, 100 percent positive predictive value and 91.6 percent negative predictive value.

COLOR DOPPLER HYSTEROSALPINGOGRAPHY

Transvaginal color Doppler hysterosalpingography is a safe and efficacious method for evaluation of fallopian tube patency without exposure to radiation or contrast dyes. The cost of the procedure is significantly lower than for X-ray HSG and it gives immediate results. It is advisable that all the scans are recorded on vide-recorder and/or polaroid films.

Further advantages of transvaginal sonosalpingography include the possibility of performing the procedure on an outpatient basis. This has significantly altered the need for inpatient facilities at some infertility departments. Similar to X-ray HSG bleeding, pregnancy and presence of adnexal masses on pelvic or ultrasound examination are contraindications for color Doppler HSG.

Equipment needed to perform color Doppler HSG includes an ultrasound unit with color Doppler capability and an intrauterine catheter. The intrauterine cannula is placed into the uterus. One balloon is placed on the level of the internal cervical os, while another one is fixed in the external cervical os. A tiny tubal catheter with a metal end is introduced after exploration of the uterine cavity. Approximately two to five ml of sterile saline is instilled into the uterine cavity (Figs 23.1A to C). After the observation of the morphology of the uterus end endometrial lining, the color Doppler is directed at the cornual region where the tubal catheter with a metal end should be located. The exact placement of the catheter is sonographically controlled. Color signals passing through the fallopian tube indicate its patency, while the absence of such signals is interpreted as tubal occlusion. [6, 27] Accumulation of the fluid in the cul-de-sac on the side of injection controlled by transvaginal color and pulsed Doppler is an accurate indicator of the ipsilateral tubal patency. Selective tubal injection increases the accuracy of the procedure and appropriateness of the interpretation. The procedure is repeated for the contralateral side (Figs 23.2A and B).

Difficulty in making the diagnosis of tubal occlusion arises in those patients with dilated hydrosalpinges because flow through the dilated fallopian tube may stimulate spillage on the Doppler ultrasonography screen. To avoid this error, we should perform careful observation of both adnexa before the procedure. Since the tubal architecture is not demonstrated with color Doppler HSG. This method is not useful in preoperative salpingoplasty procedures.[28]

Using our modified technique, we compared the findings of color Doppler HSG from 47 patients with those of chromopertubation at the time of laparoscopy.[9] Forty-three out

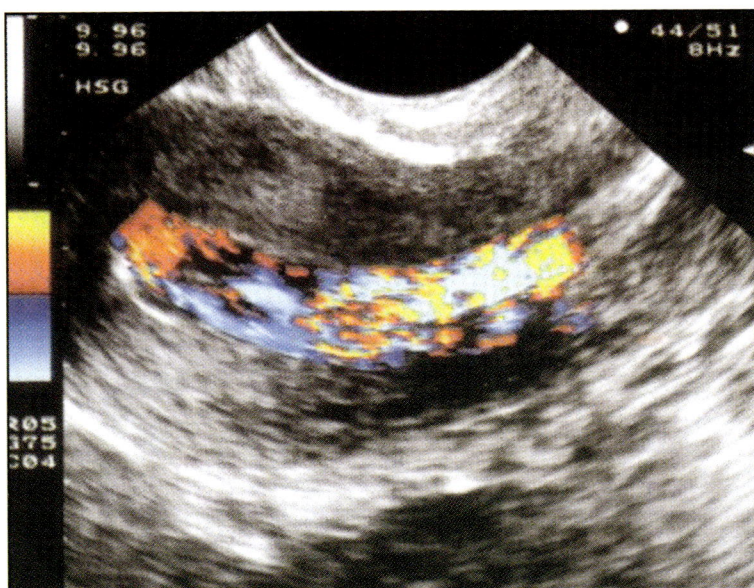

Fig. 23.1A: Transvaginal ultrasound shows the catheter and the uterine cavity after injection of isotonic saline

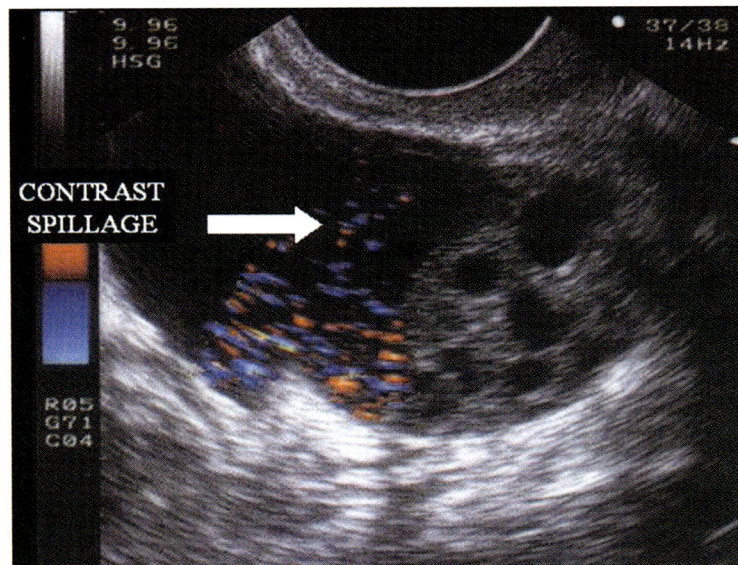

Fig. 23.2A: Transvaginal ultrasound clearly demonstrates anechoic fluid in the cul-de-sac after injection of isotonic saline

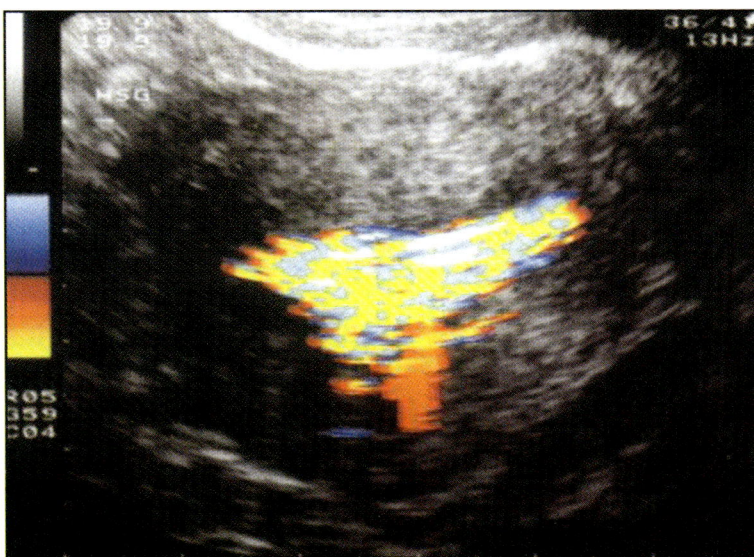

Fig. 23.1B: Transvaginal color Doppler scan of the uterus after injection of the isotonic saline solution

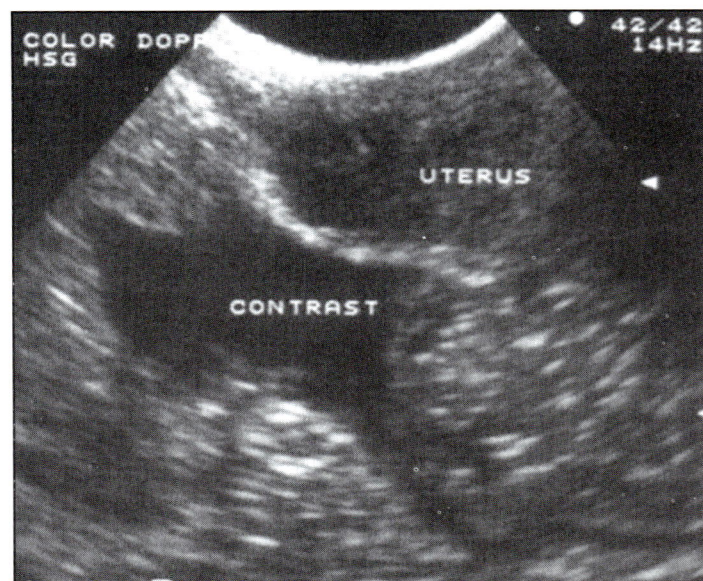

Fig. 23.2B: Transvaginal color Doppler hysterosalpingography demonstrates regular tubal patency. Note color flow signals passing through the right tube and simultaneous accumulation of the anechoic fluid in the cul-de-sac

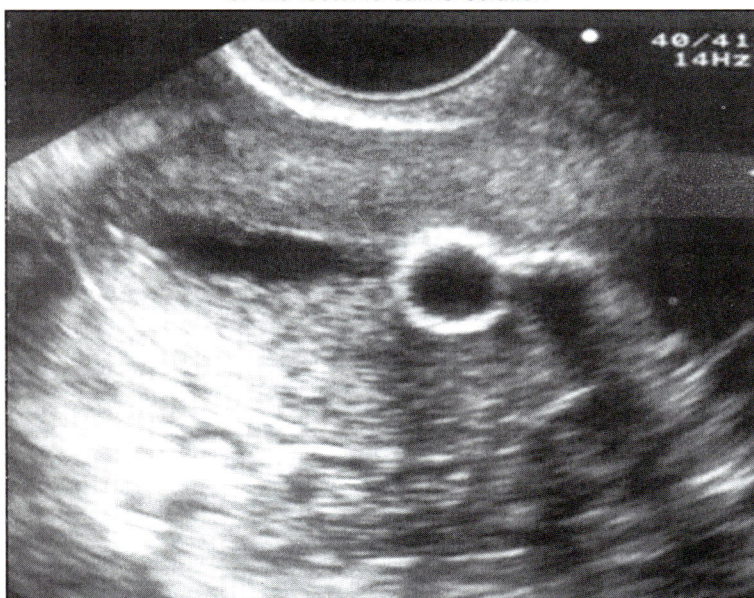

Fig. 23.1C: The triangular uterine cavity is clearly outlined by color flow imaging

of 47 (91.48%) color Doppler HSG findings agreed with observations at chromopertubation. In only one patient, in whom no patency was seen in both tubes under color Doppler evaluation, indirect diagnosis of tubal patency was performed observing accumulation of free fluid in the cul-de-sac. The increased incidence of conception during the three months after the procedure (in our study, two patients) may be an effect of a mechanical lavage of the uterus by dislodging the mucous plugs, breakdown of the peritoneal adhesions, or a stimulatory effect on the tubal cilia. No serious side effects were observed during and after the transvaginal color Doppler HSG procedure. Eighteen patients complained of pain that continued for 2 to 10 minutes after the procedure. No medication was required for these cases. The shortest time taken for the transvaginal color

Doppler hysterosalpingography was 5 minutes, while the longest time was 14 minutes. After removing the instruments, the cervix is inspected for hemostasis and pressure is applied to the tenaculum site whenever necessary.

REVIEW OF THE LITERATURE

To assess the accuracy of the diagnosis of tubal occlusion with the use of color Doppler flow ultrasonography and HSG, Peters and Coulam[6] studied 129 infertile women. When results of ultrasonography-HSG were compared with those of X-ray HSG and/or chromopertubation, 69 of 85 (81%) studies showed agreement, and 50 out of 58 (86%) ultrasound hysterosalpingography findings agreed with observations at chromopertubation. The frequency of comparable findings between X-ray HSG and chromopertubation was 75 percent.

Richman and colleagues[13] evaluated tubal patency in 36 infertile women. They compared ultrasound findings with conventional hysterosalpingograms, which had been obtained simultaneously. Ultrasound demonstrated bilateral occlusion with a sensitivity of 100 percent, and showed tubal patency with a specificity of 96 percent.

Tüfekci and colleagues[20] studied 38 women with infertility complaints. The results obtained from transvaginal sonosalpingography and laparoscopies were completely consistent for 29 cases (76.32%), and partially consistent for eight cases (21.05%). Only one case showed inconsistent result. Complete consistence means that the passage through both fallopian tubes is identical by both methods. Partial consistence indicated identical results for only either the left or the right tube. Transvaginal sonosalpingography correctly indicated tubal patency or non-patency in 37 of 38 cases.

Heikkinen and coworkers[29] evaluated the advantages and accuracy of transvaginal sonosalpingography in the assessment of tubal patency with regards to laparoscopic chromopertubation. Sixty-one fallopian tubes were examined by both techniques, resulting in concordance of 85 percent. By transvaginal sonosalpingography, 45 tubes were found to be patent and 16 occluded. In chromopertubation, 50 tubes were patent and 11 were occluded. Bilateral tubal patency was found by transvaginal sonosalpingography in 17 cases and by laparoscopy in 22 cases. Bilateral occlusion was found in three cases using either technique. Transvaginal sonosalpingography with the combination of air and saline is a low-cost, reliable, safe and comfortable examination method and it can be used for the primary investigation of infertility on an outpatient basis.

Jeanty et al[30] assessed the use of air as a sonographic contrast agent in the investigation of tubal patency by sonohysterography.

They examined 115 women assessed for infertility. After saline sonohysterography, small amounts of air were insufflating and the tubal passage of bubbles was monitored. Air-sonohysterography and laparoscopy with chromopertubation show agreement in 79.4 percent. In 17.2 percent of patients, the tubes were considered no visualized by air-sonohysterography when they were patent. The sensitivity was 85.7 percent and specificity 77.2 percent. In conclusion, air sonohysterography is a comfortable, simple, and inexpensive first line of tubal patency investigations yielding high accuracy.

Battaglia and coworkers[31] found that correlation between color Doppler HSG and roentgenogram HSG with chromolaparoscopy occurred in 86 percent versus 93 percent of all women studied.

Boudghene et al[32] compared the efficiency of air-filled albumin microspheres (Infoson) with saline solution in determining fallopian tube patency during Hy-Co-Sy. HyCoSy was performed with a 7 MHz transvaginal probe using both B-mode and color Doppler and tubal patency was demonstrated by the appearance of contrast agent in the peritoneal cavity near the ovaries. Infoson enhanced Hy-Co-Sy provided a significantly larger number of correct diagnoses (20/22 fallopian tubes) than did saline Hy-Co-Sy (12/24 fallopian tubes) and the same number as that achieved by HSG. A positive ultrasound contrast agent appears to be more efficient than saline solution at determining fallopian tube patency in infertile women by means of Hy-Co-Sy and as efficient as an iodinated contrast agent in the same population explored by HSG.

Stern and colleagues[8] administered saline transcervically during transvaginal color Doppler sonography in 238 women. Traditional X-ray HSG was performed in 89 women. Laparoscopy with chromopertubation was performed in 121 women. Forty-nine women had all three procedures performed. Correlation between color Doppler HSG and X-ray findings with chromopertubation occurred in 81 percent versus 60 percent ($p = 0.0008$) of all women studied. In forty-nine women who had all three procedures performed, color Doppler HSG results correlated with chromopertubation more often than X-ray HSG (82% versus 57%, $p = 0.0152$). In their previous report,[6] discrepancies between color ultrasound hysterosalpingography and chromopertubation findings involved a diagnosis of unilateral patency. They recommend repeating color ultrasound HSG before making a diagnosis of unilateral occlusion.

Allahbadia[33] reported a 92.6 percent agreement between color Doppler HSG compared with X ray HSG and laparoscopy. The same author described the so-called *Sion* procedure or *hydrogynecography*. This procedure takes about 15 minutes as compared to the 5 to 6 minutes for sonosalpingography. After accomplishing sonosalpingography, sterile normal saline is injected until approximately 350 ml have flooded the pelvis. With the adnexa and uterus submerged in a fluid medium, the rescanning of the pelvis is repeated. If there is a bilateral tubal block and reflux of the saline is seen in the stem of the Foley's catheter, filling up the pelvis by alternative means is applied. The saline fills up the pelvis and delineates all sorts of adhesions. All the patients undergoing this procedure are given prophylactic antibiotics.

Contrary to optimistic results of different ultrasound techniques for evaluation of tubal patency, Balen and colleagues[34] found ultrasound contrast HSG using both sterile saline and Echovist contrast media insufficiently accurate and inferior to conventional X-ray HSG. False-positive rates in the range of 9 percent and false-negative rates in the range of 20 percent have been reported in the diagnosis of tubal obstruction by color Doppler HSG.[8] Therefore, all abnormal hysterosalpingograms studies deserve laparoscopic or hysteroscopic follow-up.

Normal X-ray or color Doppler HSG does not rule out the need for diagnostic laparoscopy. While X-ray HSG is the most accurate method of diagnosing intramural or intraluminal abnormalities of the fallopian tube, color Doppler HSG is the only available noninvasive method for analyzing the tubal motility.

To obtain maximum information, a well-trained physician who is familiar with the color Doppler investigation and who is capable of manipulating the instruments, the patient's reproductive tract and the rate of injection should perform the procedure.

In the recent study from Sueoka et al[35] the authors developed the linear everting (LE) catheter to safely guide a falloposcope into the entire length of fallopian tube in order to observe the tubal lumen. This catheter may also be useful therapeutically for the recanalization of occluded tubes. On the basis of tubes attempted, the LE catheter successfully accessed 85.3 percent (87/102). A follow-up hysterosalpingogram was completed 1 to 3 months following the falloposcopic tuboplasty (FT) procedure, which revealed an overall patency rate of 79.4 percent (81/102). In their study, FT has been established as a highly useful, less invasive and novel treatment for tubal infertility.

THREE-DIMENSIONAL HYSTEROSONOSALPINGOGRAPHY

Recently, large technological efforts have been invested in promoting the capability to demonstrate the third dimension, although there is no doubt about the diagnostic value of two-dimensional ultrasound in obstetrics and gynecology. The three-dimensional (3D) ultrasound image is generated by superimposing the programmed volume box over the two-dimensional ultrasound scan image of the uterus.[36] The volumetric rotor is set into operation. The vaginal transducer then performs a sweep of transversal sections that are to be stored in the computer. The computer integrates the images and enables the sonographer to view three planes simultaneously. Once the perpendicular plane to the transducer is obtained, the calculated 3D image with the complete volume scan is stored in a removable computer disk. This scanning procedure lasts between 2 and 10 seconds. The examination of the patient is complete, while later sonographer can analyze selected sections. Three-dimensional images are generated only when the three planes are integrated and displayed on the screen. It is possible to rotate and translate any plane of the volume stored. To generate a final 3D image of the uterine cavity, a threshold has to be defined up to which echogenicity should be taken for reconstruction of the uterine cavity.[36] Depending on the structure to be studied, different 3D modes can be elaborated. The surface reconstruction mode allows study of the outer contour or profile of the uterus. The transparent maximum/minimum mode reveals objects with high echogenicity in the interior of a uterus. The basic structural information provided by conventional scans in the longitudinal and transverse planes now can be augmented by new 3D ultrasound that provides an additional view of the coronal or "c" plane, which is parallel to the transducer face (Fig. 23.3).[37] The computer generated scan is displayed in three perpendicular planes. The presentation of three perpendicular planes on one screen allows free scrolling of an endless amount of frames through the volume of interest. The coronal or "c" plane view allows more detailed analysis of the uterus and, for the first time, the endometrial cavity between the uterine angles can be visualized (Figs 23.4A and B). Translation or rotation can be carried out in one plane while maintaining the perpendicular orientation of all three. The images produced by transvaginal ultrasound are superior to those produced by transabdominal ultrasound because vaginal transducers are in closer proximity to the tissues.[37] Because of that, higher frequencies are used and artifactual echoes caused by multiple reflections from intervening tissues are minimized.

Demonstration of the coronal plane is mandatory for the diagnosis of uterine pathology, such as septate, arcuate or bicornuate uteri and also provides the most exact measurement of the endometrial width when transected in a midperpendicular manner. During 3D hysterosonography the typical triangulated uterine cavity appears in its full shape (Fig. 23.3).[38] Surface

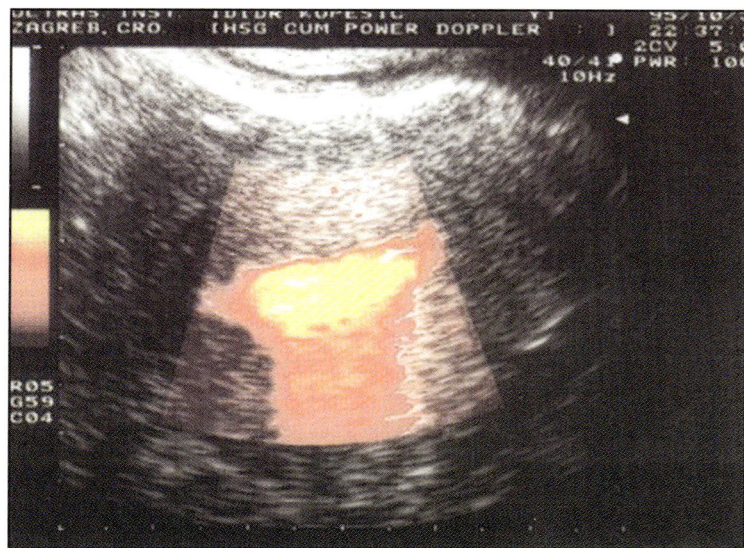

Fig. 23.3: Multiplanar image of the uterus after injection of echogenic contrast medium as obtained by power Doppler ultrasound. This modality facilitates visualization of normal uterine cavity in three orthogonal projections, while triangular shape of the uterine cavity is best imaged in frontal section

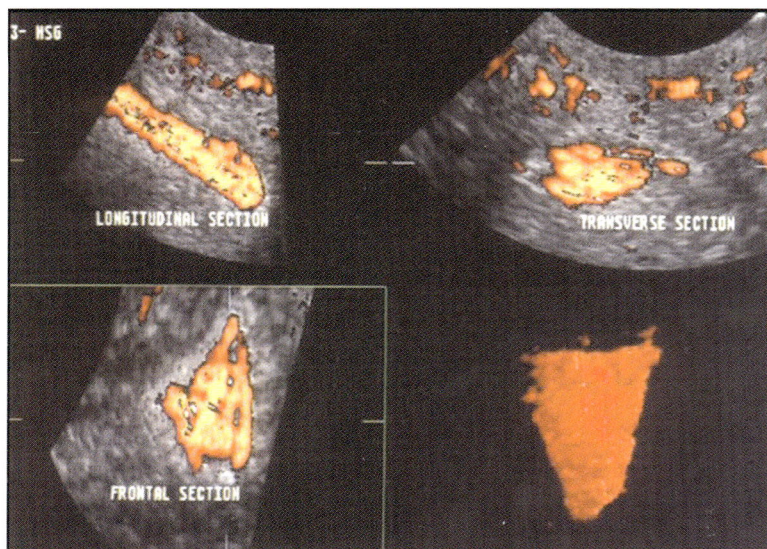

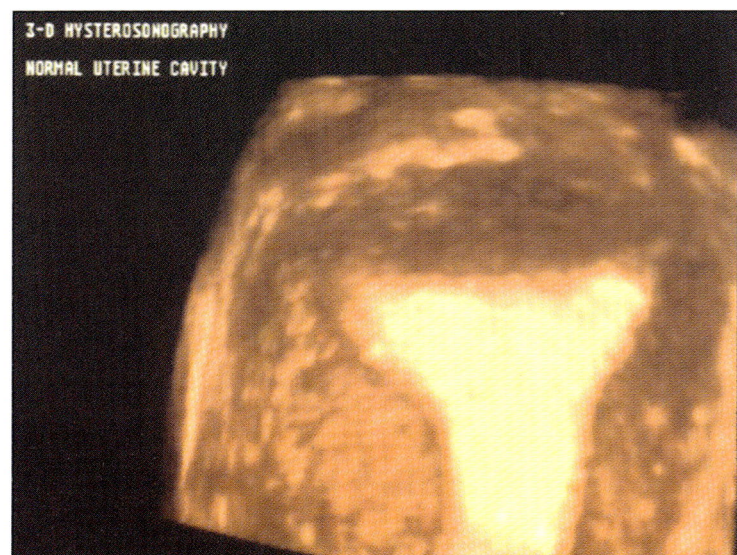

Figs 23.4A and B: Three-dimensional power Doppler hysterosalpingography enables detailed analysis of the uterine cavity shape and continuity between the endometrial cavity and uterine angles

rendering, maximal/minimal or X-ray renderings provide even more information on uterine findings, such as anatomy of the uterine cavity and its content. There are two techniques to accomplish this goal: "native" approach, and the use of echogenic contrast medium that is especially useful for demonstrating the uterine cavity shape. Uterus is due to its dual consistency of endometrium and myometrium, an excellent ultrasonic medium. Those two media have different acoustic impedance that permits visualization of the size and shape of the uterus and its cavity. In addition, contrast medium is mandatory in cases where a thin endometrium or pathologic content of the uterine cavity precludes its visualization.

The negative contrast medium, normal saline, is used for demonstration of the entire uterine cavity, its shape, pathology, and the frame of the myometrial mantel, whereas for demonstrating the permeability of the fallopian tubes a positive contrast medium (Echovist) is used.

Weinraub and Herman[38] were first to evaluate the findings of different pathology of uterus anatomy and pathological content of uterine cavity on 3D hysterosonography. Using three perpendicular planes on one screen, where the left upper plane is coronal and is termed "a", the right upper plane is sagittal and is termed "b," and the left lower plane is transverse and is termed "c" one can detect numerous causes of infertility. Looking at the fundal region in "a" it is very important not to overlook a small indentation, if it is present, in the case of septate uterus. The maximal endometrial width could be easily measured in sagittal plane. If the transverse section shows separated uterine cornua, finding is typical for arcuate uterus. Clear concavity in the middle of the uterine fundus dividing the uterine cavity creates a bicornuate uterus.

Hydrosonography is very useful in demonstration of intracavitary pathologies, such as: adhesions, myomas, endometrial polyps, endometrial carcinoma, or location of intrauterine devices (IUDs). Using 3D surface rendering in the cases of intrauterine adhesions and myomas, it is possible to present the spatial orientation and the correlation of the adhesions with the surrounding uterine walls, also round and smooth surface of the myomas giving the feeling of depth inside the uterine cavity.[38]

Hydrosonography, as well as 3D rendering is especially important for diagnosis of an endometrial polyp. Despite the fact that the cut in the coronal plane goes through the endometrial polyp it is not demonstrated on "a" plane and could be easily missed. When hydrosonography is used, the polyp or any other intracavitary lesion is easily examined in all three planes throughout the volume.[38]

Fallopian tubes can be demonstrated on ultrasound only when they contain fluid (hydrosalpinx, pyosalpinx, bleeding ectopic pregnancy, or a contrast medium). In the case of hydrosalpinx, the fluid-filled fallopian tube is demonstrated in "a", "b" and "c" sections, in each plane resembling different shape due to its tortuosity. In "d" section, 3D rendering is shown. There are a number of difficulties in tubal visualization by 2D Hy-Co-Sy.[37] Due to its tortuosity, the tube can rarely be seen completely in a single scanning plane and the echo-contrast medium is, therefore, observed in small sections. The position of the tube is very variable and distended bowel may prevent the visualization of the distal parts of the tubes. Therefore, usually only the tubal ostia and proximal parts of the tubes are visualized by gray scale 2D ultrasound imaging. Free spread of the dye is frequently difficult to visualize because the surrounding bowel can also produce strongly echogenic signals. Instead of visualizing the echo contrast with gray scale ultrasound, Sladkevicius and colleagues[39] used 3D power Doppler technology which is sensitive to slow flow. If the tube is patent, Doppler signals should be obtained from flow along the tube and free spill from the fimbrial end should be identified (Figs 23.5A and B). The aim of the their study was to evaluate the feasibility of three-dimensional power Doppler imaging (3D-PDI) in the assessment of the patency of the fallopian tubes during Hy-Co-Sy. Hysterosalpingo-contrast sonography using contrast medium Echovist was performed on 67 women. Findings on the 2D gray scale scanning and 3D-PDI were compared. The first technique visualizes positive contrast in the fallopian tube; the second demonstrates flow of medium through the tube. Contrast medium Echovist produced prominent signals on the 3D-PDI image. Free spill from the fimbrial end of the fallopian tubes was demonstrated in 114 (91%) tubes using the 3D-PDI technique and in 58 (46%) of tubes using conventional Hy-Co-Sy. The mean duration of the imaging procedure was less with 3D-PDI, but the operator time, which included postprocedure analysis of the stored information, was similar. A significantly lower volume of contrast medium (5.9 +/- 0.6 mL) was used for 3D-PDI in comparison with that (11.2 +/- 1.9 mL) used for conventional 2D Hy-Co-Sy. The authors concluded that color coded 3D-PDI with surface rendering allowed visualization of the flow of contrast through the entire tubal length and free spill of contrast was clearly identified in the majority of cases. The 3D-PDI method appeared to have advantages over the conventional Hy-Co-Sy technique, especially in terms of visualization of spill from the distal end of the tube, which was achieved twice as often with the 3D ultrasound technique. Although the design of the investigation did not allow the side effects of the two techniques to be compared, the shorter duration of the imaging and lower volume of the contrast medium used suggested that the 3D-PDI technique might have a better side

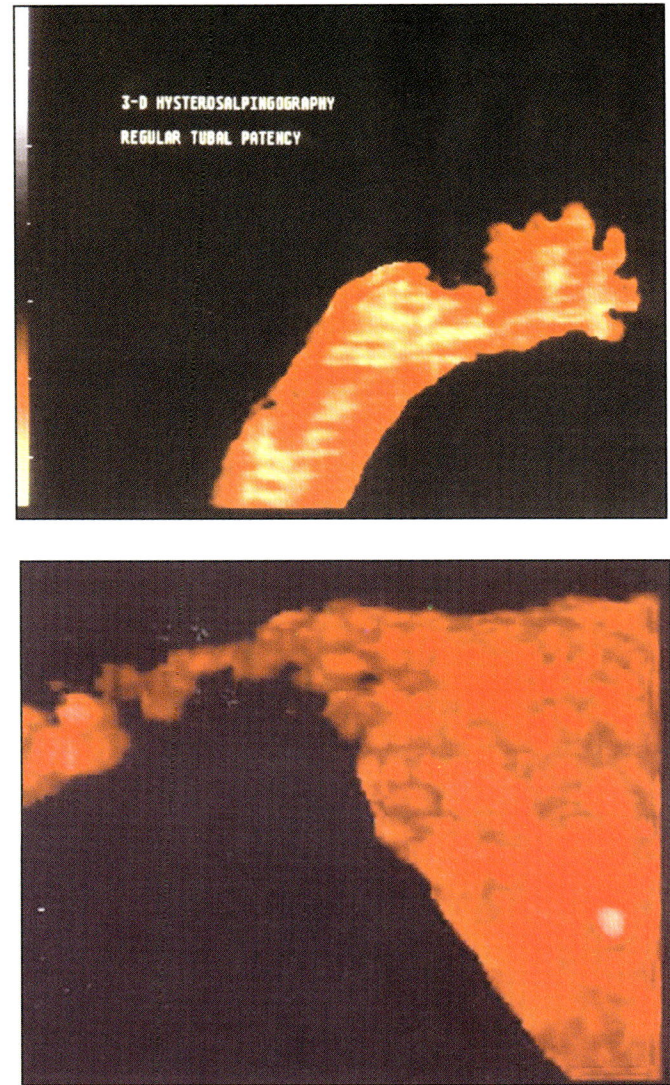

Figs 23.5A and B: Three-dimensional power Doppler image of the entire tubal length and spillage of the contrast medium through the fimbrial end as demonstrated by echo-enhanced 3D PD hysterosalpingography

effect profile. The 3D-PDI technique allowed better storage of the information for re-analysis and archiving than conventional Hy-Co-Sy.

Similarly, our group found that power Doppler visualization of echo-contrast flow is better than conventional imaging of the contrast media.

Ayida and colleagues[40] compared conventional 2 and 3D ultrasound scanning of the uterine cavity with and without saline contrast medium. The 2D scanning suggested cavity abnormalities in 4 of 10 women (fibroids, 3; hyperechoic thick endometrium, 1). The 3D scanning confirmed these and revealed one additional abnormality suggestive of a uterine septum. The 2D scanning with saline injection diagnosed abnormalities in 5 of 10 (uterine septum, 1; fibroids, 3; endometrial polyp, 1). The 3D contrast scanning with saline did not add any further information to 2D contrast scanning with saline. In this pilot study, 3D scanning to assess the uterine cavity appeared to offer no advantages over conventional 2D contrast sonography.

Weinraub and colleagues[41] have demonstrated the feasibility of combined 3D ultrasound and saline contrast hysterosonography. Since volume sampling has a short pick-up time of a few seconds, the examination is over almost immediately after the uterus is reasonably distended. In this uncomfortable examination such an advantage should not be underestimated. Evaluation of the uterine cavity at a later time allows the operator to manipulate the data at leisure and scrutinize findings in desired planes, which were not available during the initial examination. Simultaneous display of the three perpendicular planes offers a more comprehensive overview of the examined area and gives access to planes unobtainable by conventional 2D examination. Surface rendering may confirm the presence of pathological findings in equivocal cases, and characterize their appearance, size, volume and relationship to the surrounding structures. Surface rendering of the polypoid structures shows echogenic masses on a pedicle protruding into the uterine cavity. Submucous fibroids appear as mixed echogenic sites bulging into the cavity. Intrauterine synechiae appear as bands of varying thickness traversing the uterine cavity. This can be useful when deciding on treatment options, such as conservative management vs. surgery, and can be a valuable tool in surgical procedures carried out under ultrasonographic guidance.

Kiyokava et al[42] evaluated 25 unselected infertile patients for tubal patency and uterine cavity by 3D Hy-Co-Sy with saline as a contrast medium. The efficacy of the procedure was compared with X-ray HSG as reference. The positive predictive value, negative predictive value, sensitivity, and specificity of predicting tubal patency by 3D Hy-Co-Sy were 100, 33.3, 84.4, and 100 percent, respectively. The full contour of the uterine cavity was depicted in 96 percent of cases by 3D Hy-Co-Sy and 64 percent by X-ray HSG ($P < 0.005$). The uterine cavity area measured on 3D Hy-Co-Sy correlated well with the volume of contrast medium required on HSG. Three-dimensional Hy-Co-Sy provided advantages of better assessment of uterine cavity over HSG. Compared with conventional HSG, the efficacy of 3D Hy-Co-Sy to assess tubal patency was acceptable. In addition, the procedure of 3D Hy-Co-Sy appears to be better tolerated, requiring no sedation or anesthesia and a reduced examination time. Thus, 3D Hy-Co-Sy with saline as a contrast medium is feasible and could comprise a routine outpatient procedure in the initial evaluation of infertile women.

Unterweger et al[43] introduced a new method, three-dimensional dynamic magnetic resonance–hysterosalpingography (3D dMR-HSG) for imaging of the uterine cavity and fallopian tube patency. The authors evaluated whether, by using a higher viscosity contrast solution, 20 ml of gandolium-polyvidone, direct visualization of the fallopian tubes may be achieved. Three-dimensional dynamic magnetic-resonance-hysterosalpingography represents a new and promising imaging approach to female infertility causing less pain and avoiding exposure of the ovaries to ionizing radiation. By using a higher viscosity MR-contrast agent it allows not only visualization of the uterine cavity and fallopian tube patency but also direct visualization of the fallopian tubes.

CONCLUSIONS

Color Doppler and 3D hysterosalpingography are safe and efficacious methods for evaluation of fallopian tube patency without exposure to contrast dyes or radiation. These procedures allow the physician to know the results immediately and are carried out on outpatient clinic basis.

Three-dimensional technique offers the possibility of simultaneous presentation of the uterine cavity and corresponding tube, shortening the procedure and the discomfort of the patient. Transvaginal 3D ultrasound examination time is not less than that needed for 2D sonography, but some parts of the examination, like measurements, reconstruction of the planes of interest and surface rendering can be performed off-line. The acquired volumes of the most appropriate planes of interest can be stored on removable hard disk for additional reevaluations and documentation. Ultrasonic tomography can be performed using one panel control, producing parallel sections in increments of less than 1 mm. The ability of 3D ultrasound systems to produce serial scans that can be stored for subsequent analysis, 3D reconstruction, accurate assessment of volume, and coronal plane with more detailed analysis of the uterus and endometrial cavity between uterine angles is superior to conventional 2D ultrasound.

REFERENCES

1. Hill ML. Infertility and reproductive assistance. In Neiberg DA, Hill LM, Bohm-Velez M, Mendelson EB (Eds): Transvaginal Ultrasound, St. Louis: Mosby Year Book. 1992; pp.43-6.
2. Arronet GM, Aduljie SY and O'Brien IR. A 9-year survey of fallopian tube dysfunction in human infertility: diagnosis and therapy. Fertil Steril 1969; 20: 903-18.
3. Page H. Estimation of the prevalence and incidence of infertility in a population: A pilot study. Fertil Steril, 1989;71: 571-4.
4. Kerin JF, William DB, San Roman GA, Pearistone AC, Grundfest WS, Sucrey ES. Falloposcopic classification and treatment of fallopian tube disease. Fertil Steril 1992; 57: 731-5.
5. Thurmond AS, Rosch J. Non-surgical fallopian tube recanalization for treatment of infertility. Radiology 1990; 174: 371-4.
6. Peters JA, Coulam CB. Hysterosalpingography with color Doppler ultrasonography. Am J Obstet Gynecol 1991;164:1530-2.
7. Volpi E, Zuccaro A, Patriarca S, Rustichelli, Sismondi P. Transvaginal sonographic tubal patency testing air and saline solution as contrast media in a routine infertility clinic setting. Ultrasound Obstet Gynecol 1996; 7: 43-8.

8. Stern J, Peters AJ, Coulam CB. Color Doppler ultrasonography assessment of tubal patency: a comparison study with traditional technique. Fertil Steril 1992; 58: 897-900.
9. Kupesic S, Kurjak A. Gynecological vaginal sonographic interventional procedures – what does color add? Gynecol Perinatol 1994; 3: 57-60.
10. Deichert U, Schlief R, van de Sandt M, Daume E. Transvaginal hysterosalpingo-contrast sonography for the assessment of tubal patency with gray scale imaging and the additional use of pulsed wave Doppler. Fertil Steril 1992; 57: 62-7.
11. Rubin I. Differences between the uterus and tubes as a cause of oscillations recorded during uterotubal insufflation. Fertil Steril, 1954; 5: 147-53.
12. Nannini R, Chelo E, Branconi F, Tantini C, Scarselli GF. Dynamyc Echohysteroscopy. A New Diagnostic Technique in the Study of Female Infertility. Acta Europ Fertil 1981;12: 165-71.
13. Richman TS, Viscomi GN, deCherney A, Polan ML, Alcebo LO. Fallopian tubal patency assessed by ultrasound fluid injection. Radiology 1984; 152: 507-10.
14. Randolph JR, Ying YK, Maier DB, Schmidt CL, Riddick CH. Comparison of realtime ultrasonography, hysterosalpingography and laparoscopy/hysteroscopy Fertil Steril 1986; 46, 828-32.
15. Davison GB, Leeton J. A case of female infertility investigated by contrast-enhanced echogynecography. J. Clin. Ultrasound 1988; 16: 44-7.
16. Allahbadia GN. Fallopian tubes and ultrasonography. The Sion experience. Fertil Steril 1992; 58: 901-7.
17. Broer KH, Turanli R. Überprüfung des Tubenfaktors mitels Vaginalsonographie. Ultraschall Klin Prax 1992; 7: 50-3.
18. Bonilla-Musoles F, Simón C, Sampaio M Pellicer A. An assessment of hysterosalpingosonography (HSSG) as a diagnostic tool for uterine cavity defects and tubal patency. J Clin Ultrasound 1992; 20: 175-81.
19. Deichert U, Schlief R, van de Sandt M, Junke I. Transvaginal hysterosalpingo-contrast sonography (Hy-Co-Sy) compared with conventional tubal diagnostics. Hum Reprod 1989; 4: 418-22.
20. Tüfekci EC Girit S, Bayirli MD, Durmusoglu F, Yalti S. Evaluation of tubal patency by transvaginal sonosalpingography. Fertil Steril 1992; 57: 336-40.
21. Gramiak R, Shah PM. Echocardiography of the aortic root. Invest Radiol 1968; 3: 356-66.
22. Meltzer RS, Tickner G, Sahines TP, Popp RL. The source of ultrasound contrast effect. J Clin Ultrasound, 1980; 8: 121.
23. Suren A, Puchta J, Osmers R. Fluid instillation into the uterine cavity. In Osmers R and Kurjak A (Eds): Ultrasound and The Uterus. Carnforth, UK: Parthenon Publishing 1995;pp.45-51.
24. Schlief R. Ultrasound contrast agents. Radiology 1991; 3: 198-207.
25. Deichert U, van de Sandt M. Transvaginal hysterosalpingo-contrast sonography (Hy-Co-Sy). The assessment of tubal patency and uterine abnormalities by contrast enhanced sonography. Advances in Echo-Contrast. 1993; 2: 55-8.
26. Ayida G, Chamberlain P, Barlow D, Kennedy S. Uterine cavity assessment prior to in vitro fertilization: comparison of transvaginal scanning, saline contrast hysterosonography and hysteroscopy. Ultrasound Obstet Gynecol. 1997; 10: 59-62.
27. Peters JA, Stern JJ, Coulam CB. Color Doppler hysterosalpingography. In Jaffe R, Warsof SL (Eds): Color Doppler in Obstetrics and Gynecology New York: McGraw Hill 1992;pp.283.
28. Groff TR, Edelstein JA, Schenken RS. Hysterosalpingography in the preoperative evaluation of tubal anastomosis candidates. Fertil Steril. 1990; 53: 417-20.
29. Heikkinen H, Tekay A, Volpi E, Martikainen H, Juppila P. Transvaginal salpingosonography for the assessment of tubal patency in infertile women: methodological and clinical experiences. Fertil Steril 1995; 64: 293-8.
30. Jeanty P, Besnard S, Arnold A, Turner C, Crum P. Air- contrast sonohysterography as a first step assessment of tubal patency. J Ultrasound Med 2000; 19(8):519-27.
31. Battaglia C, Artini PG, D'Ambrogio G, Genazzani AD, Genazzani AR, Volpe A. Color Doppler hysterosalpingography in the diagnosis of tubal patency. Fertil Steril 1996; 65: 317-22.
32. Boudghene FP, Bazot M, Robert Y, Perrot N, Rocourt N, Antoine JM, Morris H, Leroy JL, Uzan S, Bigot JM. Assessment of fallopian tube patency by HyCoSy: comparison of a positive contrast agent with saline solution. Ultrasound Obstet Gynecol 2001; 18(5):525-30.
33. Allahbadia GN. Fallopian tube patency using color Doppler. Int J Gynecol Obstet 1993; 40: 241-4.
34. Balen FG, Allen CM, Siddle NC, Lees WR. Ultrasound contrast hysterosalpingography — evaluation as an outpatient procedure. Br J Radiol 1993; 66: 592-9.
35. Sueoka H, Asada S, Tsuchiya N, Kobayashi M, Kuroshima Y, Yoshimura. Falloposcopic tuboplasty for bilateral tubal occlusion. A novel infertility treatment as an alternative for in-vitro fertilization? Hum Reprod 1998; 13: 71-4.
36. Raga F, Bonilla-Musoles F, Blanes J, Osborne NG. Congenital Müllerian anomalies: diagnostic accuracy of three-dimensional ultrasound. Fertil Steril, 1996; 65: 523-8.
37. Kyei-Mensah A, Zaidi J, Pittrof R, Shaker A, Campbell S, Tan SL. Transvaginal three-dimensional ultrasound: accuracy of follicular volume measurements. Fertil Steril 1996; 65: 371-6.
38. Weinraub Z, Herman A. Three-Dimensional Hysterosalpingography. In Merz, E. (Ed). 3-D Ultrasonography in Obstetrics and Gynecology Lippincott Williams & Wilkins, Philadelphia 1998;pp 57-64.
39. Sladkevicius P, Ojha K, Campbell S, Nargund G Three-dimensional power Doppler imaging in the assessment of fallopian tube patency. Ultrasound Obstet Gynecol. 2000; 16(7): 644-7.
40. Ayida G, Kennedy S, Barlow D, Chamberlain P. Conventional sonography for uterine cavity assessment: a comparison of conventional two-dimensional with three-dimensional transvaginal ultrasound: a pilot study. Fertil Steril 1996; 66: 848-50.
41. Weinraub Z, Maymon R, Shulman A, Bukovsky J, Kratochwil A, Lee A, Herman A. Three-dimensional saline contrast hysterosonography and surface rendering of uterine cavity pathology. Ultrasound Obstet Gynecol 1996; 277-82.
42. Kiyokawa K, Masuda H, Fuyuki T, Koseki M, Uchida N, Fukuda T, Amemiya K, Shouka K, Suzuki K. Three-dimensional hysterosalpingo-contrast sonography (3D-HyCoSy) as an outpatient procedure to assess infertile women: a pilot study. Ultrasound. Obstet Gynecol 2000; 16(7):648-54.
43. Unterweger M, De Geyter C, Fröhlich JM, Bongartz G, Wiesner W. Three-dimensional dynamic MR-hysterosalpingography: a new, low invasive, radiation-free and less painful radiologic approach to female infertility. Hum Reprod 2002; 17(12): 3138-41.

**MA Pascual, S Kupesic,
A Kurjak, PN Barri, JM Carrera**

24 Ectopic Pregnancy

INTRODUCTION

Ectopic pregnancy represents implantation of the fertilized ovum outside the uterine cavity. In 95 percent of the cases it is localized in the fallopian tube (95%), but sites like abdominal cavity, ovary, intraligamentous location, cornual, intramural or cervical sites are not unusual.[1-4] The exact cause of blastocyst implantation and development outside the endometrial cavity is not fully understood. Increased incidence of ectopic pregnancy was found during the last decades[5,6] mainly attributed to greater degree of socially acceptable sexual behavior, which led to increased incidence of the pelvic inflammatory disease (PID). Fortunately, the fatal outcomes have been reduced up to 75 percent for the reason of early diagnosis and less invasive treatment techniques. Mechanical factors predisposing pathomorphological site of implantation are: low-grade pelvic infection (main cause for the faulty implantation), peritubal adhesions (result of the previous PID), and salpingitis with the partial or total destruction of the tubal mucosa. It has been reported that ectopic pregnancies do occur in totally normal tubes, suggesting that abnormalities of the conceptus or maternal hormonal changes may act as etiological factors.[7,8]

Risk factors for ectopic pregnancy are STD-PID (sexually transmitted diseases-pelvic inflammatory disease)[9,10] assisted reproductive techniques, abnormalities of the conceptus, maternal hormonal changes, surgical procedures in pelvis[11] IUD (intrauterine device)[12] previous ectopic pregnancy, fibroids, uterine malformations, cigarette smoking, etc. In addition to providing an accurate description of the sites of implantation of ectopic pregnancy some authors showed that current IUD use 'protects' against interstitial pregnancies, which are the most

difficult to manage and that subsequent fertility tends to be higher in women with distal EP.[13] It is essential to identify risk factors so we can provide patients with adequate information, diagnose and treat an ectopic pregnancy early, and possibly to develop preventive strategies.[14-16]

The main problem of ectopic pregnancy is clinical presentation.[17] Symptoms can vary from vaginal spotting to vasomotor shock with hematoperitoneum.[18, 19] The classic triad of delayed menses, irregular vaginal bleeding and abdominal pain is most commonly not encountered, but the exact frequency of clinical symptoms and signs is hard to assess.[1] Both typical and atypical clinical presentation can mimic all kinds of diseases, which have no connection with pathology of reproductive system, such as appendicitis, diverticulitis, non-specific mesenterial lymphadenitis, or diseases of the urinary system. In most cases ectopic pregnancy is confused with an early spontaneous abortion because of the similar symptoms in both processes (delayed menses, enlarged and softened uterus and bleeding). Other conditions that should be considered in differential diagnosis of ectopic pregnancy are: normal intrauterine pregnancy, salpingitis, torsion or rupture of the ovarian cyst, adnexal torsion, bleeding corpus luteum, endometriosis, appendicitis, gastroenteritis, diverticulitis, conditions affecting urinary tract, etc. Therefore, early and reliable diagnosis of ectopic pregnancy is major challenge for every clinician. Significance of early diagnosis lays in the possibility for application of the conservative methods of treatment, which are crucial for preserving further reproductive capability, and in severe cases the life itself.[20] Diagnostic procedures are divided into two groups:

Noninvasive: History, general clinical and gynecological examination, hormonal and other laboratory markers and ultrasound diagnostics.

Invasive: Culdocenthesis[21] curettage[22] and laparoscopy.

ROLE OF BIOCHEMICAL MARKERS IN ECTOPIC PREGNANCY

Beta hCG (human chorionic gonadotropin) is the glycoprotein hormone released into circulation by human placental trophoblastic cells. From the 8th day after conception its concentration in blood rises 1.7 times every day.[23] As soon as implantation occurs the trophoblast starts producing beta hCG. Common urine beta hCG tests react at concentrations higher or equal to 1000 IU/l of urine, which means that they become positive 10 to 14 days after conception.[1] Falsely-positive results are mainly obtained in the case of proteinuria, erythrocyturia, gynecological tumors, tuboovarian abscess,[24] or some drug intake (e.g. tranquilizers). Embryo in cases of an ectopic pregnancy usually disappears, gets resorbed and we normally visualize an empty gestational sac producing smaller amounts of beta hCG. Normal levels of beta hCG could be found only in cases of a still living embryo which occurs in 5 to 8 percent of ectopic pregnancies.[23] For the reason of low concentrations of human chorionic gonadotropin only 40 to 60 percent of ectopic pregnancies have the positive urine test, therefore the more sensitive blood test should be performed, which becomes positive already 10 days after conception.[23] Absolute value of beta hCG levels in circulation are much lower than the levels of the same hormone in normal intrauterine pregnancies of the same gestational age.[25, 26] Dynamics of the titer show slower increase of circulating concentrations and prolongate the time for doubling its values. The most important use of the quantitative beta hCG determination in conjunction with ultrasonography is that of understanding the value of "discriminatory zone" of beta hCG. The discriminatory zone represents the level of beta hCG above which all normal intrauterine chorionic sacs will be detected by ultrasound. There is now almost a consensus in considering the discriminatory zone to be about 1000 mIU/ml with the use of transvaginal probe of at least 5 MHz.[27-30]

ROLE OF ULTRASOUND IN THE DIAGNOSIS OF ECTOPIC PREGNANCY

With recent technological development ultrasonography (but more precisely, transvaginal sonography) has become the "gold standard" diagnostic modality for the effective and fast detection of ectopic pregnancy. An important advantage of most currently used transvaginal transducers is the ability to perform simultaneous and spectral Doppler studies, allowing easy identification of the ectopic peritrophoblastic flow. In comparison to transvaginal sonography, transabdominal ultrasound, as a method for detecting ectopic gestation is restricted for a very small number of oddly located ectopic pregnancies, mainly high up in the pelvis—outside the effective reach of 5 MHz vaginal probe.[31]

Transabdominal Ultrasound

The absence of gestational sac inside the intrauterine cavity at 6th week of gestation raises the suspicion of an ectopic pregnancy. Transabdominal ultrasonography cannot reliably diagnose ectopic pregnancy, except when a live fetus is demonstrated in the abdominal cavity. In only 3 to 5 percent of the cases an ectopic gestational sac with embryonic echoes and clear heart activity can be demonstrated.[32] Probe with frequency of 3.5 MHz and large contact area is used for transabdominal ultrasonographic imaging and full bladder plays a role of an acoustic window. Resolution of this probe is somewhat lower, but the penetration is much deeper than one of the transvaginal probe.

The best results in confirming the intrauterine pregnancy are achieved using following criteria:
1. Normal size, shape and location of the gestational sac in the uterine cavity.
2. Double ring surrounding the gestational sac.
3. Embryonic parts with eventual.
4. Heart action.

Signs for ectopic pregnancy could be divided into uterine and extrauterine, some of them being diagnostic or just suggestive.

Diagnostic signs include: absence of the intrauterine gestational sac surrounded with double ring, absence of the yolk sac and/or fetal structures inside the gestational sac and presence of extraovarian adnexal structure. Suggestive signs are: uterine enlargement with thickened endometrium and blood or coagulum in the retrouterine space.[32]

Low sensitivity, specificity, positive and negative predictive values for detection of ectopic pregnancy are shortcomings of transabdominal ultrasound.[33,34] This modality still has some value in successful detection of a small proportion of ectopic pregnancies with bizarre location, such as high in the pelvis.

Transvaginal Ultrasound

In comparison with transabdominal approach, transvaginal ultrasound enables much better image of the morphological features in pelvis thanks to higher frequencies and probe location in immediate vicinity of the examined area. Sensitivity of transvaginal sonography was found to be 96 percent, the specificity reached 88 percent, the positive predictive value 89 percent and the negative predictive value 95 percent.[35] Intrauterine gestational sac surrounded with double ring with clear embryonic echo is considered to be strong evidence against ectopic pregnancy because heterotopic, pregnancy (intrauterine and ectopic), coincide rarely, but shouldn't be so easily ignored (Fig. 24.1), especially in the patients undergoing some of the methods of assisted reproduction.[36]

Intrauterine sonographic findings in women with ectopic pregnancy are variable. These include:

1. Empty uterus, with or without increased endometrial thickness,
2. Central hypoechoic area, or a sac like structure inside the cavity – the so called pseudogestational sac, and
3. Concurrent intrauterine pregnancy.

Early intrauterine pregnancy and recent spontaneous abortion may present themselves on transvaginal sonography with empty uterus (Fig. 24.2) and endometrial layer variable in thickness.[3] Therefore, they are considered to be suggestive signs. Pseudogestational sac can be demonstrated in 10 to 20 percent of patients with ectopic pregnancy[3] as a mixed echo pattern of endometrium that results from a decidual reaction, fluid, or both (Fig. 24.3). Careful examination of the uterine cavity usually allows a reliable distinction to be made between the pseudogestational sac and normal gestational sac. The pseudogestational sac is detected in the middle of the uterine cavity, its shape changes, owing to myometrial contractions. In differentiating a real gestational sac from a pseudogestational one, transvaginal color and pulsed Doppler ultrasound proved to be very useful.

Adnexal sonographic findings in women with ectopic pregnancy are variable. Gestational sac located inside adnexa with clear embryonic echo and heart activity directly proves ectopic pregnancy, but is seen in only 15 to 28 percent of the cases (Figs 24.4 and 24.5). Less rare is visualization of an adnexal gestational sac with or without embryonic echo (without heart action)[37] (Figs 24.6 to 24.10). Such a finding is detected in 46 to 71 percent of reported cases if tube is unruptured[38] while the most common finding is an unspecific adnexal tumor (Figs 24.11 and 24.12). Free fluid in the retrouterine space is seen in 40 to 83 percent of cases.

Accurate ultrasound diagnosis of ectopic pregnancy depends strongly on examiner's experience. Adnexal abnormalities may be difficult to identify because of confusion with loops of bowel or other pelvic structures.[39]

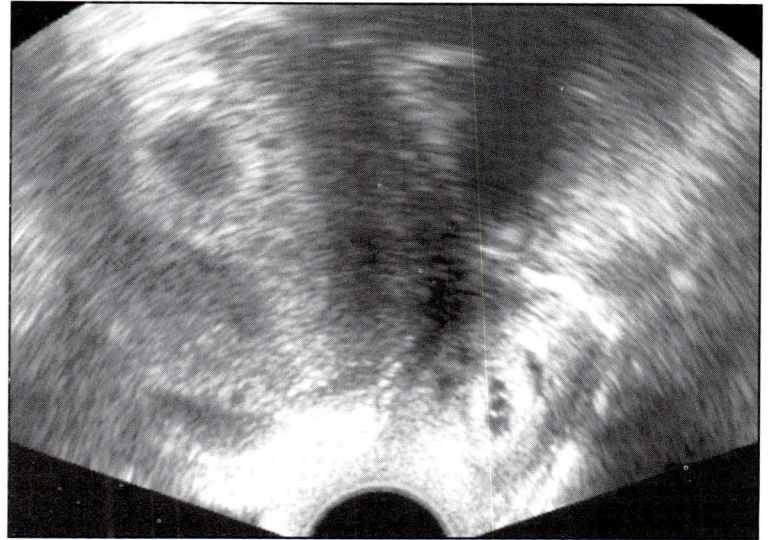

Fig. 24.1: Transvaginal sonogram showing an heterotopic pregnancy. Note the gestational sac correctly placed and another gestational sac with yolk sac in the cervix

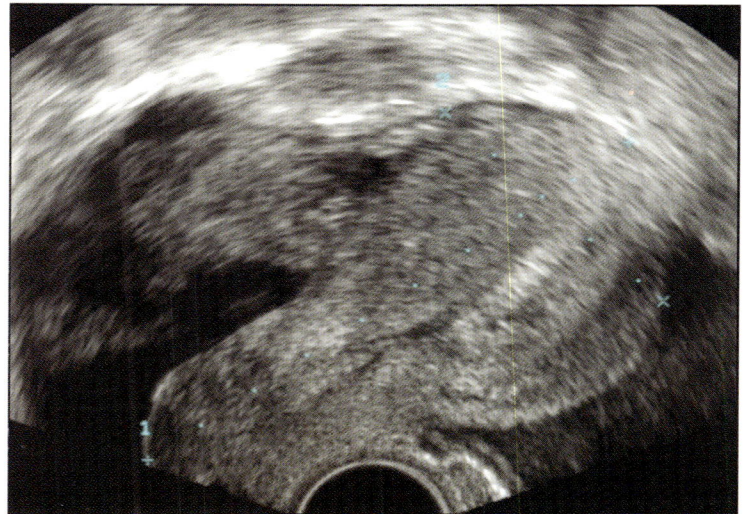

Fig. 24.2: Transvaginal sonogram of the uterus in a patient with ectopic pregnancy. Note the absence of intrauterine gestational sac and the free fluid was visualized in the pouch of Douglas, signal ruptured ectopic pregnancy

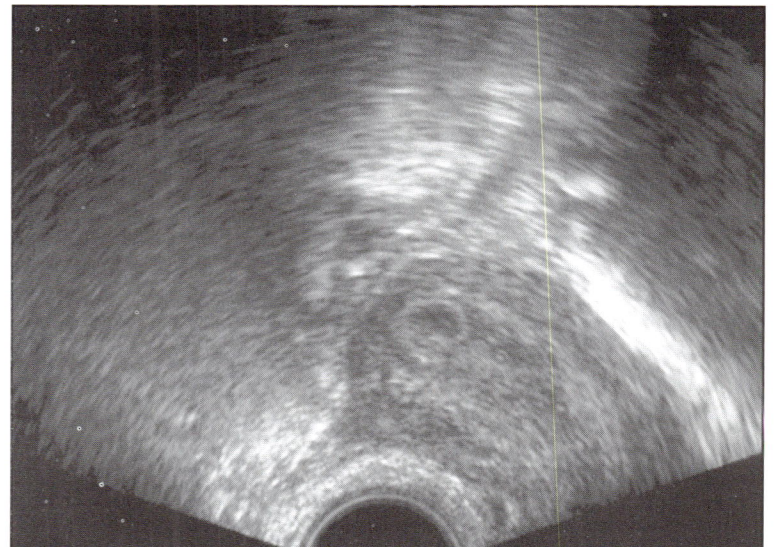

Fig. 24.3: Tranvaginal sonogram showing a hypoechoic structure representing a decidual reaction and collection on intracavitary blood. This is typical of a pseudogestational sac

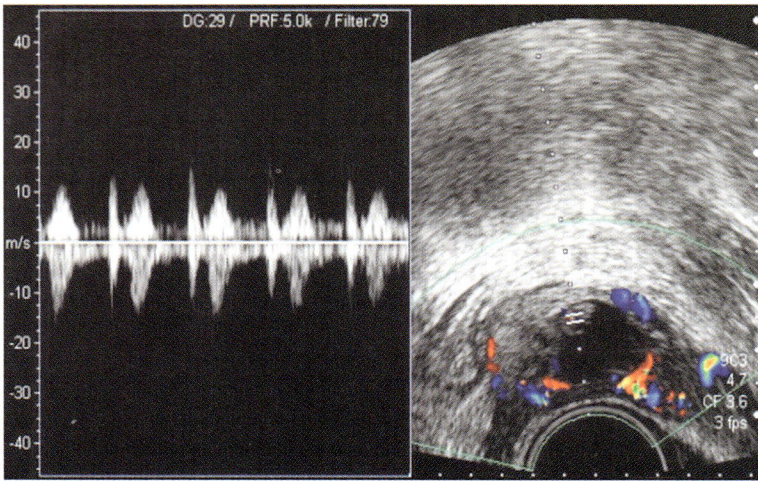

Fig. 24.4: Color Doppler transvaginal scan showing gestational sac located inside right adnexa with clear embryonic echo and heart activity

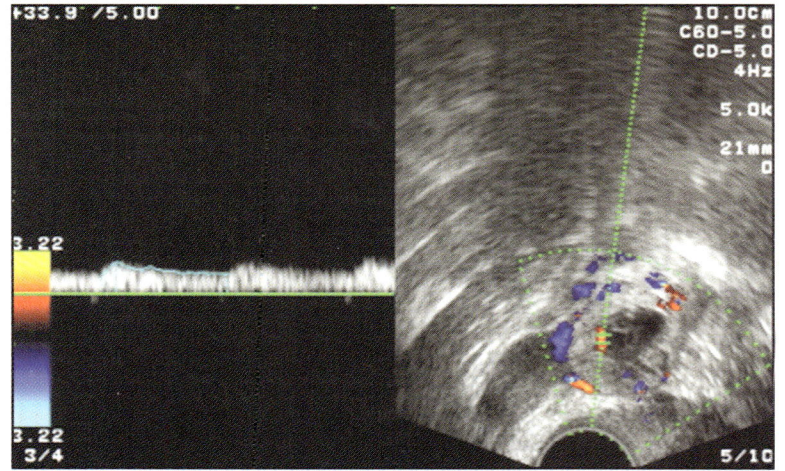

Fig. 24.7: Tranvaginal color Doppler showing a gestational sac with yolk sac. Pulsed Doppler shows a low vascular resistance (RI = 0.42)

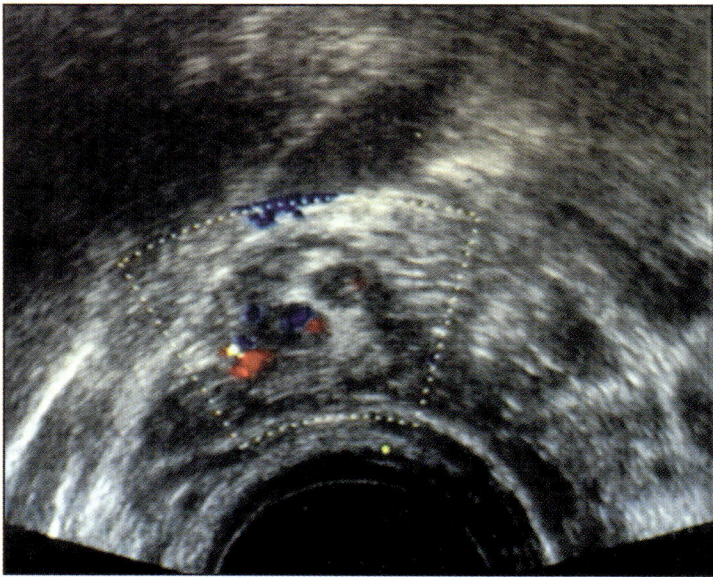

Fig. 24.5: Transvaginal color Doppler showing a twins ectopic gestation whitin the fallopian tube. Note the blood flow signals obtained from the peritrophoblastic area. Laparoscopy cofirmed twins ectopic pregnancy

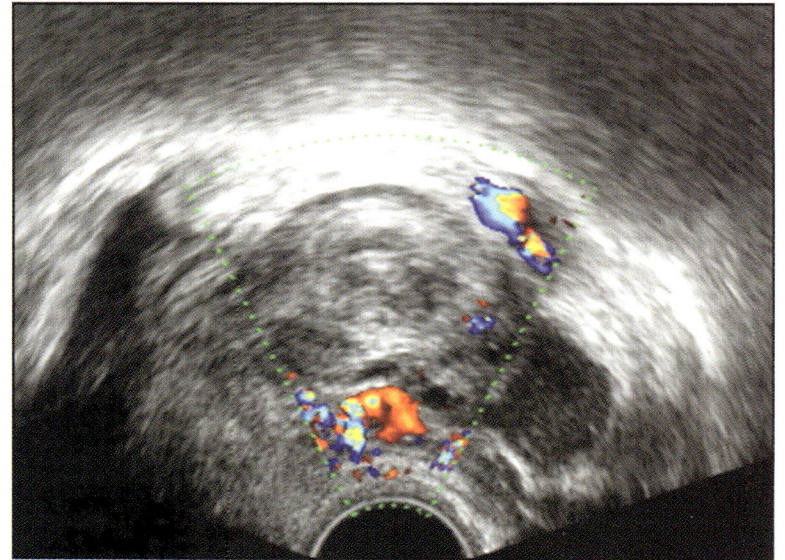

Fig. 24.8: The same patient as in Figure 24.1. We can see a solid mass free liquid surrounded suspected to be an ectopic gestation

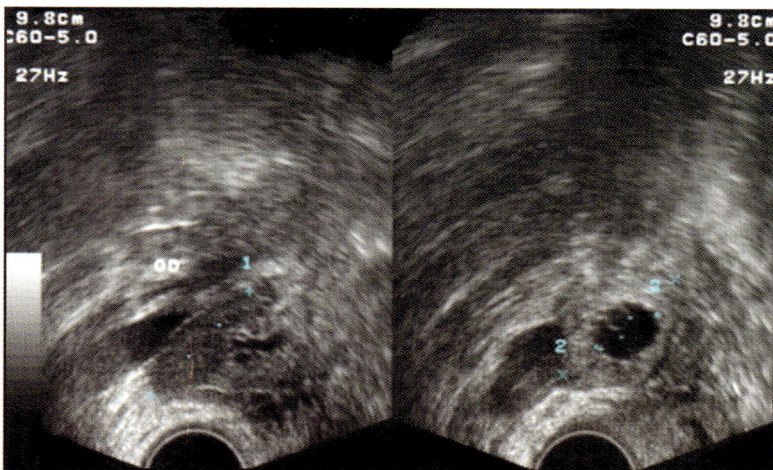

Fig. 24.6: Transvaginal scan demonstrating the right ovary a near we can see an ectopic gestation 15 mm larger with yolk sac

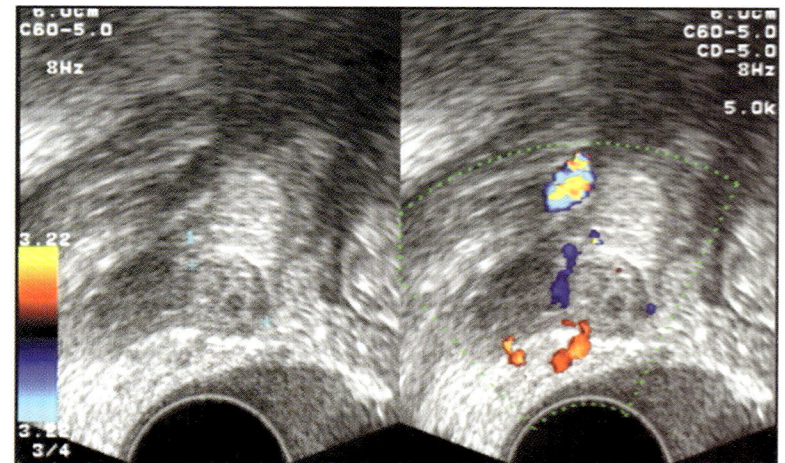

Fig. 24.9: Tranvaginal color Doppler showing a small (13 mm) ectopic gestation close to the left ovary

There are four adnexal structures that may resemble an ectopic pregnancy and should be correctly identified.[40] One is the corpus luteum (Fig. 24.13), which is eccentrically located within the ovary, surrounded by ovarian tissue and possibly creating the impression of a sac-like structure. About 85 percent of ectopic pregnancies are formed on the same side as the corpus luteum.[41] This is important to bear in mind while trying to distinguish tubal pregnancy from the ipsilateral corpus luteum.

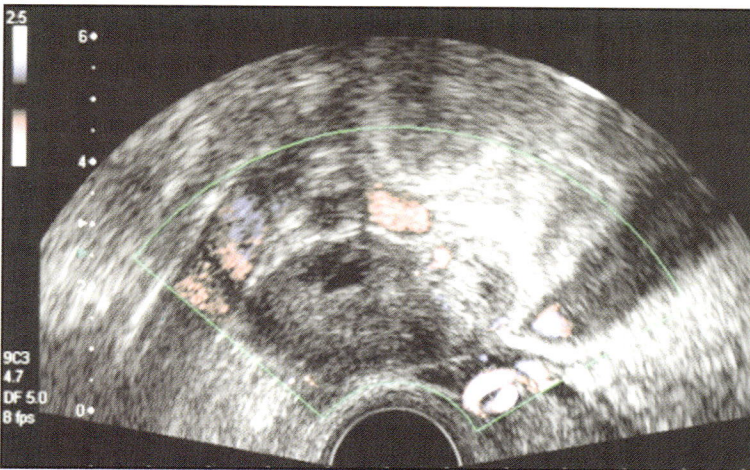

Fig. 24.10: Transvaginal dynamic flow showing a small ectopic pregnancy next to the right ovary

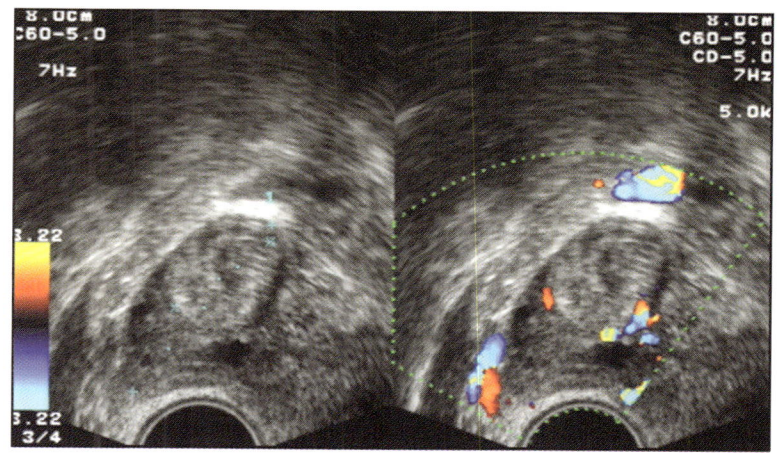

Fig. 24.11: Transvaginal scan of a complex adnexal mass occupying the pouch of Douglas in a patient with increased serum β-hCG concentration. Laparoscopy confirmed ectopic pregnancy

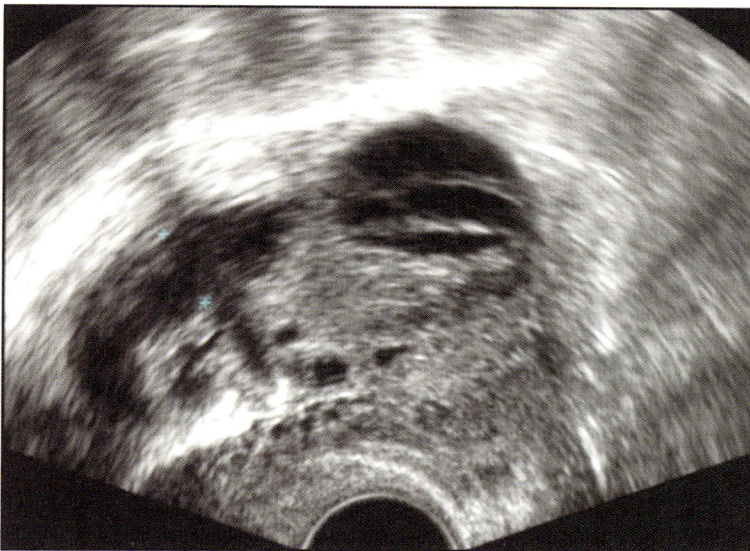

Fig. 24.12: In the left of the picture we can see a smaller (11 mm) gestational pregnancy in close proximity to the ovary. In the right of the picture transvaginal scan demonstrating an intrauterine device correctly placed

Corpus luteum is found in the ovary and its echogenicity is slightly (or at times even substantially) lower than that of trophoblastic

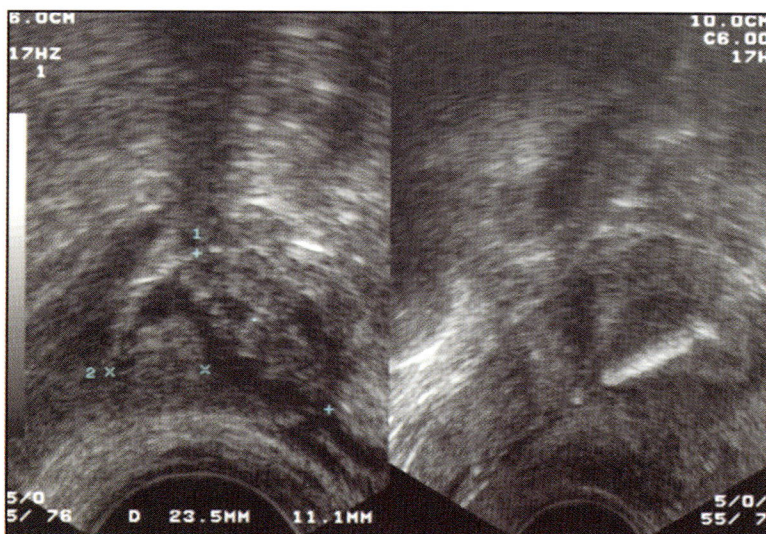

Fig. 24.13: Transvaginal color Doppler showing a corpus luteum of the ovary. This is an other cause of false-positive of ectopic pregnancy

tissue of the tubal ring. Furthermore, hemorrhagic corpus luteum usually shows a hypoechoic rather than a cystic central region.[42] Other three conditions than need to be correctly differentiated from an ectopic gestation are a thick-walled ovarian follicle, the small intestine, and tubal pathology conditions, such as hydrosalpix containing fluid (Fig. 24.14).

Using the protocol of combination of clinical examination, serum beta hCG assay and transvaginal ultrasound examination it is possible to diagnose ectopic pregnancy with a sensitivity of 100 percent and specificity of 99 percent.[43]

Another problem in detection of an ectopic pregnancy in adnexal region arises in patients undergoing assisted reproductive procedures or simple hormonal superovulation. Besides the increased risk for ectopic pregnancy in these patients, a large number of artificial corpora lutea will be seen that resemble the tubal ring of an ectopic pregnancy. Sometimes cystic adnexal masses (ovarian cystadenoma, cystadenofibroma, endometrioma, teratoma and pedunculated fibroids) may also rise differential diagnostic problems.

Free intraperitoneal fluid is seen in 40 to 83 percent the women with ectopic pregnancy, but also in up to 20 percent of normal intrauterine pregnancies.[38] In case of tubal abortion echogenic echoes suggesting the presence of blood clots are demonstrated, while tubal rupture is associated with a homogeneous, hypoechoic retrouterine echo that represents blood collection (Figs 24.15 and 24.16). The possibility of an ectopic pregnancy increases if the amount of fluid is moderate to large, but the absence of blood does not exclude its diagnosis.

Serial serum beta hCG assay may rise a suspicion on ectopic pregnancy at a very early gestation, while transvaginal ultrasound scan may not be able to demonstrate the site of the pregnancy (Fig. 24.17). Under these circumstances sometimes it is necessary to perform laparoscopic examination to exclude the possibility of ectopic pregnancy. However, even laparoscopic

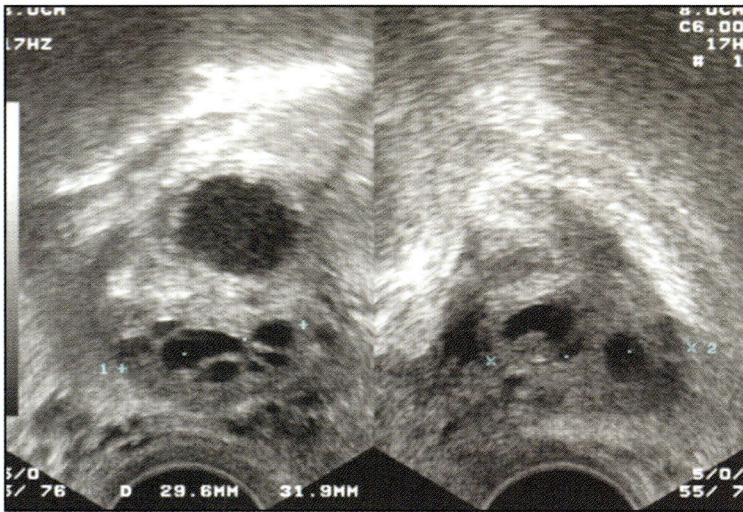

Fig. 24.14: Transvaginal sonogram showing a pelvic inflammatory disease. These findings are cause of false-positive of ectopic pregnancy

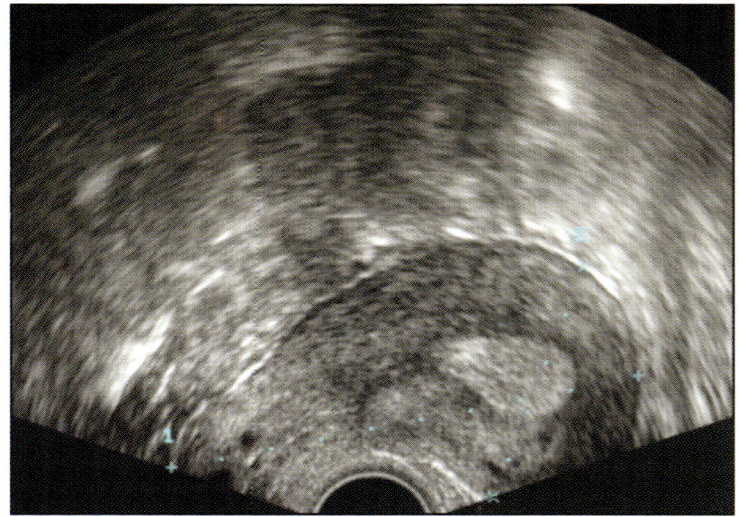

Fig. 24.15: Transvaginal scan showing blood and organized clot in pericolic recess. This is an indirect sign of ectopic pregnancy

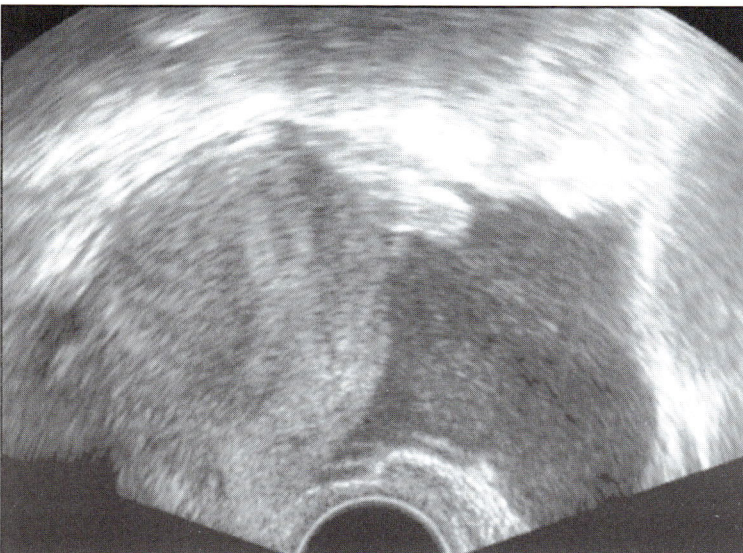

Fig. 24.16: Another example of ruptured ectopic pregnancy. We can see the empty cavity and blood fluid free

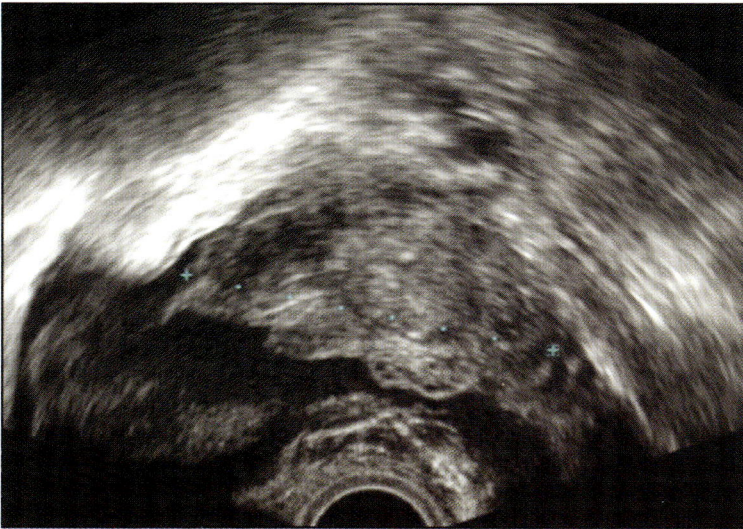

Fig. 24.17: Transvaginal scan of the uterus in a patient with increased serum β-hCG concentration. Note a decidual reaction. This is an indirect sign of ectopic pregnancy

adhesions or fibroids. Some reports demonstrated that laparoscopic ultrasound can facilitate the diagnosis of the site of ectopic pregnancy intraoperatively, even if it is as small as 3.9 mm.[44] The number of negative laparoscopies can be decreased and repeat laparoscopy avoided. Therefore, laparoscopic ultrasound should be used when the site of ectopic pregnancy cannot be determined or is obscured by other pathologies during laparoscopic examination.

Color Doppler Facility

Ultrasound machine with color Doppler facility is an excellent guide in search for blood flow signals within the entire pelvis. The color flow pattern associated with ectopic pregnancy is variable. It usually presents randomly dispersed multiple small vessels within the adnexa, showing high-velocity and low impedance signals (RI = 0.36 0.45) clearly separated from the ovarian tissue and corpus luteum. The sensitivity of transvaginal color and pulsed Doppler in diagnosis of ectopic pregnancy reported in several studies ranges from 73 to 96 percent, and specificity from 87 to 100 percent. [3,4,38,45]

Visualization of ipsilateral corpus luteum blood flow may aid in diagnosis of ectopic pregnancy. The RI of luteal flow in the cases of ectopic pregnancy has been reported to be 0.48 ± 0.07, which is between the values of the non-pregnant women (0.42 ± 0.12) and those with normal early intrauterine pregnancy (0.53 ± 0.09).[46] In majority of patients with proven ectopic pregnancy, luteal flow is detected on the same side as the ectopic pregnancy. This observation could be used as a guide in searching for ectopic pregnancy (Fig. 24.18).

The between-side difference in tubal artery blood flow was also documented. There was a significant increase in the tubal artery blood flow on the side of tubal gestation. The mean

examination may not be able to achieve a precise diagnosis, especially when the ectopic pregnancy is very small or when there are co-existing pathologies such as hydrosalpinges,

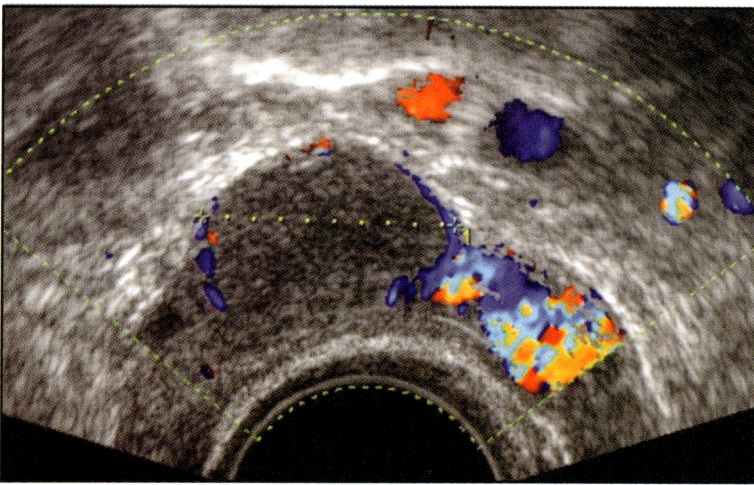

Fig. 24.18: An ipsilateral corpus luteum is demonstrated laterally to the ectopic gestational sac

reduction of the RI on the side with the ectopic pregnancy compared to the opposite side was 15.5 percent.[4] These changes appear to be due to trophoblastic invasion, and showed no dependence on gestational age. Bright color on the screen while using the pulsed Doppler facility is due to very high speed of the peritrophoblastic blood flow and low impedance (Figs 24.19 to 24.23). It should be stressed out that the patients with tubal abortion demonstrate significantly higher vascular impedance of peritrophoblastic flow (RI > 0.60), and less prominent color signals (Fig. 24.24).

The main diagnostic importance of transvaginal color and pulsed Doppler is in differentiating the nature of nonspecific adnexal masses. Doppler blood flow indices in the uterine, spiral arteries and corpus luteum arteries in ectopic and intrauterine pregnancies showed that the mean uterine and spiral artery RI decreased with increased gestational age of the intrauterine pregnancies, but remained constantly high in ectopic pregnancies.[47] The peak systolic blood flow velocity in the uterine artery increased with increasing gestational age in intrauterine pregnancies, and the values were significantly higher than in ectopic pregnancies.[48] The difference in peak systolic velocity reflects a decreased blood supply to the ectopic pregnancy. Intrauterine gestational sac shows prominent peritrophoblastic vascular signals (RI = 0.44 to 0.45), while pseudogestational sacs do not demonstrate increased blood flow (Fig. 24.25). It has been suggested that velocities below 21 cm are diagnostic for pseudogestational sac and can successfully rule out trophoblastic flow of a normal intrauterine pregnancy.[49]

The intravascular ultrasound contrast agent has a recognizable effect on Doppler ultrasonographic examination of the adnexal circulation. It appears to be helpful when the finding in color flow imaging is ambiguous. The use of the contrast agent may also facilitate localization of trophoblastic tissue in hemorrhagic adnexal lesions.[50]

As with other diagnostic methods, transvaginal color and pulsed Doppler studies include both, false-positive and false-negative findings. A false-positive diagnosis arises predominantly from the corpus luteum, but in exceptional cases some adnexal lesions may mimic ectopic pregnancy. A false-negative result may arise from technical inadequacy, lack of experience or patients' non-compliance. The other possibility of fault diagnosis is non-vascularized ectopic gestation, as these are associated with low beta hCG values.

Some authors compared technical errors with improper setting of color flow parameters.[51] The color velocity scale, color priority, color gain, color sensitivity and color wall filter should be adjusted to optimize color flow information. Technical errors may result in false diagnosis of ovarian torsion, malignancy and ectopic pregnancy.

The diagnosis of ectopic pregnancy still remains a challenge to the clinician despite advances in ultrasound and biochemical technology. Frequently the diagnosis remains uncertain until laparoscopy or D and C are performed. With the increasing tendency towards conservative therapy, the distinction between ectopic pregnancies that will resolve spontaneously and those that will rupture is essential.[52] Usually patients without acute symptoms and with declining beta hCG values are treated conservatively.[53] However, secondary ruptures have been reported in patients with low initial beta hCG concentrations.[54] The differentiation between viable ectopic pregnancies with trophoblastic activity and dissolving tubal abortions could facilitate the decision to proceed with conservative or operative treatment.

After implantation in the mucosa of endosalpinx, the lamina propria and then the muscularis of the oviduct, the blastocyst grows mainly between the lumen of the tube and its peritoneal covering.[55] Growth occurs both parallel to the long axis of the tube and circumferentially around it. As the trophoblast invades surrounding vessels, intensive blood flow and/or intraperitoneal bleeding occur. The intensive ring of vascular signals could be a criterion for viability of an ectopic pregnancy that can be determined rapidly and easily and seems to be independent of beta hCG values.[56] In patients with a viable ectopic pregnancy who demand a conservative treatment, this method could provide an aid, in addition to beta hCG values; for supervising the efficiency of treatment, especially in those cases where beta hCG levels slowly normalize. In this way duration of hospitalization could be shortened, the patients uncertainty diminished, and the cost of the treatment reduced. In cases of persisting high beta hCG levels after operative removal of the ectopic, color Doppler sonography can provide evidence for the presence of viable trophoblast remnants. On contrary, in asymptomatic patients with hypoperfused and/or avascular ectopic gestational

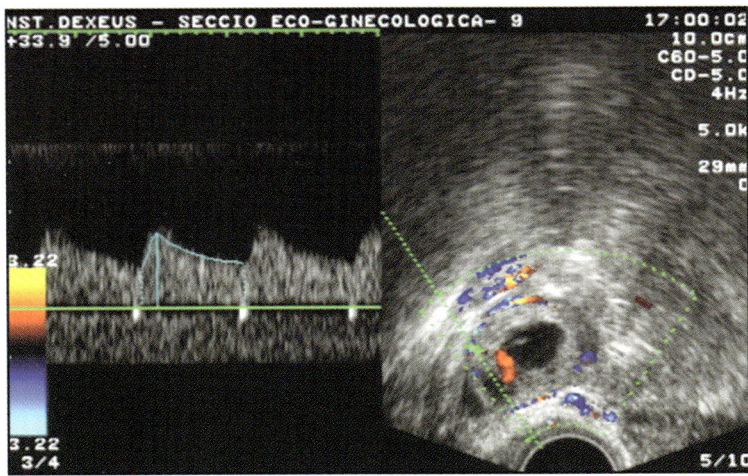

Fig. 24.19: Blood flow waveforms depicted from the area of peritrophoblastic flow show low vascular resistance (RI = 0.47)

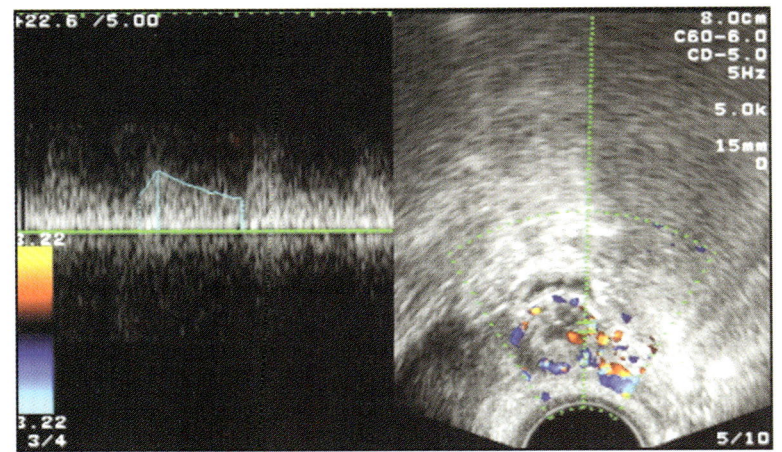

Fig. 24.22: Transvaginal color Doppler scan of a small gestational sac. Note the "ring of fire" and a low vascular resistance (RI = 0.48)

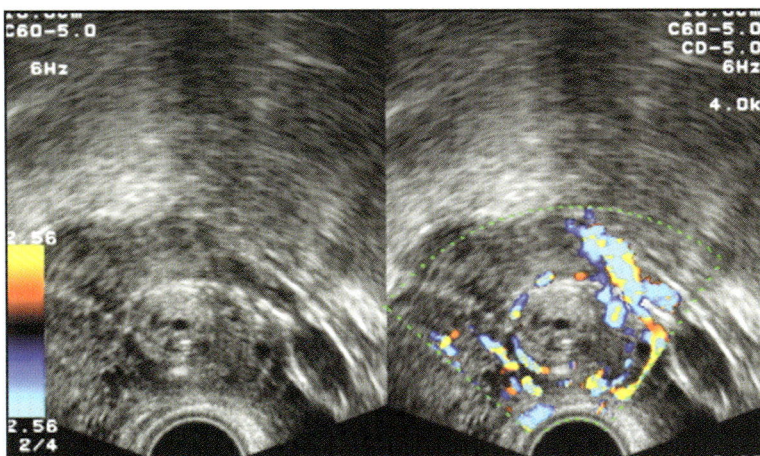

Fig. 24.20: Transvaginal color Doppler demonstratres the "ring of fire" typical of ectopic pregnancy. This finding guides the sonographer to the location of the ectopic pregnancy and shortens the diagnostic process

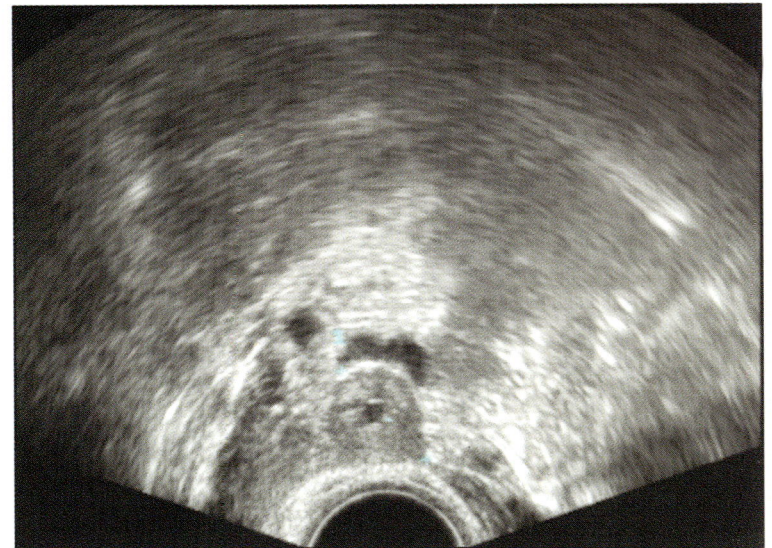

Fig. 24.23: Transvaginal sonogram demonstrating a concentric gestational ring 18 mm larger, in close proximity to the ovary. This is a typical finding of ectopic pregnancy

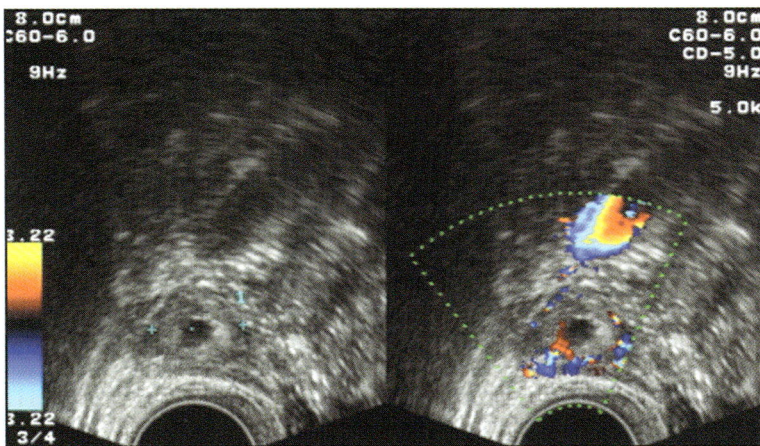

Fig. 24.21: Transvaginal color Doppler scan of a small gestational sac in the adnexal region. Note the "ring of fire"

sac and decreased values of beta hCG expectative treatment can be established.

3D Ultrasound in the Assessment of Tubal Ectopic Pregnancy

Three-dimensional (3D) ultrasound technology offers some advantages over conventional two-dimensional (2D)

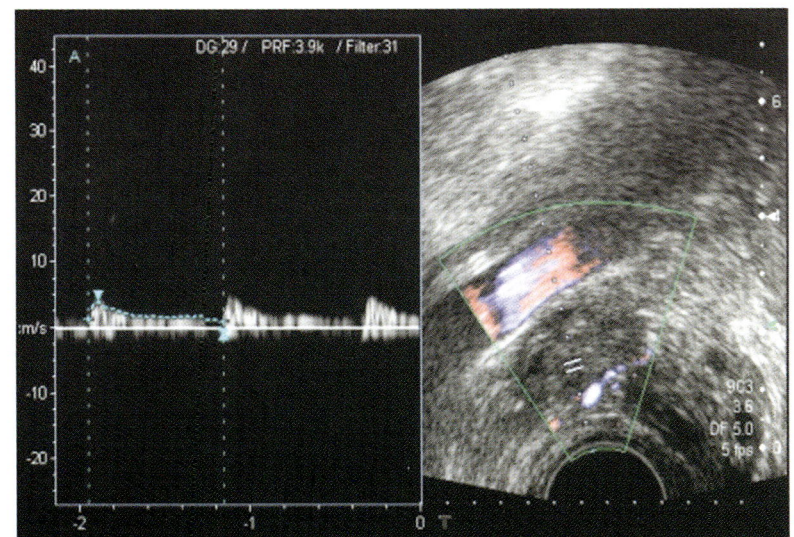

Fig. 24.24: Gestational sac measuring 14 mm visualized in the right adnexal region. Color Doppler depicts a small area of angiogenesis by a high resistance index (RI = 0.78). This finding is indicative of tubal abortion

sonographic imaging.[57,58] Modern systems are capable of generating surface and transparent views depicting the sculpture-

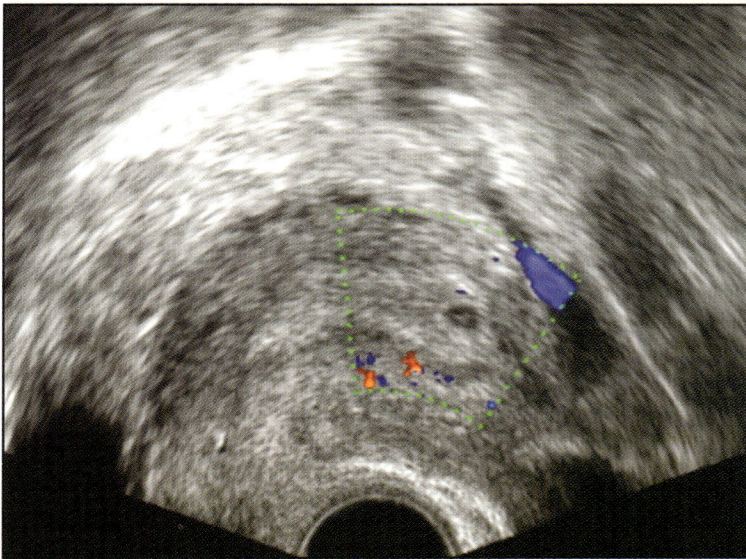

Fig. 24.25: Transvaginal color Doppler sonogram of the uterus in a patient with ectopic pregnancy. Note the hypoechoic avascular area representing a pseudogestational sac

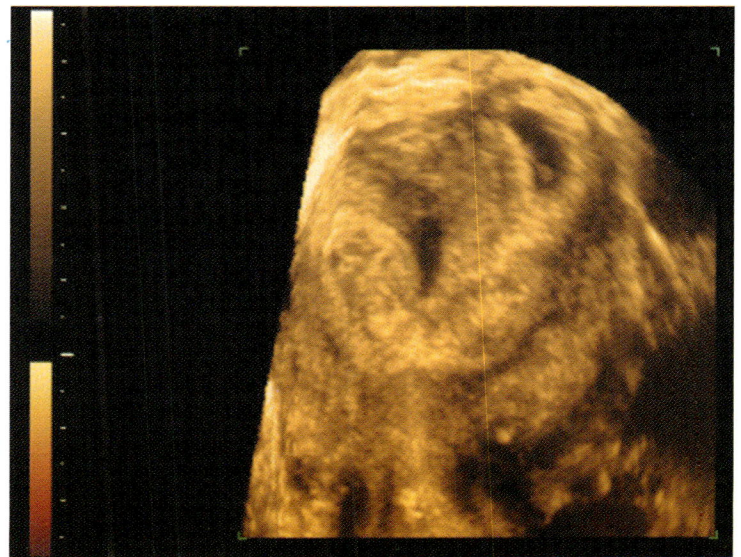

Fig. 24.26: Three-dimensional ultrasound showing a septate uterus, with ectopic gestation in the left horn. We can see the yolk sac

like reconstruction of surfaces or the transparent images structure's content (Fig. 24.26).

Planar mode tomograms are helpful in distinguishing the early intraendometrial gestational sac from a collection of the fluid between the endometrial leaves (pseudogestational sac).

A prospective follow up study was conducted in order to evaluate the potential utility of 3D ultrasound to differentiate the intrauterine from ectopic gestations.[59] Fifty-four pregnancies with a gestational age < 10 weeks and with an intrauterine gestational sac < 5 mm in diameter formed the study group. The configuration of the endometrium in the frontal plane of the uterus was correlated with pregnancy outcome. After exclusion of three patients with a poor 3D image quality, the endometrial shape was found to be asymmetrical with regard to the median longitudinal axis of the uterus in 84 percent of intrauterine pregnancies, whereas endometrium showed symmetry in the frontal plane in 90 percent of ectopic pregnancies. Intrauterine fluid accumulation may distort the uterine cavity, thus being responsible for false-positive, as well as false-negative results. The evaluation of the endometrial shape in the frontal plane appeared to be a useful additional mean of distinguishing intrauterine from ectopic pregnancies, especially when a gestational sac was not clearly demonstrated with conventional ultrasound. Similarly, preliminary data of other authors suggested that 3D sonography is an effective procedure for early diagnosis of ectopic pregnancy in asymptomatic patients before 6 weeks of amenorrhea.[60]

The possible use of 3D power Doppler is the monitoring of the vascularity of ectopic pregnancy. The hypoperfusion, quantified by indices of vascularity (VI) and flow (FI), could indicate that the ectopic pregnancy is spontaneously being resolved, and that laparoscopy should be postponed. This way, the conservative approach to ectopic pregnancy would rely on more precise and easily obtainable data. Vice versa, in case of hyperperfusion, the patients should be subjected to laparoscopy or medical treatment immediately.

Shih and colleagues[61] described the use of 3D color/power angiography in two cases in which an arteriovenous malformation of mesosalpinx was diagnosed following involution of an anembryonic ectopic gestation. The diagnosis of arteriovenous malformations has traditionally been made by arteriography. Recently, it has also been diagnosed by non-invasive methods such as contrast enhanced CT, MRI and color Doppler ultrasound. The advantage of 3D reconstruction of color/power angiography images is better spatial and anatomic orientation and quick demonstration of the vessels, usually within one minute, especially in the areas where complex structures are present. Therefore, unlike MRI, digital subtraction angiography or contrast enhanced CT, 3D color/power angiography allows the physician to examine vascular anatomy immediately and without radiation exposure.

Most tubal gestations are not ongoing viable gestations. They are usually in the involutional phase of abortion within a confined area which results in the extrusion of products of conception through a ruptured site or fimbriae. In the two reported cases, the serum assays of beta hCG in both patients increased to significant levels which precluded intrauterine missed abortion.[61] Besides, there were neither retained products of conception in utero nor heavy vaginal bleeding (indicating process of abortion in progress) prior to the diagnosis of arteriovenous malformation. Therefore, authors speculated that there might be an ectopic gestation occurring somewhere, although they could find only a pelvic arteriovenous malformation rather than an adnexal gestational sac.

The major difference between uterine implantation and tubal gestation is that endosalpingeal stroma usually falls to undergo decidualization. The chorionic villi of the tubal implantation may than invade into the tubal wall and mesentery (mesosalpinx) more directly and rapidly. The vascularization within the ectopic pregnancy is an analog of placenta increta.[62] In such situations cytotrophoblast may invade the contiguous artery and vein of mesosalpinx with destruction of these vessels' walls, and thus may induce an arteriovenous malformation in situ or nearby. Possibly, the secretion of angiogenic factors (by trophoblast) and the increasing afterload of an arterioventricular shunt existing in the tubal gestation can induce the rapid growth of a small pre-existing congenital arteriovenous malformation. However, two unusual cases of adnexal arteriovenous malformations associated with "vanishing" ectopic gestation where congenital etiology seemed unlikely have also been reported.[61] B-mode ultrasound and color Doppler provided information on the hemodynamics of the vascular tumor and led to the diagnosis of arteriovenous malformation. Three-dimensional color/power angiography further improved understanding of the complex vascular anatomy and refined the diagnosis.

Even though the exact role of 3D ultrasound in the pathology of early pregnancy is yet to be established, a promising results of already published papers are encouraging. Unlimited numbers of sections are easily obtained without the need for excessive manipulation with the probe. Additional progress has been made, owing to the permanent possibility or repeated analysis of previous stored 3D volumes and Cartesian elimination of surrounding structures and artifacts. Three-dimensional reconstruction of stored image without any degradation is the most impressive benefit of 3D scanning.

OTHER SITES OF IMPLANTATION

About 5 percent of ectopic pregnancies implant in sites other than the tubes.[1] These are at times more difficult to detect and some, owing to strategic sites of implantation, may cause rupture, significant bleeding and higher morbidity and mortality than the tubal gestations.

Interstitial Pregnancy

It occurs in 1.1 to 6.3 percent of all ectopic pregnancies.[1,63] This location of ectopic pregnancy usually occurs following in vitro fertilization (IVF) and previous salpingectomy[63] but in most cases there are no apparent risk factors. Interstitial pregnancy clinically presents with abdominal pain and a tender asymmetrically enlarged uterus. The major problem of this location lies in late diagnosis, because it is commonly diagnosed after the rupture of the cornu has occurred and this may result in massive hemorrhage. Previously, interstitial pregnancies were diagnosed only at laparotomy following the rupture. For the reason of major hemorrhage, hysterectomy rate was as high as 40 percent.[60] In recent years, the routine use of ultrasound for the assessment of women with early pregnancy complications has enabled a non-invasive diagnosis of interstitial pregnancy to be made (Figs 24.27 and 24.28). Earlier diagnosis made before serious complications, allows the use of more conservative management, such as medical treatment or laparoscopic surgery.

A viable interstitial pregnancy may occasionally be misinterpreted as a normal intrauterine pregnancy. Therefore, it is important that strict diagnostic criteria are used in every case[64]:
1. Empty uterine cavity, and
2. Chorionic sac that is seen separately and more than 1 cm from the most lateral edge of the uterine cavity and surrounded by a thin myometrial layer.

It is worth to mention that approximately 15 percent of patients with interstitial pregnancy have heterotopic pregnancy.[64] In these cases, intrauterine findings may be misleading and should be interpreted with caution, rather than being used as primary diagnostic criterion. Visualization of the interstitial part of the tube in close proximity of the endometrium and depiction of the trophoblastic tissue improves the diagnosis of interstitial pregnancy.[65] It also confirms that pregnancy is located outside the uterine cavity, facilitating the differential diagnosis between an interstitial pregnancy and unusual forms of intrauterine pregnancy such as angular pregnancy or pregnancy in the cornu of an anomalous uterus. This sign is particularly helpful in women with small intramural fibroids located in vicinity of the interstitial part of the tube (Figs 24.29 and 24.30), which may be misinterpreted as a solid interstitial pregnancy.[66] In women with fibroids, the intramural part of the tube is displaced and can be visualized bypassing the mass, thus preventing the false-positive diagnosis of the interstitial pregnancy. Color Doppler facilitates the diagnosis of a cornual pregnancy by exposing low resistance peritrophoblastic flow (Figs 24.31 to 24.33).

Three-dimensional ultrasound has the advantage of providing views of the uterus, which can rarely be obtained by conventional 2D ultrasound scan.[67] In the coronal section, the position of the interstitial pregnancy in relation to the uterine cavity can be studied in detail. Visualization of the proximal section of the interstitial tube is also facilitated, which increases diagnostic confidence.[65] It is believed that 3D ultrasound is a helpful diagnostic tool in women with suspected interstitial pregnancy and should be considered in the cases where the diagnosis is not certain on conventional 2D transvaginal ultrasound scan.[68]

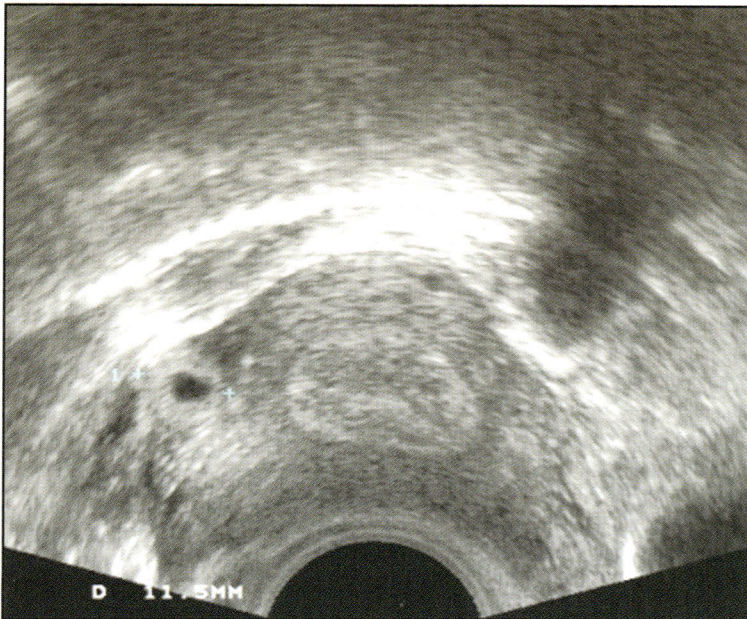

Fig. 24.27: Tranversal scan of the uterus showing a smaller (11 mm) ectopic pregnancy, in a patient with previously salpingectomy. Laparoscopy confirmed the ectopic pregnancy in a residual portion of fallopian tube

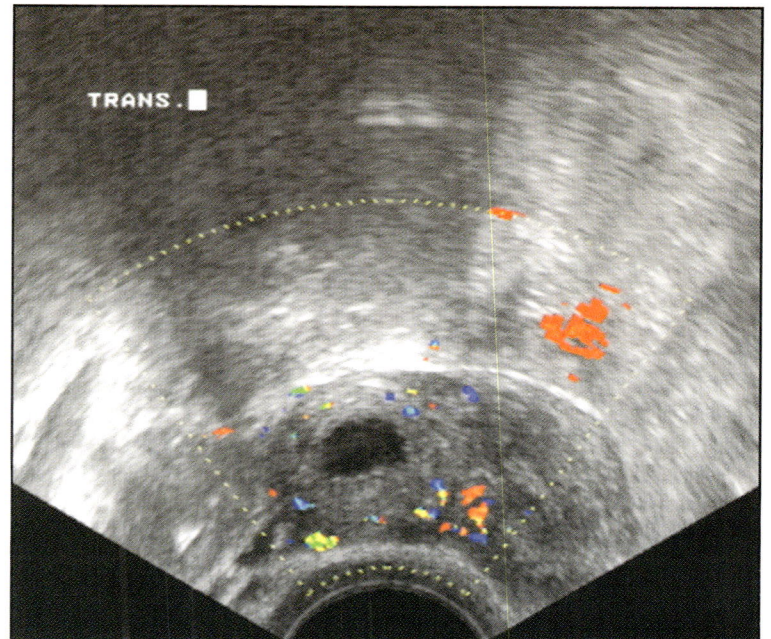

Fig. 24.28: The same patient as in Figure 24.19. Color Doppler depicted area of peritrophoblastic tissue

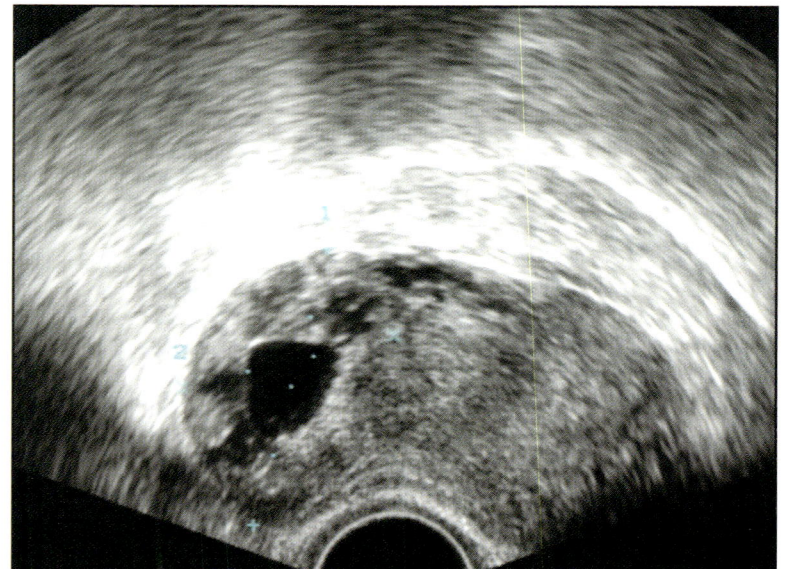

Fig. 24.29: Tranvaginal sonogram showing a necrotic myoma in the right horn, mistaken an ectopic gestation

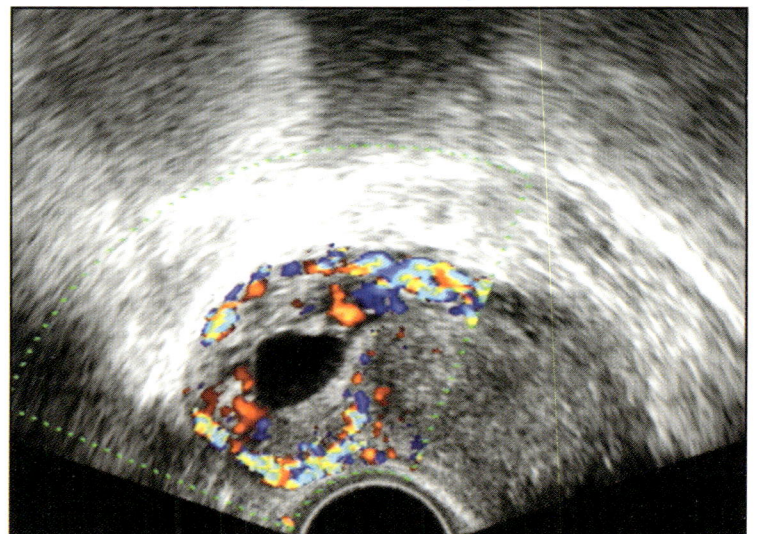

Fig. 24.30: The same patient as in Figure 24.21. Color Doppler shows peripheral vascularization

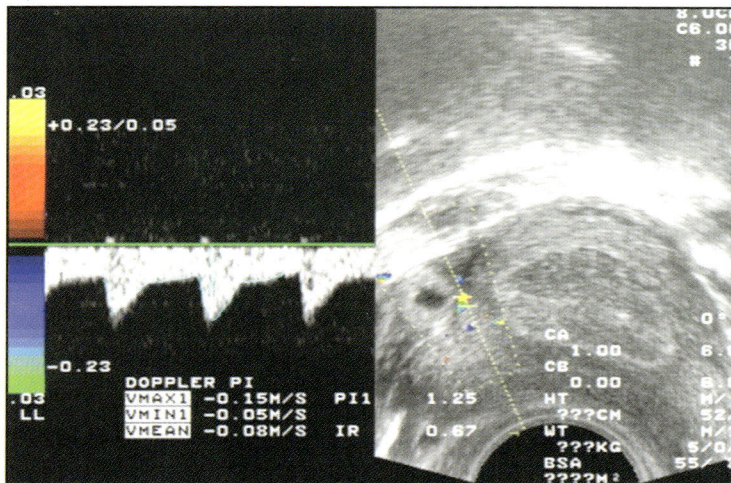

Fig. 24.31: Transvaginal sonogram showing an ectopic gestation in a right horn

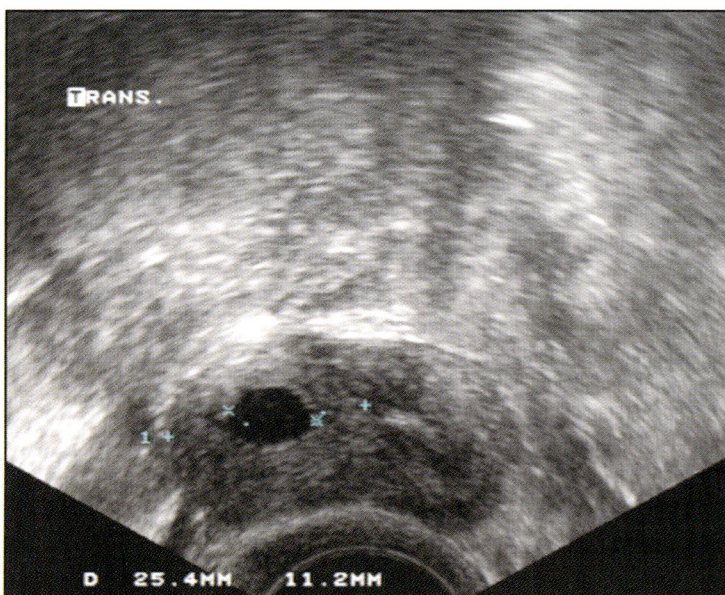

Fig. 24.32: The same patient as in Figure 24.31. Color Doppler demonstrates the "ring of fire" typical of ectopic pregnancy

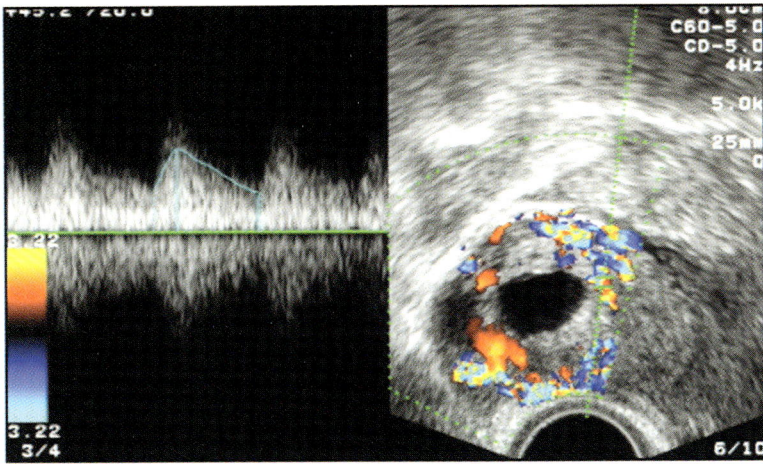

Fig. 24.33: The same patient as in Figures 24.31 and 24.32. Pulsed Doppler waveform analysis obtained from the area of angiogenesis demonstrates low-moderate resitance (RI = 0.53)

Most cornual/interstitial ectopic pregnancies are treated by laparoscopy and laparotomy using various surgical procedures (excision, suturing, etc.). Lately, transvaginal sonographic puncture and local injection of methotrexate, has been used to treat both viable and non-viable interstitial pregnancies.[64,65] There have been very few reported side-effects after treatment with low-dose local injection of methotrexate.[69] Data reported in the literature suggest the superiority of local therapy, with regard to both safety aspect and the success rate. In general, a likely explanation for the increased effectiveness of local injection is in higher concentration of therapeutic agent achieved in the target tissue. Although absorption of methotrexate into the circulation occurs after both local and systemic administration, a lower dose of methotrexate is used locally, leading to lower systemic levels and therefore fewer side effects.[70] Color Doppler plays an extremely important role providing an aid in approaching the cornual pregnancy from the medial aspect and traversing the thicker myometrial layer so rupture or bleeding are less likely to occur.[71] In these cases, color Doppler guidance during the instillation of methotrexate enables better visualization of blood vessels and avoidance of intraprocedural complications.

Viable heterotopic/interstitial pregnancies are often treated by local injection of potassium chloride, as this is not teratogenic. All six reported cases of heterotopic pregnancies in the literature were successfully treated in this way, with three (50%) intrauterine pregnancies progressing normally to full term.[4]

Expectant management of the interstitial pregnancy has also been reported.[64,66] All three non-viable interstitial pregnancies managed in this way were resolved spontaneously without any need for intervention. Expectant management can therefore, be useful option in selected cases.

Cervical Pregnancy

Cervical pregnancy is defined as the implantation of the conceptus below the level of the internal os. It is the rare condition that occurs in one in 50,000.[4] Intrauterine adhesions, uterine anomalies, previous cesarean sections, fibroids, previous therapeutic abortions and IVF treatment have all been associated with cervical implantation. Traditionally the diagnosis of cervical pregnancy was based solely on clinical findings and history reports after hysterectomy. Therefore, it is likely that only the most severe cases were diagnosed, and a number of cervical pregnancies went undiagnosed or were treated as incomplete miscarriages. In the past two decades, ultrasound has become the method of choice for diagnosis of early pregnancy disorders and certainly contributed to the recent increase in number of reported cervical pregnancies.

The diagnosis of cervical pregnancy can be made on the following criteria:

1. No evidence on intrauterine pregnancy.
2. An hour glass uterine shape with ballooned cervical canal.
3. Presence of a gestational sac or placental tissue within the cervical canal, and
4. Closed internal os.

Early diagnosis may also explain the milder clinical symptoms and better prognosis of cervical pregnancy today as compared to pre-ultrasound era.

Transvaginal ultrasound approach has become the accepted standard for the examination of patients with suspected early pregnancy abnormalities. Apart from providing superior images of pelvic anatomy, addition of color Doppler enables simultaneous visualization of the pelvic blood vessels (Figs 24.34 and 23.35). The level of the insertion of the uterine arteries should be used to identify the internal os and thus facilitate the diagnosis of cervical pregnancy.[71] The extensive vascular blood supply to the trophoblastic tissue originating from the adjacent maternal arteries at the implantation site (within the cervix) is easily visualized by transvaginal color Doppler. The products of conception in transit through the cervix after the failure of a normally implanted pregnancy are detached from their implantation site and maternal vascular supply. It is therefore impossible to detect any peritrophoblastic blood flow in these cases.[72] Conversely, even a small amount of placental tissue in a true cervical pregnancy remains highly vascularized on color Doppler examination.[73] This facilitates the differential diagnosis between the cervical pregnancy and incomplete miscarriage. Color Doppler analysis may also improve selection of the patients for primary surgical removal of cervical pregnancy and assist in

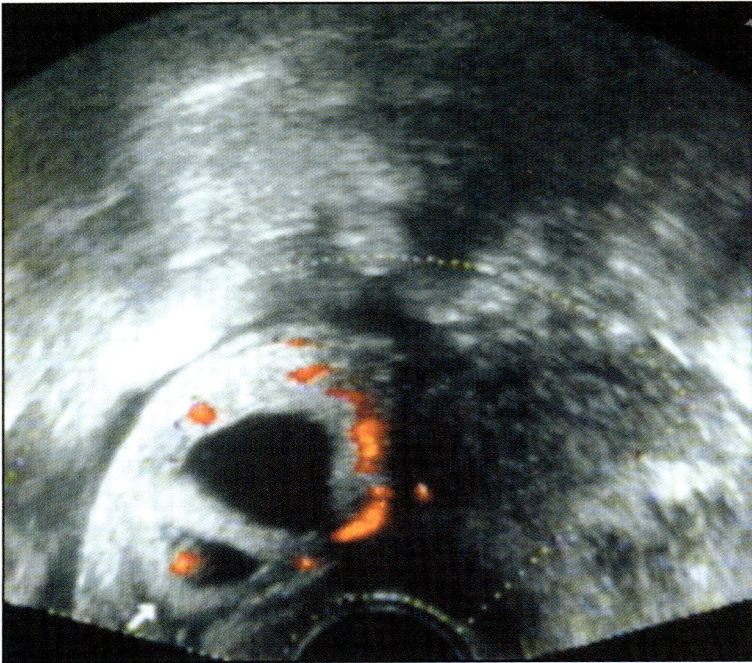

Fig. 24.34: Transvaginal power Doppler sonogram of the cervix in a patient with twin cervical pregnancy

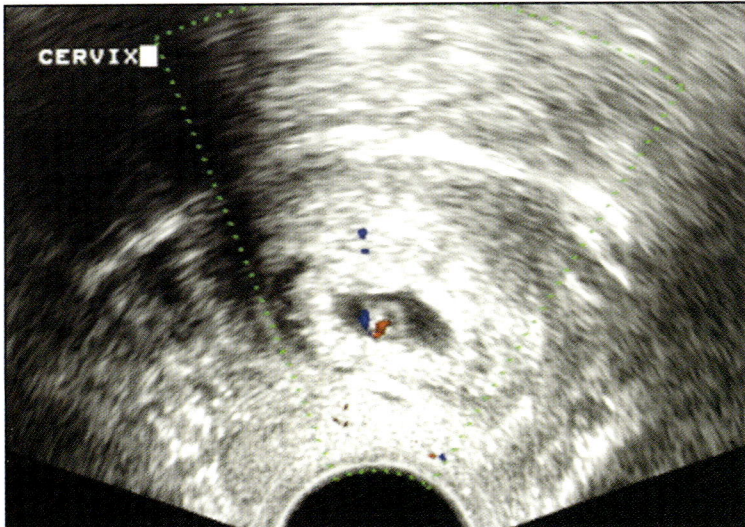

Fig. 24.35: Transvaginal scan showing a detail of the cervix, note the vessels in a yolk sac

planning D and C following medical treatment. It is necessary to stress out the potential of 3D sonography in diagnosis of cervical gestation and include: better anatomic orientation and multiplanar sections of the investigated area.

Local injection of methotrexate or potassium chloride appears to be most effective way of treating an early viable cervical pregnancy regardless of the gestational age. There are no data on the use of local injection in non-viable pregnancies, and it is uncertain whether the treatment would be as effective as in viable pregnancies. Systemic treatment in these cases is simple and highly effective and local injection would offer a very little advantage.

The regiments and dosages of methotrexate used for systemic therapy have varied considerably. There is no clear correlation between the dose and therapeutic success, and it is therefore logical to use as little methotrexate as possible to minimize side effects. The usual regiment should be two intramuscular injections of 1 mg/kg methotrexate followed by folic acid. For local injection, 25 mg methotrexate into gestation sac appears to be sufficient. Potassium chloride 3 to 5 mEq is equally successful and less likely to cause side effects.[4]

The place of surgery should be limited to those cases where medical treatment has failed. Dilatation and curettage in combination with cervical cerclage or the insertion of a Foley's catheter is probably the best choice for a general gynecologist and is as effective as more complicated and expensive methods for the prevention of uncontrollable hemorrhage.[71]

Ovarian Pregnancy

The sonographic diagnosis of ovarian pregnancy is extremely difficult to establish. It has been calculated that ovarian pregnancy accounts for less than 3 percent of ectopic pregnancies.[1,2] The sonographic diagnosis is made upon the finding of a hyperechoic trophoblastic ring detected within ovarian tissue, and the fact that it is impossible to separate the ectopic gestational sac from the ovary by transabdominal pressure from either examiner's hand or transvaginal ultrasound probe.[2] Color Doppler facilitates detection of the peritrophoblastic flow, which can speed up the entire diagnostic procedure.

Intra-abdominal Pregnancy

Intra-abdominal pregnancy is a rare condition, constituting only 1 percent of all ectopic gestations.[74] Its complications, however, can be devastating. These include massive hemorrhage due to disseminated intravascular coagulation (DIC) and placental separation complicating fetal demise, or infection with abscess formation. The outlook for the fetus is even worse, and perinatal mortality may reach 75 percent with up to 90 percent of the surviving infants having serious malformations.[75] The diagnosis of the abdominal pregnancy is not easy, especially in the early stages. Characteristically, patients present with abdominal pain, vaginal bleeding and gastrointestinal complaints. Ultrasonography together with beta hCG estimations have made early diagnosis easier. The problem still exists, however, as a patient subgroup with an ambiguous presentation remains.[76]

Ultrasound seems to be the most valuable diagnostic tool to localize this rare type of ectopic pregnancy.[2] Primary abdominal pregnancy is condition where fertilized egg implants itself directly into the peritoneal surface of abdominal cavity. If, however, an early tubal pregnancy dislodges and aborts into the pelvis, adhering to peritoneal surface, it is termed a secondary abdominal pregnancy through the secondary nidation. The sonographic presentation of abdominal pregnancy is no different from any other ectopic pregnancy, i. e. showing a hyperechoic ectopic gestational sac containing embryonic/fetal structures and extraembryonic structures with or without active heart beats. Oligohydramnion is the rule and there is no uterine mantle around the fetus.

Surgery is a time-honored treatment for abdominal pregnancy following its diagnosis, with placenta left in situ. This is mainly because, in many instances, the placenta is attached to the vital organs or vascular sites, which could be seriously damaged during placental separation. No serious complications occur when it is left in situ.[77] An additional important factor is that most abdominal pregnancies are diagnosed relatively late in pregnancy, when the placenta and its area of attachment are larger. Recently, abdominal pregnancies have been diagnosed earlier and in one case the diagnosis was made at 6 weeks of amenorrhea.[74] This made it possible for these pregnancies to be removed laparoscopically. The possible advantages of such therapeutic approach include lower morbidity and mortality, as well as better fertility outcome. However, only a limited number of cases of abdominal pregnancy have been reported early in pregnancy and the safety of operative laparoscopy can be guaranteed only in appropriately selected cases.[74] Similar cases demonstrate further the importance of first-trimester ultrasound examination in diagnosing early pregnancy complications. The importance of sonographic imaging in cases of acute abdomen in pregnancy cannot be over-stressed.[78]

Although there are no available data on the use of color Doppler and 3D ultrasound in this field, we believe that these modalities may add additional information on the implantation site and attachment of the placenta to surrounding structures.

THERAPY

Throughout the years, the treatment of ectopic pregnancy has been emergency laparotomy, including salpingectomy. In order to preserve fertility, alternatives to laparotomy and salpingectomy include observation, laparoscopic removal of ectopic pregnancy and systemic or local use of methotrexate or other feticidal agents. As medical therapy for ectopic pregnancy becomes a common practice, familiarity with its side effects may lead to greater success rates. The decision to abandon medical treatment and proceed with surgery should be based on defined guidelines, such as development of peritoneal signs, decreasing hemoglobin levels, or hemodynamic instability.[79]

Methotrexate may be administered systemically,[80] locally[81,82] or in combination (Figs 24.36 to 24.39). Local application is performed either laparoscopically or transvaginally under ultrasound needle puncture.[40] In the latter approach, methotrexate is injected directly into the gestational sac. The success rate of systemic, single-dose methotrexate (83 to 96 percent) is similar to that of local administration under laparoscopic guidance (89 to 100%), but the success rate of methotrexate under ultrasound guidance seems to be lower (70 to 83%).[83] Local injection of methotrexate under control of color Doppler imaging may increase the success rate.[4] The use of color and pulsed Doppler enables visualization of the trophoblastic adnexal flow with high-velocity and low impedance pulsed Doppler (RI<0.40). The needle can be inserted into the area of maximum color signal, which marks trophoblastic invasiveness and vitality.

Pharmacological management of an unruptured, size-appropriate ectopic pregnancy is now an established standard of care. The present protocol recommends systemic use of methotrexate in a single-dose.[84] This form of methotrexate has proven to be successful and cost-effective alternative to traditional surgical management of ectopic pregnancy.[85] In view of the risk of standard therapy and patients desire for fertility, methotrexate treatment may be a therapeutic alternative in cervical pregnancy as well. Recent reports have affirmed that ectopic pregnancy has become, a medical rather than a surgical disease.[2,4,69,72,79,83,84,86,87]

Puncture injections are valid and reasonable alternative to a traditional surgical approach, especially in patients with an interstitial, cervical or heterotopic pregnancy. In these particular cases, puncture procedures guided by transvaginal ultrasound can efficiently replace surgical treatment and save the patient from unnecessary hysterectomy.

Early diagnosis is the key to effective non-surgical treatment. Diagnostic algorithms using serial beta hCG measurements and transvaginal ultrasound examinations make definitive diagnosis possible without laparoscopy. As stated before, with help of color Doppler it is possible to identify the activity, invasiveness and vitality of trophoblast. These represent the most important characteristics for making the decision for more selective management of ectopic pregnancy. Three-dimensional ultrasound seems to be an even more effective procedure for early diagnosis of ectopic pregnancy in asymptomatic patients, even before 6 weeks of amenorrhea.[59]

Laparoscopic salpingostomy, the surgical gold standard, is an effective therapy in patients who are hemodynamically stable and wish to preserve their fertility. The reproductive performance

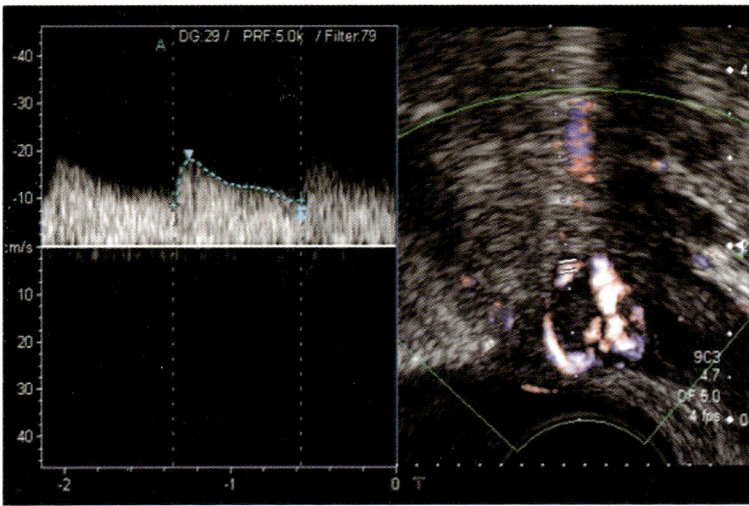

Fig. 24.36: Transvaginal color (dynamic flow) Doppler scan showing a concentric gestational ring in close proximity to the ovary. Prior to systemic methotrexate treatment, low resistance to blood flow (RI = 0.47) was detected in the peritrophoblastic area

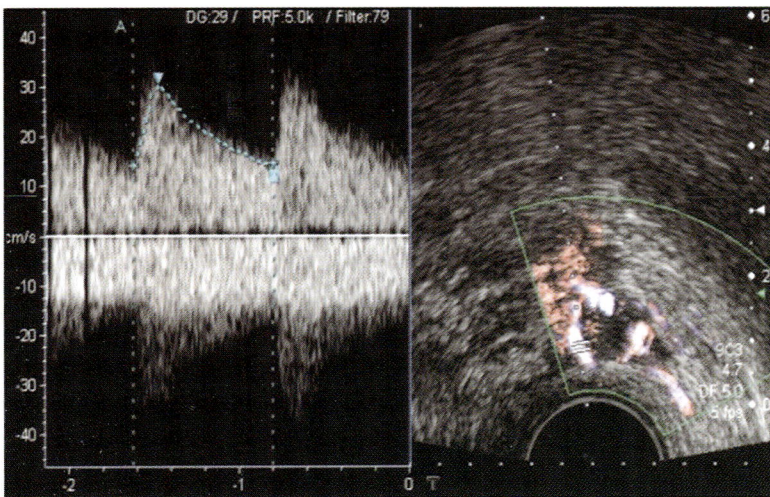

Fig. 24.37: The same patient as in Figure 24.36. Three days after methotrexate treatment was introduced, blood flow signals from the periphery of the gestational sac demonstrated increased resistance (RI = 0.52)

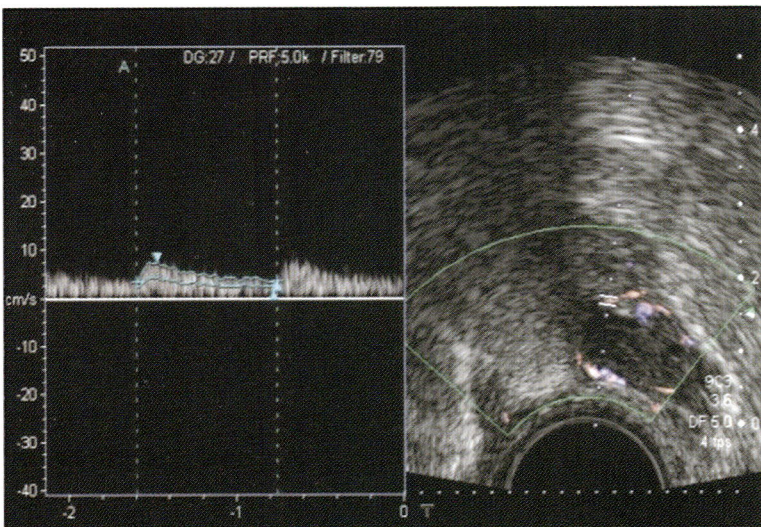

Fig. 24.38: The same patient as in Figures 24.36 and 24.37 Eleven days after methotrexate treatment color Doppler shows a few vessels from the periphery of the gestational sac and moderate-to-high resistance (RI = 0.52)

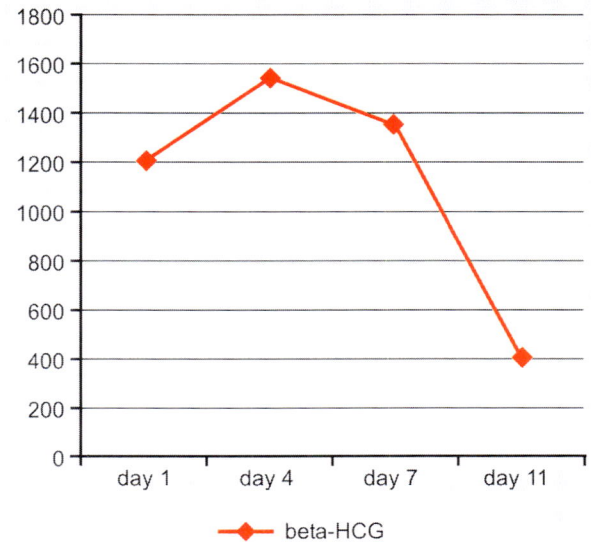

Fig. 24.39: Graph showing the evolution of serum β-hCG concentration, when methotrexate treatment was introduced. Note the increased level in the first's days after administration (due to the destruction of trophoblast)

after salpingostomy appears to be equal to, or better than salpingectomy, but the recurrent ectopic pregnancy rate is slightly higher.[3] A variable systemic dose of methotrexate produces outcomes close to those of laparoscopic salpingostomy in similar patients.[88] Methotrexate treatment is recommended in the asymptomatic patient with serum beta hCG levels of less than 2000 IU/ml, a tubal diameter of < 2 cm, and absence of fetal heart activity. The patient's understanding of her condition and compliance are mandatory. However, in many cases, ectopic pregnancy does not meet suitable medical criteria and still requires surgery. In cases suspicious of tubal abortion with a high impedance signal (RI>0.55) and beta hCG below 1000 IU/ml, local administration of methotrexate is not advised.

CONCLUSIONS

The introduction of beta hCG testing and transvaginal ultrasound has changed our approach to the patient suspected of ectopic pregnancy. An important advantage of the most currently used transvaginal transducers is the ability to perform simultaneous color and spectral Doppler studies, allowing easy identification of the ectopic peritrophoblastic flow. Therefore, color should be applied whenever a finding is suggestive of ectopic pregnancy.

Further progress in diagnostic procedures was made when 3D ultrasound was introduced. Transvaginal 3D ultrasound enables the clinician to perceive the true spatial relations and thus easily distinguish the origin of an adnexal mass, while 3D power Doppler allows detailed analysis of the vascularization.

Transvaginal color and pulsed Doppler imaging may be potentially used for detection of the patients with less prominent tubal perfusion, suitable for the expectant management of ectopic pregnancy. It is expected that increased sensitivity of the serum beta hCG immunoassay and the quality of transvaginal B-mode, color Doppler ultrasound and more recently 3D with color and power Doppler facilities will allow even earlier detection and conservative management of ectopic pregnancies. Furthermore, it seems that fertility outcomes and number of women attempting to conceive after ectopic pregnancy will further increase.

REFERENCES

1. Ectopic pregnancy. In Speroff L, Glass RH, Kase NG (Eds): Clinical Gynecologic Endocrinology and Infertility. London: Williams and Wilkins, 1999:1149-67.
2. Timor-Tristch IE, Monteagudo A. Ectopic pregnancy. In Kupesic S, de Ziegler D (Eds). Ultrasound and infertility. UK: Partenon Publishing group, 2000:215-39.
3. Kurjak A, Kupesic S. Ectopic pregnancy. In Kurjak A (Eds). *Ultrasound in Obstetrics and Gynecology.* Boston: CRC Press, 1990:225-35.
4. Kupesic S, Kurjak A. Color Doppler assessment of ectopic pregnancy. In Kurjak A. Kupesic S. (Eds). An Atlas of Transvaginal Color Doppler. London: Parthenon Publishing, 2000:137-47.
5. Boufous S, Quartararo M, Mohsin M, Parker J. Trends in the incidence of ectopic pregnancy in New South Wales between 1990-1998. Aust N Z J Obstet Gynaecol 2001;41:436-8.
6. Rajkhowa M, Glass MR, Rutherford AJ, Balen AH, Sharma V, Cuckle HS. Trends in the incidence of ectopic pregnancy in England and Wales from 1966 to 1996. *BJOG* 2000;107:369-74.
7. Nederlof KP, Lawson H W, Saftlas AF, Atrash HK, Finch EL. Ectopic pregnancy surveillance. Morbid Mortal Weekly Rep 1990;39:9.
8. Strandell A, Thorburn J, Hamberger L. Risk factors for ectopic pregnancy in assisted reproduction. Fertil Steril 1999;2:282-6.
9. Kamwendo F, Forslin L, Bodin L, Danielsson D. Epidemiology of ectopic pregnancy during a 28 year period and the role of pelvic inflammatory disease. Sex Transm Infect 2000;76:28-32.
10. Barlow RE, Cooke ID, Odukoya O, Heatley MK, Jenkins J, Narayansingh G, Ramsewak SS, Eley A. The prevalence of Chlamydia trachomatis in fresh tissue specimens from patients with ectopic pregnancy or tubal factor infertility as determined by PCR and in-situ hybridisation. J Med Microbiol 2001;50:902-8.
11. Brown WD, Burrows L, Todd CS. Ectopic pregnancy after cesarean hysterectomy. *Obstet Gynecol* 2002;99:933-4.
12. Bouyer J, Rachou E, Germain E, Fernandez H, Coste J, Pouly JL, Job-Spira N. Risk factors for extrauterine pregnancy in women using an intrauterine device. Fertil Steril 2000;74:899-908.
13. Bouyer J, Coste J, Fernandez H, Pouly JL, Job-Spira N. Sites of ectopic pregnancy: a 10 year population-based study of 1800 cases. Hum Reprod 2002;17:3224-30.
14. Mol BW, van der Veen F, Bossuyt PM. Symptom-free women at increased risk of ectopic pregnancy: should we screen? Acta Obstet Gynecol Scand 2002;81:661-72.
15. Kalinski MA, Guss DA. Hemorrhagic shock from a ruptured ectopic pregnancy in a patient with a negative urine pregnancy test result. Ann Emerg Med 2002;40:102-5.
16. Mertz HL, Yalcinkaya TM.J Early diagnosis of ectopic pregnancy. Does use of a strict algorithm decrease the incidence of tubal rupture? Reprod Med 2001;46:29-33.
17. Sagaster P, Zojer N, Dekan G, Ludwig HA. Paraneoplastic syndrome mimicking extrauterine pregnancy. Ann Oncol 2002;13:170-2.
18. Hick JL, Rodgerson JD, Heegaard WG, Sterner S. Vital signs fail to correlate with hemoperitoneum from ruptured ectopic pregnancy. Am J Emerg Med 2001;19:488-91.
19. Birkhahn RH, Gaeta TJ, Bei R, Bove JJ. Shock index in the first trimester of pregnancy and its relationship to ruptured ectopic pregnancy. Acad Emerg Med 2002;9:115-9.
20. Wong E, Suat SO. Ectopic pregnancy—a diagnostic challenge in the emergency department. Eur J Emerg Med 2000;7:189-94.
21. Dart R, McLean SA, Dart L. Isolated fluid in the cul-de-sac: how well does it predict ectopic pregnancy? Am J Emerg Med 2002;20:1-4.
22. Barnhart KT, Katz I, Hummel A, Gracia CR. Presumed diagnosis of ectopic pregnancy. Obstet Gynecol 2002;100:505-10.
23. Sheppard RW, Patton PE, Novy MJ. Serial beta hCG measurements in the early detection of ectopic pregnancy. Obstet Gynecol 1990;7:417-20.
24. Levsky ME, Handler JA, Suarez RD, Esrig ET. False-positive urine beta-HCG in a woman with a tubo-ovarian abscess. J Emerg Med 2001;21:407-9.
25. Dumps P, Meisser A, Pons D, Morales MA, Anguenot JL, Campana A, Bischof P. Accuracy of single measurements of pregnancy-associated plasma protein-A, human chorionic gonadotropin and progesterone in the diagnosis of early pregnancy failure. Eur J Obstet Gynecol Reprod Biol 2002;100:174-80.
26. Poppe WA, Vandenbussche N.Eur Postoperative day 3 serum human chorionic gonadotropin decline as a predictor of persistent ectopic pregnancy after linear salpingotomy. J Obstet Gynecol Reprod Biol 2001;99:249-52.
27. Timor-Tristch IE, Rottem S, Thale I. Review of transvaginal ultrasonography: description with clinical application. Ultrasound Q 1988;6:1-32.
28. Peisner DB, Timor-Tritsch IE. The discriminatory zone of beta hCG for vaginal probes. J Clin Ultrasound 1990;18:280-5.
29. Fossum GT, Dvajan V, Kletzky DA. Early detection of pregnancy with transvaginal ultrasound. Fertil Steril 1988;49:788-91.
30. Bernascheck G, Euaelstorfer R, Csaicsich P. Vaginal sonography versus serum human chorionic gonadotropin in early detection of pregnancy. Am J Obstet 1988;158:608-12.
31. Albayram F, Hamper UM. First-trimester obstetric emergencies: spectrum of sonographic findings. J Clin Ultrasound 2002;30:161-77.
32. Kurjak A, Zalud I, Volpe G. Conventional B-mode and transvaginal color Doppler on ultrasound assessment of ectopic pregnancy. Acta Med 1990;44:91-103.
33. Rubin GL, Petersin HB, Dorfman SF. Ectopic pregnancy in the United States 1970-1978. J Am Med Assoc 1983;249:1725-9.
34. Bolton G, Cohen F. Detecting and treating ectopic pregnancy. Contemp Obstet Gynecol 1981;18:101-4.
35. Hopp H, Schaar P, Ertezami M. Diagnostic reliability of vaginal ultrasound in ectopic pregnancy. Geburtshilfe Frauenheilkd 1995;55:666-70.
36. Hertzberg BS, Kliewer MA. Ectopic pregnancy: ultrasound diagnosis and interpretive pitfalls. South Med J 1995;88:1191-8.
37. Thoma ME. Early detection of ectopic pregnancy visualizing the presence of a tubal ring with ultrasonography performed by emergency physicians. Am J Emerg Med 2000;18:444-8.
38. Nyberg D. Ectopic pregnancy. In Nyberg DA, Hill LM, Bohm-Velez M, (Eds). Transvaginal Sonography. St. Luis: Mosby Year Book, 1992:105-35.
39. Wojak JC, Clayton MJ, Nolan TE. Outcomes of ultrasound diagnosis of ectopic pregnancy. Dependence on observer experience. Invest Radiol 1995;30:115-7.
40. Timor-Tritsch IE, Yeh MN, Peisner DB, Lesser KB, Slavik TA. The use of transvaginal ultrasonography in the diagnosis of ectopic pregnancy. Am J Obstet Gynecol 1989;161:167-70.
41. Pellerito JS, Taylor KJW, Quedens-Case C. Ectopic pregnancy: evaluation with endovaginal color flow imaging. Radiology 1992;183:831-3.
42. Fleischer AC, Pennell RG, McKee MS. Ectopic pregnancy: features at transvaginal sonography. Radiology 1990;174:375-8.
43. Bernhart K, Mennuti MT, Benjamin D, Jacobson S, Goodman D, Contifaris C. Prompt diagnosis of ectopic pregnancy in an emergency department setting. Obstet Gynecol 1994;84:1010-5.
44. Leung TY, Ng PS, Fung TY. Ectopic pregnancy diagnosed by laparoscopic ultrasound scan. Ultrasound Obstet Gynecol 1999;13:281-6.
45. Kurjak A, Zalud I, Shulman H. Ectopic pregnancy: transvaginal color Doppler of trophoblastic flow in questionable adnexa. J Ultrasound Med 1991;10:685-9.
46. Zalud I, Kurjak A. The assessment of luteal blood flow in pregnant and non-pregnant women by transvaginal color Doppler. J Perinat Med 1990;18:215-21.
47. Jurkovic D, Bourne TH, Jauniaux E, Campbell S, Collins WP. Transvaginal color Doppler study of blood flow in ectopic pregnancies. Fertil Steril 1992;57:68-73.
48. Wherry KL, Dubinsky TJ, Waitches GM, Richardson ML, Reed S. Low-resistance endometrial arterial flow in the exclusion of ectopic pregnancy revisited. J Ultrasound Med 2001;20:335-42.
49. Dillon EH, Feyock AL, Taylor KJW. Pseudogestational sacs: Doppler US differentiation from normal or abnormal intrauterine pregnancies. Radiology 1990;176:359-64.
50. Orden MR, Gudmundsson S, Helin HL, Kirkinen P. Intravascular contrast agent in the ultrasonography of ectopic pregnancy. Ultrasound Obstet Gynecol 1999;14:348-52.
51. Pellerito JS, Troiano RN, Quedens-Case C, Taylor KJW. Common pitfalls of endovaginal color Doppler flow imaging. Radiographics 1995;15:37-47.
52. Lurie S, Katz Z. Where a pendulum of expectant management of ectopic pregnancy should rest? Gynecol Obstet Invest 1996;45:145.
53. Stovall TG, Link WF. Expectant management of ectopic pregnancy. Obstet Gynecol Clin North Am 1991;18:135-44.
54. Laurie S, Insler V. Can the serum beta hCG level reliably predict likelihood of a ruptured tubal pregnancy? Isr J Obstet Gynecol 1992;3:152-544.
55. Budowich M, Johnson TRB, Genadry R. The histopathology of developing tubal ectopic pregnancy. Fertil Steril 1980;34:169-73.
56. Kemp B, Funk A, Hauptmann S, Rath W. Doppler sonographic criteria for viability in symptomless ectopic pregnancies. Lancet 1997;349:1220-1.
57. Baba K, Stach K, Sakamoto S, Okai T, Shiego I. Development of an ultrasonic system for three dimensional reconstruction of the fetus. J Perinat Med 1989;17:19-24.
58. Fredfelt KE, Holm HH, Pedersen JF. Three dimensional ultrasonic scanning. Acta Radiol Diagn 1995;25:237-40.

59. Rempen A. The shape of the endometrium evaluated with three-dimensional ultrasound: an additional predictor of extrauterine pregnancy. Hum Reprod 1998;13:450-4.
60. Harika G, Gabriel R, Carre-Pigeon F, Alemany L, Quereux C, Wahl P. Primary application of three- dimensional ultrasonography to early diagnosis of ectopic pregnancy. Eur J Obstet Gynecol Reprod Biol 1995;60:117-20.
61. Shih JC, Shyu MK, Cheng WF, Lee CN, Jou HJ, Wang RM, Hseih FJ. Arteriovenous malformation of mesosalpinx associated with a vanishing ectopic pregnancy: diagnosis with three-dimensional color power angiography. Ultrasound Obstet Gynecol 1999;13:63-6.
62. Mazur MT, Kurman RJ. Disease of the fallopian tube. In Kerman RJ, (Ed): Blaustein's Pathology of the Female Genital Tract, 4th edn. New York: Springer – Verlag, 1994:541-3.
63. Agarwal SK, Wisot AL, Garzo G, Meldrum DR. Cornual pregnancies in patients with prior salpingectomy undergoing in vitro fertilization and embryo transfer. Fertil Steril 1996;65:659-60.
64. Timor-Tritsch IE, Monteagudo A, Matera C, Veit C. Sonographic evaluation of cornual pregnancies treated without surgery. Obstet Gynecol 1992;79:1044-9.
65. Ackerman TE, Levi CS, Dashefsky SM., Holt SC, Lindsay DJ. Interstitial line: sonographic finding in interstitial (cornual) ectopic pregnancy. Radiology 1993;189:83-7.
66. Hafner T, Aslam N, Ros JA, Zosmer N, Jurkovic D. The effectiveness of non-surgical management of early interstitial pregnancy: a report of ten cases and review of the literature. Ultrasound Obstet Gynecol 1999;13:131-6.
67. Jurkovic D, Geipel A, Gruboeck K, Jauniaux E, Natucci M, Campbell S. Three-dimensional ultrasound for the assessment of uterine anatomy and detection of congenital uterine anomalies. A comparison with hysterosalpingography and two dimensional sonography. Ultrasound Obstet Gynecol 1995;5:233-7.
68. Lawrence A, Jurkovic D. Three-dimensional ultrasound diagnosis of interstitial pregnancy. Ultrasound Obstet Gynecol 1999;14:292-3.
69. Ben-Sholmo I, Eliyahu S, Yanai N, Shalev E. Methotrexate as a possible cause of ovarian cyst formation: experience with women treated for ectopic pregnancies. Fertil Steril 1997;67:786-8.
70. Schiff E, Tsabari A, Shalev E, Maschiach S, Bustan M, Weiner E. Pharmacokinetics of methotrexate after local tubal injection for conservative treatment of ectopic pregnancy. Fertil Steril 1992;57:688-90.
71. Timor-Tritsch IE, Monteagudo A, Mandeville EO, Peisner DB, Parra-Anaya G, Pirrone EC. Successful management of viable cervical pregnancy by local injection of methotrexate guided by transvaginal ultrasonography. Am J Obstet Gynecol 1994;170:737-9.
72. Jurkovic D, Hacket E, Campbell S. Diagnosis and treatment of early cervical pregnancy: a review and a report of two cases treated conservatively. Ultrasound Obstet Gynecol 1996;8:373-80.
73. Jauniaux E, Taidi J, Jurkovic D, Campbell S, Hustin J. Comparison of color Doppler features and pathological findings in complicated early pregnancy. Hum Reprod 1994;9:2432-7.
74. Morita Y, Tsutsumi O, Kurmochi K, Momoeda M, Yoshikawa H, Taketeani Y. Successful laparoscopic management of primary abdominal pregnancy. Hum Reprod 1996;11:2546-7.
75. Ahmed B, Fawzi HW, Abushama M. Advanced abdominal pregnancy in the developing countries. J Obstet Gynecol 1996;16:400-5.
76. Angtuaco TL, Shah HR, Meal MR, Quirk JG. Ultrasound evaluation of abdominal pregnancy. Crit Rev Diagn Imaging 1994;35:1-59.
77. Bajo JM, Garcia FA, Huertas MA. Sonographic follow-up of a placenta left in situ after delivery of the fetus in abdominal pregnancy. Ultrasound Obstet Gynecol 1996;7:285-8.
78. Zaki ZMS. An unusual presentation of ectopic pregnancy. Ultrasound Obstet Gynecol 1998;11:456-8.
79. Thoen LD, Crenin MD. Medical treatment of ectopic pregnancy with methotrexate. Fertil Steril 1997;68:727-30.
80. Lipscomb GH, Meyer NL, Flynn DE, Peterson M, Ling FW. Oral methotrexate for treatment of ectopic pregnancy. Am J Obstet Gynecol 2002;186:1192-5.
81. Haimov-Kochman R, Sciaky-Tamir Y, Yanai N, Yagel S. Conservative management of two ectopic pregnancies implanted in previous uterine scars. Ultrasound Obstet Gynecol 2002;19:616-9.
82. El-Lamie IK, Shehata NA, Kamel HA. Intramuscular methotrexate for tubal pregnancy. J Reprod Med 2002;47:144-50.
83. Yao M, Tulandi T. Current status of surgical and non-surgical management of ectopic pregnancy. Fertil Steril 1997;67:421-33.
84. Powell MP, Spellman JR. Medical management of the patient with an ectopic pregnancy. J Perinat Neonat Nurs 1997;9:31-43.
85. Luciano AA, Roy G, Solima E, Ann NY. Ectopic pregnancy from surgical emergency to medical management. Acad Sci 2001;943:235-54.
86. Morlock RJ, Lafata JE, Eisenstein D. Cost-effectiveness of single-dose methotrexate compared with laparoscopic treatment of ectopic pregnancy. Obstet Gynecol 2000;95:407-12.
87. Pascual MA, Ruiz J, Tresserra F, Sanuy C, Grases PJ, Tur R, Barri PN. Cervical ectopic twin pregnancy: diagnosis and conservative treatment. Hum Reprod 2001;16:584-86.
88. Tulandi T, Sammour A. Evidence-based management of ectopic pregnancy. Curr Opin Obstet Gynecol 2000;12:289-92.

Index